GNRS

A Core Curriculum in Advanced Practice Geriatric Nursing

4th Edition

Geriatric Nursing Review Syllabus

EDITORS-IN-CHIEF ■ Ellen Flaherty, PhD, APRN, AGSF ■ Barbara Resnick, PhD, CRNP, FAAN, FAANP, AGSF

AGS Geriatrics Healthcare Professionals

Leading Change. Improving Care for Older Adults.

As new research and clinical experience broaden our knowledge of medicine, changes in treatment and drug therapy are required. This publication is intended only to facilitate the free flow of information of interest to the medical community involved in the care of older adults.

No responsibility is assumed by the editors or the American Geriatrics Society, as the Publisher, for any injury and/or damage to persons or property, as a matter of product liability, negligence, warranty, or otherwise, arising out of the use or application of any methods, products, instructions, or ideas contained herein. No guarantee, endorsement, or warranty of any kind, express or implied (including specifically no warranty of merchantability or of fitness for a particular purpose) is given by the Society in connection with any information contained herein. Independent verification of any diagnosis, treatment, or drug use or dosage should be obtained. No test or procedure should be performed unless, in the judgment of an independent qualified physician, it is justified in light of the risk involved.

Inclusion in this publication of product information does not constitute a guarantee, warranty, or endorsement by the American Geriatrics Society (the Publisher) of the quality, value, safety, effectiveness, or usefulness of any such product or of any claim made about such product by its manufacturer or an author.

The *GNRS4* reflects care that can be provided to older adults in all settings. The words patient, resident, and older adult have been used interchangeably, as have the words provider, clinician, and primary care provider. Given the continually ongoing changes in health care today, some of the guidelines around reimbursement may have changed since publication.

The Chief Editors were Ellen Flaherty, PhD, APRN, AGSF, and Barbara Resnick, PhD, CRNP, FAAN, FAANP, AGSF; Editors were Marie Boltz, PhD, RN, GNP-BC, Elizabeth Capezuti, PhD, RN, FAAN, Deirdre M. Carolan, CRNP, PhD, Elizabeth Galik, PhD, CRNP, and Laurie Kennedy-Malone, PhD, GNP-BC; Medical Editor was Susan E. Aiello, DVM, ELS; Indexer was L. Pilar Wyman; and Managing Editor was Andrea N. Sherman, MS.

Many thanks to Fry Communications for all production work including typesetting, graphic design, and printing. With more than 70 years in the information industry, Fry offers printing and ancillary services to publishers and other content providers.

Citation: Flaherty E, Resnick B, eds. *Geriatric Nursing Review Syllabus: A Core Curriculum in Advanced Practice Geriatric Nursing*. 4th ed. New York: American Geriatrics Society; 2014.

Geriatric Nursing Review Syllabus: A Core Curriculum in Advanced Practice Geriatric Nursing. 4th edition. Cataloging in publication data is available from the Library of Congress.
Library of Congress Control Number: 2013951990

ISBN Number: 978-1-886775-29-9

Printed in the United States of America

10 9 8 7 6 5 4 3 2 1

TABLE OF CONTENTS

***GNRS4* Editorial Board** . . . ix
Original *GRS8* Editorial Board and Authors . . . xi
Authors of Original *GRS8* Chapters . . . xi
Contributing Question Authors . . . xv
Acknowledgments . . . xvii
Preface . . . xix
Introduction . . . xix
Program Information . . . xx

CURRENT ISSUES IN AGING

Chapter 1—Demography . . . 1
Global Aging Trends . . . 1
Demography of Aging in the United States . . . 1
References . . . 7

Chapter 2—Biology . . . 8
Theories of Aging . . . 8
Organ System Changes with Aging . . . 11
Normal Aging Versus Age-Related Pathologies . . . 16
Homeostasis and Aging . . . 16
References . . . 17

Chapter 3—Psychosocial Issues . . . 18
Stressors . . . 18
Mediators . . . 21
Moderators . . . 23
References . . . 25

Chapter 4—Legal and Ethical Issues . . . 26
Introduction to Medical Ethics . . . 26
Decisional Capacity . . . 27
Decisions Near the End of Life . . . 30
Special Ethical Issues in Dementia . . . 33
References . . . 34

Chapter 5—Financing, Coverage, and Costs of Health Care . . . 35
Medicare . . . 35
Financing of Care at Different Sites . . . 41
Changes in the Federal Financing of Health Care . . . 46
References . . . 47

APPROACH TO THE PATIENT

Chapter 6—Assessment . . . 48
The Routine Office Visit . . . 48
Patient-Clinician Communication . . . 48
Physical Assessment . . . 49
Medication Assessment . . . 51
Cognitive Assessment . . . 51
Psychologic Assessment . . . 51
Social Assessment . . . 52
Quality of Life . . . 52
Assessing the Older Driver . . . 52
Acute Functional Decline . . . 53
References . . . 53

Chapter 7—Multimorbidity . . . 54
Approach to the Older Adult with Multimorbidity . . . 54
Guiding Principles . . . 54
Controversies and Challenges . . . 56
References . . . 56

Chapter 8—Cultural Aspects of Care . . . 58
Doorway Thoughts in Cross-Cultural Health Care . . . 58
Use of Language and Nonverbal Communication . . . 59
History of Traumatic Experiences . . . 60
Issues of Immigration . . . 60
Acculturation, Tradition, and Health Beliefs . . . 60
Unspoken Challenges . . . 61
The Interface Between Culture and Religion . . . 61
Approaches to Decision Making . . . 61
Attitudes Regarding Disclosure and Consent . . . 62
Gender Issues . . . 62
Advance Directives and End-of-Life Care . . . 62
Approaches: The ETHNICS Mnemonic . . . 62
References . . . 63

Chapter 9—Physical Activity . . . 64
Benefits of Physical Activity . . . 64
Recommended Amounts of Physical Activity . . . 65
Promotion of Physical Activity . . . 67
References . . . 69

Chapter 10—Prevention . . . 70
Cancer Screening Tests . . . 70
Other Screening Tests . . . 74
Healthy Lifestyle Counseling . . . 76
Geriatric Health Issues . . . 77
Immunizations . . . 78
Chemoprophylaxis . . . 79
Counseling on Cancer Screening and Preventive Health . . . 79
References . . . 80

Chapter 11—Pharmacotherapy . . . 81
Age-Associated Changes in Pharmacokinetics . . . 81
Age-Associated Changes in Pharmacodynamics . . . 83
Optimizing Prescribing . . . 84
Adverse Drug Events . . . 85
Drug Interactions . . . 87
Drug-Disease Interactions . . . 87
Principles of Prescribing . . . 88
Discontinuing Medications . . . 88

Nonadherence 89
References 89

Chapter 12—Complementary and Alternative Medicine 90
Safety Issues 91
CAM Efficacy for Managing Illness 92
References 96

Chapter 13—Mistreatment of Older Adults 97
Risk Factors and Prevention 97
History 97
Physical Assessment 98
Psychological Assessment 98
Financial Assessment 99
Self-Neglect 100
The Role of the Older Adult 100
Institutional Mistreatment 100
Intervention 100
The Medical-Legal Interface 101
References 101

Chapter 14—Perioperative Care 102
Preoperative Assessment and Management 102
Perioperative and Postoperative Management of Selected Medical Problems 106
References 110

Chapter 15—Palliative Care 111
Overall Care Near Death 111
Ethnographic Data 111
Palliative Care and Hospice 112
Quality Indicators for Palliative Care 113
Communication 113
Palliation of Symptoms 114
References 118

Chapter 16—Persistent Pain 119
Assessment 119
Assessing and Treating Pain in Cognitively Impaired Older Adults 121
Treatment 122
References 129

CARE SYSTEMS

Chapter 17—Hospital Care 130
Assessing and Managing Hospitalized Older Patients . 130
Daily Evaluation of Older Hospitalized Patients 137
Systems of Care for Older Hospitalized Patients 137
Nurses Improving Care of Health System Elders (NICHE) 138
Alternatives to Hospital Care 138
References 138

Chapter 18—Rehabilitation 139
Conceptual Model for Geriatric Rehabilitation 139
Sites of Rehabilitation Care 139
Teams and Roles 142
Impact of Comorbid Conditions 142
Rehabilitation Approaches and Interventions 144
Comprehensive Assessment 144
Stroke 145
Hip Fracture 146
Total Hip and Knee Arthroplasty 147
Amputation 149
Mobility Aids, Orthotics, Adaptive Methods, and Environmental Modifications 149
References 152

Chapter 19—Nursing-Home Care 153
The Nursing-Home Population 153
Nursing-Home Availability 154
Nursing-Home Financing 155
Staffing Patterns 155
Factors Associated with Nursing-Home Placement . . . 156
The Interface of Acute and Long-Term Care 156
Quality Issues and Legislation Influencing Care in the Nursing Home 156
Medical Care Issues 158
Clinician Practice in the Nursing Home 159
References 160

Chapter 20—Transitional Care 161
The Treachery of Suboptimal Care Transitions 161
Barriers to Safe Transitions 162
Strategies to Improve Transitional Care 163
References 165

Chapter 21—Community-Based Care 166
Home Care 166
Community-Based Services Not Requiring a Change in Residence 169
Community-Based Services Requiring a Change of Residence 170
References 172

Chapter 22—Outpatient Care Systems 173
Geriatric Specialty Care 173
Geriatrics in Primary Care 173
Patient Selection for Outpatient Interventions 176
References 176

SYNDROMES

Chapter 23—Frailty 177
Evidence-Based Findings 177
Evidence as to Cause 179
Assessment of Frailty 179
Prevailing Management Strategies 180
Potential Approaches to Prevention of Frailty 181

Frailty and Failure to Thrive 181
Frailty and Palliative Care 182
References 182

Chapter 24—Visual Impairment 183
Common Eye Conditions in Older Adults 183
Refractive Error and Cataracts 186
Age-Related Macular Degeneration (ARMD) 187
Diabetic Retinopathy 188
Glaucoma 189
Anterior Ischemic Optic Neuropathy 190
Low-Vision Rehabilitation 191
References 191

Chapter 25—Hearing Impairment 192
Normal Hearing and Age-Related Changes in the Auditory System 192
Epidemiology 192
Presbycusis 193
Clinical Presentation and Screening 193
Evaluation of Suspected Hearing Loss 194
Treatment 194
References 198

Chapter 26—Dizziness 199
Classification 199
Evaluation 201
Management 203
References 203

Chapter 27—Syncope 204
Natural History: Diagnosis and Prognosis 204
Pathophysiology 204
Evaluation 205
Treatment 207
References 208

Chapter 28—Malnutrition 209
Age-Related Changes 209
Nutrition Screening and Assessment 210
Nutrition Syndromes 212
Nutritional Interventions 213
Legal and Ethical Issues 214
References 215

Chapter 29—Eating and Feeding Problems 216
Swallowing in Health and Disease 216
Feeding 217
References 219

Chapter 30—Urinary Incontinence 220
Prevalence and Impact 220
Risk Factors and Associated Comorbid Conditions 221
Pathophysiology 221
Evaluation 222
Treatment and Management 223
Evaluation and Management of UI in Nursing-Home Residents 225
Catheters and Catheter Care 226
References 227

Chapter 31—Gait Impairment 228
Epidemiology 228
Conditions that Contribute to Gait Impairment 228
Assessment 229
Interventions to Reduce Gait Disorders 231
References 233

Chapter 32—Falls 234
Prevalence and Morbidity 234
Causes 234
Treatment and Prevention 238
Clinical Guidelines 240
References 242

Chapter 33—Osteoporosis 243
Epidemiology and Impact 243
Bone Remodeling and Bone Loss in Aging 244
Pathogenesis 244
Diagnosis and Prediction of Fracture 246
Prevention and Treatment 249
Vertebral Fracture Management 254
References 255

Chapter 34—Dementia 256
Epidemiology and Societal Impact 256
Etiology 256
Risk Factors and Prevention 257
Assessment and Differential Diagnosis 257
Differentiating Types of Dementias 259
Treatment and Management 262
References 266

Chapter 35—Behavioral Problems in Dementia 267
Clinical Features 267
Assessment and Differential Diagnosis 268
Treatment Approach 269
Treatments for Specific Disturbances 270
References 275

Chapter 36—Delirium 276
Incidence and Prognosis 276
Diagnosis and Differential Diagnosis 276
The Spectrum and Neuropathophysiology of Delirium 278
Risk Factors 278
Delirium and Dementia 279
Postoperative Delirium 279
Evaluation and Management 279
Quality Measures and Consensus Guidelines 283
References 284

Chapter 37—Sleep Problems 285
Epidemiology 285
Changes in Sleep with Aging 285
Evaluation of Sleep 286

Common Sleep Problems 286
Changes in Sleep with Dementia 289
Sleep Disturbances in the Hospital 290
Sleep in the Nursing Home 290
Management of Sleep Problems 291
References 295

Chapter 38—Pressure Ulcers and Wound Care . 296
The Wound Healing Cascade 296
Pressure Ulcers 297
References 307

PSYCHIATRY

Chapter 39—Depression and Other Mood Disorders 308
Epidemiology 308
Clinical Presentation and Diagnosis 308
Treatment 311
References 318

Chapter 40—Anxiety Disorders 319
Classes of Anxiety Disorders 319
Comorbidity 321
Pharmacologic Management 322
Psychologic Management 323
References 323

Chapter 41—Psychotic Disorders 324
Schizophrenia and Schizophrenia-Like Syndromes . . . 324
Psychotic Symptoms 326
Syndromes of Isolated Hallucinations 327
References 328

Chapter 42—Personality and Somatic Symptom Disorders 329
Personality Disorders 329
Somatic Symptom and Related Disorders 333
References 335

Chapter 43—Addictions 336
Definitions of Substance Abuse 336
Magnitude of the Problem 337
Risks and Benefits of Substance Use 338
Identifying Substance-Use Disorders 339
Treatment 339
References 343

Chapter 44—Intellectual and Developmental Disabilities 344
Prevalence 344
Diagnostic and Treatment Issues 345
Psychiatric and Mental Disorders in Aging Adults with Intellectual Disability 346
Medical Disorders 348
Social Conditions 349
Developmental Disabilities and Comorbidity 349
References 349

DISEASES AND DISORDERS

Chapter 45—Dermatologic Diseases and Disorders 350
Aging and Photoaging 350
Inflammatory and Autoimmune Skin Conditions 350
Ulcers 355
Infections and Infestations 356
Benign Growths 358
Skin Cancer 359
References 361

Chapter 46—Oral Diseases and Disorders 362
Aging of the Teeth 362
Dental Decay 362
Diseases of the Periodontium 363
Toothlessness 364
Salivary Function in Aging 365
Common Oral Lesions 365
Chemosensory Perception 368
Common Medical Considerations in Dental Treatment of Older Adults 369
References 370

Chapter 47—Respiratory Diseases and Disorders 371
Age-Related Pulmonary Changes 371
Common Respiratory Symptoms and Complaints 371
Major Pulmonary Diseases 372
Intensive Care of the Critically Ill 377
References 377

Chapter 48—Cardiovascular Diseases and Disorders 378
Epidemiology 378
Effects of Aging on Cardiovascular Function 378
Cardiovascular Risk Factors 379
Coronary Artery Disease 380
Acute Coronary Syndromes 380
Chronic Coronary Artery Disease 382
Valvular Heart Disease 384
Heart Failure 385
Cardiac Arrhythmias 385
Peripheral Arterial Disease 391
Venous Thromboembolic Disease 392
References 394

Chapter 49—Heart Failure 395
Epidemiology 395
Etiology and Pathophysiology 395
Clinical Features 395
Diagnosis 396
Management 396
Recurrent Hospitalization 400
Prognosis 401

End-of-Life Care 401
References 401

Chapter 50—Hypertension 402
Epidemiology and Physiology 402
Clinical Evaluation 403
Treatment 403
Special Considerations 407
References 407

Chapter 51—Gastrointestinal Diseases and Disorders 408
Esophagus 408
Stomach 411
Colon 412
References 419

Chapter 52—Kidney Diseases and Disorders 420
Monitoring Kidney Function 420
Electrolyte Disorders 420
Nephrotic Syndrome 423
Renovascular Disease 424
Acute Kidney Injury 424
Chronic Kidney Disease 426
End-Stage Kidney Disease 428
References 430

Chapter 53—Gynecologic Diseases and Disorders 431
History and Physical Examination 431
Treatment of Menopausal Symptoms 432
Urogenital Atrophy 432
Vulvovaginal Infection and Inflammation 433
Disorders of the Vulva 433
Disorders of Pelvic Floor Support 434
Postmenopausal Vaginal Bleeding 435
References 436

Chapter 54—Prostate Disease 437
Benign Prostatic Hyperplasia 437
Prostate Cancer 439
Prostatitis 444
References 445

Chapter 55—Disorders of Sexual Function 446
Female Sexuality 446
Male Sexuality 448
References 452

Chapter 56—Musculoskeletal Diseases and Disorders 453
Diagnostic Approach to Musculoskeletal Complaints in Older Adults 453
Evaluation of Regional Musculoskeletal Complaints 455
General Management Strategies 457
Approach to Specific Rheumatologic Diseases 458
References 464

Chapter 57—Back and Neck Pain 465
Back Pain 465
Systemic Causes 465
Nonsystemic Causes 465
Assessment 467
Management 469
Neck Pain 469
References 470

Chapter 58—Diseases and Disorders of the Foot 471
The Role of the Primary Care Clinician in Foot Care 471
Common Deformities of the Foot 471
Skin and Nail Disorders 476
Systemic Diseases Affecting the Foot and Ankle 478
References 479

Chapter 59—Neurologic Diseases and Disorders 480
Cerebrovascular Diseases 480
Headaches 483
Movement Disorders 484
Epilepsy 489
Motor Neuron Disease 490
Myelopathy 492
Radiculopathy 492
Peripheral Neuropathy 492
Myopathy 493
Restless Legs Syndrome 493
References 493

Chapter 60—Infectious Diseases 494
Predisposition to Infection 494
Diagnosis and Management of Infections 495
Prevention of Infections 497
Infectious Syndromes 497
Fever of Unknown Origin 505
References 505

Chapter 61—Endocrine and Metabolic Disorders 506
Thyroid Disorders 506
Disorders of Parathyroid and Calcium Metabolism 510
Hormonal Regulation of Water and Electrolyte Balance 513
Disorders of the Adrenal Cortex 514
Testosterone 516
Estrogen Therapy 518
Growth Hormone 518
Melatonin 519
References 519

Chapter 62—Diabetes Mellitus 520
Pathophysiology of Diabetes in Older Adults 520
Diagnosis and Evaluation 521
Management 522
Education and Self-Management Support 528
References 529

Chapter 63—Hematologic Diseases and Disorders 530
Hematopoiesis 530
Anemia 531
Vitamin B_{12}, Folate, and Homocysteine 537
Platelets and Coagulation 537
Chronic Myeloproliferative Disorders 538
Hematologic Malignancies, Lymphomas, and Multiple Myeloma 539
References 539

Chapter 64—Oncology . . . .
Cancer Biology and Aging . . . .
Principles of Cancer Management . . . .
Specific Cancers . . . .
Principles of Management . . . .
References . . . .

Normal Laboratory Values . . . .

Index of Question Numbers by Primary

Questions . . . .

Questions, Answers, and Critiques . . . .

***GRS8* Editorial Board** . . . .

Contributing Chapter Authors . . . .

Contributing Question Authors . . . . . .

Disclosure of Financial Interests . . . . .

GNRS4 EDITORIAL BOARD

GNRS4 EDITORIAL STAFF

The *Geriatric Nursing Review Syllabus*, 4th edition, is based upon the *Geriatrics Review Syllabus*, 8th edition, which was developed by the below editorial board and authors. For a complete listing of the *GRS8* contributors and their professional affiliations, please **see p. 672**

ORIGINAL *GRS8* EDITORIAL BOARD AND AUTHORS

AUTHORS OF ORIGINAL *GRS8* CHAPTERS

CURRENT ISSUES IN AGING

Demography	Jennifer L. Wolff, PhD
Biology	Neal S. Fedarko, PhD
	Matthew K. McNabney, MD
Psychosocial Issues	Joseph E. Gaugler, PhD
Legal and Ethical Issues	Margaret A. Drickamer, MD
Finance	Richard G. Stefanacci, DO, MGH, MBA, AGSF, CMD

APPROACH TO PATIENT

Assessment	Thomas M. Gill, MD
Multimorbidity	Cynthia M. Boyd, MD, MPH
	Matthew K. McNabney, MD
Cultural Aspects of Care	Seema S. Limaye, MD
Physical Activity	Peter G. Snell, PhD
Prevention	Mara A. Schonberg, MD, MPH
Pharmacotherapy	Todd P. Semla, MS, PharmD, BCPS, FCCP, AGSF
Complementary and Alternative Medicine	Marc R. Blackman, MD
	Julie C. Chapman, PsyD
Mistreatment of Older Adults	Terry Fulmer, PhD, RN, FAAN, AGSF
Perioperative Care	Colleen Christmas, MD
	James T. Pacala, MD, MS, AGSF
Palliative Care	Grace A. Cordts, MD, MPH, MS
Persistent Pain	Vyjeyanthi S. Periyakoil, MD

CARE SYSTEMS

Hospital Care	Edgar Pierluissi, MD
	Margarita Sotelo, MD
Rehabilitation	Cynthia J. Brown, MD, MSPH
	Kathleen T. Foley, PhD, OTR/L

Nursing-Home Care	Suzanne M. Gillespie, MD, RD, CMD, FACP
	Paul R. Katz, MD, CMD, AGSF
Transitional Care	Alicia I. Arbaje, MD, MPH
Community-Based Care	Robert McCann, MD, AGSF
Outpatient Care Systems	Steven R. Counsell, MD, AGSF

SYNDROMES

Frailty	Linda P. Fried, MD, MPH, AGSF
Visual Impairment	JoAnn A. Giaconi, MD
	David Sarraf, MD
	Anne L. Coleman, MD, PhD
Hearing Impairment	Priscilla F. Bade, MD, FACP, CMD
Dizziness	Aman Nanda, MD
Syncope	Sushmitha Patibandla, MD
	Win-Kuang Shen, MD
Malnutrition	James S. Powers, MD, AGSF
Eating and Feeding Problems	Colleen Christmas, MD
Urinary Incontinence	Catherine E. DuBeau, MD
Gait Impairment	Neil B. Alexander, MD
Falls	Sarah D. Berry, MD, MPH
	Douglas P. Kiel, MD, MPH
Osteoporosis	Kenneth W. Lyles, MD, AGSF
	Loren Martinez Wilkerson, MD
Dementia	Cynthia Barton, RN, MSN
	Kristine Yaffe, MD
	Alexander W. Threlfall, MD, MA
Behavior Problems in Dementia	Melinda S. Lantz, MD
Delirium	Edward R. Marcantonio, MD, SM
Sleep Problems	Cathy A. Alessi, MD, AGSF
Pressure Ulcers and Wound Care	Courtney H. Lyder, ND, GNP, FAAN

PSYCHIATRY

Depression and Other Mood Disorders	Gary J. Kennedy, MD
Anxiety Disorders	Judith Neugroschl, MD
Psychotic Disorders	Susan W. Lehmann, MD
Personality and Somatic Symptom Disorders	Marc E. Agronin, MD
Addictions	David W. Oslin, MD
	Donovan Maust, MD
Intellectual and Developmental Disabilities	Mark H. Fleisher, MD, FAPA

DISEASES AND DISORDERS

Dermatologic Diseases and Disorders	Jane M. Grant-Kels, MD
Oral Diseases and Disorders	Kenneth Shay, DDS, MS
Respiratory Diseases and Disorders	Margaret Pisani, MD, MPH
	Kathleen M. Akgün, MD
Cardiovascular Diseases and Disorders	Michael W. Rich, MD, AGSF
Heart Failure	Michael W. Rich, MD, AGSF
Hypertension	Ihab Hajjar, MD, MS, FACP
Gastrointestinal Diseases and Disorders	George Triadafilopoulos, MD, DSc
Kidney Diseases and Disorders	Sanjeevkumar R. Patel, MD, MS
	Jocelyn E. Wiggins, MA, BM, BCh, MRCP
Gynecologic Diseases and Disorders	G. Willy Davila, MD
Prostate Disease	Lisa J. Granville, MD, AGSF, FACP
Disorders of Sexual Function	Angela Gentili, MD
	Thomas Mulligan, MD, AGSF
Musculoskeletal Diseases and Disorders	Allan C. Gelber, MD, MPH, PhD

Back and Neck Pain	Leo M. Cooney, Jr, MD
Diseases and Disorders of the Foot	Douglas A. Albreski, DPM
Neurologic Diseases and Disorders	Daniel L. Murman, MD, MS, FAAN
Infectious Diseases	H. Keipp Talbot, MD, MPH
	Kyle Widmer, MD
Endocrine and Metabolic Disorders	David A. Gruenewald, MD
	Alvin M. Matsumoto, MD
	Anne M. Kenny, MD
Diabetes Mellitus	Caroline S. Blaum, MD, MS
Hematologic Diseases and Disorders	Gurkamal S. Chatta, MD
	Roy E. Smith, MD
Oncology	Supriya Mohile, MD, MS

CONTRIBUTING QUESTION AUTHORS

R. Morgan Bain, MD
Angela Catic, MD
Rebecca Boxer, MD
Rachelle Bernacki, MD, MS
Kenneth Brummel-Smith, MD, AGSF
Morgan Carlson, PhD
Susan Charette, MD
Carl I. Cohen, MD
Leo M. Cooney, Jr, MD
Mary Ellen Csuka, MD
William Dale, MD, PhD
Ann R. Datunashvili, MD
Nancy Neveloff Dubler LL.B.
Shahrooz Eshaghian, MD, FACP
David V. Espino, MD, FAAFP, AGSF, CAQ-Geriatrics
Mark H. Fleisher, MD
Daniel E. Forman, MD, FACC, FAHA
Susan M. Friedman, MD, MPH, AGSF
Steven R. Gambert, MD, FACP, AGSF
Nalaka Gooneratne, MD
Angela Gentili, MD
Shelly L. Gray, PharmD, MS
Debra Greenberg, MSW, PhD
Blaine S. Greenwald, MD
Namirah Jamshed, MD
Theodore M. Johnson II, MD, MPH
Fran E. Kaiser, MD, AGSF, FGSA
Helen Kao, MD
Catherine McVearry Kelso, MD, MS
Anne Kenny, MD
Mary B. King, MD
Tia Kostas, MD
Stephen Krieger, MD
Lorand Kristof, MD, MSc
Larry W. Lawhorne, MD
Sei J. Lee, MD, MAS
Eric Lenze, MD
Michael C. Lindberg, MD, FACP
Hannah I. Lipman, MD, MS
Vera P. Luther, MD
Mary Ann McLaughlin, MD
Daniel Ari Mendelson, MS, MD, FACP, AGSF
Diana V. Messadi, DDS, MMSc, DMSc
Karen L. Miller, MD
Alison A. Moore, MD, MPH
Karin M. Ouchida, MD
Joseph G. Ouslander, MD, AGSF
James T. Pacala, MD, MS, AGSF
Kourosh Parham, MD, PhD
Donna J. Parker, MD
Birju B. Patel, MD, FACP
Claire Peel, PT, MS, PhD
Edgar Pierluissi, MD
Emaad Abdel-Rahman, MD, PhD, FASN
Anitha Rao-Frisch MD, MA
Julie Robison, PhD
Mitchell H. Rosner, MD
Amy E. Sanders, MD
Alessandra Scalmati, MD
Gary J. Schiller, MD
Jodie Sengstock, DPM
David Sengstock, MD, MS
Jagat Shetty, MD
Winnie Suen, MD, MSc
Gwen K. Sterns, MD
Dennis H. Sullivan, MD, AGSF
George Taler, MD
John A. Taylor, III, MD, MS
Helen Torabzadeh, DDS
Dennis T. Villareal, MD, FACP, FACE
Louise C. Walter, MD
Debra Kaye Weiner, MD
Barbara E. Weinstein, PhD
Peter J. Whitehouse, MD, PhD
G. Darryl Wieland, PhD, MPH
Michi Yukawa MD, MPH
Fariba S. Younai, DDS
Phyllis C. Zee, MD, PhD
Richard Zweig, PhD

ACKNOWLEDGMENTS

As the chief editors, it is our great pleasure to acknowledge the many people who have made the *Geriatric Nursing Review Syllabus: A Core Curriculum in Advanced Practice Geriatric Nursing, 4th Edition* (*GNRS4*) possible. We express our gratitude to our Co-Editors: Marie Boltz, PhD, RN, GNP-BC, Elizabeth Capezuti, PhD, RN, FAAN, Deirdre M. Carolan, CRNP, PhD, Elizabeth Galik, PhD, CRNP, and Laurie Kennedy-Malone, PhD, GNP-BC. We especially thank the contributing *GRS8* authors of chapters and questions for lending us their expertise to this publication. We thank Andrea Sherman, MS, *GRS* Managing Editor, for her guidance, organization, and coordination overseeing the administrative, and editorial aspects of the program. Thanks also to Susan E. Aiello, DVM, ELS, our medical editor, and to L. Pilar Wyman for her comprehensive index.

We wish to express our appreciation for the support of the AGS Board of Directors and AGS staff members Jennie Chin Hansen, RN, MS, FAAN, Chief Executive Officer; Nancy Lundebjerg, MPA, Deputy Executive Vice President, Chief Operating Officer; Elvy Ickowicz, MPH, Associate Vice President, Product Development and Marketing; Linda Saunders, MSW, Senior Director, Professional Education and Special Projects; and Dennise McAlpin, Senior Manager, Professional Education and Special Projects.

Finally, we thank our patients, who continually inform, inspire, challenge, and sustain us.

Ellen Flaherty, PhD, APRN, AGSF
Barbara Resnick, PhD, CRNP, FAAN, FAANP, AGSF
GNRS4 Editors-in-Chief

PREFACE

The American Geriatrics Society (AGS), with almost 6,000 members, works to improve the health, independence, and quality of life of all older adults. The AGS is committed to increasing the number of healthcare professionals employing the principles of geriatrics by supporting the expansion of geriatric education in nursing and all applicable health professions. The AGS recognizes the critically important role that nurses play as members of the team providing care to older adults, and in 2003, created the *Geriatric Nursing Review Syllabus* (*GNRS*) for advanced practice nurses. The *GNRS* provides current and comprehensive clinically relevant information to nurse practitioners preparing for certification exams as adult/gerontological, adult/gerontology acute care nurse practitioners or family nurse practitioners. It is an essential on-the-shelf or online resource for all providers to quickly access during their clinical day. In addition to being of value to students and nurse practitioners in practice, the *GNRS* is an invaluable resource for faculty. The comprehensive content of this new *GNRS* edition provides learners, faculty, and practicing nurse practitioners with information on diagnosis, management, and prevention of all major health problems commonly encountered when caring for older adults as well as on the social and legal issues related to health care in the United States. Having access to the information in this book will promote our current goal of providing high-quality and affordable care to all older adults.

We are releasing the fourth edition of the *Syllabus* as advance practice nursing education enters a new era that will require all nurse practitioners who focus on caring for adults to have expertise in caring for older and frailer adults. The *GNRS*, given its focus on the complexities of caring for those with multiple comorbidities, can help to support the nursing profession's efforts to ensure that the entire nursing workforce is prepared to care for the increasing numbers of older adults.

Ellen Flaherty, PhD, APRN, AGSF
Barbara Resnick, PhD, CRNP, FAAN, FAANP, AGSF
GNRS4 Editors-in-Chief

Jennie Chin Hansen, RN, MS, FAAN
Chief Executive Officer, American Geriatrics Society

INTRODUCTION

The *Geriatric Nursing Review Syllabus, 4th edition* (*GNRS4*) is modified from the *Geriatrics Review Syllabus, 8th edition* (*GRS8*) and contains 64 chapters and references that allow the interested reader to pursue topics in greater depth, 125 case-oriented, multiple-choice questions, and the repeated questions with answers and supporting critiques to aid learner self-assessment.

The Syllabus is divided into six sections—Principles of Aging, Approach to the Patient, Care Systems, Syndromes, Psychiatry, and Diseases and Disorders. *GNRS4* particularly highlights developments in geriatrics since publication of the second edition. When discussing specific drugs, the authors and editors verified that the information provided was up to date at the time of publication. Any mention of uses not specifically approved by the U.S. Food and Drug Administration (so called "off-label" uses) are tagged as OL.

Multiple Choice Questions

The questions are designed to complement material in the Syllabus chapters. The questions draw on the entire knowledge base of geriatrics, rather than just material from the Syllabus text. We recommend that participants prepare for answering these questions by first reading through the Syllabus chapters. Material addressed in the questions that is not discussed in the chapters is discussed in the critiques. The questions have been developed independently of any specialty board and will not be a part of any secure board certification examination.

We hope the *GNRS4* will meet our goal of enhancing participants' knowledge base and practice patterns when caring for older adults by providing a self-study tool that is current, concise, scholarly, and clinically relevant. We encourage your comments and suggestions, as the AGS continually strives to better serve its members and the older adults they treat.

Learning Objectives

The learning objectives for this activity have been designed to address participant knowledge, competence, performance, and patient outcomes. At the conclusion of this program, participants should be able to:

- Describe the general principles of aging and the biomedical and psychosocial issues of aging (knowledge);
- Discuss legal and ethical issues related to geriatrics (knowledge/competence);
- Evaluate the financing of health care for older adults (knowledge/competence);
- Identify the basic principles of geriatric medicine, including assessment, geriatric pharmacotherapy, prevention, exercise, palliative care, rehabilitation, and sensory deficits (knowledge/ competence);
- Use state-of-the-art approaches to geriatric care while providing care in hospital, office-practice, nursing-home, and home-care settings (performance);
- Diagnose and manage geriatric syndromes, including dementia, delirium, urinary incontinence, malnutrition, osteoporosis, falls, pressure ulcers, sleep disorders, pain, dysphagia, and dizziness (performance);

- Apply relevant information from the fields of medicine and nursing to the care of older patients (performance);
- Adjust patient care in the light of evidence-based data regarding the particular risks and needs of ethnic, racial, and sexual patient groups (patient outcomes);
- Use quality indicators to assess and improve the care of older adults in their own practices (performance/patient outcomes); and
- Employ evidence-based data to increase the effectiveness of teaching geriatrics to all health professionals (performance).

Additional American Geriatrics Society Resources

GNRS Teaching Slides are available as a subscription through www.geriatricscareonline.org. The slide presentations in Microsoft® Power Point® are based on each of the *GNRS* chapters and suitable for faculty and students. Each presentation is designed for approximately a 1-hour seminar and may be used as a stand-alone lecture or as a complement to one's own personal teaching materials.

Geriatrics Review Syllabus, 8th edition (*GRS8*) is available as a 3-volume set of books and online. The Syllabus offers 64 chapters covering the prevailing management strategies and recent research findings in geriatric medicine with references that allow the interested reader to pursue topics in greater depth. It also provides 333 case-oriented, multiple-choice questions and supportive critiques that can be used for self-assessment and also to earn continuing education credits.

The *GRS8* self-assessment program provides participants with the option of applying for 90 Continuing Medical Education (CME) credits through the American Medical Association.

Geriatrics at Your Fingertips, published annually, provides practical, up-to-date information for clinicians in a pocket-sized format.

Doorway Thoughts: Cross-Cultural Health Care for Older Adults is a three-volume series that helps the health practitioner to understand host best to care for an increasingly multicultural patient population.

GRS8 Audio Companion includes 30-minute audio discussions on 64 topics based on the *GRS8* content with chapter authors and experts in the field. Continuing education credits can be obtained by successfully completing 35 multiple-choice questions derived from the audio content. The program offers 35 AMA PRA Category 1 Credits™. Available at: http://www.grsaudio.com.

These and other publications, including resources and clinical practice guidelines, are available at www.geriatricscareonline.org. For more information on the American Geriatrics Society, visit www.americangeriatrics.org.

PROGRAM INFORMATION

CONGRUITY OF CONTENT BETWEEN SYLLABUS AND QUESTIONS

Because the Syllabus chapters and the questions with critiques are written by different authors, questions may not always correlate directly with the *Syllabus*. In the event that a question's content is not addressed in the correlating chapter, its answer is fully supported in the question critique.

REVIEW QUESTIONS

The *GNRS4* review questions are provided as learning aids but not as practice items for the Adult/Gerontological Advanced Practice Nurse Examination for the American Nurses Credentialing Center or the American Academy of Nurse Practitioners.

SELF-ASSESSMENT PROGRAM

For self-assessment testing, answer sheets are available for download at: http://www.geriatricscareonline.org/.

USER EVALUATION

The AGS would appreciate participants' comments about the *GNRS4* program through the User Survey located at: http://www.geriatricscareonline.org/. Comments and suggestions will be taken into consideration by those planning the next edition.

UPDATES AND ERRATA

Important updates, such as medication alerts, will be posted as necessary on the AGS Web site.

Please report any errata to: info.amger@americangeriatrics.org, Attention: GNRS Managing Editor. Identified errata will be posted on the AGS Web site also.

CHAPTER 1—DEMOGRAPHY

KEY POINTS

- The composition of the older United States' population is far from static. The large and growing numbers of aging baby boomers are becoming more racially and ethnically diverse. With increasing longevity, greater numbers of older adults are surviving to the oldest ages.
- Relative to their predecessors, older Americans today are generally more educated, better off financially (although racial and ethnic minority populations lag behind white Americans), increasingly live alone or in alternative residential settings, and are less functionally impaired.
- The population of older adults is characterized by heterogeneity across measures of health status, functioning, and socioeconomic position.
- Among older adults, heart disease, cancer, and stroke remain the leading causes of death, while other age-related conditions such as Alzheimer disease are becoming more common.

GLOBAL AGING TRENDS

As a result of declining fertility and mortality rates, the world today is experiencing pervasive, unprecedented population aging. According to the United Nations, the proportion of older adults (≥60 years old) comprised 8% of the worldwide population in 1950 but will represent 21% of the global population by 2050, at which time they will exceed the number of young for the first time in history. The number of people ≥60 years old was estimated at 759 million in 2010, and is projected to rise to 2 billion by 2050. The pace of aging varies by region and age group, and is much faster in developing countries and among the oldest-old age groups. The share of the global population of older adults living in less developed regions is anticipated to increase from 65% in 2010 to 80% by 2050.

Given the pace of population aging, developing countries will have less time to prepare for consequences associated with demographic change in their age structure. Financing health and long-term care services (particularly in more remote or rural areas) and maintaining economic security in old age will be particularly challenging in developing countries, although multigenerational households are more common. Three-fourths of people ≥60 years old live with children and/or grandchildren in developing countries, as compared with just one-fourth of older adults in more developed regions. In some parts of the world, skipped generation households have become common, when older adults assume responsibility for childrearing due to health-related issues (eg, HIV/AIDs in Africa) or employment-related migration of parents. Older adults' workforce participation rates tend to be higher in developing countries where pension systems are less established. For example, in 2008, labor force participation among men ≥65 years old was 37% in less developed regions as compared with 15% in more developed regions. Trends in labor participation and retirement also vary tremendously across countries. As of 2009, the age of statutory retirement varied from 50 years to 67 years. Retirement ages are generally younger in developing countries, although in most developed countries the effective actual age of retirement falls below the statutory retirement age. Less than 20% of older adults worldwide are covered by a public pension.

DEMOGRAPHY OF AGING IN THE UNITED STATES

In 2009, approximately 40 million people, or one in every eight Americans living in the United States was ≥65 years old. In light of declining birth rates and increases in longevity, the number of older adults is anticipated to comprise a greater proportion of the population, reaching one of every five Americans by 2030. This major demographic shift has prompted numerous concerns regarding U.S. social and health policy in recent years. Not only will the sheer number of older adults increase dramatically, but the composition and characteristics of the older population will also change. Although clinicians primarily attend to the needs of individual patients, some of the attributes that an older patient brings to the patient-clinician relationship are a function of the cohort to which he or she belongs. Aging baby boomers (the generation born between 1946 and 1964) will influence the health and social service systems of the United States, although the exact nature of this impact remains unclear.

During the 20th century, the U.S. population <65 years old tripled, while the group ≥65 years old increased by a factor of more than 11, growing from 3.1 million in 1900 to 39.6 million in 2009. This group is anticipated to more than double again by the middle of the 21st century, to 82 million people, with most of this growth occurring between 2010 and 2030. The United States is not unique in its growing numbers of

Table 1.1—Years of Life Expectancy at Birth and at Ages 65 and 85 by Gender and Race, 2009

	White			Black		
	Both sexes	*Male*	*Female*	*Both sexes*	*Male*	*Female*
At birth	78.8	76.4	81.2	74.5	71.1	77.6
Age 65	19.1	17.7	20.4	17.8	15.8	19.3
Age 85	6.6	5.8	7.0	6.8	5.9	7.2

SOURCE: Data from *National Vital Statistics System* as reported in Table 14b. Available at: http://www.agingstats.gov/agingstatsdotnet/Main_Site/Data/Data_2012.aspx (accessed Oct 2013).

older people. At present it is surpassed by many other developed countries, including Italy, Japan, Germany, Sweden, and the United Kingdom, where the proportion of people ≥60 years old already comprise 20% or more of the overall population.

Older adults are not evenly distributed across geographic regions of the United States. In 2009, more than half of older adults resided in eleven states, led by California (4.1 million), Florida (3.2 million), New York (2.6 million), and Texas (2.5 million). More than four in five older adults live in metropolitan (urban or suburban) areas. Residential mobility is more limited among older adults; <5% of older adults move in a given calendar year. Of older adults who move, two-thirds remain within the same county. The older U.S. population is predominantly white but is becoming increasingly diverse. Minority populations comprised approximately 20% of the adults ≥65 years old in 2009 and are expected to represent 39% by 2050. While the older black American population is anticipated to increase by 50% during this period, the older Asian American and Hispanic American populations are anticipated to triple. The number of older Hispanic Americans is projected to exceed that of older black Americans by 2050.

Life Expectancy

In the United States, the average life expectancy is currently highest for white women, followed by that for black women and white men, who have nearly identical life expectancies, and that of black men (Table 1.1). Women who survive to age 65 can, on average, expect to live to age 84, and those surviving to age 85 can expect to live to age 91. Up to age 85, the life expectancy of white American men and women exceeds that of their black counterparts. At age 85, these racial differences in life expectancy largely disappear. There is disagreement about whether these findings reflect errors in documenting age (for older black Americans) or are a true cross-over in mortality rates. The exact number of centenarians in the United States is difficult to gauge, but was estimated at approximately 0.2% of the overall population ≥65 years old in 2009. Their numbers are growing and are expected to exceed 800,000 by 2050.

Socioeconomic Status and Employment

Improvements in the Social Security system and the adoption of Medicare have had an important impact on the economic well-being of older adults in the United States. In the early 1960s, 35% of people ≥65 years old had incomes below the federal poverty level, and only 70% received Social Security pensions. By the early 1970s, over 90% of older people received Social Security retirement benefits, and 97% were covered by Medicare. Today, the percentage of older people with incomes below the poverty line is about 10%. A total of 26% of older adults are classified as "low income," based on income below 200% of the federal poverty level. For impoverished seniors (generally having an income well below the poverty line), Medicaid plays a key role in filling in the gaps in Medicare by covering nursing-home and other long-term care services, other healthcare services not covered by Medicare, as well as paying for Medicare premiums and cost-sharing. In 2007 (the most recent year for which statistics are available), approximately 5.5 million older adults were enrolled in both Medicare and Medicaid (ie, "dual eligibles").

Although the overall economic position of older people in the United States has improved significantly over the past three decades, these gains have not been shared by all. Poverty rates among older people are higher among blacks (20%) and Hispanic Americans (18%), and women (11%) versus men (7%). The poverty rate among older adults who live alone is approximately three times as high as older adults who live with others (16% versus 5%). Poverty rates in some groups of older adults are much higher—nearly half (45%) of older Hispanic American women and one-third (33%) of older black women living alone are poor, for example.

While labor force participation of older adults declined throughout most of the past century, this trend has reversed during the last 20 years, and growth in employment among older adults is expected to continue. In 2009, an estimated 6.5 million (17.2%) older adults were either working or actively seeking work—approximately 3.6 million (22%) older men and 2.9 million (14%) older women. Labor force participation is influenced by a variety of factors relating to economic

Table 1.2—Marital Status of Community-Dwelling Older Americans by Age, 2010 (individuals as a percentage of column total)

	All (%)			Male (%)			Female (%)		
	65–74	75–84	85+	65–74	75–84	85+	65–74	75–84	85+
Marital Status									
Married	66.2	52.8	32.0	78.0	73.2	58.3	55.9	38.1	18.0
Widowed	15.8	36.5	59.6	6.4	17.2	34.6	24.0	50.4	72.9
Other	18.0	10.7	8.4	15.5	9.6	7.1	20.1	10.5	9.3

SOURCE: Data from *Current Population Survey*, 2010; as reported in Tables 3 and 5a Available at: http://www.agingstats.gov/agingstatsdotnet/Main_Site/Data/Data_2012.aspx (accessed Oct 2013).

necessity (eg, declines in defined benefit pension plans, the increase in the full retirement age for Social Security benefits, the high costs of health insurance), as well as personal choice. Higher levels of education and improvements in health have afforded greater numbers of older adults the opportunity to continue to work.

Education and Literacy

One of the most dramatic changes in the older U.S. population has been in regard to levels of educational attainment. Between 1965 and 2008, the percentage of people ≥65 years old who completed high school increased from 24% to 77%, and the percentage with a bachelor's degree or more increased from 5% to 21%. Education is closely related to lifetime economic status, and many studies have shown that individuals with more education generally enjoy better health and lower rates of disability than those with low levels of educational attainment. Despite gains in education, education and literacy levels of older adults lag far behind those of working-age adults. According to Healthy People 2010, health literacy is "the degree to which individuals have the capacity to obtain, process, and understand basic health information and services needed to make appropriate health decisions." In one national survey, just 3% of adults ≥65 years old were deemed as having "proficient" health literacy skills; 29% were classified at "below basic" skill level. Given the greater availability of health and medical information via the Internet and mainstream media (eg, direct-to-consumer advertising) and older adults' high prevalence of chronic health conditions and health service use, the relevance of health literacy is arguably more important for older adults today than ever before.

Marital Status and Living Arrangements

Although approximately half of older adults live with a spouse, living arrangements vary dramatically by age, gender, and race/ethnicity subgroups. For example, older women are nearly twice as likely than older men to live alone (37% versus 19% in 2010) or with relatives other than a spouse (17.9% versus 5.9%). Not surprisingly, given older women's longer life expectancy, older men are far more likely to be married than are older women. For example, among older adults ≥85 years old, 58% of men were married versus 18% of women. Conversely, widowhood is common among older women; 50% of women 75–84 years old and 73% of women ≥85 years old are widows, compared with 17% of men 75–84 years old and 35% of men ≥85 years old (Table 1.2).

Trends in Health, Functioning, and Mortality

The burden of disease and disability is greater for older people than working-age adults and children. In fact, the vast majority of older adults have one or more chronic conditions. In 2007–2008, the most common self-reported conditions included hypertension (56%), arthritic symptoms (51%), heart disease (30%), cancer (24%), and diabetes (20%) (Figure 1.1). There is great heterogeneity in health status among older adults. Data on self-assessed health, which have been shown to correlate highly with mortality and risk of functional decline, illustrate this. Among white non-Hispanic Americans 65–74 years old, 82% regarded their health as "excellent," "very good," or "good" as compared with 67% of black non-Hispanic Americans and 66% of Hispanic Americans (Table 1.3). As might be expected, the percentages who viewed their health as only fair or poor increases with age. The proportion of older adults who reported their health to be "fair" or "poor" is higher in all age groups among black and Hispanic Americans than among white Americans. Physical functioning is closely associated with both gender and age. For example, the proportion of older adults who are unable to perform five basic physical activities increases from 19% of women 65–74 years old to 53% of women ≥85 years old, and from 13% of men 65–74 years old to 40% of men ≥85 years old (Figure 1.2). Older women exhibit a higher percentage of limitations in functioning at all ages than older men.

Deaths of older people comprise nearly 75% of all deaths in the United States. About 30% of all deaths occur at age 85 or older, which, given broader demographic trends, is likely to grow. For many decades,

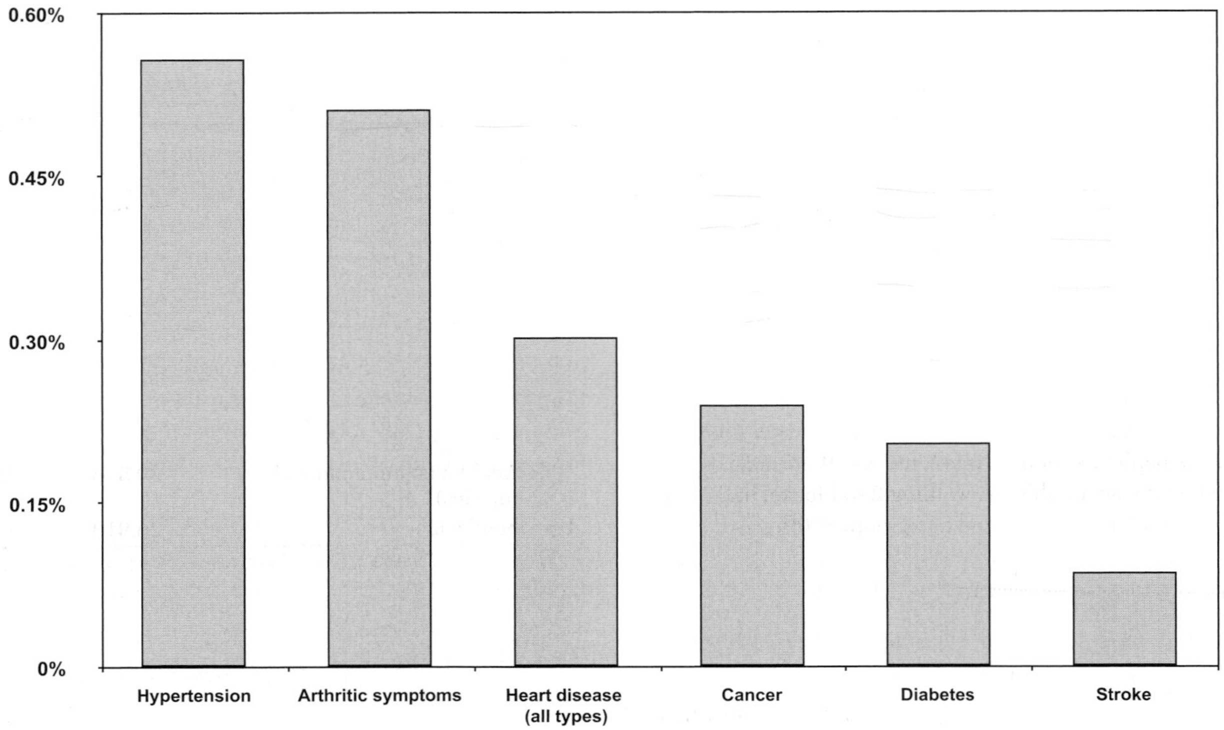

Figure 1.1—Prevalence of selected self-reported chronic conditions among adults ≥65 years old, all races.

SOURCE: Data from the *National Health Interview Survey* as reported in Table 16a. Estimates for 2009–2010. http://www.agingstats.gov/agingstatsdotnet/Main_Site/Data/Data_2012.aspx (accessed Oct 2013).

Table 1.3—Perceived Health of Older Adults by Age and Race/Ethnicity, 2008–2010

	White, non-Hispanic (%)			Black, non-Hispanic (%)			Hispanic (%)		
	65–74	75–84	85+	65–74	75–84	85+	65–74	75–84	85+
Men									
Good to excellent	80.9	75.3	68.2	67.9	57.8	54.0	67.0	60.8	54.9
Fair or poor	19.1	24.7	31.8	32.8	42.3	46.0	33.0	39.3	45.1
Women									
Good to excellent	82.7	76.7	70.7	66.7	55.9	54.3	64.4	59.0	49.9
Fair or poor	17.3	23.4	29.9	33.3	44.1	45.7	35.6	40.8	50.2

SOURCE: Data are based on a 3-year average from 2008–2010 from the *National Health Interview Survey*, NCHS Vital and Health Statistics, Table 18. Available at: http://www.agingstats.gov/agingstatsdotnet/Main_Site/Data/Data_2012.aspx (accessed Oct 2013).

heart disease, cancer, respiratory diseases, and stroke have been the leading causes of death among people ≥65 years old, accounting for 6 of 10 deaths (Table 1.4). Causes of death vary by race, ethnicity, and gender, however. For example, Alzheimer disease ranked fifth among all causes of death but is more prominent among white non-Hispanic older adults and less prominent among black non-Hispanic and Hispanic older adults. Some causes of death usually associated with younger people also are of concern in the older population. In the United States, the death rate from motor vehicle accidents is high among older adults, largely because of greater susceptibility to injury. Rates of suicide deaths among people ≥65 years old is approximately 14 per 100,000 versus 11 per 100,000 in the general population. Approximately 85% of suicides in older adults occur among men. The highest suicide rates among older people occur among white non-Hispanic men ≥85 years old; their rate of suicide death approaches 50 per 100,000 persons.

Trends in Disability

Disability dynamics have been an area of active research, in part because of the relevance of disability to public programs such as Medicare and Medicaid. Increases in life expectancy have led to debate over whether additional years of life gained will be achieved

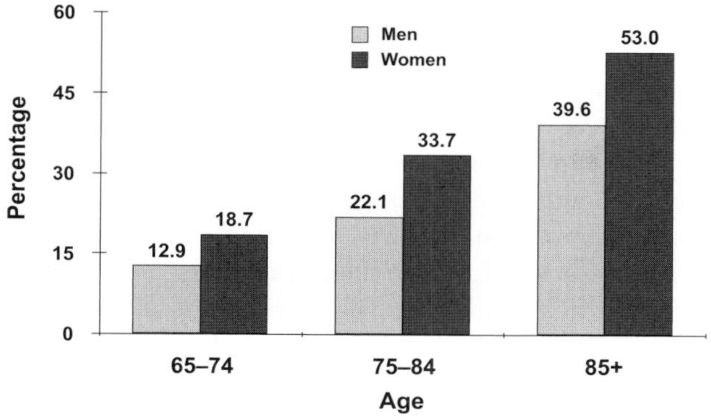

Figure 1.2—Percentage of Medicare enrollees ≥65 years old who are unable to perform any one of five physical functions (stooping, kneeling, reaching over the head, writing/grasping small objects, walking 2–3 blocks, and lifting 10 pounds) by gender and age group, 2009.

SOURCE: Data from *Medicare Beneficiary Survey*, 2009 as reported in Table 20d. http://www.agingstats.gov/agingstatsdotnet/Main_Site/Data/Data_2012.aspx (accessed Oct 2013).

Table 1.4—Leading Causes of Death and Death Rates, for Adults ≥65 Years Old, 2009

Rank	Cause of Death	Number of Deaths	Rate
	All causes	1,762,494	4,454
1	Diseases of heart	479,046	1211
2	Malignant neoplasms	391,855	990
3	Chronic lower respiratory disease	117,048	296
4	Cerebrovascular disease	109,055	276
5	Alzheimer disease	78,058	197
6	Diabetes mellitus	48,811	123
7	Influenza and pneumonia	43,433	110
8	Nephritis, nephrotic syndrome, and nephrosis	40,341	102
9	Accidents (unintentional injuries)	39,316	99
10	Septicemia	26,810	68

SOURCE: *National Vital Statistics Reports* Vol 59, No 4 (Table 7). Available at: www.cdc.gov/nchs/data/nvsr/nvsr59/nvsr59_04.pdf (accessed Oct 2013).

free of disability, or whether these incremental years of life gained will be borne in a disabled state. Studies of active life expectancy, which use mortality and disability estimates to project disability-free years, suggest an advantage for people with more education. Because of their greater total life expectancy, older women experience both greater active life expectancy and more years of disability than do older men. It has been suggested that if there is a limit to increases in life expectancy, increases in disability-free years could produce a *compression of morbidity*, with the period of disability before death gradually compressed as active life expectancy (or disability-free years) increases.

Over the last several decades, several longitudinal studies of older adults have indicated aggregate declines in disability, although the magnitude of decline across types of disability and subgroups of older Americans is more controversial. For example, estimates from the National Long-Term Care Survey suggest that the proportion of chronically disabled or institutionalized older adults declined between 1984 and 2004 (the last year the survey was fielded), with the majority of disability reduction being attributed to lower rates of disability in instrumental activities of daily living (IADLs). While the trend toward a decline in IADL disability and general stability in disability in activities of daily living (ADLs) has been substantiated by a number of national surveys, variability in sampling strategy and measurement of disability challenge definitive conclusions regarding the magnitude of such findings. For example, the extent to which questions explicitly assess respondents' use of assistive devices (eg, remote devices, canes, walkers) or the built environment (eg, growth in residential settings that have adopted universal design) may influence disability estimates. The National Health and Aging Trends Survey was designed to provide insight on late-life disability trends, and results will be available in the coming years.

Whether the benefits of greater literacy and increased longevity have been universally experienced by all subgroups of older Americans in terms of improved functioning is not clear. Recent studies substantiate the existence of disparities in disability across racial and ethnic subgroups and by education. For example, the proportion of older adults who reported no difficulty with any of six IADLs varies from 59% of older black Americans to 67% of white non-Hispanic Americans ≥65 years old. A parallel trend is observed in trends of severe disability. The proportion of older adults with three or more ADL limitations varies from 11% of white Hispanic and black non-Hispanic adults to 7% of white non-Hispanic Americans. The reasons for such disparities are multifaceted, reflecting a lifetime of behavior and experience, environmental exposure, and access to and use of medical care.

Disability Accommodation

Individuals may use a variety of approaches to compensate for a physical disability, including assistive technology, personal care, environmental modifications, or change in residential setting. Use of assistive technology is widespread and increasing among disabled older adults, with mobility-related devices, such as canes and walkers, being used most commonly. Among community-dwelling older adults with limitations in ADLs in 2007, 38% relied on assistive technology alone, an additional 22% relied on both assistive technology and personal care, and just 6% relied exclusively on personal care alone.

Individuals who rely on personal care alone tend to be most highly disabled and often have both physical and cognitive impairment. The vast majority of older adults who receive personal care rely on help from a family member or a friend ("family caregiver"). Although few disabled older adults receive help from a paid caregiver, the likelihood of receiving paid help increases with age. Family caregivers for chronically disabled older adults are predominantly spouses or adult children who live either with one another or in close proximity. While family caregivers commonly assist with household and personal-care task assistance, they are also frequently involved in providing or coordinating older adults' medical care. For example, family caregivers commonly assist with wound care, medication management, and coordination of care between clinicians or across settings of care; approximately 2 in 5 older adults are routinely accompanied to office visits by a family member or friend.

Residential-Care Facilities

Residential-care facilities are a relatively new but rapidly growing residential setting in the United States. This type of facility provides greater supervision and assistance than is typically available in a private home, while allowing more autonomy and freedom than traditional nursing-home facilities. According to recently published estimates from the first national survey of such facilities (the National Survey of Residential Care Facilities conducted in 2010), approximately 972,000 residential-care facility beds exist within 31,000 facilities. The availability and mix of facilities vary by region; approximately half of residential-care facilities are small in size (4 to 10 beds). Larger facilities are more likely to be chain-affiliated and to have a wider range of service offerings, such as occupational and physical therapy. Evidence suggests that residential-care facilities serve primarily a private-pay population, although Medicaid is gradually increasing in its financing for services in such settings. Residents are thought to move to residential-care facilities from a variety of settings. More than half move from their own private apartment or residence, with the remainder being about equally distributed from other personal-care homes, assisted-living residences, hospitals, nursing homes, or other private residence, such as an adult child's home. The average length of residency is thought to be approximately 2 years.

Nursing Facilities

Over the course of the past 20 years, nursing facilities have increasingly developed skilled-nursing capabilities to provide postacute care to individuals transitioning out of the acute hospital setting. However, nursing facilities continue to play an important role as a provider of long-term care to a particularly vulnerable segment of the population, caring for older adults with cognitive or physical impairment, or both, and with considerable ongoing medical needs. Not surprisingly, nursing-home use rates vary considerably by age group. Approximately 0.5% of working-age adults have a nursing-home level of impairment as indicated by receiving help with three or more ADLs as compared with 3.5% of adults ≥65 years old. Of approximately 1.3 million long-term nursing-home residents, the vast majority (1.1 million) are ≥65 years old. There is some indication that rates of nursing-home use have declined. This trend is likely a manifestation of improvements in older adults' health and functioning as well as increases in system-wide community supports and the growth of alternative residential arrangements, such as assisted-living facilities and continuing-care retirement communities. Regardless, the net effect is that the nursing-home population has become older and more disabled. For example, the proportion of residents ≥85 years old increased from 35% to 45% between 1977 and 2004. Nursing-home residents have a high degree of medical comorbidity and often are expected to follow complex treatment regimens; in 2004, nearly one-half of all nursing-home residents took nine or more medications. Half of all nursing-home residents require help with five or six ADLs. There is some indication that the composition of the nursing-home population is becoming more racially diverse. One study found that between 1999 and 2008, the number of nursing-home residents ≥65 years old who were Hispanic or Asian increased by more than 50% and the number of black residents increased by 11%, while the number of white residents decreased by 10%. To what extent the shifting racial composition of the nursing-home population is the result of greater numbers of minority older adults overall, or reflects disparities in access to home and community-based alternatives, is unclear.

Future Issues

Older adults are among the most heterogeneous of United States' population subgroups, encompassing the entire spectrum of health and functioning, from the bedridden Alzheimer patient to the marathon runner. One of the important unresolved questions is whether gains in longevity after age 65 are accompanied by gains or declines in years of disability-free life. It is unlikely that one answer will fit this large and diverse group. There are many questions in other areas as well. Will the increasing numbers of better-educated, longer-lived older adults contribute to the larger society, and in what ways? Will the sheer numbers of older people strain to the breaking point the medical care system and public programs that finance health care and retirement, as some analysts fear? Or will improvements in health behavior, medical breakthroughs, and financial prosperity diminish these threats? Under any scenario, chronic illness will remain a constant in the lives of many older people. Clinicians treating this population face the challenge not only of treating chronically ill adults but also in assisting the prevention of chronic disease onset.

REFERENCES

- Administration on Aging, U.S. Department of Health and Human Services. *A Profile of Older Americans: 2010*. Available at: www.aoa.gov/aoaroot/aging_statistics/Profile/2010/docs/2010profile.pdf (accessed Oct 2013).
- Federal Interagency Forum on Aging-Related Statistics. *Older Americans 2010: Key Indicators of Well-Being*. Washington, DC: U.S. Government Printing Office; July 2010. Available at: www.agingstats.gov/agingstatsdotnet/Main_Site/Data/2010_Documents/Docs/OA_2010.pdf (accessed Oct 2013).
- Kaye H, Harrington C, LaPlante M. Long-term care: who gets it, who provides it, who pays, and how much? *Health Aff (Millwood)*. 2010;29(1):11–21.
- Kochanek KD, Xu J, Murphy SL, et al. *Deaths: Preliminary Data for 2009*. National Vital Statistics Reports, Volume 59, Number 4. Hyattsville, Maryland: National Center for Health Statistics. March 16, 2011. Available at: www.cdc.gov/nchs/data/nvsr/nvsr59/nvsr59_04.pdf (accessed Oct 2013).

CHAPTER 2—BIOLOGY

KEY POINTS

- *Aging* is a loss of homeostasis, or a breakdown in maintenance of specific molecular structures and pathways; this breakdown is the inevitable consequence of the evolved anatomic and physiologic design of an organism.
- Evolutionary theories of aging address the "*why*" of aging.
- Psychosocial theories of aging address the "*who*" of aging.
- Physiologic theories of aging address the "*how*" of aging.
- The many theories of aging are not competing or mutually exclusive; rather, the theories reflect our current understanding of the multiple maintenance and homeostasis mechanisms that allow us to live as long as we do.
- Some of the molecular and cellular changes that occur with aging are unique to the specific cellular and tissue context of the organ, while others occur across a number of organ systems with a common effect on functional capacity when systems are stressed.

The most visible imprints of aging are loss of hair and pigmentation of hair; diminished height and muscle and bone mass; and increasingly wrinkled, thinned skin. These progressive and accelerating changes have a biologic basis in altered molecular and cellular structure and function. The biology of aging represents evolutionary aspects, behavioral and social facets, molecular mechanisms, and organ system changes of aging. The onset, rate, and extent of the aging process is extremely heterogeneous. Thus, biologic age, based on an individual's functional capacity (and not chronologic age), is the metric for the biology of aging. Functional capacity is a direct measure of the ability of cells, tissues, and organ systems to function properly and optimally and is influenced by both genes and environment. Within this context, aging is defined as the progressive decline and deterioration of functional properties at the cellular, tissue, and organ level that lead to a loss of homeostasis, decreased ability to adapt to internal or external stimuli, and increased vulnerability to disease and mortality.

The science of aging includes the study of the "why" of aging (evolutionary theories), the "who" of aging (psychosocial theories), the "how" of aging (physiologic theories), and the "what and where" of aging (the molecular, cellular, and organ system changes associated with increasing age). Inherent in these multiple approaches to investigating aging is the definition of what aging is. For some gerontologists, aging is a normal physiologic outcome, part of the process of being and persistence through time, manifested by simple wear and tear. For others, aging is a pathologic outcome that results from the complex cumulative interplay of multiple diseases brought about by genetic mutations, environment, and time. Underlying these two perspectives is the question of whether the goal of understanding the biology of aging is adding years to life (life extension) or life to years (improving quality of remaining years).

Aging is characterized by progressive changes in cells, tissues, and organs of the body that lead inexorably to death. These changes are the consequences of the inability to maintain cells, tissues, and organ systems indefinitely. Aging is due to the eventual breakdown of maintenance processes—an inevitable consequence of the evolved anatomic and physiologic design of the organism.

THEORIES OF AGING

Evolutionary theories of aging explain historical and evolutionary aspects of aging, addressing why aging exists in living things and how aging may have evolved as a process. *Psychosocial theories* of aging explain behavioral, cognitive and social features of aging. *Physiologic theories* of aging explain structural and functional age changes.

Evolutionary Theories of Aging

Evolution deals with the impact of natural selection (selective pressure) on the reproductive fitness of a species. There are currently two main evolutionary theories of aging: mutation accumulation theory and antagonistic pleiotropy theory.

Mutation Accumulation Theory

Mutation accumulation theory views aging as a nonadaptive trait, a by-product and inevitable result of the declining force of natural selection with age. Because no selective pressure is brought to bear on organisms expressing a mutation at older postreproductive ages (which has minimal effects on fitness), these late-acting genes accumulate over time and they yield the aging phenotype.

Antagonistic Pleiotropy Theory

Pleiotropy is when a single gene controls or influences multiple traits. The antagonistic pleiotropic theory considers aging an adaptive trait, in which genes that can influence several traits are selected for and affect individual fitness in opposite (ie, antagonistic) ways at different stages of life. Pleiotropic genes have beneficial effects on early fitness components in the young but harmful effects on late fitness components, and yet are nevertheless favored by natural selection. There is, for example, an evolutionary trade-off between reproductive capacity and longevity.

Psychosocial Theories of Aging

Psychosocial theories attempt to explain aging in terms of individual changes in behavior, cognitive function, coping ability, relationships, roles, and social interactions. As people age, there are changes in behavior, social interactions, and chosen activities. Five of the more common psychosocial theories are briefly described below.

Disengagement theory posits that with increasing age, the quantity and quality of relationships between a person and other members of society diminish. *Activity theory* highlights the maintenance of and alterations in regular activities, roles, and social pursuits. *Life-course theory* views aging as the progressive adjustment of older individuals to declining health and physical strength, retirement and reduced income, the death of a spouse or family members, new living arrangements, as well as to the pleasures of aging (increased leisure time, playing with grandchildren). *Continuity theory* states that older adults may seek to use familiar strategies in familiar areas of life to preserve and maintain internal and external structures as an adaptive strategy to deal with changes that occur during normal aging. *Gerotranscendence theory* holds aging as part of a natural progression toward a goal of achieving maturation and wisdom, with a shift in perspective from materialistic and rational view to more cosmic and transcendent view.

Physiologic Theories of Aging

Physiologic theories address how we age. A great deal of information on changes during aging at the organ system, cellular, molecular, and genetic levels has been gathered over the past few decades. The major physiologic theories with special emphasis on available supporting evidence are described below.

Target Theory of Genetic Damage

Underlying the genetic theories of aging is the idea that aging is heavily influenced or caused by genes. The genome is the repository for all genetic material, and the integrity of this information is essential for reproductive fitness and survival. DNA is subject to a number of insults, including spontaneous chemical changes, environmental damage by ionizing radiation, aflatoxin, and alkylating agents, all of which modify DNA structure. Mechanisms of repair rely on the efficiency of many enzymes that in turn depend on fidelity of the information in the DNA. Thus, the target theory of genetic damage states that genes are susceptible to hits from radiation or other damaging agents that alter function of structural, signaling and/or repair molecules, and that these cumulative hits give rise to an aging phenotype.

Mitochondrial DNA Damage Theory

Mitochondrial DNA (mtDNA) is not protected by proteins (eg, histones, chromatin) as nuclear DNA is, and mtDNA is attached to the inner mitochondrial membrane, where free radicals are produced. Thus, mtDNA damage occurs 10–20 times faster than nuclear DNA damage. In addition, mtDNA cannot repair itself, and some damaged mitochondria replicate faster than undamaged mitochondria, which gives rise to expansion of aberrant mitochondria. As a consequence, genes encoded within the mitochondria are more likely to lose their integrity over time. The damaged mtDNA has more deleterious effects than does damage to nuclear DNA, because each cell translates almost all its mtDNA genes but only 7% of its nuclear DNA. Nearly any adverse change in mtDNA will have deleterious effects on mitochondrial function. These effects include less energy production, more free-radical formation, reduced control of other cell processes, and accumulation of damaged harmful molecules, leading to aging and certain age-related diseases. The mitochondrial DNA theory of aging is closely allied with the free radical theory of aging (see below).

Telomere Theory

Telomeres are specialized sequences found at the ends of linear chromosomes. With every DNA replication event, there is progressive shortening of telomeres unless cells express enough telomerase (the enzyme that maintains sufficient length of telomeres to enable repeated replication). Once telomeres are reduced beyond a threshold length, cells enter a nonreplicating state in which their gene expression changes. Somatic cells express minimal levels of the enzyme, and cellular (replicative) senescence is triggered when cells acquire critically short telomeres. Telomere length provides a mechanism for Leonard Hayflick's mid-20th century observation that mammalian cells are limited in the number of times they can divide ("Hayflick's limit"). The telomere hypothesis of aging proposes that telomere shortening causes aging and that telomerase will prevent aging. Evidence supporting the telomere theory includes observations that telomere length is directly proportional to cell age, telomeres are lost faster from individuals with progerias, and immortal cells such as cancerous cells have a constant telomere length, while restoring telomerase enzyme in somatic cells in vitro caused an increase in replicative life span of these cells. Evidence that is not supportive includes observations that telomere length is not related to life span (mouse telomeres are much longer then those in people), and telomerase protects against replicative senescence but not cellular senescence triggered by other pathways.

Error Catastrophe Theory

This theory holds that damage is not to the genes themselves but to RNA and proteins (that read the genes and carry out their instructions). The damaged molecules spread, increasing the number of mistakes and loss of molecular function causing biologic changes that are seen as "aging." For RNA, there may be issues with RNA transcriptional accuracy, proofreading, mismatch repair, splicing, and transport. For proteins, errors in translating RNA to the correct amino acid sequence or in polypeptide folding and conformation have deleterious effects on protein function. Error catastrophe theory holds that cumulative errors in subsets of proteins involved in transfer of information from DNA to protein are normally below a threshold, so a steady state exists with random perturbations. Critical errors can destabilize the machinery for protein synthesis, causing an irreversible increase in the error level and accelerating loss of function as the organism ages.

These predictions have been tested experimentally, and this theory has equivocal support.

Free Radical Theory

Free radicals are extremely reactive and unstable and are produced in mitochondria, in oxidative enzymes in the endoplasmic reticulum, in peroxisomes, and by phagocytes. Free radicals are normally policed by enzymes that inactivate them (superoxide dismutase, catalase, glutathione peroxidase), antioxidants that neutralize them (α-tocopherol, ascorbic acid, uric acid), sulfhydryl-containing compounds (cysteine, glutathione, bilirubin, ubiquinol, and carnosine), and β-carotene.

Evidence in favor of this theory include that positive correlations have been observed between metabolic rate and free radical production, age and rate of free radical formation, and age and amount of free radical damage, while inverse correlations have been observed between longevity and free radical production, age and free radical defenses, and that abnormal mitochondria increase during aging. Evidence against this theory includes that antioxidant treatment does not reproducibly increase life span and that cells have effective defenses against radicals. Free radicals can act as causative agents in other physiologic theories of aging, including DNA damage, mitochondrial DNA, protein error, and protein modification theory.

Accumulation Theories

This group of theories posits that aging is associated with the accumulation of cellular and extracellular components with altered structure that compromise cellular function. The components can be *molecular* as in the clinker theory in which lipofuscin (an oxidized lipid), for example, accumulates in lysosomes compromising the organelle's capacity for catabolism. These components can be *macromolecular*, as in the protein modifications theory in which, for example, collagen cross-links in skin and bone, neurofibrillary tangles and plaque formation in the brain, and advanced glycation end products in multiple organ systems alter cellular and tissue functional capacity. Finally, components can be damaged organelles such as mitochondria, peroxisomes, and cell membranes, and the inability to remove functionally compromised organelles through autophagy leads to further loss of function.

Rate of Living Theory

The rate of living theory holds that aging is determined by the rate of metabolism, because aerobic metabolism causes damage, primarily through the production of oxygen-free radicals. This theory predicts that the higher the rate of metabolism, the faster the rate of aging and the shorter the life span. While most animals follow this prediction, two major exceptions are mammals and birds, which have life spans longer than their rates of metabolism would predict.

Epigenetic Theory

Most cells in the human body are somatic cells. A major mechanism maintaining these cells' appropriate, differentiated phenotype is epigenetic, dependent on DNA-protein interactions, DNA methylation, and histone acetylation. The epigenetic theory posits that phenotypic drift arising from inappropriate epigenetic modifications leads to altered gene expression and cellular function and the aging phenotype. In general, DNA methylation increases with age, but within a tissue there can be variation. The degree of hypermethylation depends on multiple factors, including age, diet, and exposure to environmental agents/insults (eg, carcinogens, epimutagens, toxins). Epigenetic silencing of repressive transcription factors may contribute to differentiated cells switching to a senescent phenotype.

Endocrine Theory

With increasing age, the synthesis and secretion of a number of hormones change. In addition, cell receptors on target organs can change in number and functional signal transduction. The circadian cycles of certain hormones also become irregular. The endocrine theory of aging posits that the occurrence of changes in hormone levels and signaling are a major cause of loss of homeostasis. This theory views aging as arising from dysregulated hormones. For example, deficits in growth hormone or sex steroid hormones impact target organs' size and ability to repair and maintain functional capacity.

Immune Theory

Relatively slow-growing organisms must confront infection by rapidly growing pathogens or parasites, and the immune system has evolved to do this. Homeostasis of the immune system is maintained by innate or nonspecific mechanisms such as humoral mechanisms (complement) and cellular mechanisms (macrophage, neutrophils, natural killer cells), as well as by the specific, acquired immune response involving humoral mechanisms (antibodies) and cellular mechanisms (T and B lymphocytes). The well documented gradual decline in the immune system maintenance ("immunosenescence") contributes significantly to increased morbidity and mortality in late life. The immune theory of aging posits that immunosenescence contributes to aging by limiting systemic defensive and repair responses that impact the functional capacity of other organ systems. An elevated pro-inflammatory state has been observed in older individuals as marked by increased levels of cytokines (such as interleukin-6) and macrophage activation markers. Failure to resolve the repair and remodeling program of inflammation results in an altered tissue structure and cellular organization that can negatively feedback on cellular and organ system function.

Stem Cell/Progenitor Cell Theory

Adult stem cells in the brain, bone marrow, and circulation maintain homeostasis by replenishing depleted reserves. Examples include satellite cells that contribute to muscle mass and repair of muscle tissue, and osteoprogenitor cells that replenish osteoblasts and form bone. Over time, precursor cells become depleted either by phenotypic dr[illegible] illness, or environmental challe[illegible] bone mesenchymal stem cells can [illegible] osteoblastic, myoblastic, or adipocy[illegible] associated with osteopenia, sarcopenia [illegible] in fat content in bone marrow and mus[illegible] related changes may arise from a shift [illegible]y commitment of bone mesenchymal stem [illegible] (away from bone and muscle cells) toward the adipocytic cell line.

ORGAN SYSTEM CHANGES WITH AGING

The many theories of aging should not be viewed as competing or mutually exclusive. Rather, the theories reflect our current understanding of the individual maintenance pathways and homeostatic mechanisms that allow us to live as long as we do. The theories also provide pathways for investigating interventions that modify aging. For example, caloric restriction, which increases life span in organisms from worms to mice, may be acting through modulation of energy metabolism, defense against free radicals, and clearance of defective components (autophagy). Similarly, exercise, which can modify the rate and extent of aging, may act through pathways involving energy metabolism, autophagy, and defense against injury. Physiologic theories elaborate a framework for translating the "what" and "where" of aging from molecules to organ system and homeostasis. Aging nerves, muscle, skin, hair, cartilage and bone, vasculature, and other organs exhibit changes at the molecular and cellular level. Some molecular changes with aging are shared between tissue types and organ systems, while others are unique. For example, in skin, bone, and cartilage, increases in cross-links (both enzymatic and nonenzymatic) alter compressibility and resiliency, and decreases in structural components (eg, proteoglycans and glycosaminoglycans) alter tissue hydration and function. In contrast, changes in the immune system (eg, diminished ability of dendritic cells to present antigen) are unique to the specific cell type, organ system, and function. A brief overview of significant age-related changes in the major organ systems follows below and in Table 2.1. These changes represent biologic processes common to everyone, although they progress at different rates.

Nerves

With increasing age, both the number and functioning of sensory neurons decline. Age-related changes in somatic motor functioning include changes in somatic cell number, action potentials, and transmission rates.

Table [illegible]1—Physiologic Changes of Aging

Body System	Change	Consequences
Nervous	↓ Number of neurons ↓ Action potential speed ↓ Axon/dendrite branches	↓ Muscle innervation ↓ Fine motor control
Muscle	Fibers shrink ↓ Type II (fast twitch) fibers ↑ Lipofuscin and fat deposits	Tissue atrophies ↓ Tone and contractility ↓ Strength
Skin	↓ Thickness ↑ Collagen cross-links	Loss of elasticity
Skeletal	↓ Bone density Joints become stiffer, less flexible	Movement slows and may become limited
Cardiovascular		
Heart	↑ Left ventricular wall thickness ↑ Lipofuscin and fat deposits	Stressed heart is less able to respond
Vasculature	↑ Stiffness ↓ Responsiveness to agents	
Pulmonary	↓ Elastin fibers ↑Collagen cross-links ↓ Elastic recoil of the lung ↑ Residual volume ↓ Vital capacity, forced expiratory volume, and forced vital capacity	↓ Effort dependent and independent respiration (quiet and forced breathing) ↓ Exercise tolerance and pulmonary reserve
Eyes	↑ Lipid infiltrates/deposits ↑ Thickening of the lens ↓ Pupil diameter	↓ Transparency of the cornea Difficulty in focusing on near objects ↓ Accommodation and dark adaptation
Ears	↑ Thickening of tympanic membrane ↓ Elasticity and efficiency of ossicular articulation ↑ Organ atrophy ↓ Cochlear neurons	↑ Conductive deafness (low-frequency range) ↑ Sensorineural hearing loss (high-frequency sounds)
Digestive	↑ Dysphagia ↑ Achlorhydria Altered intestinal absorption ↑ Lipofuscin and fat deposition in pancreas ↑ Mucosal cell atrophy	↓ Iron absorption ↓ B_{12} and calcium absorption ↑ Incidence of diverticula, transit time, and constipation
Urinary	↓ Kidney size, weight, and number of functional glomeruli ↓ Number and length of functional renal tubules ↓ Glomerular filtration rate ↓ Renal blood flow	↓ Ability to resorb glucose ↓ Concentrating ability of kidney
Immune	↓ Primary and secondary response ↑ Autoimmune antibodies ↓ T-cell function, fewer naive and more memory T cells Atrophy of thymus	↓Immune functioning ↓ Response to new pathogens ↓ T lymphocytes, natural killer cells, cytokines needed for growth and maturation of B cells
Endocrine	↑ Atrophy of certain glands (eg, pituitary, thyroid, thymus) ↓ Growth hormone, dehydroepiandrosterone, testosterone, estrogen ↑ Parathyroid hormone, atrial natriuretic peptide, norepinephrine, baseline cortisol, erythropoietin	Changes in target organ response, organ system homeostasis, response to stress, functional capacity

The number of somatic motor neurons decreases, reducing the number of cells that can be stimulated, decreasing the maximal strength of contraction that muscles can produce. The speed of action potentials in their axons decreases slightly, such that impulses arrive over an increasingly long period and contractions of muscle cells are spread out over a longer period; the slower transmission results in further delay in starting a motion. Neurons remaining in the brain have less fluid and stiffer cell membranes, internal membranes that become irregular in structure and accumulate lipofuscin, and tangled neurofibrils. The ability of neurons to grow branches of both axons and dendrites decreases, reducing fine motor control.

Changes in motor neuron cell membranes, myelin, or blood vessels within the nerves reduce blood flow in nerves, decreasing the supply of nutrients and the elimination of wastes, which contribute to the slower action potentials and spreading of muscle cell contraction. The slower contraction, lower peak strength of contraction, and slower relaxation reduce maximal muscle strength when performing quick movements.

Muscle

Lean body mass decreases, caused in part by loss of muscle tissue (atrophy). The rate and extent of muscle changes seem to be genetically determined. Average rates of muscle mass decline are 15% per decade at ages 50–60 and increase to 30% after age 60. Lipofuscin (the oxidized lipid "age pigment") and fat are deposited in muscle tissue. There is selective loss of type II (fast twitch) muscle fibers, and remaining muscle fibers shrink. Muscle tissue is replaced more slowly, and lost muscle tissue may be replaced with a tough fibrous tissue. This is most noticeable in the hands, which may appear thin and bony. Changes in muscle tissue, combined with normal aging changes in the nervous system, lead to reduced muscle tone and contractility. Muscles can become rigid with age and can lose tone even if exercised regularly, leading to changes in strength and endurance.

Skin

Cellular changes in the skin include thinning of the epidermis with a reduced mitotic rate in epidermal basal cells, shortened and attenuated rete ridges, reduced epidermal appendages, and fewer fibroblasts and capillaries in the dermis. Melanocytes in both exposed and unexposed skin decrease with age, while those remaining become larger but produce less melanin. At the molecular level, the dermal thickness decreases as the collagen content per unit area of the skin decreases. Loss of skin elasticity (caused by increased collagen cross-links and decreased elastin) leads to skin sagging and wrinkling. Hair follicles atrophy, and hair density and color decrease uniformly in both men and women. Hair turns gray because melanocytes are lost at the base of the hair follicles. Eyebrows, ear, and nasal hair coarsen and get longer, especially in men. Linear nail growth slows, and nail thickness and strength decrease. Nails become brittle, dull, opaque, and yellowish.

Bone

Bone mass or density is lost, especially in women after menopause, and bones become more brittle and can break more easily. Height decreases, primarily caused by shortening of the trunk and spine as the intervertebral discs gradually lose fluid and become thinner, and vertebrae lose some of their mineral content, making each bone thinner. The spinal column becomes curved and compressed. The foot arches become less pronounced, contributing to slight loss of height. The long bones of the arms and legs, although more brittle because of mineral losses, do not change length, making the arms and legs look longer in relation to the shortened trunk. The joints become stiffer and less flexible. Fluid in the joints may decrease, and the cartilage may begin to rub together and erode. Minerals may deposit in some joints. Hip and knee joints may begin to lose structure due to degenerative changes. The finger joints lose cartilage, and the bones thicken slightly. Inflammation, pain, stiffness, and deformity can result from breakdown of the joint structures. The posture can become progressively stooped, and the knees and hips more flexed. The neck may become tilted. The shoulders may narrow while the pelvis may become wider. Movement slows and may become limited. The gait becomes slower and shorter. Walking may become unsteady, with less arm swing.

Cardiovascular System

The heart increases in size and weight. The increasing thickness of the left ventricular wall is thought to be a compensatory mechanism in the face of increased afterload caused by increased aortic diameter, decreased central arterial compliance, and increased peripheral resistance. The size of the left ventricular cavity does not change, although the left atrium dilates. The myocardium thickens and these changes, in addition to lipofuscin deposits, fatty infiltration, and fibrosis, result in ventricular stiffness. The endocardium undergoes diffuse thickening, and valves may become thickened and calcified. Fibrosis, myocyte hypertrophy, and calcium deposition can impact the rest of the conduction system, which may manifest as prolongation in the PR and QRS intervals on electrocardiography and right bundle-branch block.

Pacemaker cells are lost at a rate of 10% per decade and can result in sinus arrest or tachy–brady syndrome. Despite these changes of normative aging, resting cardiac function remains unchanged throughout life in the absence of disease. Resting heart rate, left ventricular ejection fraction, cardiac output, cardiac index, and stroke index do not change with age. Heart rate variability is diminished, and hypertrophy, especially in older women, may actually result in an increased (hyperdynamic) resting ejection fraction.

The arteries become dilated, and the vessels increase in length, become more rigid, and lose their sensitivity to receptor-mediated agents. The intima and basement membrane progressively thicken, while endothelial cells become irregular in size and shape. Smooth muscle cells and blood-derived macrophages infiltrate, followed by increased matrix synthesis (ie, intimal sclerosis). In the media, internal elastic lamina becomes thinner and straighter, and elastin fibers are replaced by collagen, causing decreased elasticity; calcification increases, and lipids accumulate intra- and extracellularly.

Pulmonary System

The costal cartilages undergo calcification, there is kyphosis, and the compliance of the chest wall decreases. The bronchial mucous glands increase. Elastin fibers in the parenchymal framework decrease with increasing cross-linkage between these fibers, which decreases elastic recoil of the lungs. Decreased recoil can lead to reduced intrathoracic negative pressure and airway collapse. Collagen levels also decrease. Alveolar duct volume increases at the expense of the alveolus (ductectasia). The surface area of the lung decreases, residual volume increases by 20 mL/year, vital capacity decreases, and forced expiratory volume and forced vital capacity decrease by 30% by 80 years of age. Effort-independent respiration (ie, quiet breathing) decreases due to decreased elastic recoil and airway collapse in the lower lung zones. Effort-dependent respiration (ie, forced breathing) decreases with decreasing respiratory musculature. All the above factors can contribute to decreased arterial partial pressure of oxygen, exercise tolerance, and pulmonary reserve.

Eyes

Loss of periorbital fat produces sunken eyes and laxity of eyelids. Transparency of the cornea decreases as lipid infiltrates/deposits (ie, arcus senilis) accumulate. The anterior chamber becomes progressively shallower because of the thickening of the lens. Pupil diameter decreases progressively. Increasing fibrosis of the iris reduces accommodation and slows dark adaption. The eye needs double the illumination every 13 years to maintain recognition in subdued light. The lens increases in size and becomes more rigid because of the constant formation of new central epithelial cells at the front of the lens. Consequences of these changes include presbyopia (ie, difficulty in focusing, especially on near objects due to lens rigidity), general decline in transparency with an increase in yellow pigment, reduced metabolic activity, and increased cataract formation (due to a progressive increase in the annular layers of the lens and a compression of central components that become hard and opaque).

In the retina, rods constantly produce pigment membranes, but with age less phagocytosis of the pigment membranes leads to buckling and kinking of rods. Cones show a major deterioration of membranes with age, and a decline in numbers that is particularly marked after age 40. Pigment epithelial cells (captive macrophages) become full of debris that they try to extrude through Bruch's membrane, forming yellow or white plaques (termed drusen) that are visible through an ophthalmoscope. Macrophages migrate in and break up Bruch's membrane, allowing blood vessels to invade, which can lead to visual impairment. The lens, cornea, and macula exhibit increased yellow pigment with increasing age.

Ears

The pinna continues to grow, and ear wax accumulates and hardens. In the middle ear, the tympanic membrane thickens, with a loss of both elasticity and efficiency of ossicular articulation. These changes may lead to conductive hearing loss, which affects predominately low-frequency sounds. In the inner ear, a gradual bilaterally symmetrical sensorineural hearing loss predominately affects high-frequency sounds. With aging, the extent of hearing loss varies greatly. Significant hearing loss is defined as presbycusis. The multiple forms of presbycusis include sensory (atrophy of the hair cells in the organ of Corti), neural (loss of cochlear neurons in the basal part of the spiral ganglion), metabolic (patchy atrophy of the stria vascularis over the middle and apical regions of the cochlea, restricting blood supply to the neurosensory receptors), and mechanical (changes in the motion mechanics of the cochlear duct, such as that caused by increasing stiffness of the basilar membrane). The auditory canal narrows progressively.

Digestive System

The tongue develops varicosities, and decreased saliva production predisposes the mouth to oral infections. An increase in nonperistaltic spontaneous contractions of the esophagus produces difficulty in swallowing (ie, dysphagia). Normal swallowing is not often followed by the primary peristaltic wave, nonpropulsive contractions increase relaxation, and the lower esophageal sphincter is uncoordinated resulting in presbyesophagus. Diverticulae and herniation are common in older adults. In the stomach there is variable atrophy of the mucosa and muscularis mucosae, and inflammation and loss of gastric glands. The incidence of achlorhydria increases; pepsin activity decreases while plasma gastrin levels increase. Gastric emptying is delayed after fatty meals.

The proximal jejunal villi become broader and shorter. Cell production in jejunal crypts decreases, incidence of diverticula increases, and chronic intestinal ischemia due to atheroma in supply vessels also increases. Intestinal fat absorption is delayed and reduced because of delayed gastric emptying and decreased lipase production. Vitamin B_{12} absorption and calcium absorption decrease; iron absorption also decreases in the presence of achlorhydria. In the pancreas, there is duct hyperplasia, increased cyst formation, deposition of lipofuscin granules in acinar cells, and increased fatty deposition. In the large intestine, mucosa cells atrophy. There is cellular infiltration of the lamina propria and mucosa and hypertrophy of the muscularis mucosae. Atrophy of other muscle layers leads to an increase in connective tissue, development of diverticula, increased transit time, and constipation.

Urinary System

Kidney size and weight decrease. The number of functional glomeruli decreases, and the number of abnormal and sclerotic glomeruli increases. The number of functional renal tubules decreases, and these tubules decrease in length. These changes lead to an increase in tubular diverticula and an increase in tubular basement membrane thickness; impaired permeability decreases the ability to resorb glucose. The glomerular filtration rate (GFR) declines. Renal blood flow falls as a consequence of altered vascular pattern, atherosclerotic changes, altered arteriole-glomerular flow, and focal ischemic lesions. Filtration fraction (GFR/renal plasma flow) increases; therefore, renal plasma flow must decline relatively more than GFR. The concentrating ability of the kidney declines. In the bladder, there is edema, lymphocyte infiltration, trabeculae and diverticula, prolapse, and urethral mucosal atrophy.

Immune System

The general effects of aging on the immune system include a variable but gradual average decline in immune functioning. The immune system requires more stimulus and more time to become activated, produces less primary and secondary responses, and loses memory cells faster. Autoimmune antibodies also increase. T-cell function decreases gradually, and fewer naive and more memory T cells reduce the ability to mount an immune response when new exposures to pathogens occur. B-cell function decreases gradually, as does the response by naive B cells to newly introduced antigens. Aging B cells also increase production of abnormal antibodies. Atrophy of the thymus reduces function and production of T lymphocytes, proliferation of natural killer cells, and production of cytokines needed for growth and maturation of B cells. Loss of self-renewal capacity by hematopoietic stem cells contributes to immune-cell dysfunction.

Endocrine System

Age-related changes in the endocrine system vary with the individual gland and can involve changes in hormone levels, in receptor numbers on target cells, or in signal-transducing pathways. The pituitary gland exhibits minimal changes. Growth hormone exhibits a variable but average decline in pulsatile secretion pattern, contributing to a decrease in size of structures and in lean body mass to fat ratio. Prolactin also decreases nocturnal pulsatile secretion. In the pineal gland, a reduced diurnal melatonin rhythm can contribute to altered sleep patterns and a deficit in free-radical defenses. Norepinephrine secretion increases, and an altered responsiveness contributes to age-associated changes in systemic vasoconstriction and decreased cardiac function. Epinephrine levels and metabolism do not change.

The thyroid gland atrophies with increased fibrosis and nodule formation. T_4 production declines with very old age, but blood concentrations of thyroxine are normal because the clearance rate of T_4 decreases. There is an evolving debate over whether thyrotropin levels do not change with normal aging, or whether levels associated with hypothyroidism in older adults reflect a change in the set point of this hormone. Total serum calcitonin levels decrease, although bioactive calcitonin levels remain unchanged. The parathyroid glands show increased fat deposition but no atrophy. In women >40 years old, parathyroid hormone levels increase and its metabolism decreases, associated with decreased 1,25(OH)D serum concentrations and changes in bone mineral homeostasis.

The adrenal glands do not atrophy but show an increase in fibrous tissue. A moderate decrease in aldosterone secretion can contribute to orthostatic hypotension. Cortisol secretions also decrease, although the steady-state levels of circulating cortisol stay the same. Adrenocorticotropic hormone (ACTH) secretion (unstimulated and stimulated), cortisol secretion, and circadian rhythms remain unchanged, although negative feedback is delayed after a stressor, resulting in a delayed restoration of ACTH and cortisol to unstimulated levels. The adrenals also produce androgens and estrogens, although the adrenal contribution is usually masked by the testes and ovaries. However, after menopause, androgen secretion and masculinization arise from the adrenals. There are minimal changes in the pancreas, and an age-related decline in insulin signaling occurs at the target cell level, where decreased receptors and cellular glucose transporters contribute to reduced sensitivity. In the heart, atrial natriuretic peptide (ANP) levels increase, renal responsiveness to ANP decreases, and the hypotensive response to infused ANP increases. The thymus atrophies with age, and thymosin levels

Table 2.2—Organ System Age-Related Pathologies

Body System	Pathologies or Diseases that Increase in Incidence with Increasing Age
Nervous	Cerebrovascular accident, dementias
Muscle	Sarcopenia
Skin	Decubitis ulcers, fungal infections (especially toenails) Neoplasms (basal and squamous cell carcinomas, melanoma)
Skeletal	Osteoporosis Rheumatoid arthritis, osteoarthritis
Cardiovascular	Hypertension, thrombosis, anemia
Heart	Congestive heart failure, myocardial infarction
Vasculature	Coronary artery disease, atherosclerosis, varicose veins, hemorrhoids
Pulmonary	Chronic bronchitis, emphysema, pneumonia, pulmonary embolism Sleep apnea, stertorous breathing Lung cancer
Eyes	Entropion, ectropion, cataracts, age-related macular degeneration, glaucoma Diabetic retinopathy
Ears	Presbycusis Tinnitis, dizziness, vertigo
Digestive	Esophageal strictures, hiatal hernia Atrophic gastritis, acute gastritis, peptic ulcer, diverticulitis Fecal incontinence, cirrhosis, gallstones, pancreatitis Cancer
Urinary	Urinary incontinence Benign prostatic hyperplasia
Immune	Autoimmune disorders (multiple sclerosis, myasthenia gravis) Leukemias
Endocrine	Diabetes Grave disease

decrease as does immune function, contributing to an age-related increase in risk of infection and cancer.

In the kidneys, the response of antidiuretic hormone to osmotic stimuli increases, and the response of vasopressin to volume change decreases. Erythropoietin secretion increases in both the mid-aged and old as its metabolic clearance rate also increases. Circulating renin levels decrease as a consequence of decreased renin synthesis and impaired renin release. In the gonads, dehydroepiandrosterone (DHEA) and its more abundant sulfated form, DHEA-S, decrease, as do pregnenolone levels. Testosterone exhibits an average decrease in level and diurnal rhythm, which contributes to changes in skin, hair, muscle, and bone. In women, a large decrease in estrogen and progesterone is associated with altered skin, increased low-density lipoprotein levels, and decreased bone mineral. Leptin levels (produced by adipose tissue) decrease in women >70 years old, concomitant with decreases in body fat. Leptin levels increase in older men despite decreasing body fat because of an age-associated decrease in testosterone levels. A number of hormones exhibit an altered two-hormone synchrony. For example, older men secrete luteinizing hormone (LH) and testosterone more irregularly and jointly more asynchronously. Other hormone pairs that exhibit age-related asynchronous secretion include insulin and growth hormone, ACTH and cortisol, LH and prolactin, and LH and follicle-stimulating hormone.

Normal Aging Versus Age-Related Pathologies

All of the above changes accompany advancing age but occur at different rates in individuals. Variability in onset, rates, and extent of aging suggest complex interactions between genetic predisposition, environmental exposure, and biologic and behavioral coping mechanisms in the etiology of aging. Despite these age-related changes, the different organ systems continue to maintain function, although their ability to maintain homeostatic conditions under times of stress diminishes. These changes may also be magnified by the impact of organic disease. The greater incidence of certain pathologies or diseases with increasing age (Table 2.2) reflects, in part, diminution of immune and other defense systems, increased exposure to disease-causing factors, and greater time for the development of slow-progressing pathologies. Age-dependent increases in frequency of diseases such as diabetes, atherosclerosis, thrombosis, hypertension, cancer (especially of the breast, prostate, and colon), coronary heart disease, stroke, osteoporosis, and Alzheimer disease may characterize a synergy between aging and chronic disease in dysregulating homeostasis. While age-related chronic disease can be viewed as promoting an advanced biological age, a distinction between normal aging and pathology is that in disease, compromised function is evident in the resting (nonstressed) state. Normal aging involves cumulative diminution in molecular and cellular properties and processes that exhibit physiologic effects only when internal or external stressors, or both, perturb homeostasis.

Homeostasis and Aging

The changes that occur with aging contribute to systems-wide dysregulation and loss of maintenance. Additionally, the complexity in the dynamics of interacting physiologic systems decreases with age, resulting in a loss of integrated physiologic homeostasis. The physiologic parameter of body temperature maintenance can be used to explore systems-wide aging effects. With increased age, biologic changes to structures (loss of fat and thinning of skin, loss of sweat glands, decreased number of blood vessels and blood flow to skin surface, decreased muscle mass) have discrete molecular correlates and contribute to decrements in the functional capacity to maintain body temperature. Also, with increased age, biologic changes to negative feedback pathways (eg, nervous system changes such as fewer nerve cells that monitor/sense temperature and weakly functioning remaining nerve cells) also impinge on thermal regulation. Thus, aging is associated with a decreased detection and response to thermal variance, placing individuals at greater risk of hypo- and hyperthermia.

Geriatric syndromes such as delirium, dementia, depression, dizziness, failure-to-thrive, malnutrition, falls, functional dependence, and gait disorders are composites of dysregulation in multiple domains. For example, with malnutrition, in addition to the well-known, age-related changes in the digestive system that affect nutrition (eg, decreased absorption of vitamins A, D, and K, and zinc in the small intestines, decreased vitamin D production by skin and activation by kidneys causing reduced calcium), and age-related changes in other organ systems also contribute. Aging in the nervous system leads to a decreased sense of smell; altered flavor preferences lead to an altered diet. Decreased sensory function and coordination, muscle weakness, changes in cartilage and in bone mobility and stability can make it more difficult to obtain, prepare, and eat nutritionally adequate food. In the circulatory system, thicker blood vessels reduce blood flow through the digestive system, causing reduced digestion and absorption of various nutrients. In the respiratory system, decreased compliance and capacity can also lead to difficulty in obtaining, preparing, and eating a proper diet. Similarly, domains contributing to the geriatric syndrome of gait impairment include age-related changes in cartilage, bone, muscle, nerves, circulation, and vision.

Thus, the biologic changes that occur with aging act across multiple systems and create expanding perturbations to homeostasis and functional capacity. The challenge for the geriatrician is to provide care to an ever-increasing older patient population in the context of numerous subtle and not-so-subtle primary aging-related physiologic changes, along with increasing comorbid medical conditions, frailty and other geriatric conditions, and disability.

REFERENCES

- Ljubuncic P, Reznick AZ. The evolutionary theories of aging revisited—a mini-review. *Gerontology*. 2009;55(2):205–216.
- Ludlow AT, Roth SM. Physical activity and telomere biology: exploring the link with aging-related disease prevention. *J Aging Res*. 2011 Feb 21;2011:790378.
- Manor B, Costa MD, Hu K, et al. Physiological complexity and system adaptability: evidence from postural control dynamics of older adults. *J Appl Physiol*. 2010;109(6):1786–1791.
- Zaslavsky O, Woods N, Fugate, et al. Trajectories of change in frailty in frailty research: Methodological perspectives. *Commun Nurs Res*. 2011;44:169–169.

CHAPTER 3—PSYCHOSOCIAL ISSUES

KEY POINTS

- Psychosocial issues influence the health of individuals throughout the aging process and are important to consider during the course of various chronic or acute disease trajectories. When these issues are viewed within a stress framework, clinicians and researchers can identify how specific stressors can be modified to improve key psychosocial outcomes.
- A range of life events or transitions can exacerbate stress in older adults, including caregiving, loss and grief, and social transitions such as work-force changes. The way older adults adapt to these life events can lead to positive or negative health outcomes.
- Healthy behaviors are among the most potent factors that can modify stress in adult development and aging.
- Other factors that could "buffer," or protect, older adults against the negative implications of stress include active social networks and positive interpersonal relationships.

While the emphasis of clinical geriatric care may often focus on the cellular, organic, or functional mechanisms of illness, it is important to consider the psychosocial context of aging when diagnosing, treating, and managing the health of older adults. Health in adult development and aging is a complex process that must consider the dynamic interplay between biological, psychosocial, and social domains. When health during individuals' later years is viewed in this framework, geriatricians or gerontologists can begin to understand how treatment of a given condition often extends beyond direct pharmacologic or biomedical intervention to include other factors to provide more appropriate and effective management.

Stress is a state of arousal that can interfere with or deplete an individual's resources to the extent that he or she can no longer adapt to a given situation. "Arousal" can range from emotional, physiological, or behavioral responses to demands that are perceived as threatening. Classic research has consistently emphasized how stressful experiences are associated with adverse outcomes across the life span and, if stressors are not modified, a number of negative outcomes can result for older adults, impacting physical, psychosocial, or social well-being. Due to the pervasive influence of stressors, researchers and clinicians have attempted to examine how the occurrence of stress results in negative outcomes and whether intervention strategies can effectively alleviate such stress. Specifically, comprehensive "stress process models" have been developed to determine how stressors (eg, adverse life events), internal or external resources of individuals, and outcome are empirically related. A complex interaction of physical and psychosocial factors shapes the outcomes of stressors confronting older adults.

This chapter will examine the following: 1) some of the more common stressors that older adults experience; 2) stressors that are modifiable, because these factors are the likely targets of effective clinical interventions; 3) behavioral and social science research that has explored stress in older adults and how various subgroups respond to particular stressors; and 4) the "mediators" or "moderators" of stress, or those personal and social resources that may mitigate the spread of stress and negative life events. Mediators involve the older adult's perceptions of and responses to the stress situation. Moderators—which may be constituents of an older adult's environment or behaviors in which the individual engages—can be thought of as acting on the stressor itself to lessen its intensity or buffer its effect; they also affect an individual's ability to respond to the stressor. Identifying potential mediators and moderators and influencing them through clinical intervention often serves as the fulcrum of effective geriatric care.

STRESSORS

The study of stress is a multidisciplinary endeavor involving the biological breakdown of organisms and social readjustment to life events. Studies of social class and mental illness, as well as social stress and psychosocial distress, laid the foundation for more complex studies of stress as a process across the life span.

Older adults may face different types of stress, including life events on one end of a stress continuum (also "acute" stressors) and continual chronic stressors on the other end. Life events are discrete and observable and represent a significant change in the life of an older adult; examples include widowhood or disease diagnosis. In contrast, chronic stressors do not necessarily begin as a discrete event but develop slowly and progressively, continue over a longer period of time, and often do not have a discernible end point; examples include pain, inadequate sleep, or worry and caregiver strain. Clearly, major life events and chronic stressors are significant stressors. However, relatively minor stressors that characterize everyday life (eg, misplacing one's keys or being late for an appointment) and that are fairly innocuous if they occur only occasionally can "accumulate" in the presence of life events or chronic stress and also trigger negative health outcomes such as depressive or other psychological symptoms.

Factors associated with the onset of these stressors, as well as factors that exist after specific stressors occur, are often modifiable and thus susceptible to clinical intervention. These include specific behaviors over which the person may have some control, or social networks that can offer appropriate and desired support when the person is attempting to navigate the course of stressors. Other risk factors (such as gender and race) are not mutable and may even interact with stressors to exacerbate chronic stress. For example, the increasing prevalence of chronic diseases in older adults may mean a concomitant need for clinicians to develop approaches to help older adults and their families effectively manage chronic stressors that may result in such instances.

Caregiving

An area of geriatric research and care that has received considerable attention is family care for older adults who suffer from disability or health impairments, or "caregiving." There is no one consistent definition of *caregiving*, but in its broadest sense, caregiving refers to attending to an individual's health needs. More specific definitions emphasize that caregiving exceeds the bounds of normative care to include providing assistance with one or more activities of daily living (eg, bathing, dressing, transferring). Approximately 50 million people provide informal (ie, unpaid) care to a family member. The typical family caregiver is a 46-year-old woman caring for a mother (widowed) who does not live in the same household. Thirty percent of family caregivers are >65 years old.

Given the prevalence of chronic diseases among older adults, caregiving research has tended to focus on specific disease contexts, most prominently Alzheimer disease (AD). AD is now the fifth leading cause of death in adults ≥65 years old in the United States; 5. 3 million Americans currently suffer from AD. Because older adults with AD rely heavily on family members for care, the potential influence of increasing prevalence rates of AD may have a staggering effect on families. For example, 87% of adults with AD are cared for by a family member, and 10.9 million individuals provided unpaid care to a person with dementia. In the AD context, caregiving can extend to the management of dementia-related symptoms such as memory loss and behavioral disruptions. The typical AD caregiver in the United States is a 48-year-old woman (suggesting, in addition to caregiving, other roles and responsibilities such as employment) providing assistance to a relative who is, on average, 78 years old.

Various effects on family AD caregivers have been well established. For example, AD caregivers often report decreased physical health (perhaps due to impaired immune system response as a result of accumulated stressors related to AD care) (SOE=A). They also appear to engage in fewer preventive health behaviors, suffer from more chronic illnesses (eg, heart disease), and are more likely to use medications. Family AD care also has financial ramifications: providing family care costs approximately $324 per month for AD caregivers compared with $124 per month for non-AD caregivers; 60% of caregivers indicate some adjustment in employment to provide assistance to a relative with AD. Providing AD care can also affect the social well-being of family members. Reduced social time, a lack of pleasant activities, and relationship degradation with the person with AD as well as other family members may occur. Another well-studied phenomena in AD caregiving is the psychological risk of this role; for example, prevalence rates of depression range from 14% to 60% among those who provide care to a person with AD—a rate that often exceeds that of age-matched noncaregivers (SOE=B).

As evidence accumulated that demonstrated the physical, financial, social, and psychological risks of AD family care, a series of intervention strategies were developed and evaluated to test whether certain aspects of AD caregiving could be modified (eg, enhancing caregiver strategies to manage AD-related symptoms such as behavior problems, bolstering resources through either enhanced social support or provision of relief/respite from daily AD care). This could lead to improved AD caregiving outcomes, including decreased caregiver stress and depressive symptomatology, and delayed nursing-home admission for the person with AD. In general, AD caregiver interventions that adopt a family level/family systems approach or those that train AD caregivers in the management of behavior problems tend to show the most promise. More specifically, evidence-based syntheses of meta-analyses and systematic reviews of AD caregiver interventions have found that multidimensional intervention protocols, such as the New York University Caregiver Intervention or the Resources for Alzheimer's Disease Caregiver Health II, are effective. These often include combinations of individual consultation, family sessions and support, and ongoing assistance to help AD caregivers navigate the disease trajectory (with its various transitions) (SOE=A). Although less consistent in their positive effects, support-group strategies and respite services such as adult day programs may also offer skills training and relief, respectively, to enhance AD caregiver outcomes. As noted by experts in AD family care and clinical intervention, positive effects require successful and carefully planned research designs and study outcomes (including type and timing of measures). In this regard, the evaluation of AD caregiver interventions should mirror the primary aim of effective clinical care, identifying risk factors, outcomes, and interventions for each individual caregiver.

Caregivers need training, information, and support as well, as a positive alliance with the person's healthcare providers. They cannot be expected to be able to assume or to be effective in their various roles just because they have a relational bond with their family member. Acknowledgement of the role, provision of information about AD, guidance and instruction regarding the work the caregiver needs to be able to do, and referral to appropriate professionals and/or health educators are all essential. Caregivers should be regularly observed for signs of the known stressful effects of caregiving. Appropriate referrals—for direct help for themselves, for help in the home, and for respite—are all important. Caregiving also can have positive benefits for the caregiver: relationships can be strengthened, and caregivers can experience a sense of satisfaction for a job well done and an obligation fulfilled. Such rewards can be pointed out and affirmed. Attention to family dynamics may also be useful in identifying issues contributing to stressors that can be modified. A number of intervention programs (eg, those providing education, counseling, and cognitive-behavioral therapy) have proved effective in ameliorating the stress associated with caregiving. There is some evidence that religious involvement buffers the stress of caregiving (SOE=B). Disease-specific support activities offer only modest relief but may be the conduit for more focused help.

Various organizations, such as the Administration on Aging (AoA), have supported initiatives to implement evidence-based AD caregiver services throughout the United States. This is largely in response to the increasing prevalence of AD, the unmet need of family caregivers, and the call from community service providers to implement more systematic and rigorous AD caregiver support strategies. These translational efforts by AoA and other organizations, such as the American Psychological Association, have resulted in several comprehensive Web sites that provide detailed information on the delivery and evaluation of interventions for AD caregivers (see www.aoa.gov).

Federal and statewide policies designed to support caregiving families and their disabled older relatives are also available.

Loss and Grief

A common life event that occurs for many older adults is widowhood or death of other close family members or friends. More than 1.5 million spouses will be widowed annually by 2030. U.S. census data from 2004 to 2005 reported 726,000 men and 2,888,000 women between the ages of 65 and 74 as widowed; these numbers increase substantially to 1,347,000 widowers and 5,844,000 widows who are ≥75 years old (www.census.gov/prod/2004pubs/04statab/pop. pdf). Widowhood has received extensive attention in gerontologic research; for example, bereaved spouses are more likely to suffer from negative mental health as well as have higher mortality (ie, the "widowhood effect"). Despite the negative effects of widowhood, some widows and widowers are able to regain their prebereavement levels of function and psychological well-being, while others experience bereavement as more of a chronic stressor. A systematic review of psychiatric morbidity in widowed individuals found that, in the first year after the death of a spouse, major depressive disorders and anxiety disorders were significantly greater than among those who have not suffered from such losses. Up to a year after the death of a spouse, 22% of widows or widowers were diagnosed with major depressive disorder and 12% with post-traumatic stress disorder (SOE=B).

Specific treatment of the depressive or anxiety disorders related to widowhood may help individuals better adapt to the death of a spouse or loved one in the year after the loss. Large-scale descriptive studies suggest that improved social engagement during the immediate loss period may help widows or widowers stave off some of the negative effects of losing a spouse. A general review of clinical interventions directed toward those suffering from widowhood emphasizes the importance of targeting those at high risk; because most widows and widowers appear to adapt to the loss of a spouse fairly well on their own, the efficacy of psychotherapeutic, group-based, or home-based visiting programs is moderate to weak (SOE=A). A well-rounded assessment protocol to target an array of intervention strategies to widows or widowers is necessary for maximal outcome and cost benefit.

Role Loss and Acquisition

With age comes a number of life events that could result in not only positive psychosocial benefits but also stressors ranging from daily hassles to chronic upheaval. The number of Social Security beneficiaries ≥65 years old rose from 32.9 million in 2001 (a year in which 2 million Americans turned 65) to 34.5 million in 2006 (a 4.7% increase). Given the size of the "baby boomer" cohort, these numbers will increase substantially in the coming decades (to the extent that Social Security will pay out more in benefits than it receives from the U.S. workforce). There is also a concurrent increase of older workers; from 1996 to 2006, while the total U.S. workforce was growing by 13.1%, there was a 59.4% increase in workers ≥55 years old (an additional 46.7%

increase in this cohort is expected to occur from 2006 to 2016). Of note, a 68.7% increase was seen in female workers in this age group in the 1996–2006 period. The average age of retirement has been declining steadily, dropping to slightly under 62 years of age in 1995–2000 (down more than 5 years since 1950–1955). Other roles may include grandparenthood or, in more extreme cases, the need to raise grandchildren. One in 12 children are living in households headed by grandparents; 2.4 million grandparents have primary responsibility for caring for their grandchildren, often with the parents of these children not living in their household. While close grandparenting relationships can have a range of positive influences on the development of grandchildren, particularly when grandchildren have unstable situations in their immediate family, older grandparents are also at risk of negative physical and mental health outcomes because of increased childrearing responsibilities.

Several areas to enhance clinical services and interventions for custodial grandparents have been suggested (SOE=C). In many instances, there is a temporary or permanent loss of a parent, and children may suffer feelings of bereavement, thus requiring greater support and resources from a custodial grandparent. In these situations, custodial grandparents may have to manage their feelings about the loss of their own child as well as their grandchildren's emotional upheaval. Parent-skills training programs for grandparents should include information about mental health care for their grandchildren as well as themselves, education about sexually transmitted diseases, school violence, drug abuse, and peer pressure. Suggested content includes parenting skills related to appropriate discipline, communication skills with grandchildren, legal advocacy on one's rights as a custodial grandparent, and navigating feelings of grief. Support groups for custodial grandparents may also help to reinforce the content provided in individualized skills-training programs.

Social Status

In the United States, three factors are consistently associated with a broad range of negative psychosocial and physical outcomes: being nonwhite, female, and poor or poorly educated (usually a surrogate for being poor). They should serve as warnings for clinicians, because the presence of one or more of these factors can add to the person's stress load. They can also affect the kinds of coping mechanisms the person has available. Lack of disposable income, for example, may exclude the use of some formal services or involvement in community activities that charge a fee.

Race has a direct bearing on health stresses and longevity in old age. A 65-year-old black American man can expect to live nearly 2 years less than a 65-year-old white American man (a pattern mirrored among black American and white American women). Ethnic or cultural background and community context can substantially affect a person's outlook on a situation, the kinds of moderating activities he or she deems acceptable, and the importance he or she places on various outcomes. Older adults may understand disease through frameworks specific to other cultures, and treatment may need to include or rely principally on culturally centered options. A concept such as autonomy, which has become so central in issues of patient choice and advance directives, has a different weight and value in cultures in which choice belongs more to the community as a whole (as with some Native American groups) or to a community or family leader (eg, in Hmong societies). Choices like hospice care may be viewed in some cultures as tantamount to wishing for and bringing about the death of the person. A procedure like autopsy can strongly violate cultural or religious beliefs. The clinician is advised to proceed attentively in cross-cultural situations (see "Cultural Aspects of Care," p 58).

The need for clinicians to consider the cultural context of family caregivers and, by extension, patients when assessing needs and devising care plans has been emphasized (SOE=C). A "hierarchical model" of health care is not as effective as a "horizontal model," in which collaborative strategies are used in working with ethnically and racially diverse patients. In particular, the horizontal model offers a better understanding of the community contexts in which culturally diverse patients and families reside, and so sources of care or stress can be identified in these contexts to improve treatment regimens. For example, geriatric care providers may incorporate community care resources (eg, lay care providers, civic groups, religious organizations) into their care plans. Such resources can serve as effective links between the geriatric care provider and patients or families, and efficient provision of information and services must often be arranged with these resources to have maximal benefit. See also "Cultural Aspects of Care," p 58.

MEDIATORS

Mediators shape a person's responses to stress and influence the relationships between different types of stress. Mediators "are the internal and external resources the person can use to assess and interpret the stress, to assess his or her own capacities for addressing it, and to formulate a coping response to it." Many key mediators can be modified through psychosocial intervention (eg, in AD caregiving). Instruction and information can affect the person's understanding of a situation. Various forms of psychoeducation have been shown to be effective in increasing an older adult's sense of mastery within a stress situation and his or her awareness and use of formal services. Family counseling and therapy can strengthen the involvement of older adults with their social network.

Self-Efficacy Beliefs

A number of constructs have been studied that relate to a person's sense of his or her own ability to manage situations. The concept of self-efficacy is comparable to concepts such as mastery, internal locus of control, resilience, and competence; although it is singled out here, self-efficacy resembles these in representing a key personal quality to be considered when dealing with an older adult facing any stress situation. Self-efficacy is an important consideration in the mental and physical health of older adults for two reasons:

First, there is a relationship between strong or positive self-efficacy and a number of important health and mental health outcomes (Table 3.1) (SOE=B). A large number of longitudinal studies—most notably a study of "successful" or healthy aging—have produced a coherent set of conclusions about self-efficacy. Others have identified a link between memory, self-efficacy, and cognitive function or demonstrate an empirical association between self-efficacy and health among older adults (SOE=B). The way a person approaches a situation—whether it be a specific threat (eg, the onset of an acute condition) or a more pervasive one (eg, change of life roles or decline in physical performance)—affects the eventual outcome. Of particular note is the broad range of effects of strong self-efficacy beliefs, which influence physical and mental health as well as overall function (Table 3.1). In addition, self-efficacy seems to contribute to a person's ability to be actively engaged in life, an important moderating factor.

The second reason self-efficacy is important is that it can change. It can be weakened by repeated assaults and poor outcome, but it can also be strengthened. Among the strategies effective for strengthening self-efficacy are the following:

- performance accomplishment (seeing oneself succeed in a series of increasingly difficult tasks)
- vicarious learning and social modeling (seeing others like oneself succeed in a targeted area)
- encouragement (being persuaded to undertake a targeted activity)
- reinforcement (experiencing pleasure from success)

A number of training programs aimed at improving specific performance (eg, reducing the fear of falling or increasing adherence to an exercise regimen after a heart attack) have succeeded by working to strengthen participants' self-efficacy beliefs in the targeted area. Strong self-efficacy beliefs appear to be better predictors of performance than measures of physical ability. In falls prevention studies, for example, those with strong self-efficacy beliefs related to falling were found to show reduced fear of falling, despite low objective measures for risk of falling. Self-efficacy appears to play an important role in coping and overall well-being in older adults. Clinicians should assess the older adult's sense of his or her own competence and intervene, when possible, to strengthen it.

Table 3.1—Physical and Mental Health Impacts of Self-Efficacy Beliefs

Strong self-efficacy beliefs
- Buffer the effects of stress exposure on physical and mental health
- Contribute to overall physical performance, independently of ability
- Help maintain good function
- Slow functional decline among those with poor physical performance
- Contribute to good choice making, good performance, and persistence of effort (especially in women)
- Contribute to increased productivity

Weak self-efficacy beliefs
- Are associated with declines in functional status, especially in those with decreased physical performance

Coping Strategies

A number of theorists have studied the manner in which older adults meet and address the accumulated challenges of aging. Cultivating an emotional response to a stressor can mediate its effect and result in a better outcome. Thus, invoking confidence and optimism in the face of bad news helps a person to meet the challenge and strengthens the likelihood of a positive outcome. One strategy older adults can use consists of selection, optimization, and compensation. In this strategy, as people age, they begin to hone down the number and kinds of things in which they engage in on the basis of what they believe they do well, selecting activities in which they are more likely to succeed. They also reframe the way they judge their own performance, eg, by looking at people their own age or older for a source of comparison. They do the selected things more, and they derive a sense of accomplishment for doing them. As losses continue and performance diminishes, people use compensatory strategies that allow them to use their remaining performance abilities in the best way possible. A person known for preparing elaborate dinners might, for example, choose a simpler main course (selection) that he or she does well and has prepared many times (optimization) and surround it with several simple courses and side dishes as a way of favorably setting it off (compensation). Other coping strategies (eg, assimilation, accommodation, immunization, or resilience) also build essentially on the notion of reframing one's performance to provide positive reinforcement and to reinforce self-esteem. Clinicians should attempt to learn how their patients typically form successful responses to challenges and help them to address new challenges in these same terms. For example, a randomized controlled trial of a coping improvement intervention for HIV-infected older adults found that developing and implementing adaptive problem- and emotion-focused coping skills and optimizing coping efforts through the use of interpersonal supports resulted in reduced depressive symptoms than a usual care control (SOE=B). A group intervention to improve proactive coping among individuals 50–75 years old also found that proactive coping was significantly improved over that of controls, and these results were maintained over a 3-month period (SOE=B).

A particular clinical approach that has demonstrated effectiveness in building coping skills and treating negative mental health in general among older adults is psychotherapy. Psychotherapy generally refers to an array of individualized intervention strategies, including approaches designed to change thoughts, appraisals, and feelings, including cognitive-behavioral therapy, brief psychodynamic therapy (problem-focused and oriented around providing patients with necessary insights to solve immediate problems), interpersonal therapy (focus on relationship issues and can include role-playing or recounting interpersonal events), and reminiscence/life review. In a range of high-quality syntheses of evidence, psychotherapeutic approaches have shown that cognitive-behavioral therapy and group psychotherapy are effective in the treatment of depression among older adults, with cognitive-behavioral therapy in particular being highly effective (SOE=A). Moreover, psychotherapy for older adults has shown similar effectiveness as that for younger adults (SOE=A).

Social Involvement

Like people at all ages, older adults are faced with developmental tasks and challenges. In Erikson's theory of staged development, the task of old age is integration—putting the pieces together in a way that both celebrates and continues to act on the learning and accomplishments of life. In this conception, and consistent with many other findings, involvement (sometimes termed *productivity*) plays an important role. Becoming more involved, actively seeking out ways to contribute to and participate in the broader world, even engaging in paid work are all mediators that can lead to better outcomes. Taking part and making a contribution—through volunteering, productive (sometimes paid) labor, active family roles (especially child care), and participation in group activities—are all associated with older adults' continued well-being.

In terms of the framework of factors affecting health outcomes, social involvement can be understood as a positive, problem-focused coping response, a way of filtering the effects of a stressor by strengthening the connection of the person to the community (affirming the person's value in the community). Older theories of normal aging saw disengagement—the systematic withdrawal of ties to the social world—as normative. In current thinking, however, such disengagement is not encouraged and might even be considered an abnormal behavior. At the very least, there is an association between lack of social involvement and affective disorders such as depression.

MODERATORS

Moderators are components of a person's life or behaviors in which the person engages that act to affect the demands of the various stressors he or she faces. Moderators may be in place before the onset of a stressor, or they might be developed in response to it. A person who has a long history of exercise already has a good base of conditioning to deal with an emergent condition affecting mobility (eg, arthritis). Alternatively, making a decision to begin to exercise, to control diet or alcohol consumption, to seek help to improve sleep, or to cease smoking is a possible—and healthy—response to stressors ranging from the onset of illness to a realization that one has slowed down. These healthy behaviors directly moderate the effect of the threat or demand and contribute to better physical and mental health outcomes. Having a strong social network and calling on it in a time of crisis (rather than withdrawing) can help moderate age-related demands (eg, the loss of a loved one).

Three major activities moderate stress or demand and appear to contribute to healthy aging: social networks, spiritual or religious involvement, and healthy behaviors. Older adults' activities in these areas should be regularly assessed and encouraged.

Social Networks

The older adult's social network is a critical resource for overall well-being, and social isolation is a powerful risk

Table 3.2—Physical and Mental Health Impacts of Robust Social Networks*

- Reduced mortality risks
- Better physical health outcomes
- Better mental health outcomes
- Reduced risk of ADL disability or decline
- Increased likelihood of ADL recovery
- Buffered impact of major negative life events
- Promotion of strong self-efficacy beliefs
- Assistance that does not preclude self-care but that can increase risk of new or recurrent ADL disability (especially in men)

*SOE=A

factor for broad declines and mortality. The effect of a social network on an older adult's overall well-being has been extensively studied, with conclusive results (Table 3.2) (SOE=B). The literature points to the importance of quality over quantity but does not discount the latter. The closeness of social relationships is most important; thus, a well-functioning marital or familial relationship—a relationship that provides a person with a confidante—offers the kinds of support and protection suggested in Table 3.2. Dysfunctional close relationships—those characterized by negative and conflict-filled interactions—appear to work in the contrary direction. The size of an older adult's social network appears to work in both directions. Although having a larger social network offers the opportunity for greater involvement and contribution, it also presents the likelihood of experiencing a greater number of losses within the network (because of death or increased disability).

A robust social network both mediates and moderates age-related stresses. Social networks provide emotional and instrumental help in times of crisis. Families help older adults, for example, cope with the death of a spouse or close friend, but they also provide direct and indirect help when more functional losses occur. The social network can provide a person under stress with a context within which to envision and frame responses to various demands. Social networks seem to exert a positive effect on older adults by strengthening their self-efficacy beliefs (the person feels valued within the social network, which contributes to a sense of self-worth). It also provides opportunities for taking action to address demands (eg, calling on family for specific functional assistance, spending more time with children after the death of a spouse, increasing time spent with friends after retirement).

Provision of such help is positive and contributes to recovery, unless it sends the wrong message. Too much instrumental assistance provided to older adults (particularly men) by the social network can contribute to continued disability. Rather than being encouraged to work toward restored function, a person may receive too much help or not be encouraged to engage in self-care; therefore, he or she may accept a modifiable condition as permanent. Thus, although assistance from the social network should be encouraged, it should be done with attention to promoting maximal function by the person receiving the help.

Spiritual or Religious Involvement

There is a developing but as yet incomplete understanding of the role of religion and spirituality in the lives of older adults and of the effect of the presence or absence of these involvements on health and well-being. Studies consistently demonstrate that religion plays a more important part in the lives of the current cohort of older adults than in the lives of younger persons. More than 50% of older adults report frequent attendance at religious events (with little variation by gender or race), and this has been a lifelong practice—rather than a late-life development (SOE=A). A number of studies have demonstrated positive associations between religiousness, typically measured as regular attendance in organized religious activities, and a variety of markers of health (eg, blood pressure) and mental health (eg, depression). There is evidence that regular attendance at religious services is associated with a lower composite measure of allostatic load among older women but not men (SOE=B). The literature suggests that religious participation may be beneficial, in part, because it promotes social interaction; however, one study suggests evidence that the effect is independent of social interaction. In addition, a number of studies have found that the beneficial effects of religious participation are not universal, and there is a suggestion that it may be most beneficial for those with the least social resources, eg, women and minorities (SOE=B).

One benefit of this growing body of literature is an increasing clarity of the distinction between the two elements. While religion and spirituality are in no way mutually exclusive, neither do they necessarily overlap. In particular, the literature emphasizes the individualized quality of spirituality, portraying it in terms of practices through which a person seeks to establish or strengthen a link with a higher power or truth. In studies that have focused more on spirituality, findings generally indicate that such practices (eg, meditation or daily spiritual experiences) also are associated with better health and mental health (SOE=B). One study characterized the distinction between religion and spirituality as having positive associations for well-being related, in the case of religiousness, to positive social linkages and a sense of community service and, in the case of spirituality, to a sense of personal growth.

Overall, issues of religiousness and spirituality can provide clinicians with another dimension for assessing older adults. Ascertaining whether an older adult is engaged in a religious community or with religious practice and/or is involved in spiritual practices can provide insights about strengths that can be called on or areas in which resources are lacking.

Healthy Behaviors

Implementing positive behaviors (eg, exercising; controlling intake of food, tobacco, and alcohol; improving sleep; and participating in active relaxation or stress-reduction techniques) has positive effects on overall well-being, regardless of age when the behaviors are begun. Although these are physical behaviors, they often rely on and benefit from strong psychosocial mediators, particularly self-efficacy and social networks. Clinicians should use these mediators when proposing that older adults begin or strengthen healthy behaviors. It can help to invoke a person's understanding of benefits and appreciation of his or her own proven ability to make changes, while at the same time offering suggestions about how the targeted behavior might contribute to a strong social network (eg, "you could walk every day with your daughter," "you and your husband could take the healthy cooking class together").

One example in which positive health behaviors could influence chronic stress is sleep disorders among older adults. Instead of a normal phenomenon of aging, sleep disorders often have a direct, negative influence on a range of outcomes (SOE=A). Evidence-based strategies that have shown effectiveness for a range of sleep disorders in older adults (eg, insomnia, sleep apnea) include cognitive-behavioral therapy, combinations of sleep hygiene and education, relaxation therapy, exercise, and sleep restriction/compression. Given the importance of adequate sleep and health, incorporating and emphasizing healthy lifestyle behaviors along with providing more intensive, individualized intervention such as cognitive-behavioral therapy can effectively manage sleep problems in older adults. See "Sleep Problems," p 285.

REFERENCES

- Bloom HG, Ahmed I, Alessi CA, et al. Evidence-based recommendations for the assessment and management of sleep disorders in older persons. *J Am Geriatr Soc.* 2009;57(5):761–789.
- Gaugler JE. *An Evidence-Based Synthesis of Dementia Caregiver Interventions.* Minneapolis, MN: School of Nursing, University of Minnesota; 2010.
- Onrust S, Smit F, Willemse G, et al. Cost-utility of a visiting service for older widowed individuals: Randomised trial. *BMC Health Serv Res.* 2008 Jun 12;(8):128.
- Qualls SH, Zarit SH, ed. *Aging Families and Caregiving.* Hoboken, NJ: John Wiley & Sons, Inc.; 2009.
- Wilson KC, Mottram PG, Vassilas CA. Psychotherapeutic treatments for older depressed people. *Cochrane Database Syst Rev.* 2008 Jan 23;(1):CD004853.

CHAPTER 4—LEGAL AND ETHICAL ISSUES

Key Points

- Four guiding ethical principles of American medical practice are respect for autonomy, nonmaleficence, beneficence, and justice. These principles are competing, and none are absolute.
- Decisional capacity is situation specific and changes over time. A consent-assent model is often useful for decision making for individuals with different degrees of incapacity.
- Substituted judgment is the process of constructing what a person would have wanted (ie, autonomy based). Beneficence is the weighing of benefits and burdens of an intervention for the individual as he or she experiences them in the present. Its basis is a discussion of how much that individual would be willing to go through for what chance of what outcome.
- Patients and their surrogates have the right to decline treatment whether that treatment is already in place or has not yet been started.
- Respect for the patient's autonomy may come in conflict with our duty to keep an incapacitated patient safe, and with the safety of others and the public health.

Introduction to Medical Ethics

Normative ethics is the inquiry into the standards of what we see as right or wrong action. It focuses on the question "What *ought* I to do?" Medical ethics is based on a utilitarian ethical structure; that is, it is not based on deontologic overarching moral imperatives, as a religious ethic would be. Rather, it seeks the answer to the *ought* question through the principles that are applied in the context of the clinical situation. The goal of medical ethical deliberation is to maximize good consequences and minimize bad consequences (beneficence). These principles are tied to values and perspectives that are unique to each culture and that may also differ depending on whether one is addressing a specific case (situational ethics) or public policy.

The four guiding principles of American medical ethics most often cited are respect for autonomy, nonmaleficence, beneficence, and justice. How each of these principles guides the practice of medicine is different today from even 50 years ago. These principles and their application also differ widely within various subcultures within the wider American culture.

The primacy of individual autonomy is a foundation of American culture, from the early pioneers to modern medical practice. Respect for individuals' autonomy should include respect for their right to subjugate their individualism to family, culture, or religion. In many cultures, family structure dictates who will be the decision maker for individuals within that family, and that person is deferred to even when the individual involved has the cognitive ability to make his or her own decisions. However, it is unethical to defer decision making to an adult child of an older patient who is capable of making decisions for him or herself if that is not the cultural practice of the patient and family, or not the patient's wish.

Beneficence, doing more good than harm, is largely determined by each individual's reactions and needs as well as culture. See "Cultural Aspects of Care," p 58. The weighing of benefits, risks, and burdens (ie, how much would someone be willing to go through for what chances of what outcomes) is the mainstay of decision making in older adults whose wishes are unclear or unobtainable.

Nonmaleficence is often interpreted as "do no harm" but would be better represented by the phrase "do not intend to do harm." Definitions or perceptions of harm differ widely between cultures and between individuals within cultures. The most frequently cited medical conflict between mainstream culture and subculture perspectives is blood transfusions for a Jehovah's Witness. For a Jehovah's Witness, blood transfusion may be thought to cause more harm than good, even if the outcome of not having the transfusion might be death. Understanding the values of subcultures within our society may provide clues to the spectrum of values that underlie an individual's perspective on harm.

Finally, the concept of justice in the context of health care in our society remains ambiguous. There is not a recognized right to health care in the United States. The distribution of healthcare benefits and the use of healthcare technologies continue to be uneven and reflect biases regarding gender, age, race, and ethnic origin. Researchers have frequently excluded older adults in their study populations, and the lack of knowledge on the relative effectiveness of interventions when they are used for older adults can lead to the under- or overuse of interventions in this age group. Furthermore, assumptions that equate age with chronic illness and comorbidity can deny beneficial treatment to healthy older adults. Patients from groups that have long been denied many of the benefits of our society, especially our healthcare dollars, may be more reluctant than more historically privileged patients to step back from aggressive treatments because of a perception of continued prejudice.

It is important to keep these differences in mind when considering the following discussions of ethical decision making and its application to individual patients. The discussions that follow are, in a true utilitarian sense, guiding principles, not moral imperatives.

Decisional Capacity

Because of the nature of diseases affecting older adults, clinicians are often called on to assess a person's decision-making capacity and to use other sources of decisional authority when that capacity is impaired. Although the focus of much of the literature has been on clinicians' assessments of patients' capacity to make medical decisions, clinicians are also asked to render opinions on patients' ability to make decisions about other matters, such as managing money, writing a will, continuing to drive, possessing firearms, and even the everyday decisions involved in activities of daily living. It is important to use the correct terminology in discussing the clinician's responsibility. A clinician may evaluate a patient's capacity to make decisions, but *competence* and *incompetence* are legal terms, and they imply that a court has taken action.

Assessment of Decisional Capacity

Assessing the patient's ability to understand the consequences of a decision is the overarching principle used in making a judgment of decisional capacity. To make a medical decision, the patient must be able to understand basic information about his or her condition, the probable progression and outcomes of the disease, and the effects of various potential interventions. This requires the ability to understand the disease process; the proposed therapy and alternative therapies; the advantages, adverse events, and complications of each therapy; and the possible course of the disease without intervention. The patient also needs to be able to understand the broad consequences of accepting, deferring, or rejecting a proposed intervention. Admittedly, even clinicians cannot predict the full implications of complex medical decisions, because they can rarely know all the consequences of an intervention or the precise natural history of an illness in any individual. The patient should be allowed to make decisions that are based on his or her beliefs and values. Therefore, it is often most helpful for the clinician to explore a patient's hopes and fears and to help the patient clarify his or her goals so that the treatment options offered are compatible with these goals.

Cultural differences between clinicians and patients who are members of different ethnic groups can make assessing decision-making capacity an even more difficult task. Capacity assessment involves abstract concepts not easily translated into another language. It also involves the interpretation of values and the judgment of what is considered reasonable, which may differ according to culture. Because of this, it is important to ascertain the need for a translator. In emergency situations, this may have to be a family member or a staff member, but it is always preferable to offer the services of a professional interpreter. Issues of privacy arise when using a family member or a member of a small ethnic community who may have other connections with the patient. Family members may filter or modify what is being said out of embarrassment, lack of familiarity with medical terminology, or other motivations (conscious or unconscious). Patients may be unwilling to share sensitive information. In all such situations, confidentiality is lost. A professional interpreter can often accurately translate the nuances of language as well as act as a cultural broker when explanations need to be made. On the other hand, clinicians must avoid making assumptions based solely on ethnic background and evaluate each patient as an individual.

The capacity to make a living will is similar to that of being able to make treatment decisions, although it is somewhat more complicated because the patient is being asked to think in the abstract with a "what if?" frame of reference. The ability to choose a healthcare proxy (see below) is much less complex, and even fairly impaired patients are often able to choose someone to make decisions for them.

The requirements are even less stringent for testamentary competence (the ability to make a last will and testament). In general, a person's ability to decide how he or she wishes to dispose of belongings after death is felt to be preserved even when the person is severely cognitively incapacitated in other ways. As long as the person can identify the individuals involved, is not delusional or in other ways so psychiatrically ill that their judgment is impaired (eg, paranoia), and is capable of understanding the consequence of signing the will, he or she is considered to have testamentary competence.

For a summary of the elements of decisional capacity in each of these four areas, see Table 4.1.

Standardized Tests of Decisional Capacity

Traditional tests of cognitive function have some, but limited, use in determining decisional capacity. An overall score on the Folstein Mini–Mental State Examination (MMSE) of ≤10 indicates such diminished cognitive ability that it is unlikely that

Table 4.1—Elements of Decisional Capacity

Medical decisions
- Ability to understand relevant information
- Ability to understand consequences of the decision
- Ability to communicate a decision

Decisions of self-care
- Ability to care for oneself
- Ability to accept needed help to keep oneself safe

Finances
- Ability to manage bill payments
- Ability to appropriately calculate and monitor funds

Last will and testament
- Ability to remember estate plans
- Ability to express logic behind choices

the person retains decisional capacity. Some deficits uncovered by the use of the MMSE may be relevant (eg, immediate memory, attention, word finding, understanding simple verbal or written instructions, and ability to express simple ideas in writing); others are not (eg, calculation and visuospatial relationships). As we come to appreciate the influence of frontal lobe dysfunction on a patient's capacity to function, especially to perform complex instrumental activities of daily living, we are also coming to appreciate the influence that the cognitive domains of executive function have on decisional capacity. Executive functions include problem solving, planning (including appreciating consequences of an action), initiation, capacity to monitor one's own behavior, and inhibition of inappropriate behaviors. The Executive Interview 25-item examination of executive function correlates well with subjective measures of decisional capacity. Observation of the patient while completing tasks on the examination may reveal poor insight, impulsivity, the intrusion of irrelevant material, poor self-monitoring, and impaired ability to form and follow through on a plan. Clinicians can make similar observations by observing a patient draw a clock.

Specific tests of decisional capacity have been developed, but most deal in hypothetical situations, thereby requiring a greater degree of abstraction than does real-time decision making. The MacArthur Competency Assessment Tool for Treatment tests the person's ability to make a specific decision and has the advantage of dealing with decisions that are currently facing the individual, but it has not found a practical niche. Tools for the assessment of executive functioning or structured interviewing can be helpful for determining decision-making capacity, but there is no substitute for critical observation of the process itself. The Aid to Capacity Evaluation (ACE) has been found to be helpful in structuring observations of patients' abilities to make decisions and is particularly useful for trainees and primary care clinicians.

Table 4.2—Hierarchy of Decision-Making Strategies

Patient's current wishes
- If the patient has decisional capacity, this **always** takes precedence

Substituted judgment
- Done by the surrogate decision maker only when the patient is not fully capable of making the decision
- Based on the patient's prior values and wishes
- Advance directive is used as guide
- Patient input is used when possible, even if the patient is not fully capable of making the decision

Beneficence
- Done by the surrogate decision maker when the patient lacks decisional capacity and evidence does not exist for substituted judgment
- Weighing of benefits and burdens as based on the patient's present indications of pleasures and burdens
- Input from caregivers is very important

Principles Governing Decision Making for Patients Who Lack Decisional Capacity

The hierarchy of decision-making strategies for those making the decisions for incapacitated patients is as follows: 1) respect their last capable indication of their wishes, 2) use of substituted judgment, and 3) determination of their best interests (ie, an analysis of benefits versus burden). Table 4.2 summarizes the hierarchy.

The last competent indication of wishes is most relevant in cases when patients are able to foresee that they will become incapacitated and can know what decisions may need to be made. Patients entering the terminal phase of an illness who know that at some point they will become confused or unconscious can give clear advance directives (also called *advance care plans* in some contexts) that state their preferences for care. As long as the circumstances remain substantially as predicted, other individuals should not be allowed to reverse these decisions.

Substituted judgment is the process of constructing what the person would have wanted if he or she had been able to foresee the circumstances and give directions for care. In theory, those who know the person best and understand what his or her fears, pleasures, values, and goals were (ie, what the patient's rationale for a decision would have been) can provide substituted judgment. This is usually, but not always, the next of kin. A patient can appoint someone to hold durable power of attorney for health affairs (designating that person as what is also referred to as a *healthcare agent* or *proxy*). The patient should choose the person who can best represent him or her. Any such surrogate makes decisions only if the patient has become incapable of making decisions. The person granted durable power of attorney takes precedence over the next of kin, and a conservator of person takes precedence over all others.

The best-interest standard, or the principle of beneficence, means making medical decisions for an incapacitated patient on the basis of the benefits and burdens an intervention poses for that patient. When there is no expressed wish by the patient and no one to offer substituted judgment, then the surrogate decision maker must weigh the benefits and the burdens of treatment for that patient to make a decision. Such analysis is best done by someone who is knowledgeable about what gives that patient pleasure; what causes agitation, fear, pain, or discomfort; and how the patient reacts to a change in setting, use of restraints, and similar matters. They can then weigh these in deciding how substantial the chance of a wanted outcome will be in light of how much the person will have to go through in the way of tests, treatments, and changes in environment.

In honoring patients' decision making, it is incumbent upon the healthcare system to find ways in which these wishes are translated into appropriate orders across settings. Do-not-resuscitate ("DNR") bracelets and forms such as Physician Orders for Life-Sustaining Treatment (POLST) have been adopted by many states and are an important step toward more seamless care in our complex healthcare system.

Conservatorships and Living Wills

In the absence of next of kin or durable power of attorney for a patient lacking decisional capacity, the court may appoint a conservator (called a *guardian* in some states). There are usually two types of conservatorship: conservator of finance and conservator of person. Incompetence in matters of finance is usually determined either by the demonstrated incapacity of the patient to manage financial matters (eg, unpaid bills, uncashed checks), or through specific testing by either an occupational therapist or a neuropsychologist. A conservator of person is required when individuals have demonstrated that either they can no longer make personal decisions (such as medical decisions), or they are both unable to care for themselves to the point that they endanger themselves through neglect or risk of injury and they cannot understand and accept the need for help.

Living wills are advance directives that attempt to demonstrate what decisions a person would make under certain circumstances. Most living wills address a couple of hypothetical clinical situations (eg, vegetative state, terminal illness) and four possible treatment options (cardiopulmonary resuscitation, respirator therapy, artificial food and hydration, and dialysis).

Table 4.3—The Five Wishes

1. The person I want to make healthcare decisions for me when I can't make them for myself
2. My wish for the kind of medical treatment I want or don't want
3. My wish for how comfortable I want to be
4. My wish for how I want people to treat me
5. My wish for what I want my loved ones to know

SOURCE: *Aging with Dignity*. 2011. Available at www.agingwithdignity.org/forms/5wishes.pdf (accessed Oct 2013). Reprinted with permission.

A living will has limited use because of its vagueness and because it cannot be generalized to the decisions that most commonly need to be made. Some living wills offer a detailed set of hypothetical case scenarios and treatment decisions, but these can be difficult for patients to understand and may not add information about the patient's rationale for decisions. Also, an individual's reaction to a hypothetical event may differ from how he or she will deal with reality. Nonetheless, a living will can be used as evidence of preferences when one is trying to construct how a patient who lacks decisional capacity might have felt about an intervention. The Five Wishes (see Table 4.3), developed by the Aging with Dignity Commission with the help of the Robert Wood Johnson Foundation and the United Health Foundation, have become a popular guide to help individuals think about their wishes and preferences.

The Role of the Incapacitated Patient in Decision Making

Even when patients are not capable of making complex decisions, they can still participate in decision making about issues of lesser complexity. A task assessment of decision-making ability around a specific issue is always appropriate. A patient with little cognitive ability can still give some indication when something causes discomfort or displeasure or when something brings pleasure. The surrogate decision maker must consider these expressions when analyzing the benefits and burdens of an intervention. This consideration of the patient's indications of preference is supported by case law.

The perceived relative burden of an intervention can vary from one person to the next because of differences in mental status and ability to cope with change or disability. A demented patient who is accustomed to one environment will have a much harder time adjusting to hospitalization and may need restraints to undergo something as simple as intravenous antibiotic therapy. The relative benefit of this therapy should be weighed against the burden of hospitalization for such a patient. In less incapacitated patients, an assent-consent model of decision making may be appropriate. Performing certain interventions is nearly impossible without the cooperation of the patient. For instance, if a conservator has consented to a cataract operation but the patient refuses to cooperate, it is doubtful that the procedure can be performed. In this case, the conservator may consent, but the patient must assent to be treated. In other situations, patients may be able to understand the consequences of their decision well enough to give consent, but because of memory impairment, frontal lobe dysfunction, or other cognitive deficit, the clinician may wish to have the family assent as well.

Temporary Loss of Decisional Capacity

Patients can temporarily lose the ability to make decisions during acute confusional states, acute psychotic episodes, periods of unconsciousness from anesthesia or illness, or during an acute CNS event. Although the patients may be expected to regain this ability over time, the rules described above still apply. Decisions that the patient has made before becoming temporarily incapacitated should be respected. A patient may reverse his or her do-not-resuscitate status while undergoing anesthesia with the understanding that it can be reinstated after the procedure. However, a patient who has stated that he or she would never agree to resuscitation should not have this reversed by a family member during a temporary confusional state due to a concurrent illness.

When using either substituted judgment or the best-interest standard in surrogate decision making for a patient with a transient loss of decisional capacity, the decision maker should err on the side of more aggressive intervention if there are situations when the patient's wishes are not known or the circumstances are substantively different from what the patient had anticipated.

Informed Consent for Research

The new emphasis on the quality of consent obtained for participants in research must extend to the vulnerable populations of older adults. Still, it is imperative that researchers study dementia and related problems so that the care of these patients can be improved. The two most vulnerable populations are patients with cognitive impairment, by virtue of their inability to understand the study or their role in it, and institutionalized patients, who may feel coerced to consent. Research involving vulnerable populations needs to be particularly well designed and focused on issues of importance to that population and have a potential to benefit the individuals involved.

For guidelines developed by the American Geriatrics Society for informed consent for research on cognitively impaired older adults, see Table 4.4.

Table 4.4—American Geriatrics Society Guidelines for Research Using Cognitively Impaired Persons as Subjects

- The research must be justified on scientific, clinical, and ethical grounds but can be focused on conditions other than dementia itself.
- The capacity to give consent should be assessed for each individual for each research protocol because decision-making capacity is task specific, and some cognitively impaired individuals will be able to give consent.
- Advance consent to participate in research given before the loss of decisional capacity should, in general, be respected.
- The traditional surrogates for decision making can be used to obtain consent.
- Research protocols that involve more than minimal risk or that do not have a likelihood of direct benefit for the subjects should be offered only to individuals who are able to consent or who have an advance directive consenting to participate in research. Exceptions might be made for exceptionally promising treatments, but this should be reviewed at a national level.
- Surrogates can refuse participation or withdraw the individual from participation if the surrogate determines that the research protocol is not what the individual intended to consent to or is not in the individual's best interest, even if there is advance consent.
- Only in very unusual circumstances would the refusal to participate of even an incapacitated individual be overridden.

SOURCE: Data from AGS Ethics Committee. Informed consent for research on human subjects with dementia. *J Am Geriatr Soc.* 1998;46(10):1308–1310.

DECISIONS NEAR THE END OF LIFE

Although the issues discussed in this section focus on the period near the end of life, the decision-making process and ethical principles described are the same for all medical decisions. All patients make decisions, consciously or subconsciously, concerning treatment of minor conditions, adherence with medical regimens, and related issues by weighing competing values and needs. When a person is faced with a terminal illness or a chronic, disabling, or progressive disease, decision making becomes more acute and focused. Patients, families, and clinicians must attempt to balance benefits and burdens when making many healthcare decisions. This difficult task is further complicated by the fact that only probabilities of the benefits and burdens can be known, not certainties.

For more information on end-of-life decision making and care, see "Cultural Aspects of Care," p 58; and "Palliative Care," p 111.

Forgoing and Discontinuing Interventions

A patient's right to refuse unwanted treatment was confirmed by the Supreme Court of the United States in the 1991 case of *Cruzan* v. *Director, Department of Health of Missouri*. This refusal can occur before the intervention has been started or after it is in place. There is no ethical or legal distinction made between these two situations, often referred to in the more value-laden terms of *withholding* or *withdrawing* therapies. For example, in the case of uremia, a patient with kidney failure can decline to begin dialysis, thus increasing the risk of death from uremia. Alternatively, a patient can try dialysis for a period of time, even years, and then choose to stop this treatment and die from uremia. This same principle holds for discontinuing ventilatory support for a patient who will die from his or her underlying respiratory disease whether ventilatory support is never started or if it is discontinued. The act of extubating a patient with the expectation that he or she will die is difficult for many clinicians because of the proximity of the act performed by the clinician and the death of the patient, but the decision is informed by the same ethical principles as is the decision to discontinue dialysis or to decline other medical interventions.

Clinicians and families often feel uncomfortable when a patient declines tube feeding and intravenous fluids. Case law, as well as the *Cruzan* case, characterizes these methods of delivering food and fluid as medical interventions; therefore, they are subject to the same ethical right of refusal that applies to any other medical intervention. Many people worry that the terminally ill patient will suffer without these interventions, but accumulated experience in hospice care has shown that it is usually easier to make someone comfortable without them: intravenous and nasogastric administration of food and fluid can cause discomfort through decreased gastric emptying and gastric distention, the need to replace intravenous lines or nasogastric tubes, and fluid overload as membranes become more permeable. These interventions can dampen or eliminate some of the physiologic comfort measures that occur, such as the release of endorphins.

Interventions That Can Hasten Death

Palliative care, defined here as interventions that are given to relieve discomfort or suffering without intent to cure, can at times have the unintended effect of hastening death. We have come to accept that there may be two effects of such a treatment: one (intended) effect of palliation, and the other possible (unintended) effect of hastening death. This is sometimes referred to as *the rule of double effect*. The intention of the application of the medical intervention is not to hasten death, but to palliate symptoms. Aggressive management of pain or dyspnea, when respiratory depression is foreseeable but not intended, is considered an ethical practice. Furthermore, most evidence shows that gradually increasing narcotic or benzodiazepine dosage does not hasten death. The rule of double effect has been extended by some to cover the use of terminal sedation (without hydration) in cases in which any level of consciousness will constitute continued suffering, as is frequently the case in death from head and neck cancer, for example. See "Palliative Care," p 111.

Physician-assisted suicide and euthanasia occur when an intervention is made with the clear intention of ending the patient's life. The underlying motivation of patients who wish to hasten death varies. In population-based surveys, people commonly cite fear of pain and other suffering (such as shortness of breath, anorexia, nausea, constipation, insomnia, and anxiety) as the reason for considering physician-assisted suicide. In the United States, fear of being dependent or a burden to others is mentioned at least as often. In the United States, unlike in some other countries that have addressed this issue, only physician-assisted suicide (and not euthanasia) has been legalized or is being considered for legalization. Because suicide is an act committed by the person who will suffer the consequences, it is felt that such a death is more clearly voluntary than a death that results from another person's administration of a lethal intervention. Although the Supreme Court has ruled that there is not a constitutional right to physician-assisted suicide, it did not rule that it is unconstitutional. Each state has been left to make its own laws in this regard. Some states have yet to act; many have made physician-assisted suicide explicitly illegal. Oregon has had legalized physician-assisted suicide since 1997, and Washington and Montana (by judicial ruling) since 2009; many other states are currently considering legalization. Experience in Oregon has shown that relatively few terminally ill patients request physician-assisted suicide. In the 13 years since the law was enacted, there has been an average of 40 deaths by physician-assisted suicide a year (annual death rate of about 10,000), with >90% reporting that autonomy and <25% reporting that pain issues were the driving reason for availing themselves of physician-assisted suicide.

Ability to Predict Time of Death

Webster's Dictionary defines the verb *predict* as "to assert on the basis of theory, data, or experience but in advance of proof." Despite increasingly sophisticated prediction models, especially for patients who are critically ill, patients still rely on their clinician's judgment for most assessments of prognosis. Instruments such as the third version of the acute physiology and chronic health evaluation scoring system (the APACHE III), which uses a combination of age, diagnosis, cause of acute illness, and a scale of physiologic parameters to predict mortality risk in acute illness, are unable to address issues of the burden of treatment or the patient's quality of life. Long-range predictions for patients with slowly deteriorating conditions are even more difficult. Physicians must certify that a patient has ≤6 months to live for that patient to qualify for the Medicare hospice benefit. Similarly, the Oregon Death with Dignity Act asks physicians to predict, using reasonable judgment, whether a terminal illness will result in death within 6 months. The National Hospice and Palliative Care Organization guidelines make an attempt to help with such prognostication, as do several Web sites, but are not well studied. Patients often seek a precise prognosis from their clinicians as they weigh the benefits and burdens of interventions and consider quality-of-life issues as well as survival. Unfortunately, neither clinician judgment nor prediction rules have proved to be very accurate in predicting prognosis under these circumstances.

The Continuum of End-of-Life Decisions Based on Goals

Decisions near the end of life are not all-or-nothing choices. The absence or presence of do-not-resuscitate orders (more accurately referred to as do-not-attempt-resuscitation orders) is often misinterpreted as instruction to the clinician either to do everything to maintain life or to stop all forms of medical treatment. This dichotomy is false.

Other medical interventions for seriously ill patients with similar prognoses can have very different outcomes. For example, a patient with New York Heart Association Class 4 or American Heart Association Stage D heart failure from a cardiomyopathy may ask not to receive cardiopulmonary resuscitation but might choose to accept placement of an automatic implantable cardiac defibrillator. A patient who is dying of lung cancer might weigh the relative burdens and benefits of antibiotic treatment for pneumonia before deciding whether to be treated for an infection. The benefits and burdens of enteral feeding are highly influenced by the condition being treated. Most studies that have been done on the utility of enteral feeding for patients who aspirate have grouped all patients with feeding tubes together, which may not be appropriate. Many variables should be considered, for example:

- Patient 1 has had surgery for a localized pharyngeal cancer followed by radiation. The procedure has left the patient freely aspirating, making it difficult for him to take sufficient calories by mouth. The patient's overall prognosis is still uncertain.
- Patient 2 has Parkinson disease and still functions well. His pharyngeal muscle coordination is slow, and he recurrently chokes on his food, especially thin liquids.
- Patient 3 has end-stage Alzheimer disease. Although she has evidence of aspiration on a swallowing examination and has had two documented pneumonias that are probably related to aspiration, she is comfortable when she eats. One of her only remaining discernible pleasures is eating.

The balance between benefits and burdens is very different for each of these patients. Enteral feeding may or may not prolong their lives, and restrictions on eating could have a different meaning for each. The recommendations by clinicians for each patient or patient's surrogate might include everything from placing a feeding tube to avoiding oral intake to oral intake as tolerated for pleasure, using antipyretic medications for fevers caused by the aspiration, and allowing nature to take its course. Before a choice is made, the patient or family must first clarify their priorities. The clinician can then decide how different approaches can best meet these goals. See "Eating and Feeding Problems," p 216.

Treatment Decisions in the Extended-Care Setting

Until policymakers and clinicians paid attention to the resuscitation status of patients in skilled-nursing facilities, residents were assumed not to be candidates for attempted resuscitation; it was rarely, if ever, attempted. Studies that have looked at the outcomes of attempted resuscitation of patients in long-term care facilities show that it is used infrequently and associated with low long-term survival (SOE=A). However, the number of patients in long-term care settings for short-term recuperation and rehabilitation has grown, which may change the statistics concerning the utility of attempted resuscitation of patients in skilled-nursing facilities.

Staff perceptions of the utility of resuscitation efforts differ by profession. Nursing staff strongly prefer to limit interventions in this setting, especially for older patients and those with cognitive impairments (SOE=C). On the other hand, physicians tend to overestimate the benefit of interventions for these patients (SOE=C). Patient participation in the process is variable. Federal legislation requires the systematic inquiry into advance directives for all patients in institutions receiving federal funds. With the advent of this more systematic approach to discussions about treatment status, skilled-nursing facilities have transferred fewer patients to acute-care settings without a decline in patient and family satisfaction.

Some regulatory agencies have encouraged enteral feeding of patients in nursing homes to prevent nutritional deficits in patients who may not be getting enough nourishment by eating. Although the motives for enacting these regulations were compassionate, the usefulness of enteral feeding, especially for patients with advanced dementia, is questionable. Also, it is not ethical to use enteral feedings for a patient capable of taking oral sustenance but who may not be getting enough nutrition because a facility fails to provide patients with the help they need in eating. See "Malnutrition," p 209.

Special Ethical Issues in Dementia

Although most of the topics discussed above involve the ethics of caring for cognitively impaired persons, some areas of particular concern for patients with dementia merit further discussion.

Truth Telling

The ethics of truth telling has evolved considerably through the last half of the 20th century in mainstream American culture, breaking with the longstanding tradition of paternalism in medicine that advocated withholding bad news from patients to "do no harm." In many other cultures, telling bad news is still not felt to be appropriate. In the United States, however, telling a patient that he or she has a dementing illness may be the last area of controversy about truth telling. Increasingly in the United States, both professional and lay people agree that patients with dementia should be given a chance to understand what is happening to them. The opportunity for the older adult with early dementia to prepare legal documents (powers of attorney, a will, advance directives), to address personal issues, and to make plans is important. As therapies become available and research advances, patients with dementia should be informed of their options and given the opportunity to voice their preferences, even though they may no longer be fully capable of giving informed consent.

Autonomy

Ensuring personal safety and avoiding harm to others are important concerns in caring for patients with dementia. Because of the very nature of the disease process and its effect on recent memory, insight, and judgment, patients may not perceive how they have changed; they may not be able to recognize when their problem interferes with their ability to make decisions. Some patients with cognitive impairment may not understand the consequences of their actions and may have difficulty planning because of frontal lobe dysfunction. This puts them at risk of behaviors that can endanger themselves or others, including unsafe driving, the continued possession of firearms, wandering, and socially inappropriate behaviors. Their care needs can exceed what their caregivers can provide, and they may be unable to understand the rationale for having help at home, day care, or nursing-home care. The clinician plays a crucial role in being able to objectively recognize when this has happened, explain it to the family and if possible the patient, and help the family or others take the necessary steps to protect the patient and others.

Physicians face complex ethical problems when caring for older adults who endanger themselves and others by driving. The conflicting interests are powerful: respect for the patient's autonomy, duty to protect the patient from harm, duty to protect others from predictable danger, and respect for patient-doctor confidentiality. Educating the patient and family members is often the key to developing a practical solution. Legal requirements regarding physician reporting of unsafe older drivers vary from state to state. In some states, physicians are required to report patients who may be unsafe; in other states they are permitted to do so; and in a few states, reporting may be considered a violation of patient-physician confidentiality. (See also the older driver in "Assessment," p 48.)

Another area of controversy is the use of physical and chemical restraints. The use of physical restraints in the long-term care setting has become closely regulated and monitored. Studies have shown that using physical restraints has little, if any, value in preventing injuries from falls (SOE=B). Less restrictive alternatives are usually available. Clinicians and patients' surrogates must consider several factors in deciding whether to use restraints. If the patient is engaging in activities that might harm other residents or staff, and when intervention is ineffective or the patient's surrogate refuses it, then the institution's responsibility to protect others may require that it send the patient elsewhere. In medical settings, restraints are often used to protect medical devices. Because of the dire physical, cognitive, and psychologic consequences of restraints, it is incumbent on clinicians to assess the necessity of such devices and to find the least restrictive way of protecting those that are deemed absolutely necessary. The use of sitters and other interventions to keep the patient safe, as well as the prevention and treatment of delirium, allow the patient to be treated with dignity and respect his or her autonomy as much as possible.

Definition of Personhood and Advance Directives

Adults with intact decisional capacity not only have the right to make their own decisions but also always have the right to change their minds. If their last competent statements were made close to an event that rendered them incapable of decision making, the likelihood is low that their rationale for the decision or that their goals, fears, and pleasures had changed significantly.

If life experiences do mold their thinking, or if new interventions or approaches to problems occur, they can alter their directive to fit with these changes. A person with a progressive cognitive disorder can change substantially over time. What brings pleasure and what causes fear or pain can change substantially from year to year; almost certainly a patient's perceptions change greatly as the disease progresses. The demented person is unable to comprehend the future and slowly becomes more and more disconnected from the past. In some ways, the patient with advancing dementia becomes suspended in time: he or she loses his or her connection to previous and future selves, the essence of what many define as personhood. A demented person is connected to the decisions and perceptions of a previous self who he or she may not even remember. The decisions made by this prior "self" can inform current decision making, even though that person did not know what he or she would need or want at this time. Therefore, conflict can arise between the previous directives made by that person and what is best for the demented patient in the here-and-now (ie, what gives the patient pleasure and what may disturb him or her).

Sexuality and the Cognitively Impaired Individual

Expressions of sexuality and sexual desire do not end with aging or disappear with cognitive impairment. Certain aspects of cognitive impairment, specifically the disinhibition sometimes seen in frontal lobe dysfunction, can increase individuals' expression of their sexuality. Medications, particularly hormonal therapies and anti-Parkinson medications can also increase expressions of sexuality and sexual desire.

Although patients with cognitive impairment should not be denied pleasure through sexual gratification, there are ethical concerns regarding their sexual activity that need to be addressed. As certain cognitive areas become affected by disease, the individual may no longer recognize social boundaries and engage in lewd behavior toward others or in public autoerotic acts. Beyond the fact that such behavior is disturbing to others, it is behavior that the person would likely have been mortified by before the onset of dementia. Such behaviors need to be forestalled, but all such pleasures should not be forbidden or ever punished. The person should be allowed some privacy if this is possible. Families may be uncomfortable with this, because it may not be consistent with their image of their parent (rightly or wrongly). Institutions are often uncomfortable with expressions of sexuality, because staff may find it offensive and be concerned that families will be upset.

Cognitively impaired individuals can be vulnerable to unwanted and unpleasurable sexual activity as well. This can be everything from sexual abuse by a cognitively intact family member or caregiver to incidental sexual contact by another demented individual. Cognitively impaired individuals may perceive sexual abuse when none was intended, eg, they may not have the ability to understand why someone would be undressing them when having a bath or a physical examination. Demented individuals may engage in sexual activity that is pleasurable but under a misapprehension as to who they are with or where they are. Protecting vulnerable individuals from harm obviously depends on how one defines harm but is still a fundamental responsibility of social institutions and caregivers.

REFERENCES

- Appelbaum PS. Clinical Practice. Assessment of patients' competence to consent to treatment. *N Engl J Med.* 2007;357(18):1834–1840.
- Beauchamp TL, Childress JF. *Principles of Biomedical Ethics.* Oxford University Press; 2009.
- Sessums LL, Zembrzuska H, Jackson JL. "Does this patient have decisional capacity?" *JAMA.* 2011;306(4):420-427.
- Snyder, L, for the American College of Physicians Ethics, Professionalism, and Human Rights Committee. American College of Physicians Ethics Manual: Sixth Edition. *Ann Intern Med.* 2012;156(1 Part 2):73–104.

CHAPTER 5—FINANCING, COVERAGE, AND COSTS OF HEALTH CARE

KEY POINTS

- Medicare comprises four benefits: Medicare Part A, B, C, and D.
  - ☐ Medicare Part A covers hospital, skilled nursing-home, home-health, and hospice services.
  - ☐ Medicare Part B covers physicians, nurse practitioners, social workers, psychologists, therapists, laboratory tests, and durable medical equipment.
  - ☐ Medicare Part D covers some of the cost of prescription medications.
  - ☐ Medicare Part C provides the benefits offered under Medicare Parts A and B through Medicare Advantage (MA) plans, which are managed care plans. Most MA plans also offer Medicare Part D benefits.
- Medigap supplemental insurance plans are available that cover Medicare Part A and Part B deductibles and co-insurance costs, as well as preventive care and other health-related goods and services.
- Medicaid is a joint federal and state program that provides health insurance (including long-term custodial care in nursing homes) to people of all ages who have low incomes and limited savings.
- While the details of healthcare reform will evolve over the next several years, the movement toward coordination of care and delivery systems that operate in an efficient and effective manner is taking shape. Systems such as Accountable Care Organizations and Medical Homes are playing a role in care delivery.

The Affordable Care Act (ACA) of 2010 laid out several changes to the financing, coverage, and costs of health care for older adults. And while the details of healthcare reform will evolve over the next several years, the movement toward coordination of care and delivery systems that operate in an efficient and effective manner has already begun to take shape. The 2,801 pages of legislation and even more of regulation and guidelines will undoubtedly cause major changes. Some of the major areas being affected follow:

- Creation of the Center for Medicare and Medicaid Innovation (CMI), which has been charged with testing and implementing new care and payment models such as the Accountable Care Organization and the Patient Centered Medical Home.
- Partial closure of the coverage gap in the Medicare Part D prescription drug benefit; starting in 2011, 50% of the cost of branded pharmaceuticals will be covered during the coverage gap.
- Extended coverage for preventive care services, as well as elimination of the co-payment requirements for some services.
- Expansion of Medicaid (beginning in 2014), in which many more Medicare beneficiaries will be qualified as dually eligible, eliminating much of their out-of-pocket expenditures.
- Changes in provider reimbursement, including decreases for Medicare Advantage Plans and increases in reimbursement to primary care providers.

To appreciate these changes requires an examination of the foundation of the current healthcare system for older adults. This foundation began in 1965, the year that the U.S. government passed legislation designed to improve access to acute health care for old, disabled, or poor people. During the decades that followed, the resulting Medicare and Medicaid programs expanded, evolved, and spawned thousands of supplemental commercial insurance plans. Today, a complex and often confusing array of personal payments, public programs, and private insurance plans (Figure 5.1) pays for and thereby determines much of the health care that older Americans receive.

MEDICARE

Medicare is a federal insurance program run by the Centers for Medicare and Medicaid Services (CMS), which pays health professionals and organizations to provide acute health care for Americans who are ≥65 years old, disabled, or suffering from end-stage renal disease. As originally enacted, Medicare comprises two separate fee-for-service (FFS) plans (Part A and Part B), each of which pays predetermined amounts for specified health-related goods and services that are needed by its beneficiaries. More than 47 million Americans are covered by both plans, which is 15% of the total U.S. population.

Parts A and B

The Medicare fee-for-service program, the nation's largest health insurance plan, is administered by

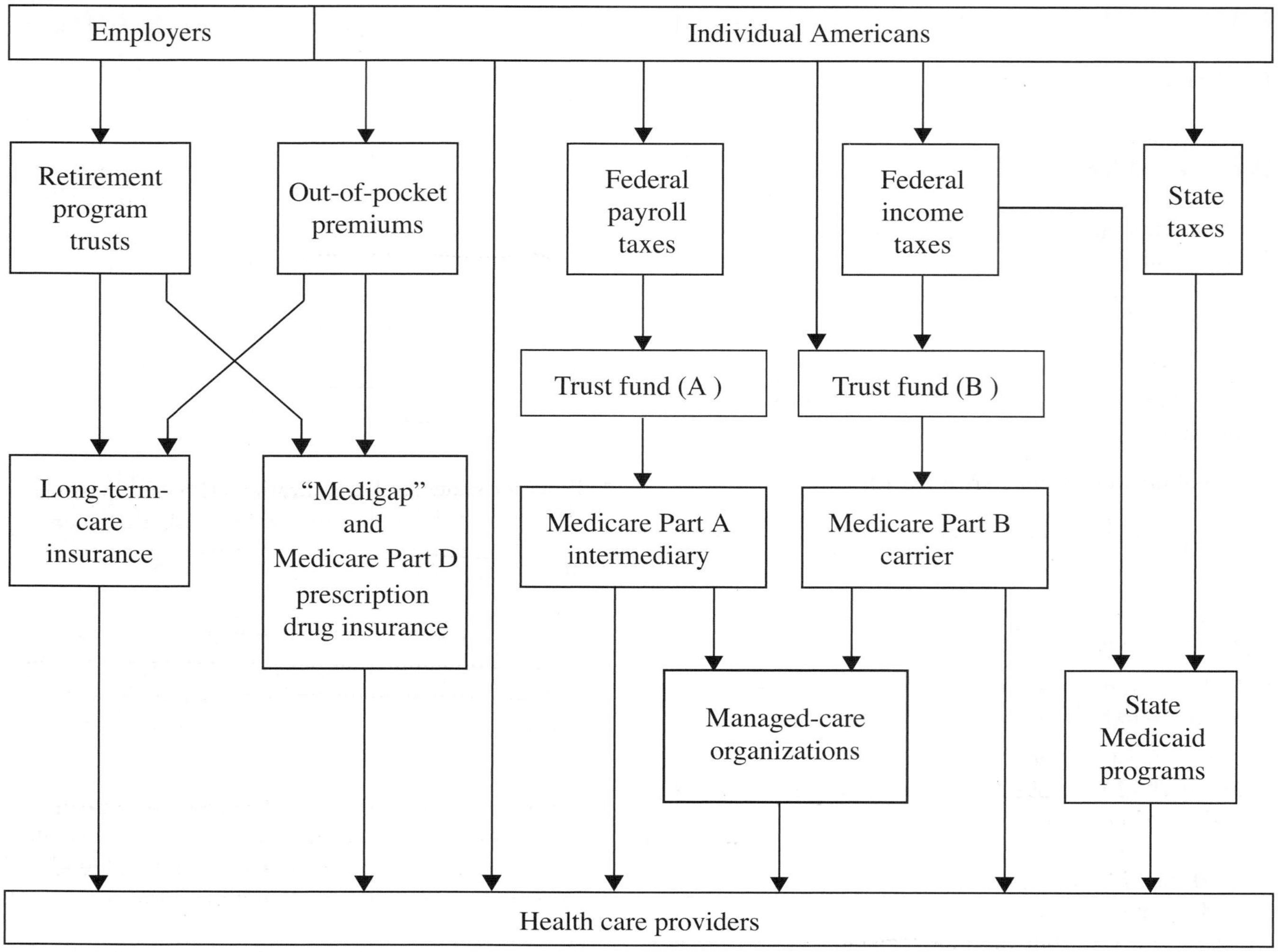

Figure 5.1—The Flow of Funds for the Health Care of Older Americans

private organizations under contract to the CMS. Called Medicare Administrative Contractors, they enroll providers, educate them about coverage and appropriate billing, answer beneficiary and provider inquiries, and detect fraud and abuse. Their primary task, however, is prompt and accurate payment of the 1.2 billion claims submitted yearly for Medicare-covered services.

Older Americans (and their spouses) who have had Medicare taxes deducted from their paychecks for at least 10 years are entitled to coverage through Part A without paying premiums. Others may be able to purchase Part A coverage (for up to $451/month in 2012, depending on how long they had Medicare taxes deducted from their paychecks).

Medicare Part B uses other regional insurance companies ("carriers") to pay physicians, nurse practitioners, social workers, psychologists, rehabilitation therapists, home-care agencies, ambulances, outpatient facilities, laboratory and imaging facilities, and suppliers of durable medical equipment for the Medicare-covered goods and services they provide. At age 65, older adults become eligible for Part B coverage if they are entitled to Part A coverage or if they are citizens or permanent residents of the United States. To obtain this coverage, eligible older adults must enroll in Part B and pay premiums ($99.90/month in 2012); higher-income beneficiaries may pay more, usually by agreeing to have these amounts deducted from their monthly Social Security checks.

Providers must choose among three options for participating in the FFS Medicare program: participation, nonparticipation, and private contracting. For each Medicare-covered service provided, a participating provider submits a claim to the Part B carrier, accepts Medicare's fee for the service (80% of its preestablished "allowed" amount), and bills the patient or the patient's secondary insurer for no more than a 20% co-insurance payment. Providers electing nonparticipation status can bill patients directly for up to 15% more than 95% of Medicare's allowed amounts. The patients pay the providers and then submit their requests to Medicare for partial reimbursement (ie, for

80% of 95% of the allowed amounts). For services not covered by Medicare, the provider may bill the patient, if the patient agrees in advance in writing.

Neither Part A nor Part B of the Medicare program covers routine dental or foot care, hearing aids, eyeglasses, orthopedic shoes, cosmetic surgery, care in foreign countries, or custodial long-term care at home or in nursing homes. Part B covers some preventive services (Table 5.1).

Beneficiaries pay out-of-pocket for the following (rates are for 2012):

- monthly premiums for Part B (standard premium is $99.90 but can be as high as $319.70 depending on income)
- annual deductible for Part B ($140)
- the deductible for Part A ($1,156 per benefit period)
- co-insurance payments (usually 20%) for goods and services for which Medicare or other insurance pays only a portion
- the full cost of those goods and services that are not covered by Medicare or other insurance

While most retirees who signed up for Medicare Part B in 2012 paid $99.90 each month, premiums for wealthier retirees ranged from $139.90 for individuals earning between $85,000 and $107,000 annually to $319.70 monthly for single tax filers with income over $214,000 annually. These income thresholds typically increase each year, but the new legislation freezes the income thresholds from 2011 through 2019 at 2010 levels meaning that each year more individuals will be required to pay these higher premiums.

Part C

As an alternative to traditional FFS Parts A, B, and D, Medicare beneficiaries can instead elect to enroll in a Medicare managed-care plan, an option known as Part C or Medicare Advantage (MA). MA plans, operated by private insurers, hold contracts with CMS specifying that, for each Medicare beneficiary they enroll, they will provide at least the standard Medicare Part A, B, and D benefits in return for fixed monthly capitation payments. Plans operate on a risk-adjusted basis for each member based on the ICD-9 diagnoses that are provided. As a result, plans are paid more for individuals with more diagnoses that require a higher level of care.

To attract enrollees, most MA plans also cover additional benefits and charge low or no premiums, deductibles, and co-payments. The plans achieve cost savings by managing their enrollees' use of services within their networks of providers, with whom they negotiate price discounts in return for patient volume. Each January, MA plans have the option of changing their premiums, benefits, and provider networks—or of discontinuing their plans altogether.

There are several types of MA plans:

- Medicare Health Maintenance Organizations (HMOs)—insurance companies that accept capitation payments from CMS and provide or purchase Medicare-covered health services
- Preferred provider organizations (PPOs)—alliances of providers that accept capitation payments and deliver Medicare-covered health services to their enrolled patients
- Provider-sponsored organizations (PSOs)—partnerships of physician groups and hospitals that accept capitation payments and deliver Medicare-covered health services to their enrolled patients
- Private FFS plans—plans that may charge beneficiaries a premium, that pay providers more liberally than the original Medicare FFS program does, and that allow providers to charge their patients co-payments of up to 15%
- Special needs plans—plans designed for patients with certain chronic diseases or other special needs, such as people who have both Medicare and Medicaid or people who live in certain institutions
- Medical savings accounts—accounts into which Medicare beneficiaries can make tax-deductible contributions and out of which they can withdraw funds to purchase routine health-related goods (including medications) and services (including long-term care insurance) from any Medicare provider; linked to the medical savings account is a catastrophic insurance policy that limits the individual beneficiary's out-of-pocket expenses for health care to $6,000/year.

Between October 15 and December 7, beneficiaries covered by Medicare Part A and Part B have the option of joining any MA plan operating in their area; they cannot be denied enrollment because of any health problems except end-stage renal disease. Between January 1 and February 14, beneficiaries enrolled in an MA plan can switch to original Medicare. In addition, Medicare beneficiaries can enroll at any time during the year in a 5-star MA program. Enrollees must continue to pay their monthly Medicare Part B premiums to Medicare, plus any additional premium that the MA plan charges to cover additional services, and they must obtain their healthcare services from the plan's provider network. They have the option of

Table 5.1—Health Insurance Coverage for Older Americans 2012

	Fee-for-Service Medicare		Supplemental Coverage			
	Part A	**Part B**	**Medicaid**[a]	**Part D**	**Medigap Insurance**	**Medicare Advantage Insurance**[b] **(Part C)**
Covers the cost of:						
Hospitals	100%[c]	—	$1156 [c]	—	$550–$1100	100%
Postacute care in skilled-nursing facility	100%[d]	—	—	—	—	100%
Hospice	100%[e]	—	—	—	—	—
Home care ("medically necessary")	100%	100%	—	—	—	100%
Durable medical equipment	80%[f]	80%[f]	20%	—	20%	100%
Diagnostic laboratory tests	—	100%	—	—	—	100%
Diagnostic imaging tests	—	80%	20%	—	20%	100%
Physicians, nurse practitioners	—	80%	20%	—	20%	100%
Outpatient PT, OT, ST	—	80%	20%	—	20%	100%
Outpatient services, supplies	—	80%	20%	—	20%	100%
Emergency care	—	80%	20%	—	20%	100%
Ambulance services	—	80%	20%	—	20%	100%
Preventive services	—	[g]	20%	—	20%	[g, h]
Outpatient mental health care		50%	50%	—	50%	100%
Custodial care in nursing home	—	—	100%	—	—	—
Hearing, vision services	—	—	[i]	—	[i]	[i]
Outpatient medications	—	—	[i]	50%–95%[j]	[i]	[i]
Additional costs to patient:						
Deductibles	$110[k]	$155[l]	—	$320	[i]	[i]
Monthly premiums	—	$96–$354	—	$31 [m]	[i]	[i]

NOTE: PT = physical therapy; OT = occupational therapy; ST = speech therapy

[a] Under the Balanced Budget Act of 1997, state Medicaid programs were given the option whether or not to pay deductibles and co-insurance costs.

[b] Some Medicare Advantage plans require members to pay deductibles and co-payments.

[c] After the beneficiary or secondary insurer pays the Part A deductible of $1156, plus $239 per day for days 61–90 of each benefit period

[d] For the first 20 days of care in a skilled-nursing facility after a hospital stay of at least 3 days: $144.50 per day for days 21–100 of each benefit period

[e] Patient makes co-payments of $5.00 per outpatient prescription and 5% of cost of respite care.

[f] When patient is receiving Medicare-covered home care

[g] 100% of allowed cost of fecal occult blood test, Pap smear interpretation, prostate-specific antigen test, blood tests for diabetes and cardiovascular disease, and influenza and pneumococcal vaccinations; 80% of allowed cost of mammograms and clinical examination of breast and pelvis (no deductible applies); after the annual Part B deductible has been paid, 80% of allowed cost of a general physical examination at age 65, glaucoma screening, sigmoidoscopy or colonoscopy or barium enema, digital rectal examination (men), measurement of bone mass, hepatitis B vaccination, and diabetic education and equipment (coverage subject to change by health reform legislation)

[h] Some Medicare Advantage plans cover additional preventive services.

[i] Benefits and costs vary widely among medigap insurance plans, state Medicaid plans, prescription drug plans, and Medicare Advantage Plans.

[j] Starting in 2011, the coverage gap ("doughnut hole") will gradually be closed over the next 10 years. In 2012, beneficiaries will pay 50% of the cost of brand name medications and 93% of the cost of generic medications while in the coverage gap.

[k] Per benefit period (first 60 days after hospital admission)

[l] Annually

[m] Basic premium for 2012; premiums vary by plan. In addition, there is an additional program required for those with individual incomes >$85,000 (joint >$170,000), which is an additional payment on top of the standard monthly premium of between $11.60 and $66.40 depending on income.

leaving the plan at any time and returning to the FFS Medicare program.

The ACA cut $145 billion over 10 years from Medicare Advantage, partly to correct a problem with overpayments to the plans. These cuts start off modestly in 2012 and build up. Insurers are expected to shift the burden to beneficiaries in the form of fewer services and higher out-of-pocket costs, triggering an exodus back to traditional Medicare. The impact of Medicare Advantage cuts is initially being softened by providing quality bonuses.

Part D

In 2003, the U.S. Congress passed and President George W. Bush signed a sweeping Medicare reform bill that included an option (Medicare Part D) for beneficiaries to purchase insurance coverage for outpatient prescription medications. The Part D option is open to all Medicare beneficiaries, whether enrolled in traditional FFS or MA. Part D benefits can be purchased as stand-alone policies or as sponsored by MA plans. For most Medicare beneficiaries, there is a dizzying array of plans from which to choose, with premiums, deductibles, co-payments, and formularies differing from plan to plan. CMS has set up a Medicare Prescription Drug Plan Finder (www.medicare.gov/find-a-plan/questions/home.aspx [accessed Oct 2013]), in which enrollees can enter their location and medications to compare Part D options available to them.

Part D coverage policies as set by law are also confusing to many beneficiaries, because different levels of coverage apply to cumulative yearly prescription drug expenditures. Many plans have a relatively small deductible; the maximal allowable deductible by law in 2013 is $325. After the deductible is paid, Part D plans usually cover 75% of the ensuing drug costs up to a specified amount ($2,970 in 2013), after which there is a gap in Part D coverage (the so-called "doughnut hole"), until the individual's spending for prescription drugs reaches a predetermined catastrophic amount, and Part D coverage resumes.

The "doughnut hole" existed for a variety of reasons, including lowering the overall price tag of the prescription drug benefit and ensuring that beneficiaries have an interest in avoiding inappropriate prescription drug spending. In 2009, an estimated 3.4 million beneficiaries entered the coverage gap, while only 15% spent enough to hit the catastrophic limit and regain drug coverage. Included in the ACA of 2010 was legislation to immediately start closing this coverage gap. In 2010, the federal government provided beneficiaries a one-time $250 rebate check on hitting the coverage gap. Beginning in 2011, when beneficiaries hit the coverage gap, pharmaceutical manufacturer(s) pay for 50% of the cost of brand drugs while the beneficiary is in the coverage gap, and the beneficiary will pay the remaining 50%. Moving forward, the coverage gap cost-sharing levels for the beneficiary will be reduced annually until 2020, when the level is then set at 25%, which is consistent with cost-sharing levels of coverage before hitting the gap.

In 2013, the cost of medications for beneficiaries who qualify for Medicaid is $2.65 for generic products and $6.50 for branded ones. The dual-eligible beneficiaries have no premium or coverage gap; in fact, beneficiaries who are nursing-home eligible have no out-of-pocket expense for any Part D–covered medication.

It is important for prescribers to appreciate that the standard Medicare Part D benefit changes each year. Some aspects like the initial deductible and period of time before getting to the catastrophic point change such that patients experience an increase in their out-of-pocket expense. This could result in adherence issues as patients are forced to pay more out of pocket at different times during the year. Changes are also occurring such that patients are paying less during the coverage gap as the Affordable Care Act moves to fill in the coverage gap from 100% out of pocket to just 25% slowly over the next several years. For Medicare Part D Comparison (2006–2013), see www.q1medicare.com/PartD-The-2013-Medicare-Part-D-Outlook.php (accessed Oct 2013).

Medigap

Medigap supplemental plans fill some of the holes in the insurance coverage provided by Medicare Part A and Part B. Private insurance companies offer FFS medigap plans of 12 types (A through L), classified according to the benefits they offer. For new Medicare beneficiaries at age 65, the premiums for A-level (basic) plans across the United States vary considerably. These policies cover a person's Part A and Part B co-insurance costs, eg, 20% of Medicare's allowed fees for durable medical equipment and health care providers' services. (In Minnesota, Wisconsin, and Massachusetts, A-level medigap policies are required by law to cover more than just the costs of Medicare co-insurance.) B-level plans cover Part A and Part B co-insurance, plus the Part A deductible. Each successive level of medigap policy provides additional benefits and costs more. J-level plans cover co-insurance, deductibles, care in foreign countries, and preventive services. Less expensive medigap coverage can be obtained by purchasing plans that require the insured to pay high deductibles (F- and J-level plans only) or plans that cover the services of only selected providers and hospitals ("Medicare SELECT" policies). Medigap policies do not cover long-term care, dental care, eyeglasses, hearing aids, or private-duty nursing. They also do not cover out-of-pocket costs for MA plans.

Within 6 months of their initial enrollment in Medicare Part B, beneficiaries are entitled to purchase any medigap policy on the market at advertised prices. After this open enrollment period, medigap insurers can refuse to insure individual beneficiaries or charge them higher premiums because of their past or present health problems.

Medicaid

Medicaid is a joint federal and state program that provides health insurance to people of all ages who have low incomes and limited savings. The exact criteria for Medicaid eligibility and the benefit packages provided by Medicaid programs vary considerably from state to state. Most programs pay Medicare Part B premiums, and some pay Medicare deductibles and co-insurance costs. Most important, Medicaid pays for long-term custodial care in nursing homes for those who qualify. Several states have begun offering fixed capitation payments to managed-care organizations that are willing to provide Medicaid and Medicare benefits to residents who are dually eligible (ie, for Medicaid and Medicare).

The ACA extends the opportunity for States to expand Medicaid coverage to all nonelderly individuals with incomes below 133% of the federal poverty level in 2014. Under the new law, the federal government will pay 100% of the cost for newly eligible individuals from 2014 through 2016. The reimbursement rate to states declines to 95% in 2017 and will be reduced gradually to 90% after 2019. This is expected to increase Medicaid enrollment nationwide by 17 million over what it would have been under current law, according to estimates by the Congressional Budget Office. However, this number may be less since The Supreme Court ruled that this expansion of Medicaid is optional rather than mandatory for states.

Dual Eligibles

Medicare and Medicaid, which were initially developed in 1965 as two distinct programs, jointly provide benefits to 9 million individuals commonly referred to as *dual eligibles* because their circumstances qualify them for both programs. Despite the notable differences between Medicare and Medicaid, the line separating the programs has become blurred over the years. For example, Medicaid used to provide prescription drug coverage for dual eligibles, but the Medicare Part D provision of the Medicare Modernization Act of 2003 shifted that responsibility to Medicare as of January 2006.

While eligible for benefits, many low-income individuals do not receive Medicaid. Some do not meet their state's income and asset eligibility criteria, and others are likely eligible but have trouble navigating the application process. Poor health literacy is an especially common problem among older adults, and focus groups have demonstrated that dual eligibles often do not understand their plan or its benefits.

Women, African Americans, Hispanics, and disabled Medicare beneficiaries <65 years old make up a relatively large share of the dual-eligible population. Dual eligibles tend to have more functional and cognitive limitations and correspondingly greater medical need than beneficiaries enrolled in Medicare or Medicaid alone. As a result, they account for a disproportionate share of Medicare and Medicaid spending. Constituting just 15% of the Medicaid population, dual eligibles account for 39% of total Medicaid spending. They make up 21% of the Medicare population, yet are responsible for 36% of Medicare spending.

Considering the significant level of need and the limited resources of dual eligibles, it is perhaps not surprising that long-term care expenses account for an overwhelming share of medical expenses on behalf of this population, with dual-eligible individuals spending 70% of their Medicaid dollars on long-term care services in 2007.

Despite the high level of need that dual eligibles typically have, they are all too often subjected to uncoordinated payment systems in Medicare and Medicaid. To address this dysfunction and to improve coordination between Medicare and Medicaid, the ACA established the Federal Coordinated Health Care Office within the CMS. The ACA also created the CMI to develop and implement innovative payment and service delivery models for recipients of Medicare, Medicaid, and the Children's Health Insurance Program, including those who are dual eligibles.

A goal of the reform efforts being undertaken is to improve coordination of care for dual-eligible individuals. This includes identifying potential areas of reform in how care for dual eligibles is provided and paid for that can be incorporated into new models of care integration, along with ongoing efforts by the CMI to develop other payment and delivery systems for Medicare.

One possible approach to integrating Medicaid and Medicare financially is to give each state a yearly block grant that is intended to fund all services used by state residents who are enrolled in either or both of the programs. States that spend less on Medicaid and Medicare services than the amount funded through the block grant would be permitted to keep the difference, but states that spend more on Medicaid and Medicare services than the amount of the block grant would be obligated to make up the difference. Another suggested approach is to have Medicare bear full financial responsibility for dual-eligible beneficiaries.

While the Federal Coordinated Health Care Office has only recently begun its work, other measures and programs have been enacted with the purpose of improving care for dual eligibles. For example, Section 3309 of the ACA contains provisions for eliminating cost-sharing for certain full-benefit, dual-eligible individuals. In addition, effective January 1, 2012, all cost-sharing under Medicare Part D will be waived for full-benefit, dual-eligible individuals who would require institutionalization if not for access to home- and community-based services.

Extensive information about all the options is available to consumers at each state's medical assistance office, at 1-800-MEDICARE (1-800-633-4227) or 1-877-486-2048 for hearing impaired TTY users, and at the Medicare Personal Plan Finder (www.medicare.gov) (accessed Oct 2013).

Veterans Administration (VA) Benefit

The VA provides a medical benefits package to all enrolled veterans. This comprehensive plan provides a full range of preventive outpatient and inpatient services within the VA healthcare system. Also, once enrolled in the VA's healthcare system, veterans can be seen at any VA facility across the country.

Those VA facilities include a system comprising 153 medical centers, 773 ambulatory care and community-based outpatient clinics, 260 vet centers, 136 nursing homes, 45 residential rehabilitation treatment programs, and 92 comprehensive home-based care programs—all providing medical and related services to eligible veterans. These facilities provide inpatient hospital care, outpatient care, laboratory services, pharmaceutical dispensing, rehabilitation for a variety of disabilities and conditions, mental health counseling, and custodial care. They also employ about 200,000 full-time–equivalent employees, including over 13,000 physicians and nearly 55,000 nurses. While the VA system is a closed system—meaning that all care is provided through VA facilities and providers—there are some exceptions. Veterans who are Medicare beneficiaries can use the Medicare system as well. In addition, the VA is increasing partnering with outside providers to extend the services available to veterans.

FINANCING OF CARE AT DIFFERENT SITES

This section describes, through the eyes of both patients and providers, how the various programs influence the day-to-day care of older adults. It illustrates their effects during a year in the life of Mrs. Rose Murat, an imaginary 79-year-old retired schoolteacher who lives with her 83-year-old husband in a small, older home. Mrs. Murat has hypertension, coronary artery disease, and mild heart failure, for which she takes hydrochlorothiazide, metoprolol, lisinopril, and nitroglycerin. She is covered by traditional Medicare Parts A and B. Mrs. Murat has also purchased a Part D drug plan, for which she pays annual premiums ($383), deductibles ($325), and co-insurance (25% of her remaining medication expenses = $298). As a result, her total out-of-pocket medication costs were reduced 34% from $1,500 to $991 per year (from $125 to $83 per month). For the primary advantages and disadvantages of each of Mrs. Murat's coverage options, see Table 5.2.

Outpatient Care

Mrs. Murat sees her primary care provider quarterly for monitoring of her chronic conditions.

Fee for Service

Under the Medicare FFS system, providers obtain the fairest possible reimbursement by understanding and following CMS's payment system, which is based on evaluation and management (E&M) codes.

For each Medicare-covered service provided, the provider submits to the regional Medicare carrier the appropriate E&M code and the international classification of disease (ICD) code that indicates the diagnosis for which the service was provided. Entries in the medical record, which are subject to audit, must document that the data collection and medical decision-making aspects of the service conform to standards established for the E&M code submitted. By providing and documenting services efficiently, providers can maximize their FFS reimbursements within the limits imposed by the Medicare fee schedules.

Were Mrs. Murat newly enrolled in Medicare, she would be eligible for a preventive visit. The "Welcome to Medicare" preventive visit is offered free of any charges to all new Medicare beneficiaries within their first 12 months of Medicare as a means for individuals to develop a personalized plan to prevent disease, improve their health, and help stay well. During this visit, her primary care providers are responsible for the following:

- Recording and evaluating medical and family history, current health conditions, and prescriptions
- Checking blood pressure, vision, weight, and height to get a baseline for care
- Making sure each patient is up-to-date with preventive screenings and services, such as cancer screenings and shots
- Ordering further tests, depending on general health and medical history

After Mrs. Murat has been enrolled in Medicare Part B for longer than 12 months, she is eligible for a yearly wellness visit to develop or update a prevention plan based on current health and risk factors. This visit is covered once every 12 months.

At the end of her quarterly office visit, Mrs. Murat asks for advice on joining a managed care organization that has been marketing an MA plan in her county. She is impressed by the MA plan's offer of free eyeglasses, hearing aids, and preventive check-ups, all of which she has purchased out-of-pocket in the past. Her options are as follows: staying with traditional FFS Medicare as her only coverage, keeping FFS Medicare and applying for either Medicaid or supplemental (medigap) coverage, or exchanging her FFS Medicare coverage for membership in the MA plan (Table 5.2). Depending on the Murats' income, savings, and state of residence, they may also qualify for a Medicare assistance program that pays for some combination of their Medicare premiums, deductibles, and co-insurance costs. Some older Americans may have additional health insurance

Table 5.2—Advantages and Disadvantages of Four Types of Health Insurance

Type of Insurance	Primary Advantages	Primary Disadvantages
Fee-for-Service Medicare (Parts A, B, and D)	Traditional Medicare benefits, choice of any provider that participates in the Medicare program, partial coverage for prescription medications	Cost of co-insurance, deductibles, noncovered goods and services (eg, eyeglasses, hearing aids)
Medicaid	Coverage of co-insurance, deductibles, and some benefits[a] not covered by Medicare	Choice of providers restricted to a single network in some states
Medigap insurance	Coverage of co-insurance, deductibles, and some benefits[b] not covered by Medicare	Out-of-pocket monthly premiums may be expensive, depending on the coverage provided by the policy purchased
Medicare Advantage plan (ie, Part C)	Traditional Medicare benefits plus coverage of additional goods and services[b]	Choice of providers restricted to a network; potential for changes in premiums, co-payments, deductibles, benefits, and providers at the discretion of the plan

[a] Benefits vary from state to state.

[b] Benefits vary from plan to plan.

options through the federal Department of Veterans Affairs or through their (or their spouses') present or previous employer or union.

Managed Care

Mrs. Murat's primary care provider, knowledgeable about her health and prognosis, can help her to choose the plan(s) that will cover the goods and services that she needs, both now and in the future. If she can obtain what she is likely to need from the MA plan's network of providers, joining the plan might be her best option, because it will likely cover eyeglasses, hearing aids, and preventive services, and she can avoid paying the usual Medicare deductibles and co-insurance. Data about the quality of care and the satisfaction of other enrollees in all the local MA plans are available at the Medicare Personal Plan Finder.

If Mrs. Murat needs health care that is not available from the MA plan's network, or if she is reluctant to change providers, retaining the flexibility of her traditional FFS Medicare coverage (which covers her use of any provider that participates in the Medicare program) might be a better choice, especially if she also qualifies for Medicaid or buys a medigap policy. Information from Medicare's information line or from the Medicare Personal Plan Finder would help her compare the prices and coverage of the medigap policies available in her area.

The primary care provider's recommendations to Mrs. Murat are likely to be influenced by the characteristics of the different plans she is considering. For instance, if the primary care provider is not in the MA plan's service network, he or she would likely point out to Mrs. Murat that her enrollment in the MA plan would require her to select a new primary care provider. If the primary care provider is in the MA plan's network, Mrs. Murat's enrollment might change (ie, probably reduce) the payment for her care. The payments would depend on the type of plan involved (Table 5.3). If it is a group or independent practice association model, the MA plan may pay providers "discounted FFS," ie, possibly less than Medicare Part B would pay for each service. Or it may pay primary providers a fixed capitation amount each month to cover specified services. If these services are limited to primary ambulatory care, the capitation amount will be relatively small. Plans may choose to reward primary care providers with bonus payments for efficient and effective use of resources for the patients for whom they are responsible. If the covered services also include specialty and inpatient care, the capitation amounts will be considerably larger, and the provider will have incentives to use these services judiciously because he or she will have to pay for them, at least in part.

Regardless of the payment mechanism, the crucial question is whether the amount of payment suffices to support high-quality care. For example, if capitation rates are below the aggregate cost of the services they are intended to cover, the provider will feel pressure to take on more patients and to limit the amount of service that each patient receives. Similarly, if FFS amounts are too small, the provider will feel pressure to schedule more visits and procedures and to reduce the time devoted to each patient. Each provider should, therefore, monitor carefully and continually the many changing elements in the practice environment (eg, payment schedules, covered services, expenses, patients' and families' expectations, population demographics) to help determine the numbers and types of services that are appropriate for each older patient.

Inpatient Care

Four months later, Mrs. Murat awakes dysarthric and unable to feel her left hand. Her face is asymmetric,

Table 5.3—How Medicare Advantage Plans Pay Healthcare Providers

	Type of Medicare Advantage Plan		
	Staff Model	***Group Model***	***Independent Practice Association Model***
Providers	Employees	One large group practice	Many small independent practices
Method of payments	Salary	Fee-for-service or capitation[a]	Fee-for-service or capitation[a]

[a] The services covered by the capitation payments range from "primary care only" in some plans to "medications and all acute care" in others.

and her left arm and left leg are weak. Her husband calls 911; the ambulance rushes her to the nearest emergency department, where the physician on duty diagnoses a right hemispheric stroke and admits her to the hospital. Mrs. Murat may qualify for the Community Care Transitions Program, which provides transition services to high-risk Medicare beneficiaries. In addition, she may fall under a program monitoring hospital readmissions. This program directs CMS to track hospital readmission rates for certain high-volume or high-cost conditions, while using financial incentives to encourage hospitals to undertake reforms needed to reduce preventable readmissions.

Fee for Service

If Mrs. Murat had retained traditional Medicare as her only health insurance, she would have to pay Medicare's required deductibles (in 2012, $140 per year under Part B for the ambulance and the emergency medical care, plus $1,156 under Part A for the hospital admission) and co-insurance amounts (20% of Medicare's allowed charges by physicians and the ambulance service). She would also have to pay any ambulance charges in excess of Medicare's approved fee. If she had supplemented her Medicare coverage, her Medicaid or private medigap coverage would cover some of these deductibles and co-insurance payments, and she would not be transferred to another hospital for insurance reasons.

When Mrs. Murat is admitted to a hospital, the hospital would submit its claim for emergency and inpatient care, which would be based on the diagnosis-related group (DRG) of her discharge diagnosis, to Medicare's Part A regional intermediary insurance company. The involved physicians and the ambulance service would submit their E&M-coded claims to Medicare's Part B regional insurance carrier. The intermediary and the carrier would pay their shares of these costs and, if Mrs. Murat had supplemental coverage, they would forward requests for payment of the balances to the state Medicaid program or to Mrs. Murat's medigap insurance company. Ultimately, CMS would reimburse the intermediary from the Medicare Part A Trust Fund and the carrier from the Medicare Part B Trust Fund.

Managed Care

If Mrs. Murat had joined the MA plan, the MA plan would pay for the ambulance, emergency, and physician services; in most cases, it would pay the hospital a prenegotiated lump sum or a per diem fee to cover all of her inpatient care. The amount of this lump sum would be determined by the DRG of her discharge diagnosis, in this case, stroke. If the admitting hospital had no contract with her MA plan, Mrs. Murat would probably be transferred to a hospital in the plan's provider network as soon as she was medically stable. Depending on the MA plan's benefit package, she might be responsible for co-payments and deductibles for some of these services.

Postacute Rehabilitation

After 4 days of stabilization, evaluation, and rehabilitation, Mrs. Murat is deemed stable enough for discharge from the acute-care hospital. She has improved somewhat, but she is still mildly hemiparetic and dysarthric, and she is apathetic and easily fatigued. Because her days in the hospital are fewer than the average number of hospital days associated with the DRG of her discharge diagnosis (ie, 5.9 days), CMS regards her "early" discharge as a "transfer." This permits CMS to reduce the amount it pays the hospital for her care. The consulting neurologist advises Mrs. Murat and her husband that her progress during the next few weeks will determine her potential for functional recovery. Mr. Murat asks the neurologist to recommend a rehabilitation facility for his wife.

Fee for Service

If Mrs. Murat could participate in rehabilitative therapy, Medicare Part A would pay for 20 days of postacute rehabilitation, in either a rehabilitation facility or a transitional (postacute) care unit of a nursing home. Mrs. Murat's admission to either type of postacute care unit would be reimbursed by Medicare under the Prospective Payment System (PPS). The Medicare PPS was implemented under the Balanced Budget Act of 1997 to control the increasing costs of subacute care. The PPS payment rates are adjusted for case mix and geographic variation in wages and cover all costs of providing covered skilled-nursing facility services (routine, ancillary, and capital-related costs). Per diem payments for each admission are case-mix adjusted using a resource utilization group system (RUGS) based on data from resident assessments and relative weights developed from staff time data. In addition, rates are based on geographic adjustment—the labor portion of the federal rates is adjusted for geographic variation in wages using the hospital wage index as well as an annual update; payment rates are increased each federal fiscal year using a skilled-nursing facility market basket index.

Mrs. Murat's RUGS category would determine the daily rate that Medicare Part A would pay the facility for the first 2 weeks of her care as long as she was demonstrating progress in rehabilitation. After 2 weeks, a nurse would reevaluate her status, update her plan of care, and adjust her RUGS category, thereby adjusting Medicare's payments to the facility for the next 2 weeks. Under this prospective payment system, the facility would be responsible not only for Mrs. Murat's nursing, rehabilitative, and social services but also for the costs of her medications, laboratory tests, and visits to an emergency department not resulting in admission to the hospital.

Using nursing-home rates, Medicare Part B would pay 80% of the allowed charges for the postacute medical care provided by Mrs. Murat's primary care provider. Any postacute care related to an inpatient surgical procedure would be the responsibility of the surgeon, who would receive a "global fee" to cover the surgery and all postoperative surgical care. The Murats would need to satisfy Medicare Part B's $140 annual deductible and then make 20% co-insurance payments for the provider's care. Their out-of-pocket expenses would be reduced or eliminated by any Medicare supplements in effect, such as Medicaid, medigap, or long-term care coverage.

Managed Care

If Mrs. Murat had joined the MA plan, her insurance coverage would include postacute rehabilitative care, probably at a nursing home in the MA plan's provider network rather than at a rehabilitation facility. Some nursing homes concentrate such high-acuity patients in transitional (or postacute) care units and provide them with coordinated rehabilitative (physical, occupational, and speech), social, and nursing services. Most homes, lacking such units, offer only custodial care supplemented by rehabilitative services as needed. The MA plan would also cover the primary care provider's postacute services, but the Murats may be responsible for a deductible and co-payments.

More than 3 million Americans have long-term care insurance policies, but these policies pay for <2% of all nursing-home care. The high premiums for these policies, combined with consumers' uncertainty about needing long-term care in the future and their doubts about the policies' ability to cover the costs of long-term care in the future, have limited the growth of the long-term care insurance sector. Many middle-aged Americans believe they will retain good health and independence into old age; they appear to be relying on a combination of good fortune, social insurance (ie, Medicaid), and their personal assets to see them through their later years.

Home-Health Care

During the first 10 days of rehabilitative therapy, Mrs. Murat regains her ability to speak, and her left arm becomes stronger. During the next 8 days, however, she makes few additional gains. After 18 days, she is still unable to walk, cook, bathe, or dress herself without help. Her lack of continued progress toward functional independence will probably make her ineligible for coverage of additional rehabilitative services in either the MA plan or the FFS Medicare program. The Murats will have to pay for any future physical therapy or occupational therapy on their own.

To obtain long-term care for Mrs. Murat's functional deficits, the Murats will need to choose between a home-health agency and a custodial nursing home. If Mrs. Murat returns home, neither the FFS Medicare program nor the MA plan will be likely to pay for a home-health aide unless she is homebound and requires the services of a registered nurse or rehabilitation therapist. Local community agencies, however, may be able to offer assistance. The Murats' choice of a home-health agency could be informed by comparisons of their local agencies' recent clinical performance, available at Home Health Compare (www.medicare.gov/HomeHealthCompare/search.aspx [accessed Oct 2013]).

Fee for Service

In the FFS environment, if Mrs. Murat were homebound and dependent on skilled professional services, then traditional Medicare Part A would pay any Medicare-certified home-health agency a fixed fee to provide her with the services and equipment necessary to treat her primary diagnosis. Medicare Part B would pay her primary care provider 80% of the allowed charges for house calls, office visits, and care plan oversight services. In addition, Medicare Part B would pay her provider for home-health certifications and recertifications. The Murats would be responsible for the Part B annual deductible ($140) and the 20% co-insurance payments, unless they had supplemental coverage through Medicaid, a medigap policy, or a long-term care policy. See also "Community-Based Care," p 166.

Table 5.4—Eligibility and Coverage for Nursing-Home Services

	Eligibility	Room and Board	Physician Services	Medication
Subacute	For Medicare beneficiaries requiring skilled-nursing care after a 3-day acute hospitalization	Part A	Part B or C	Part A or C
Nursing care	ADL/IADL needs	Medicaid, long-term care insurance, private payment	Part B or C	Part D

SOURCE: *Medicare & You Handbook* 2012. http://www.medicare.gov/publications/pubs/pdf/10050.pdf (accessed Oct 2013).

Managed Care

If Mrs. Murat's condition made her homebound and dependent on skilled professional services, her MA plan probably would pay a home-health agency a fixed fee to provide her with the services and equipment necessary to treat her primary diagnosis. The MA plan would also provide her with the services of a primary care provider.

Program for All-inclusive Care of the Elderly

If a healthcare organization in the area had contracted with CMS and the state Medicaid agency to create a Program for All-inclusive Care of the Elderly (PACE), it could provide community-based long-term care for "dually eligibles" (people eligible for both Medicare and Medicaid) whose disabilities qualified them for custodial care in a nursing home. (See also "Community-Based Care," p 166.) If she were eligible for Medicaid and she enrolled in PACE, Mrs. Murat would attend an adult day healthcare center several days each week and receive comprehensive outpatient, inpatient, acute, and long-term care from a salaried interdisciplinary team composed of a physician, a nurse practitioner or physician assistant, a nurse, a social worker, rehabilitation therapists, and other members of the PACE staff.

Nursing-Home Care

Three months after Mrs. Murat returns home, Mr. Murat, now 84 years old, suffers a myocardial infarction and is no longer able to care for his wife at home. Their daughter logs on to Nursing Home Compare (www.medicare.gov/NursingHomeCompare/search.aspx [accessed Oct 2013]) to shop for a nursing home. After comparing the local facilities' nurse-to-resident ratios, results of recent quality-of-care inspections, and rates of pressure ulcers and behavior problems, she arranges for her mother to enter a high-quality nursing home in her neighborhood, at least until Mr. Murat recovers.

Fee for Service

The FFS Medicare program would pay 80% of the allowed charges submitted by Mrs. Murat's primary care provider for visits to the nursing home. The Murats would be responsible for the Medicare Part B annual deductible ($155) and the 20% co-insurance payments. Medicare would not cover any of the nursing home's per diem charges. See Table 5.4.

Managed Care

If Mrs. Murat had joined the MA plan, one of the MA plan's providers would provide her primary care in the nursing home. Unless she was covered by Medicaid or a long-term care policy, however, she and her husband would be responsible for the nursing home's per diem charges for room, board, and other basic services (about $200/day). After "spending down" their savings at this rate, the Murats might become sufficiently impoverished to qualify, if they had not qualified previously, for Medicaid coverage. If the Murats owned their house, some states would put a lien on it to recover some of its payments to the nursing home when the house was eventually sold.

End-of-Life Care

After residing in the nursing home for 6 months, Mrs. Murat suffers a massive stroke that leaves her physiologically stable but in a persistent vegetative state. Her husband reports that she had always said she would not want to go on living in such a condition if there were little hope of recovery. Mrs. Murat is unable to swallow thin liquids, and her husband says she would not want to be fed through any sort of tube. Her provider says that, with oral feeding, she is likely to live for several weeks. Her husband agrees to enroll Mrs. Murat in a hospice program with the understanding that she will receive palliative care without life-prolonging interventions.

Optimally, a discussion of end-of-life care should occur before this change in condition. In fact, since the Patient Self-Determination Act (PSDA) was passed by the U.S. Congress in 1990, hospitals, nursing homes, home-health agencies, hospice providers, HMOs, and other healthcare institutions are required to provide information about advance healthcare directives to adult patients on their admission to the healthcare facility.

Despite this, clinicians can still provide discussions regarding advance directive planning as part of any physical examination, and healthcare facilities are required under PSDA to include this information on entry into their facilities.

After an end-of-life discussion, Mrs. Murat can be enrolled in hospice. Enrollment in hospice would require the traditional FFS Medicare program (Part A) to pay a Medicare-certified hospice program a daily fee that would cover all care for the terminal diagnosis, including home care, medications, equipment, respite, counseling, and social services even if Mrs. Murat had enrolled in (and remained in) the MA plan.

If she had remained in the FFS Medicare program, Part B would pay her primary care provider 80% of the allowed charges for home or office visits and care-plan oversight services. Mr. Murat would be responsible for the 20% co-insurance and small co-payments for outpatient prescription medications, as well as for respite care.

Changes in the Federal Financing of Health Care

The complex and evolving combinations of coverage and programs create difficult choices for older Americans and powerful incentives for the providers of their health care. The U.S. Congress and CMS continue to revise the Medicare program, making it important to stay alert for changes.

The Balanced Budget Act of 1997 (BBA 97)

BBA 97 required CMS to adjust capitation amounts according to enrollees' risk of requiring expensive health care. This results in higher capitation payments for high-risk enrollees and lower payments for low-risk enrollees. This risk-adjustment method is based on the diagnoses associated with beneficiaries' health care during a recent 12-month period. If a hospital or outpatient provider designates as a reason for providing a healthcare service a diagnosis included in CMS's list of "selected significant disease" groups, CMS increases the amount of its capitation payment for that beneficiary during the following year. For example, if a beneficiary received care for heart failure during the 12 months from July 2010 to June 2011, CMS would adjust its capitation payments for the beneficiary during 2012 to provide the extra funds typically needed to care for people who have heart failure. To make this risk-adjustment system cost-neutral, CMS offsets the diagnosis-related increases in capitation payments by reducing its capitation payments for beneficiaries who have not received care for diagnoses in the selected significant disease groups during this 12-month period.

BBA 97 provisions for improving the quality of health care for older Americans include the following:

- the Quality Improvement System for Managed Care (QISMC)
- the Healthcare Employers' Data Information System (HEDIS), which requires MA plans to monitor and report to CMS their rates of compliance with selected processes and outcomes of health care (eg, mammography and immunization against influenza)
- the Medicare Health Outcomes Survey, which requires MA plans to contract with third parties to survey a sample of their members and report information to CMS about their health status, functional ability, and satisfaction with their recent health care

CMS summarizes the information generated by all three systems and makes it available at the Medicare Personal Plan Finder to help older Americans make informed choices about Medicare's FFS program and its various managed care options.

Balanced Budget Revision Act of 1999

Within the first 18 months of the enactment of BBA 97, the quality of health care for older Americans began to erode, and the decreases in the payments to providers proved to be steeper than projected. For example, Medicare payments for home-health care decreased by 45% between 1997 and 1999. In response, Congress passed the Balanced Budget Revision Act at the end of 1999. This legislation restored some of the budget cuts made 2 years earlier, including $4.5 billion to MA plans.

Medicare Modernization Act of 2003

The Medicare Prescription Drug Improvement and Modernization Act of 2003 required dramatic changes in the nature and scope of the Medicare program, including the following:

- The creation of the Medicare Part D program covering prescription medications
- Subsidies for employers who continue to provide their retirees with insurance that covers prescription medications
- Elimination of coverage for prescription medications by Medicaid
- Competition between traditional FFS Medicare and MA plans
- Higher premiums for Medicare Part B to be paid by beneficiaries with higher incomes
- Expanded coverage for preventive services

- Increased reimbursement rates to providers and hospitals in rural areas

The American Recovery and Reinvestment Act

As part of the American Recovery and Reinvestment Act of 2009, funds were allocated with an aim to modernize the U.S. healthcare system through a new federal healthcare information technology leadership structure. Through incentive payments, providers are eligible for maximal payments of $63,750 for those primarily involved in Medicaid and of $44,000 for those in Medicare to adopt, implement, upgrade, or demonstrate certified electronic health record technology. To qualify, the electronic health record must meet or exceed the "Meaningful Use" standard, which includes clinical decision support, e-prescribing, exchange of health information, and quality reporting.

The Affordable Care Act of 2010

The areas of the ACA that affect older adults and those providing their care primarily is focused on increasing access and changing the current FFS reimbursement system. In the area of access, the ACA increases access to Medicare beneficiaries by eliminating out-of-pocket expenditures for many preventive screening studies, reducing the Medicare Part D coverage gap, and expanding Medicaid coverage, which will increase the number of dual-eligible older adults. The ACA also is moving to change reimbursement from the current FFS system to systems that improve outcomes such as those delivered through coordination of Medicare and Medicaid for the dual eligible, bundling reimbursement, and pay-for-performance. The new CMI is dedicated to developing and implementing these new payment systems, which are likely to be delivered through organizations such as Accountable Care Organizations and Patient Centered Medical Home models. In the end, the ACA should increase access for older adults while at the same time making changes to reimbursement, all in an effort to improve outcomes and lower costs.

The Future of Medicare and Medicaid

The CMI is evaluating many programs designed to improve the quality and outcomes of care for beneficiaries with chronic conditions. In most of these, CMS is paying provider and managed-care contractors capitated monthly fees for providing case-management or disease-management services to beneficiaries with specified chronic conditions, such as heart failure, diabetes mellitus, or other "special needs." Many of these are based on the principle of "pay for performance," which stipulates that CMS will pay the capitation fees only to the extent that the contractor attains pre-agreed on standards of performance, eg, performing certain diagnostic tests, reducing Medicare's overall FFS payments, and satisfying beneficiaries with the services they provide.

Another Pay-for-Performance program is the Physician Quality Reporting System (PQRS). Physicians and other healthcare providers who report data about the quality of their care when they submit their bills to their Medicare carriers may earn bonuses of up to 1.5% of their total Medicare payments. CMS also sends them personal reports comparing their PQRS data to that of peers nationwide. In 2012, there were 317 quality measures that could be reported, but some are specific to certain specialties. Additional information is available at www.cms.gov/PQRS/ (accessed Oct 2013).

The aging of the baby-boom generation, technology-driven increases in healthcare spending, and a decline in the number of workers per Medicare beneficiary will contribute to serious financial challenges for the Medicare program in the years ahead. Similarly, imminent sharp increases in the number of older Americans with serious disabilities will soon surpass states' ability to pay for their long-term care. To meet these challenges, the nation needs visionary geriatric providers able to develop and implement efficient and effective delivery systems to care for our older adults.

References

- Centers for Medicare and Medicaid Services, Department of Health and Human Services. *Medicare and You Handbook.* Available at: www.medicare.gov/Publications/Pubs/pdf/10050.pdf (accessed Oct 2013).
- Centers for Medicare and Medicaid Services. *2012 Medicare Costs.* http://www.medicare.gov/Publications/Pubs/pdf/11579.pdf (accessed Oct 2013)
- Kaiser Family Foundation. Medicare Spending and Financing. Available at: www.kff.org/medicare/upload/7305-07.pdf (accessed Oct 2013).
- Kaiser Family Foundation. *Medicaid Benefits.* Available at: http://medicaidbenefits.kff.org/index.jsp?CFID=95532007&CFTOKEN=19095903&jsessionid=60309405f8deeedf36bf72793674d57f3e45 (accessed Oct 2013).
- Q1Group LLC. *2012 Medicare Part D Outlook. Medicare Part D Comparison (2006–2013)* www.q1medicare.com/PartD-The-2013-Medicare-Part-D-Outlook.php. (accessed Oct 2013).
- Stefanacci RG. Improving the care of "dual eligibles"—what's ahead. *Clin Geriatr.* 2011;19(9):28–32.

CHAPTER 6—ASSESSMENT

KEY POINTS

- Geriatric assessment is a multifaceted approach to the care of older adults, with the goal of promoting wellness and independent function.
- Assessment of function includes the physical, cognitive, psychologic, and social domains.
- Time-efficient, valid tools are available for use in a variety of settings to evaluate the status of older adults in all these domains.
- Time tends to be a less important element than the skills of the clinician in successful communication with older adults.

Geriatric assessment is a multifaceted approach to the care of older adults, with the goal of promoting wellness and independent function. Function is defined broadly to encompass the physical, cognitive, psychologic, and social domains. The scope of the assessment of any individual domain depends on the goals of care, the site of care, the patient's level of frailty, time constraints, and the availability of a multidisciplinary team. The essential aspects of geriatric assessment should be performed routinely in all sites of care, including the ambulatory setting, the emergency department, the hospital, the nursing home, and the home. Whenever possible, assessments should be performance based. An informant, ideally a caregiver or family member who lives with the patient, is often required to provide or to verify pertinent historical information about the older adult's day-to-day functioning. *Try This*, a publication of the Hartford Institute for Geriatric Nursing, covers a series of geriatric assessment tools and describes their use. Examples include The Geriatric Depression Scale, Predicting Pressure Ulcer Risk, the Geriatric Oral Health Assessment Index, and Decision Making and Dementia. Each of the more than 40 *Try This* issues can be downloaded from www.ConsultGeriRN.org.

For comprehensive geriatric assessment, see "Outpatient Care Systems," p 173; and "Hospital Care," p 130.

THE ROUTINE OFFICE VISIT

Incorporating geriatric assessment into routine office practice requires use of efficient strategies. One such strategy entails rapid screening of targeted areas (Table 6.1), followed by comprehensive assessment in areas of concern. Many of the initial screens can be completed by trained office staff; some can be completed by the patients themselves while seated in the waiting area or at home before the visit. The use of a "rolling" assessment, which targets at least one area for screening during each office visit, should be considered. Finally, in the absence of specific target symptoms, parts of the routine examination, such as auscultation of the chest and palpation of the abdomen, can be replaced by aspects of geriatric assessment, such as observation of gait, balance, and transfers. Office-based screening for common geriatric conditions, however, has not been shown to improve patient outcomes (SOE=A).

PATIENT-CLINICIAN COMMUNICATION

Because of the demands of a busy clinical practice, the time available for office visits is often constrained. Time tends to be less important, however, than the skills of the clinician in successful communication. For several simple strategies that can be used to enhance communication, see Table 6.2. See also the table on communication in "Hearing Impairment," p 192. To accommodate the high prevalence of sensory deficits among older adults, particular attention should be given to the environment of the examination room. The use of simple, inexpensive amplification devices with lightweight earphones can be especially effective, even for those with severe hearing impairment. During the course of the interview, the clinician should go beyond the customary clinical inquiries by asking open-ended questions such as, "What would you like me to do for you?" Finding out what the patient wants can be a prime mechanism for solving potential problems, generating trust, and improving mutual satisfaction in the patient-clinician relationship. The National Institute on Aging has developed a booklet that offers practical strategies to facilitate communication with older patients. This invaluable resource is available at http://www.nia.nih.gov/health/publication/talking-your-older-patient (accessed Oct 2013).

Effective communication can be compromised by low health literacy—the diminished ability to obtain, process, and understand basic health information and services needed to make appropriate health decisions. Increasing evidence suggests that low health literacy, which has been documented in about one of every four community-living older adults, has deleterious effects on health and survival, at least in part because of deficiencies in self-management skills, poor adherence, and inadequate use of preventive services (SOE=A). Helpful information on low health literacy, including strategies to enhance communication, is available at http://www.reynolds.med.arizona.edu/html/ElderCare.html (accessed Oct 2013).

Table 6.1—Rapid Screening Followed by Assessment and Management in Key Domains

Domain	Rapid Screen	Assessment and Management
Functional status	Answers "Yes" to one or more of the following: Because of a health or physical problem, do you need help to: • shop? • do light housework? • walk across a room? • take a bath or shower? • manage the household finances?	Assess all other ADLs listed in Table 6.3. Evaluate cognitive function and mobility using performance-based tests. Assess social support. Consider use of adaptive equipment.
Mobility	"Timed Up and Go" test: unable to complete in <20 sec	Treat underlying musculoskeletal or neurologic disorder. Refer to physical therapy.
Nutrition	Unintentional weight loss of ≥5% in prior 6 months (*or* BMI <20 kg/m^2)	See "Malnutrition," p 209.
Vision	If unable to read a newspaper headline and sentence while wearing corrective lenses, test each eye with Snellen chart; unable to read greater than 20/40	See "Visual Impairment," p 183.
Hearing	Acknowledges hearing loss when questioned *or* unable to perceive a letter/number combination whispered at a distance of 2 feet	See "Hearing Impairment," p 192.
Cognitive function	3-item recall: unable to remember all 3 items after 1 min	Administer Folstein Mini–Mental State Examination or a nonproprietary instrument such as the Montreal Cognitive Assessment.
Depression	Answers "Yes" to either of the following: In the past month, have you often been bothered by: • feeling down, depressed, or hopeless? • having little interest or pleasure in doing things?	Administer 15-item Geriatric Depression Scale or 9-item Patient Health Questionnaire (see "Depression and Other Mood Disorders," p 308).

Table 6.2—Effective Strategies to Enhance Communication

- Use a well-lit room and avoid backlighting.
- Minimize extraneous noise and interruptions.
- Introduce yourself to establish a friendly relationship.
- Face the patient directly, sitting at eye level.
- Address the patient, using his or her last name.
- Speak slowly.
- Inquire about hearing deficits; raise the volume and lower the tone of your voice accordingly.
- If necessary, write questions in large print.
- Allow sufficient time for the patient to answer.
- Touch the patient gently on the hand, arm, or shoulder during the conversation.
- Provide patient education materials that are appropriate for individuals with low health literacy.

PHYSICAL ASSESSMENT

The importance of a complete, appropriately detailed physical examination cannot be overstated. Many older adults cannot see well enough to report signs of disease, or have cognitive impairment that prevents them from being able to accurately report symptoms. The clinician cannot assume that "no news is good news" in the care of older adults.

Functional Status

Functional status refers to the person's ability to perform tasks that are required for living. These tasks, usually referred to as activities of daily living (ADLs), are listed in Table 6.3. When assessing

Table 6.3—Activities of Daily Living

Self-care	
Bathing	Toileting
Dressing	Grooming
Transferring from bed to chair	Feeding oneself
Instrumental	
Using the telephone	Doing laundry
Preparing meals	Doing housework
Managing household finances	Shopping
Taking medications	Managing transportation
Mobility	
Walking from room to room	
Climbing a flight of stairs	
Walking outside one's home	

function, ask whether the patient is independent or requires the help of another person to complete the tasks. Bathing is typically the self-care ADL with the highest prevalence of disability, and disability in bathing is often the reason why older adults receive home aide services (SOE=A). Disability in ADLs may occur when there is a gap or mismatch between personal capabilities (eg, balance, muscle strength, cognition) and environmental demands. For example, an older adult with quadriceps weakness might require personal assistance to stand from a deeply cushioned, low-lying chair but have no difficulty standing from a hard-back kitchen chair. To identify patients with "preclinical" disability, ie, those who do not yet require personal assistance but who are at risk of becoming disabled, ask about perceived difficulty with the tasks and whether the patient has changed the way he or she completes the task because of a health-related problem or condition (SOE=A). Assess the use of any assistive devices, such as a cane or walker, as well as duration and circumstances of use.

Outside of a rehabilitation setting, performance-based testing of most of the self-care and instrumental ADLs is not practical. Hence, performance-based testing of functional status focuses primarily on mobility, including transfers, gait, and balance. Ask the patient to stand from the seated position in a hard-backed chair while keeping his or her arms folded. Inability to complete this task suggests leg (hip flexor/extensor and knee flexor/extensor) weakness and is highly predictive of future disability (SOE=A). Once the patient is standing, observe him or her walking back and forth over a short distance, ideally with the usual walking aid. Abnormalities of gait include path deviation; diminished step height or length, or both; trips, slips, or near falls; and difficulty with turning. The tasks of rising from the chair, walking 10 feet (3 meters), turning around and returning to the chair, turning, and then sitting back down in the chair make up the "Timed Up and Go" test. Individuals who can complete this sequence of maneuvers in <10 sec have intact mobility; those who take ≥20 sec clearly require further evaluation (SOE=B).

If time permits completion of only one performance test, measure gait speed, which is the single strongest predictor of future disability and death (SOE=A). A gait speed of 0.8 meters/sec allows for independent community ambulation; a speed of 0.6 meters/sec allows for community activity without use of a wheelchair. These norms indicate that patients who can walk 50 feet in an office hallway in ≤20 sec should be able to walk independently in normal activities. See "Gait Impairment," p 228.

Balance can be tested progressively by asking the patient to stand first with his or her feet side by side, then in semitandem position, and finally in tandem position. Difficulty with balance in these positions predicts an increased risk of falling (SOE=A). Although standardized instruments, such as the Performance-Oriented Mobility Assessment, can be used to quantify impairments in gait and balance, a qualitative assessment is usually sufficient to make recommendations about the need for an assistive device, such as a cane or walker. When assessing gait and balance, particularly in older women, clinicians should observe for the use of proper footwear, ie, flat, hard-soled shoes.

Clinicians can also glean useful functional information by observing older adults as they complete simple tasks such as undressing or dressing, picking up a pen and writing a sentence, touching the back of the head with both hands, and climbing up and down from an examination table.

Assessing life space offers a complementary strategy for distinguishing among different levels of mobility, not only in community-living older adults but also in nursing-home patients. Life space can be viewed rather simply as a series of concentric areas radiating from the room where a person sleeps to more distant locations, such as beyond one's town for community-living older adults or to outside the facility for nursing-home patients. The frequency of movement to various locations and the need for assistance are also assessed by formal life space instruments. For older adults with low life space, the ability to get in and out of a bed should be assessed.

Nutrition

Poor nutrition in older adults can reflect concurrent medical illness, depression, dementia, inability to shop or cook, inability to feed oneself, or financial hardship. Aside from visual inspection for signs of malnutrition, older adults should have their weight and height measured routinely. Unintentional weight loss of ≥5% in 6 months or a low BMI (ie, kg/m^2 <20) suggests poor nutrition and requires further evaluation (SOE=A). See "Malnutrition," p 209.

Vision and Hearing

Although visual impairment from cataracts, glaucoma, macular degeneration, and abnormalities of accommodation usually worsens with age, older adults are often unaware of their visual deficits. Asking about difficulty with driving, watching television, or reading may uncover a problem with vision. As a brief performance-based screen, an older adult can be asked to read (using corrective lenses, if applicable) a short passage from a newspaper or magazine (SOE=C). Significant visual impairment can be confirmed through the use of a Snellen chart or Jaeger card; visual acuity worse than 20/40 is the standard criteria for visual impairment. See "Visual Impairment," p 183.

The high prevalence of hearing loss among older adults and its association with depression, dissatisfaction with life, and withdrawal from social activities make it an important target for assessment. Hearing loss is usually bilateral and in the high-frequency range. In the absence of cerumen impaction, older adults who acknowledge hearing loss when questioned should be referred directly for formal audiometric testing. If hearing loss is denied, further screening with the whisper-voice test is indicated (SOE=B). Inability to perceive a letter/number combination whispered at a distance of 2 feet is considered abnormal and warrants a discussion about referral for formal audiometric testing. See "Hearing Impairment," p 192.

Medication Assessment

Time should be dedicated at each office visit to review both prescribed and OTC medications. Polypharmacy, which is common in older adults, can be the cause of many adverse reactions and contribute to the onset of new symptoms. Suspected treatment failure may be related to medication nonadherence. Exploring issues around nonadherence is important for the clinician to discern whether the cause is financially related, fear of being over-medicated, or lack of understanding of the need for a new medication regimen.

Cognitive Assessment

The prevalence of dementia doubles every 5 years after the age of 65 and approaches 40%–50% at age 90. Most patients with dementia do not complain of memory loss or volunteer symptoms of cognitive impairment unless specifically questioned. Older adults with cognitive impairment, even in the absence of dementia, are at increased risk of accidents, delirium, medical nonadherence, and disability. Therefore, an important feature of every assessment of an older adult, especially those ≥75 years old, is a brief cognitive screen (SOE=C). Before cognitive testing, clinicians should determine the patient's native language and be aware of any hearing deficits.

Because short-term memory loss is typically the first sign of dementia, the best single screening question is recall of three words after 1 min. Anything other than perfect recall should lead to further testing. For many years, the most commonly used instrument for formal testing of cognition has been the Folstein Mini–Mental State Examination (MMSE), which assesses orientation, registration and recall, attention and calculation, language, and visual-spatial skills. Although scores on the MMSE need to be interpreted in the context of educational attainment, race, and age, scores <24 generally warrant further evaluation for possible dementia.

An often overlooked area of cognition, which is essential for proper goal-directed behaviors, is executive function. As a quick screen, ask the patient to name as many four-legged animals as possible in 1 min. Fewer than 8 to 10 animals or repetition of the same animals is abnormal and suggests the need for further evaluation. The clock-drawing test is valuable because it assesses executive control and visual-spatial skills, two domains of cognition that are not tested or incompletely tested by the MMSE. In the clock-drawing test, the patient is asked to draw the face of a clock and to place the hands correctly to indicate 2:50 or 11:10. The clock-drawing test is combined with the three-item recall in the Mini-Cog Assessment Instrument for Dementia, a validated screening test that takes about 3 min to administer. The Mini-Cog has an advantage over the MMSE of being relatively uninfluenced by level of education or language differences. Because the MMSE is now proprietary and has several limitations, other validated tools are being used more commonly to assess cognition, including the Montreal Cognitive Assessment (MoCA) and Saint Louis University Mental Status Examination (SLUMS). See also "Dementia," p 256.

Psychologic Assessment

Although the prevalence of major depressive disorder among community-dwelling older adults is only about 1%–2%, the rate is much higher—up to 10%—in those seen in primary care settings. A large number of older adults, moreover, suffer from significant symptoms of depression below the severity threshold of major depression as defined by the *Diagnostic and Statistical Manual of Mental Disorders, 4th Edition, Text Revision.* These subthreshold depressive symptoms, which often include somatic complaints such as poor sleep and fatigue, increase the risk of physical disability and slower recovery after an acute disabling event (SOE=A). They are also associated with a significant increase in the cost of medical services, even after accounting for the severity of chronic medical illness (SOE=A). Hence, clinicians should have a high index of suspicion for depressive symptoms and a low threshold for treatment. The best single question to ask is, "Do you often feel sad or depressed?" An affirmative response warrants further evaluation of other depressive symptoms, perhaps through the use of a standardized instrument such as the 15-item Geriatric Depression Scale (SOE=B). The PHQ-2 is a very short, validated instrument for depression screening as well. See "Depression and Other Mood Disorders," p 308.

Anxiety and worries are also important symptoms in older adults and are often a manifestation of an underlying depressive disorder. Finally, because older adults are particularly likely to experience the loss of a loved one, special efforts should be made to recognize and manage the consequences of bereavement. See "Depression and Other Mood Disorders," p 308.

SOCIAL ASSESSMENT

A social assessment consists of several elements, including ethnic, spiritual, and cultural background; the availability of a personal support system; the need for a caregiver, his or her role, and presence of caregiver burden; the safety of the home environment; the patient's economic well-being; the possibility of mistreatment of the older adult; and the individual's advance directives. Although a comprehensive social assessment may not be feasible in a busy office practice, clinicians caring for older adults should be mindful of these aspects of their patient's lives. Clinicians can uncover important clues to unmet needs by inquiring about the availability of help in case of an emergency. For frail older adults, particularly those who lack social support, referral to a visiting nurse or physical therapist may be helpful in assessing home safety and level of personal risk. See "Psychosocial Issues," p 18; "Cultural Aspects of Care," p 58; and "Mistreatment of Older Adults," p 97.

QUALITY OF LIFE

During the past two decades, *quality of life* has been embraced as a convenient "catch phrase" to denote important patient outcomes other than death and traditional physiologic measures of morbidity. Although a gold standard does not exist, most instruments designed to measure quality of life include various aspects of physical, cognitive, psychologic, and social function. Perhaps the most commonly used instrument is the Short Form-36 Health Survey (SF-36), which includes 36 items organized into 8 domains: physical function, role limitations due to physical health, role limitations due to emotional health, bodily pain, social functioning, mental health, vitality, and general health perceptions. The SF-36 has been tested extensively among community-living adults and hospitalized patients, but it may not be suitable for use among the oldest-old group, especially those who are frail, because of floor effects and insensitivity to clinically important changes in health status.

When assessing quality of life, ask about patient preferences regarding medical care and goals of care. Goals can be multiple, diverse, and sometimes conflicting. Older adults exhibit striking heterogeneity with respect to physiologic function, health status, belief systems, cultural and ethnic backgrounds, values, and personal preferences. The successful management of chronic conditions, such as diabetes mellitus, arthritis, and heart failure, requires that patients, families, and clinicians work collaboratively to define the specific problems, to elicit personal preferences, and to establish the goals of care. Patients' cultural and ethnic heritages have an important role in their understanding of their illness, its meaning in their lives, and their response to it. It is crucial, therefore, for the clinician to have an appreciation of that heritage and the role it plays in the patient's understanding of health and illness. See "Cultural Aspects of Care," p 58. Treatment plans that include patient preferences enhance adherence and increase satisfaction, and they have the potential to improve patient outcomes.

ASSESSING THE OLDER DRIVER

Evaluating the older driver is a difficult challenge. The automobile is the most important—and often the only—source of transportation for older adults. Yet a variety of age-related changes, chronic conditions, and medications place the older adult at risk of automobile accidents. Although the absolute number of crashes involving older drivers is low, the number of crashes per mile driven and the likelihood of serious injury or death are higher than for any age group other than those aged 16–24 years old.

The vast majority of older adults make prudent adjustments in their driving behaviors by avoiding rush hour or congested thoroughfares or by not driving at night or during adverse weather conditions. Nonetheless, impaired older adults who continue to drive are a hazard not only to themselves but also to other drivers, passengers, and pedestrians. Pertinent risk factors for automobile accidents include poor visual acuity (less than 20/40) and contrast sensitivity; dementia, particularly deficits in visual-spatial skills and visual attention; impaired neck and trunk rotation; and poor motor coordination and speed of movement (SOE=A). Alcohol and medications that adversely affect alertness, such as narcotics, benzodiazepines, antihistamines, antidepressants, antipsychotics, sedatives, and muscle relaxants, can impair driving skills and increase crash risk. Hence, caution is warranted when starting or adjusting the dosage of these medications, and patients should be warned about potential adverse effects on driving safety.

Any report of an accident or moving violation should trigger an assessment of an older adult's driving

DISABILITY

ability. Safety concerns should be discussed honestly with the older driver, and ideally with a partner or other family member as well, particularly when the older driver lacks insight into his or her driving limitations. Alternative modes of transportation should be considered. Recommendations to stop driving, however, should not be proffered lightly, because driving cessation can lead to a decreased activity level and increased depressive symptoms (SOE=B). Referral for a formal driving evaluation by a skilled occupational therapist may be helpful in confirming unsafe driving behaviors, or perhaps in suggesting interventions such as adaptive equipment to correct for specific physical disabilities. In the interest of public safety, clinicians should know their state's law on reporting impaired drivers. In most states, clinicians are encouraged, and in some states mandated, to report their concerns to the licensing agency. See also driving in "Legal and Ethical Issues," p 26. To assist clinicians caring for older drivers, two excellent resources have been developed by the American Medical Association in cooperation with the National Highway Traffic Safety Administration: *The Physician's Guide to Assessing and Counseling Older Drivers* and *Medical Fitness to Drive: Is Your Patient at Risk?*, a Web-based educational course.

ACUTE FUNCTIONAL DECLINE

An acute decline in functional status is usually precipitated by an illness or injury. Most new disability episodes are attributable to illnesses or injuries leading to hospitalization (SOE=A). The most severe forms of disability commonly arise from a relatively small number of acute conditions, including hip fracture, stroke, heart failure, and pneumonia. The adverse functional consequences of hospitalization reflect not only the disabling effects of these and other serious conditions but also the hazards of immobility and hospital-acquired complications. Up to 20% of new disability episodes are attributable to less serious illnesses or injuries that lead to restriction of activity but not to hospitalization. These restrictions are usually caused by several concurrent health-related problems, although a fall or injury is most likely to result in disability. Among older adults who are physically frail, about a third of new disability episodes occur insidiously, ie, in the absence of a discernable illness or injury. These episodes may be attributable to relatively subtle perturbations in physiologic status or to the loss of compensatory strategies among highly vulnerable older adults with relatively little reserve capacity. Contrary to conventional wisdom, most older adults who become newly disabled recover independent function within 6 months (SOE=A). However, these individuals are at high risk of subsequent disability.

REFERENCES

- Carr DB, Ott BR. The older adult driver with cognitive impairment: "It's a very frustrating life". *JAMA*. 2010;303(16):1632–1641.
- Ellis G, Whitehead MA, O'Neill D, et al. Comprehensive geriatric assessment for older adults admitted to hospital. *Cochrane Database Syst Rev*. 2011 July 6;(7): CD006211.
- Kresevic DM. Assessment of physical function. In: Boltz M, Capezuti E, Fulmer T, et al. *Evidence-Based Geriatric Nursing Protocols for Best Practice*. 4th ed. New York: Springer Publishing Company; 2012: 89–104.
- Studenski S, Perera S, Patel K, et al. Gait speed and survival in older adults. *JAMA*. 2011;305(1):50–58.

CHAPTER 7—MULTIMORBIDITY

KEY POINTS

- Over 50% of older adults have three or more chronic diseases, referred to as "multimorbidity."
- Multimorbidity is associated with increased rates of death, disability, adverse effects, institutionalization, use of healthcare resources, and decreased quality of life.
- Older adults with multimorbidity are heterogeneous in terms of illness severity, functional status, prognosis, personal priorities, and risk of adverse events, necessitating more flexible approaches to care in this population.

One of the greatest challenges in geriatrics is providing optimal care for older adults with multiple chronic conditions, or "multimorbidity." Over 50% of older adults have three or more chronic diseases, with distinctive cumulative effects for each individual.

Multimorbidity is associated with increased rates of death, disability, adverse effects, institutionalization, use of healthcare resources, and decreased quality of life. Comprehensive strategies and interventions for common syndromes and organization of care in this population show promise, but the best clinical management approaches remain unclear.

Most clinical practice guidelines (CPGs) focus on the management of a single disease, but CPG-based care may be cumulatively impractical, irrelevant, or even harmful for individuals with multimorbidity. CPG deficiencies are not based solely on shortcomings of guideline development and implementation. Older adults with multimorbidity are regularly excluded or under-represented in trials and observational studies. This translates to less focus on older adults in meta-analyses and systematic reviews and guidelines, and affects appropriate interpretation of results.

Clinical management is defined here as representing all types of care for chronic conditions, including pharmacologic and nonpharmacologic treatment and interventions (eg, referral to specialists, physical and occupational therapy, use of pacemakers), screening, prevention, diagnostic tests, follow-up, and advanced illness care. Currently, the best strategies for prioritizing specific aspects of this management spectrum in a particular older adult with multimorbidity are unknown.

Clinicians need a management approach that will consider the issues particular to each individual, including the often limited available evidence, interactions among conditions or treatments, the patient's own preferences and goals, prognosis, geriatric issues and syndromes, and the feasibility of each management decision and its implementation.

Older adults with multimorbidity are heterogeneous in terms of illness severity, functional status, prognosis, personal priorities, and risk of adverse events, even when diagnosed with the same pattern of conditions. Not only the individuals themselves but also their treatment options will differ, necessitating more flexible approaches to care in this population.

APPROACH TO THE OLDER ADULT WITH MULTIMORBIDITY

Clinicians treating older adults with multimorbidity face many challenges, including complex clinical management decisions, inadequate evidence, and time constraints and reimbursement structures that hinder the provision of efficient quality care. For a useful approach for optimal management of these individuals, see Figure 7.1.

Five domains are relevant to the care of older adults with multimorbidity:

1. Patient preferences
2. Interpreting the evidence
3. Prognosis
4. Clinical feasibility
5. Optimizing therapies and care plans

The five domains apply at various steps, which can be taken in other sequences with equal validity, because approaches for addressing this population have not been compared. For example, patient preferences are often best elicited in the context of the individual's prognosis.

GUIDING PRINCIPLES

The guiding principles below are intended to help guide the clinician in management of older adults with multimorbidity to improve health care and outcomes in this population. Patients should be evaluated, and care plans should be designed and implemented according to the individual needs of each patient. However, studies have not rigorously evaluated all approaches related to these guiding principles. Therefore, just as failure to strictly adhere to CPG for single diseases should not imply medical liability or malpractice, nor should failure to adopt these principles.

Patient Preferences Domain

The guiding principle of this domain is to elicit and incorporate patient preferences into medical decision-making for older adults with multimorbidity.

Care provided in accordance with CPGs may not adequately address patients' preferences, a key aspect of medical decision-making. Older adults with multimorbidity should be presented the opportunity to evaluate choices and prioritize their preferences for care, within personal and cultural contexts.

Interpreting the Evidence Domain

The guiding principle of this domain is to recognize the limitations of the evidence base, and to interpret and apply the medical literature specifically to older adults with multimorbidity.

CPGs evaluate the best current evidence from many types of studies, but most focus on only one or two clinical conditions and address comorbidities in limited ways, if at all. Different conditions coexisting within the same patient may interact, however, changing the risks associated with each condition and its treatments. Consequently, determining whether the individual will benefit from a particular treatment is complicated.

Thoughtful standardized approaches for the interpretation of the medical literature ("evidence-based medicine") provide tools for clinicians to evaluate the evidence base. However, one element of such methodologies that must not be neglected is whether the information applies to the individual under consideration. Clinicians should be aware that significant evidence gaps exist concerning condition and treatment interactions, particularly in older adults with multimorbidity.

Prognosis Domain

The guiding principle of this domain is to frame clinical management decisions within the context of risks, burdens, benefits, and prognosis (eg, remaining life expectancy, functional status, quality of life) for older adults with multimorbidity.

Clinical management decisions for this population necessitate the evaluation of prognosis to inform patient preferences and to adequately assess risks, burdens, and benefits, including remaining life expectancy, functional disability, and quality of life. Clinicians also need to evaluate risks for specific conditions (eg, GI hemorrhage with aspirin use for primary prevention of cardiovascular disease in men) as prognosis is considered.

The prognosis for each patient informs, but does not dictate, clinical management decisions within the context of his or her preferences. As stated above, the time horizon to benefit for a treatment may be longer than the individual's projected life span, raising the risk of polypharmacy and drug-drug and drug-disease interactions, particularly in older adults with multimorbidity. Screening tests (eg, colonoscopy) may also be nonbeneficial or even harmful if the time horizon to benefit exceeds remaining life expectancy, especially because associated harms and burdens increase with age and comorbidity.

A discussion about prognosis can serve as an introduction to difficult conversations, facilitating decision-making and advance care planning, while addressing patient preferences, treatment rationales, and therapy prioritization. For example, the prognosis of a cancer patient with a solid tumor and poor performance status usually worsens with chemotherapy. At the same time, progression through

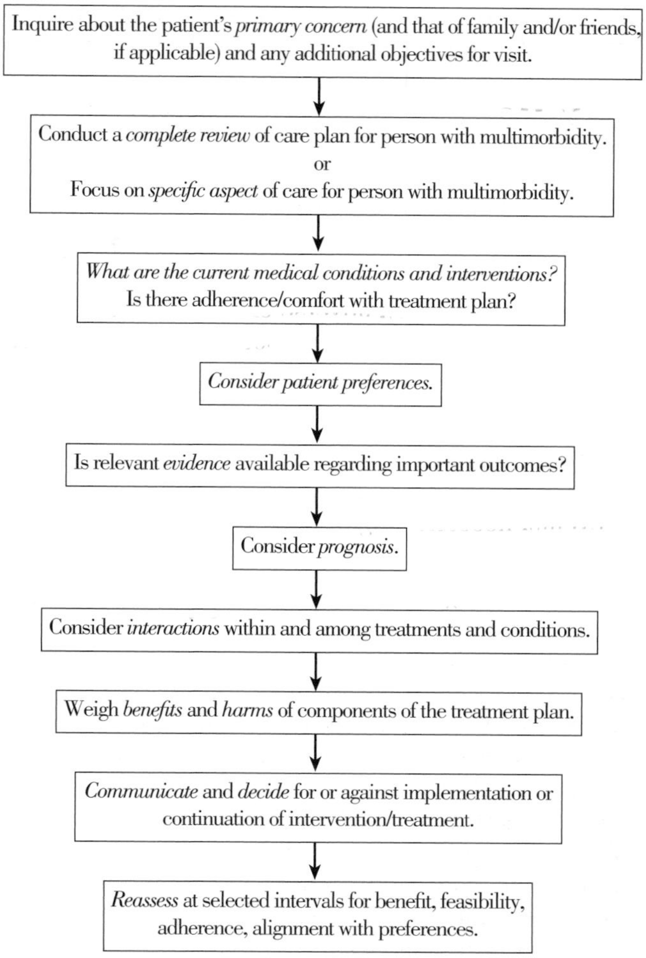

Figure 7.1—Approach to the Evaluation and Management of the Older Adult with Multimorbidity

SOURCE: American Geriatrics Society Expert Panel on the Care of Older Adults with Multimorbidity. Guiding Principles for the Care of Older Adults with Multimorbidity: An Approach for Clinicians. *J Am Geriatr Soc.* 2012;60(10):E1–E25.

first- and second-line therapies predicts a low likelihood of treatment response. A discussion about hospice, however, offers patients and families options of improved home support, better quality of life, and possibly prolonged survival.

Clinical Feasibility Domain

The guiding principle of this domain is to consider treatment complexity and feasibility when making clinical management decisions for older adults with multimorbidity.

Some guideline organizations, such as the Grading of Recommendations Assessment, Development and Evaluation working group (GRADE), now encourage routine consideration of burden when making recommendations for clinical management. The definition of these concepts, however, has been inconsistent.

A framework has been described by Nolan et al to break down treatment complexity and burden into individual components such as steps in the task, number of choices, duration of execution, informed consent, and patterns of intervening distracting tasks (which may be useful when attempting to simplify individual components of care plans). The Medication Regimen Complexity Index also identifies factors that need to be considered when assessing medication regimen complexity.

The more complex a treatment regimen, the higher the risk of nonadherence, adverse reactions, decreased quality of life, increased economic burden, and increased strain and depression among caregivers. Medication adherence also changes according to situational factors and perceptions of need, cost, or current symptoms.

Education and assessments must be ongoing, multifaceted, and individualized, and delivered via a variety of methods and settings, because patients generally do not recall discussion with clinicians. Cognitive impairment frequently impacts on adherence.

Optimizing Therapies and Care Plans Domain

The guiding principle of this domain is to use strategies for choosing therapies that optimize benefit, minimize harm, and enhance quality of life.

Older adults with multimorbidity are at risk of polypharmacy, suboptimal medication use, and potential harms from various interventions. Treatments and interventions must be prioritized to optimize adherence to the most essential pharmacologic and nonpharmacologic therapies, minimize risk exposure, and maximize benefit. Polypharmacy is associated with therapeutic omissions, reduced benefit from otherwise beneficial medications, and even harm in this population. Nonpharmacologic interventions (eg, implantable cardiac electronic devices) may prove more burdensome than beneficial if inconsistent with patient preferences.

Older adults with multimorbidity take more medications and have greater likelihood of adverse drug reactions, exacerbated by age-related changes in pharmacokinetics and pharmacodynamics. Reducing the number of medications, particularly high-risk medications, can lower the risk of adverse drug reactions.

CONTROVERSIES AND CHALLENGES

Implementing this patient-centered approach in older patients with multimorbidity is challenging, especially with the dynamic health status of such individuals and use of multiple clinicians and settings. Even with appropriate decision tools and good communication, the need to make multiple simultaneous decisions makes it difficult to explain information and uncertainties about benefits and harms. This prevents individuals, families, and friends from fully participating in treatment decisions, communicating preferences, and prioritizing outcomes. Satisfactory evidence for clinical management of individuals with multimorbidity is scarce, as are reasonable prognostic measures; different prognostic tools often yield contrasting results for the same patient. Treatments meant to improve one outcome (eg, survival) may worsen another (eg, function).

Many clinical management regimens are also simply too complex to be feasible in this population, but as clinicians attempt to reduce polypharmacy and unnecessary interventions, they may fear liability regarding underuse of therapies. Clinicians therefore may benefit greatly from the strategies put forth in this chapter. Finally, such patient-centered approaches may simply be too time-consuming for the already overwhelmed clinician within the current reimbursement structure and without an effective interdisciplinary team and require continued efforts to address these resource issues.

REFERENCES

- American Geriatrics Society Expert Panel on the Care of Older Adults with Multimorbidity. Guiding Principles for the Care of Older Adults with Multimorbidity: An Approach for Clinicians. *J Am Geriatr Soc*. 2012;60(10):E1–E25.

- American Geriatrics Society Expert Panel on the Care of Older Adults with Multimorbidity. Patient-Centered Care for Older Adults with Multiple Chronic Conditions: A Stepwise Approach from the American Geriatrics Society. *J Am Geriatr Soc.* 2012;60(10):1957–1968.
- Boyd CM, Darer J, Boult C, et al. Clinical practice guidelines and quality of care for older patients with multiple comorbid diseases: Implications for pay for performance. *JAMA.* 2005;294(6):716–724.
- Nolan TW. System changes to improve patient safety. *BMJ.* 2000;320:771–773.
- Yourman LC, Lee SJ, Schonberg MA, et al. Prognostic indices for older adults: A systematic review. *JAMA.* 2012:307(2):182–192.

Chapters

CHAPTER 8—CULTURAL ASPECTS OF CARE

KEY POINTS

- Clinicians should develop a nuanced understanding of the role that culture and religious beliefs play in promoting the health of older adults.
- Clinicians should remain alert to the differences among individual patients from a given culture or religious tradition and guard against stereotyping on the basis of ethnic, cultural, or religious affiliation.
- Communication and clinical care are enhanced when the patient and healthcare provider make an effort to simplify medical messages and negotiate a common understanding of causation, diagnosis, and treatment, while maintaining respect for the beliefs and constructs of both individuals.

As the cultural and religious diversity of older Americans continues to grow, it is increasingly important for clinicians to develop an approach to working with older adults from a broad range of cultural and religious groups. It is expected that by 2050, one out of three older Americans will be of "minority" status. In addition, it is currently estimated that more than one in three Americans has low health literacy.

There is no single or standard definition of cultural competence. Most definitions emphasize a careful coordination of individual behavior, organizational policy, and system design to facilitate mutually respectful and effective cross-cultural and interfaith interactions. Cultural competence combines attitudes, knowledge base, acquired skills, and behavior. It is an approach, not a technique or form of "political correctness." Ideally, it is a nuanced understanding of the determining role that culture plays in all of our lives and of the impact culture has on every healthcare encounter, for both the clinician and the patient.

This chapter aims to assist clinicians in developing and improving their communication skills and enhancing their awareness during cross-cultural and interfaith patient encounters. Readers are also referred to the *Doorway Thoughts* series, published by the American Geriatrics Society (see the annotated references), which demonstrate how the general approaches outlined here in each topic relate to working with patients from a variety of cultural or religious groups. It is very important to keep in mind when using the *Doorway Thoughts* series that, although the information offered in each chapter is accurate *in general,* the beliefs, traditions, customs, and preferences of individuals in all cultural and religious groups vary widely. Clinicians should never assume that any person's cultural or religious background will dictate his or her health choices or behavior. They should remain alert to the differences among individual patients and families from a given culture or religious tradition, and guard against stereotyping older adults on the basis of their cultural or religious affiliation.

Clinicians are encouraged to view each cross-cultural and interfaith encounter as an opportunity to learn more, not only about the individual patient and his or her culture or religion, but also about themselves. It is recommended that clinicians continually learn more about the impact of cultural and religious beliefs on healthcare decisions. Additionally, clinicians are urged to work with the entire interdisciplinary healthcare team, including administrators, to promote cultural competence in the healthcare organizations in which they practice.

DOORWAY THOUGHTS IN CROSS-CULTURAL HEALTH CARE

The key concepts discussed in this chapter are "doorway thoughts"—factors that the practitioner should reflect on before walking through the doorway of any examining, consultation, or hospital room. These factors can shape intercultural and interfaith healthcare encounters and relationships both positively and negatively. Cultural, spiritual, and historical facts and issues relating to the members of an entire minority group can be in play in any cross-cultural or interfaith encounter or relationship. The practitioner should be sensitive to the possibility that they may affect their relationships with individual patients and families and may also affect patients' willingness or ability to understand, accept, and adhere to prescribed regimens.

The quality of any encounter between a clinician and a patient from different religious or cultural backgrounds depends on the clinician's skill and sensitivity. Questions about the individual patient's attitudes and beliefs should be worked naturally and carefully into the clinical interview. The clinician must remember that no culture or religious tradition is monolithic; attitudes and beliefs vary widely from one individual to another within a single group. Prior familiarity with a patient's background will not suffice, for it is inaccurate to assume that a person's outlook is inflexibly determined by his or her cultural or religious heritage. The concepts presented here are intended to serve as guidelines in formulating appropriate questions, and not as a rigid list of attributes or clinical scenarios.

Use of Language and Nonverbal Communication

Preferred Terms for Cultural or Religious Identity

The terms referring to specific cultural, ethnic, or religious groups can change over time, and individuals in any one group do not always agree on appropriate terminology. It is important to learn the term that the individual patient prefers for his or her cultural or religious identity, and to use that terminology in conversation with the patient, as well as in his or her health records.

Formality

Attitudes regarding the appropriate degree of formality in a healthcare encounter differ widely among cultural groups. Learning a new patient's preferences with regard to formality and allowing those preferences to shape the relationship is always advisable. Initially, a more formal approach is likely to be appropriate.

Addressing the Patient: The patient's correct title (eg, Dr., Reverend, Mr., Mrs., Ms., Miss) and his or her surname should be used unless and until he or she requests a more casual form of address. Another important issue is to determine the correct pronunciation of the person's name, as well as the appropriate ordering of names; in a variety of countries, the family name is given first, followed by the individual's given name.

Addressing the Healthcare Provider: It is also important to learn how the patient would prefer to address the clinician and to allow his or her preference to prevail. For example, in some cultures, trust in the clinician depends on his or her assuming an authoritative role, and informality would undermine the patient's trust. This is an aspect of the clinical relationship in which the clinician's personal preferences may be relinquished.

Language and Literacy

- What language does the patient feel most comfortable speaking? Will a medical interpreter be needed?
- Does the patient read and write English? Another primary language? If so, which one(s)?
- If the patient has low health literacy, does he or she have access to someone who can assist at home with written instructions?

It is worthwhile to consider these questions early in the healthcare relationship to determine whether interpretation services are needed and to make certain that communication with the patient is effective. Even those who speak English fluently may wish to discuss complicated issues in their native language. It is the clinician's responsibility to explain medical terms and to ask the patient for explanations of any cultural or foreign terms that are unfamiliar.

Health Literacy: One commonly accepted definition of health literacy is "The degree to which individuals have the capacity to obtain, process, and understand basic health information and services needed to make appropriate health decisions." While only a few studies support screening all patients for low health literacy, clinicians should consider simplifying their verbal communication with *all* patients.

Key Communication Techniques:

- Use a teach-back method. This method can be useful to confirm the patient's understanding of the medical visit by asking the patient to recall or explain in his or her own words what has been discussed. Consider use of demonstration skill, if needed. For example, the clinician may say "I always ask my patients to repeat things back to me to make sure I explained it clearly. I'd like you to tell me how you're going to take the new medicine we discussed today."
- Use plain language, and explain things clearly.
- Emphasize 1 to 3 key points during the visit, and repeat those ideas throughout the visit.
- Encourage patients to ask questions; use an open-ended approach.
- Write down important information for the patient.

Use of Medical Interpreters: Medical interpreters are trained professionals who can facilitate the communication between clinicians and patients (and families) who speak different languages. Interpreters relay concepts and ideas between languages in a culturally sensitive way by listening attentively and then repeating the original message accurately and completely in another language. They are ethically bound to repeat everything and are obligated to maintain patient privacy and confidentiality.

Strategies to work effectively with medical interpreters include the following:

- Look and speak directly to the patient, not the interpreter.
- Speak in short sentences and pause. Allow the interpreter to repeat what has been said.

- Speak at an even pace and in a normal tone of voice.
- Some patients may understand some English, and all patients respond positively to a calm tone of voice and respectful body language.

Respectful Nonverbal Communication

Body position and motion is interpreted differently from one cultural group to another. Specific hand gestures, facial expressions, physical contact, and eye contact can hold different meanings in different cultures. The clinician should watch for particular body language cues that appear to be significant and that might be linked to cultural norms that are important to the patient, in an effort to cultivate sensitivity to the conditions that facilitate and improve communication.

Conservative body language is advisable early in a relationship with a patient or when in doubt about a patient's background or preferences; assume a calm demeanor and avoid expressive extremes (eg, very vigorous handshakes, a loud and hearty voice, many hand gestures, an impassive facial expression, avoidance of eye contact, standing at a distance). The clinician should remain alert for signals that the patient is comfortable or uncomfortable. Directly asking the patient questions about body language may also help. Making negative judgments about a patient that are rooted in unconscious cultural assumptions about the meaning of his or her gestures, facial expressions, or body language should be avoided.

The distance from others that individuals find comfortable varies, depending in part on their cultural background. The clinician should determine what distance seems to be the most comfortable for each patient and, whenever practicable, allow the patient's preference to establish the optimal distance during the encounter.

History of Traumatic Experiences

Is the patient a refugee or survivor of violence or genocide? Are family members missing or dead? Have patients or family members been tortured? Such experiences could negatively affect the healthcare encounter without the clinician's knowledge unless relevant questions are included among standard questions about the patient's history. Clinicians should remember that in some historical periods and jurisdictions, healthcare providers have participated in torture and genocide (eg, Nazi medical personnel in World War II). The methods and tools of torture used have sometimes resembled legitimate clinical procedures and tools. Patients who have survived such experiences may not feel safe in medical or governmental settings, and contact with any clinician may invoke feelings of vulnerability, fear, panic, or anger. Great sensitivity is necessary in providing health care for these individuals.

Issues of Immigration

Immigration Status

Some individuals may be living in North America without appropriate immigration documents. Clinicians may wish to assure each patient that information given within the medical encounter will be kept confidential.

History of Immigration or Migration

The history of the movements of a large portion of a religious or cultural group can affect the attitudes and behavior of an individual in that group even when he or she has not immigrated to North America from another country. In addition, understanding an individual's specific migration history often provides insight into the key life transitions informing his or her outlook. Knowing how a person came to live in North America can be important. The time and effort the clinician invests in learning more about a cultural or religious group's history and current situation can be repaid not only in a better relationship with the individual patient but also in an enhanced appreciation of the factors affecting clinical relationships with other patients from that group.

Acculturation, Tradition, and Health Beliefs

Acculturation is a process in which members of one cultural group adopt the beliefs and behaviors of another group. Acculturation of a group may be evidenced by changes in language preference, adoption of common attitudes and values, evolution of religious practices, or gradual loss of separate ethnic identification. Although acculturation typically occurs when a minority group adopts the habits and language patterns of a dominant group, acculturation may also be reciprocal between groups.

It is essential to keep principles of acculturation in mind during any cross-cultural or interfaith health encounter. Beginning by determining how long a person has lived in North America and whether he or she was born here is helpful. However, remember that the degree to which the person is acculturated to North American customs and attitudes is the consequence of many factors and not just of the number of years since he or she immigrated. Older adults who follow the traditions of their cultural or religious group may have been born outside of the United States, may be recent arrivals to the continent, or may even be lifelong North American residents.

A patient's level of cultural or spiritual shifting can impact not only his or her health behavior but also preferences in end-of-life planning and decision making. Acculturation can also be an issue dividing family members, and a person's resistance to or ease of acculturation may be a matter of pride or of shame and guilt. Developing sensitivity about the issues of acculturation for one's older minority patients is a key element in effective cross-cultural health care. Asking patients directly about their adherence to cultural and spiritual traditions can be useful.

People from a variety of cultural groups may not conceive of illness in North American terms. Some may have highly developed concepts of the causes of health and disease that are incompatible with the concepts that form the foundations of North American medicine. Some other paradigms of wellness and illness include beliefs that illnesses have spiritual causation, are the result of imbalance among bodily humors, or are caused by a person's actions in past lives, to name but a few.

In addition, patients from any cultural background may be using alternative remedies (eg, rituals, herbal preparations) that they do not mention. Therefore, it is prudent to routinely ask all patients about the use of complementary and alternative treatments as part of their history. It is unrealistic to expect that a patient will simply "adapt" to North American approaches to health and health care, just as it is impractical to expect the clinician to accept a new conception of wellness and disease. Clinical communication and efficacy will be enhanced when patients and healthcare providers make an effort to negotiate a common understanding of causation, diagnosis, and treatment for a specific health problem, while maintaining respect for the beliefs and constructs of both individuals.

UNSPOKEN CHALLENGES

Clinicians should remain alert to the possibility of issues that are critical to the success of the healthcare encounter that the patient may not voice. Examples include the following:

- lack of trust in healthcare providers and the healthcare system
- fear of medical research and experimentation
- fear of medications or their adverse events
- unfamiliarity or discomfort with the Western biomedical belief system

Some patients may feel uncomfortable or uneasy in customary North American healthcare settings for a variety of reasons, including lack of familiarity with Western practices, dissatisfying previous encounters with the healthcare system, or the belief that insensitivity or discrimination is inevitable for anyone in the cultural or religious group. Such feelings may result from having been stereotyped or treated insensitively or even unfairly by clinicians in the past. Sensitive exploration of these issues with patients is often both worthwhile and necessary. In general, sensitivity to the possibility that such issues are in play is advised in all patient encounters.

THE INTERFACE BETWEEN CULTURE AND RELIGION

In some cultural groups, most individuals share one religious heritage; in others, there is a great deal of religious and spiritual diversity. As a result, the relative impact of religion and culture on health behavior and decision making for older adults may be subtle and complex, warranting respectful exploration on the part of the clinician.

Several studies have documented that most patients either prefer or would accept clinicians asking them about their spiritual beliefs and what impact such beliefs might have on their world view, health behavior, and health decision making (SOE=A). Questions regarding religion and spirituality should be incorporated sensitively and early in the patient-provider relationship and reexplored when significant health problems arise.

APPROACHES TO DECISION MAKING

Western bioethics emphasizes individual autonomy in all health decisions, but for many other cultures, decision making is family or community centered. Autonomy principles allow competent individuals to involve others in their health decisions or to cede those rights to a proxy decision maker. The clinician should ask patients if they prefer to make their own health decisions or if they would prefer to involve or defer to others. Some may wish to assign the decision-making authority wholly to another individual or a group. In some cultures, the definition of family may include fictive kin. In families in which the degree of acculturation of the generations differs, the older adult may defer to or depend on younger relatives, even though the tradition might suggest that the reverse would occur.

Many studies have documented the impact of religious and spiritual beliefs on preferences regarding end-of-life practices and decision making. Some religious traditions characterize health outcomes as divinely willed and emphasize acceptance in the face of adversity. Other traditions stress the religious obligation for individuals to save or extend life at almost any cost.

Establishing an understanding of each patient's decision-making construct and preferences early in the clinical relationship will, in most instances, promote better communication and avoid the difficulties inherent in trying to address the issues at a time of crisis. When the patient's and clinician's cultural or religious backgrounds differ, careful exploration of the issues is all the more important because the clinician cannot proceed if he or she and the patient are not starting from common assumptions.

Attitudes Regarding Disclosure and Consent

Cultural attitudes toward truth telling and disclosure of terminal diagnoses vary widely. In some cultures, it is commonly believed that patients should not be informed of a terminal diagnosis, because this may be injurious to health or hasten death. Obtaining informed consent from patients with this belief may prove difficult. There is no consensus in bioethics concerning the rigorous application of full clinical disclosure in every situation. However, it is generally agreed that incorporating a patient's beliefs concerning disclosure and truth telling into clinical planning whenever possible is desirable. Some patients may prefer not to know if they are terminally ill and ask that family members or other caregivers receive all diagnostic information and make all treatment decisions. It is advisable to explore each patient's preferences regarding disclosure of serious clinical findings early in the clinical relationship and to reconfirm these wishes at intervals. See "Legal and Ethical Issues," p 26.

Gender Issues

Culture and religion intertwine in describing traditions and structures with regard to gender roles. Societies seemingly based on the same patriarchal or matriarchal model may vary widely in their expressions of the model. A person's gender influences the sorts of experiences he or she has had, not only within the family but also in the community and healthcare system. Another level of complexity may be added to healthcare encounters when an older adult's group struggles with conflicting traditional and contemporary views on gender roles. Cultural norms for men and women can influence their health behavior, and such norms for the genders vary widely from one culture to another. Gender-based norms may also affect how patients choose a healthcare provider and make health decisions, as well as how they form their preferences for disclosure and consent.

The clinician is strongly advised to explore each patient's attitudes regarding the interplay among gender, choice of healthcare provider, autonomy, and personal decision making early in the patient-provider relationship; to confirm his or her preferences at intervals; and to follow the individual patient's wishes whenever possible.

Advance Directives and End-of-Life Care

Cultural, religious, and spiritual beliefs are an important influence in a person's formation of his or her attitudes toward supportable quality of life, approach to suffering, and beliefs about medical feeding, life-prolonging treatments, and palliative care. Some cultures and religious traditions value a direct struggle for life in the face of death, and both patients and families expect an intensive approach to treatment. Others avoid personal confrontation of death and dying and prefer to leave such decisions to the clinician. Still others take a direct approach to death and dying but reject too aggressive an approach.

Research has shown that clinicians and patients from shared cultural and religious backgrounds have similar values in these areas (SOE=B); the implications of such findings for clinicians and patients from differing backgrounds are obviously important. Both clinicians and patients bring their own attitudes and beliefs to any clinical encounter. Clinicians should be aware of their personal views, cultural values, and religious beliefs when discussing end-of-life plans with patients, and respect patients' beliefs and preferences even when they are different from their own.

In negotiating end-of-life decisions with a patient whose background is different from his or her own, the clinician must listen especially carefully to the patient's goals and concerns and exert every effort to avoid making assumptions that do not apply. For example, the assumption that "no one would want to live in that condition" or that "everyone would want treatment in this situation" is likely to be faulty. To ensure that end-of-life plans and decisions reflect an individual's rights and wishes, the clinician must strive to understand the older adult's overall approach to life and death and, as far as possible, provide care that is consistent with that approach.

Approaches: The ETHNICS Mnemonic

The ETHNICS mnemonic is a tool to facilitate effective health interviews and care planning in cross-cultural settings. Rather than serving as a prescribed outline of questions to ask, the ETHNICS mnemonic (below) provides a framework in which to ascertain a wide variety of information and to negotiate effective therapeutic next steps, all within a routine 15-minute clinical session.

- **Explanation:** Ask patients to describe what they think is happening to them in their own words.
- **Treatments:** Inquire as to which treatments patients have used for their health problem(s) before the interview. Clinicians should specifically ask about biomedical interventions, as well as any complementary and alternative treatments patients may have used.
- **Healers:** Respectfully inquire about other healers involved in a patient's care; many patients seek treatment from alternative practitioners or traditional healers, as well as from conventional healthcare providers. Incorporating this information into the healthcare encounter is important to overall care planning and efficacy.
- **Negotiate:** Negotiate with each patient and/or his or her designated caregiver(s) as to which treatments the patient will accept and participate in.
- **Intervene:** Put together a care plan that is acceptable from the perspectives of both the provider and the patient. This frequently incorporates a blending of "scientific" explanations of wellness and disease, as well as each individual patient's concept of his or her health status and acceptable approaches to addressing concerns.
- **Collaborate:** Focus on building a trustful and resilient relationship with each older patient. Incorporating formal and informal caregivers into a broader team alliance is also critical to the success of health care for all older adults.
- **Spirituality:** Inquire respectfully about patients' spiritual beliefs, and how these might impact their healthcare preferences and behavior, particularly at the end of life.

REFERENCES

- American Geriatrics Society, Ethnogeriatrics Committee. *Doorway Thoughts: Cross-Cultural Health Care for Older Adults.* Volumes 1–3. Boston, MA: Jones and Bartlett; 2004, 2006, 2008.
- Ko E, Cho S, Bonilla M. Attitudes toward life-sustaining treatment: the role of race/ethnicity. *Geriatr Nurs.* 2012;33(5):341–349.
- Stanford Geriatric Education Center Web site (http://sgec.stanford.edu/).
- Yeo G. How will the US healthcare system meet the challenge of the ethnogeriatric imperative? *J Am Geriatr Soc.* 2009;57(7):1278–1285.

CHAPTER 9—PHYSICAL ACTIVITY

KEY POINTS

- Regular physical activity provides numerous and substantial health benefits for older adults.
- The health benefits of physical activity accrue independently of other risk factors. Greater amounts of physical activity have greater health benefits.
- To obtain substantial health benefits of physical activity, older adults are commonly recommended to do at least 150 minutes of moderate-intensity aerobic activity each week. If they cannot do this amount of activity, they should do the amount that is possible according to their abilities, so as to avoid inactivity. Doing at least 30 minutes of moderate-intensity aerobic activity on ≥5 days each week is an appropriate way for older adults to be active.
- Older adults should also engage in muscle-strengthening activity on ≥2 days each week and include balance training regularly.
- When possible, obese people and those with osteoarthritis or balance problems should perform aerobic and resistance exercise using water.
- Promoting physical activity is one of the most important and effective preventive and therapeutic interventions in older adults. The clinician's recommendation for exercise (and other lifestyle habits) for their patients carries more weight than any other source of advice. Counseling by a healthcare provider is an important way of promoting physical activity in clinical settings. Referral of patients to community resources, particularly evidence-based programs, is also important.

Physical activity in the context of public health refers to all muscular activity either at work or during leisure time, ranging from light to high vigorous as shown in Table 9.1. Its benefits arise from the adaptation of multiple body systems to the muscular demand for oxygen, and generally these benefits may be considered proportional to the absolute intensity of the exercise or the mass of muscle activated by the exercise coupled with the duration of the exercise. The term *relative exercise intensity* refers to the percentage of the individual's maximal capacity that is utilized. Thus, a weaker person will activate fewer muscle fibers than a stronger person at the same relative intensity. In this sense, being physically fit allows the individual to perform more vigorous physical activity.

Another important concept is the exercise volume, which in population studies is defined as the product of exercise intensity in METS and duration in hours. Thus, a person who walks briskly (4 to 5 METS) for 30 minutes 4 times a week achieves an exercise volume of 8–10 MET-hours, which is considered medium volume. See Table 9.1.

BENEFITS OF PHYSICAL ACTIVITY

Preventive Health Benefits

Regular physical activity in adults and older adults improves cardiorespiratory and muscular fitness (SOE=A). It reduces the risk of many diseases, including coronary heart disease, stroke, hypertension, some lipid disorders, type 2 diabetes, colon cancer, breast cancer, osteoporosis, and depression (SOE=A). It also reduces the risk of unhealthy weight gain and assists in weight loss (SOE=A). In older adults, physical activity reduces the risk of falls (SOE=A) and sarcopenia, and regularly active older adults have a lower risk of hip fracture (SOE=B). The evidence that physical activity reduces the risk of cognitive impairment is growing and substantial (SOE=B). There is some evidence that physical activity can reduce the risk of lung cancer, endometrial cancer, osteoarthritis, sleep problems, and anxiety disorders (SOE=B).

Consistent with its broad physiologic effects, regular physical activity decreases both cardiovascular and noncardiovascular mortality in older adults. This benefit is large. The risk of premature mortality is estimated to be 40% less in adults who are active ≥7 hours each week than in those who are active for <0.5 hours each week (SOE=B). While this estimate is based on cohort studies that determined amounts of physical activity from questionnaires, one study of older adults determined level of physical activity objectively using doubly labeled water. In this study, adults in the highest tertile of energy expenditure per day had a 67% lower mortality rate than adults in the lowest tertile of energy expenditure (SOE=B).

In general, greater amounts of physical activity have greater health benefits, although the relationship between the amount of physical activity and the amount of benefit appears nonlinear for many health conditions. That is, the absolute increase in benefit is greatest at low levels of activity, and less at high levels of activity. The "dose-response" relationship varies by disease in a manner that is incompletely understood. Risk of cardiovascular disease decreases with amount of aerobic activity over a wide range of dose. Blood pressure shows little dose-response effect, with most of the effect of

Table 9.1—Exercise Intensity and Exercise Volume

Exercise intensity, in METS	
Light	= 2.5; walking (approx 2.2 mph)
Moderate	= 4–5; brisk walking (3.4–3.9 mph)
Mod-vigorous	= 6.5; jogging (4 mph)
High vigorous	= 8.5; running (5.4 mph)
Duration of physical activity (also known as exercise volume, ie, intensity × duration), in MET-hours per week	
Inactive	<3.75
Low volume	3.75–7.5
Medium volume	7.6–16.5
High volume	16.6–25.5
Very high volume	>25.5

1 MET = 3.5 mL O_2/kg/min = 210 mL O_2/kg/hr = 1 kcal/kg/hr (1 L O_2 = 5 kcal)

physical activity on blood pressure occurring at low to medium levels of activity.

The health benefits of physical activity accrue independently of risk factors. For example, sedentary smokers experience health benefits of increasing physical activity even if they continue to smoke. The health benefits of physical activity are also generally independent of body weight: overweight and obese adults obtain benefits from physical activity even if it does not promote weight loss.

Strong, consistent observational evidence indicates that regularly active older adults are at reduced risk of moderate or severe functional limitations and role limitations (SOE=B). One review estimated that moderate amounts of aerobic physical activity reduced risk of functional decline by 30%. There appears to be a dose-response relationship, with greater amounts of physical activity producing more benefit.

Therapeutic Benefits

Physical activity is commonly recommended in clinical practice guidelines as therapy for specific conditions. Clinical practice guidelines identify a substantial therapeutic role for physical activity in coronary heart disease, peripheral vascular disease, hypertension, type 2 diabetes, osteoarthritis, osteoporosis, some lipid disorders, obesity, claudication, and COPD. Physical activity also has a role in the management of depression, anxiety disorders, pain, heart failure, syncope, sleep disorders, stroke, dementia, back pain, and constipation, and in prevention of venous thromboembolism.

In a systematic review, there was solid evidence from controlled trials that physical activity has a beneficial effect on functional limitations in older adults with existing mild, moderate, or severe limitations (SOE=A).

Economic Benefits

Regularly active adults are consistently reported to have lower medical expenditures than sedentary adults (SOE=B). In one study comparing older adults who remained sedentary with those who became active ≥3 days each week, medical expenditures of the active group were lower by about $2,200 per year. In one managed-care plan that offered a physical activity benefit consisting of paying per-visit costs for Medicare-eligible enrollees who participated in an exercise program called EnhanceFitness, participants adjusted total costs were $1,186 lower per year than those of nonparticipants by year two.

Recommended Amounts of Physical Activity

A public health recommendation for ≥20 minutes of vigorous aerobic activity on ≥3 days per week was developed in the 1980s. In 1995, the CDC and the American College of Sports Medicine (ACSM) developed a moderate-intensity recommendation: "Every US adult should accumulate 30 minutes or more of moderate-intensity physical activity on most, preferably all, days of the week." In 2007, the ACSM and the American Heart Association (AHA) updated the 1995 recommendation by issuing separate recommendations for adults and for older adults. In 2008, the U.S. Department of Health and Human Services issued the first national guidelines for physical activity, the *2008 Physical Activity Guidelines for Americans*. For recommended types and amounts of physical activity, see Table 9.2.

Aerobic Activity

An older adult can achieve recommended levels of aerobic activity by doing either moderate-intensity aerobic physical activity for at least 150 minutes each week, or vigorous-intensity activity for at least 75 minutes each week. Doing a combination of moderate- and vigorous-intensity activity is also acceptable. Aerobic activity should be spread throughout the week, preferably on ≥3 days per week. Doing at least 30 minutes of aerobic activity on ≥5 days each week remains an appropriate way for older adults to obtain the health benefits of activity.

Several comments help clarify this recommendation. First, episodes of moderate-intensity activity of ≥10 minutes count toward meeting the recommendation. Second, the recommendation does not refer to just leisure activity or exercise. Occupational activity (eg, carpentry), domestic activity (eg, mowing the grass), and transportation activity (eg, walking to the store) all count toward meeting recommendations. Third, participation

Table 9.2–Recommended Types and Amounts of Physical Activity

Type of Exercise	Frequency/Duration	Examples of Activities	Examples of Targeted Conditions
Aerobic	≥150 minutes of moderate-intensity activity each week, spread throughout the week; ≥75 minutes of vigorous-intensity activity each week, spread throughout the week	Walking, running, swimming, bicycling, rowing, or aerobic exercise machines (eg, ellipticals, stair steppers); walking 30 minutes/day, 5–6 days/week, or 10,000 steps/day using a pedometer	Many conditions, including cardiovascular disease, cancer, diabetes, osteoarthritis, and depression; low physical work capacity
Muscle strengthening	≥2 days each week for 20–30 minutes	Resistance training (eg, using weight machines) or floor exercises using body weight against gravity (eg, abdominal "crunches," push-ups off knees or against a table, climbing stairs); pool exercises against water resistance	Falls, frailty, sarcopenia, osteoporosis
Flexibility	10 minutes stretching daily to maintain range of motion	Stretching, gentle yoga, Pilates	Osteoarthritis, joint stiffness
Balance training	≥3 days/week	Backward walking, heel-to-toe walking, Tai Chi exercise, standing on one foot	Falls, osteoporosis

in physical activity above the minimum recommended levels results in greater health benefits. Some physical activity is clearly preferable to none for those who are unable to meet these targets. Older adults should be strongly encouraged to avoid an inactive lifestyle, even if they do not (or cannot) obtain recommended amounts of activity. Finally, as indicated earlier, the recommended activity is in addition to routine (baseline) activity of light-intensity or of short duration (<10 minutes). This is supported by a large clinical trial in which men and women ≥60 years old had a 14% lower risk of all-cause mortality with 15 minutes of moderate exercise per day. Each additional 15 minutes of exercise a day reduced the risk by a further 4%. This finding may reduce the barriers to individuals who attempt to meet the recommendation of 30 minutes a day of moderate exercise in the *2008 Physical Activity Guidelines for Americans*.

Muscle-Strengthening Activity

ACSM/AHA recommendations and the *2008 Physical Activity Guidelines for Americans* state that older adults should perform muscle-strengthening activities of the major muscle groups (arms, shoulder, legs, hip, back, chest, and abdomen) on ≥2 days each week. A typical routine for older adults involves 2 or 3 nonconsecutive days each week. These activities can be done at home; popular exercises include sit-ups and push-ups, modified to reduce the strength required to perform them. For example, push-ups may be done off the knees or against a wall, and sit-ups may be done in reverse by lowering the torso to the point where it can be raised again without excessive strain.

For adults who choose resistance training (eg, weight machines), one set of 8 to 10 different exercises is sufficient, with 10 to 15 repetitions per set. Moderate-intensity or high-intensity training is recommended, in which level of effort of moderate intensity is 5 or 6 on a 0 to 10 scale (0=no movement and 10=maximal effort). High-intensity is 7 or 8 on the same scale.

Flexibility Activity

Flexibility activity is recommended for older adults as a means of maintaining the range of motion needed for regular physical activity and daily life. Stiffness of ligaments, tendons, and other connective tissue occurs after soft-tissue injury and through the gradual glycosylation of collagen fibers with age. This process can be ameliorated with regular stretching to the point of tightness and holding the position for a few seconds. Yoga is a good activity for older adults because it combines strengthening and stretching, and classes for all abilities are widely available. Caution is advised to avoid injury by trying to achieve positions that may be too difficult.

Balance Training

Balance training is recommended for all older adults especially those at risk of falls, including adults with frequent falls or mobility problems. They can be done throughout the day in a variety of situations. Backwards walking, and standing on one foot for several seconds and then the other while taking a shower, are simple examples. Balance can be thought of as any other motor skill, which requires practice, muscle coordination, and adequate strength.

Several effective interventions to prevent falls included balance training on ≥3 days per week have been studied. Hence, it is preferable that older adults do standardized balance exercises from a program demonstrated to reduce falls. There is moderate evidence that Tai Chi exercise is effective in fall prevention, although the optimal amount and forms of Tai Chi are unclear (SOE=B).

Management of Body Weight

Most weight-loss studies conclude that exercise enhances the effectiveness of dietary restriction in achieving a healthy body weight beyond what might be expected from calculations of caloric balance. The amount of exercise to metabolize the 3,500 kcals of energy in a pound of fat is substantial. Walking a mile at 1.5–4 mph requires about 1.25 kcals/kg body weight/mile, or 100 kcal for a person weighing 175 lbs. Therefore, 5 miles of daily walking, which for most older adults would take 2 hours, is required to lose 1 lb of fat per week. This fact emphasizes the need for other forms of energy expenditure throughout the day, and especially to minimize the time spent sitting.

A reasonable approach for physical activity and weight management in older adults is to follow the *2008 Physical Activity Guidelines for Americans*. Overweight and obese older adults should first achieve minimal recommended levels of physical activity (150 minutes of moderate-intensity aerobic activity per week). If a healthy weight is not achieved with this level of activity, then caloric intake should be controlled, physical activity increased gradually, and body weight monitored. Physical activity can be increased to the point that is individually effective in controlling weight. If an older adult is not capable of sufficiently high amounts of activity, then additional dietary restriction is necessary.

When older adults lose weight, they lose not only fat mass but also muscle mass and bone mass. Because physical activity, particularly muscle-strengthening activity, acts to preserve bone and muscle mass, older adults should not attempt to lose weight by diet alone.

Screening

For older adults, especially those with chronic conditions, the ACSM/AHA recommends development of an activity plan in consultation with primary care providers. The activity plan should integrate public health preventive recommendations (summarized above) with any therapeutic use of physical activity recommended, eg, by clinical practice guidelines. Older adults should understand if, and how, chronic conditions limit the amounts and types of activity they can do.

This recommendation changes screening guidelines. Rather than advise older adults to consult a healthcare provider before starting to increase physical activity, ACSM/AHA recommends that healthcare provider consultation about physical activity should occur regardless of whether an adult currently plans to increase physical activity. One quality of care measure for older adults ascertains whether older adults discuss physical activity with a healthcare provider at least once a year. At the time of a consultation about physical activity, the clinician should ensure that the patient does not have any undiagnosed symptoms and is up-to-date on preventive care, and that medical conditions are stable. Further, the clinician should assess if and how the patient should limit his or her activity because of chronic conditions.

Thus, "screening" older adults can be used to match them to an activity plan appropriate for their abilities. Most, if not all, studies of exercise in people with disabilities have assessed potential participants to ensure the exercise intervention is appropriate. These study populations have included adults with osteoarthritis, lower limb loss, cerebral palsy, multiple sclerosis, muscular dystrophy, Parkinson disease, spinal cord injury, stroke, traumatic brain injury, dementia, intellectual disability, and mental illness. A review concluded that the benefits of physical activity for such people with disabilities clearly outweigh the risks.

It is appropriate for providers of exercise programs to ask new participants (who are not referred after an examination by a healthcare provider) to complete a symptom checklist. People with undiagnosed symptoms should seek medical care before starting an exercise program.

The Physical Activity Guidelines Advisory Committee concluded, after a systematic review of the literature, that "the protective value of a medical consultation for persons with or without chronic diseases who are interested in increasing their physical activity level is not established." The U.S. Preventive Services Task Force does not recommend any type of routine preexercise screening of healthy asymptomatic adults. Specifically, for adults at increased risk of coronary heart disease, the Task Force finds insufficient evidence for routine screening with resting ECG, exercise treadmill test, or electron-beam CT scanning for coronary calcium. For adults at low risk of heart disease, the Task Force recommends against screening with these tests.

Promotion of Physical Activity

The public health approach to promotion of physical activity is based on a socioecologic model that recognizes the interrelationship that exists between the individual and his or her environment. This involves action at all levels of society: individual, interpersonal, organizational, community, and public policy. To illustrate the logic of the model, consider that counseling an older adult to walk regularly (individual level intervention) is more effective if the person lives in a neighborhood with good access to parks and other safe places to walk (a community level intervention). A referral to an exercise program (an individual level intervention) is more likely to succeed if the costs of the exercise program are subsidized by a health plan (organizational level intervention). Physical activity promotion in clinical settings occurs in this broader context. The Task Force on Community Preventive Services has identified eight evidence-based community approaches for promoting physical activity (www.thecommunityguide.org) [accessed Oct 2013].

Clinical Settings

A system is needed in each clinical setting for routinely assessing levels of physical activity in patients, for providing patients with a recommendation about physical activity, for helping patients achieve recommended levels, and for evaluating the effectiveness of the system in promoting physical activity. An example of an evidence-based system is the Green Prescription in New Zealand. In brief, after their level of physical activity has been assessed, patients are given the option of requesting a prescription from a primary care provider. The provider provides a written "green" prescription, typically for walking or other home-based activity. A copy is faxed to the local sports foundation, which contacts patients and offers them assistance by telephone or face-to-face counseling, or peer group support. In a randomized trial of this approach, the intervention group averaged 35–40 more minutes of physical activity each week (SOE=A).

Assessing Physical Activity

The importance of routine assessment of physical activity is emphasized by the Exercise is Medicine Initiative of the ACSM. This initiative advocates for physical activity as a vital sign to be checked each visit. Tools have been developed to provide quick assessments of the physical activity level of older adults, such as the Rapid Assessment of Physical Activity, a 9-item questionnaire in which patients self-rate their strength, flexibility, and frequency and intensity of exercise. Both the amount of aerobic activity and the amount of muscle-strengthening activity should be assessed.

Emerging evidence indicates that how we spend our time during physical activity may be important. In a large prospective study of U.S. adults enrolled by the American Cancer Society, time spent sitting was independently associated with total mortality, regardless of physical activity level.

Providing an Activity Prescription

In the ACSM/AHA recommendations, the activity prescription is considered part of a broader approach of developing the physical activity plan. The plan considers individual preferences, individual abilities and fitness, chronic conditions and activity limitations, risk of falls, strategies for decreasing risk of injury, and behavioral strategies to increase adherence to the plan. Essentially, the plan provides specific guidance on how to meet physical activity guidelines. A resource for developing the plan is ACSM's *Exercise Management for Chronic Diseases and Disabilities*. This book covers issues in exercise management for some 40 different conditions. Some guidelines for developing a plan include the following:

- The plan will commonly emphasize walking, which is a popular and safe activity in older adults. However, for many people with knee osteoarthritis, swimming, pool exercise, and non-weight-bearing activities such as cycling and rowing, which can be done on machines, may be preferred.
- The plan should emphasize the importance of gradually increasing physical activity over time (see below). It can be appropriate for older adults to spend weeks or months at activity levels below recommended levels.
- The less active an adult is currently and the less experience he or she has with physical activity, the more appropriate it is to recommend starting in a supervised, evidence-based program (see below).
- Providing social support for physical activity is important. Social support can be provided by classes, formal mall walking groups, telephone counseling, and informal arrangements in which people simply meet to go for a walk.

Providing Assistance in Increasing Physical Activity

In 2002, the U.S. Preventive Services Task Force concluded that the evidence is insufficient to recommend for or against behavioral counseling in primary care settings to promote physical activity. However, some clinic-based systems of promoting physical activity have been carefully studied and reported to increase physical activity, such as the "Green Prescription" system mentioned above. A reasonable conclusion is that a clinic can implement either an existing evidence-based approach, or implement and evaluate a new approach tailored to the clinical situation based on principles of behavior change and building on existing approaches. The many negative studies of physical activity counseling in clinical settings emphasize the importance of evaluating any new approaches.

Particularly for adults with some functional limitations, an appropriate way to provide assistance is to make a referral to an evidence-based program. Resources, such as the National Council on Aging Web site (www.ncoa.org), can help identify evidence-based programs that have been tested in research studies and translated into versions that work in the community. For example, Active Living Every Day, and Active Choices are two programs that were originally tested in research studies and subsequently translated into programs appropriate for community settings. A recent study demonstrated that the community versions of these programs were effective in large samples of older adults who were substantially more ethnically, economically, and functionally diverse than the samples in the original research studies.

A longstanding resource for older adults from the National Institute on Aging is *Exercise: A Guide from the National Institute on Aging*. This publication is updated periodically.

Management of Risks of Physical Activity

The most important recommendation for avoiding activity-related injuries is to increase physical activity gradually over time (SOE=B). Observational evidence is strong that the risk of injury is directly related to the size of the gap between a person's usual level of activity and their new level of activity. A series of small increments in activity, each followed by a period of adaptation, is associated with lower rates of musculoskeletal injury. The safest method for increasing activity has not been established by intervention studies. For reasonably healthy adults, adding a small amount of light- to moderate-intensity activity (eg, walking 5–15 minutes per session, 2 to 3 times per week) has low risk of musculoskeletal injury and no known risk of sudden cardiac events (SOE=B).

In contrast, during vigorous-intensity activity, all individuals are at higher risk of sudden adverse cardiac events. However, regularly active adults are at much less risk than inactive adults who abruptly engage in vigorous activity.

In older adults, cardiovascular adaptation to a target level of physical activity can take as long as ≥20 weeks. This suggests that activity levels should be increased once per month instead of once per week.

Other factors also affect injury risk. The risk of injury is higher with vigorous exercise, with greater amounts of exercise, and with activities that involve frequent contact (eg, soccer, basketball) or purposeful collision (eg, football). The risk of injury is less with a higher level of fitness, supervision, protective equipment such as bike helmets, and in well-designed environments. To illustrate the safety of walking, one community-based study estimated 0.2 injuries per 1,000 hours of walking for transportation. In contrast, in 1,000 hours of participation, dancing had 0.7 injuries, gardening 1.0 injuries, and running 3.6 injuries.

Older Adults with Low Fitness or Low Functional Ability

In the lifestyle interventions and independence for elders (LIFE) pilot study, a randomized trial in which older adults (70–89 years old) with chronic diseases and reduced functional ability who were at substantial risk of mobility disability were enrolled, regular exercise improved measures of physical function without appreciably increasing risk of adverse events. This trial affirmed that older adults with functional impairments can achieve benefits from exercise (SOE=A). Similarly, an older study of resistance exercise in frail nursing-home residents demonstrated improvements in strength and function (SOE=A).

Regardless, in such older adults with low fitness or low functional ability, it is more challenging to match abilities with types and amounts of activity. Sometimes referrals can be made to specific rehabilitation programs, such as pulmonary rehabilitation, for assessment, exercise prescription, and medically supervised exercise. Assessment by a physical therapist is generally appropriate, and the therapist can design and tailor an exercise program to the specific limitations of the patient. This assessment can also confirm a patient is capable of participating in a specific community exercise program (eg, a water exercise program designed for adults with arthritis). Given that the care of such patients often involves a geriatric team and consultants, methods should be in place to ensure the activity recommendation is communicated to all the healthcare providers.

REFERENCES

- Chale-Rush A, Guralnik JM, Walkup MP, et al. Relationship between physical functioning and physical activity in the lifestyle interventions and independence for elders pilot. *J Am Geriatr Soc*. 2010:58(10):1918–1924.
- Rejeski WJ, Brubaker PH, Goff DC Jr., et al. Translating weight loss and physical activity programs into the community to preserve mobility in older, obese adults in poor cardiovascular health. *Arch Intern Med*. 2011;171(10):880–886.
- Tse MM, Wan VT, Ho SS. Physical exercise: does it help in relieving pain and increasing mobility among older adults with chronic pain. *J Clin Nursing*. 2011:20(5–6):635–644.
- US Department of Health and Human Services. 2008 physical activity guidelines for Americans. http://www.health.gov/paguidelines/pdf/paguide.pdf (accessed Oct 2013).
- Wen CP, Wai JP, Tsai MK, et al. Minimum amount of physical activity for reduced mortality and extended life expectancy: a prospective cohort study. *Lancet*. 2011;378(9798):1244–1253.

ᴄHAPTER 10—PREVENTION

KEY POINTS

- It is important to consider a patient's remaining life expectancy, comorbidities, and cognitive and functional status when deciding which preventive health measures to offer.
- Many preventive health measures are underused among older adults, including immunizations (eg, flu shots, pneumococcal vaccinations), exercise counseling, depression screening, and counseling on geriatric health issues (eg, safety, falls prevention, incontinence), while cancer screening tests are overused among older adults in poor health.
- Tools are available to help clinicians estimate life expectancy to appropriately target cancer screening to those with adequate remaining life expectancy.
- Medicare is increasingly covering preventive services and wellness visits.

Many preventive health measures are available to older adults, including screening tests (eg, colonoscopy), counseling about a healthy lifestyle (eg, exercise) and/or geriatric health issues (eg, incontinence), immunizations (eg, flu shot), and chemoprophylaxis (eg, aspirin). Ideally, older adults should receive preventive health measures from which they are most likely to benefit based on their health and remaining life expectancy. In this era of patient-centered practice, recommendations should incorporate patient preferences as well.

Remaining life expectancy decreases uniformly with age, but it can vary from one individual to the next according to illness burden and functional status. Predicted remaining life expectancy, cognition, and function are important determinants to consider when offering preventive services to older adults. In vulnerable older adults, screening and prevention should focus on evidence-based interventions that minimize functional limitations and increase the number of healthy years lived.

This chapter reviews the preventive health measures available to older adults and discusses which measures are appropriate based on remaining life expectancy. Table 10.1 provides an overview of all measures available and their recommended use in different populations of older adults, including robust individuals with ≥5 years remaining life expectancy, frail individuals with <5 years remaining life expectancy, those with moderate dementia, and those at the end of life. The recommendations given in Table 10.1 are based on reports from geriatric expert panels, as well as on guidelines from the American Geriatrics Society (AGS) and the United States Preventive Services Task Force (USPSTF), and include information on whether each service is cost-effective. A service that costs less than $50,000 per life-year saved is generally considered cost-effective, while those costing more than $100,000 per life-year are generally not considered cost-effective. This chapter focuses mainly on primary (ie, disease avoidance) and secondary (ie, early detection and treatment of asymptomatic disease) prevention rather than on tertiary prevention (ie, preventing functional decline from established illness). Finally, the chapter discusses effective ways to counsel older adults about preventive health measures and tools available to help clinicians estimate patient life expectancy.

Several criteria should generally be met before recommending disease screening: 1) The condition being screened for must be serious and prevalent in the population being tested. 2) The disease should have a significant asymptomatic phase that can be detected by the screening test. 3) The screening test must be safe, sensitive, and specific to limit false-positive and false-negative tests. 4) Effective treatment must be available for use early in the natural course of the disease that results in a better prognosis than treatment given after symptoms develop. 5) The costs of screening should be acceptable. 6) Ideally, the screening test should have been found effective in a randomized controlled trial (RCT). Few older adults have been included in RCTs that evaluate screening measures, especially frail older adults; therefore, recommendations are often based on indirect evidence. Clinicians are encouraged to consider the effect of preventive health measures not only on quantity of life but also on quality of life, satisfaction with life, and in maintaining independence. Preventive health recommendations for older adults need to be individualized based on patient health, function, environment, and preferences.

CANCER SCREENING TESTS

The main potential benefit of screening is reducing cancer mortality experienced by individuals whose cancer is detected early and that otherwise would have resulted in serious morbidity or death if the cancer was not treated early. The potential harms of screening include complications from screening tests or diagnostic evaluations after false-positive test results, false reassurance from false-negative test results, detection and treatment of disease that never would have become clinically significant during a person's lifetime, and psychological distress.

Cancer screening research is subject to three main types of bias: lead time, length, and selection biases. These biases can make a test appear to be effective when it actually is not. Lead-time bias occurs when screening results in earlier identification without altering the time to death. Thus, the person spends more time as a patient, but the course of the disease is basically unaltered.

Length bias occurs when screening increases the number of identified clinically slowly progressive or nonprogressive diseases that would never have become a symptomatic problem. Screening for prostate cancer is affected by length bias. Increased levels of prostate-specific antigen can detect cancers that may never cause the patient's death. This leads to overdiagnosis, or the detection of "disease" that is of no consequence, also called *pseudodisease*.

Selection bias is based on the observation that people willing to be screened for cancer may not reflect the population as a whole. Volunteers may be more health conscious or have other personal habits that favorably influence prognosis. Thus, their outcome from screening may be better than what would be seen in a random population.

Controlled prospective randomized trials are the only method of documenting the value of screening while effectively eliminating these sources of bias. Study populations must be followed for many years to document the cancer cause-specific survival advantage, if any, for the screened group. For instance, no RCTs have been done that support screening for cervical cancer, and data that support screening individuals ≥70 years old for colorectal or breast cancer are limited.

Breast Cancer

Because the mammography screening trials did not include women >74 years old, it is unknown whether screening mammography helps women ≥75 years old live longer. The USPSTF states that there is insufficient evidence on whether to screen women ≥75 years old. The AGS recommends screening mammography every 1–2 years for women with ≥5 years remaining life expectancy up until age 85 and for women >85 years old with excellent health or functional status, or for patients who feel strongly that mammography will benefit them. The recommendations are based on 5-year remaining life expectancy, because cancer-specific survival did not significantly differ between the screened and unscreened groups in RCTs until at least 5 years from enrollment (SOE=A). The risk of finding clinically insignificant disease increases as women age. To help determine who should be screened for breast cancer among the oldest populations, investigators have divided the U.S. population into 5-year age categories and into quartiles of life expectancy and then examined the number needed to screen (NNS) for at least one person to benefit in each age and life expectancy category. Although no threshold NNS has been defined, the higher the NNS, the less chance a screening test will benefit a patient and the greater chance the test may cause harm. The NNS with mammography ranges from 176 for women 75–79 years old in the top quartile of remaining life expectancy to 1,361 for those in the lowest quartile of remaining life expectancy. As for breast self-examination (BSE) and clinical breast examinations (CBEs), two large RCTs of women of all ages found no benefit of BSE compared with no breast cancer screening, and no trials have compared CBE alone to no screening. The AGS recommends that CBEs be performed periodically and neither endorses nor discourages BSEs. Similarly, the USPSTF found insufficient evidence to recommend for or against CBEs and recommends against teaching BSE, because BSE may lead to unnecessary biopsies and is not associated with a survival benefit (SOE=B).

Colon Cancer

Adenomatous polyps develop in 30%–50% of Americans >50 years old; 1%–10% of these polyps will progress to cancer in 5–10 years. Fortunately, several tests are considered effective for colon cancer screening among adults 50–75 years old, including colonoscopy every 10 years, home-based high-sensitivity fecal occult blood tests (FOBT) annually, and flexible sigmoidoscopy every 5 years with high-sensitivity FOBTs every 3 years. Although air-contrast barium enemas every 5 years were previously considered for screening, this test has not been subject to screening trials, has lower sensitivity than other screening strategies, and is thus not commonly used. Colonoscopy is the most sensitive and cost-effective screening test for colon cancer and has specificity similar to that of flexible sigmoidoscopy. Serious complications (eg, major bleeding, perforation, death) from colonoscopy occur in 25 per 10,000 procedures and are higher for older adults. The likelihood that detection of adenomas and early intervention will yield a mortality benefit declines after age 75 because of slower growth of an adenoma into invasive cancer and competing risks of mortality. Also, before screening older adults with FOBT, clinicians should be sure to ask if the patient is willing to consider colonoscopy, because one study found that 58% of veterans ≥70 years old did not receive a complete colon evaluation within 1 year after a positive FOBT. In 43% of these cases, there was a lack of acknowledgement of the positive FOBT, 26% refused colonoscopy, 10% were in poor health, and the others had scheduling difficulties or difficulties with the prep. Decisions about first-time screening after age

Table 10.1—Preventive Health Measures Available for Older Adults and Recommended Use

Procedure	Robust (≥5 years remaining life expectancy)	Frail (<5 years remaining life expectancy)	Moderate dementia (2–10 years remaining life expectancy)	End of life (<2 years remaining life expectancy)	SOE	Cost-effectiveness
Cancer screening						
Mammography	Every 2 years	Not recommended	Consider	Not recommended	A/C[a]	Somewhat cost-effective for women <80 years old, may be cost-effective for women ≥80 years old in top quartile of life expectancy.
Pap smear	May stop after age 65	Not recommended	Not recommended	Not recommended	B	Cost-effective to stop
Prostate-specific antigen	Discuss pros/cons if life expectancy >10 years, may stop at age 75	Not recommended	Not recommended	Not recommended	B	Uncertain
Colon cancer screening					A/C[b]	Cost-effective
Fecal occult blood test	Yearly, may stop at age 75	Not recommended	Not recommended	Not recommended		
Colonoscopy	Every 10 years, may stop at age 75	Not recommended	Not recommended	Not recommended		
Other screening tests						
DEXA screening for osteoporosis	At least once after age 65, or age 60 if high risk	Consider	Not recommended	Not recommended	A	Cost-effective
Blood glucose	Screen those with sustained blood pressures >135/80 mmHg or when results would affect cardiovascular disease prevention (lipids, aspirin use)[c]	Not recommended	Not recommended	Not recommended		Uncertain
Cholesterol screening	Consider for those with additional risk factors[d]	Not recommended	Not recommended	Not recommended	C	Uncertain
Ultrasonography for abdominal aortic aneurysm	Once for men 65–75 years old who ever smoked	Not recommended	Not recommended	Not recommended	A	Cost-effective
Thyrotropin	Every 2–5 years	Every 2–5 years	Every 3 years	Consider	C	Uncertain
HIV	Annually for those at high risk	Annually for those at high risk	Annually for those at high risk	Not recommended	A	Cost-effective
Blood pressure	Consider each visit	Consider each visit	Consider each visit	Consider each visit	A	Uncertain
Height	Once a year	Once a year	Not recommended	Not recommended	C	Uncertain
Weight	Each visit	Each visit	Each visit	Each visit	C	Uncertain
Immunizations						
Influenza	Annually	Annually	Annually	Annually	A	Cost-effective
Pneumococcal	Once after age 65[e]	Once after age 65[e]	Once after age 65[e]	Once after age 65[e]	A	Cost-effective
Tetanus	Booster every 10 years	Booster every 10 years	Booster every 10 years	Booster every 10 years	C	Cost-effective (a single booster at age 65)
Herpes zoster	Once after age 60	Once after age 60	Once after age 60	Once after age 60	A	Uncertain

Healthy lifestyle counseling						
Smoking cessation	Every visit	Every visit	Discuss with caregiver	Not recommended	A	Telephone quit lines and counseling are cost-effective.
Exercise	Annually	Annually	Consider annually	Consider	C	Uncertain
Alcohol misuse	Annually	Annually	Annually	Recommended initially, then if symptomatic	A	Screening and brief behavioral counseling interventions for alcohol abuse are cost-effective.
Driving assessment	Consider	Consider	Routinely	Consider	A	Uncertain
Sexual function	Annually	Annually	Consider annually	Not recommended	D	Uncertain
Geriatric health issues						
Urinary incontinence screening	Annually	Annually	Annually	Annually	C	Uncertain
Visual acuity testing	Consider annually	Consider annually	Consider annually	Not recommended	C	Population screening is not cost-effective; however, targeted screening of high-risk groups may be.
Hearing impairment screening	Consider annually	Consider annually	Consider annually	Not recommended	C	A simple systematic screen, using an audiometric screening instrument, may be cost-effective for those 55–74 years old.
Cognitive impairment screening	If symptomatic	If symptomatic	If symptomatic	If symptomatic	C	Uncertain
Gait and balance screening	Annually	Annually	Annually	Annually	C	Uncertain
Depression screening	Annually	Annually	Annually	Annually	C	Uncertain
Falls risk assessment	Annually	Annually	Annually	Annually	C	Uncertain
Advance directives completion	Complete and update as needed	Complete and update as needed	Complete and update as needed	Complete and update as needed	C	Uncertain
Chemoprevention						
Aspirin	See below[f]	See below[f]	See below[f]	See below[f]	A	
Calcium	Recommended[g]	Recommended[g]	Recommended[g]	Recommended[g]	A	
Vitamin D	Recommended[g]	Recommended[g]	Recommended[g]	Recommended[g]	A	
Multivitamin	Consider	Consider	Consider	Consider	D	
Hormone therapy (women)	Not recommended	Not recommended	Not recommended	Not recommended	A	

SOURCE: Adapted with permission from Flaherty JH, Morley JE, Murphy DJ, et al. The development of outpatient clinical glidepaths. *J Am Geriatr Soc*. 2002;50(11):1886–1901.

NOTE: FOBT = fecal occult blood test

[a] A for women up to age 74, C otherwise

[b] A for robust category, C otherwise

[c] Optimal screening interval is unknown, possibly every 3 years

[d] Examples: smoking, diabetes, hypertension

[e] If vaccinated before age 65, may vaccinate once 5 or more years later

[f] *Men*: 45–79 years old when benefit from myocardial infarction reduction outweighs risk of GI hemorrhage; coronary heart disease risk estimation tool: http://cvdrisk.nhlbi.nih.gov/calculator.asp (accessed Oct 2013)
Women: 55–79 years old when benefit from ischemic stroke reduction outweighs risk of GI hemorrhage; stroke risk estimation tool: http://www.westernstroke.org/index.php? (accessed Oct 2013)
For men and women ≥80 years old: insufficient data for recommendation

[g] If there are no contraindications

[h] Cost-effectiveness is the ratio of costs of a test/procedure compared with the benefits of the test/procedure. It is expressed as the cost per year of life saved or the cost per quality-adjusted-life-year saved. Less than $50,000 per life-year gained is considered cost-effective.

75 need to be made in the context of patient health. The USPSTF recommends against routinely screening adults ≥75 years old and against ever screening adults ≥85 years old because the risks outweigh the benefits. The American College of Physicians recommends against screening adults >75 years old or with life expectancy of <10 years. These recommendations do not apply to adults who have had previous adenomas on colonoscopy and are undergoing surveillance.

Cervical Cancer

Guidelines recommend stopping cervical cancer screening for women 65–70 years old who have been previously screened and are not otherwise at high risk of cervical cancer. These recommendations are based on evidence that shows that the incidence of high-grade cervical lesions significantly declines after middle age (SOE=A) and that the risk of false-positive tests resulting in invasive procedures is increased. Also, older women who have undergone total hysterectomy (no cervical tissue remaining) for a benign indication are not at risk of cervical cancer and should not be screened (SOE=A). An older woman of any age who has never had a Pap smear should be screened with at least two Pap smears 1 year apart. Risk factors for the development of cervical cancer (eg, new sexual partners) should be assessed on an ongoing basis and taken into consideration when deciding how often and for how long to screen older women for the development of cervical cancer.

Prostate Cancer

Two large RCTs have evaluated the effectiveness of measuring prostate-specific antigen (PSA) levels for prostate cancer screening. The Prostate, Lung, Colorectal, and Ovarian Cancer Screening Trial was a multisite U.S. trial that included men 55–74 years old without a history of prostate, colon, or lung cancer. Men randomized to the intervention were screened annually with PSA for 6 years and a digital rectal examination for 4 years. Because men in the control group received standard care, there was high contamination of the controls (approximately 50% of the controls underwent PSA screening compared with 85% of those in the intervention group), which may explain why no mortality benefit was found for PSA screening after 7–10 years follow-up. The European Randomized Study of Screening for Prostate Cancer (ERSCP) trial randomized men 50–74 years old to PSA screening every 2–4 years. In this study, the control group did not receive PSA screening. The ERSCP trial found a 20% reduction in prostate cancer mortality at 9 years for men 55–69 years old in the intervention group but no mortality benefit for men ≥70 years old and no overall mortality benefit for men of any age. The ERSCP trial concluded that 1,410 men 55–69 years old would need to be screened and 48 treated to prevent 1 prostate cancer death. However, men who were screened in this trial were more likely to be treated with radical prostatectomy than those who were not screened, which may explain the mortality benefit found. Both trials documented detection of numerous clinically insignificant tumors. The American Cancer Society and American Urological Society recommend that clinicians discuss the potential benefits of PSA screening (modest reduction of morbidity and mortality from prostate cancer) and the possible harms (false-positive results, unnecessary biopsies, overdiagnosis/overtreatment, and possible complications of treatment) among men ≥50 years old with at least 10 years life expectancy. The updated USPSTF guidelines now recommend against PSA-based screening for prostate cancer regardless of a man's age. See "Prostate Disease," p 437, for more discussion of prostate cancer screening.

Other Cancers

The USPSTF states that there is insufficient evidence to recommend whole-body skin examination by a primary care clinician for the early detection of skin cancer. Also, screening for ovarian cancer with CA-125 and transvaginal ultrasound did not reduce ovarian cancer mortality in a large RCT of women 55–74 years old at average risk.

OTHER SCREENING TESTS

Thyroid Disease

Because of the low cost of screening, the increasing risk of subclinical and clinical hyperthyroidism and hypothyroidism with age, and the low risks of treatment (particularly for hypothyroidism), screening older adults for thyroid dysfunction by measurement of thyroid-stimulating hormone every 2–5 years is recommended by some clinical experts. Screening those ≥60 years old in the clinical setting detects previously unsuspected hyperthyroidism in 0.1%–0.9% and hypothyroidism in 0.7%–2.1%. However, the USPSTF states there is insufficient evidence to recommend for or against screening for thyroid disease in high-risk patients, including older adults. Instead, the USPSTF states that clinicians should remain alert for subtle or nonspecific symptoms of thyroid dysfunction when examining older patients and maintain a low threshold for diagnostic evaluation of thyroid function.

Hypertension

Strong indirect evidence supports screening for hypertension. Randomized trials have confirmed that treatment of isolated systolic hypertension in patients >60 years old with pharmacologic therapy reduces the risk of stroke, coronary disease, and total mortality (SOE=A). In a trial reported in 2008, treatment of hypertension among adults ≥80 years old also reduced the risk of these end points. Evidence is lacking to recommend an optimal interval for screening adults for hypertension, and recommendations range from as frequently as each visit to biennially (for those with blood pressures less than 120/80 mmHg). Because of the variability in individual blood pressure measurements, it is recommended that hypertension be diagnosed only after ≥2 increased readings are obtained on at least 2 visits over a period of a week to several weeks.

Diabetes

No RCT of screening for diabetes has been performed, and the magnitude of benefit of initiating tight glycemic control during the preclinical phase of diabetes is unknown. In one RCT, intensive lifestyle modification in people with prediabetes delayed progression to clinical diabetes, but it is unknown whether early treatment affects micro- or macrovascular outcomes of diabetes or decreases mortality. Individuals with hypertension may benefit from knowing whether or not they have diabetes, because blood pressure targets are lower for diabetics than for nondiabetic individuals. The USPSTF recommends screening for type 2 diabetes in asymptomatic adults with sustained blood pressures of 135/80 mmHg (treated or untreated). Screening may also be considered when knowledge of diabetes status would help inform decisions about coronary heart disease preventive strategies (including consideration of lipid-lowering agents or aspirin). Three tests have been used to screen for diabetes: fasting plasma glucose (two fasting plasma glucose measurements of ≥126 mg/dL on two separate occasions), 2-hour post-load plasma glucose, and hemoglobin A_{1c} (≥6.5%). The hemoglobin A_{1c} assay is considered the new standard test, because it measures chronic glycemic levels.

Abdominal Aortic Aneurysm (AAA)

AAAs are found in 4%–8% of older men and in <2% of older women. Although AAAs may be asymptomatic for years, as many as one in three eventually rupture. In a meta-analysis, screening men 65–75 years old and surgical repair of those with AAAs ≥5.5 cm was associated with a significant reduction in AAA-related mortality (odds ratio 0.6 [0.5–0.7]) but no significant difference in all-cause mortality (SOE=A). Because the prevalence of AAAs was very low among men who never smoked, and because screening and early treatment are associated with significant harms (increased number of surgeries with associated clinically significant morbidity and mortality), the USPSTF concluded that the balance between the benefits and harms of screening for AAAs was too close to make a general recommendation; however, the USPSTF does recommend screening men 65–75 years old who have ever smoked. No significant reduction in AAA-related mortality was found among women, and screening is not recommended.

Osteoporosis

Four of every ten white U.S. women ≥50 years old will eventually experience a hip, spine, or wrist fracture. Over half of women ≥80 years old have osteoporosis (T score less than or equal to –2.5). No clinical trials have evaluated the effectiveness of screening older women for osteoporosis. However, age-based screening is supported by prevalence data. The NNS to prevent one hip fracture ranges from 731 for women 65–69 years old to 143 for women 75–79 years old. Routine screening (ie, measurement of bone mineral density through dual x-ray absorptiometry) is recommended by the USPSTF for all women ≥65 years old and for women ≥60 years old at high risk. An appropriate interval for screening has not been determined, but Medicare will pay for bone density testing every 2 years. When to stop screening is also a matter of controversy. Quality indicators recommend offering least burdensome treatment to vulnerable older women with >2 years life expectancy.

The USPSTF concludes that the current evidence is insufficient to assess the balance of benefits and harms of screening for osteoporosis in men. However, screening men ≥65 years old with a prior clinical fracture and all men ≥80 years old has been shown to be cost-effective, and several organizations recommend that clinicians assess older men, such as those undergoing androgen therapy, for osteoporosis risk.

Hyperlipidemia

Data are limited on the benefits of cholesterol-lowering medications for primary prevention of cardiovascular disease among adults >70 years old. However, because older adults generally are at higher absolute risk of cardiovascular events, lipid-lowering therapy is likely to be effective as long as remaining life expectancy is sufficient to allow the benefits of therapy to be realized (at least 5–7 years in high-risk patients). Although there is no agreed-upon life expectancy at which to stop screening for hyperlipidemia, most of the RCTs that evaluated statins for primary prevention showed that statins reduced cardiovascular events after 5 years in middle-aged adults. The PROSPER trial showed that pravastatin reduced cardiovascular events after 3 years in adults aged 70–82 years at high risk (SOE=A). The preferred screening tests for dyslipidemia are total cholesterol and HDL-C on nonfasting or fasting blood samples. Abnormal screening test results (HDL-C <40 mg/dL in men and <50 mg/dL in women) should be confirmed by a repeated sample on a separate occasion, and the average of both results used for risk assessment. The addition of LDL-C provides comparable information to the total cholesterol, but measuring LDL-C requires a fasting sample and is more expensive. Direct LDL-C testing, which does not require a fasting sample measurement, is available; however, calculated LDL is the validated measurement used in trials for risk assessment and treatment decisions. The optimal interval for screening is uncertain. Expert panels recommend every 5 years, with shorter intervals for people who have lipid levels close to warranting therapy, and longer intervals for those not at increased risk who have had repeatedly normal lipid levels. Repeated screenings may be less important in older adults, because lipid levels are less likely to increase after age 65.

HEALTHY LIFESTYLE COUNSELING

Physical Activity

Physical inactivity is recognized as a risk factor for many diseases (eg, coronary artery disease, diabetes, and obesity). Increasing physical activity in sedentary older adults reduces morbidity and mortality and improves psychological health, promotes functional independence, and prevents falls. Almost all older adults can engage safely in a program of moderate physical activity (such as walking) or lifestyle modification, without special screening. Stress testing is recommended for any older adult who intends to begin a vigorous exercise program (eg, strenuous cycling, jogging). Clinicians are encouraged to counsel patients about the importance of exercise, and consider patient-specific goals and barriers for exercise and expand on patients' current exercise habits. Exercise for older adults should include endurance (eg, walking, cycling), strengthening (eg, weight training), flexibility (eg, stretching), and balance training (eg, Tai Chi, dance). The exercise prescription should address the type, frequency, duration, and intensity of physical activity for each fitness component. See "Physical Activity," p 64.

Alcohol Misuse

Approximately half of the population ≥65 years old drinks alcohol, and many may experience health risks from consuming alcohol or from the combination of alcohol use with medications; approximately 2%–4% have abuse or dependence. Conversely, light to moderate alcohol consumption in middle-aged or older adults has been associated with some health benefits, such as reduced risk for coronary heart disease. Moderate drinking is defined as 1 drink or less per day for adults >65 years old.

The AGS recommends that all older adults ≥65 years old be asked annually about their alcohol use to detect abuse. Those who report alcohol use in the past year should be given the CAGE (ie, Cut down, Annoy, Guilt, Eye-opener) questionnaire or the Alcohol Use Disorders Identification Test (AUDIT), which performs better than the CAGE questionnaire, especially in women (SOE=A). Behavioral counseling interventions should be performed to reduce alcohol misuse (The "5 A's" framework may be useful: assess, advise, agree on goals, assist, and arrange follow-up). See "Addictions," p 336.

Smoking Cessation

Smoking cessation at any age decreases rates of COPD, many cancers, and coronary artery disease. Clinicians should ask all adults about tobacco use. If an adult uses tobacco, he or she should be counseled to quit. Once he or she is ready to quit, there should be documentation of a quit date, discussion of therapies to aid cessation, and follow-up in person or by phone within 3–7 days of the quit date and monthly for the first 3 months (SOE=A). See "Addictions," p 336.

Sexual Dysfunction and Sexually Transmitted Infections

Increasingly, Americans ≥50 years old are afflicted with sexually transmitted infections (STIs) and human immunodeficiency virus (HIV). Nationally, approximately 20% of patients with HIV are >50 years old. The CDC recommends routine screening of adults up to age 64 if the prevalence of undiagnosed HIV infection in the patient population is ≥0.1%. A recent cost-effective analysis found that one-time HIV screening is cost-effective for patients age 65–75 years old (<$60,000 per quality-adjusted life year gained) if the tested population has an HIV prevalence ≥0.1%, if the screened patient has a partner at risk, and counseling is streamlined (abbreviated pre-test counseling).

Although the prevalence of sexual activity declines with age (73% among adults 57–64 years old versus 26% among adults 75–85 years old) and is significantly less common among women than men, many older adults are sexually active. The USPSTF recommends high-intensity behavioral counseling to prevent STI for all sexually active adults at increased risk of STIs.

Geriatric Health Issues

Although there are little data examining the effectiveness of screening or counseling about geriatric health issues, expert panels generally recommend clinicians screen for these conditions annually. A comprehensive geriatric assessment (CGA) is recommended for frail older adults new to a primary care practice to reduce their risk of functional decline. The elements of a CGA include assessment of medications, cognitive status, functional status, nutritional status, hearing, vision, affect, social support, gait, and balance. CGA has been associated with improvements in general well-being, life satisfaction, instrumental activities of daily living, and fewer clinic visits (SOE=A). While the benefits of cancer screening tests may not be achieved for 5–10 years, the benefits of diagnosing and treating older patients with geriatric health issues can be immediate. Therefore, screening for these conditions should be of high priority in frail older adults with limited life expectancy. See "Assessment," p 48; "Outpatient Care Systems," p 173; and "Hospital Care," p 130.

Falls

Approximately 30% of noninstitutionalized older adults fall each year, and the annual incidence of falls approaches 50% in those >80 years old. Extrinsic factors that contribute to falls include poor lighting, obtrusive furniture, inadequate footwear, slippery floors, loose floor coverings, and bathrooms without handrails or grab bars. A comprehensive risk assessment for falls incorporates a review of all potential intrinsic and extrinsic factors, as well as a focused physical examination. Certain primary-care based interventions (eg, exercise and physical therapy, vitamin D supplementation) have been shown to reduce falling among community-dwelling older adults. See "Falls," p 234.

Incontinence

Incontinence is estimated to affect 30%–60% of older adults. Continence problems, which have major social and emotional consequences, are frequently treatable, but only 30%–45% of women with incontinence seek care. Because of the high prevalence of undiagnosed incontinence, older women should be specifically asked about urinary incontinence as part of a review of systems, particularly those who have had children, who have comorbid conditions associated with increased risk of urinary incontinence (ie, diabetes, neurologic disease, obesity), and who are >65 years old. The following screening questions have been suggested: Do you ever leak urine when you don't want to? Do you ever leak urine when you cough, laugh, or exercise? Do you ever leak urine on the way to the bathroom? Do you ever use pads, tissue, or cloth in your underwear to catch urine? See "Urinary Incontinence," p 220.

Cognitive Status

The USPSTF concluded that evidence is insufficient to recommend screening older adults for dementia. The AGS does not recommend routine screening but does recommend testing older adults with mild cognitive impairment for dementia because of their increased risk of developing the disease. Others recommend screening older adults on their initial visit, with repeated testing only if patients become symptomatic. Two of the more commonly used screening tools are the Mini–Mental State Exam and the Mini-Cog (clock drawing test combined with a three-item recall test). Scoring of the Mini–Mental State Exam must be adjusted for older members of minority groups and individuals with educational levels below the eighth grade. The Mini-Cog compares favorably in sensitivity and specificity for dementia, takes less time to administer, and is an effective tool for identifying unrecognized cognitive impairment in the primary care of older adults even from ethnolinguistically diverse populations. (See "Dementia," p 256.)

Depression

Studies report a 1%–2% prevalence of a major depressive disorder, 2% prevalence of dysthymia, and 13%–27% prevalence of subsyndromal depression among community-dwelling older adults. However, depression is often missed by primary care providers. The USPSTF recommends that clinicians screen adults for depression as long as they work in practice settings equipped to treat and follow patients with this disease. The Geriatric Depression Scale, the one-question screen "Do you often feel sad or depressed?", or 2 simple questions about mood and anhedonia ("Over the past 2 weeks, have you felt down, depressed, or hopeless?"and "Over the past 2 weeks, have you felt little interest or pleasure in doing things?") are effective screening tools. See "Depression and Other Mood Disorders," p 308.

Vision

The 2002 National Health and Nutrition Examination Survey estimated that 8.8% of adults ≥60 years old had impaired visual acuity (best-corrected vision of 20/40 or worse). The most common causes are presbyopia, cataracts, glaucoma, diabetic retinopathy, and age-related macular degeneration. Data from three RCTs show that screening for vision impairment in older adults in primary care settings is not associated with improved visual or other clinical outcomes. Based on these data, the USPSTF found insufficient evidence to recommend for or against visual acuity screening by primary care clinicians, and Medicare does not cover routine eye examinations. Medicare does cover annual glaucoma screening for those at high risk, although the USPSTF found insufficient evidence to recommend screening adults for glaucoma. See "Visual Impairment," p 183.

Hearing

The prevalence of hearing loss is 20%-40% in adults ≥50 years old and more than 80% for those ≥80 years old. Causes of hearing loss in older adults include presbycusis, genetic factors, exposure to loud noises or ototoxic agents, history of ear infections, and presence of systemic diseases (eg, diabetes). Although one large (N=2,305) randomized trial found that screening for hearing loss was associated with increased hearing aid use at 1 year, screening was not associated with improvement in hearing-related function.

While pure-tone audiometry is the gold standard for screening hearing, a whispered voice test at 2 feet has a positive predictive value of approximately 75%. See "Hearing Impairment," p 192.

Nutrition

The weight of older adults should be obtained each visit, and height measured annually and BMI (in kg/m^2) calculated. The USPSTF recommends that obese (BMI ≥30) adults be offered intensive counseling and behavioral interventions to promote sustained weight loss. In a 1-year, randomized, controlled trial involving obese older adults, weight loss plus exercise improved physical function and ameliorated frailty more than either weight loss or exercise alone (SOE=A). On the other end of the spectrum, malnutrition and undernutrition are common yet frequently unidentified problems in the geriatric population; 15% of older outpatients are malnourished. Nutritional health screens for use in primary care are currently being evaluated but include questions on meal frequency, unintentional weight loss, dental health, alcohol intake, money for food, and on the ability to shop, cook, and feed oneself. See "Malnutrition," p 209.

Mistreatment of Older Adults

Estimates of mistreatment of older adults range from 3% to 8%. Older adults who present with contusions, burns, bite marks, genital or rectal trauma, pressure ulcers, or BMI ≤17.5 with no clinical explanation should be asked about possible mistreatment or referred to social work for assessment. Instruments to test for abuse (eg, the Caregiver Abuse Screen) have not yet been tested in the primary care setting. See "Mistreatment of Older Adults," p 97.

Safety and Preventing Injury

Older adults should be advised to check their smoke detectors and carbon monoxide detectors, and to not set their hot water heaters >120°F–125°F. Because older adults do not adjust as well to sudden changes in temperature (sometimes due to illness or medicines that impair the body's ability to regulate its temperature), it is important to remind older adults to take precautions against heat stroke. Recommendations include drinking cool/nonalcoholic beverages, resting, taking a cool bath or shower, seeking an air-conditioned environment, and wearing lightweight clothing when the weather is hot.

In addition, older adults should be encouraged to wear seat belts and to undergo regular driving tests. One study found that 75% of adults 75–84 years old, and 70% of adults ≥85 years old were current drivers. Drivers >75 years old have more traffic violations and nonfatal collisions than younger drivers, and some states are considering legislation that would tighten license renewal requirements for older drivers. However, older adults who are forced to stop driving rely more on their families, reduce their social activities, and often become depressed. There is not currently one effective, easily administered test (or series of tests) to evaluate driving competence. However, driving refresher courses and on-the-road evaluations of older adults are available in many communities. Specific questions about driving should be included in the assessment of older adults (How did the older patient get to the primary care visit? How often and under what circumstances does he or she drive? Any traffic violations, accidents, or close calls within the past 6 months, 1 year, 2 years? Any episodes of getting lost while driving? Does the patient feel comfortable and want to continue driving?)

Older adults are also encouraged to develop an advance directive and determine a healthcare proxy.

IMMUNIZATIONS

Several immunizations are currently recommended for older adults. An annual influenza vaccination is recommended for adults ≥50 years old without contraindications (eg, egg allergy). Despite these recommendations, many older adults, especially those of racial and ethnic minorities, do not receive the influenza vaccine. Adults ≥65 years old may receive the standard or high-dose influenza vaccine; however, the intranasally administered live-attenuated influenza vaccine has not been approved for adults ≥50 years old. Although the high-dose influenza vaccine may result in increased immunogenicity, there is no stated preference for this vaccine over the standard vaccine, because there are no data demonstrating greater protection against influenza illness. Individuals ≥65 years old should also receive at least one pneumococcal vaccination in their lifetime. If the person was vaccinated before age 65, the vaccine should be repeated after 5 years. The Td (tetanus, diphtheria) booster is recommended every 10 years. Adults ≥65 years old may get the Tdap (tetanus, diphtheria, and acellular pertussis) instead. The Tdap is specifically recommended for adults ≥65 years old who have close contact with an infant <12 months old. Herpes zoster vaccine is recommended for those ≥60 years old. In an RCT, the vaccine reduced the incidence of post-herpetic neuralgia by 67% after 3 years in patients ≥60 years old (median age 69).

CHEMOPROPHYLAXIS

Aspirin

In a meta-analysis of prospective RCTs, aspirin therapy (dosage range 100 mg q48h to 500 mg q24h) reduced the risk of cardiovascular events by 12% and stroke by 17% among women with no significant effect on cardiovascular mortality. Among men, aspirin therapy reduced the risk of cardiovascular events by 14% and of myocardial infarction by 32% with no significant effects on stroke or cardiovascular mortality. Aspirin therapy increased the risk of bleeding by approximately 70% in both men and women. The USPSTF recommends aspirin for primary prevention for men with a 10-year risk of coronary heart disease of ≥4% for those aged 45–59, ≥9% for those aged 60–69, and ≥12% for those aged 70–79; and for women with a 10-year stroke risk of ≥3% for those aged 55–59, ≥8% for those aged 60–69, and ≥11% for those aged 70–79. See Table 10.1 for Web sites where individual patient data can be entered to calculate these risks. The ARR depends on the individual risks of cardiovascular disease and GI bleed for men and on individual risks of stroke and GI bleed for women. Links to calculate the ARR for an individual:

- http://www.uspreventiveservicestaskforce.org/uspstf09/aspirincvd/aspcvdrsf2.htm
- http://www.uspreventiveservicestaskforce.org/uspstf09/aspirincvd/aspcvdrsf4.htm

Calcium, Vitamin D, and Multivitamins

Calcium supplementation can prevent bone loss and mildly increase bone density (SOE=A). A meta-analysis of RCTs showed that calcium supplementation at 1,200 mg/d among postmenopausal women results in a 12% reduction in fractures of all types (SOE=A). Calcium supplements are best taken with meals and in divided doses (typically ≤500 mg at one time) to maximize absorption. However, foods should be the primary source of calcium intake. A rough method of estimating dietary calcium intake is to multiply the number of dairy servings consumed per day by 300 mg. Vitamin D can prevent bone loss and mildly increase bone density. Supplementation with 800 units of vitamin D reduces the risk of hip and nonvertebral fractures and falls, and has been shown to reduce all-cause mortality in a meta-analysis of RCTs (RR=0.93 [0.90–0.99]). Recommendations for vitamin D use range from 600 IU to 4,000 IU daily, and D_3 is the form generally recommended for long-term maintenance. While vitamin D at moderate to high doses may reduce risk of cardiovascular disease, calcium supplementation appears to have no effect. Supplementation with a multivitamin formulated at 100% recommended daily values can decrease the prevalence of suboptimal vitamin status in older adults. However, there are no RCTs demonstrating a beneficial effect of multivitamins on morbidity or mortality.

Hormone Therapy

Hormone therapy for chemoprophylaxis is not recommended, because the Women's Health Initiative Trial showed that it (ie, estrogen plus progesterone) increased the risk of ischemic stroke, coronary artery disease, venous thrombosis, pulmonary embolism, decline in cognitive function, and invasive breast cancer among older women.

COUNSELING ON CANCER SCREENING AND PREVENTIVE HEALTH

Delivery of preventive health services to older adults can be challenging for many reasons. First, many preventive health services are available, and primary care clinicians are encouraged to deliver or at least discuss most of these services. Second, there is little reimbursement for counseling about screening tests or geriatric health issues, and time during clinic visits often needs to be spent caring for older adults' acute or chronic medical conditions. Third, experts increasingly recommend that clinicians consider a patient's remaining life expectancy when deciding which screening tests to recommend; however, estimating remaining life expectancy may be difficult and discussing remaining life expectancy with patients may be uncomfortable for clinicians. Finally, many older adults suffer from concomitant disorders that encompass multiple risk factors; this presents a challenge to clinicians to synthesize the evidence and in turn make individual recommendations to patients for primary, secondary, and tertiary screening measures.

Fortunately, tools are available to help clinicians estimate patients' remaining life expectancy to guide screening decisions. One available prognostic index includes 11 questions (eg, history of diabetes, difficulty walking several blocks) that patients can answer during an office visit to help predict their risk of 5-year or 9-year mortality. In another framework, clinicians are first asked to estimate whether an individual patient is in the top quartile of health, the bottom quartile of health, or in average health, for his or her age group. Then, clinicians are referred to life expectancy tables stratified by age and health. Additional tools to help clinicians prognosticate are available at www.eprognosis.org.

When discussing cancer or other screening tests with older adults, clinicians should indicate whether any data suggest that the screening test improves older adults' quality or quantity of life. Clinicians should also discuss the risks of screening, including discomfort from undergoing the test itself, anxiety, potential complications from diagnostic procedures resulting from a false-positive test, false reassurance from a false-negative test, and overdiagnosis/diagnosis of tumors that are of no threat and that may result in overtreatment. Furthermore, clinicians may want to explain that overdiagnosis is thought to increase with age due to decreasing life expectancy, competing mortality risks, and slower-growing tumors among older adults. Patients should be asked how they view the potential benefits and harms of different screening tests, so that their values and preferences are considered in screening decisions. Health maintenance discussions among older adults with limited remaining life expectancies should focus on measures with benefits that are likely to be achieved in a short time frame (eg, counseling on home safety, falls prevention, immunizations).

Several studies have examined ways to improve health promotion for older adults in primary care but have found limited success. Recommendations include clinician education seminars, preventive health check lists, computer reminders, use of non-physician staff to screen for disease, and addressing preventive health topics at multiple visits. Medicare recently began covering wellness visits for those who have had Part B coverage for >12 months in addition to a "Welcome to Medicare" visit that must be completed within the first 6 months of enrollment. These visits offer clinicians the opportunity to discuss the pros and cons of many screening tests and health promotion with older adults and to offer appropriate preventive health measures. Patient decision aids have been shown to improve knowledge and satisfaction with screening decisions and are currently being tested to help older adults with decision-making around cancer screening.

REFERENCES

- Buys SS, Partridge E, Black A, et al. Effect of screening on ovarian cancer mortality: The prostate, lung, colorectal, and ovarian (PLCO) cancer screening randomized controlled trial. *JAMA*. 2011;305(22):2295–2203.
- Hall KT, Chun DA. *General Screening Recommendations for Chronic Disease and Risk Factors for Older Adults*. The Hartford Institute for Geriatric Nursing, NYU. 2010. http://consultgerirn.org/uploads/File/trythis/try_this_27.pdf
- Leipzig R. *Preventive Healthcare for Older Adults*. Agency for Healthcare Research and Quality. Rockville, MD. Dec 2010. http://www.ahrq.gov/news/events/conference/2010/leipzig/index.html
- Schonberg MA, Davis RB, McCarthy EP, et al. Index to predict 5-year mortality of community-dwelling adults aged 65 and older using data from the national health interview survey. *J Gen Intern Med*. 2009;24(10):1115–1121.

CHAPTER 11—PHARMACOTHERAPY

KEY POINTS

- Risk factors associated with inappropriate prescribing and overprescribing include having more than one prescriber, poor record keeping, and using more than one pharmacy.
- Evidence suggests that underprescribing of indicated medications for older adults is a bigger problem than the prescribing of inappropriate medications.
- Cardiovascular drugs, diuretics, NSAIDs, hypoglycemics, second-generation antipsychotics, anticoagulants, and antiplatelet agents are the drug classes most often associated with preventable adverse drug events.
- Age-associated changes in body composition, metabolism, and pharmacodynamics make benzodiazepine use by older adults especially hazardous.
- Collaboration with pharmacists and access to up-to-date drug information can help to minimize the total number of medications and dosages prescribed for individual patients and to avoid important drug-drug and drug-disease interactions.

Adults ≥65 years old are prescribed the highest proportion of medications in relation to their percentage of the U.S. population. Currently, approximately 13% of the U.S. population is ≥65 years old; this age group purchases 33% of all prescription drugs. These figures are expected to increase to 25% and 50%, respectively, by the year 2040.

Drugs are the most common treatment for acute and chronic diseases. They are also used to prevent many of the diseases and disorders experienced by older adults. Successful pharmacotherapy requires the correct medication at the correct dosage, for the correct disease or condition, for the correct patient. Unfortunately, achieving these goals is not simple or easy. Many other factors come into play, including the patient's other disease states, other medications, adherence, beliefs, functional status, physiologic changes due to aging and disease, and ability to afford the medication. The basic principle of prescribing for older patients—briefly, "start low, go slow"—is repeated often. However, even when this principle is adhered to, some patients will have negative outcomes from one or more of their medications.

Although the principles of pharmacotherapy have not changed significantly during the past 20 years, drug treatment has become much more complex. More medications are available every year, some with a new pharmacologic profile or mechanism of action. In addition, many available agents have expanded indications, some of which are approved by the FDA and some of which are off-label. Additional complicating factors include frequent changes in the managed-care formulary, scientific advances in the understanding of drug-drug interactions (eg, the cytochrome P-450 system), the change of many medications from prescription to nonprescription, and the boom in an unregulated third class of medications called nutriceuticals, ie, nutritional supplements, alternative medicines, and herbal preparations. Finally, very little information is available about the use of these unregulated medications in older adults—particularly, sick older patients on other medications.

AGE-ASSOCIATED CHANGES IN PHARMACOKINETICS

Pharmacokinetic studies define the time course of a drug and its metabolites throughout the body with respect to absorption, distribution, metabolism, and elimination. The effects of aging on each of these four parameters have been studied, with the resulting generalizations incorporated into the principles of prescribing for older adults.

Absorption

Aging does not affect the extent of drug absorption via the GI tract to any clinically significant degree, although the rate of absorption may be slowed. Consequently, the peak serum concentration of a drug in older patients may be lower and the time to reach it delayed, but the overall amount absorbed *(bioavailability)* does not differ in younger and older patients. Exceptions include drugs that undergo an extensive first-pass effect (eg, nitrates); they tend to have higher serum concentrations or increased bioavailability, because less drug is extracted by the liver as a consequence of decreased hepatic size and blood flow.

Factors that have a greater impact on drug absorption include the way a medication is taken, what it is taken with, and a patient's comorbid illnesses. For example, the absorption of many fluoroquinolones (eg, ciprofloxacin) is reduced when they are taken with divalent cations such as calcium, magnesium, and iron, which are found in antacids, sucralfate, dairy products, or vitamins. Enteral feedings interfere with the absorption of some drugs (eg, phenytoin). An increase in gastric pH from proton-pump inhibitors, H_2 antagonists, or antacids can increase the absorption of some drugs, such as nifedipine and amoxicillin, and decrease the absorption of other drugs, such as the imidazole antifungals, ampicillin, cyanocobalamin, and indinavir. Agents that promote or delay GI motility, such as stimulant laxatives and metoclopramide, can, in theory, affect a drug's absorption by increasing or decreasing the time spent in the segment of the GI tract necessary for dissolution or absorption. Another mechanism that can increase or decrease drug absorption is the inhibition or induction of enzymes in the GI tract (see the section on drug interactions, below).

Distribution

Distribution refers to the locations in the body a drug penetrates and the time required for the drug to reach those locations. Distribution is expressed as the volume of distribution (Vd), with units of volume (eg, liters) or volume per weight (eg, L/kg).

Age-associated changes in body composition can alter drug distribution. In older adults, drugs that are water soluble *(hydrophilic)* have a lower volume of distribution, because older adults have less body water and lean body mass. Examples include ethanol and lithium. Digoxin, which distributes and binds to skeletal muscle, has been reported to have a reduced volume of distribution in older adults because of their reduced muscle mass. Drugs that are fat soluble *(lipophilic)* have an increased volume of distribution in older adults because fat stores are greater in older than in younger people. Thus, in older adults, lipophilic drugs take longer to reach a steady-state concentration and longer to be eliminated from the body. Examples of fat-soluble drugs include diazepam, flurazepam, and trazodone.

The extent to which a drug is bound to plasma proteins also influences its volume of distribution. Albumin, the primary plasma protein to which drugs bind, is often decreased in older adults; thus, a higher proportion of drug is unbound (free) and pharmacologically active. Drugs that bind to albumin and that have an increased unbound fraction in older adults include ceftriaxone, diazepam, lorazepam, phenytoin, valproic acid, and warfarin. Normally, additional unbound drug is eliminated; however, age-related decreases in the organ systems of elimination can result in accumulation of unbound drug in the body. Phenytoin provides an example of the way an increase in unbound drug can lead to an unnecessary and potentially harmful dosage increase. A patient with a low serum albumin (≤3 g/dL) whose phenytoin dosage is increased because his or her total phenytoin concentration is subtherapeutic can develop symptoms and signs of phenytoin toxicity after a dosage increase, because the concentration of free phenytoin is increased.

Metabolism

The liver is the most common site of drug metabolism, but metabolic conversion also can occur in the intestinal wall, lungs, skin, kidneys, and other organs. Aging affects the liver by decreasing hepatic blood flow as well as by decreasing hepatic size and mass. Consequently, the metabolic clearance of drugs by the liver may be reduced in older adults. Drug clearance is also reduced with aging for drugs that are subject to the phase I pathways or reactions, which include hydroxylation, oxidation, dealkylation, and reduction. Most drugs metabolized through phase I pathways can be converted to metabolites of lesser, equal, or greater pharmacologic effect than the parent compound (eg, diazepam). Drugs metabolized through the phase II pathways are converted to inactive compounds through glucuronidation, conjugation, or acetylation (eg, lorazepam). Medications subject to phase II metabolism are generally preferred for older adults, because their metabolites are not active and do not accumulate.

Age and gender differences also have been reported. For example, oxazepam is metabolized faster in older men than in older women. The reason is unknown. Nefazodone concentrations have been reported to be 50% greater in older women, but no differences were found between older men and younger persons of either sex.

In drug metabolism, factors other than aging can exaggerate or override the effects of aging. For example, hepatic congestion due to heart failure decreases the metabolism of warfarin, resulting in an increased pharmacologic response. Smoking stimulates monooxygenase enzymes and increases the clearance of theophylline, even in older adults.

Elimination

Elimination refers to a drug's final route(s) of exit from the body. For most drugs, this involves elimination by the kidney as either the parent compound or as a metabolite or metabolites. Terms used to express elimination are a drug's *half-life* and its *clearance*.

A drug's half-life is the time it takes for its plasma or serum concentration to decline by 50% (eg, from 20 mcg/mL to 10 mcg/mL). Half-life is usually expressed in hours. Steady state is reached when the amount of drug entering the systemic circulation is equal to the amount being eliminated. For a drug administered on a regular basis, 95% of steady state in the body is achieved after five half-lives of the drug.

Clearance is usually expressed as volume per unit of time (eg, L/h or mL/min) and represents the volume of plasma or serum from which the drug is removed (ie, cleared) per unit of time. Clearance can also be expressed as volume per weight per unit of time (L/kg/h). Half-life and clearance can also refer to metabolic elimination.

The effects of aging have been studied to a greater extent on kidney function than on liver function. Glomerular filtration declines as a consequence of a decrease in renal size and blood flow and a decrease in functioning nephrons. On average, kidney function begins to decline when people reach their mid-30s, with an average decline of 6–12 mL/min/1.73 m^2 per decade. Follow-up studies (conducted in men only) over 10–15 years found three normally distributed groups: those whose creatinine clearance declined to the extent that it was clinically significant, those whose creatinine clearance declined to the extent that it was statistically but not clinically significant, and those whose creatinine clearance did not change. Renal tubular secretion also declines with age.

Serum creatinine is not an accurate reflection of creatinine clearance in older adults. Because of the age-related decline in lean muscle mass, production of creatinine is reduced in older adults. The decrease in glomerular filtration rate (GFR) counters the decreased production of creatinine, and serum creatinine stays within the normal range, not revealing the change in creatinine clearance.

The conservative approach in treating older adults is to calculate the appropriate dosage for renally eliminated medications as if the patient's kidney function actually has declined with aging. Measuring a patient's 24-hour creatinine clearance is the most accurate way to determine the appropriate dosage, but this is unrealistic because it requires an accurate 24-hour urine collection. An 8-hour urine collection time has been shown to be accurate but has not been widely accepted.

The Cockcroft-Gault equation can be used to initially estimate a patient's creatinine clearance (CrCl) (SOE=B in older adults for dosage adjustment):

$$\text{CrCl} = \frac{(140 - \text{age})(\text{weight in kg})(0.85 \text{ if female})}{72(\text{stable serum creatinine in mg/dL})}$$

Weight in kg: serum creatinine in mg/100 mL; 85% less in women

The equation is widely applied, but it has limitations. First, not all patients experience a significant age-related decline in renal function, and for them, the equation underestimates creatinine clearance. Second, for patients whose muscle mass is reduced beyond that of normal aging, the creatinine clearance is overestimated. This would apply to individuals whose serum creatinine is less than normal, ie, <0.7 mg/dL. It has been suggested that 1 mg/dL be substituted for a low serum creatinine. However, normalizing the serum creatinine has not been shown to be a precise estimate, and it generally underestimates the actual creatinine clearance.

Another method for estimating glomerular filtration rate (eGFR) is the Modification of Diet in Renal Disease (MDRD), which is endorsed by the National Kidney Foundation in its Kidney Disease Outcomes Quality Initiative (KDOQI) and the NIH National Kidney Disease Education Program for identifying and staging individuals with chronic kidney disease. The MDRD has not been validated in adults ≥70 years old or in racial or ethnic groups other than white and black Americans. A patient's eGFR value is reported when it is <60 mL/min/1.73 m^2. Because of the lower precision of the MDRD equation and creatinine assay variability, the eGFR should be reported only as "≥60 mL/min/1.73 m^2" for patients with normal renal function or Stage 1 or 2 chronic kidney disease. The routine appearance of eGFR on laboratory reports has created confusion about its use to adjust medication dosages, and it is not recommended by KDOQI for this purpose (SOE=A).

FDA-labeled dosing is based on the Cockcroft-Gault estimated CrCl and the drug's pharmacokinetic characteristics. Substituting eGFR for estimated CrCl can result in suboptimal dosing, especially in patients with Stage 2 chronic kidney disease as their GFR approaches 60 mL/min/1.73 m^2.

In cases in which the patient's kidney function may be impaired but estimates of function are uncertain, the clinician should consider the following:

- Avoid drugs that depend entirely on renal elimination and for which accumulation would result in toxicity (eg, imipenem).
- If the use of such an agent cannot be avoided, obtain an accurate measure of kidney function (eg, an 8- or 24-hour creatinine clearance).
- Monitor serum or plasma concentrations of the drug (eg, aminoglycosides).

AGE-ASSOCIATED CHANGES IN PHARMACODYNAMICS

The pharmacodynamic action of a drug—ie, its time course and intensity of pharmacologic effect—can change with increasing age. An excellent example of such pharmacodynamic changes in older adults has been demonstrated with the benzodiazepines. After a single dose of triazolam, older adults experience more sedation and lower performance on a psychomotor test than younger adults. These differences are attributed to pharmacokinetic changes, ie, to significantly higher plasma triazolam concentrations that are due to reduced clearance in older adults. However, a different pattern has been found for nitrazepam, an intermediate-acting benzodiazepine similar to lorazepam: the pharmacokinetics of nitrazepam were found to be no different in young and older individuals after a single 10-mg dose; yet, 12 hours and 36 hours after a 10-mg dose, older adults made significantly more mistakes on a psychomotor test than when they had taken placebo. Younger individuals did not demonstrate significant impairment at any time. In addition, even with short-term use, young older adults can experience impaired balance and posture after a single dose of a benzodiazepine (SOE=A).

It is uncertain whether the age-associated pharmacokinetic changes of morphine account for the increased level and prolonged duration of pain relief experienced by older adults. Morphine has a smaller volume of distribution, higher plasma concentrations, and longer clearance in older adults than in younger adults. Older adults experience pain relief at least equivalent to that experienced by younger patients at half the intramuscular dose, and the pain relief lasts longer. Thus, the dose or frequency, or both, of morphine given intramuscularly or by intravenous infusion should be lower, at least initially, in older adults.

Pharmacodynamic and pharmacokinetic changes, alone or together, generally result in an increased sensitivity to medications in older adults. In some patients, particularly those who are frail, the use of lower doses, longer intervals between doses, and longer periods between changes in dose are ways to successfully manage drug therapy and to decrease the chances of medication intolerance or toxicity. Disease- and drug-specific monitoring are also necessary to ensure a successful outcome.

Optimizing Prescribing

Optimizing drug therapy for older adults means achieving the balance between prescribing what is indicated to treat the patient's diseases and symptoms, while being consistent with the patient's goals. Overprescribing of drug therapies refers to the use of multiple medications coupled with a lack of appropriateness in medication selection, dosage, or use. In one survey, 40% of nursing-home residents had an order for at least one potentially inappropriate medication. Analyses of national medication use surveys in the ambulatory setting have consistently shown that >20% of older adults received at least one potentially inappropriate medication, with at least one potentially inappropriate medication prescribed at approximately 8% of office visits. Furthermore, nearly 4% of office visits and 10% of medical hospital admissions resulted in a prescription for one or more medications classified as "never" or "rarely appropriate" for older adults. Identification of a potentially inappropriate medication in a patient's regimen is a signal for additional prescribing problems with other medications not considered potentially inappropriate. The potential consequences of overprescribing include adverse drug events, drug-drug interactions, duplication of drug therapy, decreased quality of life, and unnecessary costs. Medications frequently deemed unnecessary based on lack of indication, lack of efficacy, or therapeutic duplication are often from the same medication classes as those considered inappropriate or overprescribed (Table 11.1). In studies in the U.S. Veterans Administration, 44% of veterans at hospital discharge and 57%–59% of outpatients had prescriptions for one or more unnecessary medications.

For factors associated with inappropriate prescribing or overprescribing, see Table 11.2. Simply limiting the

Table 11.1—Common Inappropriate/Overprescribed and Underprescribed Medications or Classes

Inappropriate/Overprescribed
Anti-infective agents
Anticholinergic agents
Urinary and GI antispasmodics
Antipsychotics
Benzodiazepines and nonbenzodiazepine hypnotics (eg, zolpidem, zaleplon, eszopiclone)
Digoxin >0.125 mg for heart failure
Dipyridamole
H_2-receptor antagonists
Fecal softeners
NSAIDs
Proton-pump inhibitors
Sedating antihistamines (H_1-receptor antagonists, eg, diphenhydramine)
Tricyclic antidepressants
Vitamins and minerals
Underprescribed
ACE inhibitors for patients with diabetes and proteinuria
Angiotensin-receptor blockers
Anticoagulants
Antihypertensives and diuretics as evidenced by uncontrolled hypertension
β-blockers for patients after myocardial infarction or with heart failure
Bronchodilators
Proton-pump inhibitors or misoprostol for GI protection from NSAIDs
Statins
Vitamin D and calcium for patients with or at risk of osteoporosis

Table 11.2—Factors Associated with Inappropriate Prescribing or Overprescribing

Patient Factors	
	Advanced age
	Female gender
	Lower educational level
	Rural residence
	Belief in using "a pill for every ill"
	Multiple health problems
	Use of multiple medications
	Use of multiple pharmacies
System Factors	
	Multiple prescribers for individual patient
	Poor record keeping
	Failure to review a patient's medication regimen at least annually

number of medications for a given patient is not always possible or desirable. For example, a patient with heart failure may be appropriately treated with three or four drugs: a diuretic, an ACE inhibitor, a β-blocker, and perhaps digoxin. If this patient has hyperlipidemia and diabetes mellitus, another two or three medications could be required. Hence, such a patient would be taking five to seven indicated medications for major medical conditions alone.

One source to identify potentially inappropriate medications has been the Beers criteria. In 2011, an interdisciplinary panel appointed by the American Geriatrics Society (AGS) updated the 2003 Beers criteria. The intent of the 2012 AGS Beers criteria is to improve drug selection and reduce exposure to potentially inappropriate medications in older adults. Recommendations are evidence based and appear in three categories: drugs to avoid, drugs to avoid in patients with specific diseases or syndromes because the drug can worsen the disease or syndrome, and drugs to use with caution. The AGS intends to update the Beers criteria annually. A detailed description of the 2012 AGS Beers criteria, including evidence tables, useful clinical tools, and patient education materials, is available at the AGS Web site (www.americangeriatrics.org).

The underprescribing of medications to older adults is also of concern. Underprescribing can result from an effort to avoid overprescribing, a complex medication regimen, or adverse events. It can also result from the thinking that older adults will not benefit from medications intended as primary or secondary prevention, or from aggressive management of chronic conditions, such as hypertension and diabetes mellitus. Underuse of medications was found in 64% of 125 veterans attending a veteran's outpatient clinic. Medications to treat cardiovascular conditions (including hypertension, anticoagulants,

Table 11.3—Risk Factors for Adverse Drug Events in Older Adults

- Age >85 years
- Low body weight or BMI
- Six or more concurrent chronic diagnoses
- An estimated CrCl <50 mL/min
- Nine or more medications
- Twelve or more doses of medications per day
- A prior adverse drug event

and lipid-lowering agents), GI conditions, diabetes, osteoporosis, and COPD were commonly omitted. For other medications often cited as underprescribed in older adults, see Table 11.1.

Investigators from the Assessing Care of Vulnerable Elders (ACOVE) project developed explicit medication quality indicators divided into four categories: prescribing indicated medications; avoiding inappropriate medications; education, continuity, and documentation; and medication monitoring. These indicators were applied to "vulnerable" older adults enrolled in two managed care organizations, and the results were reported as the percentage of eligible patients who met the indicator or "pass rate." The prescribing of indicated medications category had an overall pass rate of 50% (range 11%–94% for the 17 indicators); avoiding the prescription of inappropriate medications had an overall pass rate of 97% (range 79%–100% avoidance across the 9 indicators). The overall pass rate for education, continuity, and documentation indicators was 81% (range 10%–99% for the 8 indicators). The 9 indicators for medication monitoring had an overall pass rate of 64% (range 22%–80%). These results suggest that the prescribing of inappropriate medications is less of a problem than the underprescribing of indicated medications and the failure to monitor medications, document information about medications, maintain continuity, and educate patients.

ADVERSE DRUG EVENTS

An adverse drug event (ADE) is defined as an injury resulting from the use of a drug. Preventable ADEs are among the most serious consequences of inappropriate drug prescribing among older adults. An adverse drug reaction (ADR) is a type of ADE; it refers to harm that is directly caused by a drug at usual dosages. For a listing of risk factors for ADEs in older patients, see Table 11.3.

ADEs are estimated to be responsible for 5%–28% of acute geriatric medical admissions; the estimated annual incidence rate is 26 per 1,000 beds for hospitalized patients. One study estimated there were

Table 11.4—Common Adverse Drug Events of Selected Medications

Adverse Drug Event	Medications
Cardiovascular effects	
Decreased heart rate	Cholinesterase inhibitors, β-adrenergic blockers, diltiazem, verapamil, digoxin
Hypotension	Antihypertensives, diuretics, nitrates, phosphodiesterase type 5 inhibitors, α-blockers, tricyclic antidepressants, trazodone
CNS effects	
Delirium	Anticholinergic agents, antiparkinson agents, antidepressants, opioids, glucocorticoids, benzodiazepines, antihistamines (eg, diphenhydramine), drug withdrawal (eg, benzodiazepines, ethanol)
Depression	β-Adrenergic blockers, benzodiazepines, central-acting antihypertensives
Dizziness	SSRIs, cholinesterase inhibitors
Parkinsonism	Antipsychotics, metoclopramide
Sedation	Antidepressants, antipsychotics, antihistamines (eg, diphenhydramine), opioids, anticonvulsants, benzodiazepines
Falls	
	Benzodiazepines, antidepressants, antipsychotics, sedatives/hypnotics, anticonvulsants, opioids, diuretics, antihypertensives, anticholinergic agents, antiarrhythmics
GI effects	
Bleeding/ulceration	NSAIDs, aspirin, glucocorticoids, bisphosphonates, antiplatelet agents, anticoagulants (eg, warfarin, dabigatran, rivaroxaban)
Constipation	Opioids, iron- or calcium-containing antacids, calcium channel blockers, anticholinergic agents, cholestyramine
Diarrhea	Magnesium-containing antacids, SSRIs, cholinesterase inhibitors
Nausea/vomiting	Digoxin, cholinesterase inhibitors, bisphosphonates
Kidney or electrolyte effects	
Hyperkalemia	ACE inhibitors, angiotensin-receptor blockers, potassium supplements, potassium-sparing diuretics
Hypokalemia	Diuretics
Kidney impairment	NSAIDs, triamterene
SIADH/hyponatremia	Carbamazepine, SSRIs, diuretics
Urinary retention	Agents with anticholinergic properties, including inhaled agents in men with an enlarged prostate, opioids, calcium channel blockers, α-adrenergic agonists

nearly 100,000 emergency hospitalizations of older adults for ADEs annually in the United States. Adults ≥80 years old accounted for 48% of hospitalizations. Two-thirds of hospitalizations were attributed to warfarin, oral antiplatelet agents, insulin, and oral hypoglycemic drugs. The most common type of ADE was an unintentional overdose (67%). It has been estimated that in the nursing home, for every dollar spent on medications, $1.33 in healthcare resources is consumed in the treatment of drug-related morbidity and mortality. A cohort study of all long-term care residents in 18 nursing homes in Massachusetts demonstrated that ADEs are common and often preventable in nursing homes. During the 28,839 resident-months of observations, 546 ADEs were identified. Overall, 51% of these ADEs were judged to have been preventable. Most of the errors occurred at the ordering and monitoring stages. In a cohort study of residents of two long-term care facilities, the overall rate of ADEs was 9.8 per 100 resident-months. Second-generation antipsychotics, anticoagulants, and diuretics were the drug classes most frequently associated with ADEs.

In the ambulatory setting, the ADE rate has been reported to be 50.1 per 1,000 person-years, and the preventable ADE rate to be 13.8 per 1,000 person-years. Cardiovascular drugs, diuretics, NSAIDs, hypoglycemics, and anticoagulants are the drug classes found to be most often associated with preventable ADEs. Again, errors occurred most often at the time of prescribing or were related to inadequate monitoring. Most ADEs (≥95%) experienced by older adults are considered to be predictable. For examples of common ADRs experienced by older adults and the medications that frequently cause them, see Table 11.4.

A common pathway for ADEs and polypharmacy has been described as the "prescribing cascade." One form of this cascade occurs when a medication results in an ADE that is mistaken as a separate diagnosis and treated with more medications, which puts the patient at risk of additional ADEs and more medications. Examples that have been studied include metoclopramide-induced parkinsonism and the subsequent prescribing of antiparkinson medications, and calcium channel blockers that result in peripheral edema and the subsequent use of diuretics.

Table 11.5—Adverse Drug Interactions That Increase the Risk of Hospitalization

Combination	Risk
ACE inhibitor + potassium-sparing diuretic	Hyperkalemia
ACE inhibitor or ARB + SMX/TPM	Hyperkalemia
Benzodiazepine or zolpidem + variety of other medications	Hip fracture
Calcium channel blockers + erythromycin or clarithromycin	Hypotension and shock
Digoxin + erythromycin, clarithromycin, or azithromycin	Digoxin toxicity
Lithium + loop diuretics or ACE inhibitor	Lithium toxicity
Phenytoin + SMX/TMP	Phenytoin toxicity
Sulfonylureas + SMX/TMP, ciprofloxacin, levofloxacin, erythromycin, clarithromycin, azithromycin, and cephalexin	Hypoglycemia
Tamoxifen + paroxetine (other CYP2D6 inhibitors)	Prevention of converting tamoxifen to its active moiety, resulting in increased breast cancer–related deaths
Theophylline + ciprofloxacin	Theophylline toxicity
Warfarin + SMX/TMP, ciprofloxacin, levofloxacin, gatifloxacin, fluconazole, amoxicillin, and cephalexin	GI bleeding
Warfarin + NSAIDs	GI bleeding

SOURCE: Data from Hines L, Murphy JE. Potentially harmful drug-drug interactions in the elderly: a review. *Am J Geriatr Pharmacother*. 2011;9:364–377.
ACE = angiotensin converting enzyme, ARB = angiotensin receptor blocker, SMX/TMP = sulfamethoxazole/trimethoprim

Drug Interactions

A drug-drug interaction (DDI) is defined as the pharmacologic or clinical response to the administration of a drug combination that differs from that anticipated from the known effects of each of the two agents when given alone. DDIs are important because they may lead to ADEs. The likelihood of DDIs increases as the number of medications a patient is taking increases. Among prescription drugs, cardiovascular and psychotropic drugs are most commonly involved in DDIs. A positive correlation exists between the number of potential DDIs and the number of adverse events experienced by hospitalized older patients. The most common adverse events are neuropsychologic (primarily delirium), arterial hypotension, and acute kidney failure. For drug combinations that are reported to result in increased risk of hospitalization for older adults, see Table 11.5. Risk factors associated with DDIs include the use of multiple medications, receiving care from several prescribing clinicians, and using more than one pharmacy.

Drug interactions can take many forms. For example, absorption can be altered, drugs with similar or opposite pharmacologic effects can result in exaggerated or impaired effects, and drug metabolism can be inhibited or induced. Research focusing on the cytochrome P-450 system has proposed or studied numerous DDIs (in vivo or in vitro) involving the different P-450 isozymes. The effect of aging on the cytochrome P-450 system and the clinical implications for prescribing have not been completely determined. Cross-sectional data have shown that cytochrome P-450 content declines incrementally, once in the fourth decade and again after age 70. In vitro microsomal activity of cytochrome (CYP) 3A4 is not altered by aging, but in vivo age- and gender-related reductions in drug clearance have been found for CYP3A4 substrates erythromycin, prednisolone, verapamil, alprazolam, nifedipine, and diazepam. CYP3A4 accounts for 30% of the P-450 content in the liver and is also prominent in the intestinal tract. This isozyme is involved in the metabolism of >50% of medications on the market and can be induced by drugs such as rifampin, phenytoin, and carbamazepine, and inhibited by many drugs, including the macrolide antibiotics, nefazodone, itraconazole, and ketoconazole, as well as grapefruit juice. The isozyme CYP2D6 is involved in the metabolism of 25%–30% of marketed medications and has been associated with only minimal age-related changes. CYP2D6 is involved in the metabolism of many psychotropic drugs and can be inhibited by many agents. In addition, approximately 10% of white people are deficient in CYP2D6 and have reduced ability to clear and increased sensitivity to CYP2D6 substrates. Clinically, these patients and those taking CYP2D6 inhibitors (eg, quinidine, paroxetine, fluoxetine) cannot convert codeine and tramadol to their active metabolites and, therefore, have a reduced analgesic response to these agents.

For DDIs involving herbal preparations, see "Complementary and Alternative Medicine," p 90.

Drug-Disease Interactions

Drug-disease combinations common in older adults can affect drug response and lead to ADEs, including exacerbation of existing conditions. Obesity and ascites alter the volumes of distribution of lipophilic and hydrophilic drugs, respectively. Patients with dementia can have increased sensitivity or paradoxical reactions to drugs with CNS or anticholinergic activity. Patients with renal insufficiency or impaired hepatic function due to cirrhosis or hepatic congestion have impaired detoxification and excretion of drugs.

Table 11.6—Principles of Prescribing for Older Adults

The basics:

- Start with a low dosage.
- Titrate the dosage upward slowly, as tolerated by the patient.
- Try not to start two medications at the same time.

Determine the following before prescribing a new medication:

- Is the medication necessary? Are there nonpharmacologic ways to treat the condition?
- What are the therapeutic end points, and how will they be assessed?
- Do the benefits outweigh the risks of the medication?
- Is one medication being used to treat the adverse events of another?
- Is there one medication that could be prescribed to treat two conditions?
- Are there potential drug-drug or drug-disease interactions?
- Will the new medication's administration times be the same as those of existing medications?
- Do the patient and caregiver understand what the medication is for, how to take it, how long to take it, when it should start to work, possible adverse events that it might cause, and what to do if such events occur?

At least annually:

- Ask the patient to bring all medications (prescription, OTC, supplements, and herbal preparations) to the office; for new patients, conduct a detailed medication history.
- For prescription medications, determine whether the label directions and dosage match those in the patient's chart; ask the patient how he or she is taking each medication.
- Ask about medication adverse events.
- Note if other medications are being prescribed (by other healthcare providers) for the patient, and what the medications are and their indications.
- Look for medications with duplicate therapeutic, pharmacologic, or adverse event profiles.
- Screen for drug-drug and drug-disease interactions.
- Eliminate unnecessary medications; confer with other prescribers if necessary.
- Simplify the medication regimen; use the fewest possible number of medications and doses per day.
- Always review any changes with the patient and caregiver; provide the changes in writing.

PRINCIPLES OF PRESCRIBING

For principles of prescribing for older adults, see Table 11.6. This basic approach applies primarily to medications that are used to treat chronic conditions for which an immediate, complete therapeutic response is not necessary. Dosage adjustment may still be needed for medications used to treat conditions requiring an immediate response (eg, when prescribing antibiotics for a patient with impaired kidney function). Medications that have been newly approved by the FDA should be used cautiously in treating older adults. Such medications are likely to be more expensive, and information about their use in older adults is often limited.

Overprescribing can be prevented by reviewing a patient's medications on a regular basis and each time a new medication is started or a dosage is changed. The importance of maintaining accurate records of all medications taken by the patient cannot be overemphasized. Many patients do not consider vitamins, herbal preparations, or OTC medications (even aspirin) to be medications, so clinicians should be specific when inquiring about a patient's use of other medications.

It is best if the patient brings all medications to the review, including OTC medications, vitamins, and any herbal preparations or other types of supplements (a "brown-bag" evaluation). Examining the containers and labels and asking what each medication is for and how and when it is taken can provide insight into the patient's understanding and adherence to his or her medication regimens. Any medication for which there is no longer an indication for its continued use should be stopped. A new complaint or worsening of an existing condition should prompt consideration of whether or not it could be drug-induced. When considering treatment for a new medical condition, nonpharmacologic approaches should always be considered first. If drug therapy is still indicated, a medication that minimizes the risk of an ADE should be selected.

When initiating therapy, the basic principle should be "start low and go slow." Although the FDA requires that labeling for new medications regarding dosing in older adults not be extrapolated from another patient population (eg, patients with kidney impairment), it does not require that a drug be studied explicitly in older adults. Older adults are included in phase I and II dose tolerability and pharmacokinetic and pharmacodynamic studies of many drugs, but the older adults chosen for these studies are usually healthy and free of concomitant illnesses. Much of what is known about medications and how to use them in sick older patients, particularly those who are frail, is learned only after a medication has been available for several years.

Finally, before prescribing a new medication or renewing a prescription, the clinician should consider the patient's life expectancy, time required to achieve therapeutic benefit, goal of treatment, and treatment targets.

DISCONTINUING MEDICATIONS

Discontinuing medications is as complicated as starting a new medication, sharing many of the same tasks: recognizing an opportunity; planning, communicating, and coordinating the change; and adequate monitoring and follow-up for adverse outcomes (Table 11.4).

NONADHERENCE

Adherence is the extent that medication administration coincides with instructions. Nonadherence and poor adherence to medication regimens is a huge and often unrecognized problem. It is estimated that nonadherence among older adults may be as high as 50%. Patients may be reluctant to admit that they are not taking medications or not following directions. Because there are many possible reasons for nonadherence, there is no simple screen. Predictors of nonadherence include asymptomatic disease, inadequate follow-up, patient's lack of insight or perception of the value of treatment, missed appointments and transportation difficulties, and poor healthcare provider–patient relationship. If nonadherence is suspected, clinicians should inquire about difficulties taking medication and adverse events; they should also ask (in a nonjudgmental manner) patients to review which medications they are taking and how they are taking them. Measuring a drug's serum concentration is one way to assess adherence, but assays are available for only a small percentage of medications such as tricyclic antidepressants, lithium, and anticonvulsants. Measuring a physiologic or therapeutic response such as blood pressure, heart rate, intraocular pressure, hemoglobin A_{1c}, or a change in hormone concentration is possible for many medications to treat chronic conditions. Other measures include pill counts, refill history, and confirmation by a caregiver. All these measures have limitations, and none is foolproof. The clinician needs to consider the patient's financial, cognitive, and functional status, as well as his or her beliefs about and understanding of medications and diseases.

Prescription drug costs have increased substantially, and supplemental prescription drug benefit plans are expensive. Some plans may still leave a patient with a co-payment that he or she cannot afford or with only a fixed dollar amount for the year. Clinicians should avoid prescribing expensive new medications that have not been shown to be superior to less expensive generic alternatives.

A systematic review of interventions to improve medication compliance in older, community-dwelling adults concluded that multifaceted, tailored interventions to individual barriers were more effective than single interventions (SOE=B). Medication reviews and counseling can be used to identify individual barriers, simplify regimens, and provide education. Telephone call reminders have demonstrated improved compliance in patients with heart failure or cognitive impairment. Reminder charts and calendars have been shown to be less effective. Interactive technology is available in some areas to supervise, remind, and monitor drug adherence. This usually relies on a telephone or Internet connection, which reduces availability for many older adults. This technology has not undergone extensive scientific analysis.

Combination products, ie, medications containing more than one medication, offer the advantages of decreased pill burden and increased adherence. Potential disadvantages include exposure to higher dosages than necessary, patients not recognizing that there is more than one medication in the product, and increased cost. Before starting a combination product, it needs to be determined that both medications are necessary and that the fixed doses in the product are appropriate for the patient.

Cognitive impairment can also cause nonadherence, because patients may forget to take medications or confuse them. Simplifying the regimen and involving a caregiver to oversee medication management can be helpful approaches. Medication trays also can help with organization, and they are very useful for patients who have difficulty remembering when they last took a medication.

The older adults' ability to read labels, open containers, or pour medications or even a glass of water may be impaired, so functional assessment can be useful. Some patients may need additional education or reinforcement about the purpose of a medication, especially those used to treat conditions that are usually asymptomatic, such as hypertension and diabetes mellitus. Older adults also may need reassurance regarding the safety and possible adverse events of certain medications, particularly newly prescribed medications or those associated with serious adverse events, such as warfarin.

REFERENCES

- American Geriatrics Society 2012 Beers Criteria Update Expert Panel. American Geriatrics Society Updated Beers Criteria for Potentially Inappropriate Medication Use in Older Adults. *J Am Geriatr Soc*. 2012;60(4):616–631.
- Drepper MD, Spahr L, Frossard JL. Clopidogrel and proton pump inhibitors - where do we stand in 2012? *World J Gastroenterol*. 2012; 18(18):2161–2171.
- Guttuso T Jr. Nighttime awakenings responding to gabapentin therapy in late premenopausal women: a case series. *J Clin Sleep Med*. 2012;8(2):187–189.
- Steinman MA, Hanlon JT. Managing medications in clinically complex elders: "There's got to be a happy medium." *JAMA*. 2011;304(14):1592–1601.

CHAPTER 12—COMPLEMENTARY AND ALTERNATIVE MEDICINE

KEY POINTS

- The use of complementary and alternative medicine (CAM) appears to be on the rise in all adult age groups, including the older population.
- Healthcare providers should ask patients about CAM use at *every visit.* Most adults ≥50 years old continue to report that they have not discussed CAM use with their healthcare providers.
- Herbal products and dietary supplements are among the most frequently used complementary and alternative medicines by older adults. Because of the potential risks associated with these practices, patients should always be queried and informed about CAM use.
- Many randomized controlled trials (RCTs) of CAM interventions continue to be poorly designed, which interferes with the accumulation and interpretation of evidence. Investigators planning studies of CAM interventions should consult resources that provide specific criteria required for rigorous clinical trials, such as the Cochrane Collaboration.

Complementary and alternative medicine (CAM), as currently defined by the National Center for Complementary and Alternative Medicine (NCCAM) of the National Institutes of Health, refers to "a group of diverse medical and health care systems, practices, and products that are not generally considered part of conventional medicine." According to NCCAM, most Americans practice CAM in a "complementary" way, as an adjunct, rather than an alternative, to conventional medical treatment. This combined approach is also frequently referred to as "integrative medicine." Although scientific evidence accumulates for some CAM treatments, key questions remain that must be answered through well-designed research studies—questions such as whether certain therapies are safe and whether they work for the diseases or medical conditions for which they are used.

NCCAM conceptualizes the diversity of CAM modalities as follows:

- Natural products, which include herbal medicines, botanicals, vitamins, minerals, and other dietary supplements
- Mind-body interventions, such as meditation, yoga, acupuncture, hypnotherapy, and relaxation exercises
- Manipulative and body-based methods, which include therapeutic massage, spinal manipulation, and chiropractic/osteopathic manipulation
- Movement and energy therapies such as Pilates, therapeutic touch, bioelectromagnetic-based therapies, and indigenous healing practices specific to cultural beliefs
- Whole medical systems, such as traditional Chinese medicine, Ayurvedic medicine, homeopathy, and naturopathic medicine, which incorporate many or all of the above-noted therapies

The list of what constitutes the practice of CAM is continually evolving, as interventions that are proved to be safe and effective become adopted as components of conventional, or allopathic, medicine and as new approaches to health care emerge.

The use of CAM is increasing within the U.S. adult population, particularly among middle-aged adults. The 2007 National Health Interview Survey (NHIS), a nationally representative sample of over 31,000 U.S. adults ≥18 years old, found that 36% of those interviewed used some of 27 different CAM modalities during the previous 12 months. When CAM was defined to include self-prayer for health reasons, usage increased to 62%.

Studies consistently demonstrate that, with the exception of self-prayer, older adults use CAM less frequently than do adults 50–59 years old, the largest CAM user group. However, it is logical to predict that, as middle-aged adults grow older, they will continue the CAM practices begun in earlier decades of life. See Table 12.1 for more details.

The use of CAM by older adults is beginning to be more closely studied, in part to help design safer and more efficacious treatments specific to the needs of this rapidly expanding segment of the population. A 2010 telephone survey by the American Association of Retired Persons and NCCAM interviewed 1,013 patients ≥50 years old about their CAM use; 53% reported some lifetime use of CAM, and 47% reported CAM use within the last 12 months. Within that time period, the consumption of herbal product or dietary supplements was most frequently reported (37%), with the receipt of massage, chiropractic, or other bodywork services ranking second (22%). Of concern, 67% had not discussed CAM use with their healthcare provider, because their healthcare provider had not inquired (42%) or because the patient did not know it should be discussed (30%). Respondents reported their

Table 12.1—Complementary and Alternative Medicine Usage Patterns in Adults

Modality	Older Adults Usage (n=5,837) % / Mean (SE)	All Adults Usage (n=30,802) % / Mean (SE)	Most Frequent Users (All Adults) By Ethnicity
Self-prayer	56.20 (0.78)	42.92 (0.40)	Black
Biologically based method	15.59 (0.57)	22.01 (0.30)	Asian
Mind-body	11.68 (0.48)	18.45 (0.32)	Asian
Manipulative and body-based methods	7.57 (0.39)	10.91 (0.24)	White
Alternative medical system	1.41 (0.18)	2.74 (0.14)	Asian
Energy therapy	0.34 (0.09)	0.74 (0.06)	Asian

Data from Grzywacz JG, Suerken CK, Neiberg RH, et al. Age, ethnicity, and use of complementary and alternative medicine in health self-management. *J Health Social Behav.* 2007;48(1):84–98.
NOTE: SE = standard error

primary sources of CAM information as family/friends (26%), Internet (14%), physician (13%), magazines, newspapers or books (13%), and radio/television (7%). These data confirm and extend similar observations reported in previous small-scale studies.

CAM use can vary depending on ethnic group. A recent analysis of 2002 NHIS data by Grzywacz et al (2007) revealed the patterns shown in Table 12.1. This analysis is noteworthy because it represents a change in the prior consensus. A 2005 review by the Institute of Medicine found that most prior studies reported lower usage of CAM by individuals of various ethnic minority groups than by white Americans.

Socioeconomic status and degree of acculturation may be important factors in the use and specific choice of CAM modalities by individuals belonging to certain ethnic minority groups. For example, Mexican curanderos may be the first line of health care for impoverished individuals of Mexican descent. Curanderos are community "healers" who believe that illness can result from natural, as well as spiritual, causes. They often use herbal remedies in the form of teas, baths, or poultices, depending on the symptoms. Similarly, Native Americans may mix modern and traditional medicines, sometimes using "white man's medicine" to treat "white man's diseases." It is important to recognize that some Western pharmaceuticals were derived from Native American herbal medicines. Traditional Native American medicine covers a broad range of interventions including ceremony, fasting, sweating, herbal and/or animal medicines, or avoidance or inclusion of specific foods. See also "Cultural Aspects of Care," p 58.

SAFETY ISSUES

Most CAM practices have not been regulated, and licensure and certification among CAM practitioners can vary among practices and by geographic location. There is substantial potential for adverse reactions with the use of herbal preparations and of botanical and dietary supplements in older adults (see Table 12.2).

Approximately 67% of CAM users ≥50 years old in the United States do not discuss their use of CAM modalities with their healthcare providers. This statistic is of particular concern in the care of older adults because of the increased risk of adverse interactions between conventional drugs and various CAM biologic agents. Moreover, aging impacts the metabolism of numerous prescriptions and OTC medications, and possibly that of many herbal preparations, botanicals, and dietary supplements. Age-related alterations in hepatic and renal function contribute importantly to these phenomena, both in the absence and presence of disease.

Older adults report using herbal/dietary products and bodywork services most frequently, both of which can pose health risks. Negative outcomes from chiropractic interventions, albeit uncommon, have included stroke, transient ischemic attack, and other focal neurologic signs. Additionally, recently reported data suggest that older adults are ill informed about the dangers associated with herbal/dietary products. In one study (n=267) of older adults in the central United States, the following percentages of respondents inaccurately believed that herbal/dietary products were regulated by the FDA (60%), were routinely tested by the FDA (70%), and posed no risk to the general population (66%).

Under the Dietary Supplement Health and Education Act (DSHEA) of 1994, the FDA is not authorized to evaluate or regulate the use of dietary supplements, and manufacturers of such products are not required to prove that the advertised ingredients provide the health benefits or safety they claim. Multiple studies have found that dietary supplements often can contain little, none, or more of what the product labels claim, as well as contaminants or adulterants with unlisted products and prescription drugs. In November 2004, the FDA announced initiatives to monitor and evaluate ingredient quality, safety, and labeling of herbal and dietary products, thus attempting to assure the reliability of "what's in the bottle." However, no policy changes have followed to date.

Table 12.2—Safety Issues Related to Dietary Supplements Used by Older Adults

Supplement	Adverse Effects	Interacts With
Coenzyme Q_{10}	Infrequent nausea, emesis, epigastric pain, headaches >300 mg/day linked to increased liver transaminase	Warfarin
Dehydroepiandrosterone (DHEA)	Women: weight gain, voice changes, facial hair, headaches Men: prostatic hypertrophy, possible increase in hormone-sensitive tumors	Calcium channel blockers, sildenafil
Echinacea	Allergic reactions, hepatitis, asthma, vertigo, anaphylaxis (rare)	Immunosuppressants
Ginkgo biloba	All rare: serious bleeding, seizures, headaches, dizziness, vertigo	Anticoagulants
Glucosamine	Nausea, diarrhea, heartburn	Hypoglycemic drugs (reduce effectiveness)
Omega-3 fatty acids	Belching, halitosis, increased blood glucose	Antiplatelets, anticoagulants, antihypertensives
SAM-e	Nausea, vomiting, diarrhea, anxiety, restlessness	Tricyclics, SSRIs
Saw palmetto	All rare: constipation, diarrhea, decreased libido, headaches, hypertension, urine retention	None described
St. John's wort	Nausea, allergic reactions, dizziness, headache, photosensitivity (rare)	Anticoagulants, antivirals, SSRIs

Without the knowledge of what these products contain in their entirety, or the consequences of their use, consumers and healthcare professionals must increase communication while continued research is conducted to provide accurate evaluations. It is imperative that clinicians ask patients specifically about their use of dietary supplements and biologic products and look at the ingredients in those supplements. Older adults also consistently indicate willingness to receive more information about CAM treatments; thus, it is important for healthcare providers to disseminate such information.

CAM Efficacy for Managing Illness

The aging of the baby-boomer generation is contributing to the already established largest group of healthcare consumers—older adults. Among the most common health challenges in aged men are diseases of the circulatory, musculoskeletal and connective tissue, and genitourinary systems. In aging women, the most common health challenges are musculoskeletal, circulatory, mental health, and genitourinary disorders. Demographic considerations assure that the needs of the expanding aging population for medical services will continue to increase, and it is reasonable to predict that specific interest in, and use of, CAM modalities will expand as well.

There are numerous anecdotal reports or claims of the efficacy of diverse CAM modalities; however, scientific efficacy and safety must be established through careful study. Studies examining the effectiveness and safety of CAM interventions continue to accumulate. However, as the research efforts summarized in this chapter demonstrate, the current evidence base is hindered by studies lacking the appropriate design and methodology, number of participants, duration of investigation, and/or standardization of product or practice. Investigators planning trials of CAM modalities can improve their study design by verifying that the planned research meets the criteria for scientific quality and acceptability by reviewing resources such as those provided by the Cochrane Collaboration.

Musculoskeletal Disorders

Osteoarthritis is the most common musculoskeletal disorder and one of the most common chronic diseases affecting older adults. Evidence for short-term pain relief associated with osteoarthritis has been found for transcutaneous electrical nerve stimulation (TENS) (SOE=A), acupuncture (SOE=B), and topical capsaicin (SOE=A). A recent review of studies using glucosamine and/or chondroitin for knee osteoarthritis showed mixed results (SOE=B) for chondroitin alone, glucosamine alone, and the combination of the two. The rating for glucosamine alone was influenced by the short duration (4–6 weeks) of some of the supporting studies. Evidence for the reduction of joint space narrowing (SOE=C) for chondroitin alone and glucosamine alone was generally consistent.

Recent studies have highlighted gender and racial disparities favoring white women in the diagnosis and treatment of osteoporosis after a fracture. Over their lifetime, one in five men >50 years old will sustain an osteoporotic fracture, and their mortality rates associated with hip fracture are higher than those for women. Many of the available studies examine women's responses to interventions for osteoporosis. Phytoestrogen and soy products are increasingly used to prevent or treat osteoporosis in postmenopausal women. The inconsistent results of trials (SOE= C) likely result from the use of differing soy products (ie, food versus tablets of varying strengths and combinations therein) in various populations. At this time, evidence is insufficient to recommend their use for the prevention or treatment of osteoporosis in postmenopausal women. Moreover, there is controversy regarding the safety of their use in women with estrogen-sensitive diseases such as breast or endometrial cancer.

Dehydroepiandrosterone (DHEA) is the most abundant circulating steroid hormone in people, reaching peak levels in early adulthood and then declining progressively with age. This decline coupled with the correlation between low DHEA sulfate and osteoporosis and frailty has led to the use of DHEA supplements in an attempt to improve bone density, muscle mass, and physical functioning in older adults. Small-scale trials (SOE=C) of DHEA supplementation in older adults have produced conflicting results regarding its effects to moderately enhance bone density, and further studies are needed to determine its possible use in preventing or treating osteoporosis in older people. These same trials have shown DHEA to be without effect on muscle mass or physical performance.

Omega-3 polyunsaturated fatty acid supplementation (SOE=B) is recommended for inflammatory joint pain from rheumatoid arthritis and inflammatory bowel disease. (See also "Musculoskeletal Diseases and Disorders," p 453; and "Persistent Pain," p 119.) A recent meta-analysis of specific diet plans (vegetarian, Mediterranean, elemental, and elimination diets), including fasting, for rheumatoid arthritis pain generally found no evidence (SOE=B) of improved patient-oriented outcomes. However, the risk of bias and inadequate data reporting inherent in the reviewed studies supports the need for better designed future research. With respect to the joint and overall pain associated with inflammatory bowel diseases (eg, Crohn disease and ulcerative colitis), recent studies have found promising results (SOE=B) with seal and/or whale oils.

Acupuncture, energy modalities, and herbal medicine are all used in the treatment of lower back pain. Acupuncture appears to provide significantly better short-term relief than sham procedure for low back pain (SOE=B). With respect to longer-term back pain relief, results for acupuncture versus sham have been inconsistent. Randomized controlled trials using spinal manipulation therapy have been of low quality (SOE=B) and have produced little evidence to support this modality. Herbal medicines are also used to treat lower back pain. Short-term improvements in pain were found for *Harpagophytum procumbens* (SOE=A), *Salix alba* (white willow bark) (SOE=B), and *Capsicum frutescens* (cayenne) (SOE=C). See also "Back and Neck Pain," p 465.

Cardiovascular Disorders

Cardiovascular disease affects at least 60%–70% of adults >65 years old. Of particular relevance is the higher incidence of cardiovascular disease occurring in obese patients or those with type 2 diabetes mellitus. Healthy diet and aerobic exercise are the first recommendations to manage high blood pressure and dyslipidemia. A heart-healthy diet includes limiting sodium intake, refined sugar, and saturated fat while increasing amounts of complex carbohydrates, fruits, and vegetables. In the Dietary Approach to Stop Hypertension (DASH) trial, nearly 70% of participants following the healthy diet decreased both systolic and diastolic blood-pressure measurements.

A Cochrane Collaboration meta-analysis that examined cardiovascular metrics in 23 RCTs (SOE=C) that used omega-3 polyunsaturated fatty acids found significantly lowered levels of triglyceride (0.45% mmol/L) and very low-density lipoprotein cholesterol (0.07 mmol/L). However, low-density lipoprotein cholesterol was raised (0.11 mmol/L) overall, but not in subgroup analyses. There were no significant changes in high-density lipoprotein cholesterol or body weight. Examples of essential fatty acids are omega-3 and omega-6 acids. The omega-3 fatty acids can be found in fresh deep-water fish and in flaxseed oil. Omega-6 linoleic acid is found in raw nuts and seeds. For further reduction of the risk of developing hypertension and obesity, aerobic exercise, such as swimming or brisk walking, is advised for at least 30 minutes three times a week. Current data suggest that even mild to moderate increases in physical activity, such as walking slowly or gardening, have beneficial cardiovascular effects. Increased blood pressure can also be associated with inadequate sleep. See also "Hypertension," p 402; "Physical Activity," p 64; and "Sleep Problems," p 285.

Relaxation therapy has resulted in a small, but statistically significant, decrease in both systolic and diastolic blood pressure. However, the quality of included studies (SOE=C) was considered poor, and the authors concluded that this finding could have been due to therapeutic factors (eg, patient-provider relationship) other than the relaxation therapy.

Studies of the use of biofeedback for the reduction of hypertension have suffered from poor study design

(SOE=B) and heterogeneous treatments. In a systematic (non-quantitative) review of 52 RCTs, no difference was found between biofeedback and the comparison (placebo, no intervention, other behavioral treatments) in 24, biofeedback was favored over comparators in 16, medication or other behavioral treatments were favored over biofeedback in 4, and comparative data were not reported in 8. The term "favored" usually, but not always, referred to statistically significant results.

Psychiatric Disorders

Depression is one of the most common and debilitating major public health problems, and its incidence increases with advancing age. Although depression is more common in women, increasing attention is focused on the issue of depression in men, in whom it is more often unrecognized or untreated. There is an alarming prevalence of depression and suicide in widowed men ≥70 years old. CAM use by the aging patient may assist in the management of mild to moderate depression. However, adequate treatment of severe depression often incorporates use of psychotherapy and psychotropic medication to prevent or decrease further morbidity and mortality. Recent research suggests that depression is also a systemic disease and is accompanied by an increased incidence of sleep disorders, osteoporosis, obesity, insulin resistance, and immune dysfunction. The impact of CAM modalities on these "extrabehavioral" outcomes is unclear.

A healthy diet can be one of the first recommendations to assist with improving mood. Dietary intake that includes complex carbohydrates can improve serotonin levels. Increasing essential fatty acids and protein intake may increase alertness and mood. Of equal importance is discontinuing excess alcohol, caffeine, and tobacco, which can contribute to depression and irritability.

Aerobic exercise is also prescribed as a treatment for mild to moderate depression in aged patients. Exercise in combination with antidepressants can yield faster, more lasting results than either alone.

The botanical *Hypericum perforatum*, commonly known as St. John's wort, has received strong evidence of efficacy (SOE=A) when compared with placebo or synthetic antidepressants. Adverse effects of St. John's wort, which include GI upset, fatigue, dizziness, headache, dry mouth, and photosensitivity, are less frequently reported than adverse effects associated with standard antidepressants. Special attention should be paid to the interactions of St. John's wort with the hepatic P-450 enzyme system that induces the metabolism of many drugs, which can cause clinically significant adverse interactions and therapeutic failure with various antiretroviral, anticoagulant, immunosuppressant, antidepressant, and chemotherapeutic drugs.

S-adenosylmethionine (SAM-e) is a naturally occurring compound that is needed by the brain to adequately produce dopamine and serotonin. SAM-e is currently marketed as an antidepressant. Very few placebo comparison trials have been completed, but compared with conventional antidepressants, SAM-e has shown no difference in response rates or effect sizes (SOE=B). See also "Depression and Other Mood Disorders," p 308.

Neurologic Disorders

Some studies have investigated the use of supplements for treatment of dementia from Alzheimer disease and vascular insufficiency. Studies of *Ginkgo biloba* extract (EGb 761) for cognitive decline in older adults have produced inconsistent results (SOE=B: inconsistent) overall and no significant benefit over placebo (SOE=A: absence of effect). Brain tissue studies and spinal fluid abnormalities in Alzheimer patients also offer some rationale for supplementing with various antioxidants, including vitamins A, C, and E and selenium. However, evidence of their effect has yet to be demonstrated in clinical trials. See also "Dementia," p 256.

Studies have shown that Parkinson disease patients have reduced brain levels of glutathione, an antioxidant involved in neuroprotective functions. Parkinson patients also have deficiencies in coenzyme Q_{10}. Supplementation with these two naturally occurring substances has been shown to slow the progression of disease and reduce the severity of symptoms in very small, unblinded clinical trials (SOE=B, quality of study). Acupuncture, music therapy, and physical therapy are used by Parkinson patients to attempt to reduce disabilities and improve cognitive, emotional, and social functioning. See also "Neurologic Diseases and Disorders," p 480.

Sleep disorders are common in older adults, affecting both sleep quality and quantity. Studies suggest that abnormalities in slow-wave and rapid-eye-movement sleep may also be linked to psychologic, endocrine-metabolic, and immune system dysfunctions. Nutritional and exercise modifications are among the safest recommendations when working with older patients with sleep disorders. Milk, bananas, brown rice, and turkey are examples of foods containing tryptophan, which is a precursor of serotonin. Chamomile is an herbal tea that is claimed to be relaxing. Evidence for the use of valerian root to improve sleep quality, quantity, or next-day functioning has been mixed (SOE=B: inconsistent). Aerobic exercise in the early evening has been shown to contribute to improved sleep quality. However, exercise later in the evening can be too stimulating and hinder restful sleep. Other CAM modalities purported to improve sleep include aromatherapy combined with a warm bath and relaxing music. See also "Sleep Problems," p 285.

Menopause

Perceptions about menopause have become more realistic in recent years, with this transition becoming less frequently viewed as a pathologic process than as a natural progression in the life cycle. In addition, concerns about the safety of long-term conventional estrogen use have increased. These changes have influenced the use of alternatives, such as nutritional, nonpharmacologic supplements and exercise, for symptom management. Approximately 80% of menopausal women report using one or more CAM modalities, such as natural and plant estrogens and other herbal preparations. See also the section on estrogen replacement therapy in "Endocrine and Metabolic Disorders," p 506.

Alternative treatments under current study for menopausal symptoms consist primarily of herbal and phytoestrogen remedies. Although very popular, black cohosh (SOE=A: absence of effect) has not been found to reduce patient- or disease-oriented symptoms in good quality clinical trials. Phytoestrogens are naturally occurring sources of estrogen found in plant foods. Isoflavones, such as daidzein and genistein, are found in soy products and have been studied as alternatives to conventional estrogen therapy. The current evidence supports the efficacy of soy over placebo, especially soy extracts, but this conclusion must be tempered by methodologic concerns in some of the studies (SOE=B). Both aerobic exercise and mind-body relaxation techniques are also helpful in decreasing irritability, restlessness, and anxiety.

Urinary incontinence and vaginal dryness are common symptoms in postmenopausal women, increase with advancing age after menopause, and negatively impact quality of life. Evidence suggests that administration of systemic or local estrogens does not lessen symptoms of the former, but may improve those of the latter. Information is insufficient as to whether use of any CAM natural products or other modalities provide any relief of symptoms of urinary incontinence and vaginal dryness.

Benign Prostatic Hyperplasia

Symptomatic benign prostatic hyperplasia affects more than 40% of men ≥70 years old approximately equally among racial groups. In recent decades, men in the United States have begun to self-treat this condition with saw palmetto, which has become the fifth leading medicinal herb consumed in the United States. A review of randomized controlled trials comparing saw palmetto to placebo or other conventional medications found no evidence of efficacy. Other supplements (eg, *Hypoxis rooperi*, stinging nettle, pumpkin seed extracts, rye pollen, African plum) have been studied but need more rigorous scientific investigation. The American and European Association of Urology does not currently recommend plant extracts in the treatment of benign prostatic hyperplasia. See also "Prostate Disease," p 437.

Diabetes Mellitus

Type 2 diabetes mellitus, a major public health problem, is associated with increased incidence and prevalence of obesity, hypertension, dyslipidemia, and macro- and microvascular disease. Normal aging is associated with increased insulin resistance and glucose intolerances, and increased risk of developing type 2 diabetes mellitus. In one survey, approximately 50%–60% of diabetic patients reported the use of CAM interventions, including folk remedies in ethnic populations.

There is considerable interest in examining the potential benefit of various CAM biologic agents (eg, omega-3-fatty acids, chromium, vitamin C, other dietary antioxidants) or other modalities (eg, stress-reduction techniques), in combination with dietary modifications, exercise, and weight management, in the treatment of patients with diabetes. In this regard, omega-3 polyunsaturated fatty acids have not been shown to improve glycemic control or fasting insulin. See also "Diabetes Mellitus," p 520.

Cancer

Approximately 30%–50% of cancer patients in one survey noted that they were using CAM interventions to manage their specific cancer. Cancer CAM therapies purportedly can be used to strengthen the body's innate immune systems as well as to manage the adverse effects of conventional treatments, such as chemotherapy and radiation. One of the most important benefits for many cancer patients who use CAM modalities is the experience of being more empowered while dealing with the challenges of cancer. This has been substantiated by numerous studies examining various indices of health-related quality of life. The CAM therapies most frequently used are herbal preparations, exercise, and spiritual and energy modalities (such as qi gong, therapeutic touch, Reiki, polarity, healing touch, or Johrei).

Controversy remains regarding the role of diet as a possible risk factor for developing breast cancer. Of particular importance is the link between obesity and its associated increase in estrogen levels that are thought to contribute to de novo breast cancer development and recurrence after early-stage disease. In contrast, consumption of a high-fiber, low-fat diet with fruits, vegetables, whole grains, fish, and legumes is associated with decreased risk of disease. Biologic agents, herbal preparations, and vitamins have all been tried by patients; however, most of these modalities have not undergone much scientific study. In contrast, lifestyle changes, including exercise and stress management techniques, have been helpful in managing mood and energy changes associated with breast cancer.

Prostate cancer usually develops slowly in older men, and CAM use in combination with conventional treatment has been reported to reduce associated discomforts and improve the quality of life. Risk of death in this population is higher from heart disease than from prostate cancer per se. Exercise and healthy diet remain the safest CAM recommendations to assist with the management of adverse effects and improvement of quality of life in these patients. See also "Prostate Disease," p 437.

Lung cancer has been linked to smoking and to excess dietary intake of dairy products, red meats, and saturated fats, though these latter associations have been questioned. In addition, preliminary research has suggested that ingestion of vitamin A by those who smoke may be harmful, whereas vitamin A intake in those who do not smoke may be beneficial. Dietary changes as well as mind-body interventions may assist lung cancer patients to manage emotional distress and the adverse effects of treatment. Cancer patients using relaxation and stress-management techniques have been able to manage cravings when pursuing tobacco cessation. These mind-body techniques are also effective in managing the emotional and physical distress associated with diagnosis and with the adverse effects of treatment.

Currently, there are no herbal preparations or botanical supplements that appear to be useful in the prevention or management of patients with colon cancer. A fiber-rich diet has been postulated to possibly prevent the onset of colon cancer; however, studies are inconclusive. Lutein, which is present in broccoli, carrots, oranges, and spinach, was found in one study to be beneficial for colon cancer prevention. See also "Oncology," p 540.

References

- American Association of Retired Persons & National Centers for Complementary and Alternative Medicine Survey Report. *Complementary and Alternative Medicine: What People Aged 50 and Older Discuss With Their Health Care Providers*. Available at: http://nccam.nih.gov/news/camstats/2010. (accessed Oct 2013).
- Bolaños R, Del Castillo A, Francia J. Soy isoflavones versus placebo in the treatment of climacteric vasomotor symptoms: systematic review and meta-analysis. *Menopause*. 2010;17(3):660–666.
- Greenhalgh J, Dickson R, Dundar Y. Biofeedback for hypertension: a systematic review. *J Hypertens*. 2010;28(4):644–652.
- Lagari VS, Levis S. Phytoestrogens and bone health. *Curr Opin Endocrinol Diabetes Obes*. 2010;17(6):546–553.
- Rubinstein SM, van Middelkoop M, Kuijpers T, et al. A systematic review on the effectiveness of complementary and alternative medicine for chronic non-specific low-back pain. *Eur Spine J*. 2010;19(8):1213–1228.
- Vangsness CT Jr, Spiker W, Erickson J. A review of evidence-based medicine for glucosamine and chondroitin sulfate use in knee osteoarthritis. *Arthroscopy*. 2009;25(1):86–94.

CHAPTER 13—MISTREATMENT OF OLDER ADULTS

KEY POINTS

- Mistreatment of older adults affects 11.4% of those ≥60 years old.
- Screening for mistreatment of older adults is important and most effective when conducted in a sensitive manner.
- Indicators of mistreatment of older adults range from dramatic (eg, bruising, fractures) to subtle (eg, withdrawn behavior, dehydration).

Mistreatment of older adults is referred to by the National Research Council in its report on elder mistreatment as "(a) intentional actions that cause harm or create a serious risk of harm (whether or not harm is intended) to a vulnerable elder by a caregiver or other person who stands in a trust relationship to the elder or (b) failure by a caregiver to satisfy the elder's basic needs or to protect the elder from harm." The Center of Excellence on Elder Abuse & Neglect Web site (www.centeronelderabuse.org/) provides an evidence-based approach to the assessment and detection of elder mistreatment with cases, multimedia resources, and results from an ongoing program of research that is led by experts in the field and provides the best current resource for those practicing in geriatrics. Mistreatment can manifest itself in a variety of ways, including physical or emotional abuse, intentional or unintentional neglect, financial exploitation, or abandonment, or a combination of these. Research suggests that the U.S. national incidence of mistreatment of older adults is approximately 450,000 annually. Given these estimates, routine screening for mistreatment is an appropriate part of primary care for older adults.

Research conducted in the context of a longitudinal aging cohort study sought to determine mortality related to mistreatment. In a pooled logistic regression analysis that adjusted for demographics, chronic disease, functional status, social networks, cognitive status, and depressive symptoms, the risk of death remained higher for cohort members experiencing either mistreatment or self-neglect (SOE=A). To date, no intervention studies have evaluated the impact of screening on health outcomes, and such studies are needed. However, screening for mistreatment appears warranted, given the findings of case studies and longitudinal studies that document risk factors, as well as the information in databases of adult protective services organizations across the country.

RISK FACTORS AND PREVENTION

Risk factors for mistreatment include poverty, dependency of older adults for caregiving needs, age, race, functional disability, frailty, and cognitive impairment (SOE=B). Some factors may actually be proxies for other variables. For example, lower socioeconomic status is often associated with fewer resources to meet caregiving demands; mistreatment may be as high as 47.3% in this group. Research has shown that demented older adults who are victims of crime have the ability, in certain circumstances, to provide testimony about criminal events (SOE=B).

Frail, debilitated older adults may need a level of care that at times exceeds caregiver ability. In particular, the demented person who exhibits disturbing behaviors (eg, hitting, spitting, screaming) poses immense challenges to caregivers. Caregiver stress can give way to any of the forms of mistreatment, and a careful assessment of caregiver stress can identify opportunities to prevent mistreatment. Minority older adults may be preferentially targeted for healthcare fraud by unscrupulous home care organizations and/or durable medical equipment suppliers. For factors that indicate a risk for the development of inadequate or abusive caregiving, see Table 13.1.

HISTORY

An interdisciplinary approach to assessment and care planning is optimal. Comprehensive interdisciplinary geriatric assessment (see "Outpatient Care Systems," p 173; and "Hospital Care," p 130) that includes the physical, psychosocial, and financial domains of older adults should detect potential or any alleged mistreatment.

The mistreatment history, provided by both the older adults and caregiver(s), should be conducted in private so that all individuals can speak freely and frankly. Studies suggest that the different cultures of racial and ethnic groups may define abuse and neglect very differently; thus, cultural sensitivity is important (see "Cultural Aspects of Care," p 58). The older adult or caregiver from a culture different than the clinician's may be offended by some mistreatment screening questions; wording questions carefully can avoid alienating the older adult or caregiver, which could abolish any further opportunity to help the patient and family.

If the older adult's responses to the mistreatment questions indicate that mistreatment may be occurring, progressively focused follow-up questions are indicated. For example, the clinician might first ask, "Is there any difficult behavior in your family you would like to tell me about?" If the answer is positive, possible questions to follow include: "Has anyone tried to hurt or hit you?" "Has anyone made you do things that you did not want

Table 13.1—Risk Factors for Inadequate or Abusive Caregiving

- Cognitive impairment in patient, caregiver, or both
- Dependency of the caregiver on the older patient, or vice versa
- Family conflict
- Family history of abusive behavior, alcohol or drug misuse or abuse, mental illness, or intellectual disability
- Financial stress or lack of funds to meet new health demands
- Isolation of the patient or caregiver, or both
- Living arrangements inadequate for the needs of the ill person
- Stressful events in the family, such as death of a loved one or loss of employment

to do?" "Has anyone taken your things?" Obtaining such information requires sensitive clinical interviewing skills similar to those needed when asking about sexual orientation, alcoholism, or substance abuse.

Private interviews with caregivers can detect not only abusive or neglectful behavior but also signs of stress, isolation, or depression in the caregiver, in which case help for the caregiver can also be provided. Caregivers may be reluctant to discuss their own problems in the presence of the older adult who depends on their care. Because caregivers can range from registered professionals to well-intended neighbors, it is important to know and document the caregiver's skill level, as well as his or her understanding of the situation. The latter is an essential factor in evaluating the underlying intention of any mistreatment of a dependent older adult. For example, a registered nurse in a nursing home is held to a different level of accountability than a frail spouse providing care in the home setting.

Identification of shortcomings in the older adult's care can be the most elusive aspect of a comprehensive assessment. The symptoms and signs of incomplete, inadequate, or neglectful caregiving can be subtle (eg, when an older adult does not do as well as expected on a given regimen) or attributable to the older adult's physical or emotional disorders (eg, weight loss in an older adult with a history of depression).

Effective assessment detects mistreatment without placing undue suspicion on well-meaning caregivers or undermining a family's ability to care for an older adult with appropriate support and counseling.

For examples of symptoms and signs that indicate a particularly high level of risk of mistreatment, see Table 13.2. A number of assessment instruments have been developed to help clinicians screen for and assess mistreatment, although none has been fully validated yet, and research is ongoing.

Physical Assessment

Key signs of mistreatment include physical indicators that are incongruent with the history; examples are bruises and welts in unusual places or in various stages of healing. Bilateral bruises on the upper torso are rarely the result of falls and warrant follow-up. Other indications of possible mistreatment include frequent, unexplained, or inconsistently explained falls and injuries, multiple visits to the emergency department, delays in seeking treatment, inconsistent follow-up, or serial switching among providers. The clinician should search for unusual patterns or marks, such as bruises on inner arms or thighs; cigarette, rope, chain, or chemical burns; lacerations and abrasions on the face, lips, and eyes; or marks on areas of the body usually covered by clothes. Head injuries, hair loss, or hemorrhages beneath the scalp as a consequence of hair pulling are significant markers. Cachectic states can be the result of malnutrition that is a consequence of neglect. Unusual discharges, bruising, bleeding, or trauma around the genitalia or rectum raise concern of possible sexual abuse, prompting gynecologic and rectal examination. (See www.centeronelderabuse.org/)

The behavior of the older adult when in the presence of the suspected abuser may be significant. A victim of mistreatment may avoid eye contact, or dart his or her eyes continually. He or she may sit a distance away from an abusive caregiver, cringe, back off, or startle easily as if expecting to be struck. The caregiver may be nervous and fearful, or quiet and passive. The older adult may defer excessively to the caregiver, who may invariably answer for the older adult or even try to prevent a private interview with or examination of the older adult. Dubious explanations may be given to explain the older adult's injuries.

The emergency department is an important setting for assessment of mistreatment. The emergency department may see older adults in crisis, and every effort should be made not to simply treat and release patients whose domestic situation merits further assessment. Astute emergency personnel can identify cases in which there may be serious safety problems in the caregiving situation.

Psychological Assessment

Mistreatment is not invariably or entirely physical. Psychological abuse or neglect is generally more difficult than physical abuse to detect and confirm, but it can be equally dangerous to the dependent older adult. The behavior of both the older adult and the caregiver can provide important clues about the quality of their relationship and of the care the older adult is receiving. Factors that suggest a poor or deteriorating social and emotional situation are an important focus of assessment for mistreatment.

Table 13.2—Screening for Mistreatment of Older Adults

Assessment Domain	Key Indicators
General	■ Clothing: inappropriate dress, soil, or disrepair
	■ Hygiene (including appearance of hair and nails)
	■ Nutritional status
	■ Skin integrity
Abuse	■ Anxiety, nervousness, especially toward caregiver
	■ Bruising, in various healing stages, especially bilateral or on inner arms or thighs
	■ Fractures, especially in various healing stages
	■ Lacerations
	■ Repeated emergency department visits
	■ Repeated falls
	■ Signs of sexual abuse
	■ Statements about abuse by the patient
Neglect	■ Contractures
	■ Dehydration
	■ Depression
	■ Diarrhea
	■ Failure to respond to warning of obvious disease
	■ Fecal impaction
	■ Malnutrition
	■ Medication under- or overuse or otherwise inappropriate use
	■ Poor hygiene
	■ Pressure ulcers
	■ Repeated falls
	■ Repeated hospital admissions
	■ Urine burns
	■ Statements about neglect by the patient
Exploitation	■ Evidence of misuse of patient's assets
	■ Inability of patient to account for money and property or to pay for essential care
	■ Reports of demands for money or goods in exchange for caregiving or services
	■ Unexplained loss of Social Security, pension checks
	■ Statements about exploitation by the patient
Abandonment	■ Evidence that patient is left alone unsafely
	■ Evidence of sudden withdrawal of care by caregiver
	■ Statements about abandonment by the patient

SOURCE: Data in part from Fulmer T. Elder mistreatment assessment. *Try This: Best Practices in Nursing Care to Older Adults*. 2008;15 (www.consultgerirn.org/).

Psychological abuse includes taunting, name-calling, promoting regressive behaviors by infantilization, making painful jokes at the expense of the older adult, or other activities that are demeaning. The caregiver's style of communication can provide important clues. Impatience, irritability, and demeaning statements may indicate a pattern of verbal abuse. However, psychological neglect or mistreatment by the caregiver can also take more subtle forms. For example, not providing social or emotional stimulation, or restricting or preventing normal activities can result in total social isolation of the older adult.

The older adult's demeanor and emotional status can suggest the presence of psychological neglect or abuse. For example, ambivalence or high levels of anxiety, fearfulness, or anger toward the caregiver indicate the need for further assessment. Unexpected depression (ie, no obvious pathophysiological or psychological reason for new onset, such as death in family) or uncharacteristic withdrawal also merits follow-up. Other high-risk behaviors include lack of adherence with treatment recommendations, frequent requests for sedating medication, or frequently canceled appointments.

Cognitive impairment, dementia, and depression are prevalent in older adults referred for evaluation for possible mistreatment. It is therefore appropriate to check any older adult presenting with cognitive impairment, dementia, or depression for symptoms and signs of neglect or mistreatment. Aggressive behaviors associated with dementia can trigger abusive responses in caregivers. See also "Behavioral Problems in Dementia," p 267.

FINANCIAL ASSESSMENT

Financial exploitation includes unauthorized use of the older adult's funds, possessions, or property. Financial mistreatment by family members is estimated to have a prevalence of 5.2%. Fiscal neglect consists of the failure to use the older adult's funds and resources to provide for his or her needs. Signs that an older adult is being mistreated financially include the following (SOE=C):

- a recent marked disparity between the older adult's living conditions or appearance and his or her assets
- a sudden inability to pay for health care or other basic needs
- an unusual interest on the part of caregivers in the older adult's assets
- the sudden acquisition of expensive possessions by a caregiver who has apparently limited financial assets
- unwillingness of a caregiver to allow access to the home of an older adult

Self-Neglect

For some older adults, especially those who live in isolation or who choose to accept and endure mistreatment, self-neglect may be an issue. Self-neglected older adults reported to Adult Protective Services have multiple sociodemographic, health-related, and psychosocial characteristics that are different from those of older adults who do not get reported. Lower levels of social network and social engagement have been determined to be risk factors for self-neglect. Successful management in such cases requires an assessment of the older adult's capacity to understand the risks and benefits of the situation, as well as the consequences of allowing the circumstances to continue. (See decisional capacity in "Legal and Ethical Issues," p 26.) These are complex situations, but the older adult's right to autonomy and self-determination must be honored. Paternalistic viewpoints regarding what the older person "should do" need to be avoided. In self-neglect cases, the clinician may need support when coming to terms with the requirement to respect the decisionally capable older adult's wishes when this involves his or her choosing to remain in an abusive or neglectful situation. (The clinical dilemma resembles that confronting clinicians who treat battered women.) Intervention contrary to the decisionally capable older adult's choice is generally inappropriate, as well as being uncomfortable for the clinician. See autonomy versus protectionism in "Legal and Ethical Issues," p 26. The Diogenes syndrome, in which an older adult suffers from severe self-neglect, is still poorly understood, and evidence is primarily from case studies.

The Role of the Older Adult

The relationship of the older adult with caregivers can be very complex, and a dysfunctional relationship between a dependent older adult and a caregiver may not be entirely the fault of the caregiver. To approach such situations with the idea that the older adult is inevitably the victim infantilizes the person and is unfair to caregivers. Situations in which older adults are mistreated fall along a spectrum from victimization to mutual abusiveness to relationships in which the older adult can be viewed as a witting cause of the mistreatment. Of course, there are cases in which the older adult and his or her caregivers are making the best of a tragic situation.

To determine the best possible approach for ameliorating if not solving a dysfunctional caregiving relationship, the clinician needs to make every effort to determine the facts in the situation, including the motives of the people involved. Consultation with social workers, psychologists, or psychiatrists can be useful. Legal reporting requirements are not limited in any way by these considerations. If an older man hits his son and the son strikes back, clinicians in most states are required to report the latter hitting.

Institutional Mistreatment

Mistreatment in the setting of home care by family or friends has been the focus of much of the discussion so far, but detecting and intervening to prevent mistreatment in the institutional setting is also important. Several factors in this setting could aggravate the problem, including poor working conditions, low salaries, inadequate staff training and supervision resulting in poor motivation, and prejudiced attitudes. Disruptive or insulting behavior by the older adult can also be a factor.

The Omnibus Budget Reconciliation Act of 1987 set a new standard for care in nursing homes. (See "Nursing-Home Care," p 153.) The clinician who is alert to the possibility of abuse and neglect in any institutional setting plays an important role in protecting vulnerable older adults. Equally important is the clinician's readiness to use the resources available through the institution itself or through state regulatory agencies to investigate and intervene when appropriate. In cases of suspected institutional mistreatment, the challenge is to balance the rights of staff members with the rights of residents. State departments of public health are usually responsible for investigating cases of abuse and neglect in nursing homes. Evidence is growing (SOE=B) regarding the phenomenon of resident-to-resident mistreatment in long-term care facilities, which warrants careful attention. In such cases, residents may assault, rob, or psychologically abuse other residents, and this will be an important area for further research.

Intervention

The clinician who suspects mistreatment can use the following questions to guide intervention:

- How safe is the older adult if he or she returns to the current setting; does he or she need to be removed to a safe environment?
- What services or resources are available locally to support the care of the older adult?
- Are there any caregivers who have health problems of their own that need attention?
- Does this situation need the expertise of others (eg, in medicine, nursing, social work), and if so, who would best serve the older adult's needs?

Successful intervention in cases of mistreatment can become complex. The factors governing the clinician's course of action include the exact nature and degree of the mistreatment, whether the patient can or will cooperate with evaluation and intervention, and whether the caregiver(s) can or will cooperate with evaluation and intervention.

Local resources in support of interventions for mistreatment vary, but information is readily available. Consultation with the social work staff of the hospital, nursing home, or local health department can be a useful early step. Each state's Adult Protective Services can provide relevant information as well as direct assistance. This essential service has limitations, however, given the older adult's willingness to participate in the system and the constraints on available resources. The National Adult Protective Services Association Web site (www.apsnetwork.org) provides a convenient starting point in the search for information and resources, as does the National Center on Elder Abuse (www.ncea.aoa.gov).

The Medical-Legal Interface

It is important to know state laws applicable to cases of mistreatment of older adults; 46 states have a reporting mechanism for mistreatment, either through Adult Protective Services or state agencies associated with aging. Clinicians need to be familiar with the reporting mandates in their area. In some states, neglect by others must be reported, while reports of self-neglect are not required. Adult children can be charged with neglect of the older parent if a caregiving relationship can be proved and it can also be proved that care has been precipitously withdrawn without substitute services. In states where self-neglect is reportable, this is usually the largest intake category. Finally, states can mandate reports for self-neglect but may not provide any services unless the older adult agrees to accept them.

Clinicians are in a key position to assess and report suspected mistreatment of older adults, and most states require such reporting. Although clinicians are appropriately wary of acting precipitously, they should be willing to enlist the help of government agencies and the courts when mistreatment is clearly dangerous for an older adult. Penalties can be assessed against a nonreporter in some regions. Reports of mistreatment of older adults are confidential, and as is the case with reports of child abuse, the clinical reporter is protected from litigation unless it can be proved that the report was made maliciously. The home page for the National Center on Elder Abuse (www.ncea.aoa.gov) provides one means for reporting information.

Especially when a case is to be reported, photographs and body charts may be required to document the findings on physical examination. Risk management personnel can provide guidance in documentation and assist the clinician when evidence suggests that there may be a need for police or court action. In any case in which the clinician is called to court to discuss his or her findings, documentation is an important part of testimony. Cases of mistreatment are often extremely complicated, and it is likely that experts in several fields will need to work with clinicians and administrators to avoid under- or over-reporting of mistreatment of older adults and to provide the best outcomes for the victims of mistreatment.

References

- Acterno R, Hernandez MA, Amstadter AB, et al. Prevalence and correlates of emotional, physical, sexual, and financial abuse and potential neglect in the United States: the national elder mistreatment study. *Am J Public Health.* 2010;100(2):292–297.
- Capezuti E. Recognizing and referring suspected elder mistreatment. *Geriatr Nurs.* 2011;32(3):209–211.
- Dong XQ, Simon M, Evans D. Cross-sectional study of the characteristics of reported elder self-neglect in a community-dwelling population: findings from a population-based cohort. *Gerontology.* 2010;56(3):325–334.
- Falk NL, Baigis J, Kopac C. Elder mistreatment and the Elder Justice Act. *Online J Issues Nurs.* 2012;17(3):7.

CHAPTER 14—PERIOPERATIVE CARE

KEY POINTS

- Operative therapy is an important option for many health problems affecting older adults.
- The preoperative evaluation should include an appraisal of the patient's medical conditions, functional status, and risk of cardiac and other perioperative complications, as well as recommendations for preoperative testing and therapy to minimize surgical risk.
- Risk indices and practice guidelines for common cardiac, pulmonary, and neuropsychiatric problems assist in decision making and management of older surgical patients.
- While age is a risk factor for perioperative and postoperative complications, these problems can be minimized with appropriate proactive assessment and management.

Surgery is a common form of treatment for older adults; currently >55% of all operative procedures are done in patients ≥65 years old, and this proportion is expected to grow. Many of the chronic conditions that increase in prevalence with advancing age—cataracts, arthritis, vascular occlusions, and cancers—are amenable to surgery. Over half of all malignancies are seen in patients ≥65 years old, and the primary treatment for many tumors is surgical. Advances in surgical, anesthetic, and medical care have lowered surgical risks and shifted the risk-benefit ratio to favor surgery in increasingly older patients with more complex conditions. Nevertheless, although older patients account for just over half of all surgical procedures, they suffer three-quarters of the postoperative mortality, as well as a disproportionate majority of the postoperative morbidity.

Many of the physiologic changes accompanying normal aging impact the perioperative management of the older surgical patient. For example, altered body composition, and decreased kidney function, hepatic blood flow, and hepatic enzyme activity all contribute to changes in the pharmacokinetics of drugs. Cardiac and vascular stiffening complicate fluid management and optimization of intravascular volume. Both volume overload and volume depletion occur commonly in the perioperative setting and are poorly tolerated by many older adults. Stiffening of the thoracic cage and diminished ciliary function contribute to decreases in pulmonary reserve and heightened risk of postoperative pneumonia. Because of decreased thermoregulation, the older surgical patient is at particular risk of perioperative hypothermia. Finally, by mechanisms that are not yet fully elucidated, changes in the brain that accompany aging make older adults exquisitely susceptible to postoperative cognitive changes.

It is well recognized that the aging process is extremely variable from person to person and that within one individual not all organ systems age at the same rate, producing dramatic heterogeneity even among healthy older adults. Older individuals may have several chronic conditions that can impact on perioperative care, either directly or through the medications being used to treat those conditions. The heterogeneity in physiologic aging combined with the potential for multiple comorbidities means that older patients require a more comprehensive and individualized preoperative evaluation. They often benefit from a multidisciplinary approach to perioperative care and recovery.

PREOPERATIVE ASSESSMENT AND MANAGEMENT

Clinicians are commonly asked to perform preoperative evaluations with the goals of reducing complications and death and optimizing patient outcomes. The goal of such a consultation should not be to "clear" the patient for surgery but rather to maximize the possibility of a good outcome from surgery. This consultation should appraise the patient's medical, cognitive, and functional status, assess risk of perioperative and postoperative complications, and provide recommendations for preoperative interventions to minimize potential complications. Preoperative assessment should include evaluation of the patient's cardiovascular, respiratory, renal, metabolic, and neuropsychiatric status, as well as the patient's risk of iatrogenic problems. Usually the preoperative assessment can be accomplished with only a history and physical examination for low-risk procedures, eg, ambulatory, breast, cataract, endoscopic, or superficial surgery (SOE=B). For patients undergoing procedures that are not low risk, or in whom the history and physical examination have uncovered other potential risks, further assessment and testing are indicated.

Cardiovascular System

It is estimated that 25%–30% of postoperative deaths are from cardiac causes, and the likelihood of postoperative cardiac events is directly related to age. Cardiac risk assessment is the most fully developed and widely investigated portion of the preoperative medical assessment. The American Society of Anesthesiologists classification of patient physical status relies heavily on clinical judgment and is not specific for cardiovascular morbidity and mortality (see Table 14.1). This system has been used by anesthesiologists for years and has consistently been shown to be useful in predicting postoperative outcomes. Several indices and algorithms for specifically assessing cardiac risk in noncardiac surgery have been published since the 1970s. In 2007, the American College of Cardiology and the American Heart Association (ACC/AHA) published an algorithm for preoperative cardiac assessment (Figure 14.1). The guideline calls for consideration, in order, of the following clinical factors:

1. Urgency of surgery; if emergent, proceed to surgery if consistent with patient's overall goals (SOE=C). Depending on those goals, broaching the subject of a palliative approach may be appropriate.
2. Presence of active major cardiac risk factors, eg, unstable coronary syndromes, decompensated heart failure, significant arrhythmias, or severe valvular disease; if present, correct these conditions before reconsidering surgery (SOE=B).
3. Type of surgery; if low-risk procedure, proceed to surgery (SOE=B).
4. Patient's functional capacity; if good, proceed to surgery (SOE=B).
5. Presence of other clinical risk factors (see Figure 14.1 for definitions); if none, proceed to surgery (SOE=B).
6. Type of surgery; recommendations vary depending on number of risk factors and whether surgery is of high or intermediate risk (SOE=B).

Aside from a careful history and physical examination to determine the presence of active major cardiac risk factors and to assess functional capacity, supplemental cardiac testing or therapy should be considered in only a few specific circumstances. ECG testing is not necessary in asymptomatic patients undergoing low-risk procedures (SOE=B). An ECG can be helpful for prognostic purposes only if step 6 above is reached in the decision-making algorithm, particularly in patients with clinical risk factors undergoing high-risk (vascular) procedures (SOE=B). ECG findings suggestive of ischemia, left ventricular hypertrophy, or left bundle-branch block portend a higher risk of cardiac complications and death. Measurement of left ventricular function using echocardiography, radionuclide studies, or contrast ventriculography should be considered in patients with dyspnea of uncertain cause, current or prior heart failure and worsening dyspnea, or cardiomyopathy; an ejection fraction <35% is associated with higher rates of postoperative heart failure (SOE=C). When newly diagnosed heart failure is determined to be the cause of unexplained dyspnea, it should be maximally treated before surgery. Controversy exists as to whether asymptomatic heart failure should be sought and treated preoperatively. A recent study showed that patients who are asymptomatic but either have a low ejection fraction or diastolic dysfunction are at higher risk of postoperative cardiac events than those with normal ventricular function; however, cohort studies evaluating the benefit of screening echocardiograms to identify such patients have failed to demonstrate improved postoperative outcomes (SOE=B).

Recommendations for preoperative noninvasive cardiac stress testing have been scaled back over the past few years. Stress testing should be considered in patients with clinical risk factors who are undergoing intermediate- or high-risk procedures if the results of the stress testing will change management, eg, postponement or cancellation of surgery (SOE=B). Stress testing should be particularly considered in patients with poor exercise capacity and other clinical risk factors, who are considering vascular (high-risk) surgery. It is under comparatively rare circumstances that coronary revascularization (with coronary artery bypass graft surgery or percutaneous coronary intervention) should be performed before noncardiac surgery to decrease risk of cardiac complications (SOE=A), and as medical therapies continue to advance, the benefit of surgery relative to medical therapy even for these indications has narrowed. For indications for perioperative revascularization, see Table 14.2 (SOE=A).

Certain medications given before or after surgery reduce cardiac and vascular complications of surgery. In general, prior antiplatelet therapy can be safely continued in patients undergoing neuraxial anesthesia, cutaneous surgery, dental procedures, diagnostic endoscopy, ophthalmologic procedures, and peripheral vascular surgery (SOE=C). For patients already on an anticoagulant, its protective benefits need to be weighed against the risk of perioperative hemorrhage. Anticoagulation therapy does not need to be withheld (as long as the INR is therapeutic) for cutaneous surgery (SOE=C), dental extractions and minor oral procedures (SOE=B), or cataract surgery (SOE=C). For other surgical procedures, cessation of warfarin, with or without bridging therapy with low-molecular-weight heparin (LMWH), can be based on the patient's risk factors for thromboembolism (Table 14.3). For patients receiving bridging therapy, LMWH can generally be restarted 24 hours after surgery, longer in cases of major surgery with increased risk of major bleeding. The indications for infective endocarditis prophylaxis were dramatically reduced with the publication of new guidelines by the American Heart Association in 2007.

Table 14.1—American Society of Anesthesiologists Classification of Physical Status

Class	Description
I	A healthy patient
II	A patient with mild systemic disease
III	A patient with severe systemic disease
IV	A patient with severe systemic disease that is a constant threat to life
V	A moribund patient who is not expected to survive without surgery
VI	A declared brain-dead patient whose organs are being harvested for donor purposes

NOTE: There is no additional information to help further define these categories.

SOURCE: Data from American Society of Anesthesiologists. ASA Physical Status Classification System. Available at: www.asahq.org/clinical/physicalstatus.htm (accessed Oct 2013).

Respiratory System

Postoperative pulmonary complications, most commonly atelectasis, pneumonia, and prolonged mechanical ventilation, occur more often in older adults than in younger age groups. The impact of these complications is more costly than the cardiovascular complications of surgery in older adults (SOE=A). Pulmonary complications are predictive of increased short- and long-term mortality in older adults and have been reported to prolong the hospital stay by an average of 1–2 weeks in this age group. A comprehensive review published by the American College of Physicians (ACP) in 2006 found that age is a powerful independent risk factor for postoperative pulmonary complications (SOE=A). Other patient-associated major risk factors include COPD, ASA Class II or greater (see Table 14.1), heart failure, deficit in activities of daily living, and a serum albumin <3.5 g/dL (SOE=A). Minor patient-associated risk factors include acute confusion or delirium, alcohol use, smoking, weight loss, pulmonary findings on physical examination, and an increased BUN concentration (SOE=B). The following procedures are associated with increased pulmonary complications: emergency surgery; prolonged (>3 hour) surgery; repair of abdominal aortic aneurysm (AAA); neurosurgery; and thoracic, abdominal, head and neck, or vascular surgery (SOE=A). General anesthesia is also a risk factor (SOE=A).

In 2007, the ACP published a guideline for risk assessment and perioperative management of pulmonary complications associated with noncardiothoracic surgery. It calls for preoperative assessment of pulmonary risk by appraising the above predictive factors through history, physical examination, and modest laboratory testing. Routine chest radiography is not recommended, but imaging can be helpful for detection and management of pulmonary conditions in patients with known cardiac

Table 14.2—Major Indications for Revascularization in the Perioperative Period

- Significant left main vessel disease
- 3-Vessel disease with stable angina
- 2-Vessel disease with proximal left anterior descending stenosis, stable angina, and either left ventricular ejection fraction <50% or ischemia on noninvasive stress testing
- Acute coronary syndrome
- Acute ST-segment myocardial infarction

or pulmonary disease who are undergoing thoracic, upper abdominal, or surgery for AAA. Spirometry should be reserved for evaluating lung function in patients suspected of having undiagnosed COPD after history and physical examination, based on findings such as dyspnea or wheezing. The question of whether treatment of newly discovered COPD changes outcomes after surgery has not been well studied. Preoperative pulmonary function testing is also routine before lung reduction surgeries. In recent years, several tools to predict the risk of postoperative respiratory failure and postoperative pneumonia have been published. The type of surgery, whether the surgery is emergent, the albumin level, BUN level, functional status, presence of COPD, and age are all components of the Veterans Administration Surgical Quality Improvement Program respiratory failure risk index (SOE=B). The same group validated a risk index to predict postoperative pneumonia using largely clinical information (SOE=B).

The ACP guideline primarily recommends postoperative lung expansion therapy, which has been associated most consistently with reduced pulmonary complications of atelectasis, pneumonia, bronchitis, and severe hypoxemia (SOE=A). Lung expansion therapy can be accomplished through deep breathing exercises, incentive spirometry, and/or continuous positive-airway pressure. Use of a nasogastric tube for management of postoperative nausea and vomiting, inability to tolerate oral feeding, or abdominal distention can also be helpful for minimizing pulmonary complications (SOE=B). The evidence is also good for using short-acting neuromuscular blocking agents (as opposed to long-acting agents) to reduce complications (SOE=B). Less clear are the benefits of preoperative smoking cessation, use of laparoscopic versus open procedures, epidural versus general anesthesia, and epidural analgesia.

Kidneys and Metabolism

Glomerular blood flow decreases with age as does muscle mass, such that an apparently normal serum creatinine can be misinterpreted as indicating normal kidney function. The glomerular filtration rate (GFR) can be estimated by calculating the creatinine clearance using the Cockcroft-Gault equation or by relying on the

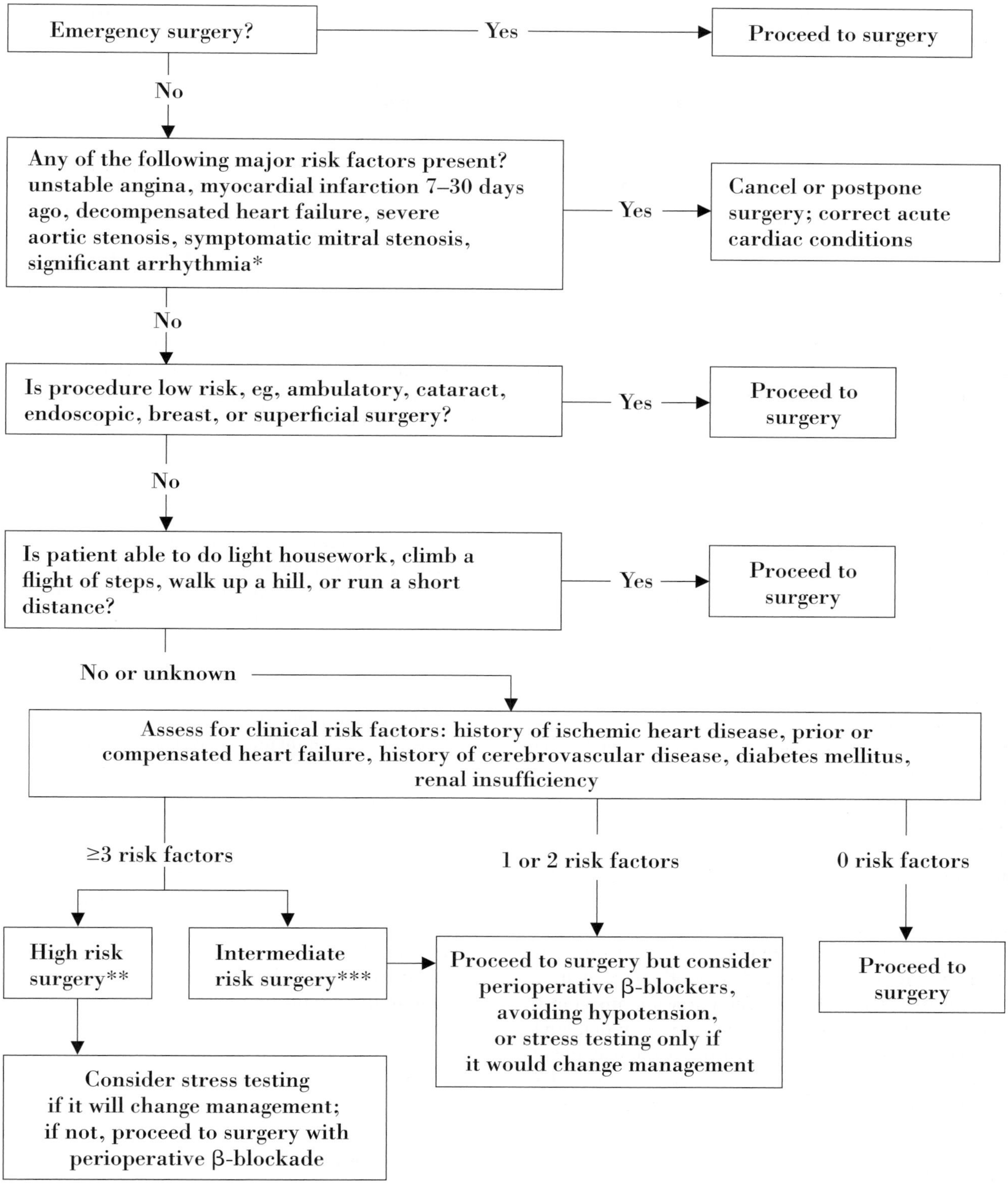

Figure 14.1—Assessing Cardiac Risk in Noncardiac Surgery

* High-grade AV block, Mobitz II AV block, third-degree AV block, symptomatic ventricular arrhythmias, supraventricular arrhythmias with resting heart rate >100 beats per minute, newly recognized ventricular tachycardia

** Open aortic or other major vascular surgery, peripheral vascular surgery

*** Intraperitoneal or intrathoracic surgery, carotid endarterectomy, endovascular abdominal aortic aneurysm repair, head and neck surgery, orthopedic surgery, prostate surgery

SOURCE: Data from Fleisher LA, Beckman JA, Brown KA, et al. ACC/AHA 2007 guidelines on perioperative cardiovascular evaluation and care for noncardiac surgery: a report of the American College of Cardiology/American Heart Association Task Force on Practice Guidelines (Writing Committee to Revise the 2002 Guidelines on Perioperative Cardiovascular Evaluation for Noncardiac Surgery). *Circulation.* 2007;116(17):e418–e499.

Modification of Diet in Renal Disease study (MDRD method) that some laboratories use to automatically calculate GFR (see the section on elimination in "Pharmacotherapy," p 81; and "Kidney Diseases and Disorders," p 420). Because many drugs administered during the perioperative period may require dosage adjustments in patients with diminished renal function, accurate estimation of GFR is important.

Also, because of decrements in the ability of the kidney to appropriately conserve salt or to maximally concentrate or dilute urine in response to intravascular volume or osmolality, the use of intravenous fluids needs to be monitored carefully. The combination of pain in a patient who is receiving nothing by mouth while receiving intravenous 5% dextrose in 0.45% normal saline may result in hyponatremia.

Neuropsychiatric Concerns

Delirium is a common event in the postoperative period. The type of surgery appears to be an important determinant of delirium, with incidence rates ranging from about 4%–5% in cataract or urologic procedures to 50%–60% in some series of patients with infrarenal AAA repair or hip fracture surgery. Both preoperative and intraoperative factors have been evaluated as risk factors for delirium. Preoperative assessment is focused on identifying factors in patients undergoing surgery that predispose to postoperative delirium, including age ≥70 years; cognitive impairment; limited physical function; a history of alcohol abuse; abnormal serum sodium, potassium, or glucose; intrathoracic surgery; and AAA surgery. Preoperative assessment should include clear assessment and documentation of mental status, so that postoperative assessments have a baseline for comparison. The most important intraoperative factor found to be associated with delirium is volume of intraoperative blood loss. Patients with a postoperative hematocrit <30% have an increased risk of delirium irrespective of the presence or absence of preoperative risk factors (SOE=B). Undertreatment of pain postoperatively is a significant risk factor for the development of delirium, at least in patients who were cognitively intact at baseline (SOE=B). When preoperative risk factors are present, the clinician can identify patients at greatest risk of developing delirium and can be vigilant about correcting fluid, electrolyte, and metabolic derangements; optimizing replacement of blood loss; maintaining circadian rhythms (by getting patients out of bed during the day and minimizing sleep interruptions at night); and prescribing medications cautiously while assuring adequate pain control. See also the section on postoperative delirium in "Delirium," p 276.

Avoiding Iatrogenic Complications

Untoward effects of well-intentioned interventions are common among older hospitalized adults. Some of the more common pitfalls to be avoided include mobility restriction, excessive use of catheters, inattention to nutrition and hydration status, and inappropriate use of medications. Few disease states benefit from bed rest. It is important to maintain mobility and function as much as possible by encouraging time out of bed and avoiding restraints. The risks of skin breakdown, muscle atrophy, joint stiffness, and bone loss can be reduced by preserving mobility (SOE=C). Although bladder catheters can sometimes be critical in accurately measuring urine output, prolonged use of an indwelling catheter carries substantial risk of infection. Indwelling catheters can also contribute to restricted mobility and should be removed as soon as possible. Restricted diets and lack of access to water can contribute to compromise in nutrition and hydration. Studies demonstrate that the traditional practice of nothing by mouth beginning the night before surgery to reduce the risk of aspiration is not more beneficial than nothing by mouth for 6 hours except water, with the latter approach more comfortable for the patient and less likely to cause volume depletion (SOE=B). Conversely, continued administration of intravenous fluids after the patient is able to maintain hydration orally can result in volume overload and impaired oxygenation. A regular review of medication administration can avoid unnecessary drug use and inappropriate dosing.

Perioperative and Postoperative Management of Selected Medical Problems

Surgery in older adults often results in destabilization of chronic, coexistent medical conditions. Additionally, because of the diminished physiologic reserve common in older adults, new medical problems can arise in the postoperative period. Some of the most common medical issues to contend with postoperatively are discussed here.

Cardiovascular Problems

The most common cardiovascular problems that arise in older adults after surgery are hypertension, rhythm disturbances, and heart failure. Postoperative hypertension should initially prompt a search for a noncardiovascular cause, such as pain or urinary retention. Next, it is important to assess volume status, review fluid administration records, and note whether antihypertensive medications were mistakenly omitted

Table 14.3–Cessation of Anticoagulation Before Surgery in Older Adults[a]

Thromboembolic Risk	Patient Conditions Determining Risk	Recommendations for Cessation of Anticoagulation
Low	No VTE in past 12 months; AF without prior TIA/stroke and 0–2 stroke risk factors[b]; bileaflet mechanical aortic valve without AF, prior TIA/ stroke, or stroke risk factors	If INR therapeutic, stop warfarin 5 days before surgery, earlier if INR is supratherapeutic or >3; bridging therapy with LMWH at prophylactic dosage is optional.
Intermediate	VTE in past 3–12 months; recurrent VTE; active malignancy; AF without prior TIA/stroke and with 3–4 stroke risk factors[b]; bileaflet mechanical aortic valve with AF, prior TIA/stroke, or any stroke risk factors	Stop warfarin 5 days before surgery and begin LMWH 3 days before surgery at therapeutic (preferred) or prophylactic (optional) dosage; give last preoperative LMWH dose at one-half total daily dosage 24 hours before surgery.
High	VTE within past 3 months; TIA/stroke within 3 months; rheumatic heart disease; AF with prior TIA/stroke and 3–4 stroke risk factors; mechanical mitral valve or ball/cage mechanical aortic valve	Stop warfarin 5 days before surgery and begin LMWH 3 days before surgery at therapeutic dosage; give last preoperative LMWH dose at one-half total daily dosage 24 hours before surgery.

VTE = venous thromboembolism; AF = atrial fibrillation; TIA = transient ischemic attack; INR = international normalized ratio; LMWH = low-molecular-weight heparin

[a] SOE=C

[b] Stroke risk factors: age ≥75 years old, hypertension, diabetes mellitus, history of heart failure

SOURCE: Data from Douketis JD, Berger PB, Dunn AS, et al. The perioperative management of antithrombotic therapy. American College of Chest Physicians Evidence-Based Clinical Practice Guidelines. *Chest*. 2008;133:299–339S.

before the procedure. To treat uncontrolled essential hypertension, parenteral formulations are available in several classes of medications: β-blockers, calcium channel blockers, ACE inhibitors, and drugs that block both α- and β-adrenergic receptors. Topical agents, such as topical nitroglycerin, could also be considered useful when the patient is unable to take medications by mouth.

Cardiac rhythm disturbances are a concern because they can lead to myocardial ischemia and heart failure. Supraventricular tachycardia, commonly seen in older adults, is associated with a history of prior supraventricular dysrhythmias, asthma, heart failure, and premature atrial complexes on a preoperative ECG. This rhythm disturbance is also more common in patients who have had vascular, abdominal, or thoracic procedures. Early restoration of sinus rhythm, or at least controlling the ventricular rate, can be attempted with an infusion of adenosine, a β-blocker, or a calcium channel blocker. If the rhythm is atrial fibrillation, conversion to sinus rhythm can be attempted with electrical cardioversion or by an infusion of amiodarone if the atrial fibrillation is poorly tolerated and the risk of thromboembolism is low. Because spontaneous reversion to sinus rhythm often occurs by 6 weeks after surgery, long-term use of an antidysrhythmic such as amiodarone may not be necessary. Persistent atrial fibrillation beyond 24–48 hours is associated with an increased risk of thromboembolism, and consideration should be given to anticoagulation therapy to reduce the risk of stroke (SOE=A).

Cardiac reserve is often compromised among older adults, especially those with chronic hypertension or coronary artery disease. Heart failure can develop as a result of excessive fluid administration, new cardiac ischemia, or a rhythm disturbance. It can be extremely challenging to ensure optimal ventricular filling pressures based on the clinical assessment of volume status in older adults by physical examination and standard laboratory parameters alone. Although some have recommended the use of pulmonary artery catheters in high-risk patients, studies have not shown a decreased mortality rate for this intervention, and most authorities advise against this approach (SOE=C).

Most older adults who are undergoing surgery or who are hospitalized for significant medical problems should receive prophylaxis for deep venous thrombosis and pulmonary embolism. See Table 14.4 for general guidelines regarding venous thromboembolism prophylaxis.

Kidney and Electrolyte Disorders

Impaired preoperative kidney function increases the risk of postoperative kidney failure. The impaired reserve makes the aging kidney more susceptible to the effects of even transient reductions of cardiac output or brief exposure to nephrotoxic medications. When kidney damage has been sustained, early clinical manifestations include oliguria, isosthenuria, and an increase in serum creatinine. When impaired renal blood flow is the cause, the urine sodium will typically be <40 mEq/L and the urine-to-plasma creatinine ratio will be greater than 10:1. In contrast, if acute tubular necrosis is the mechanism of injury, the urine

Table 14.4–Deep Venous Thrombosis/Pulmonary Embolism (DVT/PE) Prophylaxis in Older Surgical and Medical Inpatients

DVT/PE Risk	Surgeries or Medical Conditions	Thromboprophylactic Options
Low	Healthy and mobile patients undergoing minor surgery, including laparoscopic gynecologic procedures, transurethral or other low-risk urologic procedures, spine surgery, knee arthroscopy	Aggressive early ambulation after procedure
Moderate	Most general surgeries; major vascular procedures; thoracic surgery; open gynecologic and urologic surgery; medical or surgical patients admitted for heart failure or severe respiratory disease, or who are at bedrest with active cancer, previous DVT/PE, sepsis, active neurologic disease, or inflammatory bowel disease	Fondaparinux, LMWH, or unfractionated heparin[a]
High	Total hip replacement, total knee replacement, hip fracture surgery, trauma, spinal cord injury	Fondaparinux, LMWH, rivaroxaban (hip or knee replacement), or warfarin[a]

LMWH = low-molecular-weight heparin

[a] For patients at high risk of bleeding, acceptable alternative is intermittent pneumatic compression and/or use of graduated compression stockings.

SOURCE: Reuben DB, Kerr KA, Pacala JT, et al. *Geriatrics At Your Fingertips*, 15th ed. New York: American Geriatrics Society; 2013:22–23. Reprinted with permission.

sediment may have granular or epithelial cell casts, and the urine sodium will be >40 mEq/L with a urine-to-plasma creatinine ratio of less than 10:1. When acute tubular necrosis is suspected, vigorous efforts should be made to preserve kidney function by withholding all potentially nephrotoxic medications and meticulously maintaining a euvolemic state. See "Kidney Diseases and Disorders," p 420.

Another important mechanism of postoperative kidney failure is obstructive nephropathy, especially in older men with prostatic hyperplasia. The partial outflow obstruction combined with immobility, frequent constipation, and exposure to medications with anticholinergic effects compromising detrusor function can easily precipitate acute urinary retention. In addition to oliguria and an increase in serum creatinine, the bladder is typically palpable because of distention. Treatment consists of insertion of a bladder catheter to reduce the risk of hydronephrosis and lasting kidney dysfunction. Commonly, men with prostatic hyperplasia who develop postoperative obstruction are unable to void immediately after catheter removal and may need α-blocking medications and continued use of the catheter for 2–4 weeks, when another voiding trial can be attempted (SOE=C).

Gastrointestinal Concerns

Constipation is quite common postoperatively, as a consequence of the combined effects of altered diet, immobility, and frequent use of narcotics and other constipating medications. At times, ileus and obstipation can be severe and produce significant anorexia, nausea, delirium, and even vomiting. Postoperative iron therapy, commonly prescribed for anemia, is an unproven but likely contributor to postoperative constipation. Given the common co-occurrence of these risk factors for constipation in the postoperative period, a reasonable approach is to simultaneously order a laxative and a fecal softener every time a narcotic is prescribed, particularly if the patient has a history of constipation or if it is reasonably anticipated that mobility will be reduced for >1 day. Prunes or prune juice, applesauce, and bran can all also have promotility effects. For medications useful in preventing and managing constipation, see Table 51.2.

Postoperative diarrhea should raise concern for fecal impaction and antibiotic-associated or *Clostridium difficile* diarrhea in the setting of recent antibiotic use. Checking manually for fecal impaction and testing fecal specimens for leukocytes and *C difficile* toxin may be appropriate. Management must focus carefully on volume resuscitation and treating the underlying cause. Use of antimotility agents, while effective in reducing fecal incontinence from diarrhea, is very risky in older adults in the postoperative period, because they significantly increase the risk of delirium, constipation, and toxic megacolon.

Finally, nausea is not uncommon in the postoperative period, often as a result of narcotic, anesthetic, and other medications; new infection; or slowed gut motility. See the section on nausea and vomiting in "Palliative Care," p 111, for a discussion on approach to management.

Managing Common Endocrine Abnormalities

Type 2 diabetes mellitus is a common comorbid condition of many older adults. Usually, given the long half-life of oral hypoglycemic agents and the nothing-by-mouth status for surgery, oral diabetes medications are withheld the day of surgery. It may be especially important to withhold metformin, given the potential (although quite low) additional risk of metabolic acidosis arising from use of this medication during a time of stress. To optimize glucose control, an intravenous solution containing glucose can be administered at a constant rate while blood glucose by fingerstick assay is closely monitored; subcutaneous insulin should be administered as necessary to control glucose concentrations until the patient is able to resume eating. For a patient with type 2 diabetes who uses insulin, insulin should be withheld on the day of surgery and sliding-scale insulin given (SOE=C). Once the patient is able to start eating, usually half the outpatient dosage of diabetes medications are administered the first day of oral intake, with additional sliding-scale insulin coverage as needed; full doses are resumed as the patient consumes a usual diet.

Perioperative hyperglycemia among diabetic and nondiabetic patients is associated with morbidity and mortality in medical and surgical ICU patients (SOE=B), and in patients undergoing coronary artery bypass grafting (SOE=C) or carotid endarterectomy (SOE=B). Maintaining glucose concentrations of <150 mg/dL with intravenous insulin in the perioperative period for patients undergoing vascular or major noncardiac surgery with planned ICU admission has reduced morbidity and mortality (SOE=B). However, maintaining tight glycemic control (≤110 mg/dL) among ICU patients has been associated with increased occurrence of hypoglycemia and no reduction in mortality (SOE=B), so moderate glucose control in these patients is advised. The value of strict glycemic control in other surgical or medical inpatient populations has not been demonstrated.

Patients taking supplemental corticosteroids require special consideration during the perioperative period. Those taking prednisone at dosages >20–30 mg/d for longer than a week or with known adrenal insufficiency should be given "stress doses" of steroids after surgery (SOE=C). A single preoperative measurement of cortisol, if increased, is useful to assess the hypothalamic-pituitary axis (HPA) in patients who chronically use steroids when the function of the HPA is in question. If the cortisol level is not high, a 30-minute adrenocorticotropic hormone (ACTH) stimulation test may be useful. The dosage of steroids to use is debated, but some authorities advise 25 mg of hydrocortisone equivalents the day of surgery only for minor procedures, 50–75 mg of hydrocortisone equivalents daily (eg, hydrocortisone 20 mg q8h IV) for 1–2 days for moderate surgical stress, and 100–150 mg of hydrocortisone equivalents daily (eg, hydrocortisone 50 mg q8h IV beginning within 2 hours of surgery) continuing for 2–3 days after surgery for high surgical stress. Other authorities simply recommend continuing usual dosages of steroids for elective, uncomplicated surgeries, or doubling or tripling the outpatient dosage by giving hydrocortisone at dosages up to 100–150 mg/d IV for higher-risk or anticipated complicated operations.

Delirium and Postoperative Cognitive Decline

Delirium is one of the most common postoperative complications, and certainly the one for which a geriatrician is most likely to be consulted. In a randomized study, a multicomponent intervention that focused on reducing sleep interruptions, minimizing medications and immobility, enhancing sensory input, and reducing dehydration reduced the rate of developing delirium by one-third over standard care for hospitalized medical patients (SOE=A). This approach, although not specifically studied in the postoperative setting, is likely to be beneficial for these patients as well (SOE=C). For the postoperative geriatric surgical patient, undertreated pain, constipation, electrolyte abnormalities, and perioperative myocardial infarction must be particularly considered as possible precipitants of delirium.

Postoperative cognitive dysfunction, characterized by abnormalities in learning and memory, can be subtle or dramatic and is considered to be a syndrome distinct from delirium. It has been reported most commonly after cardiac surgery but is experienced by patients undergoing procedures that do not involve extracorporeal circulation. Although the symptoms are often short-lived, they persist for many months in 10%–30% of patients. Efforts to define the cause of the syndrome have not yet been successful; studies have not been able to demonstrate links with hypotension, hypoxemia, or type of anesthesia. Because a better understanding of the pathophysiology is lacking, treatment efforts are supportive. See postoperative delirium in "Delirium," p 276.

Pain Management

Management of postoperative pain remains a challenge, particularly in patients with dementia, delirium, or both. The key points to the evaluation and management of acute pain are quite similar to those discussed in "Persistent Pain," p 119; for a useful guide to tools used to help assess postoperative pain in cognitively impaired patients, see Table 16.3. The oldest-old and cognitively impaired patients appear to be at highest risk of undertreatment of pain, so they deserve particular attention. Undertreatment of pain, at least in nondemented individuals, appears to be a more powerful predictor for development of postoperative delirium than narcotic use (SOE=A).

Most postsurgical pain requires narcotic analgesia. Cognitively intact patients may have improved pain relief and overall lower use of narcotics if administered by patient-controlled analgesia pump (SOE=A). Individuals with less severe pain may be able to tolerate scheduled acetaminophen (not to exceed 4 g/d) with only as-needed use of narcotic analgesics, if they are able to ask for them. Patients with pain who are unable to communicate effectively should be given standing orders for narcotic analgesics, with guidelines as to when to withhold the medications, and should be frequently assessed for medication effect. NSAIDs are best avoided because of the potential for GI bleeding, delirium, fluid retention, nephrotoxicity, and cardiovascular risks. Because narcotic analgesics can precipitate constipation, concomitant use of laxatives and fecal softeners is generally advised. A small body of literature is accumulating supporting the benefits of "preemptive" analgesia to reduce anticipated pain and total doses of narcotic required to control pain postoperatively, but this has yet to be studied in older adults. For comprehensive, up-to-date information on pain medications and dosing, see www.geriatricsatyourfingertips.org.

Nonpharmacologic therapies, such as ice packs, heating pads, massage, and relaxation techniques, can be useful adjuncts to therapy and are often underused.

Planning for Transitions

Clinicians can significantly aid patients by anticipating and planning for transitions in care. For useful information about discharge planning and transitioning care from the hospital, see "Transitional Care," p 161.

REFERENCES

- Chow WB, Rosenthal RA, Merkow RP, et al. Optimal preoperative assessment of the geriatric surgical patient: A best practices guideline from the American College of Surgeons National Surgical Quality Improvement Program and the American Geriatrics Society. *J Am Coll Surg*. 2012;215(4):453–466.
- Devereaux PJ, Xavier D, Pogue J, et al. Characteristics and short-term prognosis of perioperative myocardial infarction in patients undergoing noncardiac surgery. *Ann Intern Med*. 2011;154:523–528.
- Douketis JD, Spyropoulos AC, Spencer FA, et al. Perioperative management of antithrombotic therapy and prevention of thrombosis. American College of Chest Physicians Evidence-Based Clinical Practice Guidelines (9th Ed). *Chest*. 2012;141(2 Suppl):e326S–350S.
- Saver C. High complication rate in older adults calls for well-planned care. *OR Manager*. 2010;26(6)10–13.

CHAPTER 15—PALLIATIVE CARE

KEY POINTS

- Palliative care is interdisciplinary care that aims to relieve suffering, optimize function, and assist with decision making for patients with advanced disease and their families, whether the patient is receiving curative treatment or not. It is distinct from hospice. Hospice is a comprehensive care system for patients expected to live ≤6 months, in which patients or their proxies have elected to enroll.
- For many older adults, dying is characterized by inadequately treated physical distress; fragmented care systems; poor to absent communication among clinicians, patients, and families; and enormous strains on family caregiver and support systems.
- Geographic variations in practice patterns and services available, religious beliefs, economic status, medical differences, gender, and cognitive status all affect the experiences of dying individuals.
- Loss of appetite is almost a universal symptom at the end of life; often it is more distressing to loved ones than to the patient.

In the United States, the overwhelming majority of deaths occur among the older adult population. Older adults typically die slowly of chronic diseases, with multiple coexisting problems, progressive dependency on others, and heavy care needs that are met mostly by family members. Many of these deaths become protracted processes for patients, family members, and clinicians, who must make difficult decisions about the use or discontinuation of life-prolonging treatments. Evidence is abundant that the quality of life during the dying process is often poor. For many older adults, dying is characterized by inadequately treated physical distress; fragmented care systems; poor to absent communication among clinicians, patients, and families; and enormous strains on family caregiver and support systems.

Although most Americans spend most of their final months at home, in most parts of the country, their deaths actually occur in the hospital or nursing home. The experience of dying, however, varies greatly from one part of the country to another. In Portland, Oregon, for example, only 35% of adult deaths occur in hospitals, but in New York City >80% occur in hospitals, a difference associated in part with differences in regional hospital bed supply and the availability of community support for the dying. Social and medical differences also account for some patterns. The need for institutionalization or paid caregivers in the last months of life is much higher among poor individuals and women. Similarly, older adults suffering from cognitive impairment and dementia are much more likely than cognitively intact older adults to spend their last days in a nursing home.

OVERALL CARE NEAR DEATH

The Hospitalized Elderly Longitudinal Project (HELP) attempted to characterize the last 6 months of life and dying in 1,266 adults ≥80 years old. Results showed that people tend to overestimate their chances of survival near the end of life (SOE=A). Patients who died within 1 year of enrollment had significant functional impairment in ADLs and expressed strong preferences for not being resuscitated and for comfort care (SOE=A). The number of patients reporting severe pain increased toward the end of life, with one in three reporting severe pain within 3 months of death (SOE=A). These results highlight the need for clinicians to talk with their patients early about their preferences, as well as to provide better symptom control and palliative measures at the end of life.

One of the challenges in providing excellent end-of-life care stems from the inability to adequately predict end of life, particularly for patients with chronic diseases such as heart failure and COPD, in whom exacerbations and remissions are common and unpredictable.

ETHNOGRAPHIC DATA

Ethnographic studies show that ethnic and cultural background influence patients' and families' response to serious illness, desire for aggressive care, death, grief, and mourning (SOE=B).

Respect for life has been shown to affect decision making in some Asian cultures. For example, cardiopulmonary resuscitation as a means of doing everything possible to preserve life is viewed as an act of respect. In the Chinese culture, filial piety implies strong devotion to the dying person, with the oldest child expected to accompany the parent through the final stage of life. Discussions of death are thought perhaps to bring it about or to bring it about sooner, so clinicians must be respectful when entering into discussion about end-of-life issues. Healthcare decisions are generally viewed as family decisions in Chinese culture, so it is important for clinicians to determine who should be present for delivery of bad news or discussion of care goals. (This is good advice regardless of ethnic and cultural background.)

A number of studies have found that, compared with white Americans, black Americans are less likely to use living wills or complete advance directives, and prefer more aggressive medical care for terminal illness (SOE=B). These preferences can conflict with hospice goals that emphasize comfort versus cure. Studies assessing attitudes and values in the context of end-of-life care have shown that black Americans are more likely than white Americans to believe that death should be avoided at all costs and to want to live as long as possible, even with terminal medical conditions. They are also less likely to want to die at home.

Studies of African Americans show that as a group, spirituality plays a dominant role in how end-of-life is experienced and interpreted (SOE=A). Data indicate that African Americans are more likely to pray for a miracle rather than accept death, to believe in the omnipotence of God, to believe that God (rather than medical treatment or the lack of it) determines the timing of death, to view the clinician as God's instrument, and to believe God is able to perform miracles (SOE=A).

Although knowledge of the tendencies of diverse ethnic groups may facilitate communication between clinicians and patients and their families regarding the end of life, it is important to remember that not all patients and families from a particular background will respond and make decisions in a similar manner; assuming patients and families will do so can often lead to misunderstanding. The clinician can better understand the patient's viewpoint by first asking "Is there anything about your culture or your beliefs that would be helpful for me to know as we plan together for the future?" See also "Cultural Aspects of Care," p 58.

Palliative Care and Hospice

Palliative care is interdisciplinary care that aims to relieve suffering, improve quality of life, optimize function, and assist with decision making for patients with advanced illness and their families. It is intended to be offered simultaneously with all other appropriate medical treatment, either by the primary medical team or in conjunction with a palliative care consultant. In contrast, hospice is specialized palliative care limited to patients with ≤6 months to live, if their disease takes its natural course; patients or their proxies have elected to focus on comfort measures and forgo curative treatment.

Hospice is the comprehensive care system for patients with limited remaining life expectancy. It can be provided at home or in institutional settings. Hospice was established as a Medicare benefit in 1982 by the federal government. Initially, hospice coverage was made available through an expanded Medicare benefit; now it is supported through both Medicare and Medicaid, and it is also a benefit of most commercial insurance policies. The benefit is a highly regulated, fully capitated healthcare arrangement, which is now implemented through >3,000 hospice agencies (most nonprofit), and is dedicated to providing comprehensive palliative care for patients with all types of terminal illnesses and their families. Hospice is primarily a home-care program, with access to inpatient hospital beds for the infrequent management of acute problems. Hospice programs receive one of four daily rates for reimbursement that are based on four levels of care: home care, inpatient level of care, continuous care (short-term, nursing-intensive crisis management of symptoms in the home), and respite care. For a summary of the services hospice provides, see Table 15.1.

Table 15.1—Hospice Services

- Care provided by an interdisciplinary team: nurse/care manager, social worker, chaplain, aides, volunteers, physical therapist, occupational therapist, speech therapist, dietitian, physician supervision and services
- Case management by a hospice nurse
- Access to a hospice physician
- Medications at no cost, as long as they are related to the terminal diagnosis and are palliative, as determined by the hospice plan of care
- Tests and other treatments at no cost, as long as they are related to the terminal diagnosis and are palliative, as determined by the hospice plan of care
- Durable medical equipment
- Bereavement services for 13 months after a death

Access to hospice is based on two conditions:

- Two physicians—the hospice medical director and the patient's primary care provider—must certify that they believe the patient has a remaining life expectancy of ≤6 months if the disease runs its expected course.

- The patient or proxy must elect hospice and thereby agree that the care plan with respect to the terminal illness will be managed by the hospice program. In effect, this indicates consent to a palliative, rather than a curative, care approach.

The patient must be recertified on a regular basis. If the patient is no longer judged to have a life expectancy of <6 months, then he or she must be discharged from hospice. The patient can revoke the hospice benefit at any time.

The referring provider, in addition to certifying that the prognosis for remaining life expectancy is ≤6 months, must decide whether to remain the provider of record or to transfer care of the patient to the hospice medical director. If the referring provider remains the provider of record, he or she continues to direct the care of the patient, becomes part of the hospice interdisciplinary team, coordinates treatment decisions related to the terminal illness with the case manager (primary nurse), and may bill under Part B of Medicare or Medicaid. On January 1, 2011, CMS enacted a new regulation on hospices requiring a "face-to-face" visit for all patients entering their third certification period (at 6 months of hospice services), and every 60-day certification period thereafter. Face-to-face visits can be done only by a physician affiliated with the hospice or by a nurse practitioner who is a W2 employee of the hospice. The purpose of this bedside evaluation is for a trained clinician to complete an assessment of a patient's ongoing eligibility for hospice services and ultimately reevaluate a patient's prognosis.

See also "Financing, Coverage, and Costs of Health Care," p 35.

QUALITY INDICATORS FOR PALLIATIVE CARE

Research demonstrates that patients want to communicate with their healthcare providers about their future medical care, including end-of-life issues (SOE=A). It is recommended that clinicians address advance care directives, identify surrogate decision makers, document patient preferences well before the onset of terminal illness, and update these preferences with cognitively intact patients regularly. This should include discussions about preferences for or against mechanical ventilation and other attempts at resuscitation, which have been identified by experts as important quality indicators.

Symptoms are a major cause of distress and suffering during the end stages of life. Studies show that clinicians often tend to underemphasize routine symptom assessment (SOE=C). Clinicians should seek to treat dyspnea, pain, and other distressing symptoms at the end of life.

Family and other informal caregivers risk financial as well as health consequences in caregiving. In one study of nearly 1,000 caregivers, 35% reported that their employment was affected, and significant time and money were spent on caregiving. Both patients and caregivers identify minimizing caregiver burden as a major concern.

A recent clinical controlled trial showed that patients with metastatic non-small-cell lung cancer who received palliative care had improved quality of life and less depression and anxiety, received less aggressive care, had resuscitative preferences documented, had longer stays in hospice, and even had longer survival (SOE=A). This study based the intervention on standards of care for palliative care. Expert opinion recommends the use of quality indicators addressing these issues in palliative and end-of-life care (SOE=D) for other disease states.

COMMUNICATION

Skillful communication by clinicians is essential in palliative care. Most patients are dying from a preexisting chronic illness like heart disease, cancer, cerebrovascular disease, chronic lung disease, dementia, or chronic liver disease. Many face repetitive exacerbations of illness and have to make difficult decisions about treatment options. To accompany patients and families through the process of diagnosis, prognosis, treatment, and eventual death, clinicians need skills in discussing serious news, prognosis, and transitions of care; clarifying goals of care; dealing with emotions of patients and families; and running family meetings. Effective communication in end-of-life care improves patients' and families' experiences of care (SOE=B).

Clinicians have historically received little formal training in communication skills. As a result, some may feel unprepared to deal with these emotionally charged discussions, and others may fear that these discussions will adversely affect the patient and the family, or the clinician-patient relationship. A systematic approach to communication can foster collaboration among the patient, the family, and the clinician (SOE=C). Effective discussions can improve the patient's and the family's ability to plan for the future, set realistic goals, and support one another emotionally.

A key skill to improve communication is recognizing and responding to emotions. Patients' emotional responses interfere with their ability to process cognitive data and thus make decisions about next steps. Patients often report not hearing anything after being told about a life-threatening condition. Responding to emotions helps patients process the emotion so they can move on to understanding the information they are given. It also signifies to patients that they are understood and that the provider is empathetic. Responding to emotions also legitimizes them and lets the patient know it is appropriate to discuss them. An approach to responding to emotions is to first recognize that the patient has had an emotional response, name the emotion to yourself, and then explicitly respond to the patient in a way that lets him or her know you recognized the response. The recognition can be verbal or nonverbal. Data show that how patients are told about serious information impacts patient outcomes (SOE=B).

Communication about serious illness is enhanced when clinicians spend sufficient time getting to know patients as people. Discussing patients' preferences and goals of care will help guide treatment and recommendations. Clinicians need to understand what is important to the patient, including determining how they want information given to them and how they want to participate in decision making about their care.

Table 15.2—Discussing Serious News: A 6-Step Framework

1. Prepare for the meeting	Have all medical facts available. Prepare an appropriate environment.
2. Establish the patient's understanding	Explore the patient's understanding of their illness. Ask "What do you understand about your illness?" or "What have the doctors told you about your illness?"
3. Determine how much the patient wants to know	Not all patients want to know about their medical situation; data suggest this may be true for certain ethnic groups. Ask "Would you like me to tell you the full details of your condition? If not, is there someone else you would like me to talk to?"
4. Tell the patient	Deliver information in a sensitive straightforward manner, avoiding technical language or euphemisms. Check for understanding. Phrasing that includes a warning helps prepare patients for bad news. For example: "The report is back, and it's not as we had hoped. It showed that there is cancer in your colon."
5. Respond to feelings	Acknowledge the patient's emotion.
6. Plan and follow-up	Organize a therapeutic plan that incorporates a follow-up visit and information on how to reach the clinician if additional questions arise.

Although most Americans say they want to be fully informed about their illnesses, a substantial minority may not want to know the full details or may prefer to have another family member informed. Data suggest that these preferences may vary among certain ethnic groups. (See also "Cultural Aspects of Care," p 58.) There is no way to know how much a given patient wants to know or wants to be involved in decision making without asking directly. Patients with serious illness and their families also may have different communication needs, and it is important to determine this early.

Discussing serious news with patients can be anxiety-producing for the clinician, and the literature offers several frameworks (all with similar steps) to do so. For one 6-step framework that can be used as a guide for these difficult conversations, see Table 15.2.

End-of-life decision-making conversations are difficult for patients and clinicians alike. Clinicians can feel like failures in treating patients with terminal conditions, and patients have to confront their mortality. It is important to determine that patients, their families, or both, understand the current medical situation. The 6-step approach for discussing serious news can help. It is important to assess patients' and families' willingness to talk about what to do next. A clinician might ask if the patient has thought about what he or she would do at this point, or what he or she is hoping for or worried about. Based on these discussions, a provider can offer to make a recommendation for care that is seen as consistent with what the patient has expressed. This often will include the suggestion to enroll in hospice or make a referral to palliative care. After making the recommendation, the clinician can explore what the patient and family think about the proposal. The provider might emphasize the expertise of a palliative care team to improve symptom management and help deal with the changes brought on by the disease. When discussing hospice, it is important to specifically describe what hospice can do to meet the patient's goals and needs. Providers should also emphasize their continued involvement with the patient regardless of hospice and or palliative care involvement. Patients and families often have misconceptions about hospice and palliative care, which should be elicited and addressed to ensure that the goals and procedures of hospice and palliative care are understood.

PALLIATION OF SYMPTOMS

Pain

For assessing and treating pain, see "Persistent Pain" p 119, which also includes a section on pain in cognitively impaired older adults, and postoperative pain management in "Perioperative Care," p 102.

Constipation

Constipation is one of the most common and distressing symptoms seen in terminally ill patients. Opioid pain medications significantly contribute to constipation, which is further exacerbated by the reduced mobility and poor fluid intake that accompanies most life-threatening illnesses. Other unwanted effects of opioids generally diminish over time, but constipation usually persists, requiring ongoing bowel management as long as opioid therapy is used (SOE=D). Patients on opioids should receive prophylactic laxatives consisting of a fecal softener (eg, docusate sodium) and a bowel stimulant (eg, senna, bisacodyl), unless diarrhea has already been a problem. If these measures are not effective, then an osmotic laxative (eg, sorbitol, lactulose, or polyethylene glycol) should be added. If there has been no bowel movement for ≥4 days, an enema should be considered. Patients presenting with constipation should be evaluated for bowel obstruction

Table 15.3—Medications for Nausea

Class	Examples	Comments
Dopamine antagonists	Haloperidol[OL] 0.5–2 mg po, IV, or SC q6h, then titrate Prochlorperazine 10–20 mg po q6h, or 25 mg pr q12h, or 5–10 mg IV q6h Promethazine 12.5–25 mg IV, or 25 mg po or pr q4–6h Perphenazine 2–8 mg po q6h	Haloperidol is an effective antinausea medication. Promethazine and perphenazine can have adverse events of sedation, urinary retention, and delirium in frail older adults.
Antihistamines	Diphenhydramine 25–50 mg po q6h Meclizine 25–50 mg po q6h Hydroxyzine 25–50 mg po q6h	Can cause adverse events of sedation, urinary retention, and delirium in frail older adults
Anticholinergics	Scopolamine 0.1–0.4 mg SC or IV q4h, or 1 to 3 transdermal patches q72h, or 10–80 mcg/h by continuous IV or SC infusion	Useful when cause of nausea is from vestibular apparatus
Serotonin antagonists	Ondansetron 8 mg po q8h Granisetron 1 mg po q24h or q12h	Effective for chemotherapy-induced nausea; expensive
Prokinetic agents	Metoclopramide 10–20 mg po q6h	Useful if nausea is secondary to dysmotility
Antacids	*H_2-receptor antagonists:* cimetidine, famotidine, ranitidine *Proton-pump inhibitors:* omeprazole, lansoprazole	Useful if nausea is caused by gastritis

or fecal impaction. In cases of impaction, manual disimpaction or enemas should be used before starting laxative therapy. See also postoperative GI problems in "Perioperative Care," p 108. Methylnaltrexone bromide is a newer agent approved for the treatment of opioid-induced constipation in patients with advanced illness in whom usual treatment has not been effective. Methylnaltrexone antagonizes opioid binding to the peripheral μ-opioid receptors in the GI tract. It does not cross the blood-brain barrier and has no effect on the central analgesic effects of opioids. It is contraindicated in known or suspected mechanical GI obstruction.

Nausea and Vomiting

The incidence of nausea and vomiting is estimated to be 40%–70% in patients with advanced cancer (SOE=B). Nausea is a subjective sensation mediated through the stimulation of the GI lining, the chemoreceptor trigger zone, the vestibular apparatus, and the cerebral cortex. Vomiting is a neuromuscular reflex. Symptoms can be caused by disease or its treatment. Because nausea involves multiple neurotransmitters, numerous agents are used for treatment, and often more than one medication is needed for control. The key to successful management involves identifying the likely cause of the nausea, selecting a medication that works on that cause, and giving around-the-clock medication if the nausea is constant (SOE=D). For medications useful in the treatment of nausea, see Table 15.3.

Diarrhea

Diarrhea affects 7%–10% of patients with cancer being admitted to hospice (SOE=C). Diarrhea is defined as the passage of more than three unformed bowel movements within a 24-hour period. The clinician should be alert to the possibility of fecal impaction that presents as watery diarrhea, particularly in immobile older adults on opioids. The treatment of impaction should begin with manual disimpaction and tap-water enemas, followed if unsuccessful by high colonic enemas. Laxatives should not be administered until the impaction is cleared because of the risk of bowel perforation. Untreated fecal impaction can be life threatening. Another common cause of diarrhea in palliative medicine is excessive laxative therapy, especially after laxative dosages have been increased to clear an impaction; this can respond to temporarily stopping laxatives and reintroducing them at a lower dosage. Radiotherapy involving the abdomen and pelvis causes diarrhea, peaking during the second or third week of therapy. This typically responds to cholestyramine at 4–12 g q8h (SOE=C). Diarrhea caused by fat malabsorption (eg, pancreatic insufficiency or small-bowel disease) responds to pancreatic enzymes such as pancreatin (SOE=B). Diarrhea after ileal resection also responds to cholestyramine.

Bowel Obstruction

The incidence of bowel obstruction can be up to 50% in ovarian and GI cancer. Patients diagnosed with malignant bowel obstruction have a poor prognosis, with a median survival of 3 months. In older adults, bowel obstruction can have multiple causes, including intraluminal obstruction from a tumor, infiltration of the bowel wall, external compression of the bowel wall, dysmotility, fecal impaction, adverse effects of radiation treatment, and adhesions from previous surgeries. The symptom burden with bowel obstruction is significant,

Table 15.4—Antisecretory and Antispasmodic Medications for Bowel Obstruction

Drug	Dosage	Comments
Glycopyrrolate	0.2–0.4 mg SC q2–4h	Antisecretory; less centrally mediated adverse events because does not penetrate blood-brain barrier.
Scopolamine	0.1–0.2 mg SC or IV q6–8h Transdermal patch every 3 days	Antispasmodic and antisecretory; transdermal patch does not have immediate effect.
Hyoscyamine	0.125 mg SL q4–8h	Antispasmodic; can cause urinary retention and confusion.
Octreotide	12.5 mcg/h SC or IV continuous infusion, or 200–600 mcg SC or IV intermittently; maximum of 900 mcg in 24 hours	Antisecretory; well tolerated and effective in decreasing GI secretions.

and can include nausea, vomiting, colic, and abdominal pain. The evaluation and management of bowel obstruction depends on the functional status of the patient, goals of care, and expected survival. Treatment approaches include surgery, stenting, and medications. There is a scarcity of randomized control trials to guide optimal treatment.

Surgical management has limited evidence for benefit in terms of quality of life and survival in most patients with bowel obstruction at the end of life. Surgery may be beneficial for patients with a good performance status, an operable lesion, and an expected survival of 2–6 months.

Advances in endoscopic techniques and self-expanding metallic stents have allowed for a nonsurgical approach to bowel obstruction. Stents are used for gastric outlet, small-bowel, and colonic obstructions. They are most useful for patients with a single point of obstruction or locally extensive disease. Stents are contraindicated in patients with perforation and peritonitis, and are not well tolerated if the lesion is within 2 cm of the anal margin.

The mainstay of treatment for bowel obstruction is medical management. In most patients, symptoms can be alleviated by combination therapy with opioids, antispasmodic medications, antiemetics, antisecretory agents, and corticosteroids (see nausea and vomiting, p 115). Opioids can be given subcutaneously, intravenously, sublingually, and transdermally, and should be titrated for relief of abdominal pain. Opioids can aggravate colic, so this needs to be assessed. For antispasmodic and antisecretory medications helpful in bowel obstructions, see Table 15.4. Corticosteroids have been used for bowel obstruction as antiemetics, as analgesics, and to reduce peritumor edema. Generally, they are given for 4–5 days and discontinued if there is no response. If medical management is not effective, a venting gastrostomy may be considered.

Nasogastric tubes are often placed if a patient is admitted to the hospital with a bowel obstruction. A nasogastric tube should be a temporary measure while a decision about surgery is considered or medications to control symptoms are started. Nasogastric tubes are associated with pain, sinusitis, aspiration, and erosions in the nose and esophagus.

Anorexia and Cachexia

Loss of appetite is almost a universal symptom of patients with serious and life-threatening illness. Anorexia in those who are actively dying and who do not express a desire to eat need not be treated. Symptoms of dry mouth can be alleviated with ice chips, popsicles, moist compresses, or artificial saliva. Lemon glycerin swabs should not be used, because they irritate dry and cracked mucosa. Megestrol acetate and corticosteroids[OL] have been found to enhance appetite, cause weight gain (primarily fat), and improve quality of life in some patients with anorexia (SOE=B). However, these agents have not prolonged survival or improved function or treatment tolerance of cancer therapies, and they are associated with their own adverse events (SOE=B). In general, patients should be encouraged to eat whatever is most appealing without regard to dietary restrictions.

Enteral feedings are often used in chronically ill and dying patients because of families' and clinicians' perceived need to provide nutrition. There is no evidence to support the use of enteral feedings in this situation. Enteral feedings are not associated with improved quality of life or survival in this context and are associated with increased aspiration and other complications. An inability to maintain oral nutrition in patients with chronic life-limiting disease is a marker of dying. There are a few situations in which enteral feeding might enhance quality and quantity of life; examples include patients with good functional status and proximal GI obstruction; patients receiving chemotherapy or radiation, or both, involving the proximal GI tract; and patients with amyotrophic lateral sclerosis. See also "Eating and Feeding Problems," p 216.

Delirium

Delirium, agitation, and confusion are common in terminally ill older patients and are often distressing to both patients and family members. Initial efforts should be directed at identifying potentially reversible causes (eg, infection, impaction, uncontrolled pain, urinary retention, and hypoxia). Antipsychotics such as haloperidol^{OL} or risperidone^{OL} in low dosages are effective treatments for both hypoactive and hyperactive delirium if medications are thought to be indicated, either to ensure the patient's safety or because the delirium appears to be causing distress. Actively dying patients who are nonambulatory and who experience terminal delirium often appear less distressed with use of sedating antipsychotics such as chlorpromazine^{OL}. Because benzodiazepines are often associated with paradoxical agitation and a worsening of the delirium in older adults, their use should be carefully considered. See also "Delirium," p 276.

Depression

Depression is under-recognized and undertreated, both in older adults and terminally ill patients. It may be underdiagnosed because of clinicians' mistaken belief that it is either a normal consequence of aging or appropriate in the context of a terminal illness. Because of underlying illness, standard vegetative symptoms described in the *Diagnostic and Statistical Manual of Mental Disorders* (insomnia, anorexia, weight change) are often not reliable indicators. Instead, clinicians should watch for change in mood, loss of interest, and suicidal ideation. Suicidal ideation should be openly discussed, including any symptoms that are contributing to the patient's suffering, which may be influencing his or her consideration of suicide. Aggressive treatment of symptoms, antidepressant therapy, cognitive-behavioral therapy, and psychiatric consultation are all appropriate initial responses. Continued discussion with the patient about a wish to hasten death often reveals a change of mind as time passes.

Standard antidepressant therapy is effective, but most agents have a delayed onset of 2–6 weeks. Psychostimulants (eg, methylphenidate^{OL}, dextroamphetamine^{OL}) are well tolerated, safe, and effective short-term treatments for medically ill depressed patients (SOE=B). Additionally, they can have a rapid onset and beneficial effect on energy, mood, appetite, and mental alertness. Methylphenidate is started at 2.5 mg in the early morning hours and given concurrently with standard antidepressants; it should be avoided in the evening hours. Finally, electroconvulsive therapy is an effective, safe method of rapidly treating depression and should be used for those who are severely depressed. The American Psychiatric Task Force Report states that electroconvulsive therapy be considered a first-line therapy when rapid response is needed (SOE=D). The presence of space-occupying CNS lesions is an important contraindication. See also "Depression and Other Mood Disorders," p 308.

Dyspnea

Dyspnea, the subjective experience of breathlessness, is one of the most distressing symptoms experienced by dying individuals. Self-reporting by the patient is the only reliable measure of dyspnea, because respiratory rates, pulmonary congestion, hypoxia, or hypercarbia do not correlate with breathlessness. Clinicians may mistakenly fear that treating dyspnea in patients close to the end of life is associated with unacceptably high risks, leading some to withhold treatment and others to prescribe inadequate dosages of medications.

Because breathlessness has many causes (eg, anxiety, airway obstruction, bronchospasm, hypoxemia, pneumonia, cachexia from advanced disease), symptomatic management should begin immediately while the underlying cause is being investigated. Like pain, dyspnea is mediated through the interaction of complex pathophysiologic processes with poorly defined psychologic factors. The optimal therapy for dyspnea is to treat its underlying cause. When this is not possible, one of a number of agents that have been evaluated for treatment of intractable dyspnea is used. The goal of treatment is the subjective improvement in breathlessness, rather than lowering the respiratory rate to normal. Often patients report improvement in breathlessness but still have a high respiratory rate. The most effective agents for the treatment of dyspnea are opioids^{OL}. Opioids are believed to act via a number of different mechanisms. These agents act centrally by decreasing the perception of dyspnea and peripherally on opioid receptors in the lung without affecting respiratory drive. In randomized controlled trials, both oral and parenteral formulations were effective (SOE=A). There is no consensus on starting dosages, but in frail opioid-naive older adults it is best to start low and titrate up. If patients are already on opioids, increasing the dosage by 25%–50% is recommended (SOC=D). Modest evidence supports the use of nebulized opioids for intractable dyspnea. Morphine has been used (although there is no evidence to support the practice), and only small studies have examined the use of fentanyl (SOE=C). The theoretical advantages of nebulized opioids include the avoidance of systemic absorption and the resulting constipation, hypotension, sedation, respiratory depression, and hypercapnia; rapid and efficient absorption because of the large surface area of the lung parenchyma; and ease of administration. This route of administration should be reserved for patients who experience intolerable adverse events from opioids administered by other routes.

Oxygen is considered by many to be an important component of any regimen for dyspnea. It is used and is paid for by hospice, regardless of patients' oxygen saturation. An international study showed that ambient air delivered by nasal cannula was just as effective in relieving breathlessness as oxygen in patients with oxygen saturation >90% (SOE=A). Cool air moving across the face (eg, from fans or an open window) can treat dyspnea by stimulating the second branch of the fifth cranial nerve, which has a central inhibitory effect on the sensation of breathlessness (SOE=C).

Benzodiazepines are beneficial in controlling anxiety associated with dyspnea, but they have not improved breathlessness in randomized controlled trials involving nonanxious persons with COPD (SOE=A). These medications should be used only in breathless patients with accompanying anxiety. Bronchodilators and corticosteroids are useful in patients with bronchospasm. Diuretics are useful in patients with pulmonary congestion.

Cough

Cough is a common symptom; its prevalence has been reported in the palliative care literature as ranging from 29% to 83%. Normal cough maintains the patency and cleanliness of the airways and thus should be treated only when distressing to the patient. Cough can be caused by the production of excessive amounts of fluids (eg, blood, mucus), inhalation of foreign material, or stimulation of irritant receptors in the airway. Additionally, patients with neuromuscular disorders may be unable to swallow saliva because of the involvement of bulbar cranial nerves, with the result that saliva causes coughing as it trickles into the larynx or trachea.

Underlying causes of cough should be investigated and treated (eg, diuretics for heart failure, antibiotics for infection, anticholinergics for aspiration of saliva resulting from motor neuron disease); however, resolving the underlying cause may be impossible. Opioids can be useful in these situations.

Dextromethorphan is structurally related to opioids and has central cough-suppressant action with few sedative effects (SOE=D). Codeine and dihydrocodeine, usually in the form of elixirs, are also good first-line choices (SOE=D). Methadone syrup can also be helpful when taken as a single daily dose because of its longer duration of action (SOE=D).

Cough due to an irritated pharynx because of local infection or malignancy can be helped by nebulized anesthetics (SOE=D). Nebulized lidocaine up to four times daily has been reported, anecdotally, to offer relief.

Loud Respiration

Inability to clear secretions from the oropharynx often results in noisy or "rattling" respirations at the end of life. This occurs as secretions oscillate up and down during inspiration and expiration. Although there is no indication that this causes discomfort for patients, it often produces anxiety in family and caregivers. Best management includes preparing the family and caregivers for its occurrence and offering anticholinergic medications to reduce secretions. Because anticholinergic agents do not dry up secretions already present, it is important to educate the family to notify clinicians at the first sign of rattling. Scopolamine^{OL} patches can be effective and also have a sedative effect. Hyoscyamine can also be administered by the sublingual route (0.125 mg), or glycopyrrolate can be given subcutaneously at a dosage of 0.2 mg q8h. When pooling oral secretions are problematic, caregivers may be able to periodically remove secretions by use of a suction device; alternatively, atropine^{OL} eyedrops can be given on or under the tongue.

REFERENCES

- Carlson MD, Lim B, Meier DE. Strategies and innovative models for delivering palliative care in nursing homes. *J Am Med Dir Assoc*. 2011;12(2):91–98.
- End of Life Online Curriculum (a joint project of the U.S. Veterans Administration and Stanford University Medical School). Available at: http://endoflife.stanford.edu/M11_pain_control/intro_m01.html (accessed Oct 2013).
- Lorenz KA, Lynn J, Dy SM, et al. Evidence for improving palliative care at the end of life: a systematic review. *Ann Intern Med*. 2008;148(2):147–159.

CHAPTER 16—PERSISTENT PAIN

KEY POINTS

- Effective management of pain begins with a thorough assessment to determine its source, severity, and impact on functioning and well-being.
- Persistent pain constitutes a distinct pathology and causes changes throughout the nervous system that may worsen over time. It has significant psychological and cognitive correlates as well.
- Multiple pain scales are available to help quantify the severity of pain. The selection of a pain scale is based on the cognitive and communication abilities of the patient.
- A stepped approach to the treatment of pain is advised, including local therapies and nonpharmacologic approaches. Often, systemic analgesics are needed in the treatment of older adults.
- Tolerance generally develops to the respiratory depression, fatigue, and sedating effects of opioid analgesics, but not to their constipating effect.
- Given persistent pain's diverse effects, interdisciplinary assessment and treatment may produce the best results for people with the most severe and long-lasting pain problems.
- Effective management of persistent pain necessitates a collaborative and ongoing partnership between the clinician, the patient, and family.

Persistent pain conditions affect at least 116 million U.S. adults at a cost of $560–635 billion annually in direct medical treatment costs and lost productivity. Relief of pain and suffering, and promotion of functional status and quality of life are primary tenets of geriatric medicine. Hospice movement pioneer Dame Cicely Saunders coined the term "total pain" and suggested that pain has psychological, social, emotional, and spiritual components that make up the "total pain" experience. In addition, the interpretation of pain is also influenced by a person's cultural beliefs and practices.

Pain is particularly common in adults ≥65 years old. Studies have revealed that 25%–50% of community-dwelling older adults and 45%–80% of nursing-home residents have substantial pain. Pain is also commonly undertreated in older adults who are cognitively impaired, who receive less analgesic medication than younger cognitively intact cohorts. The high prevalence and undertreatment of pain among the older population is probably due to a variety of factors. Some older adults tend to under-report or do not report their pain because of cognitive impairment, limited health literacy, or an erroneous perception that pain is a part of the normal aging process. Clinicians may be overwhelmed in caring for older adults who frequently have several comorbid illnesses, and thus fail to regularly and systematically assess for and manage pain. Even when pain is identified, clinicians may be reluctant to manage it effectively because of the lack of adequate knowledge of pain management strategies, as well as misperceptions about narcotic analgesic medications. Patients, too, may fear addiction to opioid analgesics and commonly choose to live with pain to avoid taking analgesics. In summary, persistent pain in older adults causes intrinsic suffering; can impair functional status; may result in depression, anxiety, and social isolation; and is often underdiagnosed and undertreated.

Pain is an unpleasant sensory and emotional experience associated with actual or potential tissue damage, or described in terms of such damage. Pain is subjective and idiosyncratic, beyond objective measure; its intensity and character are what the patient says they are. Pain is certainly a sensation in a part or parts of the body, but it is also by definition unpleasant and therefore also an emotional experience. *Acute pain* is of sudden onset and expected to last a short time and is clearly linked to a specific bodily insult or injury. *Chronic or persistent pain*, by contrast, is defined as pain without apparent biologic value that has persisted beyond the normal tissue healing time, variously defined as 3–6 months. Persistent pain endures as the pain signals keep firing in the nervous system for weeks, months, or even years after the initial insult or injury. Some people suffer persistent pain even in the absence of any past injury or evident body damage. Persistent pain can become so debilitating that it affects basic and instrumental activities of daily living, causes psychological distress, disturbs sleep, and negatively impacts social and personal relationships. For additional terms used in care of patients in pain, see Table 16.1.

Risk factors for transition from acute to persistent pain in older adults include lower socioeconomic status, vivid memory of childhood trauma, obesity, low level of physical fitness, overuse of joints and muscles, chronic illnesses, lack of social support, and abuse.

ASSESSMENT

A thorough assessment is necessary to formulate a plan to successfully treat persistent pain. The International Association for the Study of Pain (IASP) has developed taxonomy for the classification of pain that identifies five

Table 16.1—Terms Commonly Used in Care of Patients in Pain

Term	Definition
Addiction	Continued use of a substance (eg, an opioid analgesic) despite harmful consequences
Allodynia	Pain caused by a stimulus that does not normally provoke pain
Analgesia	Absence of pain in response to noxious stimulation
Central pain	Pain initiated or caused by a primary lesion or dysfunction in the CNS (eg, pain after stroke, phantom limb pain)
Dysesthesia	An unpleasant abnormal sensation, whether spontaneous or evoked
Hyperalgesia	Increased sensitivity to noxious stimulation
Hyperpathia	A syndrome in which pain-provoking stimuli produce magnified levels of pain
Hypoalgesia	Decreased sensitivity to noxious stimulation
Nociceptor	A nerve fiber preferentially sensitive to a noxious stimulus or to a stimulus that would become noxious if prolonged
Noxious stimulus	A stimulus that is capable of activating receptors for tissue damage
Pseudoaddiction	Refers to the perception by observers of drug-seeking behavior in patients who have severe pain but who have not received effective pain treatment interventions. Such patients may appear preoccupied with obtaining opioids, but the preoccupation reflects a need for pain relief and not drug addiction.
Wind-up pain	Pain sensitization caused by repetitive noxious stimulation of peripheral nerve fibers; may cause experience of a gradual increase in the perceived magnitude of pain.

axes, which are very helpful in the physical assessment of pain:

- Axis I: anatomic regions
- Axis II: organ systems
- Axis III: temporal characteristics, pattern of occurrence
- Axis IV: intensity, time since onset of pain
- Axis V: etiology

A major barrier to effective pain treatment is inadequate assessment. In addition, assessment should include an examination of effects of pain on functional status and sleep, as well as on emotional and social well-being. Because of its subjective nature, clinicians must rely on the patient's or caregiver's description of the pain and on the findings of a thorough physical examination. Assessment is complicated by several factors, including under-reporting of symptoms by many older adults, the existence of multiple medical comorbidities exacerbating the pain and impairing patient function, and the increased prevalence of cognitive impairment as people age. When assessing pain in patients with cognitive impairment, it is important to remember that they may be unable to report their pain, much less its history. They may instead present with depression or agitation, and these secondary behaviors often serve as important clues to the presence of underlying pain.

Pain intensity can be quantified using pain intensity scales. Three commonly used, validated scales are the Numeric Rating Scale, the Faces Pain Scale (Figure 16.1), and the Verbal Descriptor Scale. These scales are referred to as one-dimensional, because they ask the patient to rate the intensity of a single characteristic of the symptom, in this case the intensity of the pain. The patient is asked to rate his or her pain by assigning a numerical value (with 0 indicating no pain, and 10 representing the worst pain imaginable), a verbal description ("no pain" to "pain as bad as it could be"), or a facial expression corresponding to the pain. The choice of scale depends on the preference of a particular language or presence of sensory impairment. For example, if a patient does not speak English well, the faces scale may be the best choice, because it relies on pictures rather than on words or numbers. The Wong-Baker FACES Pain Rating Scale with Foreign Translations is useful for non-English speaking patients http://www.wongbakerfaces.org [accessed Oct 2013]. The same scale should be used at follow-up examinations to evaluate how the pain has changed since the initial assessment. Scales such as the McGill Pain Questionnaire and the Pain Disability Scale measure pain in a variety of domains, including intensity, location, and affect. Although time-intensive, scales measuring multiple domains can provide a wealth of information about the patient's unique experience of pain. However, patients in pain may be unable or unwilling to respond to scales that take time.

Before the physical examination, the patient can be asked to describe the location of the pain using a drawing of a human figure, called a pain map. The patient can indicate the locations on the figure that correspond to their own pain. Pain maps may enhance reliability in repeated assessment of pain in the cognitively intact patient.

If the patient's pain pattern is erratic and diffuse, or does not conform to an anatomic distribution, a referral to a mental health specialist may help in uncovering an underlying disorder that is complicating or contributing to the complex pain presentation.

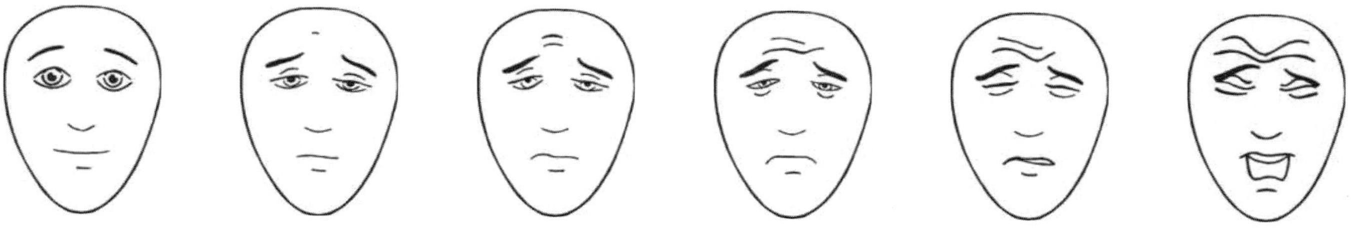

Figure 16.1— Faces Pain Scale–Revised (FPS-R)

Instruct the patient to identify which face best represents the pain he or she is feeling at that moment. Explain, "These faces show how much pain a person is feeling inside. On one end, the face is happy because the person is feeling no pain (point to the left most face). On the other end, the person is in the most pain anyone can imagine (point to the right most face). In between (point to each face from left to right), the faces show more and more pain. Point to the face that best shows the pain you are feeling now." Each face has been assigned a numerical score (0, 2, 4, 6, 8, 10). Record the score that corresponds to the face selected.

SOURCE: Hicks CL, von Baeyer CL, Spafford P, et al. The Faces Pain Scale–Revised: Toward a common metric in pediatric pain measurement. *Pain.* 2001;93:173–183. Bieri D, Reeve R, Champion GD, et al. The Faces Pain Scale for the self-assessment of the severity of pain experienced by children: Development, initial validation and preliminary investigation for ratio scale properties. *Pain.* 1990;41:139–150.

This figure has been reproduced with permission of the International Association for the Study of Pain® (IASP®). The figure may not be reproduced for any other purpose without permission.

The physical examination should include careful scrutiny of the reported site of the pain and any part of the body that may be a source of referred pain. (Occipital pain, eg, should prompt examination of the neck, and knee pain examination of hip and lumbar region. See "Back and Neck Pain," p 465.) The initial evaluation should include a complete musculoskeletal examination, recognizing the common findings of musculoskeletal disorders such as fibromyalgia, osteoarthritis, and myofascial pain, as either the primary source of pain or exacerbating processes. Accurate diagnosis of these disorders is a critical part of formulating the correct therapeutic plan (see treatment, below). Fibromyalgia may be under-recognized in older adults. It is typically characterized by multiple tender points, sleep disturbance, fatigue, generalized pain (often with a strong axial component), and morning stiffness. Myofascial pain is present in many patients with persistent pain, and is diagnosed by the presence of taut bands of muscles and trigger points (ie, pain that may radiate distally when firm pressure is applied to a muscle, as opposed to tender points, in which radiation of pain is absent).

Pain syndromes can be divided into at least three types: nociceptive, neuropathic, and undetermined (Table 16.2). Nociceptive pain describes pain due to the activation of nociceptive sensory receptors by noxious stimuli resulting from inflammation, swelling, and injury to tissues. It can be defined further as either somatic or visceral pain. Somatic pain is well localized in skin, soft tissue, and bone. It is commonly described as throbbing, aching, and stabbing. Visceral pain, often due to cardiac, GI, or lung injury, is not well localized and difficult to describe. Patients describe visceral pain as crampy, tearing, dull, and aching. Either type of nociceptive pain is often adequately treated with common analgesics.

Neuropathic pain derives from the irritation of components of the central or peripheral nervous system. Patients typically report burning, numbness with "pins and needles" sensations, and shooting pains. Common causes of neuropathic pain include diabetic neuropathy and post-herpetic neuralgia, while central pain after stroke and phantom limb pain experienced after amputation occur less often. Confusion between neuropathic pain and myofascial pain is possible, because patients may describe both as "burning." Careful physical examination will help to differentiate these disorders (ie, taut bands and trigger points with myofascial pain, and allodynia or hyperalgesia with either disorder); both may be present in the same patient. Neuropathic pain responds unpredictably to opioid analgesia; it may respond well to nonopioid therapies such as anticonvulsants, tricyclic antidepressants, and antiarrhythmic medications.

Mixed or unspecified pain is described as having characteristics of both nociceptive pain and neuropathic pain. An example of a mixed pain syndrome is chronic headache of unknown cause. Older adults often have mixed pain syndromes. Lower back pain, for example, is often a combination of spinal malalignment, myofascial pathology, and neurologic impingement. Treating these patients with trials of different medications or with combinations of medicines may be necessary.

ASSESSING AND TREATING PAIN IN COGNITIVELY IMPAIRED OLDER ADULTS

While they are able to speak, patients with mild to moderate dementia are often able to report and

Table 16.2–Types of Pain, Examples, and Treatment

Type of Pain and Examples	Source of Pain	Typical Description	Effective Drug Classes and Nonpharmacologic Treatments (SOE)
Nociceptive: somatic			
Arthritis, acute postoperative, fracture, bone metastases	Tissue injury, eg, bones, soft tissue, joints, muscles	Well localized, constant; aching, stabbing, gnawing, throbbing	Acetaminophen (A), opioids (B), NSAIDs (A) Physical and cognitive-behavioral therapies (B)
Nociceptive: visceral			
Renal colic, constipation	Viscera	Diffuse, poorly localized, referred to other sites, intermittent, paroxysmal; dull, colicky, squeezing, deep, cramping; often accompanied by nausea, vomiting, diaphoresis	Treatment of underlying cause, acetaminophen (C), opioids (B) Physical and cognitive-behavioral therapies (C)
Neuropathic			
Cervical or lumbar radiculopathy, post-herpetic neuralgia, trigeminal neuralgia, diabetic neuropathy, post-stroke syndrome, herniated intervertebral disc	Peripheral or central nervous system	Prolonged, usually constant, but can have paroxysms; sharp, burning, pricking, tingling, squeezing; associated with other sensory disturbances, eg, paresthesias and dysesthesias; allodynia, hyperalgesia, impaired motor function, atrophy, or abnormal deep tendon reflexes	Tricyclic antidepressants (A), serotonin-norepinephrine reuptake inhibitor antidepressants (A), anticonvulsants (A), opioids (B), topical anesthetics (C) Physical and cognitive-behavioral therapies (C)
Undetermined			
Myofascial pain syndrome, somatic symptom pain disorders	Poorly understood	No identifiable pathologic processes or symptoms out of proportion to identifiable organic pathology; widespread musculoskeletal pain, stiffness, and weakness	Antidepressants (B), antianxiety agents (C) Physical (B), cognitive-behavioral (B), and psychologic therapies (B)

SOURCE: Adapted with permission. Reuben DB, Herr KA, Pacala JT, et al. *Geriatrics At Your Fingertips*, 15th ed. New York: American Geriatrics Society; 2013:210.

localize their pain. Patients with severe cognitive impairment who are unable to verbally express pain pose a challenge to the clinicians who care for them. Not only are such patients unable to describe their pain and request analgesia, but clinicians may be hesitant to administer pain medications, fearing that pharmacologic treatment will worsen the patients' mental status. Clinicians must rely on observing these patients for pain-related behaviors, as well as on eliciting observations from caregivers. For common pain behaviors in cognitively impaired older adults, see Table 16.3. Validated scales such as the Hurley Discomfort Scale and the Checklist of Nonverbal Pain Indicators have been developed, but these require trained evaluators to complete properly. Experts suggest providing empiric analgesic therapy during procedures and conditions known to be painful. Trials of analgesia should also be considered for patients exhibiting potentially pain-related behaviors.

TREATMENT

Nonpharmacologic Therapy

A comprehensive review of nonpharmacologic therapies for persistent pain is beyond the scope of this chapter; however, specific therapies are worth mentioning. Many of the strategies mentioned below are appropriate considerations for all patients' treatment plans, and highlight the importance of an interdisciplinary approach to pain treatment.

Patient education and involvement in treatment decisions are essential components of all treatment plans for persistent pain. Patients should be taught how to take medications properly and how to use assessment instruments. Studies also suggest that providing partner-guided pain management training to caregivers can decrease discomfort and improve psychological and social function experienced by older adults (SOE=B).

Psychological interventions and cognitive-behavioral therapy (CBT) can be important tools for treatment of persistent pain (SOE=B). Recognizing depression, anxiety, or other mood disturbances should prompt early consultation with mental health professionals. In CBT, patients are asked to track their pain and record the thoughts that are associated with the pain experience to identify maladaptive coping strategies. By conscientiously replacing maladaptive with positive coping strategies, patients can increase control over pain and self-efficacy, leading to decreased perception of pain. CBT can be particularly useful in helping patients learn to cope with the stresses of persistent pain. When possible, family members and caregivers should be included in the therapy.

Regular physical activity has been shown to decrease pain scores, improve mood, boost functional status, and stabilize gait (SOE=A). Referral to the Arthritis Foundation or to community resources such as senior centers for exercise, Tai Chi, and hydro-aerobics (for continent patients) classes can be beneficial for many patients. Frail older adults may require closely monitored rehabilitation services. For patients with advanced illness who are bed-bound, regular repositioning, passive range-of-motion exercises, and gentle massage are key interventions. Treatment goals should include improvements in flexibility, strength, endurance, and function, with reduced pain and improved quality of life.

Referral to a pain clinic that is geared toward an interdisciplinary team approach to treatment may be useful for patients who suffer from complex pain syndromes or who have had a poor response to first-line treatments. Data support the use of many physical therapies such as massage therapy, acupuncture, heat/cold therapy, and transcutaneous electrical nerve stimulation (TENS) units (SOE=B). Interdisciplinary team members may also incorporate cognitive techniques into the treatment plan such as hypnosis, aromatherapy, biofeedback, music and pet therapy, and systematic desensitization. Finally, some patients may require referral for major interventions, such as radiation therapy for bone metastases or palliative surgical procedures for bowel obstruction. Suboptimal treatment response should not be viewed as a permanent state, but as an opportunity for input from specialists who have additional expertise in treating these difficult problems.

See also "Complementary and Alternative Medicine," p 90.

Pharmacologic Therapy

For selected analgesics, with their starting dosages and common adverse effects, see Table 16.4.

Table 16.3—Common Pain Behaviors in Cognitively Impaired Older Adults

Behavior	Examples
Facial expressions	Slight frown; sad, frightened face Grimacing, wrinkled forehead, closed or tightened eyes Any distorted expression Rapid blinking
Verbalizations, vocalizations	Sighing, moaning, groaning, grunting, chanting, calling out Noisy breathing Asking for help Verbal abusiveness
Body movements	Rigid or tense body posture, guarding Fidgeting Increased pacing, rocking Restricted movement Gait or mobility changes
Changes in interpersonal interactions	Aggressive, combative, resists care Decreased social interactions Socially inappropriate, disruptive Withdrawn
Changes in activity patterns or routines	Refusing food, appetite change Increase in rest periods Change in sleep or rest pattern Sudden cessation of common routines Increased wandering
Mental status changes	Crying or tears Increased confusion Irritability or distress

NOTE: Some patients demonstrate little or no specific behavior associated with severe pain.

SOURCE: American Geriatrics Society Panel on Persistent Pain in Older Persons. The management of persistent pain in older persons. *J Am Geriatr Soc*. 2002;50(6 Suppl):S211. Reprinted with permission.

Pharmacologic therapy for patients with persistent pain should be viewed not only as a means to reduce suffering, but also as a method to promote improved function and enhanced adherence with rehabilitation efforts. When starting pharmacologic therapy in older adults, the risks and benefits of the treatment should be considered and balanced carefully. If appropriate, nonsystemic therapies should be tried first. For example, patients with isolated knee pain might respond to intra-articular corticosteroid injections, avoiding the need for systemic analgesics. (Convincing data supporting the use of intra-articular injections for knee pain, however, are lacking.) Patients with myofascial pain often respond to local treatments such as massage, gentle stretching exercises, ultrasound, and trigger-point injections (SOE=B). Topical preparations such as capsaicin or diclofenac gel^{OL} or lidocaine patches can be effective as primary or adjunctive therapy for treating neuropathic or myofascial pain syndromes (SOE=C). If these local therapies are ineffective and a decision is made to begin systemic therapy, older adults need to be monitored closely to ensure that the treatment is effective and to minimize adverse effects.

Table 16.4 —Systemic Pharmacotherapy for Persistent Pain Management

Medication	Starting Dosage*	Usual Effective Dose (Maximal Dosage)	Titration	Comments
		NONOPIOIDS		
Acetaminophen (Tylenol)	325 mg q4h to 500 mg q6h	2–4 g/d (4 g/d)	After 4–6 doses	Reduce maximal dosage 50%–75% in patients with hepatic insufficiency or history of alcohol abuse.
Anticonvulsants				
Carbamazepine[OL] (Tegretol)	100 mg/d	800–1,200 mg/d (2,400 mg/d)	After 3–5 days	Monitor liver enzymes, CBC, BUN/creatinine, electrolytes, and carbamazepine levels. Approved only for trigeminal neuralgia and glossopharyngeal neuralgia; not approved for any other types of pain. Multiple drug interactions.
Clonazepam[OL] (Klonopin)	0.25–0.5 mg hs	0.05–0.2 mg/kg/d (20 mg)	After 3–5 days	Monitor sedation, memory, CBC.
Gabapentin (Neurontin)	100 mg hs	300–900 mg q8h (3,600 mg)	After 1–2 days	Monitor sedation, ataxia, edema. Approved for post-herpetic neuralgia; not approved for any other types of pain.
Gabapentin extended release (Gralise)	300 mg hs	(1,800 mg)		
Pregabalin (Lyrica)	50 mg hs	300 mg/d	After 7 days	Monitor sedation, ataxia, edema.
Antidepressants				
Tricyclic antidepressants:** desipramine[OL] (Norpramin), nortriptyline[OL] (Aventyl, Pamelor)	10 mg hs	25–100 mg hs (variable, but older adults rarely tolerate doses >75–100 mg)	After 3–5 days	Significant risk of adverse events in older adults; anticholinergic effects
Duloxetine (Cymbalta)	20 mg/d	60 mg/d	After 7 days	Monitor blood pressure, dizziness, cognitive effects and memory; multiple drug–drug interactions. FDA approved for diabetic neuropathy.
Milnacipran (Savella)	12.5 mg/d	50 mg q12h	See package insert for titration recommendations; discontinuation requires tapering.	Reduce dosage by 50% with CrCl <30 mL/min. Common reactions include nausea, constipation, hot flashes, hyperhidrosis, palpitations, dry mouth, hypertension. Contraindicated with MAOIs and narrow-angle glaucoma. FDA approval only for fibromyalgia.
Venlafaxine[OL] (Effexor)	37.5 mg/d	75–225 mg/d (225 mg/d)	After 4–7 days	Associated with dose-related increases in blood pressure and heart rate
Mexiletine[OL] (Mexitil)	150 mg q12h	150 mg q6–8h (variable)	After 3–5 days	Avoid use in patients with conduction block, bradyarrhythmia; monitor ECG at baseline and after dose stabilization.
NSAIDs				Use with caution in older adults, if at all.
Celecoxib (Celebrex)	100 mg/d	100–400 mg/d (400 mg/d)		Higher dosages associated with higher incidence of GI, cardiovascular adverse events. Patients with indications for cardioprotection require aspirin supplement; therefore, older adults still require concurrent gastroprotection.
Diclofenac sodium	50 mg q12h or 75 mg extended release daily	100–150 mg/d (150 mg/d)		May be associated with higher cardiovascular risk than other traditional NSAIDs owing to its relative cyclooxygenase-2 inhibitor selectivity

Table 16.4 —Systemic Pharmacotherapy for Persistent Pain Management, *continued*

Medication	Starting Dosage*	Usual Effective Dose (Maximal Dosage)	Titration	Comments
Ibuprofen	OTC: 200 mg q8h Rx: 400 mg q6–8h	400–800 mg q6–8h (3,200 mg/d)		FDA indicates concurrent use with aspirin inhibits aspirin's antiplatelet effect, but the true clinical import of this remains to be elucidated, and it remains unclear whether this is unique to ibuprofen or true with other NSAIDs.
Ketorolac	15mg q6h IV or IM 10mg q4–6h	Max 60mg/d Max 40mg/d		Not recommended; high potential for GI and renal toxicity; inappropriate for long-term use
Nabumetone (Relafen)	1 g/d	1–2 g/d (2 g/d)		Relatively long half-life and minimal antiplatelet effect (>5 days).
Naproxen sodium	OTC: 220 mg q12h Rx: 250 mg q6–8h	OTC: 440–660 mg/day (660 mg/d) Rx: 250–500 mg q8–12h (1,000 mg/d)		Several studies implicate this agent as having less cardiovascular toxicity than other NSAIDs.
Salsalate (eg, Disalcid, Mono-Gesic, Salflex)	500–750 mg q12h	1,500–3,000 mg/d (3,000 mg/d)	After 4–6 doses	In frail patients or those with diminished hepatic or renal function, checking salicylate levels during dosage titration and after steady state is reached may be important.
		OPIOIDS		
Hydrocodone (eg, Lorcet, Lortab, Vicodin, Norco, Vicoprofen)	2.5–5 mg q4–6h	5–10 mg (see comments)	After 3–4 doses	Useful for acute recurrent, episodic, or breakthrough pain; daily dose limited by fixed-dose combinations with acetaminophen or NSAIDs. NSAIDS should be used with caution in older adults, if at all.
Hydromorphone (Dilaudid) Hydromorphone extended release (Exalgo)	1–2 mg q3–4h 8 mg	Variable (variable) Variable	After 3–4 doses After 3-4 days	For breakthrough pain or around-the-clock dosing
Morphine, immediate release (eg, MSIR, Roxanol)	2.5–10 mg q4h	Variable (variable)	After 1–2 doses	Oral liquid concentrate or tablet recommended for breakthrough pain
Morphine, sustained release (eg, MSContin, Kadian)	15 mg q 8–24h (see dosing guidelines in package insert for each specific formulation)	Variable (variable)	After 3–5 days	Usually started after initial dose determined by effects of immediate-release opioid; toxic metabolites of morphine can limit usefulness in patients with renal insufficiency or when high-dose therapy is required; continuous-release formulations may require more frequent dosing if pain returns regularly at end of dose. Significant interactions with food and alcohol.
Oxycodone, immediate release (OxyIR, Percocet, Percodan, Tylox, Combunox)	2.5–5 mg q4–6h	5–10 mg (see comments)	After 3–4 doses	Useful for acute recurrent, episodic, or breakthrough pain; daily dose limited by fixed-dose combinations with acetaminophen or NSAIDs. NSAIDs should be used with caution in older adults, if at all. The specific oxycodone preparation being prescribed should be indicated to avoid toxicity from multiple analgesics.

Table 16.4 —Systemic Pharmacotherapy for Persistent Pain Management, *continued*

Medication	Starting Dosage*	Usual Effective Dose (Maximal Dosage)	Titration	Comments
Oxycodone, sustained release (OxyContin)	10 mg q12h	Variable (variable)	After 3–5 days	Usually started after initial dose determined by effects of immediate-release opioid. Although intended for 12-hour dosing, some individuals may need shorter (every 8 hours) or longer (daily) dosing.
Tapentadol (Nucynta)	50–100 mg q4–q6h	50-100 mg q4–6h prn (600 mg/d)		Avoid use of serotonergic agents (SSRIs, SNRIs, tricyclic antidepressants).
Tapentadol extended release (Nucynta ER)	50 mg q12h	100–250 mg q12h (500 mg/d)	After 3 days	
Tramadol (Ultram)	12.5–25 mg q4–6h	50–100 mg (300 mg/d)	After 4–6 doses	Mixed opioid and central neurotransmitter mechanism of action; monitor for opioid adverse events, including drowsiness, constipation, and nausea. Exert caution when used with another serotonergic drug, and observe for symptoms of serotonergic syndrome. Lowers seizure threshold.
Transdermal fentanyl (Duragesic)	12–25 mcg/h patch q72h	Variable (variable)	After 2–3 patch changes	Usually started after initial dose determined by effects of immediate-release opioid; currently available lowest dose patch (12 mcg/h) recommended for patients who require <60 mg/24-h oral morphine equivalents; peak effects of first dose takes 18–24 hours. Duration of effect is usually 3 days but may range from 48 to 96 hours. May take 2–3 patch changes before steady state blood levels are reached.

NOTE: DEA = U.S. Drug Enforcement Agency; hs = at bedtime; NA = not applicable; CrCl = creatinine clearance; MAOI = monoamine oxidase inhibitor

* Oral dosing unless otherwise specified.

** Amitriptyline is not recommended.

SOURCE: Adapted with permission from American Geriatrics Society Panel on the Pharmacologic Management of Persistent Pain in Older Persons. Pharmacological management of persistent pain in older persons. *J Am Geriatr Soc*. 2009;57(8):1331–1346.

The pain ladder from the World Health Organization (Figure 16.2) illustrates an excellent approach toward stepwise analgesic management. Choice of initial dose and rate of titration depends on the individual patient's physiology, which varies considerably among older adults. When using acetaminophen for alleviating chronic pain, it is most effective if scheduled regularly rather than as-needed. Acetaminophen provides adequate analgesia for many mild to moderate pain syndromes, particularly musculoskeletal pain from osteoarthritis, and is recommended as first-line therapy for persistent pain. No more than 4 g of acetaminophen every 24 hours should be administered to patients with normal hepatic and renal function, given the risk of hepatotoxicity at higher doses. Patients at risk of liver dysfunction, particularly those who have a history of heavy alcohol intake, should be treated cautiously; in these patients, the dosage should be decreased by 50%, or the drug should be avoided entirely. Acetaminophen should be administered every 6 hours for patients with creatinine clearance of 10–50 mL/min, and every 8 hours for patients with a creatinine clearance of <10 mL/min. Acetaminophen is commonly contained in many OTC and prescription products; therefore, knowledge of all medications that a patient is taking is critical to avoiding acetaminophen toxicity.

NSAIDs tend to be more effective than acetaminophen in chronic inflammatory pain but pose significantly higher threats to older adults. These agents must be used judiciously if they are used at all, should be used only after acetaminophen has been tried, and then only in highly select individuals. Significant adverse events, including renal dysfunction, GI bleeding, platelet dysfunction, fluid retention, exacerbation of hypertension, precipitation of heart failure, and precipitation of delirium, limit their use in the treatment of persistent pain in older adults. The FDA has issued a particular caution against using ibuprofen with aspirin, owing to an interaction that blocks the antiplatelet effect of the aspirin. COX-2 inhibitors

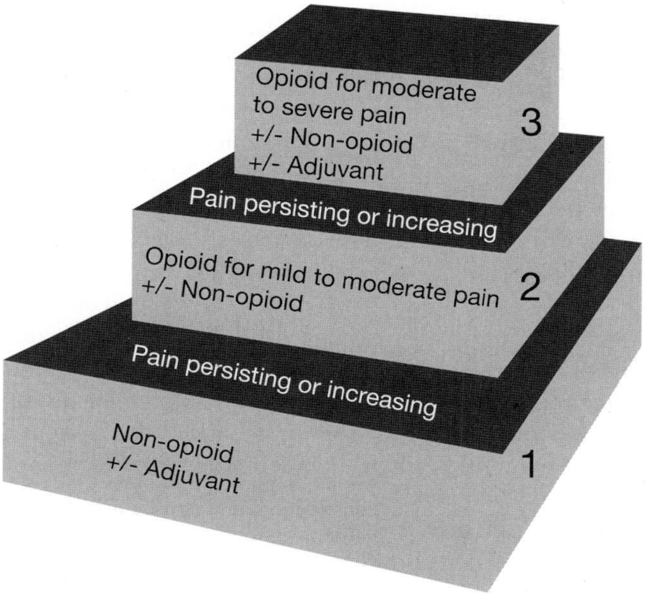

Figure 16.2 –World Health Organization's Three-Step Analgesic Ladder

Source: World Health Organization. Reprinted with permission.

were developed to decrease the risk of GI bleeding by acting on a more selective receptor, but the risk of renal complications, including hypertension, remains the same as with other NSAIDs, and the degree to which longer-term GI toxicity is reduced is not clear. Several studies have confirmed increased cardiovascular risks associated with COX-2 inhibitors, which is now believed to be a class effect. Thus, COX-2 inhibitor use should be considered with great caution—if at all—in older adults. Misoprostol, a prostaglandin analogue, or a proton-pump inhibitor can be used to reduce the risk of NSAID-induced GI bleeding, but these drugs do not reduce the risks of renal disease, hypertension, fluid retention, or delirium. Alternatively, nonacetylated salicylates such as salsalate and trisalicylate may have less renal toxicity and antiplatelet activity than other NSAIDs and therefore may be preferable in older adults, but evidence supporting this theory is sparse. Topical NSAIDs appear to be safe and effective in the short term, but longer-term studies are lacking.

Moderate to severe pain or pain that requires chronic treatment often requires opioid medications for sufficient relief, though evidence evaluating their role in managing persistent noncancer pain is scant. In general, it is prudent to start opioid therapy at the lowest dosage possible and to titrate slowly. That said, opioid dosing should not be too stingy for patients who are in a pain crisis. Rather, these patients need to be monitored closely to ensure that the dosage can be safely but aggressively increased.

Continuous pain should generally be treated with medications in long-acting or sustained-release formulations after total opioid requirements have been estimated by an initial trial of a short-acting agent. Fast-onset medications with short half-lives may be added to the long-acting regimen to cover episodes of breakthrough pain. A typical patient requires approximately 5%–15% of the total daily dose offered every 2 hours orally for breakthrough pain. In general, different opioids provide similar analgesic efficacy. Cost and route of delivery can help to guide the choice of medication.

Most opioids are metabolized by the liver and excreted by the kidneys. In renal dysfunction, the active metabolites of morphine, including morphine-6-glucuronide and morphine-3-glucuronide, can accumulate, increasing the risk of prolonged sedation and possible neurotoxicity. When using morphine to treat patients with kidney disease, the dosing intervals should be increased and the dosage decreased to reduce this risk. Hydromorphone has fewer adverse effects in patients with renal failure and, therefore, is many experts' first choice for this population (SOE=C). Some experts and limited data suggest that oxycodone is also safer than morphine in patients with kidney failure because its metabolism results in fewer active metabolites, but this remains controversial (SOE=C).

Barriers to Using Opioids in Older Adults

Older adults may have concerns about tolerance and addiction that keep them from accepting adequate treatment for their pain. They may fear that taking opioid therapy for their current level of pain will result in the medication losing its effectiveness in the future when pain becomes more severe. Fear of addiction is another major obstacle to prescribing medications for older adults. A frank discussion of these concerns may help alleviate these fears.

Physical dependence is an expected change in a patient's physiology that develops while a patient is receiving chronic, continual opioid medications. If opioids are discontinued suddenly, patients who are physically dependent experience a withdrawal syndrome that may include restlessness, tachycardia, hypertension, fever, tremors, and lacrimation. Symptoms of withdrawal can be avoided by tapering opioids carefully over days to weeks. *Tolerance* refers to a change in physiology resulting in the need to increase opioid dosages over time to achieve adequate analgesic effect. Experts note that tolerance to analgesia, as opposed to tolerance to sedation and respiratory depression, develops slowly in stable disease. If medicines must be titrated rapidly to reduce pain, a search for the cause of the exacerbation should be undertaken, and nonphysical contributors should be considered as well.

Cross-tolerance between different opioids is limited. Therefore, when switching a patient from one opioid to another (eg, morphine to oxycodone), the clinician should reduce the amount (suggested range of 50%–65%) of the theoretical equivalent dosage to reduce the risk of inadvertent overdose, but liberal as-needed doses should be made available during the transition period.

Psychological *dependence*, or true *addiction*, refers to a state defined by compulsive drug seeking and drug using with disregard for adverse social, physical, and economic consequences. It is very rare for patients who have persistent pain to become addicted to opioids, but opioid abuse can become a problem in certain individuals, and the potential for abuse should be carefully discussed in those with a prior history of addiction. Although opioid abuse is less common in older adults, clinicians should carefully monitor for misuse of this medication. Addiction must be distinguished from *pseudoaddiction*, which refers to a patient with significant unrelieved pain who adopts behaviors (eg, theatricality in their pleas for relief) similar to those of truly addicted patients.

Adverse Effects of Opioids

The most common adverse effect of opioid treatment is constipation, and unfortunately, tolerance to this toxicity does not occur. Opioid-induced constipation is due to multiple mechanisms, including dehydration, decreased GI tract secretions, and decreased intestinal motility. Because constipation usually complicates opioid use for the duration of treatment, education regarding the probable need for long-term laxative treatment is recommended for all patients when opioid therapy is started. Many experts recommend starting therapy with a stimulant laxative (such as bisacodyl or senna); however, these should be avoided in any patient with signs or symptoms of bowel obstruction. Bulking agents such as fiber and psyllium should be avoided in patients who are inactive and who have poor oral fluid intake because of the risk of causing fecal impaction and obstruction. All patients should be encouraged to exercise, as they are able, and to stay well hydrated. For patients who develop opioid-induced constipation despite laxative therapy, treatment with methylnaltrexone, a mu-opioid-receptor antagonist, may relieve constipation without precipitating withdrawal symptoms or pain crisis (SOE=B).

Nausea and vomiting are common adverse effects of opioids. These agents have a direct effect on the chemoreceptor trigger zone, the part of the brain associated with the sensation of nausea. Other common causes of nausea and vomiting in patients taking opioids include gastroparesis, constipation, and metabolic disorders such as renal and hepatic failure. Although the nausea and vomiting usually resolve spontaneously after the first few doses, some patients experience chronic nausea. After evaluation for reversible causes of nausea such as constipation, some patients benefit from changing to an alternative opioid (SOE=D). Others may need to be treated with scheduled antiemetics, recognizing the high prevalence of adverse events, including drowsiness, delirium, and anticholinergic effects, in older adults treated with these medications.

Respiratory depression is the most serious potential adverse effect associated with opioid use, but tolerance to this effect develops quickly. Older adults and individuals with a history of lung dysfunction are at particular risk when opioid dosages are increased rapidly or when another sedative is taken concomitantly. Naloxone, an opioid-receptor antagonist, can reverse opioid-induced respiratory depression; however, when given to a patient who has been treated chronically with opioids, it can precipitate a pain crisis and acute withdrawal symptoms. Experts suggest withholding naloxone unless the patient's respiratory rate decreases to <8 breaths per minute or the oxygen saturation drops to <90%. When it is needed, naloxone should be titrated carefully, using the lowest dosage possible.

Older adults can experience sedation, fatigue, and mild cognitive impairment with opioid treatment. These symptoms are common during dosage adjustment. Patients typically overcome the fatigue and sedation over days to weeks as they become tolerant to the medication. They need to be warned of the risks of increased falls and asked not to drive or operate heavy equipment when the medication is started. A small subset of patients treated with opioids experience incessant fatigue or excessive sedation that limits their function significantly. A limited course of a stimulant such as low-dose methylphenidate could reasonably be tried in this situation (SOE=D). Rotation to a different opioid is an alternative strategy used to alleviate opioid-induced fatigue.

Nonopioid Adjuvant Analgesics

Nonopioid or adjuvant medications can be used as the sole agent or in combination with opioids. These medications can be particularly useful in treating patients with neuropathic pain or mixed pain syndromes.

Tricyclic antidepressants (TCAs) are the most extensively studied medications for neuropathic pain, although none of the TCAs has been approved for the treatment of pain. Their efficacy in the treatment of post-herpetic neuralgia and diabetic neuropathy has been shown in numerous placebo-controlled studies (SOE=A). However, they are associated with significant anticholinergic adverse events in older adults, including constipation, urinary retention, dry mouth, cognitive impairment, tachycardia, and blurred vision. Of note, desipramine[OL] and nortriptyline[OL] may have fewer adverse events than amitriptyline[OL].

Clinical depression in patients with persistent pain requires treatment to achieve optimal analgesia and quality of life. Other classes of antidepressants (eg, SSRIs) have generally been less studied than TCAs as analgesics, but older adults typically tolerate these agents better than TCAs when they are used in antidepressant doses. Duloxetine, an inhibitor of norepinephrine and serotonin uptake, is approved both as an antidepressant and for the treatment of pain from diabetic neuropathy, and it may offer a more favorable adverse-event profile than the TCAs.

Anticonvulsant medications such as carbamazepine, gabapentin, pregabalin, and clonazepam[OL] are commonly used as treatments for neuropathic pain. Gabapentin and pregabalin have demonstrated clinical efficacy in the treatment of post-herpetic neuralgia, and have fewer adverse events than TCAs, but their cost is more. The main adverse events of gabapentin and pregabalin are sedation and dizziness, which frequently limit dosage increases.

Corticosteroids are useful adjuvants to treat pain associated with swelling, inflammation, and tissue infiltration, as well as neuropathic pain (SOE=C). In addition to their analgesic properties, they also can increase appetite and improve energy, although weight gained is predominantly fluid and fat rather than muscle. Adverse effects seen with short-term use of steroids include psychosis, fluid retention, hair loss, loss of skin integrity, hyperglycemia, insomnia, and immunosuppression. Corticosteroid use should be limited to treatment of inflammatory conditions and metastatic bone pain, and even then these agents should be used with caution.

Intravenous bisphosphonates can substantially reduce pain from malignant bone metastases (SOE=B). Bisphosphonates are associated with osteonecrosis of the jaw, particularly when administered to patients undergoing dental surgery.

Tramadol both binds opioid receptors and inhibits the reuptake of norepinephrine and serotonin. It can lower the seizure threshold and is therefore not recommended for patients who have a history of seizures or who take other medications known to lower the seizure threshold. Caution should also be exercised in patients taking other medications that have serotonergic properties, in order to avoid serotonin syndrome (characterized by myoclonus, agitation, abdominal cramping, hyperpyrexia, hypertension, and potentially death). Tapentadol is a synthetic, oral mu-opioid receptor agonist approved by the FDA in 2009 for the management of moderate to severe acute pain and chronic pain in adults. Tapentadol also has SNRI (serotonin–norepinephrine reuptake inhibitor) properties and is structurally and pharmacologically similar to tramadol. It is cleared by the liver and excreted by the kidney and is to be avoided in severe renal and hepatic impairment. In older adults, therapy should be initiated at the lowest recommended dosage range. For acute pain, dosage is immediate–release tapentadol at 50 mg q 4–6h as needed. For chronic pain, the extended-release formulation can be used at a dosage of 50 mg q12h and titrated to an effective dose in increments of 50 mg and no more frequently than every 3 days. Significant adverse effects include nausea, vomiting, constipation, dizziness and somnolence. Also, the extended-release formulation should be titrated off gradually to prevent withdrawal.

Medications to Avoid in Older Adults

In prescribing analgesics in older adults, it is important to start low and go slow. Most often the dosage of analgesics is limited by their adverse effects and drug-drug interactions. In older adults who live alone, it is important to regularly assess cognitive status, because this may influence their ability to take analgesics as prescribed. Mixed agonist-antagonists such as nalbuphine and butorphanol have the potential to cause restlessness and tremulousness and, therefore, should be avoided in older adults. Meperidine should also be avoided in older adults, because it can cause agitation, confusion, delirium, and disorientation,

REFERENCES

- American Geriatrics Society Panel on the Pharmacologic Management of Persistent Pain in Older Persons. Pharmacological management of persistent pain in older persons. *J Am Geriatr Soc*. 2009;57(8):1331–1346. Available at: http://www.americangeriatrics.org/files/documents/2009_Guideline.pdf (accessed Oct 2013).
- Bjoro K, Herr K. Assessment of pain in the nonverbal or cognitively impaired older adult. *Clin Geriatr Med*. 2008;24(2):237–262.
- Herr K. Pain assessment strategies in older adults. *J Pain*. 2011;12(3 Suppl 1):S3–S13.

CHAPTER 17—HOSPITAL CARE

KEY POINTS

- Adults ≥65 years old make up 13% of the population and account for 36% of acute-care hospital admissions and nearly 50% of hospital expenditures for all adults.
- Older hospitalized adults should be routinely assessed for a limited number of common geriatric problems regardless of their admission diagnosis.
- Specific system changes in providing care to hospitalized older adults have resulted in improved patient outcomes.

Older adults are at disproportionate risk of becoming seriously ill and requiring hospital care, whether it is in an emergency department, on a medical or surgical ward, or in a critical-care unit. Adults ≥65 years old make up 13% of the U.S. population but account for 36% of acute-care hospital admissions and nearly 50% of hospital expenditures for adults. The most common principal diagnoses in hospitalized older adults are congestive heart failure, pneumonia, cardiac dysrhythmia, and acute coronary syndromes.

Hospital use rates vary as much as 3-fold for Medicare beneficiaries with the same illnesses across different regions of the United States. There is no evidence that these differences in practice patterns are explained by differences in disease rates or severity. Hospital use and the use of hospital resources is much lower among those enrolled in capitated insurance plans than among those enrolled in fee-for-service plans; this difference in resource use has not been systematically linked to differences in patient outcomes.

Disparities in hospital care exist. Minority patients are significantly less likely than whites to be treated at high-volume hospitals for services for which high volume is associated with better outcomes. The differences were largest for cancer surgeries and cardiovascular procedures. Hospitals in the bottom quintile on most quality measures served a significantly higher percentage of minority patients than hospitals in the top quintile.

During hospitalization, older adults tend to receive less costly care than do younger patients. In the Study to Understand Prognoses and Preferences for Outcomes and Risks of Treatments (SUPPORT), for example, seriously ill patients in their 80s received fewer invasive procedures and less resource-intensive, less costly hospital care than similarly ill younger patients (SOE=A). This preferential allocation of hospital services to younger patients was not based on differences in severity of illness or general preferences for life-extending care and is consistent with evidence regarding outpatient care. Differences in the aggressiveness of care have not been shown to explain differences between older and younger patients in survival or other outcomes. Moreover, patients' families and clinicians commonly underestimate older patients' desire for aggressive care (SOE=A). The best guides to assessment and management in the care of any older hospitalized patient are the clinical circumstances and the patient's preferences, irrespective of age.

In a study of vulnerable older adults hospitalized on the medical service of an academic medical center, the quality of care provided was examined by measuring adherence to ACOVE-3 quality indicators. Adherence to indicators was significantly greater for general medical care (such as for heart failure or diabetes) than for geriatric conditions (such as delirium or pressure sores) (SOE=A). Yet, adherence to 16 ACOVE geriatric-specific quality indicators in the acute-care setting may be associated with lower 1-year mortality in vulnerable older hospitalized patients. This chapter is intended to assist providers in the acute setting to adhere to effective geriatric care processes, regardless of the general medical problems of their patients.

ASSESSING AND MANAGING HOSPITALIZED OLDER PATIENTS

Many of the serious illnesses disproportionately experienced by older adults require hospital care for optimal management. The benefits of hospitalization can be remarkable: correcting serious physiologic derangements, repairing vascular obstructions and broken bones, using highly technical biomedical advances in the treatment of life-threatening illnesses. However, while in the hospital, older adults also commonly experience deteriorating functional status, adverse events from medication, or delirium. A systematic approach to assessing and managing hospitalized older adults offers the best chance of reducing the risk and consequences of these common problems.

The initial assessment should include an evaluation of function at the level of the organ system, the whole person, and the person's environment. This assessment can identify needs for which targeted interventions can improve function or reduce risk of adverse outcomes. This approach complements the traditional medical assessment by highlighting problems that are common in hospitalized older patients, and it is similar in concept to geriatric assessment conducted in other settings. See "Assessment," p 48; and "Outpatient Care Systems," p 173.

Table 17.1—Systematic Assessment of Older Adults on Hospital Admission

Step	Assessments
Past medical history	■ Ask about vaccination history
Medications review	■ Assess indications for each medication, appropriateness of dosing, potential interactions
	■ Assess for medication effects contributing to acute illness
	■ Determine patient's or caregiver's method for assuring adherence (eg, pill boxes)
Social history	■ Ask about help needed (and who provides) for ADLs and IADLs
	■ Ask about social support
	■ Ask if patient feels free and safe
Review of systems	■ Ask about weight loss in preceding 6 months
	■ Ask about dietary change
	■ Ask about anorexia, nausea, vomiting, diarrhea
	■ Ask about incontinence
	■ Ask about problems with memory or confusion
	■ Ask about falls or difficulty walking
	■ Ask about difficulties with vision or hearing
Physical examination	■ Take pulse (confirm arrhythmias with ECG)
	■ Check orthostatic blood pressures in patients with falls, presyncope, syncope
	■ Assess for weight change, loss of subcutaneous fat, muscle wasting, edema, ascites, prevalent pressure ulcer
	■ Screen for cognitive function
	■ Assess vision and hearing
	■ Assess gait
	■ Use a depression screen

Table 17.2—Common Hazards and Opportunities to Address During an Older Adult's Hospital Stay

Problem	Possible Interventions
Functional impairments	Assess ADLs on admission, physical therapy, occupational therapy, engage social resources.
Immobility and falls	Avoid restraints, remove in-dwelling bladder catheters, encourage ambulation in hospital, physical therapy, avoid sedating medications.
Sensory impairment	Use eyeglasses, hearing aids; remove cerumen impaction.
Depression	Treat with pharmacotherapy, cognitive therapy, or both.
Cognitive impairment	Evaluate for dementia or delirium, assess social environment, reorientation.
Suboptimal pharmacotherapy	Review all medications at admission and discharge, modify prescriptions, involve clinical pharmacists as medical team members, consider use of explicit appropriateness criteria (see "Pharmacotherapy," p 81).
Atrial fibrillation	Begin rate control plus anticoagulation or conversion or maintain sinus rhythm plus anticoagulation, or both.
Nutrition	Supplement water, calories, protein; assess social environment and medical factors that contribute to poor oral intake.
Immunization status	Vaccinate against influenza, pneumococcus, tetanus.
Pressure ulcer prevention	Reposition frequently and use specialized support surfaces, manage moisture and incontinence, encourage ambulation.
Sleep disturbance	Address intrinsic and extrinsic causes, use nonpharmacologic protocols.
Venous thromboembolism prevention	Use prophylactic anticoagulation for patients with one or more risk factors for venous thromboembolism, mechanical thromboprophylaxis for high bleeding risk, encourage ambulation.

For suggestions on when assessment of these common geriatric problems can be incorporated into the routine of a hospital admission history and physical examination, see Table 17.1.

For commonly overlooked hazards and opportunities in older hospitalized patients, see Table 17.2. These problems have been selected based on their importance relative to other clinical issues, the quality of relevant evidence, and their specificity to older adults. Other important problems (eg, the effects of alcohol or tobacco use, pain management, and advance directives) are not specific to older adults, and some problems specific to older adults (eg, age-related decline in renal function) are widely recognized. See also "Addictions," p 336; "Palliative Care," p 111; "Legal and Ethical Issues," p 26; "Kidney Diseases and Disorders," p 420; and "Perioperative Care," p 102.

Two types of evidence suggest that these interventions are a good use of clinician time. First, for each problem, evidence supporting the proposed intervention is compelling, either because the efficacy of the intervention is well established (eg, prophylaxis of deep-vein thrombosis) or because the associated problem is common, often overlooked, and can be improved with a safe and inexpensive intervention. Second, compared with patients receiving usual care, patients receiving comprehensive geriatric assessment and management in dedicated units are more likely to be alive and living at home at 6- and 12-month follow-ups, less likely to be institutionalized, and more likely to show improvement in cognition (SOE=A). These benefits have not been demonstrated by trials using a consultation-only model.

Functional Impairments

Once hospitalized, older patients are at high risk of loss of independence and institutionalization. Among hospitalized medical patients ≥70 years old, approximately 12% decline during hospitalization in their ability to perform basic activities of daily living (ADLs) of self-care, another 23% are discharged without recovering their baseline prehospitalization abilities, and 15% of those admitted from home are discharged to a nursing home (SOE=A). Almost 50% of new-onset disability in frail older adults can be attributed to hospitalization. A recently validated clinical index identified risk factors (age, number of dependencies in instrumental activities of daily living [IADL], mobility 2 weeks before admission, number of ADL dependencies on admission, metastatic cancer or stroke, severe cognitive impairment, and hypoalbuminemia) for new-onset disability in hospitalized patients ≥70 years old. Higher risk scores predicted more severe disability, greater likelihood of nursing-home placement, and worse survival.

The ability to perform ADLs and IADLs is necessary for older adults to live independently, and functional dependence is associated with worse quality-of-life outcomes, shortened survival, and increased resource use. The older adult's ability to perform ADLs and IADLs, determined at the time of admission, can serve as a useful baseline. If functional dependence is found, the causes should be explored (eg, dependence in IADLs is often associated with dementia), and strategies to maintain and improve functional ability can be started (eg, physical and occupational therapy). These strategies may be best implemented effectively for many patients by ward staff without consultation or referral. Social work consultation and early involvement of family or other caregivers is often necessary to plan postdischarge care for those older adults who are functionally dependent. The clinician plays a critical role in educating patients and families regarding the harmful effects of limited activity and the need to engage in function-promoting activity to avoid functional decline. See also "Rehabilitation," p 139; and "Psychosocial Issues," p 18.

Immobility and Falls

It is helpful to assess the patient's gait, balance, leg strength, ability to get up from bed, cognition, and mood during the initial physical examination. Individuals able to walk independently should be encouraged to do so frequently during hospitalization. Immobility during hospitalization leads rapidly to diminished strength and subsequent difficulty walking (SOE=A). Those able to walk but unable to do so safely and independently can receive assistance from hospital staff while walking several times daily. Formal physical therapy can yield additional benefits.

The initial physical examination is also a good time to assess a patient's risk of falling by inquiring about a history of falls (SOE=A) and by careful musculoskeletal and neurologic examinations. Strategies to promote mobility and reduce falls include avoiding restraints and tethers, decluttering the environment, minimizing use of medications associated with falls, providing walking assistance for those who walk with difficulty, attending to patient's toileting needs, addressing sensory impairments, and providing physical therapy for those with weakness or gait abnormalities. A review of the effectiveness of interventions to prevent falls in older patients in the nursing-home and acute/subacute hospital settings demonstrated that multifactorial interventions targeting specific individual risk factors for falls (eg, impairment in gait, balance, strength; medications; environment; vision) significantly reduced the risk and rates of falls. The effectiveness of the interventions depended on the duration of intervention; patients in the acute/subacute hospital setting for more than a few weeks reaped greater benefits from targeted multifactorial interventions and supervised exercise. A recent randomized controlled trial of an information technology–based, nursing-led, patient education and communication falls prevention toolkit reduced both the rate of falls (3.15 versus 4.18 falls/1,000 patient-days) and the proportion of fallers (1.3% versus 1.7%) in an acute-care hospital (SOE=A).

See "Falls," p 234; "Gait Impairment," p 228; "Physical Activity," p 64; "Rehabilitation," p 139; and "Diseases and Disorders of the Foot," p 471.

Sensory Impairment

Most hospitalized older adults have impaired vision or hearing, and these sensory impairments are risk factors for falls, incontinence, delirium, and functional dependence. Of 770 patients ≥75 years old admitted to five medical wards, 48% had hearing impairment, 32% had vision impairment, and 20% had both; the combination of both sensory impairments was associated with IADL loss. Although eyeglasses or hearing aids readily correct most visual and hearing impairments, they are often forgotten or inaccessible in the hospital.

Hospitalized older adults can be screened for sensory impairment by routinely asking if they have difficulty with seeing or hearing and whether they use eyeglasses or hearing aids. Physical examination, including a test of visual acuity (eg, with a pocket card of the Jaeger eye test) and the whisper test of hearing, in which a short, easily answered question is whispered in each ear, is the next appropriate step in evaluation. For people with visual or hearing impairments, it is important to provide the appropriate assistive devices (eyeglasses or hearing aids brought from home or voice amplifiers provided by the hospital), and staff may need to be instructed in the use of appliances to communicate more effectively. See "Hearing Impairment," p 192; and "Visual Impairment," p 183.

Depression

Depressive symptoms in hospitalized older adults are common, prognostically important, and potentially ameliorable. Major or minor depression occurs in roughly one-third of hospitalized patients ≥65 years old but is often undiagnosed. The presence of depressive symptoms is associated with increased risk of dependence in ADLs, nursing-home placement, and shortened long-term survival, even after controlling for baseline function and the severity of acute and chronic illness.

It is important to assess for depression in all hospitalized older patients. Simply asking patients whether they feel down, depressed, or hopeless, or whether they have lost interest or pleasure in doing things, is a good place to start. A positive response to any one of these questions is likely sensitive to the diagnosis of depression (based on evidence from outpatients) and can be followed up by a formal assessment for an affective disorder.

Psychotherapeutic interventions are safe and often effective in the initial management of patients with suspected depression. Beginning pharmacotherapy during hospitalization for a medical or surgical condition may not be necessary, but follow-up shortly after discharge is critical. Those with persistently high numbers of depressive symptoms are especially at risk of functional decline and death in the year after discharge. If pharmacotherapy is started, SSRIs are often preferred because approximately 50% of older hospitalized patients have a contraindication to tricyclic antidepressants. See "Depression and Other Mood Disorders," p 308.

Cognitive Impairment

People >65 years old with dementia are hospitalized at over 3 times the rate of those without dementia (780 hospitalizations per 1,000 versus 234 per 1000). In one systematic review, the prevalence of dementia among older patients in the acute hospital ranged from 13% to 63%. Patients with dementia were older and more undernourished before hospitalization. In hospital, they required more hours of nursing care, had longer hospitalizations, and were more likely to suffer delirium and functional decline and to be discharged to a nursing home than patients without dementia. Preexisting cognitive impairment is also a risk factor for falls, use of restraints, nonadherence to therapy, and feeding tube placements. Despite its importance, documentation of a dementia diagnosis is often absent in hospital records. Recognizing an underlying cognitive impairment early enables the healthcare team to implement preemptive measures to prevent these hazards. Cognitive function can be assessed by use of an established test of cognitive function, such as the Mini–Mental State Examination or the Mini-Cog test. Family and caregivers should provide the medical history whenever possible. Exposure to the hospital environment may be disorienting for patients with cognitive impairment due to frequent room changes, noise, direct lighting, and poor way-finding cues. Creating a unit with a home-like ambiance that allows unrestricted mobility, provides meaningful daytime activities, encourages the presence of family, promotes sleep through nonpharmacologic protocols, and addresses nutritional needs are prudent ways of making the hospital environment safer for patients with dementia.

Cognitive impairment may complicate the assessment and treatment of pain in the hospital. As a consequence, pain is often undertreated. There is fair evidence that most patients with mild to moderate dementia can comprehend at least one pain assessment scale, but fewer than half of those with severe dementia can do so. Cognitively impaired patients may be unable to recognize their pain trajectory and or to differentiate improving pain from new or worsening symptoms. Orders for patient-controlled-analgesia pumps and as-needed pain medication should be avoided in patients with impaired recall. Scheduled analgesia (such as acetaminophen 650 mg every 6 hours in patients without contraindications) should be considered, especially if pain occurs frequently. Nonpharmacologic approaches to pain should be part of the treatment plan. Patients may be unable to report adverse effects from the analgesics, and detection of complications (eg, fecal impaction or delirium), may be delayed. Anticipating and preventing common adverse effects, for example by initiating a bowel regimen whenever opiates are prescribed, is one way of avoiding complications. When patients with dementia develop delirium, looking for untreated pain as a possible cause is appropriate.

Patients with end-stage dementia hospitalized with a hip fracture or pneumonia have poor prognoses (6-month mortality [55% and 53%, respectively]), and many hospital interventions used to treat these conditions may be particularly burdensome to those unable to understand the nature of their illness or express their needs. Clinicians should educate surrogate decision-makers of the patient's prognosis and establish treatment goals that optimize the palliation of symptoms.

Delirium

Delirium is present in 10%–15% of hospitalized older adults on admission, and it develops in up to 30% during the course of hospitalization on a general medical ward (SOE=A). Certain subgroups of hospitalized older patients have higher incidence of delirium, with rates of 15%–53% in postoperative patients and 70%–87% in patients in the ICU. The diagnosis of delirium should be considered when any of the following is observed: acute onset of change and fluctuation in mental status or behavior, inattention, disorganized thinking, and altered consciousness. Inattention, a *sine qua non* for diagnosing delirium, can be measured with 5-digit recall or serial 7's. The Confusion Assessment Method (CAM) (see Table 36.1) is a screening tool that incorporates all four of these features, with a positive screen consisting of both of the first two features plus one or both of the latter two. When a patient is noted to be confused, the first step is to determine the acuity of mental status change. Interviewing reliable informants is the key to detecting the presence of the first CAM feature. Three psychomotor behavioral subtypes are currently recognized: hypoactive, hyperactive, and mixed. Hyperactive delirious patients are restless, agitated, and hyperalert (and this diagnosis is rarely missed), while hypoactive delirious patients often have decreased movement, paucity of speech, and reduced responsiveness. Hypoactive patients are often not identified in the hospital, or misdiagnosed as having depression or dementia. Delirium arising during the course of hospitalization is associated with prolonged hospital stay, nursing-home placement, increased mortality, and worsening cognitive function. Symptoms of delirium can persist for months after hospital discharge. See "Delirium," p 276.

Prevention is the best strategy; roughly one-third of cases of delirium can be prevented by appropriately managing six risk factors for delirium: cognitive impairment, sleep deprivation, immobility, visual impairment, hearing impairment, and dehydration (SOE=A). While the benefits of interventions to prevent delirium are well established, interventions for treating established delirium have not demonstrated improved outcomes (SOE=C). Once the diagnosis is made, measures should be taken to identify the medical condition causing the delirium by reviewing recently added medications and by investigating for likely causes such as infection, electrolyte abnormalities, and ischemia. Measures to prevent or ameliorate delirium include avoiding medications associated with delirium (such as benzodiazepines, anticholinergics, and opiates), whenever possible; treating infection and fever; detecting and correcting urinary retention, fecal impaction, and metabolic abnormalities; frequently orienting patients with cognitive or sensory impairment; limiting room changes; and avoiding excessive bed rest, restraints, and unnecessary tethers (eg, in-dwelling bladder and intravenous catheters, oxygen lines, and telemetry leads). See "Delirium," p 276, for management of behavioral problems.

Suboptimal Pharmacotherapy

Pharmacotherapy involves prescribing, communicating orders, dispensing, administering, and monitoring. There is potential at each step for an error to occur. Other factors that contribute to the complexities of pharmacotherapy for the older patient in the acute-care setting include polypharmacy, multiple prescribing providers, restrictive hospital formularies that require careful medication reconciliation during care transitions, barriers to medication reconciliation, and significant turnover of the medication regimen with many old medications discontinued and new ones introduced. In one study, 40% of medications prescribed before admissions were discontinued during hospitalization, and 45% of medications prescribed at discharge were started during hospitalization. In another study, 88% of older hospitalized patients had at least one clinically significant problem related to prescribing, and 22% had at least one potentially serious and life-threatening problem (SOE=B).

Adverse drug events (ADEs) are a significant source of hospital hazard for the older patient. In one meta-analysis, the in-hospital incidence of ADEs was 6.7%. A risk index that predicts ADEs in hospitalized older patients using the risk factors of number of drugs, history of ADEs, heart failure, liver disease, presence of ≥4 conditions, and renal failure performed well in a cohort of older patients. Inappropriate medication use likely contributes to the risk of ADEs. The updated Beers criteria and the screening tool of older persons' potentially inappropriate prescriptions (STOPP) are two common sense evidence-based approaches to reducing inappropriate prescribing.

A hospital admission is an ideal time to completely review a patient's medication regimen, discontinuing or changing medications that are unnecessary, have low therapeutic value (eg, sedative hypnotics), are prescribed at the wrong dose or frequency, are duplicative, interact with another medication, or are prescribed despite a known allergy. In addition, a medication review taken at admission can evaluate whether medical conditions are maximally treated. Review of medications should include both prescription and nonprescription medications. Consultation by clinical pharmacists can improve appropriate prescribing and improve the older patient's adherence to prescribed therapy (SOE=A). These changes should be undertaken in consultation with the outpatient provider. See "Pharmacotherapy," p 81.

Sleep Disturbance

Over one-third of older patients have difficulty sleeping in the hospital. Sleep deprivation is important to prevent or to diagnose and address because it is associated with increased risk of delirium. The sources of sleep disruption in hospitalized older adults include intrinsic (eg, underlying medical illness, medications, drug withdrawal) and extrinsic factors (eg, noise, processes of care such as vital signs, phlebotomy, medication administration, and beeping medical monitors). Despite the risks of delirium, falls, hip fractures, and rebound insomnia associated with sedative hypnotics, at least one-third of older patients are prescribed these medications in the hospital. Pharmacologic treatment of insomnia has a poor benefit-to-harm ratio; the NNT for improved sleep quality is approximately 13, while the NNH for any adverse effect was 6 (SOE=A). Therefore, sleep deprivation in the hospital is best managed nonpharmacologically. One protocol using night-time noise reduction strategies, including warm drinks, soothing music, massage treatments, and rescheduled medication administration and measurement of vital signs to avoid sleep interruption, significantly reduced the use of sedative hypnotics in the hospital. See "Sleep Problems," p 285.

Pressure Ulcers

The incidence of hospital-acquired pressure ulcers (HAPU) ranges from 7% to 9%, with most (60%) acquired in the acute-care setting. The cost of treating HAPU can range from $500 to $70,000 per patient, or an estimated $11 billion nationally in 2009. As of October 2008, CMS has designated HAPU as a "never event" and no longer reimburses hospitals for the cost associated with HAPU treatment. The two most commonly used pressure ulcer risk-assessment scales are the Braden and Norton scales. Patients at risk should have their skin inspected at least daily, focusing on areas of bony prominences. In a systematic review of the evidence for pressure ulcer prevention interventions, the authors recommended use of specialized foam or sheepskin overlays and dynamic support mattresses over standard hospital mattresses. Frequent repositioning is a basic component of pressure prevention programs, but there is insufficient evidence to support a particular regimen. Attention to the nutritional status of the at-risk population may reduce incidence of HAPU. Finally, dry sacral skin is a risk factor for pressure ulcers, and the use of moisturizer is recommended as an inexpensive and harmless intervention. See "Pressure Ulcers and Wound Care," p 296.

Nutritional Deficits

Serious deficiencies of macro- and micronutrients are common in hospitalized older patients. On admission, severe protein-calorie malnutrition is present in approximately 15% of adults ≥70 years old, and moderate malnutrition is present in another 25%. Moreover, 25% of older patients suffer further nutritional depletion during hospitalization. Even after controlling for underlying acute illness, its severity, and comorbid illnesses, malnutrition is associated with increased risk of complications, dependence, institutionalization, and death.

In addition, deficiencies of vitamins (especially vitamin D) and electrolytes are common among older hospitalized patients. In one large hospital, nearly two-thirds of patients ≥65 years old were found to be vitamin D deficient; vitamin D deficiency was nearly as common in patients without a risk factor for vitamin D deficiency and in those taking multivitamins as in other patients (SOE=B). See "Osteoporosis," p 243; "Malnutrition," p 209; and "Endocrine and Metabolic Disorders," p 506.

Assessing patients' nutritional health is essential. Patients who receive nutritional assessment in the hospital are less likely to experience short-term functional decline or die 1 year after hospital discharge. Beyond considering supplements, clinicians should assess malnourished older hospitalized patients for remediable factors such as difficulty chewing, need for dentures, dysphagia, medications that impair the appetite, overly restrictive prescribed diet, or insufficient time or physical ability to eat. Another contributor to poor oral intake in the hospital is constipation. Elimination records should be reviewed regularly, and patients who have not moved their bowels in more than a couple of days may benefit from a stimulant (eg, senna) or osmotic (eg, sorbitol) laxative or from a suppository, in addition to provision of adequate fluid and fiber intake and mobility. See "Eating and Feeding Problems," p 216.

The maintenance of water and electrolyte balance requires special attention in older adults during and after fluid administration because of their decreased ability to achieve and maintain homeostasis. Initial efforts can be directed toward achieving euvolemia and correcting electrolyte abnormalities. Subsequent efforts to maintain fluid and electrolyte balance are based on estimates of daily metabolic requirements.

Immunization Status

Adults ≥65 years old should be assessed at the time of hospital admission for their vaccination status and updated accordingly. The rationale for targeting pneumococcal vaccination (PPV) for hospitalized older patients arises from studies showing that hospitalization of adults ≥65 years old is a risk factor for developing subsequent pneumococcal infection, and two-thirds of patients hospitalized with serious pneumococcal infections had been hospitalized at least once during the previous 3–5 years. Furthermore, the risk of death from invasive pneumococcal infection is highest in older adults. A recent meta-analysis found evidence that PPV prevented invasive pneumococcal disease in adults. The evidence supports the use of standing orders as an effective method of increasing PPV rates in hospitalized patients.

Influenza vaccine administered in the hospital and in the ambulatory setting was shown to be equally safe and immunogenic, and the complication associated with concurrent administration of influenza and pneumonia vaccines is noted to be mild in an older population. See also "Prevention," p 70.

Deep Venous Thrombosis (DVT) Prophylaxis

Because of diminished physiologic reserve, older adults are less able to compensate for the hemodynamic and ventilatory demands of a pulmonary embolism. Furthermore, numerous risk factors, comorbidities, and atypical presentations in older adults can lead to more challenging diagnosis of and worse outcomes from venous thromboembolic disease in this population. Older adults are less likely to present with typical symptoms such as chest pain, extremity discomfort, or difficulty ambulating, and are more likely to complain of dyspnea. Patients hospitalized for illness other than DVT who subsequently developed DVT were more likely to be elderly than nonelderly. Despite this, older patients receive DVT prophylaxis <50% of the time. The 2012 Guidelines from the American College of Chest Physicians recommend thromboprophylaxis with low-molecular-weight heparin, low-dose unfractionated heparin, or fondaparinux for acutely ill medical patients at high risk of venous thromboembolism. Risk can be assessed using the Padua Prediction Score, which takes into account increased age, previous venous thromboembolism, thrombophilia, cancer, heart or respiratory failure, reduced mobility, and use of hormonal medications. Renal function should be considered when deciding which antithrombotic to use and at what dosage. In patients with impaired kidney function, low-molecular-weight heparin and fondaparinux, both renally cleared agents, should be dose-adjusted or completely avoided; unfractionated heparin may be preferable in these patients. Mechanical thromboprophylaxis should be used primarily for patients with high bleeding risk. Ensuring proper use and maximal adherence are key to the effectiveness of mechanical prophylaxis.

Intensive Care

Adults >65 years old account for 42%–52% of the intensive care unit (ICU) admissions and for almost 60% of total ICU days in the United States. Research is ongoing in an attempt to better understand which older patients are most likely to benefit from ICU care.

Respiratory failure is the most common reason for medical ICU admission and, because advanced age is associated with higher prevalence of chronic and acute pulmonary conditions, the number of older patients admitted to the ICU requiring mechanical ventilator support is rising. Patients with acute lung injury or acute respiratory distress syndrome appear to have a higher mortality with advancing age.

Mortality in very old (>85 years) patients is 30%–70% for those with single organ and 80%–100% for those with multiple organ failure. Patients requiring renal replacement therapy have an extremely poor prognosis. Approximately 40% of older adults are alive 3 months after an ICU stay. Severe sepsis (defined as sepsis with acute organ dysfunction) increases the odds of developing cognitive deterioration and new ADL dependence in older survivors, and the postsepsis deterioration in cognition and function persists up to 8 years later.

Intensive care units now provide care at end-of-life for a significant number of decedents; 1 in 5 Americans who die receive ICU services before death. Establishing goals of care in older critically ill patients is of paramount importance. In caring for critically ill patients, it may become apparent to the patient, family, and clinician that further intervention would not likely be of substantial benefit, depending on the individual patient's goals, values, and hopes. Many older patients with life-limiting illness are most concerned about maintaining function (as opposed to prolonging physiologic life) when weighing the burdens and potential outcomes of treatment options.

Defining *futility* is often difficult. The American Medical Association recommends a standardized "fair process" rather than a strict definition of futility. This approach consists of deliberation and negotiation between all parties, steps to secure alternatives in the setting of irreconcilable differences, and a final step of closure when all alternatives have been exhausted. As much as possible, clinicians should base futility decisions on factors such as clinical efficacy of treatment, likelihood of mortality, and subsequent quality-of-life considerations rather than on chronologic age alone.

Given the well-described difficulty of clinicians to accurately prognosticate beyond hours of impending death, important decisions regarding use of life-prolonging technology in older critically ill patients should be made with humility and must incorporate the patient's goals of care. See also "Palliative Care," p 111.

DAILY EVALUATION OF OLDER HOSPITALIZED PATIENTS

Hospitalized older adults should be evaluated daily using a systematic approach to ensure that essential geriatric issues are not overshadowed by disease-specific or technologic concerns. For patients who are expected to recover mobility, progress toward that goal should be assessed. Time out of bed (eg, in a chair for meals) and ambulation (with assistance, if needed) should be encouraged. Progress on ADL recovery should be tracked, and nursing encouraged to coach patients toward functional independence.

Daily physical examination should include identifying the devices attached to, or inserted in, each patient. Many of these devices can cause injury if used inappropriately, and a daily assessment of risks and benefits is wise. Central venous catheters, for example, allow for convenient blood draws and delivery of medications and parenteral nutrition, but they are also associated with infection, restricted mobility, deep venous thrombosis, and air embolism. Indwelling bladder catheters carry a risk of urinary tract infection and delirium and should be used only when urinary retention would otherwise result, when an incontinent patient's urinary leakage may contaminate a healing wound, or for comfort in patients receiving end-of-life care. In almost all cases, urinary volume can be accurately measured without use of a bladder catheter.

Restraints constitute a hazard to both safety and personal dignity. Encouraging the bedside presence of family, "sitters," or bedside companions is far better for monitoring and assuring the safety of confused patients.

SYSTEMS OF CARE FOR OLDER HOSPITALIZED PATIENTS

Three systematic approaches have been demonstrated in controlled trials to improve hospital care of older adults. These approaches involve comprehensive multicomponent interventions, two of which were implemented on designated medical units.

Geriatric evaluation and management (GEM) units for older adults who have stabilized during an acute hospitalization were developed and pioneered in Veterans Affairs medical centers. These units incorporate comprehensive geriatric assessment (including screening for geriatric syndromes, and assessment for and treatment of functional, cognitive, affective, and nutritional problems) with interdisciplinary team-based care. In a multicenter randomized trial, ADL function and physical performance improved for veterans assigned to GEM units relative to those who received usual hospital care (SOE=A). Some measures of health-related quality of life were also superior for patients treated on GEM units. These units did not affect mortality and were cost-neutral after consideration of costs of both initial hospitalization and care after discharge.

A second approach, called Acute Care for Elders (ACE), adopted in many acute-care hospitals, involves a system of care designed to help acutely ill older patients to maintain or achieve independence in ADLs and IADLs. ACE programs adopt a proactive, "prehabilitative" approach, comprising four components:

- a prepared environment to promote mobility and orientation (eg, carpeting, raised toilet seats, low beds, clocks, calendars, and pictures to promote orientation)
- interdisciplinary, team-based, patient-centered care with nursing-initiated protocols for independent self-care, nutrition, sleep hygiene, skin care, mood, and cognition
- early planning to go home, with social work intervention to mobilize family and other resources at home
- medication review to promote optimal prescribing

This approach resulted in greater independence in ADLs at discharge, less frequent discharge to a nursing home, and somewhat shorter and less expensive hospitalization (SOE=A). In addition, ACE was associated with substantial differences in the satisfaction of patients, family members, physicians, and nurses but with only modest differences in ADL function (SOE=A). These findings demonstrate that ACE is a promising approach to improve outcomes and reduce hospital costs for acutely ill older general medical patients, but the effects of ACE on patient outcomes are likely sensitive to factors that depend on the function of the interdisciplinary team.

A third systematic approach, the Hospital Elder Life Program (HELP), involves a multicomponent intervention to prevent delirium in hospitalized older patients. The intervention consists of protocols to manage six risk factors for delirium: cognitive impairment, sleep deprivation, immobility, visual impairment, hearing impairment, and dehydration. Older patients receiving this intervention are not segregated on a special hospital ward or unit. The program makes extensive use of hospital volunteers. In one prospective controlled study, the incidence of delirium was reduced by one-third, from 15.0% to 9.9% (SOE=A). Severity and duration of delirium episodes appeared not to be affected by HELP. The intervention was also associated with significantly improved cognitive function among patients with cognitive impairment at admission and with a reduced rate of use of sleep medications among all patients. A trend toward improvement was also seen in other risk factors, including immobility, visual impairment, and hearing impairment.

Nurses Improving Care of Health System Elders (NICHE)

NICHE is a national program of the Hartford Institute for Geriatric Nursing at New York University College of Nursing, the goal of which is to improve the care of hospitalized older patients through change programs and nursing protocols.

The Geriatric Resource Nurse (GRN) Model is the foundation of the NICHE program and is based on the belief that primary nurses are most knowledgeable about the daily patterns and needs of the older adults in their units. After receiving specialized education in nursing care of older adults, the GRN receives ongoing mentorship and clinical support from an advanced practice nurse through clinical rounds and structured learning activities. GRNs serve as the unit's resource on geriatric best practices, engage in quality and research initiatives, and educate other staff regarding geriatric care.

Initially field-tested in four hospital sites, NICHE has since grown into a national hospital network for sharing lessons and collaborating in development of inpatient geriatric nursing-care resources. After implementing the NICHE GRN model, hospitals have reported improved clinical outcomes, enhanced nurse knowledge and perceptions of quality, and increased compliance with protocol application. See www.nicheprogram.org for additional information.

Alternatives to Hospital Care

It is often assumed that older adults would prefer to be treated for acute illness at home rather than in the hospital whenever possible. The safety and feasibility of this approach for some acutely ill older adults who would otherwise be hospitalized has been demonstrated. This approach, sometimes called the *home hospital*, requires intensive resources for medical and nursing care at home that are not yet widely available. See also "Community-Based Care," p 166.

Older adults' preferences for care at home rather than in the hospital vary widely. In a study of community-dwelling older adults, virtually all preferred care in the site that would provide the higher probability of survival. When home care and hospital care provide equivalent probabilities of survival, roughly half preferred care in each site, with those preferring home care more likely to be white, better educated, living with a spouse, deeply religious, and dependent in two or more ADLs. The major difference perceived by older adults between home care and hospital care was feeling safer in the hospital than at home.

Studies suggest that hospital-at-home care can provide safe, economical, and efficacious care for some older adults with selected medical conditions, eg, heart failure, community-acquired pneumonia, cellulitis, COPD (SOE=A). Common features of the home hospital models are the provision of care by a multidisciplinary team, availability of 24-hour coverage (including physician coverage), and a safe home environment. In one trial, patients with dementia in the intervention group had fewer problems with sleep, feeding, and aggression. Fewer patients were prescribed antipsychotics. There was no beneficial effect in functional ability. Patients receiving care in home hospital were more satisfied with their care than those admitted to hospital.

References

- Arora VM, Fish M, Basu A, et al. Relationship between quality of care of hospitalized vulnerable elders and postdischarge mortality. *J Am Geriatr Soc.* 2010;58(9):1642–1648.
- Boltz M, Resnick B, Shuluk J, et al. Activity restriction versus self-direction: Hospitalized older adults' response to fear of falling. *Int J Older People Nurs.* 2013; Jan 7.
- Mehta KM, Pierluissi E, Boscardin J, et al. A clinical index to stratify hospitalized older adults according to risk for new-onset disability. *J Am Geriatr Soc.* 2011;59(7):1206–1216.
- Onder G, Petrovic M, Tangiisuran B, et al. Development and validation of a score to assess risk of ADRs among in-hospital patients 65 years or older: the GerontoNet ADR Risk Score. *Arch Intern Med.* 2010;170(13):1142–1148.

CHAPTER 18—REHABILITATION

KEY POINTS

- The World Health Organization conceptual model of functioning and disability provides a useful framework for geriatric rehabilitation by taking into account the complex interactions of body functions and structures, health conditions, individual activities and participation in life situations, and environmental and personal factors.
- As rehabilitation treatments require active patient participation and long-term self-management, the patient and family are core members of the rehabilitation team.
- Factors that influence recovery after a hip fracture include prior mobility and functional status, comorbid conditions, cognitive status, and social support.
- Optimal rehabilitation outcomes depend on comprehensive assessment of the patient, coordinated interprofessional team management, multifaceted interventions, and access to appropriate and high-quality care.

Rehabilitation is a critical component of geriatric health care because of the high incidence of disabling conditions in the older adult population. Although these conditions drastically influence quality of life, they often improve with treatment. Chronic disease almost always underlies disability in older adults; for example, stroke occurs most often in people with other vascular diseases, and hip fractures occur most often in people with osteoporosis and gait disorders. Disability also worsens in progressive chronic diseases (such as osteoarthritis, Parkinson disease, or amyotrophic lateral sclerosis) or in the context of deconditioning from inactivity during acute illness. To provide the best functional recovery possible, those providing geriatric rehabilitation must do the following:

- use systematic approaches to assess the causes of disability
- be familiar with the advantages and disadvantages of all potential sites of care
- understand the role of interprofessional teams and care plans
- adapt care to comorbidities and disabilities
- be familiar with the basic requirements for rehabilitation of common geriatric conditions

CONCEPTUAL MODEL FOR GERIATRIC REHABILITATION

Geriatric rehabilitation services can be organized around a conceptual model of disability for assessing the status and needs of the patient, matching treatments with specific conditions, and evaluating rehabilitation outcomes. The World Health Organization (WHO) *International Classification of Functioning, Disability, and Health* (ICF) provides a useful framework for measuring health and disability. For an ICF guide and a discussion of the ICF model of disability, see the WHO Web site (www.who.int/classifications/icf/en/ [accessed Oct 2013]). The ICF has two main domains: "Health Condition" and "Contextual Factors." Disability and functioning are viewed as outcomes of interactions between health conditions (diseases, disorders, injuries) and contextual factors, which includes both environmental and personal. Environmental factors range from a person's most immediate environment, like furniture in the room, to the more general environment, such as access to public transportation. Personal factors include a person's age, race, gender, educational background, personality, fitness, and lifestyle.

In the WHO model, interventions can be designed to modify a person's impairments, limitations in activities, and restrictions in participation. For example, a treatment plan can be developed to improve a person's muscle strength (impairment level), but the significance of this intervention is a result of its effect on his or her physical mobility (activity) and ultimately his or her ability to return to social or physical roles (participation). The effects of gains in strength and physical mobility on participation can be modified by the person's motivation or social support. For example, if patients improve in strength and balance but their family and friends continue to "do everything for them" and do not encourage independent function, they may remain dependent. The physical environment is another powerful modifier. Even the person who achieves improved function cannot return to prior work or household roles if physical barriers to access in the community are not removed or adapted by means such as ramps or modified bathrooms. In summary, the interaction of disease and disability is particularly complex in older adults. The ICF model is useful for structuring their comprehensive rehabilitation care.

SITES OF REHABILITATION CARE

Rehabilitation services are available through Medicare Part A on a time-limited basis. These services are

Table 18.1—Rehabilitation Sites of Care and Level of Care Requirements

Rehabilitation Sites	Level of Care Requirements	Expected Intensity of Services	Payment Source
Inpatient			
Freestanding rehabilitation hospital or rehabilitation unit attached to acute hospital	24-hour availability of a physician with training or experience in rehabilitation 24-hour nursing care Relatively intense level of rehabilitation services Interprofessional team to deliver program Coordinated program of care as evidenced by team conferences at least every 2 weeks Reasonable expectation of improvement	An interprofessional team approach is required and in most cases, this calls for 3 hours of therapy at least 5 days/week; this can include physical, occupational, or speech therapy in any combination.	Medicare Part A ■ Days 1–20: full coverage ■ Days 21–100: partial coverage but co-payment ■ >100 days: no coverage
Medicare skilled-nursing facility	Physician supervision, with access 24 hours/day on emergency basis 24-hour nursing care Less intense therapy needs Interprofessional team coordination ideally will occur Maintenance of function without progress can be goal of care	Daily therapy (5 days/week) for up to 1 hour/day, as tolerated by patient; ADL assistance and/or skilled-nursing care	Medicare Part A ■ Days 1–20: full coverage ■ Days 21–100: partial coverage but co-payment ■ >100 days: no coverage
Outpatient			
Home health	Physician certifies need every 60 days Skilled need required, including either intermittent skilled nursing, physical, occupational, or speech therapy	Intermittent nursing or therapy provided; can be no more than 7 days/week or 8 hours/day; patient must have support system to meet needs of living at home	Medicare Part A
Clinic (hospital-based or independent)	Physician orders rehabilitation services to include physical, occupational, or speech therapy and reviews plan periodically Reasonable expectation of improvement with treatment	Intermittent physical, occupational, or speech therapy provided; patient must be able to get to therapy visits.	Medicare Part B There are caps on coverage, but these can be waived if medically necessary.

SOURCE: www.medicare.gov (accessed Oct 2013)

offered in both inpatient and community-based sites. Inpatient care may be provided in rehabilitation centers (freestanding hospitals or units attached to acute hospitals) or nursing facilities (Medicare skilled-nursing facilities). To receive Medicare coverage for an inpatient rehabilitation stay in either type of facility, a patient must have a hospital stay of at least 3 consecutive days for a related illness or injury. Typically reimbursed through Medicare Part B, outpatient rehabilitation services can be provided in hospital-based or independent clinics, in day hospital settings, or in the home. The patient's eligibility, the particular services provided, and costs vary across sites of care. The balance of advantages and disadvantages for the individual patient is an important factor for the clinician to consider in recommending a site for rehabilitation care. For a summary of the sites of rehabilitation, Medicare requirements and payment sources, and the expected intensity of the rehabilitation services, see Table 18.1.

Sites of Care: Coverage and Services

Medicare Part A covers intensive inpatient rehabilitation for patients who have complex needs requiring an interprofessional team approach, including multiple therapies. In most cases, this calls for a minimum of 3 hours of rehabilitation therapy services per day at least 5 days per week or 15 hours per week. Potential patients undergo a preadmission screen to evaluate their condition, need for services, and determine prior level of function. A Medicare-certified inpatient rehabilitation hospital program must demonstrate that at least a certain percentage of patients have at least 1 of 13 conditions: stroke, spinal cord injury, congenital deformity, amputation, major multiple trauma, hip fracture, brain injury, neurologic disorders (eg, multiple sclerosis, Parkinson disease), burns, three arthritis conditions for which appropriate aggressive and sustained outpatient therapy has failed, joint replacement for both knees or hips when the surgery immediately precedes admission,

Table 18.2—Functional Status and Disease-Specific Assessment Instruments

Instrument	Purpose/Description
Functional Independence Measure (www.tbims.org/combi/FIM/index.html)	■ Measures independent performance in self-care, transfers, locomotion, sphincter control, social cognition, and communication. ■ An 18-item ordinal scale with scores ranging from 0 (total assist) to 7 (complete independence); the possible total score ranges from 18 (the lowest) to 126 (highest), obtained by adding points for each item.
Barthel ADL Index (www.strokecenter.org/wp-content/uploads/2011/08/barthel.pdf)	■ Used to establish degree of independence with regard to ADLs. ■ A 10-item ordinal scale; scores vary depending on the item in question. Bathing and grooming are scored either 0 (dependent/needs help) or 5 (independent); scores for feeding, dressing, bowels, bladder, toilet use, and stairs range from 0 (dependent/unable) to 10 (independent); scores for transfers and mobility on level surfaces range for 0 (unable) to 15 (independent); the possible total score ranges for 0 (the lowest) to 100 (the highest), obtained by adding points for each item.
Stroke Impact Scale (www.chrp.org/pdf/HSR082103_SIS_Handout.pdf)	■ An 8-domain, 59-item scale that measures the aspects of stroke recovery important to patients and caregivers, as well as stroke experts. ■ Includes measures of physical domain such as strength, mobility, ADLs, and hand function, as well as the domains of memory, emotion, communication, and social participation.
Harris Hip Questionnaire (www.orthopaedicscore.com/scorepages/harris_hip_score.html)	■ Asks questions regarding pain and function, including ambulation distance, presence of a limp, ability with tasks such as public transportation or stairs, and need for an assistive device. ■ Hip deformity and range of hip motion are also included.

NOTE: Above Web sites accessed Oct 2013.

a BMI >50 kg/m^2, or age >85 years. Patients must have close medical supervision by a physician with specialized training or experience in rehabilitation, have 24-hour rehabilitation nursing care, and be managed by an interdisciplinary team of skilled nurses and therapists. Medicare prospective reimbursement is now based on case-mix groups using the Functional Independence Measure (Table 18.2).

The Medicare-approved skilled-nursing facility must provide 24-hour nursing care. Dietary, pharmaceutical, dental, and medical social services are also available. Physicians must supervise patient care and can visit the patient infrequently, but they must be available 24 hours per day on an emergency basis. Therapy services are available, and ideally interprofessional coordination will occur. In this setting, maintenance of function without progress may be the goal of care.

Medicare provides home-health benefits to patients who require nursing care or therapy services on an intermittent or part-time basis, defined as <7 days per week or <8 hours per day for all required services. Patients must also be homebound, defined as requiring considerable effort to leave home. Patients can leave home for medical treatments or for short, infrequent nonmedical reasons, including attendance at religious services. Home-health services must be prescribed and recertified every 60 days by a physician. There is no prior hospitalization requirement or limit on the number of visits a person may receive. Medicare provides care in 60-day episodes. Home-health services provide skilled nursing and home-health aides, therapy services, medical social services, and supplies. Home-health aide services require concomitant skilled-nursing or therapy visits.

The escalating expenditures for Medicare's postacute care benefits from $2.5 billion in 1986 to more than $30 billion in 1996 led to the Balanced Budget Act (BBA) of 1997, which mandated prospective payment systems rather than fee-for-service reimbursement. In skilled-nursing facilities, the BBA mandated the implementation of a per diem prospective payment system covering all costs (routine, ancillary, and capital) related to the services provided to the patients under Part A of the Medicare program. Per diem payments for each admission are case-mix adjusted by the use of a resident classification system (RUG IV) that is based on data from patient assessments (the Minimum Data Set 3) and relative weights developed from staff time data. Home-healthcare reimbursement is also under a prospective payment system. Payment rates are based on relevant data from patient assessments conducted by clinicians using the Outcome and Assessment Information Set (OASIS). The OASIS was originally developed to assess quality of care in home health. The OASIS is lengthy, encompassing sociodemographic, environmental, support system, health status, and functional status attributes; it is required for reimbursement by Medicare for home-health services. For each 60-day episode of care, national payment rates vary, depending on the intensity of care required. Home-health agencies receive less than the full 60-day episode rate if they provide only a minimal number of visits (<4) to beneficiaries.

Sites of Care and Outcomes

The effect of site of care on rehabilitation outcomes is not well established. A study of outcomes among patients with stroke and hip fracture examined rates of discharge to home and recovery of function that were based on use of inpatient or nursing rehabilitation services. When controlling for case-mix differences, the researchers found that stroke but not hip fracture patients were more likely to be discharged home and to recover activities of daily living (ADLs) if treated in an inpatient rehabilitation setting (SOE=B). In another cohort study, patients admitted for hip fracture to inpatient facilities had better 12-week functional outcomes than did patients undergoing rehabilitation at skilled-nursing facilities (SOE=B). This type of observational study is vulnerable to bias, despite adjusting the analyses, because the prognosis for recovery may influence discharge site; patients with a poor prognosis are more likely to go to the nursing home, while those with a better prognosis go to inpatient or home-health settings. Nevertheless, site of care may be an important factor in recovery.

Each site of care has advantages and disadvantages from the patient's perspective. Inpatient care is the most intense but may not be endurable for frail older patients, because it usually requires 3 hours per day of active (and fatiguing) therapy. Skilled nursing offers 24-hour care for those who cannot care for themselves or do not have a full-time caregiver. Outpatient services have clear advantages and disadvantages. Patients often prefer to return to their own homes but may not have the care support they need. Participation in day hospitals or outpatient clinics requires transportation, which can be costly and time consuming.

In summary, clinicians should be familiar with the services provided in a wide range of rehabilitation settings and with the advantages and disadvantages of each. The clinician is responsible for recommending the best match between patient needs and program services. However, under certain insurance plans, decisions about location of services can be heavily influenced by costs. More systematic evaluation of rehabilitation outcomes that is based on the structures and processes of care offered by various settings is essential for more rational use of rehabilitation programs. CMS is currently monitoring the quality of patient care using information from patient assessments.

TEAMS AND ROLES

A team approach is necessary to meet the complex rehabilitation needs of older adults. The interprofessional rehabilitation team often includes nursing, physical therapy, occupational therapy, speech language therapy, social work, psychology, nutrition services, prosthetics/orthotics, and geriatric medicine. All health professionals who work with older adults should have a basic understanding of the roles and functions of various team members (Table 18.3). Each health care professional evaluates the patient, identifies goals, and then provides discipline-specific interventions to address the patient's issues. The patient's health-related outcome is the sum of the effort of each discipline.

Multidisciplinary teamwork can be inefficient and result in duplication of services and gaps in care of the older patient. The interdisciplinary or interprofessional team is the recommended approach to providing holistic and coordinated care for the older adult. Patient-centered care is efficient and effective. Healthcare professionals complete comprehensive evaluations on the patient; however, the patient goals and the intervention plan are determined by the entire team, including the patient and his or her family. The patient and family are core members of the rehabilitation team, and their expectations and preferences must be integrated into the care plan. In collaboration, the team members should pool their skills, experience, and knowledge to work toward the patient's goals to achieve the best outcome. Because coordinating care is the function of the interdisciplinary care team, team members must be able to define roles, share tasks, and collaborate within and outside the team. Team building and continual efforts to improve team function are important issues for geriatric rehabilitation service providers to achieve positive patient outcomes.

The primary goal of the rehabilitation team is to ensure that patients receive comprehensive assessments and appropriate interventions for the disabling illness and associated comorbid conditions, as well as for the specific impairments and environmental factors that can affect activities and participation. The team must collaborate to establish common goals and a cohesive treatment plan to meet the needs of older adults.

IMPACT OF COMORBID CONDITIONS

In older patients, comorbid diseases and conditions can interrupt or delay treatment and often require the care plan to be modified. Many of the illnesses that can interfere with rehabilitation of older adults are predictable and potentially preventable. A systematic approach to assessment, prevention, and management of comorbid conditions can improve the patient's chance of receiving maximal benefit from rehabilitation services.

Older adults with reduced mobility are at high risk of skin breakdown, which can interfere with recovery and require extensive treatment. Immobility or altered weight bearing can precipitate pressure ulcers that heal poorly. Clinicians should monitor pressure and

Table 18.3—Roles of Core Healthcare Providers on Rehabilitation Team

Provider	Primary Role on Rehabilitation Team
Nursing	Provides ongoing assessment of signs and symptoms of illness, medical conditions, and affect Provides patient and family education Evaluates self-care skills
Physical therapist	Assesses joint range of motion and muscle strength Assesses gait and mobility Provides appropriate assistive devices Instructs in exercise training to increase range of motion, strength, endurance, balance, coordination, and gait Treats with physical modalities (heat, cold, ultrasound, massage, electrical stimulation) Assesses environmental barriers in planned discharge environment
Occupational therapist	Evaluates self-care skills and other ADLs Provides home assessment Provides self-care skills training; makes recommendations and provides training in use of assistive technology Fabricates splints and treats upper-extremity deficits
Speech therapist	Assesses all aspects of communication Treats communication deficits Assesses swallowing disorders Recommends changes in diet and positioning to treat dysphagia
Social worker	Evaluates family and home-care factors Assesses psychosocial factors Provides counseling
Dietitian	Assesses nutritional status Recommends dietary changes to maximize nutrition
Prosthetist	Makes and fits prosthetic limbs
Physician, nurse practitioner	Certifies rehabilitation need (physician only) Supervises patient treatment Treats medical comorbidities Provides education

weight-bearing areas and be prepared to modify footwear, wheelchairs, and bedding as needed. See also "Pressure Ulcers and Wound Care," p 296. Because thromboembolic events are also common with reduced mobility, their prevention should be a routine part of care. Length of time for prophylaxis and medication recommendations varies depending on the medical condition.

Incontinence is prevalent among older adults; causes include detrusor overactivity, obstruction, neurogenic bladder, immobility, and cognitive deficits. Indwelling catheters increase the risk of infection and are rarely appropriate in the nonacute setting. A structured approach to the assessment and treatment of bladder problems should be a basic component of any rehabilitation service. See also "Urinary Incontinence," p 220.

The risk of pneumonia is increased by inactivity and disordered swallowing, as well as by underlying lung disease. The prevention of aspiration pneumonia involves difficult tradeoffs. Awareness of aspiration has been markedly increased by routine radiologic screening, but the clinical relevance of modest aspiration detected radiologically is unknown. Conservative measures such as changing food consistency with liquid thickeners and cohesive food substances and elevating head position while eating can help alleviate the problem. Sometimes aspiration risk is addressed by discontinuing all oral feeding and placing an enteral feeding tube. This approach eliminates the fundamental human pleasure of eating and may not be successful, because oral secretions or refluxed gastric contents can still be aspirated. See also "Eating and Feeding Problems," p 216. Bleeding in the upper GI tract can occur during rehabilitation as a consequence of stress or medications and may not be preceded by typical symptoms. See also "Gastrointestinal Diseases and Disorders," p 408.

Anemia is common in older adults and has been associated with adverse outcomes, including functional impairment, decreased muscle strength, and poorer quality of life. Studies are ongoing to examine the effect of erythropoietin on exercise tolerance. See also "Hematologic Diseases and Disorders," p 530.

Mental functioning is critical for rehabilitation, which requires the ability to follow commands and to learn. Because older adults who have been acutely ill are at increased risk of delirium, clinicians should assess mental status and screen for easily reversible causes in their older rehabilitation patients. See also "Delirium," p 276. Depression is endemic in newly disabled individuals and can manifest as low motivation; formal screens for depression and early intervention are essential. See also "Depression and Other Mood Disorders," p 308. Seizures can develop after stroke, and spasticity can develop during stroke recovery. Interventions for spasticity such as physical therapy or muscle relaxants have offered only modest benefit (SOE=B). Studies have shown botulinum toxin to be effective in decreasing muscle tone and increasing range of motion (SOE=A). However, these improvements have not consistently translated into improved function (SOE=B). See also stroke in "Neurologic Diseases and Disorders," p 480.

Certain comorbid conditions common in older adults, including diabetes mellitus, heart disease, peripheral vascular disease, musculoskeletal disorders, sensory impairments, and dementia, require ongoing adaptations in rehabilitation. Activity level is a powerful factor in glucose metabolism; diabetic patients are therefore likely to experience changes in glucose levels and medication requirements during rehabilitation. Increased caloric intake during recovery can also affect medication needs. Therapy personnel should know how to assess diabetic control, use a glucometer, and intervene for hypoglycemia. See also "Diabetes Mellitus," p 520. Most abnormal gaits increase the energy requirements of walking; an abnormal gait in a patient with coronary artery disease can cause coronary symptoms to worsen. Patients with poor cardiac output may have extreme exercise limitations. Medication adjustments for heart diseases may be necessary but can cause adverse events of their own, such as orthostatic hypotension. Patients with one vascular disease often have others; peripheral vascular disease is common, often associated with insensitive or painful feet and a high risk of skin breakdown. Treatment of painful peripheral neuropathy can foster increased activity and avoid pressure ulcers. Musculoskeletal status should be monitored to avoid overuse syndromes involving increased demand on vulnerable joints. For those with vision or hearing impairment, corrections must be provided and teaching approaches adapted accordingly. In patients with dementia, rehabilitation progress is still possible, but carryover may be decreased and the need for supervision and cueing may be increased.

REHABILITATION APPROACHES AND INTERVENTIONS

The primary goals of rehabilitation treatment are restitution of function, compensation for and adaptation to functional losses, and prevention of secondary complications. Ultimately, rehabilitation should maximize the person's potential for participation in social, leisure, or work roles. Many strategies can be used to achieve these goals. Restitution of physical function usually depends on therapeutic exercises to improve flexibility, muscle strength, motor control, and cardiovascular endurance. Exercise has been shown to improve strength, endurance, and balance in well-defined populations of disabled older adults (SOE=A). See also "Physical Activity," p 64. In stroke, speech and language therapy can be used to treat aphasia. Cognitive rehabilitation might improve alertness and attention. However, research evidence is insufficient to demonstrate that speech and language therapy, or cognitive rehabilitation, improve functional deficits.

Massage, heat, cold, and ultrasound are used to decrease pain and muscle spasm. These and other pain management strategies can contribute to increased function and tolerance for further rehabilitation. There is little research evidence supporting objective benefits from these therapies, but patients commonly report symptomatic relief. See also "Persistent Pain," p 119.

Equipment for mobility, dressing and bathroom assistance, orthotic and prosthetic devices, and splints all can augment or replace the function of impaired body parts and thereby reduce limitations in activities and participation. For example, an ankle-foot orthosis can compensate for foot drop and improve safety and speed of walking. A wheelchair can provide mobility for community activities.

Repeated practice of task-specific activities such as bed mobility, transfers, and walking can improve functional mobility. Arm function improves with specific functional training activities, such as grasping, reaching, and fine manipulations. Balance training may improve balance and reduce the risk of falls. Older adults can benefit from retraining in instrumental activities of daily living (IADLs), such as cooking, managing finances, or driving a car.

Contextual factors, both environmental and personal, should be addressed to minimize restrictions on a person's activities and participation. For example, motivation can be addressed by collaborative goal setting, patient and family education, detection and management of depression, and use of support groups. Environmental modifications, such as grab bars and raised toilet seats in the bathroom or curb cutouts on public streets, can promote independent functioning.

To maintain function and enhance health status after rehabilitation, patients and families should assume responsibility for long-term self-management. Rehabilitation goals include a program to prevent worsening disability, including reintegration into social programs such as senior center programs, and health and wellness programs.

COMPREHENSIVE ASSESSMENT

Comprehensive assessment of rehabilitation patients is necessary for appropriate clinical management and evaluation of outcomes. The treatment plan should be guided by results of the initial assessment. The primary components of any assessment include patient demographics, social support, place of residence before illness, medical comorbidities, severity of current illness, and the patient's prior functional status. The rehabilitation stay is an ideal time for medication review and reconciliation, as patients transition from the hospital to the rehabilitation setting and ultimately to the community.

Impairments such as deficits in range of motion and flexibility, strength, sensory functions, balance, cognition, and depression should always be assessed. In conditions such as stroke, swallowing and language function should be evaluated. The patient's functional status is assessed with standardized measures of ADLs (eg, the Barthel ADL Index [Table 18.2]) and measures of IADLs. The patient's participation or quality of life is assessed with generic measures like the SF-36 Health Survey (available at www.sf-36.org [accessed Oct 2013]) or disease-specific measures like the Stroke Impact Scale or Harris Hip Questionnaire (Table 18.2).

STROKE

Stroke is a major cause of mortality and morbidity in the United States, particularly among adults ≥55 years old. Acute stroke occurs in >700,000 people each year, and 80% or more are likely to survive, many with residual neurologic difficulties. Stroke-related deficits are severe in approximately one-third of the survivors. Many patients with mild and moderate stroke become independent in ADLs, but other more complex dimensions of health status may still be affected. As stroke survival continues to increase, the need for comprehensive stroke rehabilitation will rise. Rehabilitation programs must address a broad range of stroke-related disabilities, including those in basic ADLs and IADLs, and participation and integration into health and wellness programs.

Goals of Rehabilitation

The overall goals of rehabilitation for older stroke patients include regaining function, compensating for or adapting to functional losses, and preventing secondary complications. Specific objectives include the following:

- preventing or recognizing and managing comorbid illness and medical complications
- assessing each patient comprehensively, using standardized assessments
- matching the patient's needs to the program capabilities
- training the patient to maximize independence in ADLs and IADLs
- facilitating the patient's and family's psychosocial coping and adaptation
- preventing recurrent stroke and other vascular conditions such as myocardial infarction
- assisting the patient in reintegrating into the community

Rehabilitation for older adults with stroke is complex because of the variability of causes, symptoms, severity, and recovery. Stroke patients present with varying symptoms, depending on the site and size of the brain lesions. The most common type of neurologic deficit is hemiparesis, but other deficits can include sensory impairment, aphasia, dysarthria, cognitive impairment, motor incoordination, hemianopsia, visual-perceptual deficits, depression, dysphagia, and bowel and bladder incontinence. The degree of initial recovery and the time needed to reach maximal recovery is affected by the number of deficits. For example, individuals who have hemiparesis, hemianopsia, and sensory deficits are less likely to ambulate independently and require a longer time to regain skills than do those with only hemiparesis.

Stroke patients usually experience some degree of recovery. This recovery is most dramatic in the first 30 days but may continue more gradually for months. In the Framingham study, improvement in motor function and self-care slowed 3 months after stroke but continued at a reduced pace throughout the first year. In a recent study of locomotor training after stroke, participants demonstrated functional improvements up to 1 year even when training was begun 6 months after the stroke had occurred (SOE=B). Language and visual-spatial function was recovered over 12 months, but cognitive function improved during only the first 3 months.

Approach to Management

Guidelines for rehabilitation after stroke have been updated by a team sponsored by the Department of Veterans Affairs and the Department of Defense (available at www.healthquality.va.gov/Management_of_Stroke_Rehabilitation.asp [accessed Oct 2013]). The guidelines offer algorithms for initial assessment and rehabilitation referral, followed by management in inpatient or community settings. The guidelines emphasize that clinical outcomes are better when patients with acute stroke are treated in a setting that provides coordinated, interdisciplinary stroke-related evaluation and services (SOE=A). Studies have confirmed that adherence to guidelines promotes better outcomes. Coordinated care reduces 1-year mortality, improves functional independence, and increases satisfaction with care (SOE=A). Stroke severity should be systematically assessed, using the NIH Stroke

Scale (www.strokecenter.org/trials/scales/nihss.html [accessed Oct 2013]).

Benefits of rehabilitation after stroke are not restricted to any particular subgroup of patients. Studies have found that racial/ethnic minorities may be more likely to receive rehabilitation and to have longer lengths of stay (SOE=B). In one study, urban-dwelling black stroke patients were more likely to be discharged to an inpatient rehabilitation facility, possibly because of the greater number and severity of stroke cases in this population. Non-Hispanic whites who undergo rehabilitation for a stroke tend to be older, and less likely to have had a hemorrhagic stroke or have Medicaid. In a large national retrospective study, non-Hispanic white patients had higher admission and discharge functional status ratings than patients in the minority groups. Despite this, whites were discharged home less frequently than blacks, Hispanics, or other minority groups (SOE=B).

In general, therapy should be started early, but later supplementary interventions can also be beneficial. There are several philosophical approaches to physical rehabilitation after strokes that are based on neurophysiologic, motor learning, or orthopedic principles. In a Cochrane review, a mixed approach was significantly more effective than no treatment or placebo (sham treatment) control for improving functional independence (standardized mean difference 0.94; confidence intervals 95%, 0.08–1.80). There is no convincing evidence that any one specific technique is superior to another.

Newer therapeutic interventions for regaining motor function are in development. Constraint-induced movement therapy discourages use of the unaffected extremity and encourages active use of the hemiparetic extremity, with a goal of improved motor recovery. In a large randomized clinical trial, constraint-induced movement therapy produced statistically significant and clinically relevant improvements in arm motor function that persisted for at least 1 year (SOE=A). Treadmill walking with partial body-weight support using a harness connected to an overhead system can improve gait velocity, balance, and motor recovery. However, this method was no better than a home exercise program managed by a physical therapist in improving functional walking ability (SOE=A). There is evidence that mirror therapy improves recovery of arm function (SOE=B). This therapy uses visual imagery by encouraging the patient to exercise both extremities symmetrically while viewing the reflection of the unaffected limb in a mirror and the affected limb occluded. It is thought that the patient experiences proprioceptive input to the affected side through the visual input. Speech and language therapy are often provided for stroke patients with aphasia. However, there is no universally accepted treatment. Although a Cochrane report states that the evidence does not support a finding of either clear effect or lack of effect, the Veterans Affairs guidelines support "good" evidence for follow-up evaluation and treatment by the speech language professional for long-term residual communication difficulties. Dysphagia (or swallowing disorders) is common after stroke, affecting up to 30% of patients. The most commonly used test to diagnose dysphagia is videofluoroscopy, which allows the speech therapy professional to observe and analyze the swallowing process and to assess for aspiration. Patients who aspirate are treated using rehabilitation exercises, changes in food consistency, and changes in posture to reduce the likelihood of aspiration. Transcranial magnetic stimulation to improve muscle function has shown promise. The guidelines also support "good" evidence for cognitive retraining for attention or visual-spatial perceptual deficits and compensatory training for short-term memory deficits. The same guidelines find "good" evidence for medication treatment for depression and emotional lability. In several studies, depression was a consistent factor adversely influencing rehabilitation outcomes. Spasticity can develop gradually after stroke and can inhibit function and interfere with hygiene. Most interventions, including surgery and medications like baclofen, have been disappointing.

The patient who has had a stroke is at high risk of recurrence: up to 7%–10% annually. The rehabilitation phase is an appropriate time to ensure that assessment and treatment for stroke prevention has occurred. Assessments for significant carotid stenosis and for atrial fibrillation should be completed. Indications for carotid endarterectomy and anticoagulation with warfarin, dabigatran, or rivaroxaban should be reviewed. Antiplatelet medications such as aspirin alone or in combination with extended-release dipyridamole or clopidogrel should be considered in many patients. Treatment with ACE inhibitors[OL] and statins[OL] has also demonstrated reduced risk of stroke. Other risk factors to be targeted for preventing stroke recurrence include hypertension and smoking (SOE=A).

In summary, the evidence for specific interventions for stroke rehabilitation is weak. The collective benefits of well-organized interprofessional care, including secondary prevention, are well established. See also cerebrovascular diseases in "Neurologic Diseases and Disorders," p 480.

Hip Fracture

Epidemiology and Surgical Care

Each year in the United States, about 300,000 older adults fracture a hip, with >90% of these fractures being the result of a fall. The risk of fracture is higher in women, whites, nursing-home residents, and in people with dementia. Mortality is about 5% during the initial hospitalization but nears 25% in the year after fracture. About 75% of survivors recover to their prior level of function, but their overall mobility is more limited; up to half still require an assistive device. About half of patients will have an initial decline requiring transient long-term care, and about 25% will still be in long-term care 1 year later.

Medical management includes interventions to relieve pain and restore bone alignment to allow fracture healing and prepare the older adult to return to their prior level of functioning. For medically stable patients, surgical repair is recommended 24–72 hours after fracture. This early repair has been associated with a reduction in 1-year mortality, as well as with a lower incidence of complications such as pressure ulcers and delirium. For medically unstable patients, delaying surgery is warranted to allow sufficient improvement to tolerate the procedure. The surgical approach is determined by the location of the fracture, the presence or absence of displacement, and the prefracture mobility. One-third of hip fractures occur at the femoral neck, and the other two-thirds are intertrochanteric, occurring lateral to the femoral neck. Prefracture mobility is used as a guide to determine the goal of surgical treatment and to allow the risks and benefits of each surgical procedure to be considered.

Femoral neck fractures, which include subcapital, transcervical, and basilar fracture locations, are more common in older adults, particularly women. A femoral neck fracture without any displacement and intact blood supply can be surgically corrected with simple screws. However, femoral neck fractures with any degree of displacement and/or poor circulation are at increased risk of nonunion or avascular necrosis and therefore are usually treated with a prosthetic femoral head (hemiarthroplasty). Patients with significant underlying bony acetabular disease and a displaced femoral neck fracture may benefit from complete hip arthroplasty. Patients are usually allowed to bear weight immediately after repair of a femoral neck fracture, regardless of type of surgical procedure. However, those undergoing a total hip arthroplasty are required to adhere to total hip precautions (described below).

For intertrochanteric fractures, the treatment of choice is open reduction and internal fixation with a compression screw or similar device. Displaced or comminuted intertrochanteric fractures commonly remain unstable, even after surgical fixation; therefore, full weight bearing is often not allowed for up to 6 weeks or until the stability of the fracture is assured. Factors that influence recovery should be assessed, including prior mobility and functional status, comorbid conditions, cognitive status, social support, type of injury, and repair and pain status. Mobility performance can be systematically assessed with numerous instruments, including the Harris Hip Questionnaire, which was developed specifically for hip fracture (Table 18.2).

Rehabilitation After Hip Fracture

Rehabilitation after hip fracture includes pain management, mobilization, and prevention of complications, such as delirium and thromboembolic events. The most important factors influencing recovery appear to be how soon mobilization is started and how frequently therapy is provided. Delay in mobilization is often driven by surgical recommendation, with proper healing of the fracture taking precedence over mobility. Partial weight bearing is difficult for many older adults to achieve. Prolonged inactivity is clearly associated with poorer functional outcomes, and early weight bearing is associated with low rates of surgical failure (SOE=A). Accelerated rehabilitation with rapid mobilization, coordinated planning, early discharge, and community follow-up has been associated with a 17% reduction in costs and no detriment to rates of recovery (SOE=B). Intensity of service clearly affects outcome, as those who receive physical therapy more than once a day during initial rehabilitation are more likely to be discharged directly to home than those who receive physical therapy once a day or less (SOE=A).

Prevention of Recurrence

Older adults who have had a hip fracture often have other comorbidities, such as osteoporosis and balance problems, that place them at risk of additional fractures resulting from falls. Efforts to diagnose and treat osteoporosis, improve balance, and reduce injury risk are a key part of treatment planning during rehabilitation. See also "Osteoporosis," p 243. The use of hip protectors for fracture prevention in older adults has been extensively studied with mostly negative results. See hip protectors in "Falls," p 234.

TOTAL HIP AND KNEE ARTHROPLASTY

Cause and Surgical Care

In the United States, joint arthroplasty is the most common elective surgical procedure performed; approximately 400,000 are done annually. The primary indications for joint replacement are progressive pain and limitation of mobility despite conservative care. Plain radiographs are the usual method for determining the severity of joint damage at both the hip and knee. Loss of cartilage is shown by joint-space narrowing, and often osteophyte formation is also present (Figure 56.1). The most common diagnosis associated with the need for hip and knee joint replacement is osteoarthrosis, followed by rheumatoid arthritis.

The long-term results of joint replacement have generally been excellent and include significant pain relief, increased motion, and improved function. Continued success rates in the 90% range are seen 10–15 years after joint replacement. The most common reason for failure of the hip or knee replacement is loosening of the implant. Joint infection is another major concern, affecting 0.2%–1.1% of total hip and 1%–2% of total knee replacements. Deep infections often necessitate removal of the implant and long-term antibiotics until there is no sign of infection, followed by ultimate replacement with a new implant. See also "Infectious Diseases," p 494.

There are various types of hip prostheses and surgical approaches for the total hip arthroplasty; the prosthetic and approach used are determined by the surgeon based on the condition of the joint and the integrity of the bone. Depending on the approach used, the patient must adhere to certain hip precautions, ie, prevention of specific movements by the affected leg for approximately 6 weeks to ensure healing and prevent dislocation. With the anterolateral surgical approach, the patient must avoid external rotation, adduction, and extension of the operated leg. With a posterolateral approach, the patient should not internally rotate or adduct the leg and not flex the hip beyond 90 degrees. Many surgeons use a minimally invasive technique for total hip arthroplasty that involves 2-inch incisions (versus the traditional 10-inch) and no detachment of muscle. Because tissue trauma is less, recovery is often quicker.

Like hip prostheses, various types of prosthetic knees are available as well; the type used depends on the joint damage. Typically, patients can begin bearing weight on the operated leg by the first day or two after surgery. However, rotation or torsion at the knee should be avoided for up to 3 months. Surgeons have also applied the concept of minimal incisions to the total knee replacement surgery and with significantly more success, including achieving greater knee flexion. This surgery, in experienced hands, decreases blood loss and length of stay (SOE=A).

Management

Anticoagulation to prevent thromboembolism and good pain control are the major goals during the immediate postoperative period for both hip and knee arthroplasty. See also "Perioperative Care," p 102. Patients who have undergone a major orthopedic procedure such as total hip or knee arthroplasty are at particularly high risk of both symptomatic and asymptomatic venous thromboembolism. For patients after total hip arthroplasty, current guidelines for prevention of venous thromboembolism recommend a minimum of 10–14 days of antithrombotic prophylaxis. (SOE=A). Pain control in the initial postoperative period is often achieved with opioids administered orally, intravenously, or by patient-controlled analgesia pumps. For both hip and knee arthroplasty, early mobilization is the standard of care, and weight bearing often begins on the first postoperative day. Patients at low risk can often be discharged from the acute care hospital within 5 days. For those at high risk, defined as being >70 years old or having two or more comorbid conditions, early inpatient rehabilitation improves functional outcomes and decreases total length of stay (SOE=B). Age alone should not be used as a criterion for eligibility for joint replacement—excellent results can be achieved even in patients >80 years old who are in good health with stable chronic conditions. In a large retrospective study of patients receiving inpatient medical rehabilitation after hip arthroplasty, non-Hispanic whites and women had the greatest functional improvement from admission to discharge. Asians had the lowest mean change in function scores. Being of nonwhite ethnicity and being male were associated with higher odds of being discharged to home (SOE=B).

Rehabilitation

To decrease the risk of dislocation after total hip arthroplasty, rehabilitation patients are taught to complete their daily activities while adhering to the hip precautions through the use of adaptive equipment and assistive devices. To prevent excessive hip flexion during toileting, a raised toilet seat is recommended for the first few months after surgery. If the patient uses a tub/shower combination at home, a tub bench is beneficial for safety in entering and exiting while maintaining hip precautions. Rehabilitation focuses on strengthening especially the abductors, which are weakened by the surgical approach, as well as on progressive range-of-motion and gait training. After total knee replacement, recovery of range of motion is the key to return of function and is often aided by the use of a continuous passive-motion (CPM) machine. Based on a systematic review, early postoperative CPM decreased the need for postoperative manipulation and, combined with physical therapy, increased active range of motion and shortened the length of stay. Postoperative swelling is common and interferes with regaining motion. However, thigh-high compression stockings, CPM, and possibly cryotherapy can be used to manage swelling.

Amputation

Epidemiology

Approximately 75,000 people undergo leg amputation each year in the United States. Most of these people have systemic vascular disease, with or without diabetes mellitus. Those with diabetes often have other end-organ disease, such as blindness, end-stage renal disease, and peripheral neuropathy. Mortality in this group approaches 50% at 2 years and 70% at 5 years. For up to one-fifth of patients, amputation of the other leg is needed within the first 2 years after the initial amputation. Most dysvascular amputees have such a burden of comorbid disease that the prosthesis is largely used for limited mobility, such as transfers and ambulation within the home.

The level of amputation and surgical approach depends on the status of the extremity; the surgery may be to remove devitalized tissue or may include reconstruction of the residual limb or stump. Common amputation levels include above or below the knee, as well as hip disarticulations.

Assessment

Key factors to assess include the patient's prior functional status, stability of comorbid conditions, cognition, and arm use, as well as the condition of the stump and the other leg. Successful prosthetic ambulation is associated with independent prior ambulation, ability to bear weight on the contralateral leg, stable medical status, and ability to follow directions. Blindness and end-stage renal disease do not necessarily preclude rehabilitation.

Rehabilitation for Amputation

Rehabilitation starts in the preoperative stage, when the patient begins with strength and flexibility exercises and is educated about the recovery process, including prosthetic preparation and training. Amputation surgery generally aims to preserve the knee, because the energy requirement for walking is much lower for the below-the-knee amputee than for the above-the-knee amputee. This decision must be weighed against risks of poor wound healing with more distal amputation.

Postoperative rehabilitation includes efforts at early mobilization, prevention of contractures, wound healing, edema control, shaping of the stump, and psychosocial support. Patients are educated on maintaining intact skin integrity through wound care, compression wrapping, desensitization, and skin inspection to prepare the residual limb for the prosthesis. Poor wound healing delays rehabilitation in about 25% of cases. Prostheses vary in weight, socket type, style of foot, and suspensions. The older amputee benefits from a prosthesis that is lightweight, stable, and easy to use. Prosthetic rehabilitation involves progressive ambulation, education about prosthesis and stump care, and stump injury monitoring.

Lastly, phantom limb pain is common after amputation, with an estimated incidence of 60%–80%; pain management influences progress with rehabilitation. Treatment remains difficult, and clear evidence-based guidelines are lacking. Because tricyclic antidepressants[OL] and sodium channel blockers such as carbamazepine[OL] are generally effective for neuropathic pain, they are often used for phantom pain despite the lack of well-controlled trials (SOE=B). Anticonvulsants, specifically gabapentin, have been effective in several randomized controlled trials but not in others (SOE=B). A number of other medication regimens, using such agents as opioids[OL] and anesthetic blocks[OL], have also had success in small trials. Although previous controlled trials using memantine showed little success, a more recent double-blinded placebo-controlled trial using memantine in the 4 weeks immediately after amputation showed a significant decrease in phantom limb pain. Thus, memantine may be useful if used shortly after amputation but not for established, chronic phantom limb pain (SOE=B).

Mobility Aids, Orthotics, Adaptive Methods, and Environmental Modifications

Assistive devices, orthotics, adaptive methods, and environmental modifications are effective for older adults with disabilities. It is important to identify the underlying causes of disability before prescribing a device or modification, because medical or surgical treatment for individual diseases and impairments may be more effective or may enhance the usefulness of these approaches.

An estimated 6.8 million Americans use assistive technology devices to enhance mobility. Unfortunately, many older adults who might benefit from the use of mobility aids do not or will not use them. There may be racial/ethnic influences in willingness to use mobility aids. Focus group studies with community-dwelling older adults of white, non-Hispanic black, and Hispanic backgrounds showed that for all groups, perceived benefits of mobility devices in maintaining independence and control produced positive attitudes. However, the association of use of mobility aids with aging and physical decline contributed to stigmatizing attitudes. Black and Hispanic participants expressed apprehension about using unsafe or inappropriate secondhand equipment, heightened concerns about

Table 18.4—Commonly Prescribed Mobility Aids

Assistive Device	Characteristics	Prescribed Conditions
Straight cane	Provide unilateral support Assist with balance and proprioception Reduce weight bearing on opposite leg	Osteoarthritis of knee or hip Peripheral neuropathy
Quad cane	Provides unilateral support More stable than straight cane Allows greater weight bearing on device	Stroke with hemiparesis
Stationary "pick-up" walker	Provides bilateral support Must be lifted and advanced requiring strength and coordination Very stable and allows non-weight bearing movement	Hip fracture in which non-weight bearing needed Unilateral amputation, before prosthesis
Two-wheeled walker	Less stable than stationary walker, but easier to advance Allows for smoother, faster gait	Deconditioning Parkinson disease
Rollator (four-wheeled walker with seat and brakes)	Less stable but allows for smoother, faster gait Requires more coordination (because of brakes) Good for outside walking because of large wheels Has seat for resting	Cardiopulmonary disease Peripheral neuropathy with balance difficulty
Manual wheelchair	Requires use of arms and some cardiopulmonary endurance Often used in nursing homes and by caregivers for ease of patient mobility	Non-ambulatory patient with cognitive impairment Low level spinal cord injury
Power wheelchair	Allows community mobility for those with limited ambulatory ability Controls do not require intact upper extremities Need cognitive ability to operate safely May need home modifications	Neurologic diseases (eg, high-level spinal cord injury, multiple sclerosis, amyotrophic lateral sclerosis) Multiple limb amputations
Scooter	Similar benefits to power wheelchair, except need to operate with upper extremities May be more acceptable to patient than power wheelchair	Cardiopulmonary disease

mobility-aid users becoming the subject of negative biases, and a preference for fashionable mobility aids. Hispanic participants expressed a preference for human assistance. Participants of all groups perceived clinicians as influencing their decision to use mobility aids.

Mobility Aids

Canes typically support 15%–20% of the body weight and are used in the hand contralateral to the affected knee or hip. A straight cane has a single tip, while a quad cane has four tips. As the number of tips increases, the degree of support also increases, but the cane becomes heavier and more awkward to use. The handle of the cane may be curved or have a pistol grip; the pistol grip offers more support. Canes can be made of a variety of materials, but most are made of wood or lightweight aluminum. The length of the cane is important for stability. Some canes are adjustable, but wooden canes must be cut to size. One of two methods can be used to evaluate the proper cane length: measuring the distance from the distal wrist crease to the ground when the patient is standing erect, and measuring the distance from the greater trochanter to the ground. Straight canes are often prescribed for patients with a single joint problem, like osteoarthritis of the knee. The cane decreases the weight bearing through the joint, thereby decreasing pain and improving ambulation. A cane can also be helpful for patients with decreased lower extremity proprioception. Proprioceptors in the hand relay vital information to the brain about where the cane and the ground are in relation to the person. Quad canes are used when a patient requires a more stable platform on which to bear weight, such as after a stroke with resultant hemiparesis. It is important when using the quad cane that all four tips are placed on the ground simultaneously, to assure the cane is stable before weight bearing (Table 18.4).

Crutches, axillary or forearm, are usually used to provide bilateral support. Axillary crutches are seldom recommended for older adults because greater arm strength and coordination are required for use. In addition, there is a risk of brachial plexus injury if the crutches are used incorrectly. Forearm crutches are more functional because a cuff secures the crutch on the patient's arm, allowing use of the hand to manipulate objects. A single crutch can be used instead of a cane if additional unilateral support is needed.

A walker is prescribed when a cane does not offer sufficient stability. A walker can completely support one leg but cannot support full body weight. Walker types include pick-up and wheeled walkers. Walkers should be adjusted so that the user maintains an erect posture and is not required to lean forward to reach the walker. The pick-up walker is lifted and moved forward by the user, who then advances before lifting the walker again; the result is a slow, staggering gait. It requires strength to repeatedly pick up the walker and cognitive ability to learn the necessary coordination. It may be the mobility device of choice when offloading one limb and maximal stability is preferred, such as after a hip fracture in a patient with a tenuous fixation in which non-weight bearing is needed to allow the bone to heal. A wheeled walker allows for a smoother, coordinated, and faster gait and takes advantage of compensated gait patterns; it is more likely to be correctly used by those with cognitive impairment. The most commonly used type is the two-wheeled walker, which brakes automatically with increased downward pressure. Patients with Parkinson disease often do well with a wheeled walker because once they start walking, they do not have to stop and start as is required with a pick-up walker. The two-wheeled walker is also easier to stop, because patients only need to lean on the device to engage the brakes.

A "rollator" is a four-wheeled walker with hand brakes, which can be locked when the patient is transferring. This type also has a platform seat for resting and a basket for carrying objects. Because of the use of the hand brakes, the rollator requires greater skill. It is preferred for outdoor use because the wheels are larger and move easier over sidewalks and slightly rough terrain. The rollator is often prescribed for patients with cardiac or pulmonary conditions and deconditioning. The ability to lean on the device increases the distance patients can travel because it decreases energy expenditure, and patients can sit to rest when fatigued.

Patients who cannot safely use or who are unable to ambulate with an assistive device require a wheelchair. A wheelchair must be fitted according to the patient's body build, weight, disability, and prognosis. Incorrect fit can result in poor posture, joint deformity, reduced mobility, pressure ulcers, circulatory compromise, and discomfort. The Rehabilitation Engineering and Assistive Technology Society of North America Wheelchair Service Guide provides detailed information for determining the most appropriate wheelchair for the patient (www.resna.org/dotAsset/22485.pdf [accessed Oct 2013]). Several factors are associated with use of a prescribed wheelchair, including age, gender, health, characteristics of the device (eg, type, size), and environmental facilitators and barriers. Often the prescribed devices do not meet the needs of the older adult. In one study, 61% of the older adults reported having difficulty with manual wheelchair propulsion. Important considerations in the evaluation for a wheelchair are cognitive status and functional ability to use the device. Manual wheelchairs are frequently used in the nursing-home setting to allow ease of mobility, either through self or staff propulsion. The most significant factor associated with manual wheelchair use was not living at home.

The demand for power mobility devices has increased substantially in recent years, and accounts for 66% of the Medicare expenses for mobility-related devices. Motorized wheelchairs can be used by mentally alert individuals with bilateral arm weakness or other neurologic disorders that limit arm use. Power wheelchairs can be controlled using a joystick or an alternative control device like a sip-and-puff switch or head control. Examples of patients who might do well with a power wheelchair include those with spinal cord injuries, multiple sclerosis, or amyotrophic lateral sclerosis. Motorized scooters offer less trunk support than motorized wheelchairs but are more acceptable to some people. Patients are more likely to use scooters rather than power wheelchairs if they have a primary diagnosis of cardiovascular and pulmonary disease and if they are living at home. Motorized scooters and wheelchairs increase patients' mobility, but there is a risk of deconditioning because patients might otherwise push a wheelchair or ambulate. The use of a wheelchair commonly requires home modifications, including ramps and widened doorways. Cars may need to be adapted with lifts.

Orthotics, Adaptive Methods, and Environmental Modifications

Orthotics are exoskeletons designed to assist, resist, align, and stimulate function. Orthotics are named by the use of letters for each joint that the device involves in its structure. Thus, an AFO is an ankle and foot orthotic device used to support weak calf or pretibial muscles (eg, for a stroke patient with leg weakness).

Adaptations to facilitate dressing may be necessary for patients with problems such as frequent soiling or diminished flexibility, coordination, and endurance. Clothing that is easy to clean and tops that fit easily over the head or fasten in the front and allow for freedom of movement are helpful. Hook-and-loop tape is usually easier to use than buttons and can be sewn on to replace buttons and zippers. When buttons are necessary, if they are sewn on with elastic thread, the need to manipulate them can be eliminated. Putting on shoes and socks is particularly difficult for older adults with decreased agility. Longer, looser socks (eg, tubular socks) are easier to put on. For patients who find that reaching the feet to put on shoes is a problem, a long-handled shoehorn may be useful. Elastic shoelaces eliminate the need for tying and untying.

Environmental modifications can have a major impact on the older adult's ability to function independently or with minimal assistance at home. A variety of assistive devices, such as reachers, special utensils, and adapted telephones, can reduce the difficulty of performing daily tasks and have a significant impact on a person's quality of life.

The bathroom is a common place for falls. Any older adult with impaired balance or leg weakness should have bars installed near the toilet and tub or shower. Raised toilet seats and bathtub benches are available to assist those with leg weakness. These are also useful for older adults with arthritis of the hips or knees because they reduce biomechanical stress on the joint. Long-handled bath brushes, hand-held shower heads, and "soap on a rope" can be helpful for older adults with arm weakness or other impairment.

REFERENCES

- Resnik L, Allen S, Isenstadt D, et al. Perspectives on use of mobility aids in a diverse population of seniors: Implications for intervention. *Disabil Health J*. 2009;2(2):77–85.
- Tyrell EF, Levack WM, Ritchie LH, et al. Nursing contribution to the rehabilitation of older patients: patient and family perspectives. *J Adv Nurs*. 2012;68(11):2466–2476.
- Sherrington C, Tiedemann A, Cameron I. Physical exercise after hip fracture: an evidence overview. *Eur J Phys Rehabil Med*. 2011;47(2):297–307.

CHAPTER 19—NURSING-HOME CARE

KEY POINTS

- Currently there are 15,700 nursing homes with 1.7 million beds, 1.4 million residents, and 2.5 million discharges each year.
- The Omnibus Budget Reconciliation Act of 1987 requires a periodic comprehensive assessment of all nursing-home residents, sets minimum staffing requirements, and fosters residents' rights by limiting the use of restraints and psychoactive medications.
- The care of nursing-home residents has become more complex over the past several years, commensurate with an increasing level of medical acuity in an environment constrained by limited resources.

THE NURSING-HOME POPULATION

Currently 1.4 million Americans live in nursing homes. Relatively speaking, this is a small portion of the 36 million Americans that are >65 years old, and <12% of nursing-home residents are <65 years old. The typical nursing-home resident is a white, unmarried woman >85 years old with limited social supports and usually widowed. Most people admitted to nursing homes are older adults, with average age at admission of 79 years. The percentage of black residents in U.S. nursing homes has increased in recent years (12.2%), approaching national population norms. In fact, black Americans 65–74 years old are more likely than white Americans to be admitted to a nursing home. Similarly, the proportion of Hispanic Americans >65 years old who reside in a nursing home is also increasing. Despite this, Hispanic Americans as well as other nonwhite populations, such as Asian Americans and Native Americans, are under-represented in nursing homes despite even higher disability rates in these groups. Existing studies of Korean American and Japanese American older adults have found that in general they are willing to use nursing-home services and plan to do so under certain circumstances. These may include poorer perceived health, having someone close to them who lived in a nursing home, and in the event of permanent disability such as dementia. Older adults with developmental disabilities constitute another unique population that is requiring increasing nursing-home care as their older parent-caregivers are lost. These individuals often require specialized care that many nursing homes have difficulty providing. See also "Intellectual and Developmental Disabilities," p 344.

Functional disability is prevalent in nursing-home residents. More than half of long-stay nursing-home residents require supervision or hands-on assistance from another person in five ADLs (ie, eating, dressing, bathing, transferring, and toileting). Cumulative disability is high, with >80% of nursing-home residents requiring assistance in three or more ADLs. Many residents are totally dependent for eating (53.5%), more than a third require a mechanically altered diet consistency (33.5%), and 5% receive tube feedings. Difficulty with bladder or bowel control, or both, is reported in nearly 60% of newly admitted and 40% of long-stay nursing-home residents >65 years old. Hearing and visual impairments are also common, with each affecting approximately one-third of nursing-home residents. Not surprisingly, most residents have communication problems, with frequent difficulty both in being understood and understanding others. In 2000, <18% of nursing-home residents ambulated independently; the number of nursing-home residents able to independently ambulate has diminished steadily since that time. Currently few residents (10%) walk without assistance or supervision, and the majority (59%) can be described as "chairfast," reflecting reliance on a chair for mobility, and an inability to take steps without extensive or constant weight-bearing support.

Today's population in the nursing home is sicker than the nursing-home population of the past. Over two-thirds of long-stay residents in skilled-nursing facilities have multiple medical conditions. More than 1 in 20 nursing-home residents have pressure sores. Nearly 40% of older adults in the nursing home are diagnosed with heart failure or ischemic heart disease. Diabetes and stroke are reported in 22% and 26% of new nursing-home admissions, respectively. COPD, hypertension, arthritis, and hip fractures are also prevalent health conditions among nursing-home residents. Although approximately 50% of older adults residing in nursing homes are diagnosed with dementia, experts estimate that as many as 70% of nursing-home residents meet the diagnostic criteria for dementia, making dementia the most commonly occurring condition in nursing homes. The prevalence of cognitive impairment is reflected in the fact that 81% of nursing-home residents are felt by nursing home staff to be impaired in their ability to make daily decisions, and two-thirds have orientation difficulties or memory problems, or both. Depression is diagnosed in 20%–25% of residents. In 39% of nursing-home residents >65 years old, both medical and psychiatric conditions have been diagnosed, reflecting a 60% increase in prevalence of comorbid physical and mental diagnoses in this population, when compared with 1999 data. Additionally, behavioral issues, such as verbal and social inappropriateness, wandering, and resistance to care, are observed in one-third of nursing-home residents.

NURSING-HOME AVAILABILITY

According to CMS, there are currently 15,700 nursing homes in the United States with 1.7 million beds and 2.5 million discharges (ie, to home, hospital, or secondary to death). Of these facilities, 67.7% are proprietary (ie, for profit), with voluntary nonprofit (26.6%) and government nursing homes (5.7%) accounting for the remainder. One-hundred and thirty-three Veteran's Administration Community Living Centers provide nursing-home care to eligible veterans. The Veteran's Administration also recognizes State Veterans Homes, which are owned, operated, and funded by all 50 states and Puerto Rico to provide long-term care services to veterans. In some states, nonveteran spouses and parents may also be eligible for care in a State Veterans Home. The average nursing home operates 107 beds, and a minority (6%) has >200 beds. A little more than half of all nursing homes are part of a chain. Nursing homes vary with respect to what ancillary services are available. Many facilities offer on-site mobile radiography services; however, challenges exist in maintaining optimal quality of images. Similarly, many nursing homes provide infusion service (42%), but results of studies have been variable with respect to the impact of the availability of the infusion service on resident hospitalization.

Most admissions to nursing facilities come from acute hospitals, followed by private residences and other nursing homes. Not surprisingly, assisted-living facilities are becoming a greater source of older adults admitted to nursing facilities, accounting for 7.9% of total admissions. Assisted-living facilities do not operate under the oversight of a single national regulatory or licensure agency. In general, assisted-living facilities have greater heterogeneity than nursing homes in services offered and are most commonly paid for with out-of-pocket funds. See "Community-Based Care," p 166.

By age 65, a person's lifetime risk of nursing-home admission is high, estimated at 46%. The risk of nursing-home admission rises steeply with age. While 7.4% of those ≥75 years old reside in nursing homes, this figure approaches 16% for those ≥85 years old. Barring breakthroughs in the treatment of dementia, the number of people ≥65 years old using nursing homes will double by the year 2030. Interestingly, the occupancy rates in nursing homes nationally have declined over the past several years and now stand at 82%. This decline has generally been attributed to the availability of other long-term care options, such as assisted living, but there are likely other causal social and financial variables that have yet to be identified. The availability and use of home-care services for Medicare-eligible patients have not been found to consistently reduce nursing-home admissions.

Postacute care is increasingly being offered in nursing-home settings, a response to the higher-care needs of older adults in conjunction with shorter hospital stays and the presence of a Medicare payment stream. Although the types of postacute services and programs vary significantly from one locale to another (eg, dialysis, orthopedic, ventilator, postoperative, rehabilitative, wound care), they remain distinct from the standard nursing-home services by integrating the features of acute medical, long-term care nursing, and rehabilitative settings. The challenge in postacute care is that of accommodating patients with varying degrees of disease severity, functional dependence, and comorbidities. Some limited studies suggest that, for selected patient populations, postacute care in the nursing home has outcomes equal to or better than postacute care in acute hospitals. Definitions as to what constitutes postacute care, however, vary widely, as do regulatory standards, which make comparison studies difficult. See also "Rehabilitation," p 139.

On any given day, residents with a length of stay of <3 months comprise 20% of the total nursing-home population. Conversely, long-stay residents, whose length of stay is ≥90 days after admission, account for 80% of the nursing-home population. Among all nursing-home residents, 25.6% have a length of stay >3 years. This diversity in nursing-home stays is reflected in a mean length of stay for those admitted to a nursing home of 835 days, with a median length of stay of only 463 days. Historically, increases in the number of residents with shorter lengths of stay coincided with increased Medicare funding of postacute care in nursing homes.

This continuum spanning subacute and long-term care in nursing homes contributes to the development of two populations of residents. Many short-stay residents are admitted for rehabilitation, targeting restoration of the functional ability and endurance that will allow them to return to community-based living settings. Others enter nursing homes for terminal care. In contrast, many of those who ultimately become long-stay residents present to nursing homes for the ongoing supportive care of progressive, chronic illnesses. Interestingly, improvement in function among long-stay nursing-home residents is quite common, further reflecting the heterogeneity of the nursing-home population. The role of the nursing home in the continuum of health care is expected to become more important as healthcare systems adapt to the need to provide high-quality, accountable care to the expanding population of older adults and disabled adults.

Nursing-Home Financing

Nursing-home expenditures currently total more than \$120 billion dollars per year. In 2010, the average cost of a private room in a nursing home was \$229 per day or \$83,585 annually. Public health programs primarily finance this cost; Medicaid and Medicare account for 64% and 14% of nursing-home care payments, respectively. With the high annual costs, those paying for nursing-home care out-of-pocket often deplete their personal funds and turn to public funding. While purchase of long-term care insurance has been increasing, at present these policies generally pay for only a small fraction of nursing-home care.

Medicare funding for nursing-home costs is available for certain limited conditions for beneficiaries who require skilled-nursing or rehabilitation services. In general, to be covered, beneficiaries must receive services from a Medicare-certified skilled-nursing home after a qualifying hospital stay. A qualifying hospital stay is a hospital stay of at least 3 days before entering a nursing home. Some groups have argued for elimination of this requirement for a 3-day qualifying hospital stay on the basis that it limits accessibility to appropriate levels of care for patients, increases cost, and unnecessarily exposes patients to hazards of hospitalization. Medicare covers only those skilled-nursing facility services rendered to help a beneficiary recover from an acute illness or injury. Medicare pays for skilled care in full for the first 20 days in a skilled-nursing facility. For days 21–100, a co-payment from the resident is required for skilled-nursing facility services; beyond 100 days, Medicare does not cover skilled-nursing facility care. As part of the Balanced Budget Act of 1997, Medicare payments to nursing homes are based on an individual's functional needs and potential for rehabilitation. This prospective payment system, also called PPS, requires careful documentation of functional gains, particularly by rehabilitation therapists. Although the PPS has not conclusively limited access to skilled-nursing care for Medicare beneficiaries, it has forced nursing homes to be more diligent with regard to their admission policies. Not unexpectedly, physical, occupational, and speech therapies are commonly prescribed in the nursing home, with half of all patients admitted to nursing homes receiving at least 90 minutes of these rehabilitation services, according to one study. The PPS requires nursing-home staff to carefully document gains in function to ensure reimbursement. See "Rehabilitation," p 139.

Supplemental increases in reimbursement are made to offset costs of caring for those with HIV/AIDS. Despite the high cost of nursing-home care, resources remain constrained. In general, psychiatric conditions are undervalued with respect to reimbursement in long-term care. Residents with active psychiatric illness often require increased care and staff time, but mechanisms do not exist for increased reimbursement for those efforts. Shortages of psychiatric specialists trained in nursing-home care, combined with relatively low reimbursement rates for care in nursing homes, add to the challenge of providing optimal mental health care in this setting.

Staffing Patterns

Resident care and evaluation in the nursing home largely depend on nurses and nursing assistants. Nursing facilities are required to provide nurse staffing sufficient to provide the care outlined in its care plans. According to federal guidelines, every nursing home must have the following on staff: a licensed nurse that acts as charge nurse on each shift; a registered nurse who is on duty at least 8 consecutive hours, 7 days a week; and a registered nurse who is designated as the director of nursing. Studies have confirmed the correlation between the provision of quality care to total nursing hours and the ratio of professional nurses (ie, registered nurses) to nonprofessional nursing staff. A 2001 Institute of Medicine report recommended increasing nurse staffing levels to enhance the quality of nursing-home care, spurring Congress to debate the merits of mandatory minimal staffing ratios. Although recommendations for minimal and optimal staffing at nursing facilities have been made by CMS based on links to quality of care, current federal regulations do not mandate specific nurse-to-resident staffing ratios. The total direct care staffing averages 4.01 hours per resident day (HPRD), or roughly 241 minutes per resident per day. Nursing assistants contribute most direct staff time, at 2.45 HPRD. Licensed nurses and registered nurses contribute 0.85 and 0.73 HPRD, respectively. Despite the increasing medical acuity and care needs of nursing-home residents, staffs ratios have been relatively stable. It has been estimated that 9 of 10 nursing homes are inadequately staffed, and nearly \$8 billion dollars would be needed to bring staffing to adequate levels. Of note, many states set staffing requirements for nursing facilities that are higher than federal recommendations.

Recruiting and retaining staff, particularly nursing assistants who constitute the bulk of the nursing-home workforce, also continues to be difficult. Turnover rates of >70% for nurse assistants and >50% each for directors of nursing, registered nurses, and licensed practical nurses have been reported. Turnover rates have been associated with increased rates of hospitalization for nursing-home residents and have been linked to the organizational culture within the nursing facility.

FACTORS ASSOCIATED WITH NURSING-HOME PLACEMENT

Although there is a significant chance of being admitted to a nursing home with increasing age, other factors, such as low income, poor family supports (especially lack of spouse and children), and low social activity have been associated with institutionalization (SOE=B). Cognitive and functional impairments have also predicted nursing-home placement. Interestingly, for patients with dementia, education and caregiver support have been shown to delay the need for nursing-home placement for up to 1 year (SOE=B). The range of long-term care services that are now available (ie, skilled nursing, home care, assisted living) further increases the complexity of placement decisions. The use of formal (ie, paid-for) community services does not necessarily reduce the likelihood of nursing-home placement for patients with severe disabilities.

THE INTERFACE OF ACUTE AND LONG-TERM CARE

Discharge to a long-term care facility is the second most common type of discharge from the hospital. The number of hospital discharges to nursing homes and long-term care settings increased 35% between 1997 and 2008. Conversely, nursing-home residents also have high rates and frequently use emergency department care. Nursing-home residents account for >2.2 million emergency department visits annually in the United States, or 1.6 emergency department visits for every nursing-home resident. Almost half of these nursing-home residents were admitted to the acute hospital.

Unfortunately, the transitions between acute and long-term care settings are often complicated by suboptimal information transfer. Illegible or nonexistent transfer summaries; omission of prescribed medications; and the lack of documentation of advanced directives, psychosocial information, and behavioral issues are but a few of the information gaps commonly reported. In 2006, almost one-fourth of Medicare beneficiaries (23.5%) discharged from the hospital to the skilled-nursing facility were readmitted to the acute hospital within 30 days at a cost to Medicare of $4.34 billion dollars. Five conditions account for most (78%) of these rehospitalizations: congestive heart failure, respiratory infection, urinary tract infection, sepsis, and electrolyte imbalances.

Recent initiatives have focused on improving transition of care to and from the nursing home. One example is the "Interventions to Reduce Acute Care Transfers" program, also known as INTERACT (http://interact2.net/ [accessed Oct 2013]). INTERACT is a quality improvement project that was developed with the support of CMS to improve the early identification, assessment, documentation, and communication about changes in the status of residents of skilled-nursing facilities with the goal of reducing the frequency of transfers from the nursing home to the acute hospital. The INTERACT II intervention, which includes communication tools, clinical care paths, and advanced care planning tools, has resulted in a 17% reduction in acute-hospital admissions in a group of community-based nursing homes. See also transitions from hospital care in "Hospital Care," p 130; and "Perioperative Care," p 102.

QUALITY ISSUES AND LEGISLATION INFLUENCING CARE IN THE NURSING HOME

In 1983, the Institute of Medicine published a report documenting significant deficiencies in the care of nursing-home residents. The findings of that report influenced the passage of the Omnibus Budget Reconciliation Act (OBRA) in 1987. As the first major revision of nursing-home legislation in over 20 years and the first detailed source of clinical expectations for nursing-home care, OBRA has had significant impacts on medical care in nursing homes. OBRA set new, higher standards for quality of care provided in nursing facilities certified for reimbursement under Medicare and Medicaid (which includes most skilled-nursing facilities) by CMS. See "Financing, Coverage, and Costs of Health Care," p 35. CMS pays Medicare claims and interprets legislation into written regulations for skilled-nursing facilities. CMS interprets federal statutes and also writes regulations for Medicaid that are administered by each state's Medicaid program. Federal regulations, including those pertaining to long-term care, are compiled in the *Code of Federal Regulations*. Each federal regulation is given a tag number, often called "F-tags." To qualify for federal reimbursement under Medicare and Medicaid, facilities must comply with these CMS regulations. OBRA regulations targeted many residents' rights issues, including setting limits on restraint use and regulating use of psychoactive medications. Assisted-living facilities do not operate under such all-inclusive mandates, which some believe contribute to the significant variability of care practices and quality of care in that setting.

OBRA also mandates comprehensive periodic assessments of all nursing-home residents. This is accomplished by the Minimum Data Set (MDS), which surveys a host of clinical issues thought to directly relate to the quality of resident care and thus considered pertinent to effective care planning. A resident's medical regimen must be consistent with the assessment compiled in the MDS. CMS also uses the MDS for individual facilities to compile nursing-facility quality measures data, which are reported publicly on the CMS Web site (www.medicare.gov/NHcompare/Home.asp). Measures include outcomes data such as prevalence of pain, pressure ulcers, weight loss, and depression, as well as rates of vaccination, restraint use, and urinary tract infection. While publication of these measures is intended to offer a route by which to compare facilities, it has been criticized for lack of standardization of data to account for the substantial variability in disability and medical acuity between different facilities. For quality measures for nursing homes that are publicly reported by CMS, see Table 19.1. The minimum data set was updated to version 3.0 by CMS in 2010 and resulted in changes in the publicly reported quality measures. Included in the measures of nursing-home quality publicly reported by CMS is the 5-star quality rating for nursing homes. This rating was developed to help consumers, families, and caregivers make comparisons about nursing homes and areas of strength or concern. The 5-star rating is based on three sources of data, the facility's health inspection survey results, staffing levels, and quality measures. Recently, several state Medicaid programs have initiated pay-for-performance programs in nursing homes where quality measures are linked to reimbursement. The measures vary according to each state's program, but often include metrics similar to those used in CMS quality ratings, consumer satisfaction, and employee retention. CMS has also recently initiated a nursing home value-based purchasing demonstration project in four states.

Adherence to regulations is assessed by mandatory site visit surveys. These surveys are mandated every 15 months but occur on average every 12 months. During traditional nursing home surveys, facility procedures and records are reviewed, and quality of care and quality of life for residents are observed. Recently, national implementation of the Quality Indicator Survey process (QIS) has been initiated by CMS. QIS is a computer-assisted, two-staged long-term survey process used to systematically review nursing-home requirements and objectively investigate any triggered regulatory areas. In the QIS, a sample of residents, developed from census, admission, and MDS data, is created and used to strategically perform interviews, observations, and chart reviews that calculate indicators of quality of care and quality of life in that facility. Those areas, as well as a group of standard facility-level tasks, are then assessed in an in-depth fashion.

Failure to meet regulatory standards for care is cited in a "deficiency." Penalties imposed for deficiencies depend on the nature and severity of the deficiency and can range from implementation of a corrective action plan to monetary fines, limits on facility admissions, or even facility closure. Inspections can also occur at any time in between mandated surveys as a result of a complaint received by the state. In 2008, nursing homes received an average of seven deficiencies during regulatory visits, with 17% of these deficiencies relating to actual harm or immediate jeopardy of residents. In the years since OBRA was instituted, the use of restraints in nursing homes has decreased significantly, registered nurse staffing has increased, and training requirements for certified nursing assistants have been established.

OBRA mandates that each individual in a nursing facility receive and be provided the necessary care and services to achieve and maintain "the highest practicable physical, medical, and psychological well-being" that can be obtained. The facility must ensure that the resident optimally improves or deteriorates only within the limits of that resident's right to refuse

Table 19.1—Quality Measures for Nursing Homes Based on the Minimum Data Set and Publicly Reported by CMS

Quality Measures
For Long-Stay Residents
Percent assessed and given, appropriately, the seasonal influenza vaccination
Percent assessed and given, appropriately, the pneumococcal vaccination
Percent whose need for help with daily activities has increased
Percent who self-report moderate to severe pain
Percent who were physically restrained
Percent who have depressive symptoms
Percent who have/had a catheter inserted and left in their bladder
Percent with a urinary tract infection
Percent who lose too much weight
Percent who experience one or more falls with major injury
Percent who received an antipsychotic medication
For Long-Stay Low-Risk Residents
Percent who lose control of their bowels or bladder
For Long-Stay High-Risk Residents
Percent who have pressure ulcers
For Short-Stay Residents
Percent assessed and given, appropriately, the seasonal influenza vaccination
Percent assessed and given, appropriately, the pneumococcal vaccination
Percent who newly received an antipsychotic medication
Percent who self-report moderate to severe pain
Percent with pressure ulcers that are new or worsened

SOURCE: Adapted from Department of Health and Human Services, Medicare. *Nursing Home Compare.* www.medicare.gov/NHcompare/ (accessed Oct 2013).

Chapters

treatments and within the influence of their illnesses and normal aging. When a resident declines (or does not improve), a survey team may investigate whether the decline was avoidable. A decline may be determined unavoidable if the resident has been given a careful and thorough assessment, which directs the resident's care plan. The interventions included in the care plan should be evaluated and revised as necessary. Documentation of a resident's reasonable prognosis and the risks versus reasonable expected benefits of treatments has an important role in care planning in the nursing home, particularly given current regulatory and liability influences.

OBRA requires that a state agency must screen and preapprove the admission of individuals with intellectual disability (mental retardation) or serious mental illness to a nursing facility (F285). This screening is done to ensure that the facility can provide appropriate programs and services to meet the individual's needs. Residents readmitted to a nursing facility from a hospital, or those admitted from a hospital with an anticipated stay of <30 days who require treatment at the nursing facility for the same problem for which they were hospitalized, are exempt from screening.

Additional regulations require medication review at regular intervals and that each resident's medication regimen includes no unnecessary drugs. Clinical documentation must demonstrate the indication for all drugs, especially psychoactive medications. Unnecessary medications are those given without indication, at excessive dosages, for excessive duration, without adequate monitoring, or when there has been a significant adverse event. Residents without a history of antipsychotic drug use should not be treated with antipsychotic medication unless the drug is required to treat a specific diagnosed condition that is documented in the medical record. For those residents receiving psychoactive medications, gradual dosage reductions and behavioral interventions are mandated unless a clinical contraindication exists and is documented in the medical record. To date, the impact on quality of care from these guidelines has not been well described in the clinical research literature.

A thorough evaluation of medication regimens, done monthly by a pharmacist, is also required. This monthly medication review is intended to minimize adverse events and unnecessary medication use and to ensure proper medication monitoring. A facility must ensure that the medication error rate is <5% and that no significant medication errors occur. No errors should occur that cause a resident discomfort or jeopardize his or her health and safety. Care in assisted-living facilities does not have the same regulations that guide care in nursing homes.

MEDICAL CARE ISSUES

The care of nursing-home residents has become more complex over the past several years, commensurate with an increasing level of medical acuity in an environment continually constrained by lack of adequate resources. Comprehensive, ongoing assessment within an interdisciplinary framework works to restore function, when possible, and to enhance quality of life.

Clinical challenges abound in the nursing home, created, in part, by the atypical and subtle presentation of illness so characteristic of residents with profound physical and psychologic frailty. In addition, limited access to biotechnology, frequent dependence on nonphysicians such as nurses and nurse assistants for resident evaluation, and the high prevalence of cognitive impairment in a setting of intense regulatory oversight all complicate the medical decision-making process. Families of nursing-home residents often remain an integral part of the overall care plan and may require specific educational and psychosocial supports. Ethical and legal concerns are also very common, particularly those regarding end-of-life, feeding, hydration, and resident rights issues. See "Legal and Ethical Issues," p 26. Finally, the heterogeneity among nursing-home residents demands an individualized, thoughtful, and reasoned approach to each individual.

Problems in nursing homes that commonly require unique diagnostic and treatment strategies include infections, falls, malnutrition, dehydration, incontinence, behavioral disturbances, the use of multiple medications, and prevention and screening. See "Infectious Diseases," p 494; "Falls," p 234; "Malnutrition," p 209; "Urinary Incontinence," p 220; "Behavioral Problems in Dementia," p 267; "Pharmacotherapy," p 81; and "Prevention," p 70. For example, determining the risks and benefits of tube feedings for frail nursing-home residents must be predicated not only on underlying illness but also on the resident's and family's value system, the resources available in the nursing facility, and staff acceptance of the intervention. Given that the evidence for and against enteral feeding in nursing-home residents is controversial (ie, benefits are not well established), therapy must be individualized. See "Eating and Feeding Problems," p 216. Many of the problems commonly encountered in the nursing home result when multiple comorbidities interact with a host of environmental factors, all of which may be only partially remediable. Unfortunately, expectations of family, as well as regulations, often do not account for these complexities and commonly engender "risk-averse" behavior that may be counter to autonomy and optimal quality of life.

Many have advocated for culture change in nursing-home care from institutional, provider-centered models to person-centered models that are driven by choice and self-determination of older adults and their caregivers. Transformed nursing-home culture would include resident direction of activities; homelike atmosphere; close relationships between staff, residents, and families; empowered staff members who are trained to respond to residents' needs; and collaborative decision making with residents about care. Several culture-change initiatives, including the Eden Alternative and the Green House Model, have been described. Evidence to date suggests these models improve resident quality of life and employee satisfaction, while preserving or improving quality of care, but additional research regarding the benefits and costs of culture change is needed.

CLINICIAN PRACTICE IN THE NURSING HOME

The medical care of nursing-home residents is challenging and fulfilling, requiring excellent clinical skills as well as sensitivity to a variety of ethical, legal, and interdisciplinary issues. Interventions, whether they are curative, preventive, or palliative, demand an individualized approach that recognizes the complex interplay among resident, family, and staff needs. Further, the evidence on which to base treatment may be nonexistent.

The comorbidity present in most nursing-home residents commonly creates the need for multiple drug therapies, with attendant risk of complications. The prevalence of nursing-home residents who were prescribed nine or more medications was reported as a quality measure for nursing facilities for many years, with 32% of all nursing-home residents falling into this group. With revisions to the MDS, this is no longer included in the regulated quality measures, in part reflecting that the use of multiple medications by nursing-home residents with prevalent comorbid illnesses cannot always be avoided. In fact, on average, nursing-home residents are prescribed between seven and eight medications. The most common health conditions found in the nursing home for those ≥65 years old, after dementia, are heart disease, hypertension, arthritis, and stroke. The approaches to these and other illnesses have evolved dramatically in recent years and complicate treatment decisions when cost-effectiveness is increasingly considered a desirable goal. Clear documentation of the rationale for a given medication or intervention is the best way to protect against potential scrutiny; frequent discussion with the facility's consultant pharmacist is also helpful. See "Pharmacotherapy," p 81.

Nurse practitioners and physician assistants have become increasingly involved in the primary care of nursing-home residents. Studies suggest that nurse practitioners and physician assistants who act in concert with the primary care physician as a coordinated team provide more intensive care to the nursing-home resident and may decrease hospitalization rates while maintaining cost neutrality (SOE=A).

Responsibilities encompass ongoing comprehensive assessment and coordination of care to ensure resident autonomy and safety as well as optimal physical and psychosocial function. Regulations mandate that the initial comprehensive visit for the purpose of certifying that a newly admitted nursing-home resident requires a skilled level of care be done by a physician. During this visit, physicians perform a thorough assessment, develop a plan of care, and write appropriate orders for the nursing-home resident. Nurse practitioners may perform initial history and physical visits for long-term care residents who do not require skilled level of care. Regulations mandate that nursing-home residents be seen for subsequent face-to-face medical visits every 30 days for the first 90 days after admission and then at least every 60 days thereafter. For these subsequent visits, a visit by a nurse practitioner or physician assistant may be substituted for every other physician visit. Additional medical visits should take place if acute medical needs or changes in condition develop. Medicare allows for physician reimbursement for evaluation and management activities for both nursing home regulatory visits and medically necessary visits to provide acute care. Availability of on-site medical providers can improve timeliness of acute medical care and decrease hospitalization rates.

Opportunities to improve medical care in nursing homes exist. Several studies have documented misdiagnoses, inappropriate interventions, and poor preventive care practices in nursing homes. Intensive research is currently being done to understand the processes necessary to integrate validated care guidelines into nursing homes in an effort to improve quality of care. Vaccination rates for eligible chronic-care nursing-home residents vary. Nationally, current vaccination rates in nursing homes are 87% for influenza and 81% for pneumococcus. Vaccination programs for long-term care employees have also been taken as a primary prevention strategy for influenza in nursing facilities. Vaccination of employees is thought to decrease the influenza incidence in residents through decreased entry of influenza virus into facilities and decreased resident-to-resident transmission through staff. Unfortunately, healthcare worker vaccination rates are generally <50%. While brief educational programs have been associated with increased acceptance of vaccines, improved understanding of the individual and operational barriers to and facilitators of optimal immunization is needed.

Strategies have been developed that may enhance the quality of care in nursing homes. The commonly used special-care units, although conceptually attractive, have not consistently been shown to enhance quality of care apart from the involvement of individual professionals. Specific consultation services in the nursing home, however, may improve care practices and condition-specific resident outcomes, such as the reduction of falls (SOE=A). In addition, interactive educational programs for physicians and nursing staff may improve practice, as has been demonstrated in programs to promote appropriate psychoactive drug use (SOE=B). Clinical practice guidelines for the care of nursing-home residents have been developed by the American Medical Directors Association (www.amda.com/) and the American Geriatrics Society (www.americangeriatrics.org).

Understanding each nursing-home resident's preference for care in the context of his or her underlying value system will undoubtedly improve overall quality. According to the CDC, 65% of nursing-home residents have at least one advance care directive on record. The most common advance directives in nursing-home residents are living wills and do-not-resuscitate orders, which are present for 18% and 56%, respectively, of all nursing-home residents. Nursing-home residents >65 years old are more likely to have advance directives than their younger counterparts. White nursing-home residents are more likely than black nursing-home residents to have a living will (20% versus 6%) and do-not-resuscitate orders (61% versus 28%). This disparity in advance directives highlights the need for long-term care research that contributes to the development of culturally sensitive approaches to advance care determination in the nursing home.

Durable power of attorney for healthcare documentation is present for 26% of nursing-home residents at admission and for 39% after 1 year of residence. Less than 5% of nursing-home residents have "do-not-hospitalize" orders, which document that the resident is not to be hospitalized even after developing a condition that is generally treated in the hospital. While ongoing discussion of care preferences appears to be present in the nursing home, there likely remain ongoing opportunities for improved understanding of nursing-home resident preferences for care. Notably, the use of hospice programs to augment end-of-life care in nursing homes has increased in recent years. When ethical dilemmas do arise in nursing-home care, institutional ethics committees can provide important guidance. The multidisciplinary nature of these committees ensures a spectrum of opinion and insight critical for nursing-home residents. See also "Legal and Ethical Issues," p 26.

REFERENCES

- Castle NG, Ferguson JC. What is nursing home quality and how is it measured? *Gerontologist*. 2010;50(4):426–442.
- Kaye HS, Harrington C, LaPlante MP. Long-term care: who gets it, who provides it, who pays, and how much? *Health Aff (Millwood)*. 2010;29(1):11–21.
- Koren MJ. Person-centered care for nursing home residents: the culture-change movement. *Health Aff (Millwood)*. 2010;29(2):312–318.
- Liu LM, Guarino AJ, Lopez RP. Family satisfation with care provided by nurse practitioners to nursing home residents with dementia at the end of life. *Clin Nurs Res*. 2012;21(3):350–367.
- Murray LM, Laditka SB. Care transitions by older adults from nursing homes to hospitals: implications for long-term care practice, geriatrics education, and research. *J Am Med Dir Assoc*. 2010;11(4):231–238.

CHAPTER 20—TRANSITIONAL CARE

KEY POINTS

- Older adults undergoing care transitions are at risk of experiencing suboptimal care and adverse events.
- Effective solutions to improve care during transitions require a team-based approach to coordinate care, and clinicians have an important role in implementing these solutions.
- Successful care transitions can result in more effective implementation of care plans, reduced adverse events, faster restoration of older adults' functioning, and improved satisfaction among older adults, caregivers, and healthcare providers.

THE TREACHERY OF SUBOPTIMAL CARE TRANSITIONS

A care transition is defined as the movement of a patient from one set of providers, level of care, or healthcare setting to another. Other terms for care transitions include "handoffs," "handovers," or "transfers." Figure 20.1 depicts typical care transitions that older adults experience within the healthcare environment. Some transitions are *within* the hospital setting, such as the transition from the intensive care unit to the floor, while others are *across* healthcare settings, such as the transition from the hospital to a skilled-nursing facility. Although care transitions are generally well intended, eg, to provide a higher level of care for an older adult who is clinically deteriorating, care transitions are a time when older adults are vulnerable to receiving suboptimal care.

Care transitions are common, complicated, and costly. Almost 40% of older adults experience two or more care transitions within 30 days of hospital discharge. A national study of Medicare beneficiaries found that about 78% of older adults stay in place over the course of a year, while 22% experience care transitions of some kind. About half of these transitions involved a single hospitalization followed by return to the original residence, but the other half involved a complex sequence of other transitions. Few predominant transition patterns were present; most patterns were unique, which makes predicting (and accommodating) the traffic flow of patient transfers difficult. This has profound implications for organizations or individuals involved in care provision. The heterogeneity of transition patterns of older adults challenges approaches to improving care transitions because it is onerous and inefficient to plan for all possible care patterns, when many apply to a small number of individuals.

Suboptimal care transitions that result in hospital readmission can be costly. One in five older adults discharged from the hospital are rehospitalized within 30 days, and one-third are rehospitalized within 90 days. The cost of unplanned rehospitalizations to the Medicare program is estimated at $15 billion annually. In addition to cost implications, suboptimal care transitions can lead to increasing risk of adverse events resulting from poor care coordination among providers and healthcare entities.

Suboptimal care transitions across care settings can also pose a significant threat to patient safety. Suboptimal care transitions from the hospital result in adverse events, medication errors, and inaccurate or incomplete information transfer. Indeed, almost half of all medication errors occur during admission or discharge, ie, care transitions to and from the acute hospital setting. Inaccurate or incomplete information is a common problem during care transitions with significant implications for patient safety, including delayed diagnosis, duplicative medical services, and reduced provider and patient satisfaction. Lack of availability of discharge summaries during follow-up clinician visits is common and can lead to duplicate testing and hospital readmission.

While suboptimal care transitions adversely affect patients of all ages for several reasons, older adults are at particularly increased risk of safety problems. Age is a strong predictor of use of hospital services, and older adults have a 4-fold higher risk of hospitalization than the general population. Older adults also have higher rates of iatrogenic complications, are more likely to be admitted through an emergency department, and have longer lengths of stay than their younger counterparts. Further, older adults are more vulnerable to the hazards of hospitalization: functional decline, delirium, adverse drug events, pressure ulcers, bowel and bladder dysfunction, malnutrition, and dehydration. See "Hospital Care," p 130. Because of these hazards, older adults are more likely to experience complications and require complex care after discharge. Older adults transition frequently across healthcare settings, are rehospitalized often, have multiple chronic conditions, and generally follow more complex therapeutic regimens than other population groups. They also have a greater prevalence of functional deficits and cognitive impairments, and some have limited health literacy, all of which further complicate their ability to participate in the care-transitions process and to understand discharge and self-care instructions. The following are

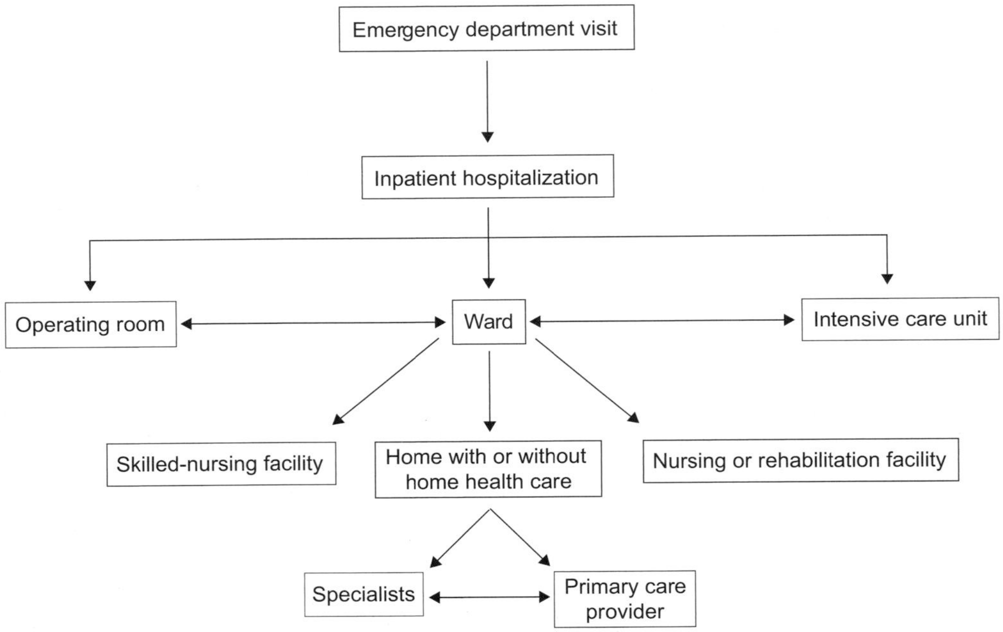

Figure 20.1—Care transitions commonly experienced by older adults in the healthcare environment

important risk factors for experiencing a suboptimal care transition:

- Limited education (less than high school)
- Unmet functional need (no help with at least one deficit in an activity of daily living)
- Limited self-management ability
- Worse self-rating of health
- Living alone
- Transition to home with home-care services
- Prior hospitalization
- Low income or Medicaid eligible
- Older age
- Five or more comorbidities
- Specific diagnoses: depression, heart disease, diabetes mellitus, cancer

Barriers to Safe Transitions

Improving care transitions for older adults, especially between hospital and home, is an attractive target for improving healthcare quality and reducing medical and liability expenditures. Older adults are among the highest users of healthcare services and account for the largest amount of government health spending. Interventions to improve care transitions are a high priority under the Affordable Care Act of 2010, which attempts to realign financial incentives to improve care transitions and reduce hospital readmission rates. Care transitions programs are now expected to be implemented in many healthcare systems. In addition, there are medicolegal liability concerns related to suboptimal care transitions. Hospital clinicians and primary care providers share the risk of liability during care transitions. Hospital medicine physicians have a duty to the patient upon discharge to assure care until the care transition is complete, including follow-up of pending tests, incidental findings, and medical treatments started in the hospital. The primary care provider has a duty to the patient to obtain hospital records if not received and ensure proper follow-up once the care transition is complete. For all of these reasons, it is important to ensure that care transitions are executed safely.

Several barriers exist to executing safe care transitions. Common ones include:

- Diverse older adult and caregiver transitional care needs depending on illness, social situation, and type of transition
- Lack of provider education and feedback on execution of care transitions, including preparation of timely and effective discharge summaries and understanding the capabilities of different types of postacute care settings
- Difficulty communicating with colleagues at the previous or next site of care
- Lack of time or financial resources; transitional care activities that involve care coordination are largely not billable in the current American reimbursement system.

STRATEGIES TO IMPROVE TRANSITIONAL CARE

Transitional care entails a broad range of time-limited services designed to ensure the coordination and continuity of health care as patients transfer between different locations or different levels of care. Transitional care contains elements of care coordination, discharge planning, and disease or case management. Many successful interventions to improve transitional care share common features, such as assigning an individual as a care transitions coach, guide, or navigator to monitor the older adult during care transitions. Optimal transitional care is focused on the highly vulnerable and chronically ill population and includes the following components:

- Accurate and timely transfer of information to the next set of providers
- Empowerment of the older adult to assert his or her own preferences
- Comprehensive assessments of older adult and caregiver needs
- Comprehensive medication review and management
- Logistical arrangements related to executing the care transition
- Education to prepare both older adults and caregivers for what to expect at the next site of care
- Support for self-management of medical conditions
- Coordination among medical and community resources
- Follow-up and support after discharge

Targeted interventions, both before and after discharge, including home-health services, older adult and caregiver empowerment, and comprehensive discharge planning, may improve transitional care and avert early readmission and other adverse outcomes. For example, although labor-intensive, meticulous discharge planning can maximize the probability that older adults maintain the clinical and functional benefits achieved by hospitalization, it also probably reduces the risk of early readmission and the use of emergency services. Discharge planning ideally begins at hospital admission, with a projection of medical, nursing, rehabilitative, and functional support required by the older adult at the time of discharge.

Discharge Destinations and Care Venues

The choice of discharge destination reflects a match between the needs of a given older adult and the services available at each setting. The array of possible settings includes home with family support, home with home-health care, custodial care (such as assisted living or "nursing home"), skilled-nursing facilities, acute rehabilitation hospitals, long-term acute care, and inpatient hospice. Home-health care works well for older adults requiring only intermittent skilled services (nursing, physical therapy, or speech therapy), and older adults with one of these needs may also receive assistance (under Medicare) from occupational therapy, medical social work, or home-health aides. Medicare requires that older adults receiving home-health care be homebound. Under Medicare, older adults appropriate for skilled-nursing facilities must also have a need for a skilled service, such as a requirement for intravenous therapy, artificial nutrition and hydration, complex wound care, ostomy care, or rehabilitation. Medicare covers all or part of skilled-nursing care for up to 100 days after a qualifying hospital stay, but coverage stops earlier if an older adult's treatment goals are met or if the older adult "plateaus" and no longer demonstrates improvement. Older adults with substantial rehabilitation needs (more than just physical therapy, occupational therapy, or speech therapy) and considerable rehabilitation potential may be appropriate for transfer to an acute rehabilitation unit, but many older adults are deemed ineligible because of an inability to participate in 3 hours per day of intense therapy. Long-term acute care, also known as "chronic hospitalization," is appropriate for the rare hospital patient who requires prolonged, hospital-level care. Long-term acute-care facilities provide care for patients requiring long-term mechanical ventilation, multiple intravenous medications, parenteral nutrition, or complex wound care, along with a need for frequent clinician monitoring.

The Discharge Medication Regimen

A critical activity near the time of hospital discharge is the preparation of the discharge medication list. This list should include an indication for each medication, stop dates (eg, for antibiotics) or tapering schedules (eg, for systemic corticosteroids) as appropriate, and clear behavioral triggers for as-needed psychiatric medications. Medications added during the hospital stay (such as analgesics, proton-pump inhibitors, or laxatives with as-needed orders) can be tapered and discontinued at this time. Finally, the discharge regimen should be formally reconciled with the preadmission regimen. Reconciliation results in clear documentation of which medications on the discharge list are new (relative to the preadmission regimen), which of the preadmission medications have been stopped, and which dosages of continued medications have been changed.

Communicating with Patient, Caregivers, and Receiving Team

The following items should be communicated to older adults (or their caregivers) who are being discharged directly home: follow-up appointments, warning symptoms or signs to watch for with instructions on whom to contact, clinical disciplines (eg, nursing, physical therapy) contracted for provision of services in the home, and the reconciled medication list. Older adults being discharged to other care venues should be oriented with respect to the nature of the new institution, the identity of a new primary care provider (if known), and the expected frequency of provider visits. Tools are available to assist older adults and caregivers with assessing care preferences, clarifying discharge instructions, reconciling medication inaccuracies, and facilitating communication across care sites at discharge (eg, see www.caretransitions.org [accessed Oct 2013]). If the provider at the receiving institution differs from the hospital clinician, then clear and prompt communication is essential. Some items of information (critical but pending study results, nuances of goals of care, or family dynamics) call for direct communication between sending and receiving clinicians. Otherwise, a brief and prompt discharge summary containing the following will suffice: summary of hospital course with care provided and results of important tests; a list of problems and diagnoses; baseline physical functional status; baseline cognitive status; physical and cognitive status at discharge; reconciled medication list; allergies; tests results still outstanding; follow-up appointments; and information related to goals, preferences, and advance directives.

Three Steps to Improve Care Transitions

Creating a strategy to improve care transitions consists of three essential steps. The first step is setting expectations for both the sending and receiving provider teams. The National Transitions of Care Coalition recommends shifting from the concept of "discharge" to that of "transfer with continuous management." The following are some questions to assist with completing this step:

- Starting with the information available on the day of admission, what needs will this older adult have after transfer?
- What are the older adult's and caregiver's preferences about the transfer plan?
- How will this older adult care for himself or herself after transfer?
- What other clinicians need to evaluate the older adult to formulate an effective care plan?
- Once the transfer plan is set, do the older adult and caregiver understand the purpose of the transfer and what to expect at the next site of care?
- Has the next site of care received, understood, and clarified discrepancies about the care plan?

The second step to creating a strategy to improve care transitions involves tailoring communication strategies to the type of information being communicated and to the type of care transition. Communication strategies vary based on specific resources and institutional arrangements. The following are some questions to assist with completing this step:

- Based on this older adult's current episode of illness, what is the most relevant information to communicate to the next site of care?
- How quickly does this information need to be communicated? Note that electronic communication is best for notification of admission, discharge, or nonurgent issues. Verbal communication is best for situations of urgency, uncertainty, or with complex social dynamics. Written communication is best for information that must be a part of the medical record or used as a reference by the older adult, caregiver, or clinical provider.
- Does the information also need to be given directly to the older adult and caregiver?

The third step to creating a strategy to improve care transitions involves focusing on specific processes or outcomes as targets for improvement, using established quality improvement methods. It is important to begin by choosing one or two measures to focus on to track progress, and then expand further once initial goals are achieved. Examples of measures that can be targets for improvement include the following:

- Communication with primary care provider before older adult's transfer
- Medication reconciliation at the time of transfer
- Older adult's, caregiver's, or receiving clinician's satisfaction with quality of care transition
- Timeliness of arrival of transfer summaries
- Inclusion of various components in transfer summaries, eg, documentation of cognitive and functional status
- Ease of scheduling of follow-up appointments
- Frequency of healthcare usage after transfer

REFERENCES

- Hansen LO, Young RS, Hinami K, et al. Interventions to reduce 30-day rehospitalization: a systematic review. *Ann Intern Med.* 2011;155(8):520–528.
- Jencks SF, Williams MV, Coleman EA. Rehospitalizations among patients in the Medicare fee-for-service program. *N Engl J Med.* 2009;360(14):1418–1428.
- National Transitions of Care Coalition (www.ntocc.org)
- Naylor MD, Aiken LH, Kurtzman ET, et al. The care plan: the importance of transitional care in achieving health reform. *Health Aff (Millwood).* 2011;30(4):746–754.
- Sato M, Shaffer T, Arbaje AI, et al. Residential and health care transition patterns among older Medicare beneficiaries over time. *Gerontologist.* 2011;5(12):170–178.

CHAPTER 21—COMMUNITY-BASED CARE

KEY POINTS

- Home care will play an increasingly important role as healthcare reform is enacted, helping to keep people living in their homes longer.
- Physicians and other providers often find home care rewarding; reimbursement charges for home visits have improved, making home visits more financially viable for clinicians.
- Community-based services that do not require a change of residence (eg, adult day care, day hospitals, home hospitals, Program of All-Inclusive Care for the Elderly [PACE], telemedicine) may be a useful alternative to inpatient services. However, the availability of these services strongly depends on financial reimbursement.
- Community-based services requiring a change of residence (eg, assisted living, group homes, adult foster care, and continuing-care retirement communities) offer a wide range of services. These are regulated at the state level and vary considerably in availability, cost, and services provided.

HOME CARE

Approximately 12 million people received home care in 2009 at a cost of $72 billion. For a large number of these people, home care has the potential to improve their quality of life and avoid unnecessary institutionalization.

Under a cost-based reimbursement system, home care grew rapidly in the 1980s and 1990s. This growth coincided with the initiation of the prospective payment system (diagnostic-related groups [DRGs]) for hospitals, which resulted in patients being discharged sooner from hospitals, and an increased need for home services. New technologies created the possibility of providing therapies in the home that were previously available only in hospitals or nursing homes. Because of an explosive increase in costs, Congress placed limits on Medicare spending as mandated in the Balanced Budget Act of 1997, which led to the development of a prospective payment system (PPS) for home-care services. Since enactment of the PPS, the number of recipients of home-care services and the number of visits for patients receiving home care have declined by >20%. Many home-care agencies have adjusted to these changes and developed more efficient, targeted home care, but hundreds have closed because of financial pressures. Rural agencies have closed at a higher rate than urban ones. The Outcome and Assessment Information Set (OASIS) is a tool that classifies patients into home-health–related groups (HHRGs). The OASIS instrument is completed by the home-care agency and tracks several domains of the patient's functional status and medical needs. Like the DRGs, the HHRGs provide the basis for agency reimbursement and are based on severity of the patient's illness, disabilities, and nursing needs; they include an adjustment for location in the United States. The instrument is also intended to provide a uniform means of measuring quality of care across all home-care agencies. Refinements to the Medicare PPS were introduced January 1, 2008. The number of HHRGs was increased to 10, and comorbid conditions are considered in the ultimate reimbursement. The OASIS assessment and the International Classification of Diseases (ICD-9) codes must be accurate to ensure that reimbursement matches the needs of the patient being served. Like other sectors of our healthcare system, home-care agencies are charged with developing cost-effective, high-quality care despite diminishing reimbursement. Another major challenge facing home-care agencies is recruiting and retaining qualified nurses and aides. Developing community-wide systems of care between hospitals, home care, nursing homes, and practitioners' offices may help meet these challenges and ensure that patients receive timely and appropriate care.

The Primary Provider's Role in Home Care

Home care often requires an interdisciplinary team that is generally composed of nurses, therapists (speech, physical, occupational, and respiratory), social workers, personal care aides, home medical equipment suppliers, and most importantly, informal caregivers. Currently, physicians certify and recertify the plan of care and need for individual therapy services for Medicare-covered home-health services.

Physicians are reimbursed for certification of the home-care plan and for oversight of complex cases in skilled home care and hospice. The documentation requirements for billing allow activities over multiple days in a month to be combined. Reimbursement can vary in different parts of the country by as much as 20% based on a Medicare adjustment called "Geographical Practices Cost Indices."

Nurse practitioners are authorized by law to provide both primary care and registered nurse services; however, reimbursement depends on the type of care provided. If the nurse practitioner provides a service described by a Current Procedural Terminology (CPT) code made necessary by an ICD-9 diagnosis to a homebound patient, then this is billable to Medicare Part B as a medical service. It does not require a physician's order and could be billed directly using the nurse practitioner's provider number. If the nurse practitioner is providing nursing care that is billable under Medicare Part A, then the nurse is working as an employee of a certified home-care agency that would bill for these services using their Medicare provider number.

House calls can add an important dimension to the primary provider's knowledge of the patient's circumstances and environment. Home evaluation can identify additional problems not readily apparent in office-based assessment. Barriers to maximal functioning can be identified and addressed. House calls have the additional benefit of reducing the burden for patients who have difficulty getting transportation. Changes in Medicare have increased reimbursement for home visits, making home visits more financially feasible for clinicians.

Patient Assessment

Homebound patients have significant functional impairment. Comprehensive geriatric assessment is particularly valuable in this setting to establish a baseline, monitor the course of illness, and evaluate the effects of intervention. However, assessment in the home has some important differences from office-based assessment.

During a home visit, the patient's daily environment can be assessed to determine whether the home is safe and supportive, given the particular patient's abilities and disabilities. Performance-based functional assessment can focus on the practical aspects of performing ADLs by directly observing the environment for bathing, dressing, and transferring. Difficulties can be identified, and the assessor can evaluate the caregiver's abilities to address the patient's needs. The caregiver's needs for counseling, training, support, and education can also be identified and addressed.

Environmental modifications can be recommended to improve function. For example, modifications of the bathtub, a hand-held shower, a shower seat, grab bars, and a bedside commode can improve the patient's quality of life and functioning. Barriers to wheelchairs and walkers (eg, door sills) can be identified and removed. Chair lifts and outdoor ramps can help patients circumvent stairs. Occupational therapy consultation can be particularly useful in identifying other personal-care and assistive devices for performing ADLs and housekeeping chores. A number of home safety checklists are available to help a reviewer assess the home. Additional technological additions to improve home safety, including necklace or wrist radio devices to call for help, can be considered. Some types of emergency response systems require that a person push a button by a specified time each day to avoid triggering an emergency response or telephone call to check on the owner of the device.

Healthcare providers are finding that home diagnostics, including radiology and electrocardiography, are available in most areas, and hand-held laboratory devices are becoming more common. These home diagnostics allow for a much more comprehensive medical evaluation to take place in the home.

Developing an Office-Based House-Call Program

Medical care in the home may be provided as part of an ongoing office-based program, as an extension of hospitalization through a postacute care program, or as a freestanding entity. Regardless of the method chosen, the organization of the home-care program must be well conceived to maximize effectiveness and efficiency and to remain financially viable. Current regulations allow house calls to be provided by physicians, nurse practitioners, and physician assistants. Regardless of the primary care medical provider, appropriate links to other providers of home-based services are necessary to develop an interdisciplinary team. Consistency and familiarity among all members of the interdisciplinary team are essential to a smoothly functioning house-call program.

Choosing the Right Patients

To qualify for Medicare home-care benefits, a patient must meet two criteria to establish homebound status. First, the patient must be absent from the home for reasons other than obtaining medical treatment infrequently (≤3 times per month) or for short periods of time. Second, leaving home must require considerable and taxing effort on the part of the patient or the caregiver, or both (eg, if the patient is bedbound or has a severe mobility impairment).

Patients who are likely to be good candidates for house calls are those with mobility impairments that make transportation to the office difficult; disruptive behaviors; terminal illnesses; and multiple medical, psychiatric, and social problems. For some patients, house calls are needed for a limited amount of time, but others require house visits on an ongoing basis. Home visits may be particularly useful for patients who are either not responding to adequate therapy or responding inconsistently. A diagnostic home visit may reveal caregiver burnout, mistreatment of the patient, or the use of medications from other sources that may be interfering with the expected response. See also

"Pharmacotherapy," p 81; and "Mistreatment of Older Adults," p 97.

Financial Considerations

House calls are now more financially feasible for clinicians; documentation is the key to receiving reimbursement. There are no specific restrictions on the number of visits, as long as sufficient justification is included in the progress notes. As with most documentation, it is necessary that the primary care provider identify historical data, physical examination findings, diagnostic test results, and an assessment that reflects all active diagnoses. Further, an evaluation of the patient's functioning, caregiver issues, and the medical plan of care are important elements to include in the house-call progress note. Physician assistants and nurse practitioners can also bill for home-care services under Medicare regulations adopted in January 1998. When visits become prolonged, time codes can be used that justify an enhanced reimbursement. Insurers sometimes demand copies of the documented visit when time codes or extended visits are billed. Reimbursement can vary in different localities, particularly where health maintenance organizations act as intermediaries for Medicare.

Caregiver Support

Family caregivers provide most of the care received by patients in the community. In the United States, three-fourths of caregivers are women, either wives or daughters. Caregiving is often intense, time consuming, and stressful. The caregiver's physical and emotional health may be affected, resulting in depression and a worsening of his or her own health problems. Attention to caregiver support and issues are essential to allow caregivers to continue to provide care. Caregiver support groups can be particularly helpful.

For discussions of specific issues concerning caregiving, see "Psychosocial Issues," p 18; "Dementia," p 256; "Behavioral Problems in Dementia," p 267; "Mistreatment of Older Adults," p 97; and "Depression and Other Mood Disorders," p 308.

Limitations of Home Care

Most older adults would prefer to remain in their own home, but certain situations and conditions arise that make institutional care a more appropriate choice than in-home care. For example, caregivers may not be available to adequately address the needs of the patient. Relatively unstable medical situations that require frequent laboratory testing, respiratory interventions, or intravenous medications can also make institutional care a better choice than home care. Caregiver burnout and stress can prevent continued safe care for the patient in the home.

Further, the home environment itself may be a barrier to continuing in-home care. Unsafe neighborhoods, ongoing household social disruptions from alcohol or drug abuse, and inadequate room for equipment or environmental modifications may make in-home care a poor or risky option.

Finally, home care can be prohibitively expensive for the patient. It is not always the least expensive alternative, and out-of-pocket expenses can make ongoing home care unaffordable. Insurance coverage is more likely to cover care provided in a nursing facility or other institutional setting.

Liability and Legal Issues

Malpractice suits related to home care are relatively uncommon. It remains important to maintain appropriate documentation for medical purposes, to support provider compensation, and to support payment requests for other providers of in-home services. In addition, physicians should be aware that inaccurate certificates of medical necessity could lead to charges of Medicare fraud. These forms should be reviewed carefully before they are signed.

It is important to be sensitive to potential conflicts of interest. Federal legislation prohibits providers from receiving financial benefit, compensation, or rebate for referring a patient to a home-care provider. Further, providers may not refer patients to home-care companies in which the physician or the physician's family has a "substantial" financial interest. Legal advice should be sought for any question of a potential conflict of interest.

Ethics and Decisions about Institutionalization

Two ethical themes arise commonly in home care. The first is the balance between patient autonomy and patient safety. The second involves issues surrounding mistreatment and neglect of older adults.

Respect for patient autonomy often dictates that the patient remain in the home as a result of the patient's (or surrogate decision maker's) choice. Conflict arises when a patient's medical care or safety cannot be adequately maintained in the home, yet the patient insists on staying at home. It is difficult to balance respect for patient autonomy with the desire to prevent patient neglect. In some situations, the outcome is likely to be terminal, regardless of whether the patient is maintained at home or in an institution. In such situations, a hospice referral can help provide additional services in the home and support for both the patient and family. In situations in which there is a clearly neglectful or abusive situation, Adult Protective Services should be contacted (see "Mistreatment of Older Adults," p 97).

Community-Based Services Not Requiring a Change in Residence

Adult Day Care

Adult day care is a community-based option that provides a wide range of social and support services in a congregate setting. Adult day care has become increasingly common. Providers of adult day care may offer a variety of services, ranging from simple nonskilled custodial care to more advanced skilled services. The availability of a registered nurse allows for on-site health services, clinical assessment and monitoring, and assistance with medication management. Adult day care is used commonly for patients with dementia who need supervision and assistance with their ADLs while primary caregivers work. Adult day care can also serve as a form of respite for caregivers. Most adult day-care centers are community based, either in churches or community centers. In general, custodial adult day care is not covered by Medicare, although some costs may be covered by Medicaid or other insurers.

Day Hospitals

Day hospitals provide a broad range of skilled-nursing care services, including parenteral antibiotic treatment, chemotherapy, and intensive rehabilitation. Most programs are housed in chronic-care hospitals or rehabilitation centers. This arrangement allows for the provider to take advantage of in-house professional expertise and resources, while allowing the patient to return to his or her own home or alternative living site after day treatment is complete. Services are covered under Medicare, with similar requirements to those surrounding home-health care.

Day hospitals are most often used for two groups of patients: those needing multidisciplinary rehabilitation and those with psychiatric illnesses. A systematic review of day hospital care found no significant differences between day hospitals and alternative sources of care with respect to death, disability, or use of health services, but that among those receiving care in a day hospital, there was a trend toward less functional decline and less hospital and institutional care (SOE=B).

The Program of All-Inclusive Care for the Elderly (PACE)

PACE is a capitated model of care that provides comprehensive care services to frail community-dwelling older adults by a single organization. The program provides all inpatient, outpatient, and long-term care services to frail older adults. See also "Financing, Coverage, and Costs of Health Care," p 35. Participants in the PACE program must be ≥55 years old and meet state-defined requirements regarding their need for a nursing-home level of care. Most will also qualify for Medicaid and Medicare; pooling funds from Medicare and Medicaid allows for comprehensive care to be planned and coordinated by the PACE interdisciplinary team. Without Medicaid and Medicare coverage, out-of-pocket expenses are high. Few private insurance plans provide a PACE benefit as part of their policies. The average PACE enrollee is 80 years old and has an average of eight medical conditions and three ADL limitations; half of PACE participants have dementia.

The goal of the PACE program is to keep the participant in the community for as long as is medically, socially, and financially feasible. The system, designed to be seamless, uses an interdisciplinary team of healthcare providers who know the patient and caregivers well and who provide care across the spectrum of hospital, home, alternative living situations, and institutional care. This team includes a physician (often a geriatrician), nurse practitioner, clinic and home-health nurses, social workers, physical therapist, pharmacist, dietician, and transportation workers. The hub of care is the PACE center, which provides adult day health care. Other care includes respite, transportation, medication coverage, rehabilitation (including maintenance physical and occupational therapy), hearing aids, eyeglasses, and a variety of other benefits. The program, at the discretion of the interdisciplinary team, has the flexibility to pay for nonmedical costs in unusual circumstances (eg, paying a person's electric or gas bill). Care by the interdisciplinary team provides for the complex social needs as well as the medical needs of the participant. PACE has been described as one of the few truly integrated systems of care in the United States.

Although the effectiveness of PACE has not been directly tested by a randomized controlled trial, research has shown that PACE provides high-quality care, albeit with significant site-to-site variation (SOE=B).

In 1997, legislation was passed that changed the status of PACE from a demonstration program to a permanent provider under Medicare. PACE is an optional program under state Medicaid. There are more than 3 million dually eligible and nursing-home–certifiable older adults in the United States that might benefit from PACE, but only a small fraction have enrolled. The growth of PACE has been slower than expected. Barriers to growth have included large start-up costs, insufficient supply of physicians, and the reluctance of patients to leave their primary care physician. The National PACE Association and CMS are evaluating modifications to the PACE model that would allow for community physician involvement as primary care providers (rather than using a PACE-paid, staff health-maintenance organization model). This change in the model may result in more significant growth of PACE, because it could allow patients to keep their primary care physician.

Managed Long-Term Care Programs (MLTC)

Many states are developing initiatives in MLTC programs with the hope of enabling older adults to live in the community and avoid nursing home placement and to decrease hospital utilization. These programs include patients with Medicare and Medicaid and those who are eligible for both ("dually eligible") who have chronic conditions that have impaired their ability to live independently. Some of these programs have been referred to as "PACE without walls" and will provide funding to test new models of care that build on the successful PACE model. States are partnering with entities such as home-care agencies, nursing homes, hospitals, and integrated delivery systems to develop these programs. These programs will provide financing through various capitated per member, per month payments. The aim of the MLTC programs will be to provide safe and cost-effective care.

Home Hospital

The home hospital focuses on providing more complex care at home to older adults who would have been hospitalized for an acute-care need. Patients receiving home-hospital care have access to nurses and physicians on a regular basis and for episodic care through an on-call system that allows problems to be addressed promptly. The concept can be viewed as an evolution of home care, which it resembles, although it is more intense. Studies conducted outside the United States suggest that care is comparable for selected patients and that patient satisfaction is high. See also "Hospital Care," p 130.

Technologic Innovations in the Home

A wide array of technologies have been developed that can assist patients with their ADLs and provide valuable information to caregivers. Older devices such as personal emergency response systems, usually worn on the wrist or around the neck, can alert care providers that help is needed. Newer systems can provide help in medication administration and tracking, monitor and transmit vital signs, and even connect patients through audiovisual telemedicine screens to care providers. Homes can be equipped with fully automated systems to adjust heating and lighting, allow doors to be opened and closed with remote devices, and monitor activity throughout the home. Home robotics are under development that will help in meal preparation and serving or assist in other ADLs and IADLs. Computers and smartphones can also be used to connect people to each other through social networks to combat isolation and loneliness. The rapid development and interconnectivity of these tools will likely become increasingly important in the safe and efficacious delivery of home-care services.

Community-Based Services Requiring a Change of Residence

Assisted Living

Assisted-living facilities continue to grow as the U.S. population ages. They have different names, including personal care homes, residential care homes, domiciliary care, sheltered care, and community residences. Even though these facilities are based on a social (not medical) model, they are caring for more frail people with significant medical needs. The transitional nature of assisted living is suggested by the average length of residency, which is about 2 years. The most common reason for discharge is need for nursing-home care.

Assisted-living residences are characterized by some level of coordination or provision of personal care services, social activities, health-related services, and supervision services in a home-like atmosphere that maximizes autonomy and privacy. The services provided under assisted living vary considerably, both within and between states.

In one national survey of assisted-living facilities, privacy options ranged from private rooms to apartment units; about half of the facilities would not admit residents with moderate to severe cognitive impairment, and about two-thirds did not have a registered nurse on staff but did provide 24-hour staff oversight, housekeeping, two meals, and personal assistance with ADLs. One example of the difference between state licensing requirements is in the area of medication administration. Depending on licensing requirements, medication administration and management can be directed by nonskilled, skilled, or fully licensed nursing staff.

In states where regulations do not require skilled care in assisted-living facilities, home-health skilled care is often provided as an external or independent service to the individual patient who happens to be living in an assisted-living facility. In this context, the boundary between assisted-living and skilled-nursing facilities often becomes blurred. Because care in assisted living is generally less costly than in a nursing home, there has been a trend to use assisted living as a lower-cost alternative to nursing-home care. Part of the reason assisted-living care is usually less expensive is that there are fewer regulations governing assisted-living facilities. However, as these facilities have come to care for more people with increasing disability and more medical needs, the pressure to regulate them has been increasing.

Costs for assisted-living residences vary greatly (from $800 to $4,000 per month) and depend on the size of units, services provided, and location. Assisted living is covered in a growing number of long-term care insurance policies. The Health Insurance Association of America reports that all 11 of the leading insurance companies that sell long-term care insurance offer assisted-living coverage. However, most people in assisted-living residences or their families pay for care themselves, because most older Americans do not carry long-term care insurance.

Assisted living is not covered by Medicare, but certain services are paid under Supplementary Security Income and Social Services Block Grant programs. Thirty-eight states reimburse or plan to reimburse for assisted-living services as a Medicaid service. In addition, states have the option to pay for assisted living under Medicaid by including services in the state's Medicaid plan or by petitioning the U.S. Department of Health and Human Services for a waiver.

Group Homes

Group homes (including domiciliary care, single-room occupancy residences, board-and-care homes, and some congregate living situations) are houses or apartments in which two or more unrelated people live together. Group homes vary in types of residents and often serve patients with chronic mental illness or dementia. Residents share a living room, dining room, and kitchen but usually have their own bedrooms. Advantages of this arrangement include a lower cost of living and socialization with peers. Independence and functional status are supported through the interdependence and relationships of the residents. Resident-to-staff ratios may be higher than in other supported-living environments. Opportunities for socialization are increased, reducing social isolation. Most group homes are run as for-profit businesses, and some states require licensing.

Adult Foster Care

Foster care homes generally provide room, board, and some assistance with ADLs by the sponsoring family or by paid caregivers, who customarily live on the premises. Perhaps the longest experience with adult foster care is in the state of Oregon, where it is used as an alternative to long-term care and institutionalization. Adult foster care has the advantages of maintaining frail older adults in a more home-like environment. Regulations for foster care vary by state, and some states require licensing. Some states provide coverage of adult foster care through their Medicaid programs.

Sheltered Housing

Sheltered housing is funded through the Older Americans Act and is offered as an option for housing subsidized through section 8, Housing and Urban Development programs for seniors and disabled residents. Often these arrangements are sheltered homes offering personal care assistance, housekeeping services, and meals. Programs may be supplemented by social work services and activities coordinators. Charges to clients are based on a sliding scale, which may cost up to 30% of income.

Continuing-Care Retirement Communities (CCRC)

More affluent seniors may choose a CCRC, which usually have a variety of living options, ranging from apartments or condominiums, to assisted living, and skilled nursing-home care. Often, residents enter the more independent living areas and progress through assisted living and into skilled care as they age.

Three financial models are common: the all-inclusive model, which provides total healthcare coverage, including long-term care; the fee-for-service model, in which payments match the level of care; and the modified coverage model, which covers long-term care to a predetermined maximum. Most CCRCs require an entry fee, which may or may not be refundable, plus a variable monthly fee to pay for rent and supportive services. Monthly fees vary, depending on the level of care being provided. Funding is largely private, although some facilities have Medicare- or Medicaid-funded beds for skilled care.

See also "Financing, Coverage, and Costs of Health Care," p 35.

REFERENCES

- American Academy of Nurse Practitioners. *Ordering Home Health Care*. http://www.aanp.org/component/content/article/68-articles/332-good-news-hr2267 (accessed Oct 2013).

- The National Association for Home Care and Hospice (nahc.org/facts/10HC_Stats.pdf) (accessed Oct 2013).

- The National Hospice and Home Care Survey 2007. Centers for Disease Control and Prevention (www.cdc.gov/nchs/nhhcs.htm) (accessed Oct 2013).

- Ornstein K, Smith KL, Foer DH, et al. To hospital and back home again: a nurse practitioner-based transitional care program for hospitalized homebound people. *J Am Geriatr Soc*. 2011;59(3):544–551.

- Program of All-Inclusive Care for the Elderly. Center for Medicare and Medicaid Services (www.cms.hhs.gov/PACE/) (accessed Oct 2013).

CHAPTER 22—OUTPATIENT CARE SYSTEMS

KEY POINTS

- Outpatient interventions that improve the quality and outcomes of care of older adults include personalized care that is provided by a team in accordance with best practice, coordination among all providers and settings of care, consideration of the resources and environment of older adults, and inclusion of older adults as active partners in their care.
- For optimal cost-effectiveness, outpatient programs need to be targeted to patients identified in advance who are likely to be active participants in an intervention that is known to better meet their specific clinical needs.
- Broad dissemination of effective models of outpatient care for older adults may be potentiated by payment reform (eg, patient-centered medical home) and initiatives to expand the geriatrics workforce.

Traditional outpatient care in the United States does not deliver the recommended standard of care to older adults for preventive services, chronic disease management, and geriatric syndromes. In addition, there are racial and ethnic disparities in preventive and chronic care. Realizing that a more proactive, patient-centered, and population-based approach is needed to improve the overall quality of geriatric care, several innovative outpatient care systems have been developed over the past two decades. This chapter describes new system approaches having evidence from clinical trials of improved processes or outcomes of care, or both, including those that involve geriatric specialty care and others that integrate geriatrics in primary care. Current methods for targeting these approaches most likely to benefit older adults are also reviewed.

GERIATRIC SPECIALTY CARE

Senior Health Clinic

The senior health clinic (SHC) care model is a specialized ambulatory clinical service center for older adults providing primary care using an interdisciplinary team approach to developing and implementing a plan of care. All SHC providers have competency in geriatrics, and care is provided and/or coordinated throughout the continuum of care, including hospital, skilled-nursing facility (SNF), assisted living, and home care. Team members work with patients, families, and caregivers, and link patients with needed community-based services and information. The chronic care model has recently offered an organized framework to provide the comprehensive resources and processes needed to deliver evidence-based primary care within an integrated healthcare system that supports the interactions between the informed, activated patient and a prepared, proactive team. Patients new to the SHC are screened for risk status, and a comprehensive geriatric-focused evaluation is completed.

The core interdisciplinary clinical practice team consists of a geriatrician, nurse practitioner, and social worker. An extended team may include other professionals, such as a pharmacist, physical therapist, dietitian, and home-health nurse. Provider teams share a common medical record and meet at least weekly to review complex care plans and discuss new or anticipated patient issues. When SHC patients are admitted to the hospital or SNF, care is delivered directly and/or coordinated by providers from the SHC.

Studies in community settings and Veterans Affairs medical centers have demonstrated that geriatric patients cared for in the SHC model have improved mental health status and better maintained health-related quality of life over time than patients in traditional care (SOE=A). Financially, SHCs may be a cost center when viewed in isolation, but these clinics are more likely revenue generators when viewed from the perspective of an integrated health system because of the associated "downstream" fee-for-service revenues generated from hospital inpatient, hospital outpatient, and professional fees (SOE=B). There exist financially viable private practice groups who provide this type of care in a fee-for-service environment; however, broad uptake of the SHC model is limited by health system administration considering the clinic in isolation and as a cost center and the limited number of specialty trained geriatrics healthcare professionals available to staff such clinics.

Program of All-Inclusive Care for the Elderly

See "Community-Based Care," p 166.

GERIATRICS IN PRIMARY CARE

Outpatient Consultation

Comprehensive geriatric assessment (CGA) is a process intended to determine a patient's medical, psychosocial, and functional capabilities and limitations, with the goal of developing an overall plan for treatment and long-term follow-up. Because CGA typically requires a highly trained team of geriatricians, geriatric nurse clinicians, physical and occupational therapists, geriatric psychiatrists, and social workers, it is expensive and time consuming. Success generally requires the geriatric team to take over the direct care of the patient. An extended period of intensive team involvement with ongoing care is essential to ensure the efficacy of the intervention. When the geriatric team assumes a purely consultative role (ie, without a role in implementing the recommendations), CGA is unlikely to be successful in improving patient outcomes (SOE=A). However, CGA coupled with an adherence intervention to improve primary care physician (PCP) and patient adherence with recommendations has demonstrated improved outcomes. In a randomized controlled trial, CGA coupled with adherence strategies was associated with less decline in physical functioning, less fatigue, and better social functioning among community-dwelling older adults with at least one of four conditions (functional impairment, falls, urinary incontinence, or depressive symptoms [SOE=A]). In this care model, patients undergo an in-depth, standardized CGA from a social worker, a geriatrics nurse practitioner/geriatrician team, and a physical therapist (when indicated by falls or impaired mobility), after which the evaluation team holds a short interdisciplinary case conference and forms its recommendations for care. The adherence intervention includes the geriatrician contacting the patient's PCP to convey the recommendations and also sending a letter describing the recommendations along with a copy of the dictated consultation and copies of full-text references specific to the patient's conditions. In addition, the patient receives a written list of recommendations at the time of the CGA and is subsequently mailed a copy of the dictated consultation and list of recommendations along with a "How to Talk to Your Doctor" booklet. Approximately 2 weeks later, a health educator telephones the patient to review the team's recommendations and help prepare the patient for discussion of the proposed recommendations with his or her PCP.

A more intensive outpatient consultation model is short-term geriatric evaluation and management (GEM). In GEM, a geriatrics interdisciplinary team diagnoses *and treats* problems, including adjusting medications, providing counseling and health education, and making referrals to other health professionals and community services. In addition, monitoring and coordination of care between visits is provided through regular telephone calls. In one trial, community-dwelling adults ≥70 years old and found to be at high risk of hospital admission by mailed screening questionnaire underwent CGA followed by interdisciplinary primary care by the GEM team (geriatrician, geriatrics nurse practitioner, nurse, and social worker) for an average of 6 months before being discharged for care by their original PCP. This GEM model prevented functional decline, improved patients' satisfaction with their health care, and lessened caregiver burden. Other trials of GEM have shown similar positive results (SOE=A). However, fully implementing the above GEM model was more expensive than usual care. Other GEM trials have produced different results on costs, some costing more than usual care, some costing the same, and some costing less.

Forms of CGA may also be attempted in the home setting. Accumulating evidence suggests that preventive home visitation programs, based on CGA with extended follow-up of patients at lower risk of death, can reduce functional decline and nursing-home placement (SOE=A).

Enhanced Primary Care

A variety of new models of primary care aimed at improving the quality and outcomes of care for older adults have been studied and share many concepts with the recently proposed patient-centered medical home (PCMH) model of practice. In 2007, four primary care organizations—The American Academy of Pediatrics (AAP), the American College of Physicians ACP), the American Association of Family Physicians (AAFP), and the American Osteopathic Association (AOA)—agreed on a set of Joint Principles of the PCMH (AAP, ACP, AAFP, AOA. Joint Principles of the Patient-Centered Medical Home, March 2007 http://www.medicalhomeinfo.org/downloads/pdfs/JointStatement.pdf). These principles include the following: 1) each patient having an ongoing relationship with a personal physician, 2) a physician-directed medical practice having a team of individuals who collectively take responsibility for care, 3) a "whole-person orientation" providing or arranging for all the patient's healthcare needs, 4) coordination of care across all elements of the complex healthcare system, 5) "quality and safety are hallmarks of the medical home" with physicians engaging in continuous quality improvement and patients participating in decision making, 6) access to care is enhanced, and 7) payment recognizes the added value provided to patients who have a PCMH (eg, enhanced fee-for-service, care management fee, and/or shared savings).

The Geriatric Resources for Assessment and Care of Elders (GRACE) model of primary care includes each of these principles and could be described as an intensive "medical home" for older patients with complex healthcare needs. GRACE provides patients with home-based CGA and long-term care management by a nurse practitioner and social worker (GRACE support team) who collaborate with the PCP and a geriatrics interdisciplinary team involving a geriatrician, pharmacist, physical therapist, mental health social worker, and community-based services liaison. Individualized care planning during weekly team meetings is guided by 12 care protocols for common geriatric conditions, including "advanced care planning" and "health maintenance" protocols used in all patients. The nurse practitioner and social worker (employees of the primary care practice) review and prioritize the care plan with the patient's PCP, and then implement the care plan in collaboration with the PCP and consistent with the patient's goals. The GRACE support team provides ongoing home-based care management, including coordination and continuity of care among all healthcare professionals and sites of care facilitated by an electronic medical record and Web-based tracking system.

The GRACE model was developed specifically to improve the quality of care of a mixed-race population of seniors who are poor (many dually eligible for Medicare and Medicaid), have multiple comorbid conditions, and receive primary care in community-based health centers affiliated with an urban safety net healthcare system. Low-income seniors enrolled in a randomized controlled trial of the GRACE intervention, compared with usual care, received better quality of care for the geriatric conditions and general health processes targeted, had improvements in health-related quality-of-life measures, and had fewer emergency department visits over 2 years. In addition, hospital admissions were significantly reduced in the second year among GRACE patients identified at baseline as being at high risk of future hospitalization (SOE=A). Cost analysis of the GRACE intervention revealed that in the high-risk group, increases in chronic and preventive care costs were offset by reductions in acute-care costs such that the intervention was cost neutral in the first 2 years. Two-year costs were higher in the low-risk group. The intervention was cost saving in the high-risk group during the post-intervention, or third, year because of continued lower hospital costs in GRACE patients than in those who receive usual care.

Replication of the GRACE model has been successful in Medicare managed-care and Veterans Administration healthcare settings and demonstrated consistent improvements in quality of care and reductions in hospital utilization. The GRACE model has been applied within a home visitation program, as a care transition intervention, and as a model for integrated medical and social services in seniors enrolled in the Medicaid Home and Community-Based Services waiver.

Other successful models of enhanced primary care demonstrating reduced acute-care utilization have also involved a geriatrics interdisciplinary team that provides ongoing care management (usually including home visitation) in support of and integrated with the PCP (SOE=A). Guided Care was designed to improve the quality of life and the efficiency of resource use for older adults with multiple morbidities. Guided Care aims to enhance primary care by infusing the operative principles of seven chronic care innovations: disease management, self-management, case management, lifestyle modification, transitional care, caregiver education and support, and geriatric evaluation and management. A specially trained registered nurse works with assigned PCPs and office staff to provide the intervention to a panel of the practice's older patients at highest risk of using health care heavily during the coming year. Preliminary results from a multisite randomized controlled trial of Guided Care demonstrated improved quality of chronic care, reduced family caregiver strain, increased patient and clinician satisfaction with care, and a trend toward less use of expensive health services in the first 8 months. Final trial results concluded that Guided Care reduced the use of home health care but had little effect on the use of other health services in the first 20 months. Interestingly, in the same trial, Guided Care was found to reduce skilled-nursing facility admissions and days among the subgroup of Kaiser-Permanente patients. Payment reform like that proposed for PCMH may offer a means for implementing models of enhanced primary care like GRACE and Guided Care on a wider scale and under traditional fee-for-service Medicare.

Disease Management

Disease management programs focus healthcare delivery around a single disease with the goal of optimizing patient care for this disease. The most effective disease management programs are those that are integrated with the patient's primary or specialty care physician, or both. Heart failure and depression interventions are examples of disease management programs that lead to better outcomes in older adults and that are potentially cost saving. One notable heart failure program that was nurse-directed and multidisciplinary (geriatrician, cardiologist, nurse, dietitian, and social worker) reduced readmission rates and costs in hospitalized older adults with heart failure (SOE=A). Key components included comprehensive education of the patient and family, a prescribed diet, social-service consultation and planning for an early discharge, a review of medications, and intensive follow-up.

In the disease management program for late-life depression called Improving Mood—Promoting Access to Collaborative Treatment (IMPACT), patients had access to a depression care manager, supervised by a psychiatrist and a primary care expert, who offered education, care management, and support of antidepressant management by the patient's PCP or a brief psychotherapy for depression. In a large multicenter clinical trial, depressed patients who received the IMPACT intervention were more likely than patients who receive usual care to be given guideline-concordant depression care and to recover from depression (SOE=A).

Finally, a collaborative care model developed for older adults with Alzheimer disease has demonstrated improvements in the quality of care and in behavioral and psychological symptoms of dementia among primary-care patients and their caregivers (SOE=A). In this program, an advanced practice nurse supported by an interdisciplinary team (psychologist, neuropsychologist, geriatrician, and geriatric psychiatrist) served as the care manager working with the patient's family caregiver and PCP. The team used standard protocols to initiate treatment and to identify, monitor, and treat behavioral and psychological symptoms of dementia with an emphasis on nonpharmacologic management.

PATIENT SELECTION FOR OUTPATIENT INTERVENTIONS

Programs described above have been developed to better address the multiple healthcare needs of older adults with chronic conditions and in response to rising costs. For these interventions to be successful, they must target patient populations having clinical needs that are addressed by the intervention, or who are at risk of high healthcare expenditures in the future, or both. Ideally, identifying individuals in advance who are also likely to engage in the intervention program is also desirable. Patient selection for intensive outpatient interventions is one of the major challenges facing healthcare organizations that serve older adults.

Three complementary approaches have been used to identify high-risk older adults: referral by clinicians, screening by mail or telephone, and analysis of administrative data (predictive modeling). The ideal system for identifying high-risk individuals would rely on multiple sources of information. Clinicians in primary care settings are perhaps well positioned to identify some high-risk older adults, especially when provided with objective criteria on which to base referral. However, they may lack the time, skills, and incentives to do so. Surveys can be administered systematically by mail or telephone to a defined population of older adults. The Probability of Repeated Admission Questionnaire (Pra) has been used extensively in managed-care settings to identify high-risk older adults upon enrollment. A risk score is calculated based on age, sex, perceived health, availability of an informal caregiver, heart disease, diabetes, physician visits, and hospitalizations. A score above a certain threshold indicates that the member is at high risk of hospital admission and use of other health-related services during the coming year. The Pra has been found to be valid in many different populations of community-dwelling older adults, including Medicaid, fee-for-service, and managed-care patients (SOE=B). Because of the associated expenses and <100% response rates, an administrative proxy has been developed as a close substitute to the Pra. The Vulnerable Elders Survey-13 (VES-13), another risk screening instrument, is a 13-item questionnaire that produces a vulnerability score from 0 to 10 based on age, self-reported health, and function. Patients with a VES-13 score of ≥3 are at four times the risk of functional decline or death over the next 2 years and are therefore defined as vulnerable (SOE=B). Finally, predictive modeling approaches use administrative data for identifying high-risk older adults and are usually proprietary and not described in the peer-reviewed literature. They typically analyze health insurance enrollment records and claims data with predictions based on age, gender, diagnoses, prior use of health services and associated costs, and pharmacy data.

REFERENCES

- Boult C, Wieland GD. Comprehensive primary care for older patients with multiple chronic conditions: "Nobody rushes you through". *JAMA.* 2010;304(17):1936–1943.
- Callahan CM, Boustani MA, Weiner M, et al. Implementing dementia care models in primary care settings: The Aging Brain Care Medical Home. *Aging Ment Health.* 2011;15(1):5–12.
- Lowery J, Hopp F, Subramanian U, et al. Evaluation of a nurse practitioner disease management model for chronic heart failure: a multi-site implementation study. *Congest Heart Fail.* 2012;18(1):64–71.
- NCQA standards: how to be certified as a Patient-Centered Medical Home (www.ncqa.org/tabid/631/Default.aspx).

CHAPTER 23—FRAILTY

KEY POINTS

- Frailty is understood to be a clinical syndrome of dysregulation of energetics and multiple physiologic systems, with definable clinical manifestations that become apparent when physiologic dysregulation reaches a critical threshold. It has recognizable causes that are associated with altered physiology and that may be reflective of underlying alterations in genetic, cellular, and molecular processes.
- A validated frailty syndrome is manifested when multiple components are present: weakness, slowed walking speed, low physical activity, low energy or exhaustion, and weight loss. Consistent with the clinical definition of a syndrome, the whole is greater than the sum of the parts.
- Frailty identifies patients at high risk of adverse clinical outcomes, including falls, disability and dependency, and mortality.
- Frailty develops along a continuum of severity. This likely includes a latent phase of vulnerability that is not clinically apparent in the absence of stressors, early stages that may be most responsive to intervention, and a late end-stage that indicates high risk of short-term mortality.
- The most effective preventive approach appears to be maintaining muscle mass and strength through resistance exercise. Supplementation of dietary protein also appears to be beneficial. Consistent with theory regarding the multisystem dysregulation of frailty, interventions that optimize multiple systems, such as exercise, are most likely to be effective for prevention or amelioration.

EVIDENCE-BASED FINDINGS

Frailty as a Core Clinical Concept

Care of frail older adults is a central focus of geriatric health care. Frail older adults are a subset of the older population who are at high risk from stressors such as extremes of heat and cold, acute infection or injury, or the stress of hospitalization or surgery. In the face of such stressors, frail older adults are more likely to have delayed recovery from illness or are more likely to fall, or both; to develop greater functional impairment, including becoming disabled or dependent; or to die. As a group, frail older adults are at high risk of needing to be hospitalized, and risk worse outcomes once hospitalized, including dependency.

Frailty is clinically observed to be a chronic, progressive condition, with a spectrum of severity. The most severely frail older adults appear to be in an irreversible, predeath phase with high risk of mortality over 6–12 months. Earlier phases may be responsive to treatment, either to prevent or ameliorate the clinical manifestations of frailty.

Frailty may result from intrinsic aging processes, ie, *primary frailty*. It also appears that a similar phenotype and vulnerability, thought of as *secondary frailty*, is associated with the end stages of several chronic diseases associated with inflammation and wasting, such as cancer, heart failure, COPD, and HIV/AIDS. The similarity of presentation between primary and secondary frailty suggests that, clinically, frailty is actually a physiologic entity unto itself that can be triggered by disparate causes and, ultimately, represents a final common pathway resulting from these causes.

Frailty and Associated Vulnerability

Frailty is associated with heightened vulnerability to adverse outcomes, and this vulnerability may most likely manifest in the face of stressors. Frailty theories suggest that, regardless of the causes, those who are frail have decreased reserves with which to compensate for, or recover from, stressors. Aggregate loss of physiologic function is the process thought to underlie the high risk of adverse outcomes. An emerging research agenda is focused on developing approaches that can identify older adults with this vulnerable physiologic status before frailty becomes clinically apparent.

Frailty as a Clinical Syndrome

Beyond the consensus that frailty is a physiologic state of heighted vulnerability, current definitions of who is frail fall into two major categories. One is that the vulnerability of frailty is the outcome of the accumulation of a number of likely unrelated diseases, impairments, and other health conditions in an individual. This state of having multiple comorbidities is associated with increased risk of mortality; the number of conditions predicts this vulnerability, ie, a large number of conditions mark an individual as frail.

The second conception of frailty is that it is a distinct physiologic process resulting from dysregulation of multiple physiologic systems; many of these systems interact with each other, and resulting impairments contribute to clinical manifestations. The aggregate impact of too many dysregulated systems is a decreased ability to maintain homeostasis in the face of stressors, resulting in vulnerability to adverse outcomes. This

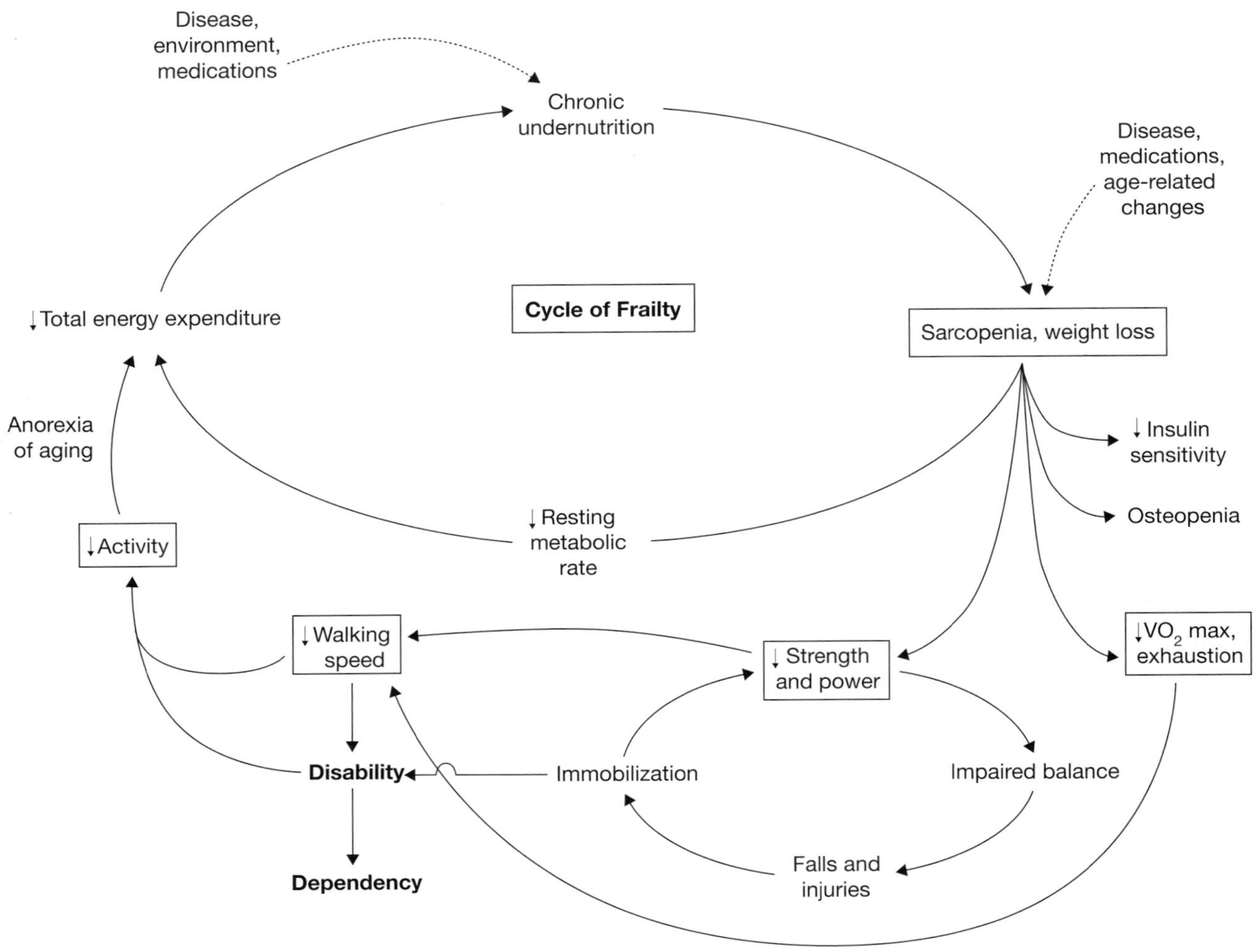

Figure 23.1–The Cycle of Frailty

SOURCE: Fried LP, Tangen CM, Walston J, et al. Frailty in older adults: evidence for a phenotype. *J Gerontol A Biol Sci Med Sci*. 2001;56(3):M146–156.

physiologic (or pathophysiologic) process appears to lead to an observable clinical phenotype. The consensus is that clinical manifestations of frailty are seen in specific domains: strength, balance, motor processing, nutrition, endurance, physical activity, mobility, and possibly cognition. A proposed phenotype has been developed and validated that links all aspects but cognition, based on the hypothesis that the clinical presentation of frailty results from a vicious cycle of dysregulated energetics, leading to the following:

- decreased muscle mass, or sarcopenia, with resulting loss of strength
- slowed motor performance (such as walking speed)
- decreased physical activity
- worsened exercise tolerance (or low energy or fatigue)
- inadequate nutritional intake (even when physical activity is low)

The latter three result in further sarcopenia and, when nutritional intake is inadequate, weight loss as well (Figure 23.1). Identifying the presence of multiple manifestations (formally defined as ≥3 of the list above) provides specificity in defining an individual as frail (Table 23.1). Research has shown this construct results in the definition of a clinical syndrome that is primarily chronic and progressive, with early stages generally predicting progression to more severe frailty; progression is not inexorable, however, because some afflicted individuals can show improvement. Early stages of frailty are likely most amenable to intervention. The first manifestations of frailty tend to be weakness, slowed walking speed, and/or decreased physical activity.

Observations to date support the concept of frailty as a clinical syndrome with definable manifestations that become apparent when physiologic dysregulation reaches a critical threshold. It has recognizable causes at the level of both altered physiology and potentially

Table 23.1—Criteria that Define Frailty (≥3 characteristics identified indicates frailty)

Characteristic	Criteria for Frailty[a]
Weight loss	Lost >10 pounds unintentionally last year
Exhaustion	Felt last week that "everything I did was an effort" or "I could not get going"
Slowness	Time to walk 15 feet (cutoff depends on sex and height)
Low activity level	Expends <270 kcal/ week (calculated from activity scale incorporating episodes of walking, household chores, yard work, etc)
Weakness	Grip strength measured using hand dynamometer (cutoff depends on sex and body mass index)

[a] For specific measures and details for determining frailty criteria, see Fried LP, Tangen CM, Walston J, et al. Frailty in older adults: evidence for a phenotype. *J Gerontol Med Sci.* 2001;56A:M146–M156.

altered genetic, cellular, and molecular processes (Figure 23.2).

EVIDENCE AS TO CAUSE

Primary Frailty

Mounting evidence suggests that frailty as a distinct clinical syndrome can be precipitated by a number of factors. Sarcopenia, or loss of lean body mass, is a central component of frailty and a key predictor of the other clinical manifestations. Predictors of loss of muscle mass and strength with aging include decreased anabolic factors such as testosterone and IGF-1, diminished physical activity, reduced nutritional intake (eg, protein, energy, vitamin D and other micronutrients), and older age itself.

While the most basic underlying cause of frailty is still unknown, the intermediate process, and precipitant of clinical manifestations, may be aging-associated dysregulation of multiple physiologic systems. Systemic abnormalities in frailty include sarcopenia, inflammation (indicated by increased IL-6 and C-reactive protein), decreased immune function, anemia, increased insulin resistance, low levels of DHEA-S and IGF-1, decreased heart rate variability, and nutritional derangements (low levels of certain vitamins and carotenoids, reduced intake of protein and energy). The number of abnormal systems is a stronger predictor of frailty than injury in any one system, and there is evidence that abnormal systems synergistically interact to increase frailty risk. It is unknown whether intervention on any one system modifies frailty risk.

Overall, research indicates that the vulnerability and clinical presentation of the frailty syndrome results from an aging-associated dysregulation of the complex biology of mutually regulating and compensating systems that maintain a robust organism. When this complex systems biology is compromised, because too many systems have ceased to function effectively, energy is dysregulated; both reserves and resilience are lost, with diminished ability to maintain homeostasis in the face of stressors.

Secondary Frailty

Inflammatory and wasting diseases independently predict frailty, potentially through inflammation and/or their effect on cardiopulmonary function (eg, heart failure, COPD), immune diseases (eg, HIV/AIDS), and chronic cytomegalovirus infection. Secondary frailty theoretically develops as a result of the core wasting process of these illnesses, perhaps precipitating an independent, final common process that leads to the frailty phenotype. Data on HIV-positive men indicate that HIV infection, even in the absence of clinical AIDS, is associated with rates of a frailty-like presentation that would be found in HIV-negative men who are 10 years older. Additionally, frailty in association with HIV/AIDS predicts a lower response to therapy and a worse prognosis than HIV positivity alone.

ASSESSMENT OF FRAILTY

The presence of frailty can be assessed by several established methods. The approach used may differ depending on the setting and goal. There is a consensus that frailty is distinct from disability, which is an outcome of frailty. In the clinical setting, screening for frailty (Table 23.1) might be appropriate to identify those at risk of adverse outcomes, to gauge severity of risks, to find those who may benefit from risk amelioration as well as treatment, or to determine eligibility for palliative care for those at end stage.

Several screening measures exist: 1) For frailty as a clinical syndrome with a distinct phenotypic presentation, characterizing the number of criteria present (out of 5) (see Table 23.1), offers a standardized approach to diagnosis and characterizing severity. 2) For frailty as a clinical composite, an instrument providing a clinical global impression of change in frailty has been validated. This draws on clinical judgment and incorporates assessment of the status of the clinical syndrome plus outcomes and precipitants into one score. 3) Walking speed has been shown to predict mortality and mobility disability which, as 1 of 3 first frailty manifestations, can serve as a marker in screening (SOE=A) and a shortened assessment of physical activity in this syndrome. 4) The cumulative number of symptoms, signs, illnesses, and disabilities present is useful to understand morbidity burden. It is proposed that multiple comorbidities, in the form of an index of accumulated deficits, identify those at high risk of mortality, presumably due to multisystem dysregulation.

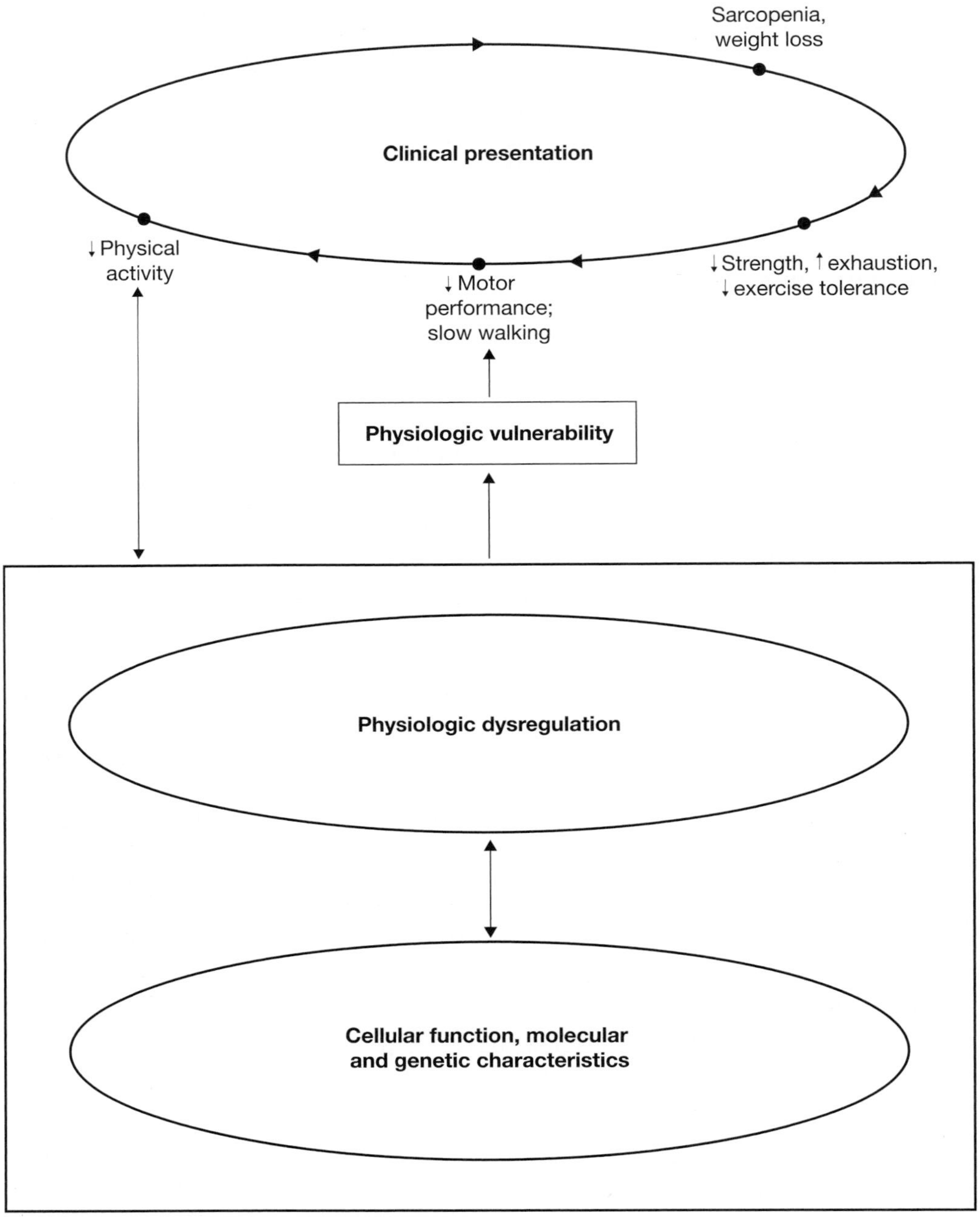

Figure 23.2—Conceptual representation of the multiple levels of contribution to the syndrome of frailty: clinical phenotype, physiologic and biologic causes, and resulting vulnerability in the face of stressors

These different definitions of frailty identify populations that overlap to a modest degree (SOE=A).

PREVAILING MANAGEMENT STRATEGIES

Comprehensive geriatric assessment and management is a clinical care model designed to optimize outcomes for frail older adults, particularly to prevent loss of independence. This team-based, multidisciplinary approach has been shown to have positive effects on polypharmacy, falls, functional status, nursing-home admission, and mortality. The assessment should include accurate longitudinal screening for frailty, including gait speed, and ongoing, expert geriatric care. The focus of care should be 1) to exclude any modifiable precipitating causes of frailty, including causes that are treatable or environmental; 2) to improve the core manifestations of frailty, especially physical activity, strength, exercise tolerance, and nutrition; and 3) to minimize the consequences of the vulnerability of frail older adults, by directing attention to environmental risks, extent of social support, falls prevention, or the risks from stressors such as acute illness or injury, hospitalization, or surgery. The impact of these stressors is worsened when homeostatic systems and resilience are compromised in frailty. Resistance, or strengthening, exercise, with added nutritional support, particularly protein supplementation, appears to be a key management approach for frailty and for its prevention. This can be supplemented by aerobic exercise and balance training. The approach that older adults use to adapt to age-related psychosocial losses and behaviors can also be applied to physical health and to frailty in particular. In the face of diminished resources or reserves, older adults must carefully choose their goals, focus on optimizing the abilities needed to reach their goals, and then compensate for diminished competencies by increased reliance on other functions or by replacement. Such compensations could include supportive services such a "meals on wheels" or home environments that offer care or meals if needed. Clinical management needs to include such approaches for care of frail older adults, as well as more standard medical approaches, as described above. Further, decreasing the stress of environments such as hospitals and maximizing supportive care during acute illness and recovery may be effective clinical approaches as well. See "Hospital Care," p 130; and "Outpatient Care Systems," p 173.

POTENTIAL APPROACHES TO PREVENTION OF FRAILTY

Points of Vulnerability and Precipitants

Exposure to any of a variety of stressors appears to put frail older adults at risk of adverse outcomes and is thought to potentially precipitate clinically apparent frailty in those already at risk. Immobility is one key precipitant, causing frailty to develop or worsen, as well as exacerbating the onset of adverse outcomes such as dependency. This holds regardless of whether immobility results from pain, illness, or in context of hospitalization. Depression may be another precipitant, given its association with decreased activity, energy, and nutritional intake, as well as with inflammation and worsened social isolation. (Depression also appears to be both an outcome of frailty and a precipitant.) Overall, attention needs to be paid to minimizing these precipitants or the stress associated with them, or both. Screening for risk assessment, diagnosis, and early detection can be done using the screening approaches described above.

Potential Pharmacologic Treatments

It has not been demonstrated that replacing deficiencies of any one hormone or repleting defects in other systems can prevent or ameliorate frailty. Theoretically, this is understandable, given that it is the number of deficits in multiple physiologic systems that most strongly predicts frailty, rather than the presence of any one deficit alone. This suggests that improving only one system may not be clinically effective. Consequently, future effective treatments will likely be ones that target multiple systems. The prototype of such approaches, comprehensive geriatric assessment and management, has been shown to decrease polypharmacy and related adverse medication events in frail older adults (SOE=A).

Behavioral Prevention or Treatment

Maintaining physical activity and muscle mass is critical in older adults at risk of frailty. Evidence is substantial that resistance, or strengthening, exercise is effective in increasing muscle mass, strength, and walking speed in frail older adults, such as nursing-home residents (SOE=A). Other forms of exercise, including stretching, Tai Chi, and aerobic exercise, are also helpful. Prevention of immobility is key. These proactive exercise regimens or prehabilitation approaches may be beneficial for frail older adults to prevent decline in physical function. Overall, exercise has notable beneficial physiologic effects on sarcopenia, inflammation, and other systems associated with frailty, making maintenance of physical activity as well as strength a cornerstone of prevention and treatment. See "Physical Activity," p 64. Importantly, recent randomized controlled trials of exercise interventions show ability to improve gait speed and functional limitations. Frail older adults may also benefit from an occupational therapy evaluation and/or biofeedback to assist with strengthening, balance, and gait training. It remains to be determined if that can prevent or ameliorate frailty and disability.

Attention to preventing nutritional inadequacy appears to be important, including supplementation of protein and micronutrients. In most studies, nutritional supplementation appears to be effective only when added to resistance exercise. Preventing and treating depression may also be important in preventing or ameliorating frailty.

FRAILTY AND FAILURE TO THRIVE

A clinical concept that is an antecedent of current conceptualizations of frailty is that of failure to thrive. In geriatrics, this was historically used as a blanket diagnosis at admission to a hospital or long-term care setting, in the setting of an older patient with nonspecific symptoms, including fatigue, poor nutritional intake, weight loss, social withdrawal, and/or decline in cognitive and physical function, often in a state of functional collapse, and without an apparent cause. It was commonly thought that depression was a key component as well. This diagnosis was observed to be associated with poor response to treatment or rehabilitation, increased rates of pressure sores, infection, diminished cell-mediated immunity, and high surgical and short-term mortality rates. Some experts have argued that the term should be abandoned because it does not assist thoughtful evaluation, while others have expressed concern that the application of a term initially used for delayed development in children appeared pejorative when applied to older adults. Nevertheless, there may well be conceptual overlap between the concept of failure to thrive and very severe, or end-stage frailty.

Frailty and Palliative Care

There is evidence that frailty leads to functional decline and dependency at the end of life. Severe frailty, with a score of 4–5 using a syndromic definition (Table 23.1), and metabolic abnormalities of low cholesterol and albumin, predict particularly high short-term mortality rates in frail older adults (SOE=B). Additionally, clinical case series suggest a poor response to treatment in those with end-stage frailty. Therefore, it may be appropriate to consider palliative approaches for these patients.

References

- Benefield LE, Higbee RL. Frailty and its implications for care. Hartford Institute for Geriatric Nursing. http://consultgerirn.org/topics/frailty_and_its_implications_for_care_new/want_to_know_more.
- Collard RM, Boter H, Schoevers RA, et al. Prevalence of frailty in community-dwelling older persons: a systematic review. *J Am Geriatr Soc*. 2012;60(8):1487–1492.
- Poltawski L, Goodman C, Lliffe S, et al. Frailty Scales-their potential in interprofessional working with older people: a discussion paper. *J Interprof Care*. 2011;25(4):280–286.
- Shega JW, Dale W, Andrew M, et al. Persistent pain and frailty: a case for homeostenosis. *J Am Geriatr Soc*. 2012;60(1):113–117.
- Theou O, Stathokostas L, Roland KP, et al. The effectiveness of exercise interventions for the management of frailty: A systematic review. *J Aging Res*. 2011 Apr 4;2011:569194.

CHAPTER 24—VISUAL IMPAIRMENT

KEY POINTS

- Visual impairment increases exponentially with age; 20%–30% of the population ≥75 years old is affected. Blindness affects 2% of the population ≥75 years old. Those ≥65 years old make up 12% of the total U.S. population but 50% of the blind population.
- Cataracts and refractive error are common; both are correctable, and correction improves quality of life.
- Age-related macular degeneration (ARMD) is common; the wet form, the major complication of ARMD leading to blindness, is treatable with a series of intravitreal antiangiogenesis injections. Antioxidant multivitamins can slow progression to the wet form.
- Glaucoma is common, and increased intraocular pressure is no longer required to meet diagnostic criteria. Screening for glaucoma should be done every 1–2 years after age 50 and more often in high-risk individuals.
- Control of blood glucose and blood pressure in type 2 diabetes reduces retinopathy. Glycemic and blood pressure control needs to be sustained to achieve significant benefit. Laser therapy is still the mainstay for treatment of complications of diabetic retinopathy.

Visual impairment has considerable impact on the medical system and older age groups. Chronic eye conditions are one of the most common reasons for office visits to health care providers among those ≥65 years old. Of all office visits by older adults, 14% are to ophthalmologists, one of the highest rates of all specialty visits. Falls and car crashes, each associated with impaired vision in older adults, consume considerable medical resources. Moreover, impaired vision has been linked to a significant deterioration in the quality of life and the ADLs of older adults.

The American Academy of Ophthalmology recommends a comprehensive eye examination every 1–2 years for adults ≥65 years old. Prophylactic and therapeutic ocular management can effectively alter the course of various conditions causing visual impairment. About one-third of all new cases of blindness can be avoided with effective use of available ophthalmologic services.

COMMON EYE CONDITIONS IN OLDER ADULTS

Older adults with eye complaints frequently first seek care from their primary care provider. Common complaints include red eye, ocular swelling or discomfort, blurred or sudden loss of vision, diplopia, and floaters. A key question to determine whether a patient can be treated by his or her primary care provider or needs an ophthalmologist is "Has your vision changed?" A decrease in vision can indicate a serious condition. For this reason, it is vitally important to check visual acuity in each eye separately with the patient's current corrective aid (eg, eyeglasses) in place for any eye complaint. Significant vision loss can also be indicated by the presence of a relative afferent pupillary defect, which can be assessed using a "swinging flashlight test." While in a dark room, the patient is asked to stare into the distance. A bright flashlight is then placed in front of one eye to check the pupillary light reflex; the other eye should also constrict because of the consensual light reflex. The flashlight is then quickly swung over to the second eye. If this eye dilates, there is an afferent pupillary defect (ie, the second eye is not detecting the light as the first eye detects it).

For serious eye conditions that require immediate attention from an ophthalmologist, see Table 24.2. All of the listed conditions are usually associated with a decrease in vision that can be profound but masked by good vision in the other eye. The symptoms of a retinal detachment include new floaters in one eye along with photopsias (the perception of flashes of light), distorted peripheral vision, or decreased vision. Ocular pain and hyperemia do not accompany a retinal detachment; the only signs a primary care provider may detect are a relative afferent pupillary defect, decreased vision, or a monocular visual field deficit. Signs and symptoms of acute angle-closure glaucoma include an injected eye with fixed, dilated pupil and cloudy cornea; the patient is often in severe pain, nauseous, and vomiting. In ischemic optic neuropathy, vision in one eye is lost suddenly, usually in the upper or lower hemifield (this can be detected on visual field testing by confrontation). Giant cell arteritis must be excluded quickly in patients with ischemic optic neuropathy to prevent bilateral blindness. Diplopia and central retinal artery occlusion can also be the result of giant cell arteritis. Bacterial keratitis usually presents with pain and a corneal infiltrate. Scleritis is frequently associated with significant autoimmune disease; symptoms include boring pain, decreased

Table 24.1—Symptoms and Treatment of Most Common Eye Diseases of Older Adults

Condition	Comments	Signs and Symptoms	Treatment
Cataracts	*Reversible* cause of blindness	Decreased vision; cause refractive shifts, reduced visual acuity, reduced contrast sensitivity, glare, monocular diplopia/ghosting	Change eyeglasses to match changing refractive error. Surgical cataract extraction when eyeglasses no longer improve vision: extremely successful in improving vision in those without other ocular pathology; can also be helpful in those with other ocular pathology.
Age-related macular degeneration	Most common cause of *irreversible* blindness		
Dry form		Slow onset, vision loss not severe, usually asymptomatic	To decrease rate of conversion to wet form: vitamin supplements (vitamins C, E, zinc, β-carotene)
Wet form		Sudden onset of vision loss or distortion of vision; central vision loss can be severe, peripheral vision maintained	Intravitreal injections of vascular endothelial growth factor inhibitors and laser
Glaucoma	Second leading cause of *irreversible* blindness	Peripheral vision lost first, but in advanced stages all vision can be lost; early glaucoma typically asymptomatic	
Open angle		Typically asymptomatic until advanced; may note contrast sensitivity loss or night vision problems	Lowering of intraocular pressure with medications, laser trabeculoplasty, and/or incisional surgery
Narrow angle	Drug warnings apply to this type of glaucoma. Avoid medications that can dilate the pupil (anticholinergic and sympathomimetic drugs, ie, those used for bladder problems, decongestants, and some antidepressant drugs)	Acute: painful, red eye, decreased vision, nausea, vomiting, headache Chronic: usually asymptomatic until vision loss advanced or central vision affected	Acute: pilocarpine 2% ophthalmic solution (2 drops in affected eye), acetazolamide 250 mg IV or po, if tolerated, and immediate laser treatment needed; may require continued medical and/or surgical treatment Chronic: lowering of intraocular pressure with medications, laser, and/or incisional surgery
Diabetic retinopathy	Vision loss is caused by macular edema and ischemia, vitreous hemorrhage, and retinal detachments.	Decreased/blurred vision, sudden loss of vision, floaters	Laser treatment and intravitreal injections; tight control of blood glucose and blood pressure

vision, and a red eye. Posterior uveitis presents with decreased vision and floaters.

Red eye is an extremely common eye complaint, the cause of which may be benign or malignant (Table 24.3). Hyperemia of the eye can accompany any inflammation or infection. Causes of red eye that require referral include corneal ulcers, which are usually accompanied by a visible white infiltrate on the cornea, anterior and posterior uveitis, herpes simplex and herpes zoster ophthalmicus, scleritis, angle-closure glaucoma, ocular surface tumors, and postoperative infections. The reason for referral is to prevent permanent vision loss, which can be the end point of any of these conditions. While it is sometimes difficult to differentiate one cause from another without a slit lamp ophthalmologic examination, signs and symptoms that should prompt referral are decreased vision, severe pain, photophobia, recent intraocular surgery, or even distant surgery (especially if glaucoma surgery).

Relatively benign causes of red eye include blepharitis or inflammation of the Meibomian glands in the eyelids, dry eye, allergic conjunctivitis, corneal exposure due to lid malposition, viral conjunctivitis, and subconjunctival hemorrhages. Blepharitis and dry eye often present together because blepharitis affects the integrity of the tear film, which then evaporates more readily. Tears serve several important functions, including corneal lubrication, debris clearance, and immune protection. With age, tear production decreases, and older adults are prone to develop keratitis sicca, characterized by redness, foreign body sensation, and reflex tearing. Patients may complain of severe eye discomfort and blurred vision, which usually improves with blinking or eye rubbing because these two maneuvers spread the remaining tear film over the cornea. Dry eye can be especially problematic in older women, in whom hormonal changes are thought to play a role. Keratitis sicca can also be associated

Table 24.2—Common Signs and Symptoms of Eye Conditions Requiring Immediate Referral to an Ophthalmologist

Condition	Symptoms and Signs
Retinal detachment	Flashes, floaters, decreased vision
Acute angle-closure glaucoma	Eye pain or headache, ocular hyperemia, dilated pupil, decreased vision, nausea, vomiting
Ischemic optic neuropathy	Sudden loss of vision (complete or partial) in one eye
Central artery occlusion or giant cell arteritis	Sudden painless loss of vision in one eye; if from giant cell arteritis, then review of symptoms may reveal accompanying jaw claudication, headache, transient diplopia, etc
Bacterial keratitis	Decreased vision, eye redness, pain, discharge
Scleritis	Eye redness, pain, decreased vision
Posterior uveitis	Floaters, decreased vision
Corneal ulcers	Eye redness, pain, decreased vision, corneal infiltrate
Uveitis	Photophobia, eye redness, decreased vision
Herpes zoster ophthalmicus	Eye redness, pain, burning, rash, decreased vision, light sensitivity

Table 24.3—Treatment of Eye Conditions Commonly Seen by Primary Care Providers

Condition	Treatment and/or Cause
Red eye	
Subconjunctival hemorrhage	Supportive treatment with artificial tears
Dry eye	Artificial tears, cyclosporin 0.2% eye drops
Blepharitis	Lid scrubs, ophthalmic antibiotic ointment qhs, oral doxycycline
Lid malposition/exposure	Ocular lubricant, refer for surgical repair
Allergic conjunctivitis	Cold compresses, allergen avoidance, topical/systemic antihistamines
Viral conjunctivitis	Supportive treatment with artificial tears; refer to ophthalmologist if vision significantly affected
Chalazion	Warm compresses, may refer for excision
Herpes simplex keratitis	Trifluridine eye drops, refer to ophthalmologist
Herpes zoster ophthalmicus	Tear drops, refer to ophthalmologist immediately
Angle-closure glaucoma	Pilocarpine 2% ophthalmic solution, refer to ophthalmologist immediately
Floaters, flashes	Refer to ophthalmologist immediately; may be retinal detachment or vitreous hemorrhage
Sudden decrease in vision	Refer to ophthalmologist immediately; may be secondary to a number of vision-threatening problems
Diplopia	
Monocular	Refractive error, cataract
Binocular	Microvascular infarct to cranial nerve, giant cell arteritis, compressive tumor

with autoimmune disease; conditions such as Sjögren's syndrome should be excluded. Management of dry eye includes tear replacement with artificial tears during the day (preservative-free tears if being used more than four times daily) and a lubricant ointment at bedtime. Topical cyclosporin A (0.2%) eye drops can be used for more severe cases of dry eye to combat the underlying ocular inflammation that affects tear production; however, caution is warranted in patients with a history of ocular herpetic infections. Treatment for accompanying blepharitis includes lid hygiene consisting of gentle scrubbing of the lash bases with nontearing baby shampoo twice daily and applying topical antibiotic ointment to the eyelids nightly. Oral doxycycline can also be a useful adjunct, especially when blepharitis is associated with acne rosacea. If symptoms continue despite these conservative measures, referral is warranted.

Viral conjunctivitis (or pink eye) is associated with severe tearing, mucous discharge, and matting of the eyelids, especially in the morning. Symptoms include eye irritation and blurred vision. Viral conjunctivitis is distinguished from bacterial conjunctivitis by history and, because it is highly contagious, patients frequently report either an upper respiratory tract infection or recent contact with someone suffering from a red eye. It is treated conservatively with warm compresses and artificial tears. Topical antibiotics are not indicated. If viral conjunctivitis is accompanied by severely reduced vision, the patient should be referred for an ophthalmologic examination, because corneal infiltrates can (rarely) develop, requiring steroid eye drops. Viral conjunctivitis is extremely contagious (by contact), and patient education is necessary to limit spread of the infection to the other eye or to contacts (including office staff).

Allergic conjunctivitis is a common benign condition; its hallmark is ocular pruritus. Patients should be advised to avoid known precipitants (eg, pet dander or cosmetics). Management of allergic conjunctivitis includes cool compresses, systemic antihistamines, topical antihistamines or decongestants, and ophthalmic corticosteroids for limited periods of time. Allergic conjunctivitis can also be an adverse event of some topical glaucoma medications. Usually, the conjunctivitis is accompanied by dermatitis of the eyelids. This problem should prompt referral to the ophthalmologist treating the glaucoma.

The use of ophthalmic corticosteroids merits comment. Ophthalmic steroid drops or ointment can have serious potential adverse events, including risks of ocular hypertension and glaucoma development (which can be asymptomatic for a long period of time), secondary infections, cataract formation, and corneal thinning if used in undiagnosed infections. Because of these risks, the prescription of ophthalmic corticosteroids is best limited to practitioners with the tools to monitor for these adverse events. The risk of adverse events increases greatly with prolonged use of steroid (months to years); therefore, prescriptions for any steroid-containing eye medication should never be refilled without ophthalmic evaluation. Ocular hypertension that can lead to glaucoma can develop within 2–3 weeks with daily use of topical steroid in susceptible individuals (those with glaucoma, either diagnosed or undiagnosed, or with a family history of glaucoma). Low-potency steroids given for 7–10 days will not be problematic for the vast majority of patients, but patients and caregivers should be warned of the risks of prolonged and unmonitored use of steroids in and around the eyes.

Lid abnormalities are a common problem for older adults. Because of the gradual loss of elasticity and tensile strength that develops with age, secondary degenerative changes can develop. Blepharochalasis (drooping of the brow) and blepharoptosis (drooping of the eyelid) can cause cosmetic deformity and, if severe, can impair vision. Lid ectropion or entropion (ie, eversion and inversion of the lid margins, respectively) can disrupt the ocular surface and cause discomfort. These conditions can be addressed by various surgical procedures. Ocular lubricant ointments (those without antibiotics) can be recommended to minimize discomfort from exposure of the globe. Older adults can also develop squamous cell and basal cell carcinomas of the eyelids. Ulcerations or chronic irritation, especially if associated with loss of eyelashes, should be evaluated by an ophthalmologist.

Herpes zoster ophthalmicus, or shingles, is a painful reactivation of varicella zoster virus that not uncommonly affects older adults. Dermatomal distribution of weeping vesicles affecting the ophthalmic branch of the trigeminal nerve is the classic presentation. Ocular involvement can be signaled by lesions on the tip of the nose (Hutchinson sign) and can include dendritic keratopathy or uveitis. Oral acyclovir can shorten the course of disease. Trifluridine eye drops are indicated for herpes simplex dendriform corneal ulcers (not for herpes zoster). Post-herpetic neuralgia can be quite debilitating; systemic medications (narcotics, tricyclic antidepressants[OL], gabapentin, pregabalin) can reduce pain, and less often, topical agents such as capsaicin and lidocaine patches can be tried (these should not be used near the eye—capsaicin can be extremely irritating to the eye, and lidocaine can anesthetize the eye, placing the patient at risk of eye injury while the eye is numb). See also "Dermatologic Diseases and Disorders," p 350.

Subconjunctival hemorrhages are very common and, despite being benign, elicit worried responses from patients. Many patients are on a blood thinner, and minor trauma such as eye rubbing, which usually is not recalled by the patient, can cause a small blood vessel to tear and bleed. Artificial tears are recommended for comfort until the hemorrhage clears. If the patient is on warfarin, checking an INR, if not done recently, may be prudent.

Other common conditions seen in older adults include cataracts, macular degeneration, glaucoma, and ischemic optic neuropathy, which are discussed more fully in the following sections.

Refractive Error and Cataracts

The leading causes of visual impairment worldwide are refractive error and cataracts, for which eyeglasses and surgical cataract extraction, respectively, are mainstays of treatment. Despite the considerable successes of these therapeutic options, many populations do not receive adequate treatment for these problems.

Refractive error can be categorized as emmetropia (neutral refraction), ametropia, or presbyopia. Three forms of ametropia exist: myopia (nearsightedness), hyperopia (farsightedness), and astigmatism (distorted vision). Typically, older adults have increasing hyperopia, unless a cataract is present, which can induce a myopic shift. Although contact lens wear and laser refractive surgery are available for myopic and hyperopic refractive errors, these forms of refractive treatment are not favored by older people. Corneal refractive surgery, such as LASIK, is not the best remedy for refractive problems in older adults who usually have some degree of cataracts. Removal of the cataract and replacement with an artificial intraocular lens, the power of which can be chosen to eliminate refractive error, is a better option in older adults. Toric intraocular lenses can correct astigmatism, and multifocal lenses can decrease the need for eyeglasses after surgery. After the age of approximately 40, emmetropic individuals begin to develop progressive presbyopia, impaired ability to focus on near objects that is caused by gradual hardening of the lens and decreased muscular effectiveness of the ciliary body. Reading glasses can be obtained OTC, or bifocal eyeglasses can be prescribed.

Approximately 20% of adults ≥65 years old and 50% of adults ≥75 years old have cataracts, a lens opacity that reduces vision. Cataracts can be associated with increased glare symptoms, decreased contrast sensitivity, and decreased visual acuity that is not correctable by glasses. The most important risk factor is increased age; other risk factors include decreased vitamin intake, light (ultraviolet B) exposure, smoking, alcohol use, long-term corticosteroid use, and diabetes mellitus.

Cataract extraction is one of the most successful surgeries in medicine (90% of patients achieve vision of 20/40 or better). Approximately 3 million cataract procedures are performed each year in the United States. The benefits of cataract surgery include not only improved vision but also a decreased rate of falls (SOE=B) and improved vision-related quality of life (SOE=A).

Indications for cataract surgery are a decrease in vision that affects ability to perform activities of daily living, such as reading, driving, and playing sports or hobbies, among others. Cataract extraction is safe and can be completed in <30 min under local or topical anesthesia. The surgery involves the breakdown of the lens by ultrasound energy and its aspiration (phacoemulsification). An artificial implant (intraocular lens) is placed in the capsular bag, which is the only remnant of the native lens retained. A secondary laser procedure (capsulotomy) may be necessary to ablate subsequent capsular opacification that can develop in ≥15% of patients.

AGE-RELATED MACULAR DEGENERATION (ARMD)

ARMD is the most common cause of irreversible blindness in older adults throughout the developed world. Increasing age is the most important risk factor, although a genetic predisposition is also contributory. Currently, there is no role for genetic screening as a clinical tool, because it is not yet clear how to use this information. Other risk factors include smoking and hypertension. Fair-skinned individuals are at greater risk of developing this disease than are black individuals, in whom pigment may serve as a protective element. Exposure to ultraviolet light is a debated risk factor. Researchers are also looking at links between ARMD and Alzheimer disease because both are common in older adults.

ARMD is classified into two forms, dry and wet. The dry form is much more common and is characterized by deposits of macular drusen. Drusen, submacular yellow lipoprotein deposits composed of metabolic by-products, do not typically cause vision loss but are a marker for the wet form of ARMD, which is characterized by angiogenesis or choroidal neovascularization (CNV). The presence of larger, more numerous drusen conveys the greatest risk of development of CNV. The Age-Related Eye Disease Study (AREDS) found that the risk of CNV development could be decreased by 25% (ARR of 8% for progression to advanced ARMD, and 6% for loss of vision of 3 lines or more) when patients with high-risk drusen are treated with high-dose oral multivitamin therapy (SOE=A).

Combination multivitamins containing β-carotene 25,000 IU, vitamin E 400 IU, vitamin C 500 mg, and zinc 80 mg are available OTC. Supplements are recommended indefinitely or until the wet form of ARMD develops, which then necessitates other treatment. This vitamin therapy, however, is contraindicated in smokers because of the higher risk of lung cancer with use of β-carotene supplements. High-dose vitamin A and β-carotene are also associated with risk of osteoporosis. The formulation of the combination multivitamins used in AREDS (listed above) is not recommended for patients with less than high-risk drusen (because they have a low baseline risk of progressing to wet ARMD). The prophylactic benefit of other vitamin A derivatives, lutein and zeaxanthine, in preventing progression to the wet type of ARMD is being assessed in a follow-up study (AREDS II). Patients with the dry form of ARMD should be examined periodically by an ophthalmologist for the development of early signs of CNV. CNV in wet ARMD is marked by the presence of subretinal fluid and blood that may appear as a gray-green membrane (Figure 24.1). The development of CNV is signaled by sudden vision loss or distortion of vision and requires urgent evaluation, because untreated CNV can lead to severe central vision loss. The natural history of CNV is progressive subfoveal growth and leakage with eventual fibrotic scarring and central blindness.

Angiogenesis inhibition has proved to be a major breakthrough in the treatment of CNV. Various inhibitors of vascular endothelial growth factor (VEGF) have been approved by the FDA for treatment of wet ARMD. Serial intravitreal injections (9 per year) of pegaptanib sodium, an anti-VEGF aptamer or mRNA oligonucleotide that inhibits mRNA synthesis, are approved for the treatment of all subtypes of wet ARMD. These injections do not typically improve vision, but they do reduce the risk of further vision loss. Another antiangiogenesis inhibitor, ranibizumab, is a fragment antibody that exhibits broad-spectrum inhibition of VEGF. In a multicenter, prospective randomized clinical trial, visual acuity improved by approximately 2 lines in patients with CNV treated with ranibizumab compared with those given sham treatments (absolute risk reduction [ARR]

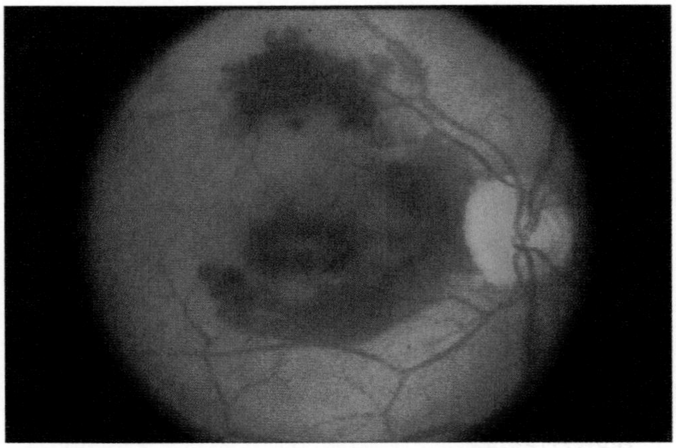

Figure 24.1—Choroidal neovascularization in the wet form of age-related macular degeneration, demonstrating a gray-green membrane associated with subretinal hemorrhage

=33%, number needed to treat [NNT] =3 [SOE=A]). Serial intravitreal injections of ranibizumab are now the gold standard of care for all subtypes of wet ARMD (ANCHOR and MARINA trials). Ranibizumab costs $2,000 per vial, and one vial is needed per eye. The manufacturer has recommended an injection every month for 2 years ($48,000). However, most clinicians are giving a monthly injection for 3–4 months per eye, monitoring, and reinjecting as needed when neovascularization recurs. Injections may be necessary indefinitely. Bevacizumab is another VEGF inhibitor related to the ranibizumab molecule that has shown promise as being equally efficacious and is significantly less expensive than ranibizumab, although it is not approved by the FDA for treatment of wet ARMD. In 2011, the Comparison of AMD Treatments Trial (CATT) sponsored by the National Institutes of Health published 1-year results from a 2-year multicenter randomized controlled trial comparing ranibizumab and bevacizumab for wet ARMD in which the primary outcome measure was visual improvement. Visual improvement was not significantly different for either group at 1 year, whether receiving monthly injections or an as-needed schedule of injections, although the as-needed bevacizumab group fared the poorest (SOE=A). Anatomically, monthly ranibizumab injections were most effective in clearing macular edema. Serious adverse events (primarily hospitalizations) occurred at a 24% rate for patients receiving bevacizumab and a 19% rate for patients receiving ranibizumab. Clinical trials of avastin for cancer used a much higher dose of avastin systemically (500 times higher than that injected into the eye for macular degeneration). The cancer trials did not report many of the adverse events seen in the CATT trial. The CATT trial adverse events may be due to the older age of macular degeneration patients and the underlying health problems that an older population tends to have, rather than to the effects of the drug per se. The number of deaths, heart attacks, and strokes were low and similar for both drugs during the study. More information will be forthcoming as the study finishes its 2-year follow-up. There is yet a fourth medication newly approved by the FDA but not yet marketed called VEGF Trap-Eye. It is a fusion protein that has greater binding affinity of VEGF-A than ranibizumab and bevacizumab. In addition to binding all forms of VEGF-A, it binds placental growth factor. The advantage of VEGF Trap-Eye will be a longer duration of action and, therefore, less frequent injections.

DIABETIC RETINOPATHY

Duration of disease, control of blood glucose, and control of blood pressure are the most important variables in the development and progression of diabetic retinopathy. After 10 years, 70% of those with type 2 diabetes have some form of retinopathy, and nearly 10% show proliferative disease. Diet control, exercise, blood pressure control (target <130/80 mmHg), and maintaining glycosylated hemoglobin concentrations at <7% are general recommendations approved by the American Diabetes Association that can be reasonably applied to older adults without preexisting vascular disease who have a remaining life expectancy of >5–7 years. The Diabetic Control and Complications Trial demonstrated that tight control of blood glucose in individuals with type 1 diabetes resulted in a long-lasting decrease in the rate of development and progression of diabetic retinopathy. The United Kingdom Prospective Diabetes Study (UKPDS) validated these results in an older population with type 2 diabetes. Tight blood glucose control was shown to decrease the need for the studies' primary outcome measures (ie, the need for laser) and the level of retinopathy; therefore, it was indirectly shown to influence and benefit vision, although some authors have questioned this surrogate measure. For example, a patient with poor control of blood glucose is more likely to progress to preproliferative and proliferative levels of retinopathy and need surgery, which is more likely to result in poor vision. The benefit of tight glucose control reduced the need for laser therapy within 3–4 years in the groups with no baseline retinopathy and within 2–3 years in the groups with mild to moderate baseline retinopathy; however, most other studies and guidelines indicate that 7–8 years of tight control are needed to show microvascular benefits. However, tight control of blood pressure (≤130/80 mmHg) is an important factor in decreasing microvascular complications, and becomes evident within 2–3 years.

More recent data from the ACCORD, ADVANCE, and VADT studies have raised the question of whether intensive glycemic control is of enough benefit to outweigh the risks of hypoglycemia. The ACCORD study was stopped early because of excessive mortality in the intensive control group (relative risk increase 20%, absolute risk increase 1.0%, number needed to harm 100) and showed no significant benefit for macro- or microvascular disease in a group of patients of average age 62 years old and longstanding diabetes. The ADVANCE study showed reductions in microvascular disease; however, the significant benefits were in reductions of albuminuria rather than retinopathy. In contrast to the ACCORD study, a follow-up of UKPDS found evidence of a "legacy effect," of benefits of intensive control early in the course of the disease. In a group of patients followed for 10 years after the end of the trial, intensive control during the trial reduced microvascular disease (in the group treated with sulfonylureas plus insulin and in the group treated with metformin) even though patients had not maintained the low target hemoglobin A_{1c} levels. The results of these studies prompted significant controversy in both the lay press and the medical literature, and led the American Diabetes Association, the American Heart Association, and the American College of Cardiology to issue a revised position statement in 2009 about the value of intensive control in type 2 diabetes mellitus. In this statement, the recommended hemoglobin A_{1c} target remains 7.5%–7.9%; however, it notes that targets should be individualized and that patients with limited life expectancy, those with longstanding diabetes mellitus, and those with preexisting vascular disease are less likely to benefit from intensive control. Many, and probably most, geriatric patients fall into the latter categories; thus, the benefits of intensive control need to be very carefully weighed against the potential for harm. The risk of hypoglycemia is significantly greater in those who are frail, demented, or otherwise unable to comply with medical regimens and merit particular attention.

Other systemic risk factors, including kidney function and serum cholesterol, can also influence the course of diabetic retinopathy and should be optimized. ACE inhibitors decrease progressive nephropathy in diabetic patients and may have similar benefits on the retina.

Patients with type 2 diabetes require baseline ophthalmologic screening at diagnosis of systemic disease and annually thereafter. Subsequent follow-up depends on the grade of retinopathy. Nonproliferative diabetic retinopathy, the earliest stage of retinopathy, can first be manifested by retinal microaneurysms. Intraretinal hemorrhages and exudates, with or without associated macular edema, can ensue. Progressive ischemia characterized by increasing hemorrhages, venous caliber changes or intraretinal microvascular abnormalities or both, and capillary nonperfusion on fluorescein angiography characterize the preproliferative stage of diabetic retinopathy. About 40% of patients with preproliferative retinopathy develop proliferative diabetic retinopathy within 1–2 years, characterized by neovascularization or new blood vessel growth of the retina or disc, or both.

Visual loss in patients with diabetes can occur as a result of macular nonperfusion or macular edema. The Early Treatment Diabetic Retinopathy Study demonstrated the benefit of focal or grid laser photocoagulation in stabilizing and improving vision in diabetic patients with clinically significant macular edema (Figure 24.2). Neovascularization (Figure 24.3) can cause severe vision loss or blindness in proliferative diabetic retinopathy as a result of vitreous hemorrhage or tractional retinal detachment. Proliferative diabetic retinopathy is amenable to treatment by panretinal laser photocoagulation to inhibit the growth stimulus for neovascularization. In the Diabetic Retinopathy Study, incidence of severe visual loss in patients treated with panretinal photocoagulation was 11%, but the incidence in those who did not receive laser during a 2-year follow-up was 26%. Pars plana vitrectomy, membrane peeling, and endolaser can address nonclearing vitreous hemorrhage or tractional macular detachment surgically.

Although not approved by the FDA for the care of diabetic retinopathy, intravitreal anti-VEGF or steroid therapy is an important adjunct to laser therapy that is not uncommonly used to treat recalcitrant or cystoid diabetic macular edema. Intravitreal bevacizumab therapy has also been used for high-risk proliferative retinopathy.

GLAUCOMA

Glaucoma is the second most common cause of irreversible blindness worldwide and, in the United States, the most common cause of blindness in black Americans. It affects more than 2.25 million Americans ≥40 years old and results in >3 million office visits each year. The financial burden is considerable because of the prevalence and chronicity of glaucoma and the debilitation that results. Glaucoma-related Medicare and Medicaid payments and disability are reported to reach as high as $1 billion.

The definition of glaucoma has evolved considerably, and it is now defined as characteristic optic nerve head damage and visual field loss. Increased intraocular pressure (IOP) is no longer considered an absolute criterion, although it is a very important risk factor. There are many different types of glaucoma, of which primary open-angle glaucoma (POAG) is the most common. Adults >50 years old should be screened for glaucoma every 1–2 years. Older adults with a family

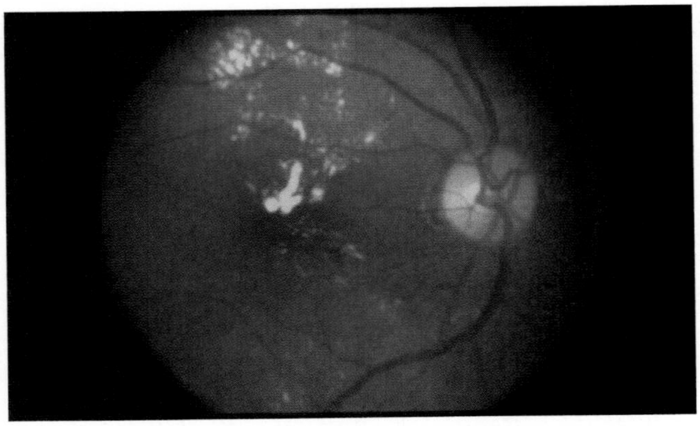

Figure 24.2—Intraretinal edema and exudate in the superior macular region consistent with clinically significant macular edema in a patient with type 2 diabetes mellitus

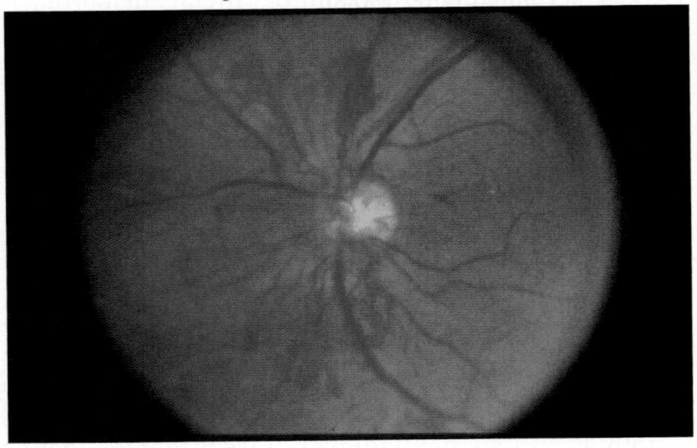

Figure 24.3—Florid neovascularization of the disc in a patient with high-risk proliferative diabetic retinopathy

history of glaucoma, black ethnicity, or other risk factors may need more frequent screening.

POAG is a chronic disease most commonly affecting older adults. The "clogged" drain of the eye impairs passage of aqueous humor out of the angle. Slow aqueous drainage leads to chronically increased IOPs. This is in contrast to acute angle-closure glaucoma, in which the eye's drain is suddenly blocked off, IOP increases precipitously, and the patient has considerable redness and pain with acute vision loss. Pain may be so severe as to cause headache, nausea, and vomiting. Emergent ophthalmologic referral is required to reverse the angle closure and decrease the IOP through the use of aqueous suppressants, miotics, and laser iridotomy. Conversely, the increase in IOP in POAG is slow and much less severe. Individuals with POAG are asymptomatic and can suffer substantial field loss before consulting an ophthalmologist, which underscores the importance of regular ophthalmologic screening of older adults.

Development of POAG is most likely multifactorial and polygenic. Initial pedigrees demonstrated linkage to the 1q locus. Subsequent investigations have more precisely defined the GLC1A gene that encodes for myocilin, the trabecular meshwork-induced glucocorticoid response protein. Several other chromosomal loci, including those mapped to chromosomes 2, 3, 7, and 10, are also associated with the development of glaucoma.

The management of POAG can be approached by the ophthalmologist in a stepwise manner. A variety of IOP-lowering medications, both local and systemic, are available. Mechanisms of action include decreased aqueous production or increased aqueous outflow. Various eye drop formulations are available; α_2-adrenergic agonists that decrease aqueous production and prostaglandin analogs that increase uveal-scleral outflow are two relatively new and effective drug types, but they may have adverse events (Table 24.4). In the face of visual field progression despite maximal medications, intolerance to medications, or inability to comply with eye drop administration (eg, because of problems such as rheumatoid arthritis or dementia), argon laser trabeculoplasty (application of laser energy to the trabecular meshwork) can be effective in lowering IOP in approximately 50% of patients for 3–5 years after treatment. Intraocular surgery involves the creation of a fistula or filtration site to allow an alternative route of aqueous egress (trabeculectomy). Adjunctive antimetabolite use with 5-fluorouracil[OL] or mitomycin-C[OL] has increased the success of this procedure in those patients at high risk of surgical failure because of fibrosis and scarring of the filtration site. Alternative surgeries for glaucoma include drainage devices or aqueous shunts. Drainage devices, which are made of a foreign material such as plastic, shunt fluid from the anterior chamber to the subconjunctival space. Cryotherapy or laser procedures to destroy the ciliary body (cyclocryoablation or cyclophotocoagulation) can be used when the prognosis for vision in the eye is poor.

The strength of evidence is high in support of treating ocular hypertension to prevent the onset of glaucoma and of treating prevalent glaucoma to slow down progression of disease. Based on a meta-analysis of the literature, 12 ocular hypertensive patients need to be treated to prevent 1 patient from developing visual field defects or optic nerve changes consistent with glaucoma (SOE=A). From a meta-analysis of literature on treatment of established glaucoma patients, the NNT to prevent 1 glaucoma patient from progressive vision damage within 5 years of treatment is 7. The ARR is 14.2%.

Anterior Ischemic Optic Neuropathy

Anterior ischemic optic neuropathy (Figure 24.4) can result in acute vision or field loss. Microvascular occlusion of the blood supply to the optic nerve can

Table 24.4—Adverse Events of Selected Eye Drops for Glaucoma

Class	Adverse Events
Aqueous suppressants	
α-Agonists (eg, brimonidine)	Allergic dermatoconjunctivitis, dry mouth/nose, mental status changes occasionally
β-Blockers (eg, timolol)	Bradycardia, dyspnea, asthma, heart failure exacerbations, impotence, exercise intolerance, hypoglycemia masking
Carbonic anhydrase inhibitors (eg, dorzolamide)	Blurry vision, stinging, bad taste in mouth, allergic dermatoconjunctivitis
Aqueous outflow facilitators	
Epinephrine (eg, dipivefrin)	Palpitations, angina, cystoid macular edema
Miotics (eg, pilocarpine)	Brow ache, blurriness, detached retina, small pupils
Prostaglandins (eg, latanoprost)	Hyperemia, increased length and thickness and darkness of eyelashes, increased iris and eyelid pigmentation, orbital fat atrophy, cystoid macular edema, exacerbation of herpetic eye disease

be attributed to atherosclerotic vascular disease or inflammation in the setting of giant cell (temporal) arteritis. The nonarteritic form typically affects patients with vasculopathic risk factors such as diabetes mellitus and hypertension; the latter, the arteritic form, tends to occur in older adults with a history of myalgias, headaches, and weight loss. An increased Westergren erythrocyte sedimentation rate and a positive temporal artery biopsy are diagnostic. Systemic corticosteroid treatment is crucial to avoid visual loss in the other eye.

Low-Vision Rehabilitation

Despite considerable advancements in the medical treatment of ocular conditions, many patients, especially those with the wet form of ARMD, can ultimately sustain permanent visual loss. Visual training and the provision of visual aids are indispensable services for those with low vision (visual acuity <20/60).

Patients with low vision can develop useful adaptive skills with proper instruction. Eccentric viewing by ARMD patients with central macular pathology uses the principle of off-center fixation. The patient can benefit from formal training to find and use the most effective eccentric viewing points. Instruction in scanning and tracking and other skills can help the patient integrate his or her visual environment.

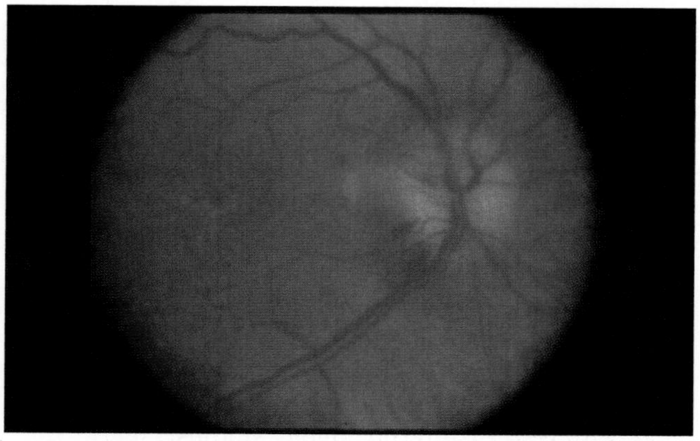

Figure 24.4—Pallid swelling of the optic nerve head in a patient with anterior ischemic optic neuropathy

Various low-vision aids are available to improve the ability to see both near and far. The fine detail required for reading is the most common indication for visual aids. Improved lighting is a simple modification that can enhance visualization of print. Selection of reading material using bold, enlarged fonts and accentuated black-on-white contrast can also be helpful. Magnification also is commonly used. Various devices such as high-plus spectacles, hand-held magnifiers, stand magnifiers, and closed-circuit television can also enhance reading. Distance magnification can be achieved with the use of telescopic devices that can be hand-held for spot viewing or spectacle mounted for continual viewing. Talking devices, which are computers used to create voice synthesis such as those used at stoplights, or Braille can be especially helpful for those who have completely lost vision.

References

- ACCORD Study Group; ACCORD Eye Study Group, Chew EY, Ambrosius WT, Davis MD, et al. Effects of medical therapies on retinopathy progression in type 2 diabetes. *N Engl J Med.* 2010;363(3):233–244.
- CATT Research Group, Martin DF, Maguire MG, Ying GS, et al. Ranibizumab and bevacizumab for neovascular age-related macular degeneration. *N Engl J Med.* 2011;364(20):1897–1908.
- Cronau H, Kankanala RR, Mauger T. Diagnosis and management of red eye in primary care. *Am Fam Physician.* 2010;81(2):137–144.
- Quantifying the effect of intraocular pressure reduction on the occurrence of glaucoma. *Acta Ophthalmologica.* 2010;88(1):5–11.
- Sharts-Hopko N. Low vision and blindness among midlife and older adults: A review of the nursing research literature. *Holistic Nurs Pract.* 2009;23(2):94–100.

CHAPTER 25—HEARING IMPAIRMENT

KEY POINTS

- Hearing loss is among the most common chronic diseases among older adults: 10% of adults 65–75 years old and 25% of those >75 years old have hearing loss.
- Treatment of hearing loss and attention to communication strategies can improve quality of life for individuals with hearing impairment.
- Important issues when considering hearing aids for an older adult with hearing loss are the nature and degree of hearing loss, the person's ability to manipulate the aid and adapt to its use, and the person's social support and financial resources.

Hearing loss is the fourth most common chronic disease among older adults. Hearing impairment is often assumed to be benign, but it has profound effects on quality of life. The psychologic effects of hearing loss include family discord, social isolation, loss of self-esteem, anger, and depression. Epidemiologic studies suggest an association between hearing loss and cognitive impairment, and between hearing loss and reduced mobility. Hearing loss can also affect an older adult's interaction with clinicians, making history taking and patient education difficult. Treatment of hearing loss and attention to communication strategies can improve quality of life for individuals with hearing impairment by facilitating interaction with family, friends, and caregivers. Studies indicate that use of a hearing aid can relieve symptoms of depression that are associated with hearing loss.

NORMAL HEARING AND AGE-RELATED CHANGES IN THE AUDITORY SYSTEM

The normal ear is an efficient transducer of sound energy into nerve impulses. Sound energy is transmitted through the external ear to the tympanic membrane and the auditory ossicles. The malleus, incus, and stapes in series transmit vibrations to the oval window of the cochlea. Fluid waves within the cochlea stimulate the outer hair cells of the scala tympani. These cells stimulate the inner hair cells, which generate impulses that are sent via cochlear neurons to the cochlear nuclei and then to auditory pathways elsewhere in the brain.

Age-related changes in the auditory system can interfere with its function. The walls of the external ear canal become thin. Cerumen becomes drier and more tenacious, increasing the likelihood of cerumen impaction. The tympanic membrane becomes thicker and appears duller in older adults than in younger people. The ossicular joints undergo degenerative changes, but this generally does not interfere with sound transmission to the cochlea. Cochlear changes include loss of sensory hair cells and fibrocytes in the organ of Corti, stiffening of the basilar membrane, calcification of auditory structures, and cochlear neuronal loss. Changes in the stria vascularis include thickening of capillaries, decreased production of endolymph, and decreased Na^+/K^+-ATPase activity. These degenerative changes occur to varying degrees in different individuals. It is currently not possible to fully correlate the degree of hearing loss with histologic changes in the aging ear.

Changes in central auditory processing also occur with aging. In one study, when competing speech stimuli were presented to each ear, the right ear had a 5%–10% advantage over the left ear in younger people (the effect of right- and left-handedness was not assessed; all the participants were right-handed). In adults 80–89 years old, this difference increased to >40%. This difference may be related to a loss of efficiency of transfer of auditory information from one side of the brain to the other through the corpus callosum.

EPIDEMIOLOGY

Hearing loss can result from dysfunction of the auditory system at any point from the external ear to the brain. This loss can be described in terms of the loss of ability to hear pure tones across the range of audio frequencies important for understanding speech, but in practical terms, impairment of the ability to understand spoken language and to perceive environmental sounds significantly affects quality of life. The prevalence of hearing loss increases with age. Ten percent of adults 65–75 years old and 25% of those >75 years old have hearing loss. In nursing homes, estimates of prevalence vary from 50% to 100%, depending on the criteria used to define hearing loss.

In addition to age, male sex is a risk factor for hearing loss. Loss of hearing in the higher audio frequencies is associated with noise exposure; higher levels of education are associated with a lower prevalence of hearing loss. Black race is associated with a lower risk of age-associated hearing loss. The association of hearing loss with cardiovascular risk factors is less clear, with results differing among studies.

Hearing loss can be caused by pathology in the external ear canal, the middle ear, the inner ear, the auditory nerve, central auditory pathways, or a combination of these.

Conductive hearing loss is caused by disease in the external ear, such as cerumen impaction or a foreign body in the canal, or by middle-ear pathology, such as otosclerosis, cholesteatoma, tympanic membrane perforation, or middle-ear effusion.

Sensorineural hearing loss is most often caused by cochlear disease. Noise is the most common factor in cochlear damage. Hearing loss is less common among people in quiet rural environments than among those in industrialized communities. Other causes of hearing loss include ototoxic medications, genotype, vascular disease, and rarely, occupational and environmental chemical exposures. Smokers have higher rates of hearing loss than nonsmokers. Autoimmune disease and auditory nerve tumors are rare causes of sensorineural hearing loss. Neuronal loss can affect the brain stem and cortical ascending auditory pathways. The resulting deficits in central auditory processing can affect perception of sound and the ability to understand speech. These deficits are not apparent on a simple audiogram.

PRESBYCUSIS

Most hearing loss in older adults is categorized as presbycusis (literally, "older hearing"). Presbycusis is a sensorineural, usually symmetrical hearing loss. It is usually due to cochlear pathology but may have central components. Many people with presbycusis can be helped by amplification, especially if speech discrimination is preserved.

Sensory presbycusis is attributed to a loss of sensory hair cells in the basal end of the cochlea. It is often slowly progressing, beginning with the higher frequencies. It can involve the higher portion of the range of frequencies in human speech. Loss of auditory acuity can begin when people are in their twenties but may not become clinically evident until later decades. People with this type of hearing loss often have trouble hearing in the presence of background noise but are able to hear adequately in quiet settings. Amplification often helps these patients, because speech discrimination is satisfactory.

Strial presbycusis results from atrophy of the stria vascularis. It typically begins between the ages of 20 and 60 years old and is characterized by mild to moderate hearing loss in most frequencies. People with strial presbycusis usually have good speech discrimination and do well with amplification.

Neural presbycusis is caused by a cochlear neuronal loss of ≥50%. Despite preserved pure-tone thresholds, which are not affected until >90% of cochlear neurons have been lost, individuals with neural presbycusis show very poor speech discrimination. Successful use of amplification is difficult for this form of presbycusis.

Cochlear conductive presbycusis is caused by changes in cochlear mechanics produced by mass or stiffness changes or spiral ligament atrophy. It has a unique audiogram, which gradually descends over at least five octaves with no more than a 25-dB difference between any two adjacent frequencies. Speech discrimination can also be impaired. Pathologically, this form is defined by the absence of histologic changes seen in the other forms of presbycusis.

Most presbycusis is probably a mixture of these forms. The shape of the audiogram and speech discrimination scores depend on the extent of injury to various components of the cochlea.

CLINICAL PRESENTATION AND SCREENING

It is common for patients with hearing loss not to bring it to medical attention. Partly because of the slowly progressive nature of hearing loss, many older adults are unaware of their hearing deficit. They may also be unaware of advances in hearing instrument technology that can help people who did not benefit from older devices. In some cases, the perceived stigma of wearing a hearing aid causes the patient to deny the problem. The hearing loss may be brought to medical attention by family members, who complain that the patient does not hear them or plays the television or radio too loudly. Clinicians may notice that the patient does not respond when spoken to by someone out of the patient's field of view, or seems to misunderstand questions. Hearing loss can also be interpreted as cognitive impairment. Caregivers and clinicians may not recognize the presence of hearing loss or may assume it is a benign component of aging.

Tinnitus, or "ringing in the ears," can be an early sign of hearing loss. Individuals with tinnitus or buzzing should be evaluated by an otolaryngologist. Medical treatment for tinnitus is often unsuccessful, but hearing aids for those with hearing loss, or the use of devices that provide background white noise, may be useful to reduce the impact of tinnitus.

Screening programs to identify hearing loss are important. Fitting hearing aids early in the course of hearing loss can help the person adjust to their use (SOE=B), and treatment can reduce psychologic morbidity related to hearing loss (SOE=A). The Hearing Handicap Inventory for the Elderly—Screening Version is a 10-item questionnaire that asks about difficulty with communication in various settings. It can be useful to determine the impact that hearing loss has on a patient's daily activities. A handheld otoscope with a tone generator can be used by primary care providers to screen for the presence of hearing loss at selected frequencies (0.5, 1, 2, and 4 kHz) and two loudness levels (25 and 40 dB hearing loss). This device should be used in a quiet environment. When set at 40 dB hearing loss, testing at 1 and 2 kHz has a sensitivity of 94% and a specificity of 82%–90% for detecting hearing loss. A similar device costs $660–$900 with accessories; the cost of using it would not be directly reimbursable by third-party payors. When a screening test is consistent with hearing loss and the patient is willing and able to pay for a hearing aid, referral to an audiologist should be discussed.

EVALUATION OF SUSPECTED HEARING LOSS

The ear canals should be examined with an otoscope to exclude the presence of obstruction or effusion before referral for audiologic testing. Medications should be reviewed for their potential contribution to hearing loss. Furosemide and salicylates can cause reversible hearing loss. Other medications, such as aminoglycosides and vancomycin, can cause irreversible sensorineural hearing loss and should be used only with caution.

Cerumen impaction can cause a clinically significant hearing loss, as much as 40 dB. If the patient has a history of tympanic membrane surgery or perforation, referral to an otolaryngologist for removal of the impaction is advisable. Otherwise, cerumen can be removed by manual extraction in cooperative patients. Cerumenolytics alone, used for several days, are effective about 40% of the time in treating cerumen impaction. Alternatively, cerumenolytics or saline can be applied to soften the wax 15–30 min before irrigating the ear with warm water. If irrigation fails, using a cerumenolytic for several days may clear the impaction or soften it enough that repeat irrigation is successful. If the impaction remains, the patient should be referred to an otolaryngologist.

The otolaryngologist will further evaluate the hearing loss and identify treatable causes. An asymmetrical hearing loss demands thorough investigation. Auditory nerve tumors are rare, but tumors of the posterior pharynx can obstruct the eustachian tube, causing a middle-ear effusion with conductive hearing loss.

The audiologist will assess hearing to determine the presence and type of hearing loss. A comprehensive audiologic assessment consists of pure-tone thresholds for both air and bone conduction, speech-recognition thresholds, speech discrimination, and middle-ear function. This information, along with the medical evaluation, is used to determine appropriate treatment. Audiologists recommend and fit hearing aids and provide auditory rehabilitation. Medicare will pay for an audiologic examination if it is ordered by a physician.

Table 25.1—Strategies to Improve Communication with Hearing-Impaired People

- ***Ask the listener what is the best way to communicate with him or her.***
- Obtain the listener's attention before speaking.
- Eliminate background noise as much as possible.
- Be sure the listener can see the speaker's lips:
  - Speak face-to-face in the same room.
  - Do not obscure the lips with hands or other objects.
  - Make certain that light shines directly on the speaker's face, not from behind the speaker.
- Speak slowly and clearly, but avoid shouting.
- Speak toward the better ear, if applicable.
- Change phrasing if the listener does not understand at first.
- Spell words out, use gestures, or write them down.
- Have the listener repeat back what he or she heard.

TREATMENT

Some causes of hearing loss are amenable to medical or surgical treatment. Paget disease of the bone can affect the middle ear, causing conductive loss, or the inner ear, leading to sensorineural loss. Bisphosphonate therapy rarely restores hearing, although it may stabilize hearing loss (SOE=C). Otosclerosis or tympanosclerosis may be correctable with surgery (SOE=C). Otosclerosis may respond to bisphosphonate therapy (SOE=C). Sudden hearing loss may be autoimmune in nature and sometimes responds to corticosteroids (SOE=B) or immunosuppressant therapy (SOE=C). Most older adults with hearing loss are treated with communication strategies or amplification, or both. Hearing aids often improve ability to understand speech, particularly soft speech and conversational loud speech (SOE=B). Almost all hearing aids currently sold use digital sound processing to limit noise to comfortable levels and to reduce feedback, and have dual microphones for reduction of background noise. They may have automatic volume control.

Surgical treatment of sensorineural hearing loss may include implantation of prosthetic devices (see bone-anchored hearing aids and cochlear implants, below).

Strategies to Enhance Communication

Hearing-impaired individuals should be encouraged to let others know about their hearing loss and to suggest strategies that will help them communicate more easily (Table 25.1). In addition to using these strategies, clinicians should provide options for patients with hearing loss, such as sign language interpreters, the use of writing materials (eg, pen and paper, dry-erase board, or computer screen), or assistive devices. Office and hospital staff should be alerted to a patient's hearing loss. Background noise from the environment can interfere with hearing and should be reduced as much as possible.

Lipreading can be a useful adjunct to listening, but it requires thoughtfulness on the part of the speaker. When speaking to a hearing-impaired person who lip-reads, it is important to face him or her and to obtain the person's attention before speaking; a gentle touch on the hand or arm will usually suffice. Each word should be spoken clearly and distinctly. Shouting not only distorts lip movements so they are harder to read but also can make the speaker sound angry even when not. It is best to speak in complete sentences; single words are hard to lip-read because the listener often needs cues from context to identify meaning. It is helpful to make certain the person knows the topic of conversation. The language used should be appropriate for the listener's educational level. Unlike deaf persons who have usually had hearing impairment all or most of their lives, most older adults with hearing loss do not know sign language. Sometimes, amplification and lipreading are not enough. Gestures can aid communication even with cognitively impaired individuals.

For patients with hearing impairment, it can also be helpful to write words down. For those with both hearing and visual impairment, large printing with a marker pen or a laptop computer screen with magnified print may be necessary. These patients may benefit from correction of the visual problem, if possible (eg, cataract removal or use of eyeglasses). In any case, providing written instructions generally improves understanding and retention of important information.

The clinician should be alert to misunderstandings, which are common. If a reply does not make sense, repeating the idea of what was said using different words can help, as can asking the patient to express what he or she heard.

Assistive Listening Devices

For some people with hearing impairment, a personal amplifier may be more useful than hearing aids. These pocket-sized devices are considerably less expensive than hearing aids and are harder to misplace. Headphones stay on the head better than earbuds and provide sound to both ears. The volume and microphone placement of the amplifier should be adjusted to find the best combination for a given user. At least one or two of these devices should be available in every healthcare facility; these devices are not personalized and so can be used by different people.

Adaptive equipment can facilitate telephone use. State agencies may provide amplified telephones, vibrating and flashing ringer alert devices, and text telephones (TTY) or captioned telephones to hearing-impaired people. This equipment can also be purchased from retailers of assistive devices. Text telephones can be contacted through telecommunications relay services by dialing 711, then the number. A communications assistant transcribes the caller's voice into text that is displayed for the listener. Captioned telephones and Web-based captioning services allow the user to hear the caller's voice and then to read a transcription of the caller's voice during the call.

Many other assistive devices are available. Television listening devices can spare others from overly loud volume levels. FM loop systems can be used for groups of people with FM receivers or telecoil switches in their hearing aids. Wireless FM transmitters and receivers are also available for indoor or outdoor use. Infrared group-listening devices are primarily useful indoors. Vibrating and flashing devices such as alarm clocks and timers, smoke alarms, doorbell alerts, and motion sensors can improve quality of life and safety for hearing-impaired people. These items can be purchased through the agencies mentioned above, or from catalog retailers of assistive listening devices.

Newer forms of electronic communication, such as text messaging and e-mail, can be helpful for patients and caregivers. However, measures to protect patient confidentiality must be considered if using these devices.

Hearing Aids

Hearing aids are the most common form of amplification. Many factors need to be considered in deciding whether to fit an individual with a hearing aid. In addition to the nature and degree of hearing loss (Table 25.2), the person's motivation and ability to adapt to use of the aid and to physically manipulate the aid (Table 25.3), the degree of his or her social support, and his or her ability to afford the aid (Table 25.4) must be considered. Although hearing aids can be purchased from numerous sources, including over the Internet, working with an audiologist or other individual who has master's level training in audiology is advisable because of his or her expertise in hearing-aid fitting and adjustment.

Not everyone benefits from a hearing aid. The pattern of sensorineural damage can be such that speech discrimination is poor even with amplification. Some individuals are unable to tolerate the presence of the hearing aid in the ear. It is important to be sure that the aid can be returned during an initial trial period, usually 30 days, without having to pay the full cost of the aid. It is equally important not to give up on the aid too soon, because the audiologist often can adjust it to improve comfort and sound quality. The audiologist should provide counseling for optimal use of the aid.

Table 25.2—Effects and Rehabilitation of Hearing Loss, by Degree of Loss

Degree of Loss	Hearing Loss (dB)	Sounds Difficult to Hear	Effect on Communication	Amplification or Other Assistance Needed
Mild	25–40	Whisper	Difficulty understanding soft speech or normal speech in presence of background noise	Hearing aid needed in specific situations
Moderate	41–55	Conversational speech	Difficulty understanding any but loud speech	Frequent need for hearing aid
Severe	56–80	Shouting, vacuum cleaner	Can understand only amplified speech	Amplification needed for all communication
Profound	≥81	Hair dryer, heavy traffic, telephone ringer	Difficulty understanding amplified speech; may miss telephone calls	May need to supplement hearing aid with lipreading, assistive listening devices, sign language

SOURCE: Data in part from *A Report on Hearing Aids: User Perspectives and Concerns.* Washington, DC: American Association of Retired Persons; 1993:2.

Table 25.3—Advantages and Disadvantages of Styles of Hearing Aids

Style	Degree of Hearing Loss	Advantages	Disadvantages
CIC	Mild to moderate	Almost invisible Less occlusion of ear canal allows more natural sound Easier to use with headphones and telephone	Dexterity may be a problem. Small size may limit available features. May cost more than canal or in-the-ear aids Shorter battery life
Canal	Mild to moderate	More cosmetic than larger aids Telecoil available in some models May be able to use with headphones	Dexterity may be a problem. Small size may limit available features.
In the ear	Mild to severe	Ease of handling Comfortable fit Available options: telecoil, directional microphone More power than CIC or canal aid	More conspicuous than CIC or canal aid May be difficult to use with headphones
Behind the ear	Mild to profound	Greatest power Available options: telecoil, direct audio input, directional microphone Earmold can be changed separately	More conspicuous May be more difficult to insert than in-the-ear aids Difficult to use with headphones
Body aid	Severe to profound	Greatest separation of microphone from receiver reduces feedback	Most conspicuous Body-level microphone is subject to noise from clothing. Microphone is on chest or at waist, but speech is usually directed at ear level.
Bone conduction aid	Mild to severe	Bypasses middle ear; used if ear canal is unable to tolerate aid or earmold, or for unilateral hearing loss	Receiver of traditional aid causes pressure on the scalp, which can be uncomfortable; does not correct sensorineural loss. Being replaced by bone-anchored hearing aids

NOTE: CIC = completely in the canal

In general, two hearing aids are more beneficial than one. The first aid provides the most gain; the second one helps with speech discrimination and with localizing the source of sounds. However, the presence of asymmetrical hearing loss or significant difficulty in understanding competing speech stimuli may mean that the use of a single hearing aid is more appropriate.

Many different styles of hearing aids are available (Table 25.3). Behind-the-ear aids hang behind the ear and are connected directly to an earmold. The earmold is usually custom made to fit each ear. Some behind-the-ear aids can be connected to assistive listening devices via a "boot," which fits over the end of the aid to provide direct audio input. Some newer models of hearing aids can be used with Bluetooth devices, including mobile telephones, remote microphones, and computers. Body aids are worn on the belt or in a pocket or harness, and they are connected to a custom-made earmold by a wire. These are rarely used. All-in-the-ear aids and canal aids usually have cases that are custom fit to the user. The smaller hearing aids may have remote controls. Selection of aid style for each individual depends on the degree of hearing loss, available features, and the person's dexterity and motivation.

The telecoil is an induction coupling coil that can be built into the hearing aid. It detects the magnetic

Table 25.4—Approximate Costs of Assistive Listening Devices and Hearing Aids

Type of Technology	Cost	Comments
Assistive listening devices (eg, personal amplifiers, telephone amplifiers, television listening devices)	$100 and up	Useful for specific situations (see text for details)
Hearing aids		
	One aid/two aids	
Digital, economy	$1,200/$2,200	Economy aids process signals more slowly and have fewer programs. Telecoils are available on request. Background noise suppression may be switched on manually. Economy aids may be very appropriate for persons with a quiet lifestyle.
Digital, value	$1,500/$2,800	Multiple programs, telecoil
Digital, mid-range	$2,100/$4,000	Multiple programs, telecoil, Bluetooth input
Digital, premium	$2,800/$5,400	Multiple features available, including multiple programs, telecoil, Bluetooth input, and more rapid signal processing

NOTE: Assistive listening devices and hearing aids are not covered by Medicare. Features of hearing aids in a given price range vary by manufacturer.

field produced by telephones that are compatible with hearing aids. The telecoil is used to listen to the telephone with less distraction from noise in the same room. It can also be used with many assistive listening devices. The amount of coupling, and therefore the volume of the signal, depends on the angle of the telecoil with respect to the magnetic field. Users may need to experiment to find the right angle. Strongly magnetic devices such as computer monitors often produce interference, which also depends on the angle and the distance of the telecoil from the device. These drawbacks aside, the telecoil is a useful feature and can be added to hearing aids at relatively low cost. Individuals with moderate to severe hearing loss should be encouraged to consider purchasing an aid with a telecoil.

Analog hearing aids were the first type available but are rarely sold now. Digital technology has allowed improved sound quality, reduced size, and increased ability to customize the amplification of the aid to the needs of the user. Programmable aids are adjusted for each individual while he or she is wearing the aid. Often, two or more programs are available within a single aid. Using a computer, the audiologist makes adjustments to gain, response in different frequency ranges, and loudness balance for each program. One program may be most useful in the presence of background noise, whereas another works better in a quiet environment, and a third works with a telecoil. Patients with Ménière disease can have their aids reprogrammed to accommodate fluctuating hearing loss. Many hearing aids automatically adjust the volume to increase amplification of soft sounds while avoiding uncomfortable loudness, reducing the need for the user to manipulate the aid. This can be helpful for first-time users, although experienced users may require time to adjust to this feature. Hearing aids may have an automatic telecoil feature that switches to the telecoil program when a hearing-aid compatible telephone is brought close to the ear. Background noise is a significant problem for hearing-aid users. Traditional hearing aids amplify sound indiscriminately, so that background noise, eg, papers rustling or water running, can be very distracting. For new hearing-aid users, this problem can be addressed by having the audiologist gradually increase the gain of the hearing aid as the listener adjusts to being able to hear environmental sounds over the course of weeks. However, background noise in the presence of speech is a problem even for experienced hearing-aid users. The use of multiple microphones in the hearing aid, combined with digital signal processing, can decrease the effects of background noise. This can significantly improve the user's ability to understand speech and increase satisfaction with the aid. Most hearing aids now include noise reduction and feedback suppression.

Unfortunately, the cost of hearing aids is often a significant barrier to their use and can affect the purchaser's choice of features (Table 25.4). The cost of a hearing aid ranges from $1,200 to $3,000 per device, or $2,200 to $5,400 for a pair. The features available in a given price range vary by manufacturer. Typically the cost of the aid includes follow-up visits to the hearing-aid dispenser through the life of the aid, although some audiologists may unbundle the follow-up visits from the original fitting and purchase. The expected life span of a hearing aid is 3–5 years, although with care, aids may last longer. Although hearing aids are covered by Medicaid in most states, the amount of reimbursement often does not cover aids with advanced features. Hearing aids are not covered by Medicare or by private health insurance in many states, except in rare circumstances. Federal programs such as the Department of Veterans Affairs may pay for hearing aids, depending on the recipient's eligibility for services. Some charitable organizations assist in providing hearing aids to low-income persons.

Table 25.5—Characteristics of Older Candidates for Cochlear Implants

Severe to profound sensorineural hearing loss in both ears
Functional auditory nerve
Short duration of severe hearing loss
Good speech, language, and communication skills
Not benefiting enough from other kinds of hearing aids
No medical contraindication to surgery (eg, active infection, inability to tolerate general anesthesia)
Realistic expectations about results
Appropriate support services available for aural rehabilitation after cochlear implant
Adequate motivation and cognition to participate in aural rehabilitation

Caring for Hearing Aids

Hearing aids should be stored with the battery compartment door open; this may be the only way to turn the hearing aid off. They should be wiped with a dry cloth daily (earmolds of behind-the-ear aids should be cleaned according to manufacturer's instructions). Wax may plug the sound outlet of a hearing aid, and the manufacturer's instructions should be consulted before trying to clean it.

Patients may need assistance to insert the hearing aid. First, it should be noted whether the hearing aid goes into the right ear (the aid may be marked with red) or the left ear (marked with blue). The battery door faces the outside of the ear. If there is a vent or a removal string, these are usually at the bottom. The following instructions apply to all except behind-the-ear aids:

The aid should first be turned on to be sure it is working. If so, a high-pitched squeal or vibration (feedback) should be heard; if no noise is heard when the volume is set at maximum, the battery should be replaced. The hearing aid should be oriented right side up, with the canal portion of the aid or earmold facing toward the canal. The wide, flat portion of an in-the-ear aid or earmold should be posterior. This part of the aid may need to be rotated so that it fits into the external ear, and the helix lifted gently to ease this part in. If there is feedback, the aid may be gently pushed to seat it more firmly into the ear. Turning the volume down may also reduce feedback.

Patients with dementia may remove and dispose of the aid. To reduce this risk, it can be helpful to order a loop attached to the hearing aid case; a piece of fishing line can be attached to the loop and the other end of the line pinned to the patient's clothing to catch the aid when the patient removes it. In long-term care institutions, a system for collecting the aids each night and placing them in the patients' ears each morning may facilitate use of the aids, while reducing the number that are lost.

Bone-Anchored Hearing Aids (BAHA)

People with unilateral hearing loss, inability to tolerate an earmold or hearing aid in the canal, or conductive/mixed hearing loss may be treated with a BAHA. A BAHA has a small post that is surgically implanted in the mastoid bone, which connects to a speech processor that converts sound into vibrations. The vibrations are transmitted through the post in the skull to the inner ear, bypassing the middle ear. BAHAs are replacing bone conduction aids.

Cochlear Implants

For patients with severe to profound hearing loss who gain little or no benefit from hearing aids yet who are motivated to participate in the hearing world, cochlear implants can provide useful hearing (Table 25.5). A cochlear implant is an electronic device that bypasses the function of damaged or absent cochlear hair cells by providing electrical stimulation to cochlear nerve fibers. A receiver-stimulator and an intracochlear electrode array are surgically implanted. A headset is worn behind the ear. The headset microphone transmits signals to the speech processor, which filters and digitizes the sound into coded signals. The coded signals are sent to the cochlear implant, which then stimulates auditory nerve fibers in the cochlea. Nerve signals are then sent through the auditory system to the brain. Patients must be able to tolerate general anesthesia and to participate in extensive pre-implant testing and post-implant training. Meningitis is a rare complication of cochlear implants.

The cochlear implant procedure is covered by most Medicare carriers and insurance companies, although prior authorization is generally required. In general, outcomes of cochlear implantation in adults ≥65 years old have been comparable to those of younger adults, with many patients obtaining excellent results by both audiologic and quality-of-life measures. Cochlear implants do not restore normal hearing, but users can sense environmental sounds and are able to understand speech more easily. Many can use a telephone, and some can even enjoy music.

REFERENCES

- Chou R, Dana T, Bougatsos C, et al. Screening adults aged 50 years or older for hearing loss: a review of the evidence for the U.S. Preventive Services Task Force. *Ann Intern Med.* 2011;154:347–355.
- Laubach G. Speaking up for older patients with hearing loss. *Nursing.* 2010;40(1):60–62.
- U.S. Food and Drug Administration Center for Products and Medical Procedures. Cochlear Implants. Available at: www.fda.gov/MedicalDevices/ (accessed Oct 2013).

CHAPTER 26—DIZZINESS

KEY POINTS

- The classification of dizziness into vertigo, presyncope, dysequilibrium, mixed, or others may be useful in guiding patient evaluation; however, precise classification is often difficult, and multiple causes of the same symptoms are common.
- Dizziness is associated with increased fear of falling, functional disability, and depressive symptoms.
- Multiple factors can contribute to chronic dizziness.
- Expensive tests like electronystagmography, rotational chair testing, posturography, and neuroimaging, such as CT or MRI, are not often needed in the evaluation of dizziness.
- Multifactorial interventions can help in ameliorating chronic dizziness.

Dizziness ranks among the most common symptoms presented by older adults to primary healthcare providers. The various and often nonspecific terms—lightheadedness, giddiness, wooziness, vertigo, spinning, floating, and imbalance—that patients typically use to describe dizziness add to the diagnostic and management challenge. Dizziness that continues >1–2 months is considered chronic. The prevalence of dizziness in adults ≥65 years old ranges from 4% to 30%. The wide prevalence range is related to differences in age, symptoms, and sample population among the various studies. The prevalence of dizziness is lower between the age of 65 and 69 years and increases as people get older. Dizziness is more common in women than in men.

Acute dizziness, which is independent of age, has causes and interventions similar to those of chronic dizziness. However, chronic dizziness, which is much more common in older adults, has a larger variety of contributing causes and requires additional skill and patience to evaluate and manage successfully. This chapter focuses on chronic dizziness in older adults, which is commonly seen with increasing fear of falling, depressive symptoms, fall risk, and general functional disability.

CLASSIFICATION

Drachman and Hart classified dizziness into four types of sensations: vertigo, presyncope, dysequilibrium, and other. A fifth type—mixed—results from a combination of two or more of the above, and is the most common type of dizziness reported by older adults (Table 26.1).

Vertigo

Vertigo is an often episodic spinning or rotational sensation; objective vertigo ("the room is spinning") versus subjective vertigo ("I am spinning") results from disturbances in the vestibular system. The most common causes of vertigo are benign paroxysmal positional vertigo (BPPV) and Ménière disease. BPPV, an inner ear disorder, is characterized by sudden onset, seconds-long bouts of vertigo precipitated by certain changes in head position (rolling over in bed, gazing up or down). BPPV probably results from changes in endolymphatic pressure during head movements resulting from dislodged otoconia in the semicircular canal. Ménière disease, an idiopathic inner ear disorder, is characterized by episodic vertigo, tinnitus, fluctuating hearing loss, and a sensation of fullness in the inner ear. Other causes of vertigo include idiopathic recurrent vestibulopathy and central vestibular lesions such as cerebrovascular disease and acoustic neuroma. Absence of spinning sensation does not exclude vestibular diseases, because patients with vestibular problems can describe dizziness as an imbalance or dysequilibrium or other sensation. Patients with cervical dizziness secondary to cervical arthritis can also present with vertigo.

Presyncope

Presyncope, a feeling of faintness or lightheadedness, usually results from a cardiovascular problem causing brain hypoperfusion through postural hypotension. There is no specific definition of postural hypotension in older adults, but it is commonly defined as a drop in systolic arterial blood pressure of at least 20 mmHg and/or a drop in diastolic blood pressure of 10 mmHg after standing up from a supine position. However, older adults commonly describe dizziness on standing from a supine position without any orthostatic changes in blood pressure. Another common condition, postprandial hypotension, is defined as a decrease in systolic blood pressure of ≥20 mmHg in a sitting or standing posture within 1–2 hours of eating a meal.

Dysequilibrium

Dysequilibrium, a feeling of imbalance or unsteadiness on standing or walking, usually results from visual or proprioceptive system abnormalities, with or without vestibular system involvement. Common contributing conditions include vision problems (eg, refractory errors, cataract, macular degeneration), musculoskeletal disorders (eg, arthritis, muscle

Table 26.1–Classification of Dizziness

Type	Common Causes or Coexisting Conditions	Diagnostic Features	Treatment
Vertigo	Benign paroxysmal positional vertigo	History of episodic vertigo; rotational nystagmus; Dix-Hallpike maneuver confirms diagnosis	Epley maneuver is treatment of choice
	Meniere disease	Episodic vertigo lasting for a few hours; tinnitus; fluctuating hearing loss; sensation of fullness in ears; audiogram reveals sensorineural hearing loss (at low more than high frequencies)	Salt restriction, diuretics; vestibular suppressants may be helpful during acute attacks; in severe cases, may need surgical interventions, including endolymphatic decompression, vestibular nerve resection, and labyrinthectomy
	Ototoxic medications, eg, aminoglycosides, diuretics, NSAIDs	Presence of nystagmus, bedside vestibular function tests (eg, head thrust test) can be abnormal	Discontinue, substitute, or reduce the dosage of offending medication
Presyncope	Cerebral ischemia secondary to orthostatic hypotension, cardiac causes, dehydration, medications, vasovagal attack, autonomic dysfunction secondary to diabetes, parkinsonism	Near fainting/lightheadedness when getting up from lying down or sitting position; orthostatic changes in blood pressure; investigations relevant to predisposing diseases	Treatment of specific cause, eg, proper hydration; dosage adjustment or removal of the offending medications; slow rising from sitting or lying down position; graduated support stockings; physical therapy and/or occupational therapy; medications (eg, fludrocortisone, midodrine) as needed
	Postprandial hypotension	Near fainting/lightheadedness when getting up from lying down or sitting position; orthostatic hypotension usually within 45–60 min of eating	Frequent small meals; avoid exertion after meals; slow rising from sitting position; avoid antihypertensive drugs with or near meal time
Dysequilibrium	Vertebrobasilar ischemia and/or cerebellar infarcts/hemorrhages	History of dizziness usually associated with slurred speech; visual changes; one-sided weakness and/or gait ataxia; truncal ataxia; CT or MRI or magnetic resonance angiography scan may be helpful	Low-dose aspirin, clopidogrel, or extended-release dipyridamole/aspirin; rehabilitation
	Cerebellopontine angle tumor, eg, acoustic neuroma	History of vertigo or dysequilibrium, unilateral hearing loss, tinnitus; audiometry reveals sensorineural hearing loss more for higher frequencies; MRI is diagnostic	Surgery
	Parkinson disease	Bradykinesia; muscular rigidity; tremor; orthostatic hypotension	Drug therapy, rehabilitation therapy
	Peripheral neuropathy secondary to diabetes; vitamin B_{12} deficiency; idiopathic, etc	Decreased vibration or position sense; gait abnormality; hyperglycemia; low vitamin B_{12} level	Treatment of the underlying disease
	Cervical spine degenerative arthritis, spondylosis	Limitation of range of motion of neck; decreased vibratory or joint position sense; signs of radiculopathy or myelopathy; cervical spine radiologic abnormalities	Cervical or vestibular rehabilitation; cervical collar; surgery if needed
Other	Anxiety, depression, or psychosomatic disorders	Usually continuous nonspecific dizziness; fatigue; poor appetite; sleep problems; somatic complaints; positive results on anxiety or depression screening scales	Psychotherapy and/or antidepressant therapy
Mixed	Medications: antianxiety drugs, antidepressants, anticonvulsants, antipsychotics, antihypertensives, anticholinergics	History of fatigue; dizziness often vague and can be continuous, postural, or associated with confusion	Discontinue, substitute, or reduce the dosage of offending medication
	Combination of any of the above causes	Combination of any of the above features	Multifactorial intervention

weakness, deconditioning after prolonged illness), proprioceptive disorders (eg, neuropathies), and gait disorders (eg, cerebrovascular stroke, Parkinson disease, cerebellar disorders).

Other Forms of Dizziness

Others include a vague feeling other than vertigo, presyncope, or dysequilibrium. The patient may describe “floating,” “lightheadedness,” “wooziness,” “spaciness,” “whirling,” or other nonspecific sensations. Patients with psychogenic dizziness commonly report anxiety or depressive symptoms. The psychiatric symptoms can primarily cause or contribute to the dizziness complaint in older adults.

Mixed Dizziness

Mixed dizziness, a combination of two or more of the above types, is the most common type of dizziness reported by older adults. It most likely results from combinations of diseases affecting the vestibular, CNS, visual, or proprioceptive systems. Systemic disorders like anemia, heart failure, diabetes mellitus, and hypothyroidism can contribute to instability or dizziness by affecting the sensory, central, or effector components. Although less commonly reported, carotid sinus hypersensitivity or carotid sinus syndrome can also cause dizziness. Patients with dementia often get fixated on being dizzy or unsteady.

Many medications can contribute to chronic dizziness through various mechanisms. Important classes of medications to consider in the dizziness evaluation include anxiolytics, antidepressants, antihistaminics, antihypertensives, aminoglycosides, anticholinergics, antipsychotics, and NSAIDs.

Research data indicate that chronic dizziness often has a multifactorial etiology. Chronic dizziness is associated with risk factors such as angina, myocardial infarction, stroke, arthritis, diabetes, syncope, anxiety, depressive symptoms, impaired hearing, and the use of medications in several classes. In a study of a large community sample and in another study in which patients attended a geriatric clinic, the complaint of chronic dizziness was associated with factors such as anxiety, depressive symptoms, postural hypotension, use of five or more medications, and impaired gait and balance (SOE=B). Complaints of chronic dizziness were more common in patients who had more than five of these risk factors than in those having less than two of these risk factors. Similar to delirium and falls, chronic dizziness can be thought of as a geriatric syndrome that prompts a multifactorial assessment and intervention strategy, which is likely more effective at alleviating symptoms than a standard disease-oriented approach.

EVALUATION

The evaluation of dizziness is challenging, and diagnostic evaluation can be extensive. Patients present with vague sensations, which generate a broad differential diagnosis. An expansive evaluation can often be avoided by taking a more detailed history and conducting a more directed physical examination.

History

The clinical history begins with helping patients to describe their symptoms as precisely as possible, which is potentially daunting for those with multiple sensations. Patients should be encouraged to use their own words to distill the symptoms into specific sensations such as spinning, imbalance or unsteadiness, or fainting. Documenting the frequency and duration of dizziness, and whether changing head position exacerbates the dizziness, is important. Establishing whether symptoms peak at any specific time of day, such as after meals or first thing in the morning, is also useful. Patients should be asked about associated symptoms such as hearing loss, ear fullness, diplopia, dysarthria, and tinnitus. It is also important to elicit the impact on the patient's quality of life. Patients with Meniere disease complain of recurrent dizziness associated with ear fullness and/or tinnitus along with fluctuating hearing loss. Patients with acoustic neuroma complain of hearing loss and tinnitus but not of ear fullness. Patients with Meniere disease, CNS diseases, and BPPV complain of recurrent dizziness, while patients with psychogenic and central dizziness usually complain of continual dizziness. Inquiring about precipitating factors such as after eating meals (postprandial hypotension), looking down or rolling over in bed (vestibular conditions), or standing from supine position (orthostatic hypotension) can suggest interventions, as well as corroborate timing of symptoms. Any evaluation must include a critical review of medications, including OTC medications.

Physical Examination

The physical examination should begin with measurements of orthostatic changes in blood pressure. Nystagmus should be evaluated; horizontal or rotatory nystagmus usually indicates a peripheral vestibular lesion, while vertical nystagmus is seen in central lesions. Hearing and vision tests should be done, and the cranial nerves examined if vertebrobasilar ischemia or infarction is suspected. The Timed Up and Go test can be performed to look for gait and balance problems (see “Gait Impairment,” p 231).

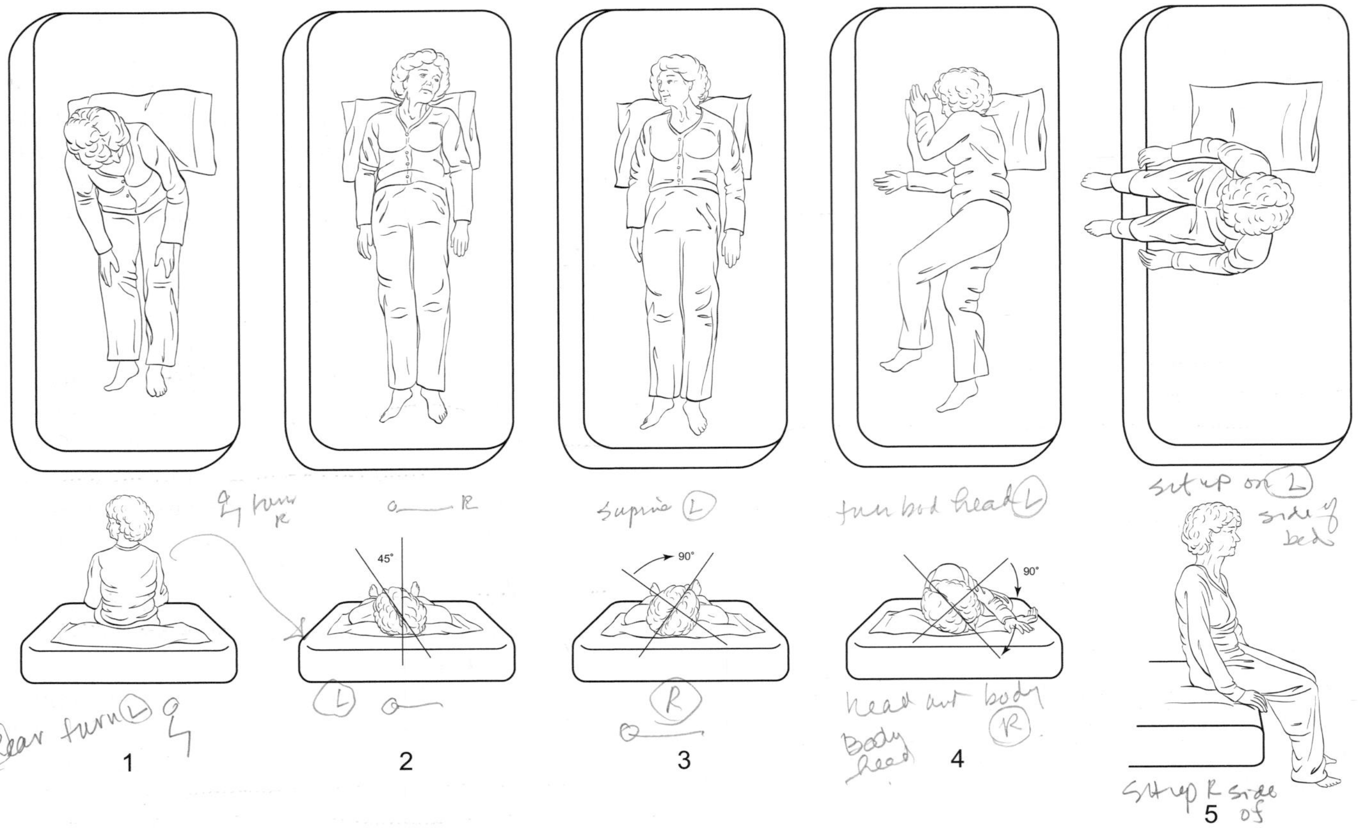

Figure 26.1 —Self-treatment of benign paroxysmal positional vertigo using Epley maneuver.

Perform the maneuver three times a day until free of positional vertigo for 24 hours. Use the positions shown here when the right ear is affected. Reverse all positions (left instead of right) when the left ear is affected. The affected ear is the ear that when turned downward during the Dix-Hallpike maneuver triggers vertigo or nystagmus, or both.

Each maneuver consists of the following steps (numbered to match the illustration):

1. Sit on the bed with a pillow far enough behind you to be under your shoulders when you lie back. Turn your head 45 degrees to the left.
2. Holding your head in the turned position, lie back quickly so that your shoulders are supported on the pillow and your head is reclined on the bed. Hold this position for 30 sec.
3. Remain supine on the bed and turn your head 90 degrees to the right. Hold this position for 30 sec.
4. Turn your head and body another 90 degrees to the right; you should now be looking down at the bed. Hold this position for 30 sec.
5. Sit up, facing to the right.

SOURCE: Data from Radtke A, Neuhauser H, von Brevern M, et al. A modified Epley's procedure for self-treatment of benign paroxysmal positional vertigo. *Neurology.* 1999;53(6):1358–1360.

The following provocative tests of the vestibular system can be done at the bedside:

Head-thrust test: Ask the patient to fixate on the examiner's nose. The examiner then rotates the head rapidly about 10 degrees to the left or right. In patients with a vestibular deficit, the eyes move away from the target along with the head, followed by a corrective saccade back to the target, while normal eyes remain fixed on the target without a saccade.

Fukuda stepping test: Draw a circle on the floor, and ask the patient to stand in the center. Blindfold the patient and ask him or her to take a few steps forward as if walking on a straight line with outstretched arms. The examiner notes the patient's body sway as the patient takes the steps. In a unilateral vestibular lesion or acoustic neuroma, the patient's body will sway by >30 degrees toward the affected side.

Dix-Hallpike maneuver: This is a useful test for the diagnosis of BPPV. Ask the patient to sit on the examination table with the head rotated 30–45 degrees to one side. Instruct the patient to fix his or her vision on the examiner's forehead. The examiner holds the patient's head firmly in the same position, and moves the patient from a seated to a supine position with the head hanging below the edge of the table and the chin pointing slightly upward. The examiner notes the direction, latency, and duration of the nystagmus, if present. The diagnostic criteria for BPPV include 1) paroxysmal vertigo along with a rotatory nystagmus, 2) latency for 1–2 sec between the completion of the maneuver and the onset of vertigo and nystagmus, and 3) fatigability (decrease in the intensity of the vertigo and nystagmus with repeated testing).

Diagnostic Testing

A small battery of laboratory tests, including hematocrit, glucose, electrolytes, BUN, vitamin B_{12}, folic acid, and thyrotropin, should be performed on all patients with chronic dizziness. An ECG should be done if a cardiac cause is suspected, and a Holter and event monitor only if suspicion of arrhythmia is strong. Tilt-table testing should be done only for select patients with postural hypotension or syncope. Audiometry assists in the evaluation of patients with tinnitus or hearing loss, and helps differentiate between acoustic neuroma and Meniere disease.

Suspected vestibular disorders can be evaluated with vestibular function tests such as electronystagmography, rotational testing, and dynamic posturography. These tests are not needed in every patient.

Likewise, neuroimaging is not needed in all patients with dizziness. MRI provides better resolution than CT for posterior fossa lesions. However, in a community-based study of adults ≥65 years old, the similar prevalence of MRI abnormalities in the dizzy and nondizzy group led to the conclusion that routine MRI will not identify a specific cause of dizziness in most patients (SOE=B).

MANAGEMENT

Medical therapy of acute dizziness depends on its cause, and patients with chronic dizziness, especially older adults, can have multiple comorbid conditions or impairments. Given the multifactorial nature of dizziness, it has been suggested that dizziness may be a geriatric syndrome. Therefore, a multifacted approach to interventions can help treat chronic dizziness and reduce the impact on day-to-day functioning. Treatment of coincident symptoms from depression, anxiety, hearing loss, and vision loss can help reduce the disability arising from dizziness. Dizziness from medication responds to dosage adjustment or to withdrawal of the offending medication.

Vestibular suppressants, including antihistamines (eg, meclizine), provide effective symptomatic relief for vertigo but generally do not provide benefit in management of chronic dizziness or dysequilibrium. Long-term use of meclizine should be avoided because it suppresses central and vestibular adaptation and can thus eventually worsen or exacerbate dizziness.

Vestibular rehabilitation therapy (VRT) can help suppress symptoms in patients with peripheral and central vestibular causes of dizziness. VRT includes different exercises such as vestibulo-ocular reflex adaptation exercises and habituation exercises. Vestibulo-ocular reflex adaptation exercises help the CNS to adapt to a change or loss in input of the vestibular system. Habituation exercises include a combination of exercises designed to provoke dizziness; the movements are repeated until they can no longer be tolerated. Initially, the exercises can worsen the dizziness, but over time (weeks to months) movement-related dizziness improves, likely because of central adaptation. VRT has been shown to improve dizziness as well as quality of life (SOE=B).

The canalith repositioning procedure, introduced by Semont as well as Epley, can provide quick relief for those patients with BPPV (Figure 26.1).

A small subset of patients need surgical intervention. Surgical excision remains the treatment of choice for cerebellopontine angle tumors. Surgery should be reserved for disabling unilateral peripheral disease that is unresponsive to medical therapy. Surgical procedures are ablative or nonablative. Surgeons select ablative procedures, including transmastoid labyrinthectomy and partial vestibular neurectomy, for uncontrolled Meniere disease. Nonablative procedures, such as posterior canal occlusion, provide benefit to those patients whose BPPV remains refractory to repeated attempts of canalith repositioning procedures.

REFERENCES

- Alrwaily M, Whitney SL. Vestibular rehabilitation of older adults with dizziness. *Otolaryngol Clin No Am.* 2011;44(2):473–496.
- Gray-Miceli D, Ratcliffe SJ, Liu S, et al. Orthostatic hypotension in older nursing home residents who fall: are they dizzy? *Clin Nurs Res.* 2012;21(1):64–78.
- Sloane PD, Coeytaux RR, Beck RS, et al. Dizziness: state of the science. *Ann Intern Med.* 2001;134(9 Pt 2):823–832.

CHAPTER 27—SYNCOPE

KEY POINTS

- The incidence of syncope increases with age.
- In older adults, the cause of syncope is often multifactorial. In nearly one in five cases, the cause of syncope is not determined, but in those patients the prognosis is generally favorable.
- Although many diagnostic procedures are available to search for the cause of syncope, most are expensive and have a low yield unless findings from the history or physical examination suggest a particular cause.
- Bradycardia is the single most common cardiac cause of syncope in older adults.
- Treatment of syncope often requires treatment of multiple possible underlying causes in geriatric patients.

Syncope is a symptom complex composed of a sudden and transient loss of consciousness resulting from a temporary interruption of global cerebral perfusion. It is a common reason for evaluation in both outpatient clinics and emergency departments, and for hospital admission. Annually it accounts for approximately 3% of emergency department visits and 2%–6% of hospital admissions. Incidence of syncope increases with age; incidence doubles in those ≥70 years old, and the rate among those ≥80 years old is three to four times that seen among younger people. Approximately 80% of patients hospitalized for syncope are ≥65 years old.

Syncope is a clinically important condition that is challenging to evaluate. Its potential causes range from those that are benign and self-limiting to those that are life threatening. In older adults, the cause of syncope can often be multifactorial, adding to the diagnostic difficulty. Because syncope encompasses a wide range of potential causes, its diagnostic evaluation can be complex and expensive.

NATURAL HISTORY: DIAGNOSIS AND PROGNOSIS

Causes of syncope in older adults are often multifactorial. Decreases in cardiac output or peripheral vascular resistance, or both, resulting in decreased systemic blood pressure and cerebral perfusion are common mechanisms of syncope. In addition to many medical conditions affecting cardiac output or peripheral vascular resistance, adverse events of drugs must be considered during evaluation of syncope in older adults. Thus, the common causes of syncope in older adults are:

- Neurally mediated
- Cardiac rhythm disturbances
- Decreased intravascular volume due to blood loss or dehydration
- Alterations in the peripheral vasculature due to arterial vasodilation or increased venous pooling
- Medication related

Localized atherosclerotic diseases, such as vertebral basilar insufficiency and subclavian steal, can result in syncope without alteration in systemic blood pressure. These causes are uncommon.

Epileptic seizure, a common cause of transient loss of consciousness, is no longer categorized as a cause of syncope because seizure is not mediated by a decrease in cerebral perfusion. Nevertheless, differentiation of seizure from syncope as a cause of transient loss of consciousness is clinically relevant, because both conditions are common and have overlapping clinical features in the older population.

The prognosis of syncope depends on the underlying cause. The major issue is whether the cause is cardiac. The 1-year mortality for patients with syncope due to cardiac causes is 18%–33% (deaths are chiefly due to underlying disease, not syncope), while that for patients with syncope due to noncardiac causes is approximately 6%. Neurally mediated or vasovagal syncope, which has a benign prognosis in the young, was once thought to be an unusual cause of syncope in older adults. However, reports from syncope evaluation centers have found vasovagal mechanisms as the cause of syncope in approximately 30%–50% of patients >65 years old (SOE=A). It has not been established that vasovagal syncope in older adults has the same benign prognosis as in younger individuals as there has been some suggestion that vasovagal syncope in older adults is often associated with comorbid illness that can increase overall mortality (SOE=B). In approximately 20% of syncopal patients, no cause can be found. The prognosis for these patients is no worse or better than that of the general population (SOE=C).

PATHOPHYSIOLOGY

The integrity of a number of control mechanisms is crucial for maintaining adequate perfusion of the brain and cerebral oxygen delivery after sudden changes in blood pressure. These mechanisms include the following:

- Carotid and aortic baroreceptors increase the autonomic sympathetic outflow, causing vasoconstriction and increased heart rate.
- Sympathetic renal stimulation of renin-angiotensin and vasopressin results in vasoconstriction.
- The veno-arteriolar axon reflex, which is a local response at dependent sites, increases the vasoconstriction of the resistance vessels; the myogenic reflex increases the smooth muscle contraction of the resistance vessels, thereby increasing venous return.
- The abdominal-respiratory pump facilitates venous return and increases preload.

In aging, many of these reflex mechanisms are less responsive. For example, the arterial baroreceptor reflex and cardiac response to β-adrenergic stimulation (cardiac acceleration and increased contractility) decrease with advancing age. In addition, comorbid conditions that can affect postural reflex responses, such as diabetes mellitus and Parkinson disease, are common among older adults. Medications such as α-blockers, β-blockers, calcium channel blockers, ACE inhibitors, and tricyclic antidepressants can also impair postural reflexes. Because the ability to increase heart rate in response to sympathetic stimulation is decreased in older adults, maintaining blood volume and vasoconstriction become more important in maintaining postural blood pressure. Thus, older adults can be particularly sensitive to the effects of dehydration, diuretics, and vasodilator medications. These three factors—age-related decline in adaptive reflexes, comorbid conditions, and medications—may be present in combination in older adults, resulting in syncopal events.

EVALUATION

History

An accurate recall of the syncopal event is frequently inadequate because of the high prevalence of cognitive dysfunction in the older population. The medical history, if possible from a witness to the event, in combination with a physical examination play a key role in the initial evaluation. It is important to establish whether the patient suffered a true syncopal event, as opposed to dizziness (dysequilibrium) or falls. Falls are common in older adults (estimated annual incidence up to 30% in ambulatory community-dwelling older adults); it is important to differentiate accidental falls from syncope causing falls. Key elements to obtain from the history are:

- Was there a precipitant? Could the patient's activities around the time of the event have triggered it? Such activities include eating, urinating, coughing, using medication, and experiencing emotional stress. Syncope occurring while sitting or supine suggests a profound hemodynamic disturbance and should raise a concern about a significant cardiac arrhythmia. Syncope occurring during physical exertion should raise the possibility of myocardial ischemia or aortic stenosis. A history of syncope after turning motions of the head should raise the possibility of carotid sinus hypersensitivity.
- Were there prodromal symptoms before the event? Chest pain, palpitations, or shortness of breath suggests a cardiac or pulmonary cause. Diaphoresis, presyncope, and GI symptoms, such as nausea or vomiting, can be associated with vasovagal syncope. Sudden onset of syncope with <5 sec of warning is characteristic of syncope due to a cardiac arrhythmia and should be evaluated as such. However, in older adults, vasovagal syncope can present with short or no prodrome because of inability to precisely recall the event. Thus, if the initial evaluation for arrhythmia in an older adult with syncope without a prodrome is unrevealing, a vasovagal mechanism should also be considered.
- What medications are being used? It is important to establish how medications were taken with relationship to meals and other activities, and whether the medication regimen was recently changed. Specifics about dosage times should be obtained. Many antiarrhythmic medications and other commonly used medications can increase the propensity for ventricular arrhythmias by prolonging the QT interval (for a full current list, see www.qtdrugs.org).
- What did witnesses observe? They should be queried about the duration of the event and the appearance of the patient during the event. Patients with cardiac causes of syncope are generally flaccid in tone and motionless while unconscious, unless the event lasts for >15 sec, when myoclonic jerks and truncal extension can be seen. In contrast, increased body motion, tone, and head turning to one side with loss of consciousness are more common with seizure activity.
- Are there significant comorbid conditions? A history of coronary artery disease or its associated symptoms is particularly important. Approximately 5% of myocardial infarctions present as syncope. Sustained ventricular tachycardia resulting in syncope is most common in patients with prior myocardial infarction. Patients with diabetes mellitus are at increased risk of coronary atherosclerosis, as well as autonomic dysfunction predisposing to syncope.

Table 27.1–Evaluation of Guidelines in Syncope Study (EGSYS) Score: Predictors of Cardiac Syncope

Variable	Score[a]
Palpitations preceding syncope	4
Heart disease or abnormal ECG	3
Syncope during effort	3
Syncope while supine	2
Precipitating or predisposing factors, or both[b]	−1
Autonomic prodromes (nausea/vomiting)	−1

[a] Scores ≥3 are associated with higher rates of cardiac syncope and higher mortality.

[b] Warm or crowded place, prolonged orthostasis, fear, pain, or emotional distress

SOURCE: Data from Del Rosso A, Ungar A, Maggi R, et al. Clinical predictors of cardiac syncope at initial evaluation in patients referred urgently to a general hospital: the EGSYS score. *Heart*. 2008;94(12):1620–1626.

A scoring system has been useful in distinguishing cardiac from noncardiac syncope (Table 27.1). The probability of cardiac syncope increases with higher scores, with scores of ≥3 being associated with 95% sensitivity and 61% specificity. Mortality was 17%–21% in those with a score ≥3, and 2%–3% in those with a score <3 after 600 days of follow-up (SOE=B).

Physical Examination

A physical examination should focus on elements raised by the history. Blood pressure should be measured in both arms, as well as with postural changes. The pulse should be taken with the patient in both supine and standing positions. Blood pressure with the patient in the standing position should be obtained after 1 min and 3 min of standing. Although any definition of postural hypotension is arbitrary, a decrease in systolic blood pressure of >20 mmHg is the definition used most frequently (SOE=C).

The character of the carotid pulse should also be assessed for the delayed upstroke and low volume characteristic of significant aortic stenosis. The presence of a carotid bruit, a history of cerebrovascular disease, and recent myocardial infarction are relative contraindications to carotid sinus massage. Even in the absence of contraindications, carotid sinus massage should be performed only under continuous ECG monitoring (to detect induced sinus pauses, atrioventricular [AV] block, or other arrhythmias) in a setting where resuscitation equipment is available.

The physical examination of the patient with syncope should include cardiac examination for evidence of murmurs characteristic of valvular abnormalities or extra heart sounds suggestive of cardiomyopathy. Fecal examination for occult blood and neurologic examination for focal deficits are also important.

Several clinical characteristics and diagnostic approaches are particularly important for evaluation of syncope in older adults:

- Postural hypotension is not always reproducible in older adults (particularly medication- or volume-related). Therefore, orthostatic blood pressure assessment should be repeated, preferably in the morning, after meals, and/or promptly after syncope.
- In evaluation of neutrally mediated syncope in older adults, tilt testing is well tolerated and safe.
- Twenty-four hour ambulatory blood pressure recordings can be helpful if intermittent instability of blood pressure is suspected (eg, medication or post-prandial).
- An implantable loop recorder can be useful in older adults to assess infrequent unexplained syncope.

Ambulatory Electrocardiographic Monitoring

An ambulatory ECG recording can establish or exclude many causes of syncope if the patient experiences syncopal or presyncopal symptoms during the recording. Unfortunately, the occurrence of symptoms during ambulatory ECG monitoring is relatively infrequent in most patients with syncope that remains unexplained after a history, physical examination, and ECG. On average, studies examining the diagnostic yield of ambulatory ECG report an arrhythmia correlating with symptoms in approximately 4% of patients. In another 15% of patients studied, an arrhythmia was excluded by the presence of symptoms during the recording, but without evidence of an arrhythmia; in approximately 14% of patients, arrhythmias were found to be present but without concomitant symptoms (SOE=B). These patients can represent a diagnostic dilemma. However, certain arrhythmias, even asymptomatic ones, such as nonsustained ventricular tachycardia, second- and third-degree AV block, and sinus pauses >3 sec, are rare in people without heart disease. Their presence, even if asymptomatic, in a patient with a history of syncope indicates the need for further evaluation.

Ambulatory external Holter monitoring devices are usually used for 24–48 hours. Because symptoms do not recur in most patients during the monitoring period, the positive diagnostic yield of Holter for syncope evaluation is low, approximately 1%–2% in unselected populations. External loop recorders have a loop memory that continuously records rhythm in single or multiple leads. When activated by the patient, typically after a symptom has occurred, 5–15 min of pre- and post-activation ECG is stored and can be retrieved for analysis. Patients are typically given the external loop recorder for 1 month. The diagnostic yield can be up to

25% in selected patients. The external loop recorder is less useful when recurrence of syncope is infrequent.

Implantable Loop Recorders

Implantable loop recorders (ILRs) are implanted subcutaneously in the prepectoral region under local anesthesia with a battery life of up to 36 months. These devices have a solid-state loop memory that stores ECG recordings, when activated either by the patient or a bystander, usually after a syncopal episode or are automatically activated in the case of occurrence of predefined arrhythmias. Some of these devices have remote (at home) telemetry capable of transmitting the signals in real time. Studies have shown that symptom–electrogram correlation ranges between 35% and 88%. Additional studies have shown that implantation of an ILR early during the evaluation was more likely to provide a diagnosis than the conventional strategy (52% vs 20%). Current guidelines recommend that the use of ILR should be considered early in patients when an arrhythmic cause of syncope is suspected but not sufficiently proved (SOE=B).

Echocardiography

In the absence of features suggestive of heart disease by history, physical examination, or ECG, two-dimensional echocardiography has a low yield (SOE=C). It is most useful in confirming a specific diagnosis suspected by other assessment. Occult coronary artery disease is also prevalent among older adults, and stress testing is often used for screening. In some patients, particularly those with the suggestion of structural cardiac abnormalities and ischemia by history, physical examination, or ECG, it is efficient to perform stress echocardiography as a single procedure.

Tilt-Table Testing

Head-up tilt-table testing results in pooling of blood in the legs and, in susceptible individuals, can trigger syncope mediated by neurocardiogenic mechanisms or to confirm postural hypotension. Tilt-table testing is useful for patients suspected of having vasovagal syncope and those with unexplained syncope who are not suspected of having a cardiac cause. Responses to tilt testing performed for evaluation of syncope tend to differ by age among adults without significant structural heart disease. Those ≥65 years old tend to have far higher rates of symptoms due to pure vasodilatation without significant change in heart rate than individuals ≤35 years old. In contrast, individuals ≤35 years old tend to have more profound cardioinhibitory responses, characterized by profound bradycardia or asystole induced by tilt testing, than those ≥65 years old. The different patterns of responses induced by tilt studies between younger and older adults suggests that different mechanisms for neurocardiogenic syncope predominate at different ages. Exaggerated autonomic response is common in younger people, whereas attenuated autonomic responses become predominant with advancing age.

Electrophysiologic Study (EPS)

The diagnostic efficacy of EPS to determine the cause of syncope greatly depends on patient selection and the degree of suspicion of an arrhythmic substrate for syncope. The development of effective noninvasive methods, ie, prolonged rhythm monitoring, has decreased the importance of EPS as a diagnostic test. Nevertheless, this test is still useful for diagnosis in suspected intermittent bradycardia, tachyarrhythmia, or in patients with bundle-branch block (suggestive of impending high-grade AV block). EPS is not recommended for patients with normal ECGs or without a history of heart disease or symptoms of palpitations.

Neurologic Testing

Neurologic testing, including imaging of the head by CT or MRI and electroencephalographic recording, is appropriate in situations when focal neurologic signs or symptoms are present or when the history suggests seizure during the evaluation of loss of consciousness. Autonomic evaluation should be considered when symptoms and signs of autonomic insufficiency are present.

TREATMENT

The goals of treatment for syncope, particularly in older adults, are to improve quality of life and prevent physical injuries. The effectiveness of therapy depends on whether a cause of syncope can be clearly established.

Reflex Syncope and Postural Hypotension

Nonpharmacologic measures with physical counter-pressure maneuvers such as leg crossing, arm tensing, hand grip, and buttock clenching are able to induce a significant blood pressure increase during the phase of impending reflex syncope so that the patient can avoid or delay losing consciousness in most cases (SOE=B). These measures in conjunction with conventional therapies have shown to reduce the recurrence by 39% (SOE=A). However, the effectiveness of these physical counter maneuvers in older adults has not been confirmed. Compression stockings and abdominal binders can be helpful in some patients with postural hypotension. Smaller and frequent meals can be effective in patients with postprandial hypotension.

Medical Management

The baroreceptor reflex plays a key role in blood-pressure hemostasis. A fall in blood pressure leads to unloading of these receptors in the aortic arch and carotid sinus, resulting in reduced traffic in glossopharyngeal and vagal afferents, activation of sympathetic outflow, and inhibition of cardiovagal neurons.

Drugs that mimic sympathetic activity such as α-agonists, including midodrine and etileferine, have been used to increase vasoconstriction. Midodrine is a useful addition to the nonpharmacologic approaches in patients with persistent postural hypotension. However, the use of an α-agonist is limited by supine hypertension, particularly in older adults with decreased vascular compliance. The use of an α-agonist for the treatment of orthostatic hypotension requires careful titration of the drug dosage and close monitoring of blood-pressure response and symptoms.

In studies that assessed the effects of pyridostigmine, an acetylcholinesterase inhibitor, on facilitating transmission of impulses from the cholinergic neurons across the synaptic cleft, both standing blood pressure and peripheral resistance were significantly increased, while orthostatic blood pressure was attenuated. Supine blood pressure increased modestly in some patients but overall was not significantly affected. Common adverse events include abdominal cramps with diarrhea from increased peristalsis and urinary urgency (SOE=C). The use of pyridostigmine in syncopal patients with orthostatic hypotension and autonomic failure should be closely supervised.

Volume expansion with added salt (liberalize diet) or fludrocortisone, or both, to increase renal sodium retention and intravascular volume can be effective in patients with persistent postural hypotension (SOE=C).

Additional and less frequently used treatments, alone or in combination, include desmopressin in patients with nocturnal polyuria, octeotride in postprandial hypotension, erythropoietin in anemia, use of walking sticks, frequent small meals, and use of compression stockings and abdominal binders.

Role of Pacemakers

Beyond the discontinuation of culprit medications, pharmacologic treatment has little place in the long-term treatment of bradycardia associated with syncope. Atropine or isoproterenol is indicated only in emergencies and temporary situations before cardiac pacing can be introduced. The mainstay of treatment for sinus node dysfunction or high-grade AV block is a pacemaker. Permanent pacing is clearly indicated when syncope or near syncope is correlated with bradycardia, regardless of the site of block. See Table 48.4.

The role of pacemaker therapy in patients with reflex syncope remains to be defined. In older adults with recurrent syncope of a vasovagal nature, pacemaker placement should be considered when a cardioinhibitory response is documented during monitoring.

REFERENCES

- Kim DH, Brown RT, Ding EL, et al. Dementia medications and risk of falls, syncope, and related adverse events: meta-analysis of randomized controlled trials. *J Am Geriatr Soc.* 2011;59(6):1019–1031.
- Task Force for the Diagnosis and Management of Syncope of the European Society of Cardiology (ESC); European Heart Rhythm Association (EHRA); Heart Failure Association (HFA); Heart Rhythm Society (HRS). Guidelines for the diagnosis and management of syncope (version 2009). *Eur Heart J.* 2009;30(21):2631–2671.
- Wahlrab L. The differential diagnosis of syncope: A guide for emergency department advanced practice nurses. *Adv Emerg Nurs J.* 2012;Oct-Dec;34(4):341–349.

CHAPTER 28—MALNUTRITION

KEY POINTS

- Aging is associated with changes in body composition such that well-standardized nutrient requirements for younger or middle-aged adults cannot be generalized to older adults.
- The Mini-Nutritional Assessment–Short Form is a brief and simple instrument useful for nutritional screening in geriatric patients.
- Identification of the presence of undernutrition or obesity can be facilitated by determining a person's BMI.
- Many medications have anorexia as a major adverse event or can reduce nutrient availability in older adults.
- Various appetite stimulants and anabolic agents are being used in older adults and are the focus of intensive investigation.

Malnutrition in older adults spans the spectrum from under- to overnutrition. Nutritional problems accompany many chronic disease processes of older adults. Moreover, age-related changes in physiology, metabolism, and function can alter the older adult's nutritional requirements. Better understanding among clinicians of the aging process and of nutritional screening, assessment, and interventions could potentially improve the health and independence of older adults.

AGE-RELATED CHANGES

Body Composition

Aging is associated with notable changes in body composition. Bone mass, lean mass, and water content all decrease, while fat mass generally increases. The volume of distribution of many medications changes as a result of these changes in body composition, and creatinine-based determinations can overestimate renal clearance in older adults. The increase in total body fat is commonly accompanied by greater intra-abdominal fat stores. The consequence of these changes in body composition is that well-standardized nutrient requirements for younger or middle-aged adults cannot be generalized to older adults. The aging process also affects organ functions, although the degree of change observed is highly variable among individuals. Decline in organ functions can affect nutritional assessment and intervention.

Energy Requirements

The reduced basal metabolic rate in older adults reflects loss of muscle mass. The basal metabolic rate is the principal determinant of total energy expenditure; energy expenditure in relation to physical activity is the most variable component. The Harris-Benedict equations can be used to predict basal energy expenditure. In any determination of energy needs for older adults, care must be taken to avoid overfeeding while still meeting basal requirements.

Macronutrient Needs

A modified food guide pyramid for older adults based on the 2010 U.S. Department of Agriculture food guidelines, now known as MyPlate, has been released. My Plate (www.choosemyplate.gov/ [accessed Oct 2013]) is a USDA initiative with helpful, culturally sensitive advice that is replacing the food pyramid formerly used. This pictorial recommendation depicts easy-to-understand examples to balance calories, avoid oversized portions, encourage lower-fat dairy and low-sodium food choices, and make half the plate fruits and vegetables and half of all grains whole grain.

The Food and Nutrition Board of the Institute of Medicine has released macronutrient guidelines that recommend a prudent diet, with 20%–35% of calories as fat, and reduced intakes of cholesterol, saturated fat, and trans-fatty acids. Carbohydrates should constitute 45%–65% of total calories; complex carbohydrates are the preferred fiber source. More specifically, the recommended daily fiber intake for those ≥60 years old is 30 g for men and 21 g for women. Protein intake is recommended at 0.8 g/kg/d at approximately 10%–35% of total calories. With stress or injury, protein requirements are typically estimated at 1.5 g/kg/d, but underlying renal or hepatic insufficiency may warrant protein restriction.

Micronutrient Requirements

Revisions of the dietary reference intakes (DRIs) include recommended dietary allowances (RDAs), defined as the average daily nutrient intake level estimated to meet the requirements of 97%–98% of the healthy individuals in a group, with more specific guidelines for older adults; those for the group ≥71 years old are shown in Table 28.1. The Food and Nutrition Board has also updated the RDAs with population-weighted estimated average requirements, defined as the average daily nutrient intake level estimated to meet the requirements of half of the healthy individuals in a group, based on updated census data. This information may be helpful for individualized recommendations to avoid overnutrification (http://www.iom.edu/ [accessed Oct 2013]).

Fluid Needs

Dehydration is the most common fluid or electrolyte disturbance in older adults. Normal aging is associated with a decreased perception of thirst, impaired response to serum osmolarity, and reduced ability to concentrate urine after fluid deprivation. A decline in fluid intake can also result from disease states that reduce mental or physical ability to recognize or express thirst, or that result in decreased access to water. In general, fluid needs of older adults can be met with 30 mL/kg/d or 1 mL/kcal ingested. Fluid needs may increase during episodes of fever or infection, as well as with diuretic or laxative therapy. Common signs of dehydration are decreased urine output, confusion, constipation, and mucosal dryness, although neither is sensitive or specific.

Table 28.1—Recommended Dietary Intakes of Micronutrients for Adults ≥71 Years Old

	Recommended Daily Allowance	
Nutrient	***For Men***	***For Women***
Calcium	1,200 mg*	1,200 mg*
Magnesium	420 mg	320 mg
Vitamin D	1,600 IU*	1,600 IU*
Thiamine	1.2 mg	1.1 mg
Riboflavin	1.3 mg	1.1 mg
Niacin	16 mg	14 mg
Vitamin B_6	1.7 mg	1.5 g
Folate	400 mcg	400 mcg
Vitamin B_{12}	2.4 mcg	2.4 mcg
Pantothenic acid	5 mg*	5 mg*
Vitamin A	5,000 IU	4,000 IU
Vitamin K	120 mcg*	90 mcg*
Iron	10 mg	10 mg
Zinc	15 mg	15 mg
Vitamin C	90 mg	75 mg
α-Tocopherol	10 IU	10 IU
Selenium	55 mcg	55 mcg
Potassium	4,700 mg*	4,700 mg*

*Adequate intake, not recommended dietary allowance.

SOURCES: Data from Standing Committee on the Scientific Evaluation of Dietary Reference Intakes, Food and Nutrition Board, Institute of Medicine, *Dietary Reference Intakes for Calcium, Phosphorus, Magnesium, Vitamin D, and Fluoride*. Washington, DC: National Academy Press; 1997; Standing Committee on the Scientific Evaluation of Dietary Reference Intakes, Institute of Medicine, *Dietary Reference Intakes for Thiamin, Riboflavin, Niacin, Vitamin B_6, Folate, Vitamin B_{12}, Pantothenic Acid, Biotin, and Choline*. Washington, DC: National Academy Press; 1999; Standing Committee on the Scientific Evaluation of Dietary Reference Intakes, Food and Nutrition Board, *Dietary Reference Intakes for Vitamin C, Vitamin E, Selenium, and Beta Carotene, and Other Carotenoids*. Washington, DC: National Academy Press; 2000; Standing Committee on the Scientific Evaluation of Dietary Reference Intakes, Food and Nutrition Board, *Dietary Reference Intakes for Vitamin A, Vitamin K, Arsenic, Boron, Chromium, Copper, Iodine, Iron, Manganese, Molybdenum, Nickel, Silicon, Vanadium, and Zinc*. Washington, DC: National Academy Press; 2000; Standing Committee on the Scientific Evaluation of Dietary Reference Intakes, Institute of Medicine, *Dietary Reference Intakes for Water, Potassium, Sodium, Chloride, and Sulfate*. Washington, DC: National Academy Press; 2004; *Dietary Reference Intakes for Calcium and Vitamin D* (2011). Available at www.nap.edu (accessed Oct 2013).

NUTRITION SCREENING AND ASSESSMENT

Anthropometrics

Anthropometric measurements are often used for nutritional assessment of older adults. An unintended weight loss of 10 pounds in the preceding 6 months is a useful indicator of morbidity; this degree of weight loss is predictive of functional limitations, healthcare charges, and the need for hospitalization (SOE=B). The Minimum Data Set (MDS-3) used by Medicare-certified nursing homes defines significant weight loss as ≥5% in the past month or ≥10% in the past 6 months. BMI, calculated by weight in kg/(height in meters)^2, is a useful measure of body size and indirect measure of body fat that does not require the use of a reference table of ideal weights. For National Institutes of Health guidelines regarding body size classification based on BMI, see http://www.cdc.gov/healthyweight/assessing/bmi/adult_bmi/index.html (accessed Oct 2013). The risk threshold for low BMI is set at 18.5 but should be interpreted in the context of the individual's lifelong habits. Other anthropometric tools include skin-fold and circumference measurements, but these have had limited practical application because of the difficulty of achieving acceptable reliability among those taking the measurements.

Nutritional Intake

Generally, inadequate nutritional intake has been defined as average or usual intake of servings of food groups, nutrients, or energy below a threshold level of the RDI. Poor intake is often an indication of illness. The limited reliability of accurately assessing dietary intake measures is well known, so thresholds of 25%–50% below the RDI have generally been selected. In one study, energy intake (<50% of calculated maintenance energy requirements) was reduced in 21% of a sample of hospitalized older adults. This subset of patients had higher rates of in-hospital mortality and 90-day mortality than did those with energy intakes above the threshold. Surveys of nutritional status conducted among chronically institutionalized older adults suggest that 5%–18% of nursing-home residents have energy intakes below their recommended average energy expenditure. However, evidence is generally lacking to

Table 28.2—Drug-Nutrient Interactions

Drug	Reduced Nutrient Availability
Alcohol	Zinc, vitamins A, B_1, B_2, B_6, B_{12}, folate
Antacids	Vitamin B_{12}, folate, iron
Antibiotics, broad-spectrum	Vitamin K
Colchicine	Vitamin B_{12}
Digoxin	Zinc
Diuretics	Zinc, magnesium, vitamin B_6, potassium, copper
Isoniazid	Vitamin B_6, niacin
Levodopa	Vitamin B_6
Laxatives	Calcium, vitamins A, B_2, B_{12}, D, E, K
Lipid-binding resins	Vitamins A, D, E, K
Metformin	Vitamin B_{12}
Mineral oil	Vitamins A, D, E, K
Phenytoin	Vitamin D, folate
Salicylates	Vitamin C, folate
Trimethoprim	Folate

support any benefits of nutritional supplementation in this population (SOE=B).

Energy intakes of men and women 65–98 years old have been estimated in a nationwide food consumption survey; 37%–40% of the men and women studied had energy intakes lower than two-thirds of the RDI, and many reported skipping at least one meal each day. Estimated intakes by consumption surveys, however, may be unreliable, because some studies suggest that older adults under-report energy intakes by 20%–30%.

Issues in obtaining food commonly contribute to inadequate nutritional intakes among older adults. It is important to ascertain whether limitations in resources, transportation, or functionality may limit access to food or the ability to prepare food.

Laboratory Tests: Albumin, Prealbumin, Cholesterol

Serum albumin has been recognized as a risk indicator for morbidity and mortality. Hypoalbuminemia lacks specificity and sensitivity as an indicator of malnutrition; however, it can be associated with injury, disease, or inflammatory conditions. As a negative acute-phase reactant, albumin is subject to cytokine-mediated decline in synthesis and to increased degradation and transcapillary leakage. Longitudinal studies of serum albumin suggest a modest decline in levels with aging that may be independent of disease. The prognostic value of hypoalbuminemia may be largely because of its use as a proxy measure for injury, disease, or inflammation. In the community setting, hypoalbuminemia has been associated with functional limitation, sarcopenia, increased healthcare use, and mortality (SOE=B). In the hospital setting, it has also been associated with increased length of stay, complications, readmissions, and mortality (SOE=B).

Other protein markers of nutritional status have clinical significance. Prealbumin has a considerably shorter half-life (48 hours) than albumin (18–20 days) and may therefore more adequately reflect short-term changes in protein status. Although prealbumin appears to have the same limitations as albumin as a diagnostic tool for nutritional status, in the absence of an inflammatory state, it can be used to measure the effectiveness of nutritional interventions or as an indicator of recovery (SOE=B). In addition to a shorter half-life, prealbumin has a small serum pool that allows for easier detection of small changes in nutritional status over a shorter time period if inflammation is not present. Serum cholesterol has also been linked to nutritional status. Low cholesterol levels (<160 mg/dL) are often detected in adults with serious underlying disease, such as malignancy. Poor clinical outcomes have been observed among hospitalized and institutionalized older adults with hypocholesterolemia. In a study of community-dwelling older adults, nutrient intakes were not different in those in the lowest quartile of serum cholesterol levels and in others. It appears likely, again, that acquired hypocholesterolemia is a nonspecific feature of poor health status that is independent of nutrient or energy intakes, and that it may better reflect a pro-inflammatory condition. Of interest is the observation that community-dwelling older adults with both hypoalbuminemia and hypocholesterolemia have higher rates of adverse functional and mortality outcomes than those with hypoalbuminemia or hypocholesterolemia alone (SOE=B).

Drug-Nutrient Interactions

Medications can modify the nutrient needs and metabolism of older adults. Certain medications, such as digoxin and phenytoin, even at therapeutic levels, can cause anorexia in older adults. Additional agents that have anorexia as a major potential adverse event include SSRIs, calcium channel blockers (eg, dihydropyridines), H_2-receptor antagonists, proton-pump inhibitors, narcotic and nonsteroidal analgesics, furosemide, potassium supplements, ipratropium bromide, and theophylline. Many medications are known to interfere with taste and smell (see "Oral Diseases and Disorders," Table 46.2, p 369), and others can reduce the availability of specific nutrients (Table 28.2). Some can reduce intake by causing inattention, dysphagia, dysgeusia, or xerostomia. Medications that precipitate constipation can also reduce appetite.

Table 28.3—Risk Factors for Poor Nutritional Status

Alcohol or substance abuse
Cognitive dysfunction
Decreased exercise
Depression, poor mental health
Functional limitations
Inadequate funds
Limited education
Limited mobility, transportation
Medical problems, chronic diseases
Medications
Poor dentition
Restricted diet, poor eating habits
Social isolation

Multi-Item Tools for Nutrition Screening

The nutritional status of older adults can be influenced by a variety of factors (Table 28.3). The absence of single assessment measures that are valid indicators of comprehensive nutritional status has prompted the development of multi-item tools. Older adults in acute- or chronic-care facilities have been extensively studied to identify indicators and predictors of nutritional status; those in the community setting have been subject to less investigation. Nutritional screening tools for older adults have been widely disseminated. Their effectiveness remains to be demonstrated—specifically, whether these tools can identify undernourished individuals whose problems are amenable to intervention.

The Nutrition Screening Initiative (a collaborative effort of the American Dietetic Association, the American Academy of Family Practitioners, and the National Council on Aging, Inc) developed three interdisciplinary tools to screen for nutrition risk and help evaluate the nutritional status of older adults. The DETERMINE checklist (http://nutritionandaging.fiu.edu/downloads/NSI_checklist.pdf [accessed Oct 2013]) was created to raise public awareness about the importance of nutrition to the health of older adults. This self-report questionnaire is composed of 10 items and is intended to identify risk but not to diagnose malnutrition. The Level I screen, intended for use by healthcare professionals, incorporates additional assessment items regarding dietary habits, functional status, living environment, and weight change, as well as measures of height and weight. The Level II screen, for use by more highly trained medical and nutrition professionals and suggested for use in the diagnosis of malnutrition, contains all the items from Level I with additional biochemical and anthropometric measures, as well as a more detailed evaluation of depression and mental status.

The Mini-Nutritional Assessment tool was developed to evaluate the risk of malnutrition among frail older adults and to identify those who may benefit from early intervention (SOE=B). This assessment tool requires administration by a trained professional and consists of 18 items, including questions about BMI, mid-arm and calf circumferences, weight loss, living environment, medication use, dietary habits, clinical global assessment, and self-perception of health and nutrition status. A shortened screening version that contains only 6 items, the short form Mini-Nutritional Assessment, is now available (www.mna-elderly.com [accessed Oct 2013]). Another nutritional assessment tool, the Simplified Nutrition Assessment Questionnaire can be answered by patients through the mail or while sitting in a waiting room; it has a sensitivity and specificity of 88.2% and 83.5% for identifying those at risk of weight loss (www.slu.edu/readstory/newslink/6349 [accessed Oct 2013]).

NUTRITION SYNDROMES

Undernutrition

Subdividing this group of nutritional syndromes, characterized by loss of weight or compromised protein status, or both, is challenging. The nomenclature used implies that these syndromes are distinct, while in practice it is often difficult to distinguish one from another, and the syndromes commonly overlap. Inflammation permeates the syndromes of cachexia, protein energy undernutrition, sarcopenia, failure to thrive, and obesity, such that an inflammatory continuum may be a more appropriate model. The presence (cachexia) or absence (wasting) of cytokine-mediated response to injury or disease is at times used, but in some situations, eg, the weight loss from AIDS, not all of the loss appears to be the result of inflammation. Some authors note that with cachexia, resting energy expenditure is increased whereas with wasting it is decreased, but this measure is not generally available to most practicing clinicians. Also confusing is the term *protein-energy undernutrition*, which is meant to encompass the spectrum of protein and energy undernutrition but is often erroneously applied to individuals with reduced albumin or prealbumin levels from an inflammatory response. Sarcopenia is defined as the age-associated loss of skeletal muscle mass and function (loss of muscle mass with limited mobility) and is a major contributor to frailty, a state of vulnerability to adverse outcomes attributable to the loss of physiologic reserve necessary to withstand minor stressors. (See "Frailty," p 177.)

Obesity

The growing prevalence of obesity in America extends to older adults in their 60s and 70s. According to

National Health and Nutrition Examination Surveys, the prevalence of obesity (BMI ≥30 kg/m^2) has climbed from 14% to 32% between 1976 and 2004. Trends were similar for all ages, both genders, and all racial or ethnic groups.

Excess body weight and modest weight gain (≥5 kg) in middle age can be associated with medical comorbidities in later life that include hypertension, diabetes mellitus, cardiovascular disease, obstructive sleep apnea, and osteoarthritis. Adverse outcomes associated with obesity include impaired functional status, increased use of healthcare resources, and increased mortality (SOE=B). A BMI ≥35 kg/m^2 is associated with increased risk of functional decline among older adults. Of interest, poor diet quality and micronutrient deficiencies are relatively common among obese older adults, especially obese older women living alone. Many homebound older adults are also obese. The National Institutes of Health has suggested: "Age alone should not preclude weight loss treatment for older adults. A careful evaluation of potential risks and benefits in the individual patient should guide management." The focus must be on achieving a more healthful weight to promote improved health, function, and quality of life. A combination of prudent diet, behavior modification, and activity or exercise may be appropriate for selected candidates. For frail, obese older adults, the emphasis may better be placed on preservation of strength and flexibility, rather than on weight reduction.

NUTRITIONAL INTERVENTIONS

Oral Nutrition and Supplements

Preventing undernutrition is much easier than treating it. Food intake can be enhanced by catering to food preferences as much as possible and by avoiding therapeutic diets unless their clinical value is certain. Patients should be prepared for meals with appropriate hand and mouth care, and they should be comfortably situated for eating. Assistance should be provided for those who need help. Placing two or more patients together for meals can increase sociability and food intake. Foods should be of appropriate consistency, prepared with attention to color, texture, temperature, and arrangement. The use of herbs, spices, and hot foods helps to compensate for loss of the sense of taste and smell often accompanying old age and to avoid the excessive use of salt and sugar. (See "Oral Diseases and Disorders," p 362.) Hard-to-open individual packages should be avoided. Adequate time should be taken for leisurely meals. Title IIIC of the Older Americans Act has provided for congregate and home-delivered meals for older adults, regardless of economic status. This service is available in most parts of the country, albeit with a waiting list in many locations. Adequate access to nutritious and appetizing food should be assured for patients of various cultural backgrounds and in all settings.

Dietary supplements have been widely used in an effort to enhance nutrient intake, especially when patients eat only small amounts. The use of such supplements often decreases food intake, but overall nutritional intake usually increases owing to the nutrient quality and density of the supplements. Standard supplements contain macro- and micronutrients. Many different oral formulations are available in both liquid and bar forms. They can be chosen based on patient preferences, chewing ability, or product cost. Oral formulas can also be selected based on their caloric density, osmolality, protein, fiber, or lactose content. Most formulas provide 1–1.5 calories/mL, and many are lactose- and gluten-free. However, it has yet to be demonstrated that any supplement is superior to regular food intake.

Interest is also growing in the use of micronutrient supplements in health promotion. Many vitamin and mineral supplements are commonly available in supermarkets and drugstores. New recommendations for older adults include higher intakes of calcium and vitamin D to prevent osteoporosis (SOE=B) (Table 28.1). Vitamin D deficiency occurs in 30% of individuals >70 years old and is associated with impaired physical performance. Screening for vitamin D deficiency with measurement of total vitamin D levels is appropriate in older patients, because repletion is associated with improved physical performance, reduced falls, improved bone healing, and response to bisphosphonates (SOE=B) (see "Endocrine and Metabolic Disorders," p 506). Folic acid, B_6, and B_{12} can lower homocysteine levels, theoretically reducing the risk of coronary artery disease and helping to prevent decline in cognitive function. However, evidence to date from randomized controlled trials with folic acid or B_6 supplementation is poor. Insufficient evidence also exists to determine whether immune function can be improved by supplementation of protein, vitamin E, zinc, or other micronutrients (SOE=C). Whether the effects of antioxidants are beneficial is also the subject of controversy. While it has previously been suggested that antioxidants can help in preventing age-related cataracts and macular degeneration, more recent evidence indicates that they may have little or no effect. Although naturally occurring dietary antioxidants can reduce cardiovascular disease and mortality, supplementation with specific antioxidants, namely β-carotene, vitamin A, and vitamin E, can increase mortality in some settings (SOE=C). In addition, vitamin E supplementation has not been

Table 28.4—Examples of Potential Pathways and Molecular Targets for Drug Treatment of Sarcopenia

Drug	Reduced Nutrient Availability
Androgen receptors	Increase muscle mass and strength
Peroxisome proliferator-activated receptor-gamma coactivator 1-α	Increase muscle oxidative metabolism
Myostatin	Increase muscle mass and strength
Peroxisome proliferator-activated receptor-delta	Increase type 1 fibers and oxidative metabolism
Insulin-like growth factor 1	Increase muscle mass and strength
β-adrenergic receptor	Increase muscle mass
Neuregulins	Increase muscle mass and enhance glucose utilization
Angiotensin-converting enzyme	Increase muscle function and physical performance
Inflammatory cytokines	Decrease catabolic effects

SOURCE: Data from Houston DK, Tooze JA, Hauseman BD, et al. Considerations in the development of drugs to treat sarcopenia. *J Gerontol A Biol Sci.* 2011;66A(4):430–436.

shown to slow the progression of Alzheimer disease or prevent cardiovascular disease, and it may be associated with higher risk of hemorrhagic stroke. Further, among individuals with diabetes or vascular disease, supplementation with vitamin E can increase risk of heart failure (SOE=C).

Because approximately 60% of older adults take self-prescribed dietary supplements, it is imperative that the clinician obtain information about the patient's use of all supplements. The appropriateness and safety of each supplement should be evaluated, because consumers are often unaware of potential risks and adverse events of many OTC supplements, and solid evidence in favor of these purported benefits is currently lacking.

Drug Treatment for Undernutrition Syndromes

A number of agents have been suggested to promote appetite or to serve as anabolic aids. Appetite stimulants include the antidepressant mirtazapine^{OL}, a serotonin norepinephrine reuptake inhibitor that antagonizes the 5-HT_3 receptor, possibly stimulating appetite by that mechanism, but proof of this effect is limited. Dosing is 7.5–30 mg po at bedtime. Caution is required for dosages 15–30 mg/d, because of hepatic or renal insufficiency, and because of more noradrenergic and serotonin effects, some of which may counteract the appetite stimulatory effects. Cyproheptadine^{OL}, a serotonin and histamine antagonist, can also enhance appetite (SOE=C), but there is the potential for confusion in older adults. It is given at a dose of 2–4 mg po with meals. Megestrol^{OL} is a progestin that stimulates appetite and is given daily at 320–800 mg po in two divided doses (see Hypoadrenocorticoidism in "Endocrine and Metabolic Disorders," p 506). Appetite and usually weight gain improve with megestrol acetate; however, this weight gain is primarily fat, and clinical benefits have not been demonstrated (SOE=A). Megestrol acetate in nursing-home populations can be associated with a higher risk of deep-vein thrombosis, fluid retention, edema, and exacerbation of congestive heart failure. Megestrol acetate during rehabilitation may negate the benefits of exercise on strength and function. Dronabinol^{OL}, a cannabinoid, can stimulate appetite at 2.5 mg twice daily before lunch and dinner (maximum 20 mg/d), but it is associated with somnolence and dysphoria in older adults.

Cytokine-modulating agents are experimental in the treatment of undernutrition syndromes, even though anticytokines have been breakthrough treatments for selected forms of disease-related cachexia. Approaches include anti–tumor necrosis factor, consisting of antibodies that can inhibit cytokine-mediated inflammation, and n-3 fatty acids and antioxidants, which can modulate cytokine production.

Anabolic agents include human growth hormone^{OL}, which induces preferential usage of carbohydrates and fats while preserving proteins and increasing muscle mass. Increased muscle strength and functional capacity, however, depend on exercise rehabilitation. Growth hormone is contraindicated in cancer states. Hyperglycemia and fluid retention can be seen, and no studies have demonstrated significant functional benefits. Oxandrolone is an anabolic steroid that increases muscle protein synthesis; it is given at 2.5–20 mg/d po in divided doses. Anabolic agents can increase muscle mass, but questions remain concerning long-term safety and cost that currently mitigate endorsement (SOE=B). Likewise, while muscle mass has consistently improved with anabolic agents, significant improvements in strength, function, or a reduction in fractures have not been demonstrated. For potential drug pathways and molecular targets for drug treatment of sarcopenia, see Table 28.4.

Legal and Ethical Issues

In the nursing home, unacceptable weight loss, as defined by the Omnibus Budget Reconciliation Act of 1987, is any loss ≥5% in the past month or ≥10% in the past 6 months. Sections of the Minimum Data Set (see "Nursing Home Care," p 153) that are related to nutritional status include those assessing cognitive function, mood and behavior, physical function, health condition, oral and nutritional status, dental status, skin condition, and special treatments and procedures, including restorative care for eating and swallowing. Care Area Assessments (formerly called Resident Assessment Protocols) ensure prompt identification of problems focused on by the MDS. The MDS uses intake of <75% of food provided as the threshold to trigger nutrition assessment. Standards of care dictate the following:

- Acceptable parameters of nutritional status such as body weight and protein levels should be maintained, unless the resident's clinical condition demonstrates that this is not possible.
- A resident should receive a therapeutic diet when there is a problem.

Food and fluid should always be offered to all patients; however, the decision to start or to discontinue artificial nutrition or hydration must be considered very carefully. Competent adults may choose to forgo artificial feeding, just as they have the right to decline any invasive procedure. Some adults have advance directives executed at a time when the individual was competent that prohibit the use of feeding tubes. These should be honored unless there is compelling evidence that the individual would have changed his or her mind in the current situation. Incompetent adults without advance directives pose a greater challenge. The decision to start or to discontinue artificial feeding should be considered carefully with the surrogate, taking into account the risks and burdens of such an action, the risks and burdens of alternative actions, and the evidence to support likely benefits of the various actions. To date, evidence supporting the use of feeding tubes in patients with end-stage cancer, dementia, and COPD are lacking (see "Eating and Feeding Problems," p 216).

After total cessation of nutrition, depending on underlying conditions, several weeks may ensue before death, and some patients who consume very little may survive much longer. Pleasure/comfort eating is always continued if the patient requests. In this setting, palliative care, including emotional support, is extremely important and complex. See "Palliative Care," p 111; and "Legal and Ethical Issues," p 26.

REFERENCES

- Amella E, Aselage M. *Meal time Difficulties: Nursing Standard of Practice Protocol Assessment and Management of Mealtime Difficulties.* http://consultgerirn.org/topics/mealtime_difficulties/want_to_know_more. Updated 2012. (accessed Oct 2013).
- ChooseMyPlate. http://www.choosemyplate.gov/healthy-eating-tips.html (accessed Oct 2013).
- Institute of Medicine, Food and Nutrition Board. *Dietary Reference Intakes for Energy, Carbohydrate, Fiber, Fat, Fatty Acids, Cholesterol, Protein, and Amino Acids (Macronutrients).* Washington, DC: National Academy Press; 2005.
- Shenkin A. Serum prealbumin: Is it a marker of nutritional status or of risk of malnutrition? *Clin Chem.* 2006;52(12):2177–2179.

CHAPTER 29—EATING AND FEEDING PROBLEMS

KEY POINTS

- Several age-related changes in older adults contribute to a slowed ability to swallow.
- Dementia is the most common cause of oral dysphagia.
- Most healthy people aspirate without any important clinical consequences.
- Aspiration pneumonia is believed to occur when contaminated oral secretions arrive in the lungs in a high enough inoculum to overcome host defenses.
- No studies demonstrate that feeding tubes reduce the occurrence of aspiration, but rather, many studies identify feeding tubes as major risk factors for aspiration.
- The assessment of swallowing function is controversial. Data correlating specific findings from any type of swallowing examination with clinically meaningful outcomes are lacking.

Swallowing is an important and complex event that can be affected by both normal aging and diseases that are common in older adults. Treatment of eating and feeding problems depends on the identified cause or causes and contributing factors.

SWALLOWING IN HEALTH AND DISEASE

Swallowing and Aging

Swallowing can be divided into three phases on the basis of anatomy. First is the preparatory or oral phase, which includes the complex activities of mastication and propelling the food bolus to the back of the mouth toward the pharynx. This stage is under voluntary control. The second or pharyngeal phase is involuntary and involves initiation of the swallow reflex with propulsion of the food bolus past the laryngeal vestibule and into the esophagus. Execution of the oral and pharyngeal phases of swallowing requires the complex coordination of five cranial nerves and a large number of small muscles in the head and neck, with regulation from cortical input to the medullary swallow center, all in the appropriate sequence, usually within 1 second. The third stage of swallowing is the esophageal phase, during which food is propelled down the esophagus by the action of skeletal muscle proximally and smooth muscle distally; this phase is regulated by its own intrinsic innervation.

Normal aging is associated with several changes in eating. With advanced age, taste sensation decreases but not taste discrimination (older adults may be able to distinguish sweet from salty but may need to add more salt to food to taste it sufficiently). Olfactory function declines with advancing age, further impairing taste sensation. Salivary function is not clearly reduced with aging, but xerostomia is a common complaint of older adults, usually because of adverse events of medication. Loss of teeth greatly reduces chewing efficiency (ie, chewing is needed for a longer period of time and with more chewing strokes to achieve the same level of food maceration), which is only partly ameliorated with dental prostheses. Sarcopenia, or age-related loss of lean muscle mass, can contribute to loss in chewing efficiency and to pharyngeal muscle weakness demonstrated on videofluoroscopic deglutition examination (VDE) of asymptomatic older adults. Whether aging alone contributes to esophageal dysmotility (so-called *presbyesophagus*) remains a subject of debate. Esophageal function is probably well preserved, except perhaps in very advanced age. In total, these changes with age result in a prolonged duration of each swallow.

Dysphagia

Dysphagia, or difficulty swallowing, can occur when a disease affects any level of swallowing function. Dysphagia is usually classified as oral, pharyngeal, or esophageal. In oral dysphagia, there is difficulty with the voluntary transfer of food from the mouth to the pharynx. This might be diagnosed, for example, when scrambled eggs are discovered in the cheeks of a demented patient shortly before lunch. The most common cause of oral dysphagia is dementia.

In pharyngeal dysphagia, there is a problem with reflexive transfer of the food bolus from the pharynx to initiate the involuntary esophageal phase of swallowing while simultaneously protecting the airway from misdirection of food. The affected person or a caregiver may notice coughing, choking, or nasal regurgitation while eating and localize the symptoms to the throat. The most common cause of pharyngeal dysphagia is stroke, but any disease that impairs the swallowing center in the brain stem or the cranial nerves involved (eg, Parkinson disease, CNS tumor), the oropharyngeal striated muscle (eg, myasthenia gravis, amyotrophic lateral sclerosis), or the local structures involved (eg, retropharyngeal abscess, tumor) can lead to pharyngeal dysphagia. Management of both oral and pharyngeal dysphagia involves treating the underlying disorder and devising an individualized, often labor-intensive, feeding program.

In esophageal dysphagia, the patient has the sensation that food has gotten "stuck" after a swallow. Dysphagia for both solids and liquids suggests an esophageal motility disorder (eg, achalasia, scleroderma), whereas progressive dysphagia for solids suggests a mechanical obstruction (eg, cancer, esophageal ring, stricture from mucosal irritation). None of these diseases is unique to the geriatric population, although older adults tend to take more medications and are therefore more likely to experience medication-induced esophagitis (which manifests initially as odynophagia, followed by dysphagia). Medications most commonly causing esophagitis in older adults are potassium, NSAIDs, oral bisphosphonates, and tetracycline-related antibiotics. See also the section on dysphagia in "Gastrointestinal Diseases and Disorders," p 408.

Aspiration

The misdirection of pharyngeal contents into the airway is termed *aspiration*. Generally, there are two major sources of aspiration: oropharyngeal flora or gastric contents. However, despite this relatively straightforward definition, controversy persists over the definition of *aspiration pneumonia*. Aspiration pneumonia is believed to occur when bacteria arrive in the lungs from the pharynx in a large enough inoculum to overcome host defenses. In the case of more virulent organisms, defenses can be overwhelmed by smaller inocula. Pneumococcal pneumonia arises from aspiration of *Pneumococcus* from a colonized oropharynx, however, and is usually not considered an aspiration pneumonia. Aspiration of gastric contents, or Mendelson syndrome, usually results in a chemical pneumonitis; the usefulness of antibiotics in this situation is questionable. Most often, local host defense mechanisms clear the lung of the offending aspirate, without serious clinical effect. Many healthy individuals episodically aspirate without any important clinical consequences.

Aspiration of contaminated oral contents or gastric contents is not prevented by placement of a feeding tube. In fact, tube feeding is universally cited as a risk factor for major aspiration, and some patients who have never previously aspirated begin to do so after a feeding tube has been placed. A review found no evidence that tube feeding of any sort would reduce the risk of aspiration pneumonia (SOE=B). A common misconception is that jejunostomy tube feeding has lower rates of associated aspiration of gastric contents than gastrostomy does. Most studies do not demonstrate reduced aspiration with jejunostomy than with gastrostomy (SOE=C). Whether hand feeding (personal assistance with oral intake) is safer than tube feeding is also unclear. In a single nonrandomized prospective comparison of hand with tube feeding in patients with oropharyngeal aspiration, hand feeding resulted in lower rates of pneumonia. No prospective randomized trials comparing hand with tube feeding to reduce aspiration have been published. An active area of clinical research is focused on the role of substance P in swallowing and aspiration and the potential benefit of ACE inhibitors (which prevent the breakdown of substance P) in patients who aspirate.

Assessment of Oropharyngeal Dysphagia

Several tools can be used to assess swallowing function when oropharyngeal dysphagia is suspected clinically. The most common are the full bedside evaluation (of which there are many variations), the videofluoroscopic deglutition examination (VDE; a variant of the modified barium swallow), and nasopharyngeal laryngoscopy performed by an otolaryngologist. There is considerable controversy regarding the relative efficacy of these tools.

VDE is usually performed by a speech-language pathologist who videotapes the patient swallowing barium-impregnated foods of several consistencies while maintaining various head positions. This can permit identification of the food consistency or compensatory mechanisms that minimize fluoroscopic evidence of aspiration. Depending on the results of the VDE, the therapist may recommend swallow therapy or diet modifications, or both. Swallow therapy may be compensatory (eg, turn head toward weaker side while swallowing), indirect (eg, exercises to improve the strength of the involved muscles), or direct (ie, exercises to perform while swallowing, such as swallowing multiple times per bolus). Dietary recommendations generally consist of altering bolus size or consistency of food or fluid, or of restricting foods of certain consistencies (Table 29.1).

Data regarding the usefulness of VDE and nasopharyngeal laryngoscopy have been derived from small, historically controlled studies rather than from larger prospective randomized trials. A systematic review of studies of dysphagia secondary to stroke published by the Agency for Healthcare Research and Quality concluded that evidence was insufficient to recommend one type of swallowing study over another and that data correlating specific findings from any type of examination with clinically meaningful outcomes are lacking (SOE=C).

FEEDING

When an older adult experiences difficulty eating, the two main therapeutic approaches are careful feeding by hand or tube. The first requires extraordinary patience and is labor intensive; the latter is an invasive

Table 29.1—Characteristics of Altered Diet Consistencies

Prescribed Consistency	Description
Solids	
Regular or whole foods	Food served as it would be at a restaurant
Cut up	No pieces larger than ½″ cubes
Chopped*	Food chopped into pea-sized pieces no larger than ¼″ cubes
Ground*	Size/consistency of cottage cheese, moist, soft
Pureed*	Smooth, like yogurt or very thick soup
Liquids	
Unrestricted	Also known as "thin" liquids with the consistency of water
Nectar	Consistency of tomato juice (usually some thickening agent added)
Honey	Liquid can be poured but slowly (most liquids require addition of thickening agent)
Pudding	Liquids cannot be poured and must be spooned

* Avoid foods that are tough to chew (eg, nuts, seeds, bacon, meat with casing, bagels, popcorn, dried fruits) for any consistency other than regular or cut-up.

intervention associated with its own risks. Data about either approach are limited, and randomized comparisons have not been done. The role of dietary supplements, if any, in augmenting the caloric intake of hand-fed older adults has not been clearly defined. One systematic review suggested that mortality was less with the use of oral protein and energy supplements in acutely hospitalized or community-dwelling adults >65 years old, although the quality of the studies reviewed were not optimal. Functional status does not appear to be improved with oral nutritional supplements in any of the studies evaluating this outcome.

The number of percutaneous endoscopic gastrostomy feeding tubes placed in patients ≥65 years old has grown at an astonishing rate over the past two decades. Low procedure-related complication rates are often cited; however, long-term studies reveal substantial mortality among tube-fed patients. Despite the popularity of feeding tubes, studies have not demonstrated improved survival, reduced incidence of pneumonia or other infections, improved symptoms or function, or reduced pressure ulcers with the use of feeding tubes of any type in demented patients who have eating difficulties. A 2009 Cochrane review of tube feeding in patients with advanced dementia found no evidence of a decrease in mortality (SOE=B). Median survival after placement of a feeding tube is well under a year, but it is unknown whether this results from tube feeding or if the need for tube feeding is a marker that death is near.

Complications described with feeding tubes are numerous and include an increased risk of aspiration pneumonia, metabolic disturbances, diarrhea, and local cellulitis. Monitoring for these complications should be meticulous. In a study that used a large administrative data set, 1-year mortality was higher in 5,266 nursing-home residents with chewing or swallowing difficulties who were fed with a tube than in those who were not, even when statistically accounting for potential confounding variables (SOE=B). No prospective randomized studies comparing tube and hand feeding have been published, and information on quality-of-life outcomes is sorely needed. Tube feedings may interfere with the absorption of some medications, eg, levodopa/carbidopa and phenytoin. Time-released medications cannot be crushed for administration through the tube.

Placement of a percutaneous endoscopic gastrostomy or jejunostomy bypasses the oropharynx and the esophagus, allowing nutrients and medications to be instilled directly into the stomach or the jejunum to be absorbed by a functioning gut. It is clear that neither gastrostomy nor jejunostomy feeding tubes reduce aspiration compared with a program of hand feeding, but no randomized trials comparing these interventions have been published. The only condition for which feeding tubes have been shown to be of clinical benefit to the patient is esophageal obstruction, such as from malignancy. For most other disease states, their use remains unproved (SOE=D).

Contraindications to gastrostomy include the inability to pass an endoscope into the stomach, uncorrectable coagulopathy, massive ascites, peritonitis, and bowel obstruction. After successful placement of a gastrostomy, tube feedings of commercially available canned nutritional supplements can be started either as slow gravity boluses for gastrostomy tubes over 30–60 minutes or as a continuous infusion for gastrostomy or jejunostomy tubes. The feeding tube should be flushed with water before and after each feeding or at least four times a day in cases of continuous feedings.

Consideration of feeding tube placement requires careful examination of the data, with a focus on whether there is evidence of clinical benefit to support this invasive and potentially burdensome approach.

Not all feeding problems, of course, are related to dysphagia, and many contributing factors are quite amenable to therapy. Other approaches to consider in older adults who demonstrate eating or feeding problems are evaluation for depression, elimination of unduly restrictive diets, consideration of individual food preferences, consideration of the environment in which the person eats to improve socialization and reduce disruptive stimuli, examination of the condition of the oral cavity, determination of the needs for personal assistance with feeding, and reduction or elimination of medications that can cause inattention, xerostomia, movement disorders, or anorexia. Small studies have documented improved clinical outcomes in nursing-home residents with the use of flavor enhancers, increased food variety, and attention to the meal ambiance.

REFERENCES

- Eisenstadt ES. Dysphagia and aspiration pneumonia in older adults. *J Am Acad Nurse Pract*. 2010;22(1):17–22.
- Hill M, Hughes T, Milford C. Treatment for swallowing difficulties (dysphagia) in chronic muscle disease. *Cochrane Database Syst Rev.* 2008;(2):CD004303.
- Sampson EL, Candy B, Jones L. Enteral feeding for older people with advanced dementia. *Cochrane Database Syst Rev.* 2009;(2):CD007209.

CHAPTER 30—URINARY INCONTINENCE

KEY POINTS

- The prevalence of urinary incontinence (UI) increases with age and ADL dependence, affecting 15%–30% of all adults ≥65 years old and 60%–70% of long-term care residents.
- UI in older adults can be caused or worsened by medical conditions, functional and cognitive impairment, and medications, with or without concomitant lower urinary tract dysfunction. Therefore, assessment of comorbidity, medications, and function are essential components of evaluation.
- Even in frailer older adults, UI is manageable through a stepped approach starting with lifestyle interventions and behavioral therapy, followed by medications and surgical interventions as appropriate.

UI is the involuntary leakage of any amount of urine. Even when UI is distinguished by type of leakage (eg, urge or stress), in older adults urinary leakage does not necessarily represent a specific diagnosis or pathophysiologic entity. In younger people, the etiology of UI often can be attributed after evaluation to specific pathophysiology in the lower urinary tract (LUT) and/or pelvic floor. In older adults, however, UI can be caused or worsened by comorbid conditions, medications, or functional and cognitive impairments, either alone or in combination with LUT dysfunction. Thus, UI is a classic geriatric syndrome, in which multiple risk factors interact with one another and other modulating factors to produce a clinical phenotype.

The most common types of UI symptoms in older adults are:

- Urge UI — occurs with urgency, a compelling and often sudden need to void; most common in both men and women
- Stress UI — leakage associated with coughing, sneezing, laughing, physical activity; second most common form in women and also seen in men after prostatectomy
- Mixed UI — leakage occurs with both urgency and activity; common in women
- UI from incomplete emptying — associated with "increased" postvoiding residual (PVR), often with symptoms of intermittent small dribbling; uncommon. The cut-off level for PVR is not well established, but the consensus is about 200 mL. The coexistence of urge UI and increased PVR (in the absence of bladder outlet obstruction) in frail patients is called detrusor hyperactivity with impaired contractility (DHIC).

UI may be accompanied by other LUT symptoms (ie, frequency, nocturia [awakening to void >1 time during sleep], slowed stream, hesitancy, sense of incomplete emptying, intermittent stream). "Overactive bladder" refers to a symptom complex of urgency, with or without urge UI, often accompanied with frequency and nocturia. These symptoms are all nonspecific and can be due to a variety of LUT conditions as well as comorbid diseases.

The terms "transient UI" and "functional UI" have been used to describe UI that is caused or exacerbated by factors beyond the LUT, such as comorbid conditions, medications, and impaired mobility. However, in many cases LUT dysfunction will be present as well, and thus correction of contributing factors may be insufficient to resolve UI. There is no widely accepted alternative term, although some authors suggest "UI due to potentially reversible factors."

PREVALENCE AND IMPACT

UI increases with age and affects women more than men (ratio 2:1) until age 80, after which men and women are equally affected. The prevalence is 15%–30% in community-dwelling adults ≥65 years old, and 60%–70% in long-term care settings. In most studies, overall rates of UI are higher in white women than in black, Hispanic, and Asian women, and stress UI is more common in white and Hispanic women than in black women. Racial and ethnic differences among older men are less clear. The few longitudinal studies in older women suggest annual UI incidence rates of 5%–11% in the community and 22% in long-term care, with remission rates that nearly match incidence.

UI significantly impairs quality of life, including emotional well-being, social function, and general health. Older adults with UI may maintain social activities, but do so with an increased burden of coping, embarrassment, and poor self-perception. Morbidity from UI includes dermatitis and cellulitis, pressure ulcers, urinary tract infections, falls with fractures, sleep deprivation, social withdrawal, depression, and sexual dysfunction. UI is not associated with increased mortality. UI increases caregiving time and burden, which may be why it remains a significant cause of long-term care placement. Estimated annual costs related to UI in older adults total more than $26 billion.

Risk Factors and Associated Comorbid Conditions

The evidence-based risk factors for UI in older patients include obesity (best demonstrated in young-old women), functional impairment, dementia, medications (estrogen and alpha blockers [in women], and cholinesterase inhibitors), and environmental barriers to toilet access. The association of vaginal delivery and parity with UI attenuates with age. These data pertain primarily to white women; much less is known about UI risk factors in other racial and ethnic populations and in men (other than prostate disease).

Especially in older adults, continence depends not only on LUT function but also on the ability to toilet, which requires sufficient physical function (mobility and manual dexterity), cognition, motivation, and available toilets. Medications and medical conditions can cause or worsen UI by their effects on toileting, LUT function, and/or urine output.

Not all older adults with a comorbid condition or taking a medication that is associated with UI will develop UI, and the presence of such factors in an individual person with UI does not imply that they are causative. The best example of this is the relationship between UI and dementia. Although older adults with dementia may have impairment in central inhibitory pathways that control urgency, impaired functional status and mobility are at least as strong or stronger predictors of UI than cognitive status. Older adults with advanced dementia may remain continent if they can transfer and ambulate with minimal to moderate assistance. Furthermore, older adults with dementia may have other types of LUT dysfunction and symptoms than urge UI: one-third of nursing-home residents with UI have stress UI or bladder outlet obstructions on urodynamic testing.

Pathophysiology

Age-related LUT Changes

A number of age-related physiologic changes in LUT function predispose older adults to UI. In both genders, bladder contractility decreases, uninhibited bladder contractions are more prevalent, diurnal urine output occurs later in the day, sphincteric striated muscle attenuates, and bladder capacity decreases and PVR increases (both modestly and without clear clinical significance). In women, urethral closure pressure decreases, and vaginal mucosal atrophy is prevalent. Benign prostatic hyperplasia and prostate hypertrophy increase in men (see "Prostate Disease," p 437). Why some older adults develop UI and others do not remains unclear; differences in LUT function and other compensatory mechanisms may play a role.

LUT Pathophysiology in UI

Specific UI symptoms and LUT pathophysiology overlap substantially. However, some general associations (with caveats) are possible:

- **Urge UI with detrusor overactivity (DO) (uninhibited bladder contractions):** Up to 40% of continent healthy older adults demonstrate DO on urodynamic testing, suggesting that urge UI requires not just DO but impaired compensatory mechanisms as well. Research now emphasizes the roles of afferent stimulation from the bladder urothelium and impaired CNS control of urgency in DO and overactive bladder. DO may be idiopathic, age-related, secondary to lesions in cerebral and spinal inhibitory pathways, due to bladder outlet obstruction, or (less commonly) result from local bladder irritation (eg, infection, stones, tumor).

- **Stress UI and impaired urethral sphincter support and/or closure:** Stress UI can result from 1) damage to pelvic floor supports (levator ani, connective tissues), which compress the urethra when intra-abdominal pressure increases; and 2) sphincter failure (usually due to surgical damage or severe atrophy or, in rare cases, subsacral spinal cord injury). DO can cause apparent "stress" UI when a cough triggers an uninhibited detrusor contraction. In such cases, leakage usually occurs after and not coincident with the cough, is large in volume, and difficult to stop.

- **Mixed UI with both DO and impaired sphincter support/function**, with the same caveats as above

- **UI with impaired bladder emptying due to bladder obstruction and/or detrusor underactivity:** The most common cause of obstruction in men is prostate hypertrophy and in women urethral surgical scarring or a large cystocele/prolapse that kinks the urethra. Detrusor underactivity can be caused by intrinsic bladder smooth muscle damage (eg, from ischemia, scarring, fibrosis), peripheral neuropathy (diabetes mellitus, vitamin B_{12} deficiency, alcoholism), or damage to the sacral cord and spinal bladder efferent nerves by disc herniation, spinal stenosis, tumor, or degenerative neurologic disease. Neurologic diseases affecting the sacral spinal cord can cause detrusor underactivity and/or neurally mediated obstruction, depending on the exact level and extent of damage.

- **Nocturia is a nonspecific symptom, even in older men, and causes other than urge UI and prostate disease should be considered.**

EVALUATION

Similar to other geriatric syndromes, UI requires multifactorial evaluation with a focus on comorbidity, function, and medications as contributing factors. Evaluation and management of UI in nursing-home residents is discussed separately below.

Screening

All older patients, especially women, should be asked at least every 2 years about UI, because 50% of affected individuals do not voluntarily report their symptoms to a healthcare provider.

Screening questions

- Do you have any problems with bladder control?
- Do you have problems making it to the bathroom on time?
- Do you ever leak urine?

If positive, screen for UI, then ask classification questions:

Do you leak urine most often: (type of UI)

- When you are performing some physical activity, such as coughing, sneezing, lifting, or exercising? (stress)
- When you have the urge or feeling that you need to empty your bladder but cannot get to the toilet fast enough? (urge)
- With both physical activity and a sense of urgency? (mixed)
- Without physical activity and without sense of urgency? (other)

History

The history should include the type(s) of UI symptoms; UI onset, frequency, volume; timing; other LUT symptoms; and amount and types of fluid intake. It is important to establish goals of care (eg, complete continence, fewer pad changes), because these may drive extent of evaluation as well as treatment.

UI may be the herald symptom of neurologic disease and cancer. "Red flag" symptoms that require prompt evaluation and referral are abrupt onset of UI, pelvic pain (constant, worsened, or improved with voiding), and hematuria.

Medical conditions and their status, medications, functional status, and access to toilets should be reviewed, including their association with onset or worsening of UI. Review of systems should include fecal incontinence, which is common in older adults with UI. Ask patients (and/or caregivers) specifically about UI-associated bother and impact on quality of life, starting with simple questions (eg, "What bothers you most about your leakage?" or "How does leakage affect your life?"), followed by more specific probes, as appropriate, regarding impact on ADLs and IADLs, social role, emotional and interpersonal relations, sexual function and relations, self-concept, general health perception, and financial burden.

Physical Examination

The initial general examination should include cognition and functional status, if not recently assessed, and focus on signs of comorbidity associated with UI. Abdominal palpation is insensitive and nonspecific for bladder distension. Rectal examination should check for masses, fecal loading, and prostate nodules or firmness. Prostate sizing by digital examination is inaccurate (see "Prostate Disease," p 437). Neurologic evaluation is especially important in patients with new onset or worsening UI, or who have motor and sensory symptoms. Tests for integrity of sacral cord (origin of the pelvic and pudendal nerves) are perineal sensation, anal "wink" (lightly scratch the perianal area and look for anal sphincter contraction), and bulbocavernosus reflex (lightly touch the clitoris or glans and look or palpate for rectal contraction). A basic pelvic examination in women should include checking for labial and vaginal lesions and marked pelvic organ prolapse (see "Gynecologic Diseases and Disorders," p 431). Uncircumcised men should be checked for phimosis, paraphimosis, and balanitis.

Depression screening is recommended because of the bidirectional association between depression and UI (see "Depression and Other Mood Disorders," p 308). Screening for sleep apnea (eg, using STOP) should be considered in patients with nocturia (see "Sleep Problems," p 285).

A clinical stress test can corroborate stress UI symptoms. The patient should have a full bladder and a relaxed perineum and buttocks, and the examiner positioned to observe or catch any leakage when the patient gives a single vigorous cough. Clinical stress testing is highly sensitive (most helpful when negative) and less specific. Sensitivity is highest when the patient is standing. It is insensitive if the patient cannot cooperate, is inhibited, or the bladder volume is low.

Additional Testing

The only recommended test for all patients is urinalysis to look for hematuria (and glycosuria in diabetic patients). In women without an acute onset of UI, dysuria, fever, or other signs of urinary tract infection, pyuria and bacteriuria likely represent asymptomatic bacteriuria (see "Infectious Diseases," p 494). Asymptomatic bacteriuria is not associated with UI and should not be eradicated with antibiotics.

Bladder diaries (also called frequency-volume charts) can help to determine whether urine volume contributes to frequency and nocturia symptoms, and can assist in evaluation of UI frequency, timing, and circumstances. Typically, a diary entails recording the time and volume of all continent voids and UI episodes for 2–3 days, including day and evening.

Measuring PVR is not routinely necessary in the evaluation of UI. Definition of an "increased" PVR is not standardized, the overall prevalence of high PVR (eg, >200 mL) is low, and there is insufficient evidence that routine PVR measurement affects outcomes. Even older men with LUT symptoms and/or known prostate disease do not require routine PVR testing (see "Prostate Disease," p 437). Measuring PVR should be considered in patients with prior urinary retention, longstanding diabetes, recurrent urinary tract infections, severe constipation, or using medications known to impair bladder emptying; and in women with marked pelvic organ prolapse or who have had prior surgery for UI (SOE=C). PVR can be measured in the office with ultrasonography or catheterization. Routine urodynamic testing is not necessary or desirable; it should be considered only if the cause of UI is unclear and knowing it would change management (eg, a man with severe urge UI who may have bladder outlet obstruction), or when empiric treatment has failed and the patient would consider invasive or surgical therapy. Cystometry can determine only bladder proprioception, capacity, and detrusor stability; carbon dioxide cystometry is unreliable. Simultaneous measurement of abdominal pressure is necessary to exclude abdominal straining and detect DHIC. Fluoroscopic monitoring, abdominal leak-point pressure, and/or profilometry are necessary to diagnose physiologic stress UI. Pressure-flow studies are required to diagnose outlet obstruction.

TREATMENT AND MANAGEMENT

Treatment should proceed stepwise, from correcting contributory factors and lifestyle modification, to behavioral therapy, medications, and then minimally invasive procedures and surgery as appropriate and consistent with the goals of care. Not all steps will be needed or appropriate for all patients, and some patients may want to proceed directly to specific therapy (eg, surgery for women with severe stress UI). Some treatments are effective for several UI symptoms (see below). Management should focus on relieving the aspect of UI that is most bothersome for the patient; eg, treatment that only decreases daytime UI episodes may not be sufficient for those most bothered by the timing of UI, nocturia, or leakage with exercise.

Patients with UI and pain, hematuria, recurrent symptomatic urinary tract infections, pelvic mass, previous pelvic irradiation, prior pelvic or LUT surgery, significantly increased PVR, significant pelvic organ prolapse, or suspected fistula should be referred for specialty management, if appropriate for goals of care.

Lifestyle Modification

Weight loss significantly reduces stress incontinence in obese, younger-old women (SOE=A). Other lifestyle interventions lack confirmatory evidence but may be helpful: avoiding extremes of fluid intake, caffeinated beverages, and alcohol; minimizing evening intake for nocturia; and quitting smoking for patients with stress UI.

Behavioral Therapies

Bladder training and pelvic muscle exercises (PMEs) are effective for urge, mixed, and stress UI, and are often used in combination (SOE=A). Prompted voiding may be effective in cognitively impaired patients with urge UI; its efficacy in other patients with UI is unknown.

Bladder training uses two principles: frequent voluntary voiding to keep bladder volume low, and urgency suppression using CNS and pelvic mechanisms. The initial toileting frequency can be every 2 hours or based on the smallest voiding interval on bladder diary. When urgency occurs, patients should stand still or sit down, do several pelvic muscle contractions, and concentrate on making the urgency decrease by taking a deep breath and letting it out slowly, or visualizing the urgency as a wave that peaks and then falls. Once patients feel more in control, they should walk to a bathroom and void. After 2 days without leakage, the time between scheduled voids can be increased by 15–30 min intervals, until the patient is dry when voiding every 4 hours. Successful bladder training usually takes several weeks, and patients need reassurance to proceed despite any initial failure.

PMEs strengthen the muscular components of urethral support and are effective for urge, mixed, and stress UI. PMEs also are effective for prevention and treatment of UI after prostatectomy (see "Prostate

Disease," p 437). PMEs require patient instruction and motivation, although simple instruction booklets alone have had moderate benefit.

To do PMEs, the patient 1) performs an isolated pelvic muscle contraction, without contracting buttocks, abdomen, or thighs (this can be checked during a bimanual examination in women), and holds it for 6–8 seconds (initially, only shorter durations may be possible); 2) repeats the contraction 8 to 12 times (one set), relaxing the pelvis between each contraction; 3) completes three sets of contractions daily at least 3 to 4 times a week, and continuing for at least 15 to 20 weeks. As patients progress, they should try to increase the intensity and duration of the contraction, perform PMEs in various positions (sitting, standing, walking), and alternate fast and slower contractions. Many experts believe biofeedback can improve bladder retraining and PME teaching and outcomes, but marginal benefit is unproved. Medicare covers biofeedback for patients who do not improve after 4 weeks of conventional instruction.

The only behavioral treatment with proven efficacy in cognitively impaired patients is prompted voiding. A caregiver monitors the patient and encourages him or her to report any need to void, prompts the patient to toilet on a regular schedule during the day (usually every 2–3 hours), leads the patient to the bathroom, and gives the patient positive feedback when he or she toilets. Patients most likely to improve are able to state their name, transfer with a minimum of one assist, void ≤4 times during the day (12 hours), and are able to accept and follow the prompt to toilet at least 75% of the time in an initial 3-day trial. Toileting routines without prompting, such as habit training (based on a patient's usual voiding schedule without prompting) and scheduled voiding (using a set schedule) are not effective.

Medications

Antimuscarinic agents are moderately effective for urge UI, overactive bladder, and mixed incontinence. They work by decreasing basal excretion of acetylcholine from the urothelium, and increasing bladder capacity; they do not decrease DO. Data are conflicting whether combined antimuscarinic and behavioral therapy is better than either alone for reducing UI; the combination is significantly better for improving quality of life. Antimuscarinics are safe and effective in men with urgency and urge UI associated with benign prostatic hyperplasia (see "Prostate Disease," p 437). Antimuscarinics are contraindicated for patients with narrow-angle glaucoma (not open-angle), impaired gastric emptying, and urinary retention. It is not necessary to routinely monitor PVR with antimuscarinic treatment. Patients complaining of worsening UI while taking antimuscarinics need to have a PVR checked, because an increased PVR decreases functional bladder capacity, thereby increasing frequency and UI.

Antimuscarinics with proven efficacy are oxybutynin (immediate release, 2.5–5 mg q6–12h; extended release 5–20 mg/d; topical patch 3.9 mg/24 hr applied twice weekly to abdomen, thighs, or buttocks; and topical gel [3% gel or 10% sachet daily]), tolterodine (immediate release 1–2 mg q12h; extended release 2–4 mg/d), trospium (immediate release 20 mg q12h or q24h; extended release 60 mg daily in AM), darifenacin (7.5–15 mg/d), solifenacin (10–20 mg/d), and fesoterodine (4–8 mg/d). Based on systematic reviews, the six antimuscarinic agents have generally similar efficacy in reducing urge UI frequency but differ in adverse events, metabolism, drug interactions, and dosing requirements. Direct drug-drug comparison trials are limited and industry supported. Although older adults have been included in antimuscarinic trials, no study has targeted vulnerable or frail older adults. A trial of an anticholinergic in targeted vulnerable older adults has been presented in abstract, but not yet published.

Anticholinergic adverse events impact both tolerability and safety. Chronic anticholinergic use increases the risk of caries and tooth loss, and patients should have regular dental care. Although anticholinergics as a class are associated with cognitive impairment, the risk, prevalence, type, and magnitude of cognitive changes from specific antimuscarinic UI medications in individual patients are unknown. A randomized study found no increase in delirium in frail nursing-home patients treated with extended-release oxybutynin 5 mg/d. Evidence is insufficient that one drug is "safer" for all patients or those with dementia, or that the cognitive risk outweighs the potential treatment benefit. Antimuscarinics should not be combined with cholinesterase inhibitors because of lack of efficacy and risk of increased functional impairment. All antimuscarinics except trospium are metabolized by cytochrome P-450 pathways, and can interact with drugs that induce CYP2D6 (eg, fluoxetine) or are metabolized by CYP3A4 (eg, erythromycin, ketoconazole). Fesoterodine is a prodrug that is metabolized to tolterodine by nonspecific peripheral esterases. Trospium is renally cleared and should be given once daily in patients with renal insufficiency; it should be taken on an empty stomach. Therefore, choice of agent for a particular patient should depend on potential adverse events to be avoided, possible drug-drug and drug-disease interactions, dosing frequency, titration range, and cost. A lack of response to one agent does not preclude response to another.

Mirabegron is a β_3-adrenergic agonist that stimulates detrusor relaxation and increases bladder capacity; it was FDA approved in 2012 for treatment of overactive bladder and urge UI. The package label carries warnings about an adverse effect of hypertension and not using in combination with antimuscarincs; mirabegron increases digoxin levels and is a CYP2D6 inhibitor that can increase levels of CYP2D6 substrates (eg, metoprolol, venlafaxine, desipramine, dextromethorphan).

There is insufficient evidence for the efficacy of propantheline, dicyclomine, imipramine, hyoscyamine, calcium channel blockers, NSAIDs, and flavoxate. Vasopressin (DDAVP) should not be used for nocturia in older adults because of the risk of hyponatremia (SOE=A).

The serotonin–norepinephrine uptake inhibitor antidepressant duloxetine decreases stress UI but is not FDA approved for this indication. Oral estrogen, alone or in combination with progestins, increases UI (SOE=A). There is insufficient evidence whether vaginal topical estrogen improves UI (cream, vaginal tablet, or slow-release ring), but it is helpful for uncomfortable vaginal atrophy and may decrease recurrent urinary tract infections (see Urinary Tract Infection in "Infectious Diseases," p 494). Oral estrogen increases UI; this has not been found to be the case so far with topical vaginal estrogen.

Minimally Invasive Procedures

Sacral nerve neuromodulation has some effect for both urge UI refractory to drug treatment and urinary retention (idiopathic and neurogenic). The mechanism of action is unknown. The procedure involves percutaneous implantation of a trial electrode at the S3 sacral root, which is connected to an external stimulator. Patients responding to the trial have a permanent lead with a pacemaker-like energy source implanted. Peroneal nerve stimulation is a less invasive form of neuromodulation that is under investigation for the same indications.

Intravesical injection of botulinum toxin is effective for refractory urge UI and is FDA approved for this indication in persons with neurologic conditions (eg, spinal cord injury, multiple sclerosis). Optimal dosing for specific patient groups is uncertain, and patients must be willing to do self-catheterization because of the risk of urinary retention.

Pessaries may benefit women with stress and urge UI exacerbated by bladder or uterine prolapse. See "Gynecologic Diseases and Disorders," p 431.

Surgery

Surgery provides the highest cure rates for stress UI in women. The most commonly used procedures are colposuspension (Burch operation) and slings (synthetic mesh, or autologous or cadaveric fascia placed transvaginally). Older women have less improvement with these procedures than younger women, but quality of life and patient satisfaction with surgery is significantly better than without surgery. Periurethral injection of collagen is a short-term (≤1 year) alternative and usually requires a series of injections. Early short-term reports suggest that suburethral sling placement may be effective in men with persistent UI after prostatectomy.

Artificial sphincters are used for refractory stress UI from sphincter damage, typically after radical prostatectomy. A cuff is placed internally around the urethra, and its inflation controlled by the patient squeezing a reservoir device placed in the scrotum. They are effective but require manual dexterity and intact cognition; an alert bracelet should be considered, because catheter insertion through a closed artificial sphincter can cause significant damage. Revision rates can be high (up to 40%). Urodynamics should assist patient selection, because outcomes are worse with severe DO and poor detrusor compliance.

Supportive Care

Pads and protective garments should be chosen based on patient gender and the type and volume of UI. For example, an absorbent sheath may be sufficient for a man with mild UI after prostatectomy. In some states, Medicaid may cover the cost of pads; Medicare and private insurance do not. Medical supply companies and patient advocacy groups publish illustrated catalogs to guide product selection. Because these products are often expensive, some patients may not change pads frequently enough.

Evaluation and Management of UI in Nursing-Home Residents

The CMS *Guidance for Surveyors for Long Term Facilities* sets the nursing-home compliance standards, known as the F-tag 315, for the evaluation and management of UI and urinary catheters. The 2006 revision of F-tag 315 changed the focus from documentation of toileting plans to an increased emphasis on screening, the process and documentation of UI assessment, and reevaluation. The Minimum Data Set requires that residents are screened for UI at admissions quarterly, and with any change in cognition, function, or urinary tract function. F-tag 315 guidance suggests an evaluation essentially equivalent to that described above. Instead of bladder diaries, toileting patterns and UI episodes are monitored over several days. Although evaluation is largely a nursing responsibility, physician input is especially important given the F-tag 315 emphasis on physical examination, evaluation of medications and comorbidity as a cause of UI, and differential diagnosis.

Nearly all studies of UI treatment in long-term care involve behavioral therapy. Evidence is strong that prompted voiding is effective in reducing daytime UI, but treatment is rarely continued long term. Interventions that combine prompted voiding with bedside exercise improve both incontinence and physical function. Prompted voiding should be tried in all eligible patients (able to state their name, can transfer with at most an assist by one), but continued only in those who are able to accept and follow the prompt to toilet at least 75% of the time in an initial 3-day trial. Long-term care residents who do not respond should be managed with "check and change." The revised F-tag 315 supports this targeted approach and the role of patient and family preferences in evaluation and treatment. Unfortunately, in most nursing homes, common practice is scheduled toileting without prompting, which is ineffective. Quality improvement efforts focused on staff organization and systems may ultimately be necessary to reduce UI in long-term care.

The only randomized studies of antimuscarinic efficacy in nursing-home residents used oxybutynin. A 4-week randomized controlled trial found no difference between extended-release oxybutynin given at 5 mg/d and placebo. Consequently, antimuscarinics are infrequently prescribed, despite evidence that patients may prefer medications over behavioral therapy and "check and change." It is reasonable to consider an antimuscarinic trial for residents with urge UI who respond to prompted voiding but are still incontinent.

It is important to remember that up to a third of nursing-home residents with UI have an underlying bladder outlet problem (stress incontinence or bladder outlet obstruction) and may be candidates for alternative medical or surgical treatment.

CATHETERS AND CATHETER CARE

Indwelling catheters cause significant morbidity, including polymicrobial bacteriuria (universal by 30 days), febrile episodes (1 per 100 patient days), nephrolithiasis, bladder stones, epididymitis, chronic renal inflammation and pyelonephritis, and meatal damage. Condom catheters also cause bacteriuria, infection, penile cellulitis and necrosis, and urinary retention and hydronephrosis if the condom twists or its external band is too tight. Indwelling catheters should be used only for short-term decompression of acute urinary retention, chronic retention that cannot be managed medically or surgically, protection of wounds that may be contaminated by urine, and terminally ill or severely impaired patients who cannot tolerate garment changes and who have an informed preference for catheter management despite risks. Inappropriate and/or poorly documented indications for catheter use are a major focus in the revised F-tag 315 guidance for nursing homes. The guidance states that catheters should primarily be used for short-term decompression of acute retention. However, F-tag 315 allows for catheter use over 14 days for patients with chronic retention (PVR volumes >200 mL who are not candidates for medical or surgical treatment or management with intermittent catheterization; have persistent UI, urinary tract infections, and/or renal dysfunction; have stage III or IV pressure ulcers for which UI impedes healing; or have terminal illness or severe impairment that makes positioning or clothing changes uncomfortable or that is associated with intractable pain).

All patients with acute retention should have decompression with an indwelling catheter while being evaluated and treated for potentially remediable causes, such as medications that impair detrusor contractility or increase urethral tone, outlet obstruction, and constipation. Duration of catheterization before voiding trial should depend on time course for reversing underlying cause. A voiding trial without catheter should follow decompression. To do so, the catheter should be removed (never clamped), the patient adequately hydrated, and a PVR checked after the first void or bladder volume checked if there is no void after about 6 hours. Studies have not confirmed any benefit of bethanechol chloride for patients with retention.

Intermittent clean catheterization is an effective alternative to an indwelling catheter for willing and able patients. Strict sterility is not necessary, although good hand washing and regular decontamination of the catheters is needed. Specialized stiff and smooth short catheters are available for use. Bacteriuria can be minimized by a frequency of catheterization that keeps bladder volume <400 mL. Sterile intermittent catheterization is preferred for frailer patients and those in institutionalized settings. See "Infectious Diseases," p 494.

Bacteriuria is universal in catheterized patients and should not be treated unless there are clear symptoms of cystitis or pyelonephritis. Routine cultures should not be done because of changing flora and difficulty in differentiating colonization from active infection. In symptomatic patients, urine for culture is best obtained by removing the old catheter and urine obtained from a newly placed catheter. Institutionalized patients with catheters should be kept in separate rooms to decrease cross-infection. Topical meatal antimicrobials, catheters with antimicrobial coating, collection bag disinfectants, and antimicrobial irrigation are not effective in preventing catheter-associated urinary tract infection.

Although antibiotics decrease bacteriuria and infection, routine use induces resistant organisms and secondary infections (such as with *Clostridium difficile)* and should not be used. Prophylactic antibiotics are recommended only in high-risk patients (eg, those with prosthetic heart valves) during short-term catheterization. For men with chronic obstruction, suprapubic catheters may be preferable to avoid meatal and penile trauma.

Catheters need not be changed routinely as long as monitoring is adequate and catheter blockage does not develop. Risk factors for blockage include alkaline urine, female gender, poor mobility, calciuria, proteinuria, copious mucin, *Proteus* colonization, and preexistent bladder stones. Changing the catheter every 7–10 days may decrease blockage in such patients. If patients cannot be monitored, changing catheters every 30 days is reasonable (SOE=D). Possible causes of persistent leakage around the catheter are large Foley balloon, detrusor overactivity, catheter diameter that is too large, bacteriuria, constipation or impaction, or improper catheter positioning. These can be addressed by trials of partial deflation of the balloon, smaller catheter, treatment of constipation, use of an anticholinergic, or treatment with pyridium.

Catheters coated with silver alloys reduce asymptomatic bacteriuria in hospitalized patients requiring short-term urethral catheterization, but their use in reducing symptomatic bacteriuria is less certain. Data are scant whether silver alloy catheters reduce asymptomatic or symptomatic bacteriuria in other settings (such as long-term care or home care) or with longer-term catheterization. See "Hospital Care," p 130.

REFERENCES

- DuBeau C, Johnson T, Kuchel G, et al. Incontinence in the frail elderly: Report from the 4th international consultation on incontinence. *Neurourol Urodynam.* 2009;29:165–178.
- Flanagan L, Jack B, Barrett B, et al. Systematic review of care intervention studies for the management of incontinence and promotion of continence in older people in care homes with urinary incontinence as the primary focus (1966-2010). *Geriatr Gerontol Int.* 2012;12(4):600–611.
- Madhuvrata P, Cody JD, EllisG, et al. Which anticholinergic drug for overactive bladder symptoms in adults. *Cochrane Database Syst Rev.* 2012;1:CD005429. DOI:10.1002/14651858.CD005429.pub2.
- www.catheterout.org (accessed Oct 2013)

CHAPTER 31—GAIT IMPAIRMENT

KEY POINTS

- Gait disorders are common in older adults and are a predictor of functional decline.
- The cause of gait impairment in older adults is usually multifactorial; therefore, a full assessment must include consideration of a number of different causes, as determined from a detailed physical examination and a functional performance evaluation.
- Various interventions, ranging from medical to surgical to exercise, can reduce the degree of impairment, although some residual impairment is often present.

Gait disorders are commonly associated with falls and disability in older adults. This chapter reviews the epidemiology of gait impairments, comorbidities that contribute to these disorders, and office-based clinical assessments and interventions to reduce their functional impact.

EPIDEMIOLOGY

Limitations in walking increase with age. At least 20% of noninstitutionalized older adults admit to difficulty with walking or require the assistance of another person or special equipment to walk. In some samples of noninstitutionalized older adults ≥85 years old, the prevalence of walking limitations can be over 50%. Age-related gait changes such as slowed speed are most apparent after age 75 or 80, but most gait disorders appear in connection with underlying diseases, particularly as disease severity increases. For example, advanced age (>85 years old); three or more chronic conditions at baseline; and the occurrence of stroke, hip fracture, or cancer predict catastrophic loss of walking ability (SOE=B).

Determining that a gait is disordered is difficult, because there are no clearly accepted general standards of normal gait for older adults. Some believe that slowed gait speed suggests a disorder; others believe that deviations in smoothness, symmetry, and synchrony of movement patterns suggest a disorder. Regardless, a slowed and aesthetically abnormal gait can in fact provide the older adult with a safe, independent gait pattern. Attributing a gait disorder to one specific disease in older adults is particularly difficult, because similar gait abnormalities are common to many diseases.

Longitudinal observational studies suggest that certain gait-related mobility disorders progress with age and that this progression is associated with morbidity and mortality. Community-dwelling older adults with gait disorders, particularly neurologically abnormal gaits, are at higher risk of institutionalization and death (SOE=B).

CONDITIONS THAT CONTRIBUTE TO GAIT IMPAIRMENT

Impaired gait may not be an inevitable consequence of aging but rather a reflection of the increased prevalence and severity of age-associated diseases. These diseases, both neurologic and non-neurologic, are the major contributors to impaired gait. (For a glossary of gait abnormalities, see Table 31.1.)

Patients in primary care report that pain, stiffness, dizziness, numbness, weakness, and sensations of abnormal movement are the most common causes of their walking difficulties. The most common conditions seen in primary care that are thought to contribute to gait disorders are degenerative joint disease, acquired musculoskeletal deformities, intermittent claudication, impairments after orthopedic surgery and stroke, and postural hypotension. Usually, more than one contributing condition is found. In a group of community-dwelling adults >88 years old, joint pain was by far the most common contributor, followed by multiple causes such as stroke and visual loss. Factors such as dementia and fear of falling also contribute to gait disorders. The disorders found in a neurologic referral population include frontal gait disorders (usually related to normal-pressure hydrocephalus [NPH] and cerebrovascular processes), sensory disorders (also involving vestibular and visual function), myelopathy, previously undiagnosed Parkinson disease or parkinsonian syndromes, and cerebellar disease. Known conditions causing severe gait impairment, such as hemiplegia and severe hip or knee disease, are commonly not mentioned in these neurologic referral populations. Thus, many gait disorders, particularly those that are classical and discrete (eg, those related to stroke and osteoarthritis) and those that are mild or may relate to irreversible disease (eg, vascular dementia), are presumably diagnosed in primary care and treated without a referral to a neurologist. Other less common contributors to gait disorders include metabolic disorders (related to renal or hepatic disease), CNS tumors or subdural hematoma, depression, and psychotropic medications. Case reports also document reversible gait disorders due to clinically overt hypo- or hyperthyroidism and B_{12} and folate deficiency.

Factors associated with slowed gait speed are also considered contributors to gait disorders. These factors

Table 31.1—Glossary of Gait Abnormalities

Term	Description
Antalgic gait	Pain-induced limp with shortened stance phase of gait on painful side
Circumduction	Outward swing of leg in semicircle from the hip
Equinovarus	Excessive plantar flexion and inversion of the ankle
Festination	Acceleration of gait
Foot drop	Loss of ankle dorsiflexion secondary to weakness of ankle dorsiflexors
Foot slap	Early, frequent audible foot-floor contact with steppage gait compensation
Freezing of gait	Sudden, short duration diminution or cessation of walking usually associated with shift in attention or movement circumstance or direction
Genu recurvatum	Hyperextension of knee
Propulsion	Tendency to fall forward
Retropulsion	Tendency to fall backward
Scissoring	Hip adduction such that the knees cross in front of each other with each step
Steppage gait	Exaggerated hip flexion, knee extension, and foot lifting, usually accompanied by foot drop
Trendelenburg gait	Shift of the trunk over the affected hip, which drops because of hip abductor weakness
Turn en bloc	Moving the whole body while turning

are commonly disease associated (eg, cardiopulmonary or musculoskeletal disease) and include decreased leg strength, vision, aerobic function, standing balance, and physical activity, as well as joint impairment, previous falls, and fear of falling. Combining these factors can result in an effect greater than the sum of the single impairments (as when combining balance and strength impairments). Furthermore, the effect of improved strength and aerobic capacity on gait speed may be nonlinear; that is, for very impaired individuals, small improvements in strength or aerobic capacity yield relatively larger gains in gait speed, whereas these small improvements yield little gait speed change in healthy older adults.

Although older adults can maintain a relatively normal gait pattern well into their 80s, some slowing occurs, and decreased stride length thus becomes a common feature in descriptions of gait disorders of older adults. Some authors have proposed the emergence of an age-related gait disorder without accompanying clinical abnormalities, ie, essential "senile" gait disorder. This gait pattern is described as broad-based with small steps, diminished arm swing, stooped posture, decreased flexion of the hips and knees, uncertainty and stiffness in turning, occasional difficulty initiating steps, and a tendency toward falling. These and other nonspecific findings (eg, the inability to perform tandem gait) are similar to gait patterns found in a number of other diseases, and yet the clinical abnormalities are insufficient to make a specific diagnosis. This "disorder" may be a precursor to an as-yet-undiagnosed disease (eg, related to subtle extrapyramidal symptoms) and is likely to be a manifestation of concurrent, progressive cognitive impairment (eg, Alzheimer disease or vascular dementia). Thus, "senile" gait disorder may reflect a number of potential diseases and is generally not useful in labeling gait disorders in older adults.

Subclinical as well as clinically evident cerebrovascular disease is increasingly recognized as a major contributor to causes of gait disorders (SOE=B). Nondemented individuals with clinically abnormal gait (particularly unsteady, frontal, or hemiparetic gait) followed for approximately 7 years were found to be at higher risk of developing non-Alzheimer, particularly vascular, dementia. Of note, those with abnormal gait at baseline may not have met criteria for dementia but already had abnormalities in neuropsychologic function, such as in visual-perceptual processing and language skills. Gait disorders with no apparent cause (also termed "idiopathic" or "senile" gait disorder) are associated with a higher mortality rate, primarily from cardiovascular causes (SOE=B). These cardiovascular causes are likely linked to concomitant, possibly undetected, cerebrovascular disease.

ASSESSMENT

Gait disorders (Table 31.1) can be assessed and categorized according to the sensorimotor levels that are affected.

Disorders that are the result of pathology of the low sensorimotor level can be divided into peripheral sensory and peripheral motor dysfunction, including myopathic or neuropathic disorders that cause weakness and musculoskeletal diseases. These disorders are generally distal to the CNS. With peripheral sensory impairment, unsteady and tentative gait is commonly caused by vestibular disorders, peripheral neuropathy, posterior column (proprioceptive) deficits, or visual impairment. With peripheral motor impairment, a number of classical gait patterns emerge. Examples of these patterns include Trendelenburg gait (ie, weight shifts over the weak hip, which drops because of hip abductor weakness), antalgic gait (weight bearing is avoided and stance shortens on one side because of pain), and foot drop (due to ankle dorsiflexor weakness and characterized by a frequently audible foot-floor contact with steppage gait compensation, ie, excessive hip flexion). These gait impairments are the result of body segment and joint deformities, pain, and focal myopathic and neuropathic weakness. In general, if the gait disorder is limited to this low sensorimotor level (ie, the CNS is intact), the person can adapt well to the gait disorder, compensating with an assistive device or learning to negotiate the environment safely.

At the middle sensorimotor level, the execution of centrally selected postural and locomotor responses is faulty, and the sensory and motor modulation of gait is disrupted. Gait may be initiated normally, but stepping patterns are abnormal. Diseases causing spasticity (eg, those related to myelopathy, B_{12} deficiency, and stroke), parkinsonism (idiopathic as well as medication induced), and cerebellar disease (eg, alcohol induced) are examples of those that cause this type of impairment. Gait abnormalities appear when the spasticity is sufficient to cause leg circumduction and fixed deformities (eg, equinovarus), when the Parkinson disease produces shuffling steps and reduced arm swing, and when the cerebellar ataxia increases trunk sway sufficiently to require a broad base of gait support. Recent attention has focused on the pathophysiology, diagnosis, and therapy of freezing of gait, found commonly in parkinsonian syndromes.

At the high or central level, gait impairments become more nonspecific. Lesions in the frontal lobe account for most gait abnormalities at this level. The severity of the frontal-related disorders runs a spectrum from difficulty with initiation of gait to frontal dysequilibrium, in which unsupported stance is not possible. Cerebrovascular insults to the cortex, as well as to the basal ganglia and their interconnections, may contribute to difficulty with initiation of gait and to apraxia.

Dementia and depression are also thought to contribute to an abnormal gait at the high or central level. With increasing severity of the dementia, particularly in patients with Alzheimer disease, frontal-related symptoms also increase. Gait impairments in this category have been given a number of overlapping descriptions, including *gait apraxia*, *marche a petits pas*, and *arteriosclerotic parkinsonism*.

More than one disease or impairment is likely to contribute to a gait disorder; one example is the longstanding diabetic patient with peripheral neuropathy and a recent stroke who is now very fearful of falling. Certain disorders can actually involve multiple parts of the nervous system, such as Parkinson disease affecting cortical and subcortical structures. Drug and metabolic causes (eg, from sedatives, tranquilizers, and anticonvulsants) can involve both central and peripheral nervous systems (eg, phenothiazines can cause central sedation and extrapyramidal effects).

History and Physical Examination

A careful medical history can help elucidate the multiple factors contributing to gait impairments in older adults. A brief systemic evaluation for evidence of subacute metabolic disease (eg, thyroid disorders), acute cardiopulmonary disorders (eg, myocardial infarction), or other acute illness (eg, sepsis) is warranted because an acute gait disorder may be the presenting feature of acute systemic decompensation in older adults. The physical examination should include an attempt to identify motion-related factors, eg, by provoking both vestibular and orthostatic responses. A focused examination, based on symptoms, should include the Dix-Hallpike test (see "Dizziness," p 199) to test for vestibular dysfunction, postural blood pressure measurements to exclude orthostatic hypotension, and vision screening at least for acuity. In addition, the neck, spine, extremities, and feet should be evaluated for pain, deformities, and limitations in range of motion, particularly regarding subtle hip or knee contractures. Leg-length discrepancies such as can occur with a hip prosthesis and either as an antecedent or subsequent to lower back pain can be measured simply as the distance from the anterior superior iliac spine to the medial malleolus. A formal neurologic assessment is critical and should include assessment of strength and tone, sensation (including proprioception), coordination (including cerebellar function), station, and gait. The Romberg test screens for simple postural control and whether the proprioceptive and vestibular systems are functional. Some investigators have proposed that one-legged stance time <5 seconds is a risk factor for injurious falls, although even relatively healthy adults ≥70 years old can have difficulty with one-legged stance. Given the importance of cognition as a risk factor, assessing cognitive function is also indicated.

Laboratory and Imaging Assessments

Depending on the history and physical examination, further laboratory and diagnostic imaging evaluation may be warranted. A CBC, serum chemistries, and other metabolic studies may be useful when systemic disease is suspected. Head or spine imaging, including radiography, CT, or MRI, are not indicated unless history and physical examination identifies neurologic abnormalities, either preceding or of recent onset, that are related to the gait disorder. However, cerebral white matter changes, often considered to be vascular (termed *leukoaraiosis*), have been increasingly associated with nonspecific gait disorders (SOE=B). Periventricular high signal measurements on MRI as well as increased ventricular volume, even in apparently healthy older adults, are associated with gait slowing. White-matter hyperintensities on MRI correlate with longitudinal changes in balance and gait, and the periventricular frontal and occipitoparietal regions appear to be most affected. Functional MRI generally supports these structural MRI findings, and diffusion tensor imaging techniques show that small-vessel disease, even in normal-appearing white matter, can affect gait. Age-specific guidelines for and the sensitivity, specificity, and cost-effectiveness of these evaluations remain to be determined.

Performance-based Functional Assessment

Technologically oriented assessments involving formal kinematic and kinetic analyses have not been applied widely in clinical assessments of balance and gait disorders in older adults. Simpler assessments using an instrumented gait mat or motion sensors, particularly portable accelerometers worn on the body, are being studied for wider clinical application. Comfortable gait speed and a related measure, distance walked (as measured by the 6-minute walk test), are powerful predictors of a number of important outcomes, such as falls, disability, hospitalization, institutionalization, and mortality (SOE=B). Gait speed is faster in individuals who are taller, who have a lower disease burden, and who are more active and less functionally disabled. Usual gait speed is frequently tested from a standing start over a distance of 4 meters. A recent pooled analysis of nine cohort studies of community-dwelling older adults found that usual gait speed predicted 5- and 10-year survival as accurately as a number of other important clinical variables such as age and chronic conditions. The likelihood of poor health and function increases at usual walking speed cut-offs of 0.8 or 1.0 meter per second (m/s) and particularly below 0.6 m/s; speeds >1.0 m/s and perhaps 1.2 m/s are associated with better functional outcomes and increased life expectancy. Several studies have found age- and disease-associated deficits in the ability to walk and perform a simultaneous cognitive task ("dual tasking," such as talking while walking), and also linked these deficits with increased fall risk (SOE=B), often using a measure of gait variability. Many investigators have also begun to test different exercise and cognitive-based interventions to improve dual-task performance. While slower gait speed can predict decreased cognition in healthy older adults, the opposite is true as well, namely that decreased cognitive function, particularly executive function, are associated with slower speed.

A number of timed and semiquantitative balance and gait scales have been proposed as a means to detect and quantify abnormalities and to direct interventions. Fall risk, for example, can be increased with more abnormal gait and balance scale scores, such as with the Berg Balance Scale or the Performance-Oriented Mobility Assessment. Perhaps the simplest battery in the clinical setting is the Timed Up and Go (TUG), a timed sequence of rising from a chair, walking 3 meters, turning, and returning to sit in the chair. One study suggests a TUG score of ≥14 seconds as an indicator of fall risk. Other investigators have found limitations in TUG in the presence of cognitive impairment and difficulty in completing the test because of immobility, safety concerns, or refusal. Another functional approach that can be useful clinically is the Functional Ambulation Classification scale, which rates the use of assistive devices, the degree of human assistance (either manual or verbal), the distance the person can walk, and the types of surfaces the person can negotiate.

Interventions to Reduce Gait Disorders

Even if a condition can be diagnosed on evaluation, many conditions causing a gait disorder are, at best, only partially treatable. The patient is often left with at least some residual disability. However, other functional outcomes such as reduction in weight-bearing pain may be equally important in justifying treatment. Functional improvement becomes the treatment goal. Comorbidity, disease severity, and overall health status tend to strongly influence treatment outcome.

Achievement of premorbid gait patterns may be unrealistic, but improvement in measures such as gait speed is reasonable as long as gait remains safe. Recent studies have estimated the extent to which a change in gait performance, such as gait speed, is clinically meaningful. For example, in cohorts that include mobility-impaired individuals, estimates range from 0.05 m/s to 0.10 m/s for small and substantial change, respectively. Using even a 0.10 m/s cut-off, however, may not coincide with perceived change in mobility in certain patient populations, such as in patients with a previous hip fracture.

Many of the older reports dealing with treatment and rehabilitation of gait disorders in older adults are retrospective chart reviews and case studies. Gait disorders presumably secondary to B_{12} deficiency, folate deficiency, hypothyroidism, hyperthyroidism, knee osteoarthritis, Parkinson disease, and inflammatory polyneuropathy improve with medical therapy.

A variety of modes of physical therapy for knee osteoarthritis can result in modest improvements but continued residual disability. For example, a combined aerobic, strength, and functionally based group exercise program increased gait speed approximately 5% in adults with knee osteoarthritis. The focus is on strengthening the extensor groups (especially knee and hip) and stretching commonly shortened muscles (such as the hip flexors). Randomized controlled trials of exercise for osteoarthritis focus primarily on the knee and can involve strengthening, walking, and aerobic training with positive outcomes on physical function that can include improved walking (SOE=A).

Regarding neurologic disorders, one review suggests unclear effects of conventional physical therapy in treating Parkinson gait disorders but that cueing, specifically audio and visual, can improve gait speed (SOE=C). For stroke patients, randomized controlled trials of fair to good quality support the use of strength training, electromyographic biofeedback, and functional electrical stimulation as adjuncts to gait training, while there is conflicting evidence to support the use of ankle-foot orthotics, treadmill training, partial body-weight support, and electromechanical-assisted training (SOE=B). Meta-analyses of several trials support a beneficial effect on gait of repetitive task-specific training and electromechanical assistance to augment physical therapy after stroke (improvements in 6-minute walk distances of 55 meters and 34 meters, respectively [SOE=A]). The quality of many trials varies, and long-term retention of the training effect is not clear.

A few studies of group exercise have shown improvements in gait parameters such as gait speed. Generally, the most consistent effects are with varied types of exercise provided in the same program (SOE=B). In a 12-week combined program of leg resistance, standing balance, and flexibility exercises, usual gait speed increased 8% in minimally impaired life-care community residents. In a similar varied 16-week format with more intensive individual support and prompting, gait speed increased 23% in selected demented older adults (Mini–Mental State Examination mean score of ≤15). A number of these studies note improvement in functional, gait-oriented measures (although not strictly gait "disorder" measures), such as the distance walked in 6 minutes by knee osteoarthritis patients undergoing either an aerobic or resistance training program.

Modest improvement and residual disability are also the result of surgical treatment for compressive cervical myelopathy, lumbar stenosis, and NPH. Few controlled prospective studies and no well-controlled randomized studies address the outcome of surgical versus nonsurgical treatment for these three conditions. A number of problems plague the available series: outcomes such as pain and walking disability are not reported separately, the source of the outcome rating is not clearly identified or blinded, the criteria for classifying outcomes differ, the outcomes may be subjective and subject to interpretation, the follow-up intervals are variable, the subjects who are reported in follow-up may be a highly select group, the selection factors for conservative versus surgical treatment between studies differ or are unspecified, and there is publication bias (only positive results are published). Many of the surgical series include all ages, although the mean age is usually >60 years old. A few studies document equivalent surgical outcomes with conservative, nonsurgical treatment.

With regard to lumbar stenosis procedures, many older adults have reduced pain and improved maximal walking distance after laminectomies and lumbar fusion surgery, although they have continued residual disability (SOE=B). In a somewhat younger cohort (mean age 69 years) and after an average of 8 years of follow-up after lumbar stenosis surgery, approximately half reported that they were unable to walk two blocks and many attributed their decreased walking ability to their back problem. Some improvement can be found in select patients >75 years old (mean age 78); in an uncontrolled study, 45% of patients with preoperative "severe" limitation of ambulatory ability had either "minimal" or "moderate" limitation postoperatively after an average of 1.5-years follow-up. Part of the problem in determining long-term gait outcomes of surgery for lumbar stenosis is other comorbidity, such as cardiovascular or musculoskeletal disease, that influences mobility. Nonoperative treatment (with a variety of interventions, including oral anti-inflammatory medications, heating modalities, exercise, mobilizations, and epidural injections) can also result in modest improvements such as in walking tolerance (SOE=B). Regarding cervical stenosis, studies involving postoperative gait outcomes in older adults are limited, but in one nonrandomized study, walking speed improved significantly in most of the postcervical myelopathy decompression patients whose mean age was 60 years old (SOE=B).

The most substantial improvements after shunt surgery for NPH are seen in gait as opposed to dementia or incontinence (SOE=B). In a noncontrolled study after shunt surgery for NPH (follow-up interval not specified), walking speed increased by >10% in 75% of the patients and by >25% in more than 57% of the patients. While there may be initial improvement after shunt placement, long-term results are often disappointing (eg, in one study, gait disorder initially improved in 65% of patients after shunt surgery, but this improvement was maintained in only 26% by 3-year follow-up). The poor long-term outcomes may be related to concurrent cerebrovascular and cardiovascular disease, a frequent cause of mortality in these cohorts. Gait outcomes after shunt surgery may be better in those in whom the gait disturbance precedes cognitive impairment and in those who respond with improved gait speed after a trial of cerebrospinal fluid removal (SOE=B).

Outcomes for hip and knee replacement surgery for osteoarthritis are better, although some of the same study methodologic problems exist. Multidisciplinary rehabilitation (versus more limited rehabilitation) after hip or knee replacement results in improved global functioning beyond walking measures (SOE=A). Other than pain relief, sizable gains in gait speed and joint motion occur, although residual walking disability continues for a number of reasons, including residual pathology on the operated side and symptoms on the nonoperated side. In one longitudinal cohort study, self-reported walking-related function was improved in patients undergoing total hip replacement for osteoarthritis versus in patients with osteoarthritis who received medical therapy (SOE=B). For joint replacements, despite rehabilitation after surgery, some residual weakness, stiffness, and slowed/altered gait and balance may remain. Simple function may be maintained after knee replacement, such as maintaining the ability to safely clear an obstacle, but usually at the expense of additional compensation by the ipsilateral hip and foot. Based on a recent meta-analysis, the effect of preoperative therapy before elective knee or hip replacement for osteoarthritis is modest, and primarily improves pain and activity, rather than gait per se (SOE=B).

Finally, the use of orthoses and other mobility aids can help reduce gait disorders (SOE=C). Although there are few data supporting their use, lifts (either internal or external) to correct for limb length inequality can be used in a conservative, gradually progressive manner. Other ankle braces, shoe inserts, shoe body and sole modifications, and their subsequent adjustments are part of standard care for foot and ankle weakness, deformities, and pain but are beyond the scope of this chapter. In general, well-fitting walking shoes with low heels, relatively thin firm soles, and if feasible, high, fixed heel collar support are recommended to maximize balance and improve gait. Mobility aids such as canes and walkers reduce load on a painful joint and increase stability. Note that light touch of any firm surface like walls or "furniture surfing" provide feedback and enhance balance. See also "Rehabilitation," p 139; and "Diseases and Disorders of the Foot," p 471.

REFERENCES

- Abellan Van Kan G, Rolland Y, Andrieu S, et al. Gait speed at usual pace as a predictor of adverse outcomes in community-dwelling older people: an international academy on nutrition and aging (IANA) task force. *J Nutr Health Aging*. 2009;13(10):881–889.
- Canavan PK, Cahalin LP, Lowe S, et al. Managing gait disorders in older persons residing in nursing homes: a review of literature. *J Am Med Dir Assoc*. 2009;10(4):230–237.
- Nutt JG, Horak FB, Bloem BR. Milestones in gait, balance and falling. *Mov Disord*. 2011;26(6):1166–1174.

CHAPTER 32—FALLS

KEY POINTS

- A fall is one of the most common events threatening the independence of older adults. Complications resulting from falls are the leading cause of death from injury in adults ≥65 years old.
- The causes of a fall often involve a complex interaction among factors intrinsic to the individual (age-related declines, chronic disease, acute illness, medications), challenges to postural control (environment, changing position, normal activities), and mediating factors (risk-taking behaviors, situational hazards).
- For patients presenting with a fall, important components of the history include the activity of the patient at the time of the fall, the occurrence of prodromal symptoms (lightheadedness, imbalance, and dizziness), and the location of the fall. Older adults with a single fall should be evaluated for gait and balance.
- For older adults with two or more falls in the past 12 months or with gait or balance abnormalities, a multifactorial falls risk assessment should be pursued.
- Interventions shown to be effective in reducing falls include medication review, exercise programs that include muscle strengthening and balance training, vitamin D supplementation, use of appropriate footwear, and multifactorial interventions including home hazards assessment for those at high risk of falls.

A fall is one of the most common events threatening the independence of older adults. A fall is considered to have occurred when a person comes to rest inadvertently on the ground or lower level. Most of the literature on falls in older adults does not include falls associated with loss of consciousness (eg, syncope, seizure) or with overwhelming trauma, because most falls are not associated with syncope or trauma.

PREVALENCE AND MORBIDITY

According to a CDC report, one of three adults ≥65 years old reports falling in the previous year. The incidence of falls is more frequent with advancing age and among nursing-home residents, such that one-half of individuals >80 years old or nursing-home residents will fall each year. Among those with a history of a fall in the previous year, the annual incidence of falls is close to 60%. Almost one-third of those who fall need medical attention related to the fall or need to restrict their activities for at least 1 day as a result of the fall. Most falls result in minor soft-tissue injury, while 10%–15% of falls result in fracture, and 5% of falls result in more serious soft-tissue injury or head trauma. Women and nursing-home residents are more likely to experience a nonfatal fall-related injury than men. Even among those who do not experience physical injury, falls are associated with subsequent declines in functional status, greater likelihood of nursing-home placement, increased use of medical services, and the development of a fear of falling. Of those older adults who fall, only half are able to get up without help, thus experiencing the "long lie." Long lies are associated with lasting declines in functional status. Fall-related injuries are not a common cause of death in older adults; however, complications resulting from falls are the leading cause of death from injury in adults ≥65 years old. The death rate attributable to falls increases with age, with white men ≥85 years old having the highest death rate (>180 deaths per 100,000 population).

The true cost of falls in healthcare dollars is difficult to ascertain. Because many falls result in injury, use of emergency department facilities among those who fall is common. In 2009, 2.2 million nonfatal falls were treated in emergency rooms, with 26% of these visits resulting in hospitalization. Thus, the direct cost of medical visits for falls and services/therapies for fall-related injuries is substantial. Indirect costs from fall-related injuries, such as hip fractures, can also be considerable.

CAUSES

Falls, incontinence, delirium, and other geriatric syndromes result from the accumulated effects of multiple impairments. In older adults, falls rarely have a single cause. Rather, there is often a complex interaction among factors intrinsic to the individual (age-related declines, chronic disease, acute illness, medications), challenges to postural control (environment, changing positions, normal activities), and mediating factors (risk-taking behaviors, or situational hazards, such as unfamiliar staff or high patient-to-staff ratios).

In multiple prospective cohort studies, several risk factors have been consistently associated with falls, including older age, cognitive impairment, female gender, past history of a fall, leg or gait problems, foot disorders, balance problems, hypovitaminosis D, psychotropic medication use, Parkinson disease, stroke, and arthritis (SOE=B). These studies differed significantly in the types of risk factors evaluated, the types of population studied (eg, past fall history was sometimes an entry criterion), and the outcome (one fall, two or more falls, rate of falls, injurious falls). The differences in risk factors found across the studies highlight the multifactorial nature of falls and suggest that there may also be unique circumstances surrounding falls that were not accounted for. In general, the risk of falling increases with the number of risk factors, although as many as 10% of falls occur in individuals with no identifiable risk factor for falls. Also, risk factors for indoor and outdoor falls differ: indoor falls tend to occur among older, frail adults with mobility disorders, while outdoor falls occur in younger, healthier persons.

Successful prevention of falls begins with knowledge of the age-related changes that increase the risk of falls. With aging, there are declines in the visual, proprioceptive, and vestibular systems. For example, the visual system has reduced visual acuity, depth perception, contrast sensitivity, and dark adaptation. The proprioceptive system loses sensitivity in the legs. The vestibular system has a loss of labyrinthine hair cells, vestibular ganglion cells, and nerve fibers.

Despite these age-related changes in sensory systems, quantifying the age-related changes in postural control that are independent of disease is difficult. In general, when postural stability is tested in young and old people with no apparent musculoskeletal or neurologic impairment, age-related differences in measured sway are most pronounced with moderately severe perturbations of stance, such as changing the support surface, changing body position, changing the visual input, or moving the support surface horizontally or rotationally. This occurs because these perturbations stress the redundancy of the sensory systems in their ability to maintain postural stability. This is borne out by the observation that gait speed deteriorates when individuals are presented with a dual task ("walking while talking"). In addition, there may be other age-related changes in the CNS that affect postural control, including the loss of neurons and dendrites, and the depletion of neurotransmitters, such as dopamine, within the basal ganglia.

Because it is difficult to find older adults without at least subtle neurologic findings, studies have been unable to determine whether some of the differences between young and old people may be due to these factors. Some of the most striking postural control differences between young and old people relate to the order or grouping of muscle activation patterns. Thus, in response to perturbations of the support surface, older adults tend to activate the proximal muscles, such as the quadriceps, before the more distal muscles, such as the tibialis anterior. This strategy may not be an efficient way to maintain postural stability. Similarly, in older adults, there may be greater co-contraction of antagonistic muscles, and the onset of the muscle activation and associated joint torque may be delayed. Finally, the ability to recover balance after a postural disturbance may be compromised by an age-related decline in the ability to rapidly develop joint torque by using muscles of the leg. All these mechanisms potentially impair maintenance of upright posture.

Another important physiologic contributor to the maintenance of upright posture is the regulation of systemic blood pressure. With advancing age, baroreflex sensitivity declines, which manifests as an inability to increase heart rate in response to everyday stresses (such as changing posture, eating a meal, or suffering an acute illness) and subsequent hypotension. Because many older adults have a resting cerebral perfusion that is compromised by vascular disease, even slight reductions in blood pressure can result in cerebral ischemic symptoms, such as falls. Finally, with aging, the amount of total body water is reduced, which places older adults at increased risk of dehydration with acute illness, diuretic use, or hot weather. Because with aging, basal and stimulated renin and aldosterone levels progressively decrease, dehydrating stresses can lead to orthostatic hypotension and a fall.

A number of age-related chronic conditions deserve special mention because of their association with fall risk. Parkinson disease, in particular, increases the risk of falls through several mechanisms, including the rigidity of leg musculature, the inability to correct sway trajectory because of the slowness in beginning movement, hypotensive effects of medication, and in some cases, cognitive impairment. Strokes can also result in an increased risk of falls secondary to visuospatial defects, impaired peripheral sensation, cerebellar dysfunction, muscle weakness, and residual dizziness. When present in the knee, osteoarthritis can affect mobility, the ability to step over objects and maneuver, and the tendency to avoid complete weight bearing on a painful joint, which may also increase the risk of falls.

One of the most modifiable risk factors for falls that has been repeatedly demonstrated in observational studies is medication use. Individual classes of psychotropic medications, such as the benzodiazepines, other sedatives, antidepressants, and antipsychotic medications, have been associated with an increased risk of falls or hip fracture. There appears to be no difference in the risk of falling with the use of older antidepressants or antipsychotics versus that of the newer SSRIs or second-generation antipsychotics. An increased risk of falling has also been associated with recent changes of a non-SSRI antidepressant, benzodiazepine, or antipsychotic medication. As might be expected, the risk of falls increases in older adults taking more than one psychotropic medication, and among older adults taking more than 3 or 4 medications of any type.

Other classes of medications may have an effect on risk of falls as well. Meta-analyses have demonstrated an increased risk of falls among those taking antihypertensives, digoxin, diuretics, type 1A antiarrhythmic agents, and NSAIDs. Acetylcholinesterase inhibitors, which are used to treat dementia, have been associated with an increased risk of syncope. Diabetic medications can also be associated with fall risk during periods of hypoglycemia. Prospective studies are needed to determine whether an independent association between these medications and falls exists, or whether these medications are simply a surrogate marker for older adults with diabetic neuropathy, a chronic risk factor for falls.

The relative importance of environmental and mediating factors on the risk of falling has not been well quantified. Most intervention studies have focused on improving the risk-factor profile of the individual or have combined individual interventions with environmental manipulation, making it difficult to isolate the contributions of the environmental factors. Nevertheless, attention to safety hazards in the home environment appears to be most worthwhile in those at high risk of falls.

History and Physical Examination

Many falls never come to clinical attention for a variety of reasons: the patient may never mention the event, there is no injury at the time of the fall, the clinician may neglect to ask the patient about a history of falls, or the patient or the clinician may make the invalid assumption that falls are an inevitable part of the aging process. The treatment of injuries resulting from falls commonly fails to include an investigation of the cause of the fall.

In the clinical evaluation of noninstitutionalized older adults who are not being seen specifically as the result of a fall, it is still important to include an assessment of fall risk in the history and physical examination. (For an overview of falls assessment and management in all older adults, see Figure 32.1.) The most important point in the history is asking whether there has been a previous fall, because this is a strong risk factor for future falls. Older adults presenting with a single fall should be evaluated for gait and balance problems. Older adults with two or more falls in the past 12 months or with gait or balance abnormalities should undergo a multifactorial falls risk assessment.

For patients presenting with a fall, important components of the history include the activity at the time of the fall, the occurrence of prodromal symptoms (lightheadedness, imbalance, dizziness), and the location and time of the fall. Loss of consciousness is associated with injurious falls and should raise important considerations, such as orthostatic hypotension or cardiac or neurologic disease. See "Syncope," p 204. Information on previous falls should be collected to identify patterns that may help determine strategies to reduce future falls. A complete medication history should focus on newly added medications, as well as the use of diuretics and psychotropic medications because of their association with falls and their common use in older adults.

In addition to inquiring about the circumstances surrounding the fall, the clinician should attempt to identify any potential contributing environmental factors. Information on lighting, floor coverings, door thresholds, railings, and furniture can add important clues. Footwear can also be an important factor. In one small study that evaluated the effect of various shoe types on balance in older men, shoes with thin, hard soles produced the best results, even though they were perceived as less comfortable than thick, soft, mid-soled shoes, such as running shoes. In another nested case control study of men and women, athletic shoes were associated with the lowest risk of falls, and shoes with increased heel height and decreased surface area between the sole and the floor were associated with a higher risk of falls.

The physical examination of the person who has fallen should focus on risk factors. Much of the examination duplicates that done in a gait assessment (see "Gait Impairment," p 228). Probably the most important part of the physical examination is an assessment of integrated musculoskeletal function, which can be accomplished by performing one or more of the following tests of postural stability. The functional reach test is a practical way to test the integrated neuromuscular base of support and has predictive validity for falls in older men. This test is performed with a leveled yardstick secured to a wall at the height of the acromion. The person being tested assumes a comfortable stance without shoes or socks and stands so that his or her shoulders are perpendicular to the yardstick. He or she makes a fist and extends the arm forward as far as possible along the wall without taking a step or losing balance. The total reach is measured along the yardstick and recorded. Inability to reach ≥6 inches is cause for concern and merits further evaluation. Another useful test of integrated strength and balance is the Timed Up and

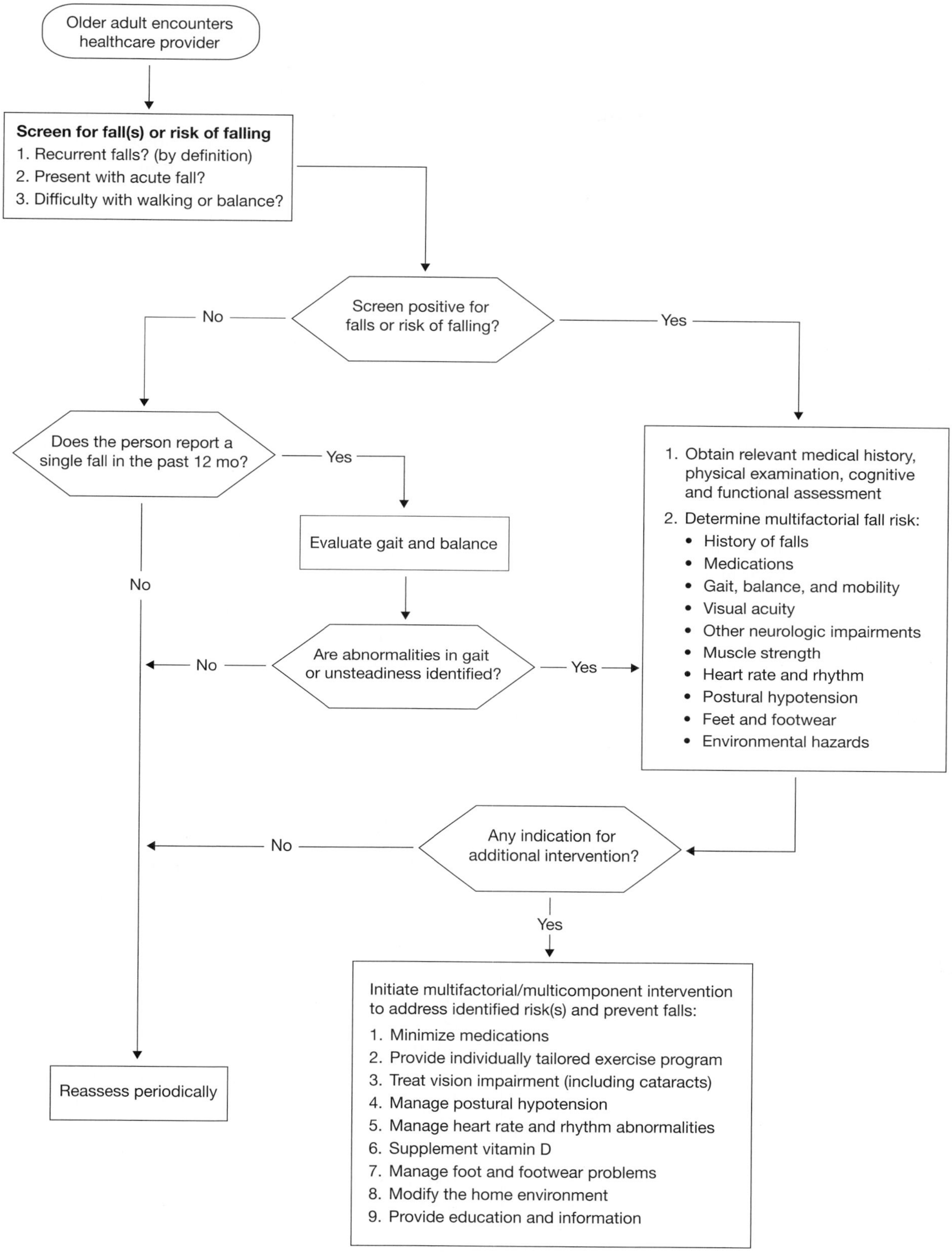

Figure 32.1—Prevention of Falls in Older Adults Living in the Community

SOURCE: American Geriatrics Society and British Geriatrics Society. Clinical Practice Guideline for the Prevention of Falls in Older Persons. New York: American Geriatrics Society; 2010.

Go test, which can be performed with or without timing. It consists of observation of an individual standing up from a chair without using the arms to push against the chair, walking across a room (about 3 meters), turning around, walking back, and sitting down without using the arms. This test can grade muscle weakness, balance problems, and gait abnormalities using a scale of 1–5, with 5 indicating severe abnormalities. This test may be timed, with failure to complete the test within 15 seconds suggesting an increased risk of falls. A third test of integrated musculoskeletal function is the Berg Balance Test. The Berg test includes 14 items of balance, including timed tandem stance, semitandem stance, and the ability of a person to retrieve an object from the floor. Berg scores <40 have been associated with an increased risk of falls. Lastly, the Performance-Oriented Mobility Assessment (POMA) tests balance and gait through a number of items, including ability to sit and stand from an armless chair, ability to maintain standing balance when pulled by an examiner, and the ability to walk normally and maneuver obstacles. POMA scores are considered abnormal if there is a 1-point deduction from two or more items, or if there is a 2-point deduction from a single item.

A number of screening tools for risk of falls have been developed for use in the acute hospital setting, including the Morse Fall Scale and the St. Thomas's Risk Assessment Tool (STRATIFY). The Morse Fall Scale, one of the more commonly used scales, comprises six items: history of falling in the past 3 months, presence of any secondary diagnosis, use of an ambulatory aid, receipt of intravenous therapy, abnormal gait, and impaired mental status. Scores range from 0 to 125, with higher numbers indicating a greater risk of falls. A cutpoint of >45 is often used to identify patients at high risk of falls.

Although these screening tools perform relatively well in predicting falls, a systematic review and meta-analysis of prospective studies suggests that they are comparable with nursing clinical judgment when predicting falls in the hospital setting. Screening tools are likely to be even less useful in the nursing-home setting, where most residents have a high risk of falls. For this reason, all nursing-home residents should be considered at high risk of falls, prompting a consideration of modifiable, individual risk factors.

Laboratory and Diagnostic Tests

There is no standard diagnostic evaluation of a person with a history of falls or a high risk of falling. Laboratory tests for hemoglobin, BUN, creatinine, or glucose concentrations can help to exclude anemia, dehydration, or hyperglycemia with hyperosmolar dehydration as the cause of falling. There is no proven value of routinely performing Holter monitoring of individuals who have fallen. Because data demonstrate that carotid sinus hypersensitivity contributes to falls and even hip fracture, some have advocated performing carotid sinus massage with continuous heart rate and phasic blood pressure measurement in older adults with unexplained falls. Similarly, the decision to perform echocardiography, brain imaging, or radiographic studies of the spine should be driven by the findings of the history and physical examination. Echocardiography should be reserved for those with cardiac conditions believed to contribute to the maintenance of blood flow to the brain. Spine radiographs or MRI can be useful in patients with gait disorders, abnormalities on neurologic examination, leg spasticity, or hyperreflexia to exclude cervical spondylosis or lumbar stenosis as a cause of falls.

Treatment and Prevention

Multiple studies of preventive interventions have been conducted over the past decade, including programs to improve strength or balance, educational programs, optimization of medications, and environmental modifications in homes or institutions. Some interventions have targeted single risk factors; others have attempted to address multiple factors by either targeting patient-specific risk factors (multifactorial intervention) or by offering the interventions to an entire population (multicomponent intervention).

A Cochrane collaboration systematic review of interventions to reduce the incidence of falling in older adults was performed. Because of the large numbers of fall intervention trials and because interventions may be more effective in certain settings, systematic reviews of fall prevention interventions were divided into two groups: those among community-dwelling adults and those among institutionalized adults. The April 2009 update of the Cochrane systematic review of fall interventions among community-dwelling adults included 111 individual trials, whereas the January 2010 review of falls interventions in the hospital and nursing-care facilities included 41 trials. The results of this systematic review demonstrated that the following falls prevention interventions are likely to be beneficial in the community setting: medication review; home hazards assessment by healthcare professionals in older adults at high risk of falling; Tai Chi, muscle strengthening, and balance training by trained professionals; vitamin D supplementation in patients with vitamin D deficiency; an antislip shoe device to be worn in icy conditions; pacemaker placement in patients with carotid sinus hypersensitivity; and multifactorial, multidisciplinary interventions. Multifactorial interventions were successful in reducing falls in the hospital setting and, when delivered by a multidisciplinary team, were marginally successful in reducing falls in the nursing-home setting. Exercise may be effective in reducing falls in the subacute hospital setting, but its effectiveness in preventing falls in the long-term care setting is unclear.

In 2009, the American Geriatrics Society and the British Geriatrics Society published clinical practice guidelines for the prevention of falls in older adults. These guidelines advocate for initiating multifactorial/multicomponent interventions to address identified risks and to prevent falls; these interventions should include an education component addressing issues specific to the intervention being provided and tailored to the individual's cognitive ability and language. Additionally, offering an exercise program to incorporate balance, gait, and strength training was suggested for older adults at risk of falls. The guidelines place these intervention measures into the following nine groups:

- **Minimize medications:** In one study of 93 community-dwelling adults, a gradual taper of psychotropic medications was associated with a decreased rate of falls (relative hazard 0.34; CI 95%, 0.16–0.74) (SOE=B). Multifactorial interventions that include education and a review of medications with cessation or dosage reduction when possible have also successfully reduced the number of falls among community-dwelling adults (SOE=B).

- **Initiate an individually tailored exercise program:** As of the 2009 Cochrane review, 43 trials tested the efficacy of exercise as an intervention to prevent falls in the community setting. Exercise classes incorporating more than one type of exercise (eg, gait training, balance, strengthening) were effective in reducing the rate of falls (14 trials; 2,364 participants; relative risk [RR] 0.83; CI 95%, 0.72–0.97) (SOE=A). In three trials of hospitalized patients, supervised exercise was effective in reducing the risk of falls (RR 0.44; CI 95%, 0.20–0.97), but there was no effect on risk of falls in seven trials of exercise in nursing-care facilities (SOE=B). Tai Chi, which combines both strengthening and balance measures, is effective in reducing the risk of falls among community-dwelling adults (RR 0.65; CI 95%, 0.51–0.82) (SOE=A).

- **Treat vision impairment:** First cataract surgery results in a decreased rate of falls (1 trial; 306 participants; RR 0.66; CI 95%, 0.45–0.95) (SOE=B). Second cataract surgery showed no benefit in reducing the rate of falls or number of fallers. Routine eye screening with correction of visual defects is considered good medical practice. It has not been demonstrated to be effective in reducing falls as a single intervention. Multifactorial interventions that include visual screening and/or treatment have had a modest effect in reducing the risk of falls.

- **Manage postural hypotension:** The sensation of dizziness is strongly associated with an increased risk of falls, and thus, treating orthostatic hypotension may be prudent among certain groups of older adults at risk of falls. Achieving better control of systolic blood pressure has been associated with a decrease in postural changes in blood pressure. It is unclear whether this might also translate into a decreased risk of falls. While no trial to date has addressed whether a single intervention to reduce orthostasis results in decreased falls, multifactorial interventions that include fluid optimization, medication review and reduction, and behavioral changes have shown a modest effect in reducing the risk of falls among community-dwelling adults (SOE=B).

- **Manage heart rate and rhythm abnormalities:** One trial demonstrated a reduction in the rate of falls among older adults with carotid sinus hypersensitivity treated with a pacemaker (175 participants; weighted mean difference –5.20; CI 95%, –9.40 to –1.00) (SOE=B).

- **Supplement vitamin D:** In 2009, a meta-analysis found that higher doses of vitamin D (at least 700–1000 IU) have been associated with a 9.5% absolute reduction in the risk of falls among community-dwelling and institutionalized older adults. While the exact mechanism is unknown, it is believed that vitamin D may reduce falls by increasing muscle strength and decreasing body sway. Vitamin D supplementation also improves bone mineral density and reduces the risk of vertebral and nonvertebral fractures (NNT=15) (SOE=A).

- **Manage foot and footwear problems:** One small trial (109 participants) demonstrated a reduction in falls among community-dwelling older adults wearing a nonslip shoe covering during icy conditions (RR 0.42; CI 95%, 0.22–0.78) (SOE=B). Footwear associated with higher heels and decreased surface area has been associated with an increased risk of falls. Although there are limited data to demonstrate that avoiding more risky types of footwear prevents falls, clinicians should advise their patients to use walking shoes with high contact surface area. In older adults with disabling foot pain, falls may be reduced by a multifaceted intervention including customized insoles, attention to shoe wear, foot and ankle exercises, and falls prevention education.

- **Modify the home environment:** When included as part of a multifactorial intervention, home environment assessments with environmental modification performed by a healthcare professional reduced the risk of falling among older adults who have fallen or are at high risk of falling because of visual impairment (2 trials; 491 participants; RR 0.56; CI 95%, 0.42–0.76) (SOE=A).

- **Provide education and information:** There is little direct evidence to demonstrate that education on falls and fall-related injuries results in a reduction in fall risk. Nonetheless, it may be prudent for clinicians to educate older adults at risk of falls on home hazards, proper choices for footwear, and the importance of regular exercise.

Additionally, several multifactorial interventions in which participants received more than one intervention were effective in reducing the rate of falls (15 trials; 8,141 participants; pooled RR 0.75; CI 95%, 0.65–0.86) (SOE=A). Because these trials were conducted in different populations and used different interventions, it is unclear which combinations of interventions are the most effective.

A number of interventions have not been effective for fall prevention, including group-delivered exercise interventions (SOE=B), nutritional supplementation (SOE=C), isolated modification of home hazards (SOE=B), cognitive-behavioral approach (SOE=B), hormone therapy (SOE=C), and individual strength training (SOE=B).

Fall prevention programs in nursing-home settings have been largely unsuccessful to date. Only a post-hoc analysis showed that multifactorial interventions, including personalized exercises provided by a multidisciplinary team, were successful in reducing risk of falls (5 trials; 1,925 participants; pooled RR 0.85; CI 95%, 0.77–0.95) (SOE=C). In the hospital setting, multifactorial interventions reduced the risk of falling in three trials (4,824 participants; pooled RR 0.73; CI 95%, 0.56–0.96) (SOE=B). A multicenter randomized controlled trial of over 10,000 acutely hospitalized adults found that a fall prevention tool kit using individual patient characteristics as ascertained from health information technology was successful in reducing the absolute rate of falls by 1.16 falls/1,000 bed days (CI 95%, 0.17–2.16). This intervention was particularly effective in reducing falls among adults ≥65 years old (adjusted rate difference 2.08/1,000 patient days; CI 95%, 0.61–3.56).

A practical approach for clinicians who are treating older adults with a high risk of or a history of falls, including nursing-home residents, targets risk factors for falls in three major domains: medications, mobility, and medical conditions (Table 32.1). Further research is needed to confirm whether successful fall prevention strategies are also effective in reducing serious sequelae of falls, such as fractures or other injuries.

Hip Protectors

Although hip protectors have been advocated as a means to reduce fracture risk in those at risk of falls, meta-analyses of studies that randomized individual patients within an institution or among older adults living at home have not shown a significant reduction in hip fractures. However, adherence to the use of hip protectors was low in these studies, which many argue could explain the lack of efficacy. In prior studies that found a benefit with hip protectors, groups of patients were randomly assigned to an intervention based on setting (eg, by ward in a nursing home). These studies were potentially susceptible to bias because unintended "co-interventions" can occur when whole units or facilities participate in trials and are allocated to use hip protectors. A multi-institutional study in which individual nursing-home residents were randomized for use of a right- or left-sided hip protector found no reduction in fractures on the protected hip (SOE=B).

At least a dozen types of hip protectors are commercially available. Many of these hip protectors have not been tested in clinical trials. Recently, a systematic testing of all commercially available hip protectors revealed significant variability in their material properties. Recently, a systematic testing of all commercially available hip protectors revealed significant variability in their material properties. Despite the lack of evidence to date to support the use of hip protectors, it is not unreasonable to consider their use in patients at high risk of hip fractures who are willing to use them.

CLINICAL GUIDELINES

For older adults who have sustained a fall, a multifactorial approach is appropriate and should consider known risk factors for falls, include a multidimensional assessment of the patient, and target interventions on the basis of these findings. For older adults who have no history of falling, it is reasonable to use traditional multidimensional geriatric assessment with targeted interventions as risk factors are

Table 32.1—Preventing Falls: Selected Risk Factors and Suggested Interventions

Factors	Suggested Interventions
General Risk	Offer exercise program to include combination of resistance (strength) training, gait, balance, and coordination training: ■ medical assessment before starting ■ tailor to individual capabilities ■ initiate with caution in those with limited mobility not accustomed to physical activity ■ prescribed by qualified healthcare provider ■ regular review and progression Education and information, cognitive-behavioral intervention to decrease fear of falling and activity avoidance Recommend daily supplementation of vitamin D (1000 IU). After supplementation, vitamin D levels may be appropriate for select patients at risk of vitamin D deficiency with the goal of achieving a 25-hydroxy vitamin D level >30 ng/mL (see "Osteoporosis," p 243)
Medication-related Factors	
Use of benzodiazepines, sedative-hypnotics, antidepressants, or antipsychotics	Consider agents with less risk of falls Taper dosage and discontinue medications, as possible Address sleep problems with nonpharmacologic interventions (see "Sleep Problems," p 285) Educate regarding appropriate use of medications and monitoring for adverse events
Recent change in dosage or number of prescription medications, or use of ≥4 prescription medications, or use of other medications associated with fall risk	Review medication profile and reduce number and dosage of all medications, as possible Monitor response to medications and to dosage changes
Mobility-related Factors	
Presence of environmental hazards (eg, improper bed height, cluttered walking surfaces, lack of railings, poor lighting)	Improve lighting, especially at night Remove floor hazards (eg, loose carpeting) Replace existing furniture with safer furniture (eg, correct height, more stable) Install support structures, especially in bathroom (eg, railings, grab bars, elevated toilet seats) Use nonslip bath mats
Impaired gait, balance, or transfer skills	Refer to physical therapy for comprehensive evaluation and rehabilitation and for training in use of assistive devices Gait training Balance or strengthening exercises If able to perform tandem stance, refer for Tai Chi, dance, yoga, or postural awareness Provide training in transfer skills Prescribe appropriate assistive devices Recommend appropriate footwear (eg, good fit, nonslip, low heel height, large surface contact area)
Impaired leg or arm strength or range of motion, or proprioception	Strengthening exercises (eg, use of resistive rubber bands, putty) Resistance training 2–3 times/week to 10 repetitions with full range of motion, then increase resistance Tai Chi Physical therapy
Medical Factors	
Parkinson disease, osteoarthritis, depressive symptoms, impaired cognition, carotid sinus hypersensitivity, other conditions associated with increased falls	Optimize medical therapy Monitor for disease progression and impact on mobility and impairments Determine need for assistive devices Use bedside commode if frequent nighttime urination Cardiac pacing in patients with carotid sinus hypersensitivity who experience falls due to syncope
Postural hypotension: drop in systolic blood pressure ≥20 mmHg (or ≥20%) with or without symptoms, within 3 min of rising from lying to standing	Review medications potentially contributing and adjust dosing or switch to less hypotensive agents; avoid vasodilators and diuretics if possible Educate on activities to decrease effect (eg, slow rising, ankle pumps, hand clenching, elevation of head of bed) and to slow rising from recumbent or seated position, grab bars by toilet and bath Prescribe pressure stockings (eg, Jobst) Optimize hydration Liberalize salt intake, if appropriate Caffeinated coffee (1 cup) or caffeine 100 mg with meals for postprandial hypotension Consider medication to increase blood pressure (if hypertension, heart failure, and hypokalemia not serious): ■ midodrine 2.5–10 mg given 3 times/day 4 hr apart ■ fludrocortisone 0.1 mg q8–24h
Visual impairment	Cataract extraction Avoid wearing multifocal lenses while walking, particularly up stairs

SOURCE: Adapted with permission from Reuben DB, Herr KA, Pacala JT, et al. *Geriatrics At Your Fingertips*, 15th ed. New York: American Geriatrics Society; 2013:106–107.

identified. For a summary of the recommendations of the expert panel on falls prevention assembled by the American Geriatrics Society and the British Geriatrics Society, see www.americangeriatrics.org.

REFERENCES

- American Geriatrics Society and British Geriatrics Society. *Clinical Practice Guideline for the Prevention of Falls in Older Persons.* New York: American Geriatrics Society; 2009 (www.americangeriatrics.org/).
- Cameron ID, Murray GR, Gillespie LD, et al. Interventions for preventing falls in older people in nursing care facilities and hospitals. *Cochrane Database Syst Rev.* 2010 Jan 20;(1):CD005465.
- Gillespie L, Gillespie W, Robertson M, et al. Interventions for preventing falls in older people living in the community. *Cochrane Database Syst Rev.* 2009 Apr 15;(2):CD007146.
- Milisen K, Coussement J, Arnout H, et al. Feasibility of implementing a practice guideline for fall prevention on geriatric wards: A multicenter study. *Int J Nurs.* 2013;50(4):495–507.

CHAPTER 33—OSTEOPOROSIS

KEY POINTS

- Osteoporosis is a common metabolic bone disorder affecting older adults that is preventable and treatable. The resultant fractures can lead to chronic pain, decreased mobility, loss of independence and function, and increased mortality.
- Bone mineral density (BMD) measurement establishes the diagnosis of osteoporosis (T-score ≤–2.5). Osteoporosis can also be defined clinically in at-risk persons who sustain a fragility or low-trauma fracture.
- Secondary osteoporosis should be excluded in men and women with osteoporosis. Common causes of secondary osteoporosis include glucocorticoid use, hyperparathyroidism, hypogonadism, hyperthyroidism, and vitamin D insufficiency.
- Screening for osteoporosis is recommended for all postmenopausal women ≥65 years old and men ≥50 years old with risk factors for osteoporosis. FRAX is a free online clinical tool that estimates the 10-year probability of osteoporotic fracture based on a patient's clinical risk factors and femoral neck BMD.
- Prevention of osteoporosis includes adequate calcium and vitamin D intake, weight-bearing exercise, and reduction of known risk factors for osteoporosis.
- Bisphosphonates are first-line pharmacologic therapy for osteoporosis. Consideration of denosumab and teriparatide as effective therapies for osteoporosis is also warranted.

Osteoporosis, the most common metabolic bone disease, is a major cause of morbidity, loss of independence, and mortality in older adults. It is a systemic skeletal disorder defined by decreased bone strength and increased risk of fracture. Bone strength is determined by both BMD and bone quality. In osteoporosis, bone density is decreased through reduced bone mass and increased loss of bone tissue while bone quality and strength are impaired by disrupted skeletal microarchitecture, accelerated skeletal turnover, and altered bone mineralization, among other factors. Osteoporosis can be categorized as primary (age-related) or secondary (result of other diseases or medications). Prevention of fractures is the main goal of any prevention and treatment program.

The World Health Organization (WHO) defines osteoporosis by a BMD measurement that is less than or equal to 2.5 standard deviations below the young normal adult reference (T-score ≤–2.5). For WHO classifications of BMD measurements, see Table 33.1. BMD measurement at the spine, hip, or forearm is achieved through dual energy x-ray absorptiometry (DXA). The basis for the WHO-defined BMD criteria is from analysis of fracture data in postmenopausal white women, with fracture risk increasing exponentially below the –2.5 T-score cut point. However, most fractures occur in patients with T-scores above this cut point. Therefore, osteoporosis can also be diagnosed clinically in at-risk individuals who sustain a fragility or low-trauma fracture, which is defined as any nonpathologic fracture that occurs from a fall from standing height or less. Specific standards for definitions of osteoporosis have not been established for men or for racial and ethnic groups other than whites, although conventional practice applies similar standards universally.

EPIDEMIOLOGY AND IMPACT

The National Osteoporosis Foundation estimates that 10 million Americans have osteoporosis by bone density criteria and that another nearly 34 million adults ≥50 years old with low bone density are at increased risk of fracture. Osteoporosis affects people of all ethnic backgrounds. Although less prevalent than the estimated 27% of white and Asian adults, 13% of Hispanics and 9% of blacks ≥50 years old have osteoporosis.

Osteoporosis is the most important cause of fracture in older adults. In 2005, osteoporosis caused more than 2 million fractures in the United States; this number is expected to rise to greater than 3 million by the year 2025. One in two postmenopausal women and up to one in five men >50 years old will have an osteoporotic-related fracture in their remaining lifetime. Increased mortality is related primarily to hip fractures, although vertebral fractures have also been associated with increased mortality, generally from associated comorbidities. An estimated 20% greater mortality occurs in older adults in the year after hip fracture with the rate of death in men nearly double that of women (SOE=B). In a recent meta-analysis, the excess mortality risk persists for at least 10 years after the hip-fracture event. Hip fractures are also associated with 2.5-fold increased risk of future fractures. Hip fracture rates in black Americans, Japanese Americans, Hispanics, and Native Americans occur at lower frequencies than that in white Americans, with the rate of hip fractures in Mexican Americans higher relative to that in other Hispanic groups.

Osteoporotic fractures can lead to permanent declines in functional status, independence, and quality of life. In patients who were previously ambulatory,

Table 33.1—WHO Bone Mineral Density (BMD) definitions

Classification	BMD	T-score
Normal	Within one SD[a] of reference mean[b]	≥–1.0
Osteopenia (low bone mass)	More than 1 but less than 2.5 SD below reference mean	Between –1.0 and –2.5
Osteoporosis	2.5 or more SD below reference mean	≤–2.5
Established osteoporosis	Below 2.5 SD of reference mean in the presence of one or more fragility fractures	<–2.5

[a] Standard deviation

[b] For young, normal adult

only approximately 40% regain their previous level of functioning after hip fracture and 20% require long-term nursing-home care. Pain, kyphosis, height loss, and other changes in body habitus can develop from vertebral fractures. Patients may be unable to bathe, dress, or walk independently. The economic costs associated with osteoporotic-related fractures are substantial. In 2005, the total direct healthcare costs were estimated at $19 billion. By 2025, this number is expected to rise to $25.3 billion. Thus, because the social and economic costs associated with osteoporotic fractures in older adults are substantial, reduction of this burden is widely seen as a healthcare policy imperative.

Bone Remodeling and Bone Loss in Aging

Bone is a dynamic tissue that undergoes active remodeling (also called bone turnover), a coupled process of bone resorption followed by bone formation throughout adult life. Bone remodeling maintains both skeletal strength through repair of microfractures and systemic calcium homeostasis. Local signals bring osteoclasts to specific areas of bone where resorption is initiated and resorption cavities are formed. Once osteoclasts move to the area, osteoblasts are recruited to the resorption lacunae and lay down osteoid, which is subsequently mineralized into new, mature bone. Under steady state conditions, bone resorption and formation is equally balanced. However, after menopause in women and with aging in both sexes, the remodeling cycle becomes unbalanced, with bone resorption exceeding bone formation, resulting in net bone loss. Menopause and estrogen deficiency are associated with an increase in the rate of remodeling, which can also lead to loss of bone tissue and disrupted bone architecture.

Osteoblast activity decreases with aging in both men and women, compounding the bone loss that results from increased resorption seen with aging and menopause. Growth factors, such as transforming growth factor β and insulin-like growth factor 1, can be impaired with estrogen deficiency or with aging, resulting in decreased osteoblast function.

Bone mass changes over the life span of an individual. In women, bone mass increases rapidly from puberty until approximately the mid-20s to mid-30s, when bone mass peaks. Contributing factors include physical activity, nutrition, and endocrine status, as well as comorbid disease processes. Once women reach peak bone mass, bone loss occurs very slowly until the onset of menopause. After menopause, the rate of bone loss is accelerated for 8–10 years. Bone loss continues in later life, albeit at a slower rate of 1%–2% per year; however, some older women may lose bone density at a higher rate. Data suggest that reducing bone loss and skeletal turnover at any time will decrease fracture risk.

Although studies thus far have focused mostly on women, it is well documented that men also lose bone with age. It is estimated that men 30–90 years old lose approximately 1% per year in the radius and spine; some men with risk factors lose as much as 6% per year (SOE=B). The pattern of bone loss differs between men and women: men lose bone mass due to trabecular thinning, while women have a decrease in total number of trabeculae. Preservation of trabeculae may in part explain the lower lifetime risk of fracture in men. Both men and women predominantly lose the inner, spongy cancellous bone, which is concentrated in the vertebral spine. Cortical bone accounts for 45%–75% of the mechanical resistance to compression of the vertebral spine, and men actually gain cortical bone with age through periosteal bone deposition. The cross-sectional area of the vertebrae of men increases by 15%–20% through adulthood, increasing maximal load levels until the age of 75 years. Subsequently, bone strength seems to be reversed by thinning of the cortical ring by age 75, the age at which men begin to present with vertebral fractures. Although bone loss at the hip has not been extensively studied in men, in cross-sectional analyses, healthy 90-year-old men have a 40% lower femoral neck BMD than 20-year-olds.

Pathogenesis

The pathogenesis of osteoporosis in men and women is complex, encompassing factors that affect the level of peak bone mass, the rate of bone resorption, and

Table 33.2—Risk Factors in Fracture Risk Assessment Model (World Health Organization)

- Current age
- Gender
- Prior osteoporotic fracture, including morphometric vertebral fracture
- Femoral neck BMD
- Low BMI
- Oral glucocorticoids (≥5 mg/d of prednisone or equivalent for ≥3 months [ever])
- Rheumatoid arthritis
- Secondary osteoporosis
- Parental history of hip fracture
- Current smoking
- Alcohol intake of ≥3 drinks/day

the rate of bone formation. Peak bone mass seems to be 75%–80% genetically determined. A number of candidate genes that may be important to osteoporosis are currently being studied, including the vitamin D receptor, estrogen receptor, transforming growth factor, interleukin-6, interleukin-1 receptor 2, type I collagen genes, and collagenases. However, it is clear from studies to date that osteoporosis in the vast majority of individuals is in part a polygenic disorder.

Estrogen Deficiency in Women

After menopause, the natural decline of estrogen levels is associated with risk of osteoporosis, with fracture risk inversely related to estrogen levels (SOE=A). Increased resorption appears to be the major factor for bone loss in estrogen deficiency. More recent evidence also suggests a role of estrogen deficiency in reducing bone formation, although both markers of bone resorption and formation are increased after menopause.

Estrogen has both direct and indirect effects on osteoclasts, the cells that are responsible for bone resorption and bone loss. It can act on cells of the osteoblastic lineage to decrease the expression of human receptor activator of nuclear factor kappa-B ligand (RANKL), the major cytokine that promotes the development and facilitates the differentiation of osteoclasts to mature forms. Estrogen deficiency also decreases production of osteoprogerin, a soluble receptor that neutralizes the effect of RANKL. It can also have direct effects on cells of hematopoietic lineage, including osteoclast precursors, mature osteoclasts, and lymphocytes.

Calcium and Vitamin D Insufficiency and Secondary Hyperparathyroidism

A major mechanism by which older men and women continue to lose bone is likely related to calcium insufficiency, which results in secondary

Table 33.3—Risk Factors for Osteoporosis

- Age (postmenopausal in women, >70 years in men)
- Female sex
- Low body weight (BMI <20 kg/m^2)
- 10% decrease in weight (from usual adult body weight)
- Physical inactivity
- Glucocorticoids
- Previous fragility fracture as adult
- White or Asian race
- Current smoking
- Low dietary calcium
- Alcohol intake ≥3 drinks a day

hyperparathyroidism. Decreased dietary calcium intake, impaired intestinal absorption of calcium due to disease or aging itself, and vitamin D insufficiency can all lead to calcium insufficiency and secondary hyperparathyroidism. Older black Americans are at particular risk of vitamin D deficiency as they age.

Aging skin and decreased exposure to sunlight reduce the conversion of 7-dehydrocholesterol to cholecalciferol (vitamin D_3) by ultraviolet light, causing vitamin D insufficiency and reduced calcium absorption. The hormonally active form of vitamin D is $1{,}25(OH)_2D_3$, or calcitriol. It is necessary for optimal intestinal absorption of calcium and phosphorus, and also exerts a tonic inhibitory effect on parathyroid hormone (PTH) synthesis. Vitamin D insufficiency not only contributes to accelerated bone loss and increasing fragility but also appears to promote muscle weakness that can increase the risk of falls.

PTH is a potent stimulator of bone resorption when chronically increased. As a result of decreased serum concentrations of calcium, PTH increases, which leads to increased bone resorption. In one study, older women (mean age 79 years) hospitalized with a hip fracture had lower 25(OH)D levels and bone formation, and higher PTH and bone resorption than women in the control group (mean age 77 years). Further, data from the Study of Osteoporotic Fractures indicate that women with low fractional absorption of calcium are at increased risk of hip fracture. Trials involving older adults at high risk of calcium and vitamin D insufficiency show that supplementation of both can reverse secondary hyperparathyroidism (SOE=A); increase bone mass (SOE=B); and decrease bone resorption (SOE=A), fracture rates (SOE=B), and possibly the frequency of falling (SOE=C). See also “Endocrine and Metabolic Disorders”, p 506 for more on disorders of calcium metabolism.

Hormonal Influences in Men

Hypogonadism is an important risk factor for osteoporosis in men. Androgens are important determinants of peak bone mass in young men and fall gradually as men age.

Table 33.4—Modifications to Reduce Risk of Osteoporosis

Exercise	Encourage regular, weight-bearing exercise at least 5 times per week for 30 min
Nutrition	Encourage adequate intake of calcium (1,200 mg/d in divided doses) and vitamin D_3 (800–1000 IU/d)
Smoking	Encourage smoking cessation
Alcohol consumption	Avoid excessive intake
Medications that can increase risk of osteoporosis—use with caution	■ Glucocorticoids ■ Anticonvulsants ■ Cancer chemotherapeutic agents ■ Long-term heparin ■ Excess thyroid hormone replacement ■ Gonadotropin releasing-hormone agonists (used for prostate cancer) ■ Aromatase inhibitors (used for breast cancer)

While total testosterone levels remain relatively stable due to an increase in sex-hormone binding globulin levels, a decline in free or bioavailable testosterone levels at a rate of approximately 1% per year has been demonstrated in observational studies. Bioavailable testosterone levels are below the normal reference range of young adult men in approximately half of men >70 years old.

Several studies have demonstrated that late-onset hypogonadism can also play a role in osteoporosis in men. Although it is evident that severe hypogonadism in men (eg, due to pituitary tumors or androgen-deprivation treatment) can cause osteoporosis, the effect of moderate decreases in testosterone levels in aging men on rates of bone loss is uncertain. In one study, >60% of men presenting with hip fracture had low testosterone levels compared with about 20% of those in the control group. In several studies in which men with low-normal testosterone levels received supplemental testosterone, femoral bone density increased in the testosterone group and leg muscle strength increased in some but not all. For more information on hypogonadism and testosterone supplementation, see the discussion on testosterone in "Endocrine and Metabolic Disorders."

Evidence for a pivotal role of estradiol in bone metabolism in men has been demonstrated in several studies. Estradiol in older men has been positively associated with BMD, and a threshold bioavailable estradiol level of 40 pmol/L (11 pg/mL) has been identified in which bone loss at the lumbar spine and femoral neck is increased below this value.

Diagnosis and Prediction of Fracture

Osteoporosis is a preventable disease; however, because bone loss is silent, it is often not diagnosed until a fracture occurs. The National Osteoporosis Foundation recommends clinical assessment of osteoporosis risk factors for all postmenopausal women and men ≥50 years old. The diagnosis of osteoporosis should be considered in any older adult with a fracture. BMD measurement is used to establish the diagnosis of osteoporosis in those at high risk clinically but without a prior fragility fracture.

Risk Factors

Clinical evaluation begins with a thorough history to uncover risk factors that may lead to increased bone fragility. Risk factors for osteoporosis and osteoporotic fracture have been identified (Table 33.3) and can be used to determine who should be placed on preventive or therapeutic regimens. Obtaining a thorough history of fracture and the setting in which the fracture occurred is important. Vertebral fractures directly reflect bone fragility and are strong predictors of future fractures. The WHO has developed a specific set of risk factors as part of its 10-year fracture risk model (FRAX) (Table 33.2). These factors are associated with an increased risk of fracture independent of bone mineral density. For a list of modifiable risk factors for osteoporosis, see Table 33.4; all of these risk factors should be addressed as part of the routine care of older adults.

Secondary Causes

The diagnosis of idiopathic or primary osteoporosis is made by BMD measurement before fracture or by incident fracture. Exclusion of other diseases that can present with fracture or low bone mass is important in evaluating women and men with osteoporosis, because different or additional interventions may be required. For the major secondary causes of osteoporosis, see Table 33.5. Certain laboratory tests should be considered for all older adults who present with acute fracture or with a diagnosis of osteoporosis by BMD measurement (Table 33.6). Idiopathic hypercalciuria, found in approximately 10% of the general population, is an important secondary cause of osteoporosis. It is diagnosed by a 24-hour urinary calcium excretion >4 mg/kg and can be treated with a thiazide-type diuretic. Primary hyperparathyroidism is a cause of

Table 33.5—Common Causes of Secondary Osteoporosis

- Male hypogonadism
- Vitamin D insufficiency
- Idiopathic hypercalciuria
- Malabsorption (often celiac disease)
- Multiple myeloma
- Glucocorticoids
- Hyperthyroidism
- Primary hyperparathyroidism
- Solid organ transplantation

Table 33.6—Recommended Initial Laboratory Testing in Those with Osteoporosis

- Fasting comprehensive metabolic panel (including albumin and alkaline phosphatase)
- Serum phosphorus
- 25(OH)D concentration
- Serum parathyroid hormone
- Thyrotropin
- 24-hour urine collection for calcium and creatinine
- CBC
- Serum testosterone

secondary osteoporosis in women with an incidence in older women as high as 1:500. The most commonly reported secondary causes of osteoporosis in men include hypogonadism and excessive alcohol use. Androgen-deprivation therapy with gonadotropin-releasing hormone (GnRH) agonists for the treatment of prostate cancer reduces BMD from 3% to 7% per year and increases the risk and rates of fracture. Men are more likely to have a secondary cause of osteoporosis than women, with up to 50% of men having a secondary cause identified based on clinical and laboratory evaluations.

Glucocorticoid use is the most common drug-induced cause of osteoporosis in both men and women. An estimated 2.5% of people 70–79 years old take an oral glucocorticoid. Glucocorticoid-induced osteoporosis is caused by an early increase in bone resorption and turnover; with prolonged exposure, osteoblastogenesis is reduced, resulting in low bone turnover and decreased bone formation. Fracture risk is greatest in the first 3–6 months of therapy due to rapid bone loss in the hip and spine. Increased fracture risk may be present at daily dosages as low as 2.5–7.5 mg/d. The risk of fracture increases with increasing glucocorticoid dosages and duration, partially independent of BMD. Stopping glucocorticoids is associated with a decrease in fracture risk, although it is unclear if it ever returns to the preexposure level. Although inhaled corticosteroids have not been as well studied, high doses of high-potency inhaled steroids can also result in bone loss. The best strategy for older adults who require long-term glucocorticoid therapy is to maximize bone health by a variety of interventions, including using the lowest possible dosage of glucocorticoids, ensuring adequate intake of calcium and vitamin D, serial monitoring of BMD, and starting prescription osteoporosis therapy (see treatment, below). Other medications that adversely affect BMD include aromatase inhibitors, excess thyroid supplementation, anticonvulsants, methotrexate, calcineurin inhibitors, and heparin. More recent studies have also implicated a negative skeletal effect of SSRIs, antiretroviral agents, and proton-pump inhibitors.

Physical Examination

The physical examination is directed toward detecting signs of fracture as well as potential secondary causes. Key elements include height, weight, posture, mobility, nutritional status, and overall build. Vertebral fractures are suggested by thoracic kyphosis, although this finding is not diagnostic. Wall-to-occiput distance >0 cm and rib-pelvis distance ≤2 fingerbreadths are findings that suggest occult spinal fracture. Height loss >4 cm in women and >6 cm in men from peak young adult height or prospective height loss of 2 cm in women and 3 cm in men is also suggestive of previous vertebral fracture.

Bone Density Measurement

BMD measurement establishes the diagnosis of osteoporosis and is the best predictor of fracture. The relative risk of fracture is 10 times greater in women whose BMD is in the lowest quartile than in women whose BMD is in the highest quartile (SOE=A).

Bone density of the hip, spine, wrist, or calcaneus can be measured by a variety of techniques. The preferred method of BMD measurement is central DXA, which measures BMD of the proximal femur and lumbar spine. Femoral neck BMD is the best predictor of hip and other osteoporotic fractures. Other methods of measuring BMD include quantitative CT, ultrasonography of the calcaneus, single radiographic absorptiometry of the calcaneus, peripheral DXA, and radiographic absorptiometry. These methods are not currently recommended in the United States, although they are used globally.

BMD is expressed in grams of mineral per square cm scanned (g/cm^2). The Z-score is the relationship between the patient's BMD to the expected BMD for the patient's age and sex, while the T-score compares it to "young normal" adults of the same sex. The lowest T-score from either the lumbar spine, femoral neck, or total proximal femur is used to make the overall diagnosis. Forearm BMD from the mid-third radius

Table 33.7—U.S. Preventive Services Task Force Guidelines: Indications for Osteoporosis Screening

Women	■ ≥65 years old without previous known fractures or secondary causes of osteoporosis ■ <65 years old whose 10-year fracture risk is equal to or greater than that of a 65-year-old white woman without any additional risk factors (according to FRAX-US, 10-year fracture risk is 9.3% for a 65-year-old white woman without any additional risk factors for osteoporosis)
Men	Not currently recommended in those without known previous fracture or secondary causes of osteoporosis

can be used for diagnosis, specifically if that from the hip or spine cannot be interpreted, the patient has a history of hyperparathyroidism, or weight is >300 pounds (thus precluding measurement of the other sites). Osteoporosis is defined as 2.5 or more standard deviations below the young adult mean (ie, T-score ≤–2.5). For every standard deviation below the young adult mean (or a 1-unit decrease in T-score), fracture risk at the spine and hip approximately doubles. For example, if a woman has a T-score of –2, her risk of fracture is four times that of a woman with normal bone density for her age (controlled for height and weight).

The U.S. Preventive Services Task Force (USPSTF) recommends BMD testing for all women ≥65 years old, regardless of risk-factor status; there are limited data to determine the frequency of screening or the age to stop screening for osteoporosis in women. Women <65 years old should be screened if their 10-year fracture risk is equal to or greater than that of a 65-year-old white woman without additional risk factors (SOE=B). There is insufficient evidence to recommend screening in men according to the USPSTF (SOE=C). For indications for BMD testing, see Table 33.7. The National Osteoporosis Foundation recommends screening all men ≥70 years old regardless of risk factors (SOE=C). DXA is also recommended in men 50–69 years old with diseases or medications known to increase risk of osteoporosis and in those with a history of fracture after age 50. Although data relating BMD to fracture risk are derived from studies of women, data also suggest that similar associations may be valid for men. Men tend to fracture at a higher BMD than women, but like women most fractures occur in men with a T-score greater than –2.5.

Interpretation of BMD involves evaluating the quality of the DXA as well as the T-scores. Several considerations are important when evaluating BMD of the spine over time. BMD of lumbar vertebrae L1–L4 should be measured when making a decision about therapy. Vertebral, arterial, or lymph node calcification as well as any scoliosis can falsely increase BMD of the anterior-posterior spine DXA. Thus, a woman with osteoporosis of the spine can have a DXA T-score that is higher than –2.5. Usually, these changes can be seen on the DXA report if the picture of the scan is included in the report. Proximal femoral neck BMD is preferred because it is more likely to be free of osteoarthritic changes and is most associated with fracture risk. Proximal femur is based on the lower measure of the total hip or femoral neck. Another important issue of DXA testing is measurement variability. It is critical to scan a patient on the same DXA machine, given that unaccountable inter-machine differences can substantially impair the ability to detect statistically different changes in BMD over time. In addition, patient positioning should be consistent on repeated measurements. The International Society of Clinical Densitometry offers guidelines and standardized training courses for technicians and clinicians acquiring and interpreting the results.

FRAX

The WHO fracture risk assessment tool (FRAX) has been the most widely adopted method to incorporate clinical risk factors and BMD. The FRAX is a free online clinical tool (www.shef.ac.uk/FRAX) that estimates the 10-year probability of fracture at the hip or major osteoporotic fracture (hip, spine, proximal humerus, or distal forearm). It is used for both women and men from different geographic settings. The data used to calculate this risk includes femoral neck BMD; patient's age, sex, height, and weight; seven clinical risk factors (previous fracture, parental history of fracture, current smoking, glucocorticoid use, rheumatoid arthritis, secondary osteoporosis, alcohol consumption of ≥3 drinks per day); and the brand of DXA scanner used. FRAX was developed through the WHO after analyzing 12 population-based cohorts of nearly 60,000 men and women with approximately 250,000 person-years of observation; this data was then externally validated in another 11 cohorts comprising 230,000 men and women with >1.2 million person-years of observation. It is most useful for patients who have a low hip BMD, because fracture risk may be underestimated if BMD is low at the spine but relatively preserved at the hip. It has not been validated in patients who have or are currently taking medications for osteoporosis or for individuals <40 years old or >90 years old. Currently in the United States, FRAX limits its algorithm to four ethnicities (white, black, Hispanic, and Asian).

Vertebral Fracture Assessment

Vertebral fracture assessment (VFA) is a technology used for the diagnosis of vertebral fractures that can be performed as part of a routine DXA measurement. Vertebral fractures are highly associated with future fracture risk and morbidity (SOE=A), but they are often not clinically apparent and can be present in patients with T-scores greater than −2.5. In addition, under-reporting of radiographic vertebral fractures by radiologists is well established. Treatment of patients with vertebral fractures, including those with T-scores greater than −2.5, reduces further fracture risk (SOE=A). For diagnosing vertebral fractures, VFA has lower resolution than CT and spine radiographs but has the advantage of less radiation, lower cost, convenience (at time of BMD), and comparable sensitivity and specificity to spine radiographs. VFA can therefore be a useful adjunct to BMD testing, particularly when results can influence clinical decision making. Risk stratification of patients at risk of fracture, who otherwise might not be considered for pharmacologic therapy, is an important benefit of this technology. The International Society of Clinical Densitometry (www.iscd.org) published a position statement in 2007 on indications for VFA.

The following are suggested indications for VFA:

- When results will influence clinical decision making (eg, regarding beginning medical therapy for bone loss)
- Documented height loss >2 cm or historical height loss >4 cm in postmenopausal women with osteopenia, or >3 cm or historical height loss >6 cm in men with osteopenia
- Long-term glucocorticoid use (≥5 mg of prednisone or equivalent for ≥3 months)
- History or findings suggestive of vertebral fracture not previously documented

Biochemical Markers of Bone Turnover

Serum and urine biochemical markers can estimate the rate of bone turnover (remodeling) and provide additional information to assist the clinician. A number of markers have been developed that reflect collagen breakdown (or bone resorption) and bone formation (proteins secreted from osteoblasts). Several markers have been associated with increased risk of hip fracture, decreased bone density, and bone loss in older adults. Markers of bone resorption and formation decrease in response to antiresorptive treatment. Two markers of bone resorption, deoxypyridinoline cross-links and cross-linked N-telopeptides of type I collagen, and one formation marker, bone alkaline phosphatase, can be used in clinical practice to provide an early assessment of treatment efficacy. A decrease in the level of these markers from baseline after 3–6 months of therapy may indicate a therapeutic response. However, the use of markers in clinical practice is controversial because of the substantial overlap of marker values in women with different bone densities or rates of bone loss. Therefore, routine measurement is not recommended.

PREVENTION AND TREATMENT

Whom To Treat

Treatment should be offered to all postmenopausal women and men ≥50 years old who meet the criteria for osteoporosis by DXA or have a history of hip or vertebral fracture. However, some individuals may be at high risk despite not meeting the BMD criteria for osteoporosis or having a fracture by history. The National Osteoporosis Foundation recommends considering treatment in patients with a 10-year probability of hip fracture ≥3% or major osteoporotic fracture ≥20%, as calculated by FRAX-US algorithm. In patients whom treatment is being considered, secondary causes should be evaluated and excluded as appropriate. All patients should have adequate calcium and vitamin D supplementation, engage in regular weight-bearing exercise, avoid excessive alcohol intake and all tobacco products, and receive falls prevention counseling.

The Role of Exercise

Weight-bearing and muscle strengthening exercises are an important component of osteoporosis treatment and prevention, although exercise alone is not adequate to prevent the rapid bone loss associated with estrogen deficiency in early menopause. Regular exercise is positively associated with BMD, and starting an exercise program even late in life can help to preserve BMD (SOE=A). The effectiveness of high-intensity strength training in maintaining femoral neck BMD as well as in improving muscle mass, strength, and balance in postmenopausal women has been demonstrated, supporting the use of resistance training in helping to maintain BMD and to reduce the risk of falls (SOE=B).

Marked decrease in physical activity or immobilization results in a decline in bone mass; accordingly, it is important to encourage older adults to be as active as possible. Weight-bearing exercise, such as walking, can be recommended for all adults. Older adults should be encouraged to start slowly and to gradually increase both the number of days as well as the time spent walking each day. See "Physical Activity," p 64.

Calcium and Vitamin D

Current recommendations for calcium intake to maintain a positive calcium balance for postmenopausal women >50 years old is elemental calcium at 1,200 mg/d. For

Table 33.8—Calcium-Containing Foods

Food	Serving Size	Calcium (mg) per serving
Dairy Products		
Milk	1 cup	290–300
Yogurt	1 cup	240–400
Swiss cheese	1 ounce (1 slice)	250–270
American cheese	1 ounce (1 slice)	165–200
Ice cream	½ cup	90–100
Cottage cheese	½ cup	80–100
Parmesan cheese	1 tablespoon	70
Powdered nonfat milk	1 teaspoon	50
Other		
Sardines in oil with bones	3 ounces	370
Calcium-fortified orange juice	1 cup	300
Canned salmon with bones	3 ounces	170–210
Broccoli	1 cup	160–180
Tofu (soybean curd)	4 ounces	145–155
Turnip greens	½ cup, cooked	100–125
Kale	½ cup, cooked	90–100
Cornbread	2 ½-inch square	80–90
Egg	1 medium	55
Other fortified foods (eg, bread, cereal, fruit juices)	1 serving	Varies; read label

men 51–70 years old, the recommendation is 1,000 mg/d and after age 70 years, 1,200 mg/d. The upper intake level for all groups is 2,000 mg/d. The average dietary intake of calcium for postmenopausal women in the United States is 500–700 mg/d; thus, most require some form of additional dairy or calcium supplementation to ensure adequate intake. For information on the amount of calcium in selected foods, see Table 33.8. Common calcium supplements are carbonate or citrate, and absorption of either supplement is best in dosages ≤600 mg at a time. Calcium citrate can be absorbed efficiently without food, while calcium carbonate is best absorbed with food. Calcium carbonate may cause adverse effects such as bloating and constipation more commonly than calcium citrate.

The recommended requirement of vitamin D is 600 IU/d for women and men 51–70 years old, and 800 IU/d for women and men >70 years old. The upper intake level for all groups is 4,000 IU/d. Dietary sources of vitamin D include liver, egg yolks, saltwater fish, and vitamin D–fortified food. Many patients may require higher levels of supplementation to achieve serum 25(OH)D concentrations of ≥30 ng/mL (75 nmol/L). Fracture risk is decreased with the combination of calcium and vitamin D (SOE=A). See vitamin D deficiency in “Endocrine and Metabolic Disorders,” p 506, for information regarding vitamin D supplementation and repletion.

Pharmacologic Options

For dosing and special considerations for the medications used to prevent and treat osteoporosis, see Table 33.9. Combination therapy is not currently recommended.

Bisphosphonates

The oral bisphosphonates alendronate and risedronate are approved for osteoporosis prevention in postmenopausal women and as treatment in both men and women. Both medications increase bone density and decrease fractures at the spine and hip in postmenopausal women with osteoporosis (SOE=A). Ibandronate, which can be taken orally on a monthly basis or intravenously every 3 months, is approved for osteoporosis prevention and treatment in postmenopausal women. Ibandronate has shown efficacy in preventing vertebral fractures only (SOE=A). These medications can be given weekly (alendronate, risedronate) or monthly (risedronate, ibandronate). In post-hoc analyses of the Fracture Intervention Trials, alendronate decreased the relative risk of hip, symptomatic vertebral, and wrist fractures in postmenopausal women up to age 85. Risedronate has been shown to decrease the relative risk of new vertebral fractures in women >80 years old with osteoporosis. Alendronate and risedronate are also approved to treat glucocorticoid-induced osteoporosis.

Zoledronic acid is an IV bisphosphonate approved for osteoporosis prevention and treatment in postmenopausal women and for patients after osteoporotic hip fracture. It is also indicated as treatment for osteoporosis in men and for the prevention of osteoporosis in men and women who are expected to receive ≥12 months of glucocorticoid therapy. In the

Table 33.9—Prescription Medications Used to Prevent and Treat Osteoporosis

Medication	Dosage	Special Considerations	Observed Beneficial Treatment Outcomes[a]
Bisphosphonates (should not be used if CrCl <30 mL/min)			
Alendronate	70 mg/wk; 35 mg/wk for prevention	Adherence to dosing instructions required; used in men and women to prevent glucocorticoid-induced osteoporosis	Vertebral fracture: ARR=7.1%, NNT=14 over 3 years Hip fracture: ARR=1.1%, NNT=91 over 3 years
Risedronate	35 mg/wk or 150 mg/mo	Adherence to dosing instructions required	Vertebral fracture: ARR=5%, NNT=20 over 3 years Nonvertebral fracture: ARR=4%, NNT=25 over 3 years
Ibandronate	150 mg/mo or 3 mg IV every 3 mo (treatment only)	Adherence to dosing instructions required	Vertebral fracture: ARR=4.9%, NNT=20 over 3 years
Zoledronic acid	5 mg/year IV; 5 mg every 2 years for prevention	Adherence to dosing instructions required	Morphometric vertebral fracture: ARR=7.6%, NNT=13 over 3 years Clinical vertebral fracture: ARR=2.1%, NNT=48 over 3 years All nonvertebral fractures: ARR=2.7%, NNT=37 over 3 years Hip fracture: ARR=1.1%, NNT=91 over 3 years
Selective estrogen-receptor modulator			
Raloxifene	60 mg/d	Also approved for breast cancer prevention	Vertebral fracture: ARR=3.5%, NNT=29 over 3 years
Calcitonin			
Nasal spray	200 IU/d	Metered spray; 1 spray gives daily dose; alternate nostrils each day to reduce adverse events	Vertebral fracture: ARR=8.1%, NNT=12 over 5 years
Injectable (SC or IM)	100 IU every other day	Injectable can be useful for acute pain syndrome related to vertebral fracture	
Estrogen	See text	Not recommended as first-line choice	See text
Parathyroid hormone			
Teriparatide	20 mcg/d SC	For use in patients who cannot tolerate other approved treatments for osteoporosis	Vertebral fracture: ARR=9%, NNT=11 over 21 months Nonvertebral fracture: ARR=3%, NNT=33 over 21 months
RANK ligand inhibitor			
Denosumab	60 mg SC every 6 months	For treatment of postmenopausal women at high risk of fractures	New vertebral fractures: ARR=4.9% Nonvertebral fractures: ARR=1.5%

[a] Patient populations were not comparable across studies, so direct comparisons of ARR (absolute risk reduction) and NNT (number needed to treat) may not be valid.

HORIZON studies, which were randomized clinical trials involving 8,000 postmenopausal women and >2,100 patients who were 3 months after surgical hip-fracture repair, zoledronic acid increased BMD at the spine and hip and decreased vertebral, spine, and nonvertebral fractures (SOE=A). Zoledronic acid has also been proved to reduce all-cause mortality when given to patients after surgical hip-fracture repair (SOE=A). Post-hoc analyses have shown a risk reduction for new clinical fracture in women ≥75 years old with treatment.

The major adverse events of oral bisphosphonates are GI symptoms, which can include abdominal pain, dyspepsia, esophagitis, nausea, vomiting, and diarrhea. Musculoskeletal pain can also rarely occur. Esophagitis, particularly erosive esophagitis, is seen most commonly in patients who do not take the medication properly, including not remaining upright for 30 minutes after administration. The absorption of oral bisphosphonates is very poor; thus, it is extremely important for patients to follow the specific and detailed instructions for taking them. Zoledronic acid has been associated with an acute-phase response (fever, myalgias, arthralgias, and headache) as soon as 6 hours and lasting up to 72 hours after infusion.

The optimal duration of treatment with bisphosphonates is unclear; however, the effects of bisphosphonates may extend for months to years after treatment is stopped. In the FLEX study, patients who took alendronate for 10 years had less decline in their BMD at the hip and spine than those who stopped the drug after 5 years. Risk of clinical (symptomatic) vertebral fractures, but not total fractures or hip fractures, was higher in those who stopped alendronate after 5 years (SOE=A). This data suggest that alendronate can be discontinued after 5 years of treatment in patients at low risk of future fracture (eg, no new fractures on therapy, T-score greater than –3.5, and T-score that has increased while on therapy). The American Association of Clinical Endocrinologists guidelines recommend a "drug holiday" of 1–2 years. After 10 years of therapy, those at highest risk of fracture should be offered a drug holiday with consideration of possible interval treatment with another agent. After 3 years of therapy with risedronate, no change in fracture risk was seen after a 1-year drug holiday, although BMD did significantly decline. Ibandronate and zoledronic acid have been proved safe and effective for up to 3 years of treatment. In the long-term care population, expert opinion recommends discontinuation of bisphosphonates when a person is no longer ambulatory or has a remaining life expectancy of <2 years. An FDA review of the clinical studies that explored the long-term benefit of bisphosphonates concluded that patients at low risk of fracture may be good candidates to discontinue treatment after 3–5 years, while those at increased risk may continue to benefit from continued bisphosphonate treatment. However, further research is needed to better understand an individual's risk of fracture after stopping bisphosphonate therapy and when and whether to resume therapy in the future.

Selective Estrogen-Receptor Modulators

The selective estrogen-receptor modulators act as estrogen agonists in bone and heart but as estrogen antagonists in breast and uterine tissue. These medications have the potential to prevent osteoporosis or cardiovascular disease without increased risk of breast or uterine cancer. Several studies have reported that tamoxifen, an agent used to treat breast cancer, has beneficial effects on bone, but because of stimulatory effects on the uterus, it is not indicated for osteoporosis treatment or prevention.

Raloxifene has been approved for the treatment and prevention of osteoporosis in postmenopausal women. Efficacy has not been proved past 4 years of treatment, although long-term beneficial effects on bone and breast cancer risk reduction have been demonstrated with treatment up to 8 years. Comparison of raloxifene with placebo in postmenopausal women with osteoporosis found that raloxifene decreases bone turnover, maintains BMD, and reduces incident vertebral fractures (SOE=A). Raloxifene has not, however, been shown to decrease nonvertebral fractures, and it significantly increases the risk of venous thromboembolism and fatal stroke (SOE=A). Additional adverse events with raloxifene include flu-like symptoms, hot flushes, leg cramps, and peripheral edema.

Another important finding with raloxifene was reduced risk of breast cancer in women who participated in the Multiple Outcomes of Raloxifene Trial, with a relative risk of developing breast cancer in women receiving raloxifene of 0.24 (95% CI, 0.13–0.44). Raloxifene is approved by the FDA for the prevention of breast cancer.

Calcitonin

Calcitonin, which inhibits bone resorption, is available as a subcutaneous injection and as a nasal spray for the treatment of postmenopausal osteoporosis in women. The nasal spray is more widely used. Although there are no direct comparisons, calcitonin appears to be less effective than other antiresorptive drugs. Compared with placebo, calcitonin modestly improves spine BMD and reduces vertebral fractures but has not been demonstrated to reduce hip or other nonvertebral fractures (SOE=B). There is some evidence that calcitonin produces an analgesic effect in some women with painful vertebral compression fractures, particularly in its subcutaneous injectable form (SOE=C). Safety and efficacy data are available for up to 5 years of treatment, and the drug is well tolerated with few adverse events.

Estrogen

Estrogen replacement therapy is an option for osteoporosis prevention (approved by the FDA; indication withdrawn as a treatment); however, it is not recommended as a first-line choice. Multiple studies have demonstrated that postmenopausal estrogen use prevents bone loss at the hip and spine when begun within 10 years of menopause (SOE=A). Decreased incident vertebral fractures were seen in a small study of postmenopausal women using a transdermal estradiol preparation. In the Women's Health Initiative

(WHI) trial, >16,000 postmenopausal women with and without low BMD were randomized to receive estrogen plus progesterone versus placebo. After a mean of 5.2 years of follow-up, hormone therapy reduced hip fracture (relative risk reduction [RRR]=34%, absolute risk reduction) and colon cancer. However, hormone therapy also increased the risk of breast cancer (relative risk increase, number needed to harm, heart disease, stroke, and venous thromboembolism). Given the WHI findings, recent USPSTF guidelines advise against the routine use of estrogen plus progesterone for the prevention of chronic conditions in postmenopausal women. The estrogen-only arm of the WHI was also stopped a year ahead of schedule and demonstrated an increased risk of stroke but not of coronary heart disease or breast cancer; estrogen alone also decreased hip fracture risk. Previously, hormone therapy was recommended for prevention of osteoporosis; however, given the results of the WHI and the availability of other effective medications for osteoporosis prevention and treatment, the FDA changed its indication for estrogen and estrogen-progestin products: "When these products are being prescribed solely for the prevention of postmenopausal osteoporosis, approved non-estrogen treatments should be carefully considered. Estrogens and combined estrogen-progestin products should only be considered for women with significant risk of osteoporosis that outweighs the risks of the drug."

Other data suggest that lower-than-usual doses of estrogen, when given with adequate calcium and vitamin D, are effective in reducing bone turnover and bone loss in older women. The effect of lower-dose estrogen on fracture incidence and other health outcomes is unknown. See also estrogen therapy in "Endocrine and Metabolic Disorders," p 506.

Parathyroid Hormone

Recombinant 1-34 human PTH (teriparatide) is the only anabolic agent approved for the treatment of osteoporosis in men and women. PTH increases both bone formation and resorption. Because formation is increased before resorption, the resultant "anabolic window" appears to result in increased bone mass, trabecular connectivity, and mechanical strength when PTH is administered in a daily pulsatile manner. This is in contrast to the chronic increases of PTH seen in primary hyperparathyroidism, which lead to increased resorption, bone loss, and osteoporosis.

Recombinant 1-34 human PTH increases spine and hip BMD in osteoporotic men and women, and reduces vertebral and nonvertebral fractures in postmenopausal women (SOE=A). In men with primary or hypogonadal osteoporosis, PTH also has been shown to increase BMD at all sites, although BMD declines when the drug is stopped. Studies have shown that using PTH for 2 years followed by bisphosphonate therapy maintains the BMD gains afforded by PTH, although the impact of this strategy on fracture risk is not known.

Teriparatide, which is given subcutaneously on a daily basis, is approved for men and women who are at risk of osteoporotic fracture and unable to tolerate or take other approved agents. It is also the preferred treatment of glucocorticoid-induced osteoporosis. It is typically reserved for those with severe osteoporosis and a higher prevalent fracture burden, although cost and parenteral administration have limited its use. Teriparatide increased the incidence of osteosarcoma in rats in drug development trials; therefore it has a "black box" warning and is contraindicated in patients with Paget disease or who have a history of skeletal irradiation, and all others who are at higher baseline risk of osteosarcoma.

RANKL Inhibitor

Denosumab is a human monoclonal antibody that binds and neutralizes RANKL, a critical mediator of bone resorption by cells of osteoclast lineage. Specifically, denosumab inhibits RANKL, which decreases bone turnover and increases BMD. It is FDA approved for postmenopausal women at high risk of fracture or in whom other therapies for osteoporosis have failed or who are otherwise intolerant of other medications. In the FREEDOM clinical trial, postmenopausal women were randomized to treatment with denosumab every 6 months for 36 months or placebo (all patients received calcium and vitamin D supplementation). Those who received denosumab had a reduced risk of vertebral, nonvertebral, and hip fractures than those who received supplements alone. Planned subgroup analyses demonstrated a reduction in vertebral fractures that persisted in women ≥75 years old. The most statistically significant adverse events associated with denosumab were eczema and serious infections.

Special Concerns

Bisphosphonate use has been observed to be rarely associated with osteonecrosis of the jaw, a necrotic area of bone more commonly found in the mandible than the maxilla. The preponderance of cases has been reported in patients receiving parenteral bisphosphonates for malignant bone disorders such as myeloma who have undergone dental procedures such as tooth extraction. There are rare reports of patients contracting osteonecrosis of the jaw on long-term conventional oral bisphosphonates for osteoporosis. Osteonecrosis of the jaw is also a reported possible effect of denosumab. There is also concern that long-term use

Chapters

of bisphosphonates could be associated with atypical femur fractures, such as subtrochanteric and diaphyseal femur fractures. Cohort studies have shown an increased risk of subtrochanteric and femoral shaft fractures with ≥5 years of bisphosphonate use as well as a drug-dose effect. However, secondary analyses of randomized trials have not found an association. Overall, the absolute risk of osteonecrosis of the jaw and atypical femoral fractures is very low and is outweighed by the benefits of bisphosphonate use in the vast majority of patients. Patients taking bisphosphonates are encouraged to report new groin or thigh pain to their health providers. When such pain is reported, radiographs of both femurs should be obtained, which can identify people who may be at risk of these atypical fractures. Further studies such as MRI or whole-body scan may be warranted in certain circumstances given the low sensitivity of plain radiographs in detecting stress fractures. Evidence is conflicting for an association between bisphosphonates and esophageal cancer. No clear association with atrial fibrillation and bisphosphonates exists.

Investigational Agents

Strontium ranelate is an anabolic agent that increases bone formation and decreases bone resorption in animals. In a randomized, placebo-controlled study in postmenopausal women with osteoporosis (at least one vertebral fracture plus lumbar spine T-score less than or equal to −2.5) at baseline, strontium ranelate increased BMD and decreased the incidence of vertebral fractures at the highest dosage tested (2 g/d). At this dosage, bone alkaline phosphatase increased, and urinary excretion of N-telopeptides of type I collagen decreased. Strontium ranelate is approved in a number of European countries but not in the United States.

Other osteoporosis treatments under study include additional bisphosphonates; cathespin K inhibitors (odanacatib) and *src* kinase inhibitors (saractinib), which impair osteoclast activity; calcium receptor antagonists (calcilytic), which pulse endogenous PTH secretion; and sclerostin antibody, which enhances osteoblast function.

Monitoring

Patients receiving treatment for osteoporosis commonly undergo serial BMD measurements at least every 2 years to assess effectiveness, an interval that is currently covered by Medicare. This interval is not a universal recommendation, and there is not sufficient evidence to date to support modifying treatment based on BMD response. Serial BMD measurement is generally used to identify patients who are losing BMD and thus may not be adhering to treatment, who have an underlying secondary cause of bone loss that is undermining therapy, or in whom the prescribed osteoporosis treatment is failing. Compliance with treatment, especially with oral bisphosphonates, should be questioned at each visit. Patients on bisphosphonates who experience GI adverse events are 50% more likely to discontinue their medication; poor compliance is associated with increased risk of fractures (SOE=A).

VERTEBRAL FRACTURE MANAGEMENT

Vertebral compression fractures are often asymptomatic and diagnosed incidentally by spinal radiographs. They most commonly occur in the thoracolumbar transition zone or midthoracic region. In affected individuals, height may decrease, kyphosis may increase, or clothes may no longer fit properly over time. Many older adults have chronic back pain caused by changes in the spine that develop with degenerative osteoarthritis or vertebral compression; distinguishing the source of the pain can be difficult. On a practical level, pain should be treated if it interferes with ADLs and quality of life, regardless of cause. However, identifying vertebral fractures is important so that future fractures can be prevented.

In the case of symptomatic vertebral compression fractures, adequate pain control is essential. The pain usually lasts 2–4 weeks and can be quite debilitating. NSAIDs, narcotics, transdermal lidocaine, and neuropathic agents are commonly effective. Calcitonin given intramuscularly or intranasally has been proved in small studies to decrease acute vertebral fracture pain. Physical therapy is an important part of osteoporosis treatment programs to manage acute and chronic pain and to provide patient education. A physical therapist can provide postural exercises, alternative interventions for pain reduction, and information on changes in body mechanics that can help prevent future falls. Back braces may also help to decrease pain and disability after a fracture. See also "Persistent Pain," p 119. Support groups for patients with osteoporosis can also be helpful.

Vertebroplasty and Kyphoplasty

Vertebroplasty and kyphoplasty are surgical options for the treatment of painful vertebral compression fractures. The number of vertebroplasty procedures has increased dramatically over the past decade in the absence of high-quality data regarding its risks and benefits. In 2009, two randomized trials of vertebroplasty were published that involved 280 patients with painful vertebral fractures. No significant differences in pain reduction were observed between the vertebroplasty and placebo (sham procedure) groups at 1–6 months of follow-up (SOE=A). Complications were rare, although the procedure may be associated with an increased risk of adjacent vertebral fractures based on the available data.

REFERENCES

- Ensrud KE, Schousboe JT. Vertebral fractures. *N Engl J Med.* 2011;364(17):1634–1642.
- Grossman JM, Gordon R, Ranganath VK, et al. American College of Rheumatology 2010 recommendations for the prevention and treatment of glucocorticoid-induced osteoporosis. *Arthritis Care Res.* 2010;62(11):1515–1526.
- Watts NB, Belizikian JP, Camacho PM, et al. American Association of Clinical Endocrinologists medical guidelines for clinical practice for the diagnosis and treatment of postmenopausal osteoporosis. *Endocr Pract.* 2010;16(Suppl 3):1–37.
- Wright WL. Quantifying fracture risk. Focus on postmenopausal women and older men. *Adv NPs PAs.* 2011;2(3):31–32.

CHAPTER 34—DEMENTIA

KEY POINTS

- Alzheimer disease, vascular dementia, and dementia with Lewy bodies are the most common forms of degenerative dementias seen in late life.
- Cholinesterase inhibitors and N-methyl-D-aspartate antagonists can be modestly helpful in delaying decline of the cognitive symptoms of Alzheimer dementia.
- Behavioral symptoms can occur with any type of dementia and tend to respond best to a combination of psychosocial and environmental modifications and medication management of symptoms.

Dementia is a general term used to describe several disorders that cause significant decline in two or more areas of cognitive functioning that are severe enough to result in functional decline. Of those who suffer from dementia, most have Alzheimer disease (AD), which affects an estimated 5 million people in the United States. Dementia also afflicts millions more caregivers and relatives, who must cope with the patient's progressive and irreversible decline in cognition, functioning, and behavior. Both caregivers and patients can misinterpret the initial symptoms of dementia as normal age-related cognitive losses; clinicians as well may not recognize early signs or can misdiagnose them. However, dementia and aging are not synonymous. As people age, they usually experience such memory changes as slowing in information processing, but these kinds of changes are minimal and do not affect function. By contrast, dementia is progressive and disabling and is not an inherent aspect of aging.

Diagnostic and treatment advances have benefited many patients. Early and accurate diagnosis of dementia and its cause can minimize use of costly medical resources and give patients and their relatives time to anticipate future medical, financial, and legal needs (SOE=B). Sustained reversal of the progressive cognitive decline of dementia is not currently possible, but psychosocial and pharmacologic treatments can improve such associated conditions as depression, psychosis, and agitation, and enhance quality of life. See also "Psychosocial Issues," p 18; and "Legal and Ethical Issues," p 26.

EPIDEMIOLOGY AND SOCIETAL IMPACT

Dementia is typically a disease of later life, generally beginning after 65 years of age. AD is the most common type of dementia, accounting for approximately two-thirds of all cases and affecting 6%–8% of those ≥65 years old. The disease prevalence doubles every 5 years after age 60; an estimated 45% or more of those who are ≥85 years old have AD. Vascular dementia is thought to cause an estimated 15%–20% of cases and often coexists with AD pathology, ie, so-called "mixed dementia." In recent years, dementia associated with Lewy bodies has received increased attention and is now thought to be the second most common cause of dementia. Frontotemporal dementia is also a more recent diagnostic category of dementia and represents a smaller percentage of cases, with a younger age of onset than seen in other dementias. Neurodegenerative diseases such as Huntington disease, Parkinson disease, or other causes such as head injury and alcoholism account for other dementia syndromes.

Dementia has a major impact on society. According to the World Report on Alzheimer's 2010, total costs for dementia were $604 billion annually, which were attributable to the direct costs of medical care, direct costs of social care, and informal care. Medicare, Medicaid, and private insurance pay much of the direct cost, but families caring for patients with dementia bear the greatest burden of expense. In 2010, the Alzheimer's Association reported family caregivers provided 17 billion hours of care, estimated to cost $202.6 billion dollars in the United States alone.

The financial costs of dementia are only one aspect of the total burden. Nearly half of primary caregivers of patients with dementia experience psychologic distress, particularly depression, and have more physical health issues. An accurate economic assessment of the problem underestimates the true cost of the disease to society unless the quality of life of both patients and caregivers is included in the analysis.

ETIOLOGY

Research into the pathophysiologic mechanisms of dementia has rapidly evolved over the last several decades. For each type of dementia, a putative protein or set of proteins has been implicated in the cause and progression of the neurodegenerative process. Whether it is the amyloid plaques/oligomers or tau neurofibrillary tangles (or both) associated with AD, the tau or ubiquitin proteins of frontotemporal dementia, or the cytoplasmic α-synuclein inclusion bodies of Lewy body dementia and Parkinson dementia, it is the accumulation of these proteins or protein aggregates within the brain that appears to set off a cascade of events that directly affect neuronal function and ultimately cell death in a disease-specific pattern. Efforts continue to better understand the genetics and environmental influences on these mechanisms, which appear to be well underway, possibly even up to 30 years, before any pathology is clinically identifiable. Therefore, current research is focusing on determining how best to analyze these pathologic processes in their earliest and most insidious stages, possibly providing us with the tools to intervene early or to prevent dementia altogether.

RISK FACTORS AND PREVENTION

The two greatest risk factors for AD are age and family history. Studies that account for death from other causes suggest that by 90 years of age, nearly half of those with first-degree relatives (ie, parents, siblings) with AD develop the disease themselves. Rare forms of familial AD beginning before age 60 have been associated with mutations in one of three genes—amyloid precursor protein (APP), presenilin 1 (PS1), or presenilin 2 (PS2)—and account for approximately 1% of individuals with AD. Most commonly, AD begins late in life, and for such late-onset cases, the apolipoprotein E gene (*APOE*) on chromosome 19 influences risk. The *APOE* gene has three alleles: *2*, *3*, and *4*. The risk increases for those carrying two *APOE4* alleles, but those with one *APOE4* allele are still at greater risk than those with *APOE2* and *APOE3*. The *APOE4* allele increases risk and decreases age of onset in a dose-related fashion, whereas the *APOE2* allele may have a protective effect. The *APOE4* allele may be less common in black Americans than in white Americans. Using *APOE* genotyping as a prognostic test for asymptomatic older adults is not currently recommended pending results from further studies, and it may be useful only in increasing the diagnostic confidence for AD if a patient already has dementia. Recently, some genome-wide association studies identified single nucleotide polymorphism genetic variants such as clusterin (CLU-C), complement component receptor 1 (CR1), and phosphatidylinositol binding clathrin assembly protein (PICALM), but their role in diagnostic practice is unclear.

Other established risk factors include a history of head trauma, cardiovascular disease and its risk factors (hyperlipidemia, smoking, diabetes, and hypertension), depression, diminished physical activity, and possibly fewer years of formal education. Head trauma is thought to disrupt neuronal synapses and predispose to β-amyloid formation. Cardiovascular risk factors are thought to increase risk by predisposing individuals to impairment in cognition through ischemic mechanisms, although there is newer evidence linking some vascular risk factors to Alzheimer pathology. Research suggests that more years of formal education can delay the onset of dementia, which may represent a confounding variable of socioeconomic status or a factor that truly provides protection by supplying a cognitive "reserve." Emerging risk factors that need further study include diet, sleep quality, and obesity.

Prevention of dementia, especially AD, is an active area of research. Drugs associated with reduced risk in epidemiologic studies include NSAIDs[OL], statins[OL], *Ginkgo biloba,* insulin, and possibly antioxidants. Several of these have been studied in randomized clinical trials but to date, none has been shown to be effective. Research in healthy older adults shows a possible protective effect of physical and intellectual activity on the risk of cognitive decline (SOE=B). The onset of dementia can also be delayed by adequate treatment of hypertension (SOE=B).

ASSESSMENT AND DIFFERENTIAL DIAGNOSIS

Most cases of dementia can be diagnosed on the basis of a general medical and psychiatric evaluation. It is important for primary care clinicians to be alert to the early symptoms, because dementia is often undetected until severe symptoms or an adverse event, such as behavioral disturbances, flags its presence. Subjective complaints are significant, and, if a patient or family member expresses concerns about cognitive decline, a mental status assessment and probably a dementia evaluation are indicated. Subtle signs of cognitive change can include displaying behavioral changes, missing deadlines or having other problems at work, increasing difficulty managing complex tasks such as finances, or giving up a hobby or interest that may have become too challenging. Several consensus guidelines are now available for the clinical diagnosis and treatment of most types of dementia.

The informant interview and clinical assessment are the most important diagnostic tools for dementia. Both the patient and a reliable informant should be interviewed to determine the patient's current condition, medical and medication history, patterns of substance use, and living arrangements. Determination of onset and nature of symptoms can help differentiate clinical syndromes. Useful informant-based instruments, such as the Functional Activities Questionnaire, can help determine whether lapses in memory or language use have occurred and assess the patient's ability to learn and retain new information, handle complex tasks, and demonstrate sound judgment. Any changes are best determined by comparing present with previous performance, because functional decline and multiple cognitive deficits support the diagnosis.

Cognitive performance is influenced by number of years of formal education. Affected patients with

Table 34.1—Screening Instruments for the Evaluation of Cognition

Instrument Name	Items Scoring	Domains Assessed	Available at (accessed Oct 2013)
Mini-Cog	2 items Score = 5	Visuospatial, executive function, recall	http://geriatrics.uthscsa.edu/tools/MINICog.pdf
St. Louis University Mental Status (SLUMS) Examination	11 items Score = 30	Orientation, recall, calculation, naming, attention, executive function	http://medschool.slu.edu/agingsuccessfully/pdfsurveys/slumsexam_05.pdf
Montreal Cognitive Assessment (MoCA)	12 items Score = 30	Orientation, recall, attention, naming, repetition, verbal fluency, abstraction, executive function, visuospatial	www.mocatest.org
Folstein Mini–Mental Status Examination	19 items Score = 30	Orientation, registration, attention, recall, naming, repetition, 3-step command, language, visuospatial	For purchase: www.minimental.com

more years of education may have normal cognitive test scores, while patients with less education may have low scores and no decline in function. This must be considered, especially in patients with more subtle deficits or subjective complaints. In addition, in tests that are most sensitive to language performance, cultural differences can lead to an over-interpretation of dementia in minority patients. One way to improve the accuracy of assessment is to perform serial evaluations (using a medical interpreter if needed), which allow determination of decline in an individual that is consistent with a neurodegenerative process. In addition, measuring changes in everyday functional abilities by evaluating a person's performance of ADLs, either by direct observation or obtaining information from a reliable informant may be helpful. A comprehensive physical examination should include a neurologic and mental status evaluation. Brief quantified screening tests of cognitive function, such as the Folstein Mini–Mental State Examination, the Mini-Cog Assessment Instrument for Dementia, the St. Louis University Mental Status (SLUMS), or the Montreal Cognitive Assessment (MoCA) (see Table 34.1), can be useful, particularly if they demonstrate change over a 6-month or 1-year follow-up period, and can provide a practical approach to acquiring a quantitative baseline against which to compare future assessments. However, these are screening tests, and full neuropsychologic testing may be necessary to accurately define the character and severity of the deficits, especially in atypical cases or when presentation may be confounded by a high level of education or subtle changes. Cognitive and functional assessments should be conducted in the patient's native language, if at all possible. (In the face of cognitive decline, it is common for dementia patients to retain the greatest fluency in their native language.)

A routine laboratory evaluation, generally including a CBC, serum sodium and calcium concentrations, BUN/creatinine, fasting glucose rapid plasma reagin test, thyrotropin, and vitamin B_{12} concentration, is recommended. Optional tests, based on clinical examination and clinical suspicion, include liver function tests, serum folic acid, serum homocysteine and methylmalonic acid concentrations, urinalysis, urine toxicology, CSF analysis, and HIV testing. In addition, the history or physical examination may indicate the need for other tests, such as an ECG or a chest radiograph, or a neurology consultation.

Although brain imaging studies are optional, they may be especially useful in the following situations:

- Onset occurs at an age <65 years old.
- Symptoms begin suddenly or progress rapidly.
- There is evidence of focal or asymmetrical neurologic deficits.
- The clinical picture suggests normal-pressure hydrocephalus (eg, onset has occurred within 1 year, gait disorder or unexplained incontinence is present).
- There is a history of a recent fall or other head trauma.

In general, a noncontrast CT head scan is adequate to exclude intracranial bleeding, space-occupying lesions, and hydrocephalus. If vascular dementia is suspected, MRI is often performed but not recommended. If performed, white-matter changes revealed by T2-weighted MRI images should not be over-interpreted. Functional brain imaging studies such as positron emission tomography (PET) may be useful when the diagnosis remains uncertain. Functional analysis with FDG-PET can reveal the characteristic parietal and temporal deficits in AD or the widespread irregular deficits in vascular dementia; however, the use of PET scans for detection of Alzheimer brain pathology is currently limited to research. CSF analysis has gained interest in helping detect AD early, but analysis

Table 34.2—Diagnostic Features and Treatment of Dementia Syndromes

Syndrome	Onset	Cognitive Domains, Symptoms	Motor Symptoms	Progression	Imaging	Pharmacologic Treatment of Cognition
Mild cognitive impairment	Gradual	Primarily memory	Rare	Unknown, 12% per year proceed to Alzheimer disease	Possible global atrophy, small hippocampal volumes	Cholinesterase inhibitors (ChIs) possibly protective for 18 months (SOE=A) in subset of patients
Alzheimer disease	Gradual	Memory, language, visuospatial	Rare early, apraxia later	Gradual (over 8–10 years)	Possible global atrophy, small hippocampal volumes	ChI for mild to severe (SOE=A); memantine for moderate to severe stages
Vascular dementia	May be sudden or stepwise	Depends on location of ischemia	Correlates with ischemia	Gradual or stepwise with further ischemia	Cortical or subcortical changes on MRI	Consider ChI for memory deficit only (SOE=C); risk factor modifiers
Lewy body dementia	Gradual	Memory, visuospatial, hallucinations, fluctuating symptoms	Parkinsonism	Gradual but faster than Alzheimer disease	Possible global atrophy	ChI (SOE=B); ± carbidopa/levodopa for movement
Frontotemporal dementia	Gradual; age <60 years	Executive, disinhibition, apathy, language, ± memory	None	Gradual but faster than Alzheimer disease	Atrophy in frontal and temporal lobes	Not recommended per current evidence

of β-amyloid and phosphorylated-tau remains only interpretable and applicable at the research level and, at this stage, provides only marginal additive value over clinical diagnosis.

In general, the diagnosis of dementia is a clinical one, and laboratory assessment and imaging are used to identify uncommon treatable causes and common treatable comorbid conditions and, when used in the setting of specialty care clinics, can help further differentiate atypical presentations.

DIFFERENTIATING TYPES OF DEMENTIAS

Dementia is defined as an acquired syndrome of decline in at least two cognitive domains, sufficient to affect daily life in an alert patient, which according to updated guidelines does not have to include memory. Diagnosis then requires further investigation to identify the cause of the dementia by determining chronology of symptoms along with the pattern and extent of deficits. A general discussion of the most common dementias is provided below; for an overview of diagnostic features, see Table 34.2.

Cognition in aging is now understood to be a continuum, ranging from the mild changes of normal aging to the significant impairments that define dementia. Although studies are not conclusive, it appears that normal aging involves some mild decline in memory, usually requiring more effort and time to recall new information. However, this decline does not impair functioning; new learning is slower but still occurs and is usually well compensated with lists, calendars, and other memory supports.

With early identification of cognitive deficits, a disorder referred to as *mild cognitive impairment* (MCI) has been identified, which includes individuals who have a subjective complaint of cognitive decline in at least one domain (memory, executive function, language, or visuospatial perception) to a degree that is noticeable and measurable, but not to a degree that causes impairment in independent living. This official set of diagnostic criteria allows for identification and possible early treatment of individuals who may convert to AD (9.4–14.3/1000 person-years). For individuals with MCI whose single domain of impairment is memory (amnestic MCI versus nonamnestic MCI), the rate of conversion to AD is predictably higher, but is not wholly predictive of AD or other dementias. Nearly half of individuals with amnestic MCI maintain a stable degree of impairment or return to a state of normal cognition over 3–5 years. While there are no accepted criteria at this point in time, the National Institute on Aging and Alzheimer's Association have designated "preclinical AD" in expectation of developing a set of biomarkers to assess for presence of preclinical brain changes that have yet to manifest into clinical signs and symptoms of cognitive impairment.

Clinically, AD is characterized by gradual onset and progressive decline in cognitive functioning; motor and sensory functions are spared until middle and late stages. Memory impairment is often a core symptom of any dementia, but in AD it is typically *the* core feature present in the earliest stages. Typically, AD patients demonstrate difficulty learning and retaining new information. In later disease stages, their ability to learn and retrieve information is compromised even more, and patients are unable to access older, more distant memories. Aphasia, apraxia, disorientation, visuospatial dysfunction, impaired judgment, and executive dysfunction are also often present. Neurologic examination is usually nonfocal.

Vascular dementia refers to cognitive deficits most often associated with vascular damage in the brain, either micro or macro in nature. It is sometimes associated with focal neurologic deficits that accompany cognitive loss, and the cognitive and neurologic impairments should correlate anatomically with the areas of ischemia, although the often diffuse nature of vascular disease may make this correlation difficult to identify. This is especially true in the case of small vessel ischemic disease, which can be found in up to 50% of the cases of vascular dementia. Small-vessel ischemic disease involves white matter damage and subcortical vessel damage, which in contrast to large-vessel disease, can present with more subtle neurologic signs, ie, pronator drift, gait instability, slowing of motor performance, and/or a neuropsychologic profile consistent with a dysexecutive syndrome of slow information processing and inattention. These changes are often seen as focal or diffuse white matters changes on MRI (T2-weighted hyperintensities) and, as a function of volume, are often associated with worsening cognitive function. Parsing the differences between AD and vascular dementia can be challenging, especially given the relatively high rate of "mixed" etiology found in AD.

For a diagnosis of dementia with Lewy bodies, both dementia and at least one of the following must be present: detailed visual hallucinations, parkinsonian signs, and changes in alertness or attention. Additional distinguishing features may include autonomic dysfunction, sleep disorder, and psychiatric misidentification syndromes. The diagnosis may overlap with AD and the dementia associated with Parkinson disease. Poor visuospatial abilities are also often out of proportion to other cognitive deficits. The chronology of symptoms and pattern of cognitive deficits allow differentiation between dementia with Lewy bodies and AD and the dementia associated with Parkinson disease. If Parkinson disease has been diagnosed or has been present for ≥2 years before cognitive symptoms are seen, the diagnosis is more consistent with Parkinson disease dementia. If parkinsonian symptoms are present at the same time as cognitive symptoms, a diagnosis of dementia with Lewy bodies should be considered.

Frontotemporal dementia is a disease often seen in patients with onset of cognitive symptoms at a younger age; these patients present most often with executive and language dysfunction and significant behavioral changes. These behaviors include social disinhibition and hyperorality, and they often have had a profound effect on the patient's social functioning. Memory deficits are often not as pronounced in these patients in the early stages as they are in patients with other dementias. The language impairments in frontotemporal dementia may be detected in neuropsychologic tests such as the Boston Naming Test and may progress even early in the course of illness much faster than other cognitive impairments. It is important to recognize the difference between frontotemporal dementia and AD with "frontal" symptoms. The latter refers to social disinhibition and behavioral impulsivity that can be seen with AD. In these patients, the behavioral problems occur much later in the course of illness, after a cognitive problem is already clearly evident. In contrast, patients with frontotemporal dementia display social disinhibition before prominent memory decline. Pick disease is a type of frontotemporal dementia characterized by rapid decline and the presence of Pick bodies, balloon-like intracellular inclusions at autopsy.

Common to all types of dementia, cognitive impairment eventually has a profound effect on the patient's daily life. Difficulties in planning meals, managing finances or medications, using a telephone, and driving without getting lost are not uncommon. Such functional impairments may first alert others that a problem is emerging. Numerous functions are maintained in patients with dementia of mild to moderate severity, including such ADLs as eating, bathing, and grooming. The behaviors of many patients remain socially appropriate during the early disease stages.

Behavior and mood changes are common, including personality changes, apathy, irritability, anxiety, or depression. During the middle and late stages of the disease, delusions, hallucinations, aggression, resistance to care, and wandering may develop. These behaviors are extremely troubling to caregivers and often result in family distress and long-term care placement. Although the course of dementia is variable, the progression of dementia often follows a sequential clinical and functional pattern of decline (Table 34.3). See also "Behavioral Problems in Dementia," p 267.

Dementia recognition can be complicated by the presence of either delirium or depression. Delirium has been defined as an acquired impairment of attention, alertness, or perception. Delirium and dementia are in some ways similar; both are characterized by global

Table 34.3—The General Progression of Dementia

Stage 1: No cognitive impairment

Unimpaired individuals experience no memory problems, and none is evident to a healthcare professional during a medical interview.

Stage 2: Very mild cognitive decline

Individuals at this stage feel as if they have memory lapses, especially in forgetting familiar words or names or the location of keys, eyeglasses, or other everyday objects. However, these problems are not evident during a medical examination or apparent to friends, family, or coworkers.

Stage 3: Mild cognitive decline

Early-stage Alzheimer disease can be diagnosed in some, but not all, individuals with these symptoms.

Friends, family, or coworkers begin to notice deficiencies. Problems with memory or concentration may be measurable in clinical testing or discernible during a detailed medical interview. Common difficulties include the following:

- Word- or name-finding problems noticeable to family or close associates
- Decreased ability to remember names when introduced to new people
- Performance issues in social or work settings noticeable to family, friends, or coworkers
- Reading a passage and retaining little material
- Losing or misplacing a valuable object
- Decline in ability to plan or organize

Stage 4: Moderate cognitive decline (mild or early-stage Alzheimer disease)

At this stage, a careful medical interview detects clear-cut deficiencies in the following areas:

- Decreased knowledge of recent occasions or current events
- Impaired ability to perform challenging mental arithmetic, eg, to count backward from 100 by 7s
- Decreased ability to perform complex tasks, such as marketing, planning dinner for guests, or paying bills and managing finances
- Reduced memory of personal history

The affected individual may seem subdued and withdrawn, especially in socially or mentally challenging situations.

Stage 5: Moderately severe cognitive decline (moderate or mid-stage Alzheimer disease)

Major gaps in memory and deficits in cognitive function emerge. Some assistance with day-to-day activities becomes essential. At this stage, individuals may:

- Be unable during a medical interview to recall such important information as their current address, their telephone number, or the name of the college or high school from which they graduated
- Become confused about where they are or about the date, day of the week, or season
- Have trouble with less challenging mental arithmetic, eg, counting backward from 40 by 4s or from 20 by 2s
- Need help choosing proper clothing for the season or occasion
- Usually retain substantial knowledge about themselves and know their own name and the names of their spouse or children
- Usually require no assistance with eating or using the toilet

Stage 6: Severe cognitive decline (moderately severe or mid-stage Alzheimer disease)

Memory difficulties continue to worsen, significant personality changes may emerge, and affected individuals need extensive help with customary daily activities. At this stage, individuals may:

- Lose most awareness of recent experiences, events, and surroundings
- Recollect their personal history imperfectly, although they generally recall their name
- Occasionally forget the name of their spouse or primary caregiver but generally can distinguish familiar from unfamiliar faces
- Need help getting dressed properly; without supervision, may make errors such as putting pajamas over daytime clothes or shoes on wrong feet
- Experience disruption of their normal sleep-wake cycle
- Need help with handling details of toileting (flushing toilet, wiping, and disposing of tissue properly)
- Have increasing episodes of urinary or fecal incontinence
- Experience significant personality changes and behavioral symptoms, including suspiciousness and delusions (eg, believing that their caregiver is an impostor); hallucinations (seeing or hearing things that are not really there); or compulsive, repetitive behaviors such as hand wringing or tissue shredding
- Tend to wander and become lost

Stage 7: Very severe cognitive decline (severe or late-stage Alzheimer disease)

This is the final stage of the disease when individuals lose the ability to respond to their environment, to speak, and ultimately to control movement.

- Frequently lose the ability for recognizable speech, although words or phrases may occasionally be uttered
- Need help with eating and toileting, and there is general urinary incontinence
- Lose the ability to walk without assistance, then the ability to sit without support, smile, and to hold up head; reflexes become abnormal, muscles grow rigid, and swallowing is impaired

SOURCE: Excerpted from www.alz.org/AboutAD/Stages.asp and reproduced with permission of the Alzheimer's Association.

cognitive impairment. Delirium can be distinguished by acute onset, cognitive fluctuations throughout the course of a day, impaired consciousness and attention, fluctuating levels of alertness, and altered sleep cycles. In hospitalized patients, delirium and dementia often occur together. The presence of dementia increases the risk of delirium and accounts in part for the high rate of delirium in older patients. A delirium episode in an older adult, therefore, should alert the clinician to search for dementia once the delirium clears. See also "Delirium," p 276.

Symptoms of depression and dementia often overlap, presenting additional diagnostic challenges. Patients with primary dementia commonly experience symptoms of depression, and such patients may minimize cognitive losses. By contrast, patients with primary depression can demonstrate decreased motivation during the cognitive examination and express cognitive complaints that exceed objectively measured deficits. Moreover, patients with primary depression usually have intact language and motor skills, whereas patients with primary dementia may show impairment in these domains. As many as half of older adults who present with reversible dementia and depression become progressively demented within 5 years. See also "Depression and Other Mood Disorders," p 308.

Treatment and Management

The primary treatment goals for patients with dementia are to enhance quality of life and maximize functional performance by improving or stabilizing cognition, mood, and behavior. Both pharmacologic and nonpharmacologic treatments are available, and the latter should be emphasized. However, research has shown only modest effects on cognition, and providers should educate patients and caregivers to have realistic expectations. Patients with dementia often develop significant behavioral symptoms that are a challenge to both family members and professional caregivers. Any acute change requires an evaluation for undiagnosed medical problems, pain, depression, infection, metabolic disturbance, or delirium. Other factors that can contribute to behavioral symptoms include interpersonal or emotional issues. Addressing such issues, treating underlying medical conditions, providing reassurance, and attending to the possible need for changes in the patient's environment can reduce agitation. See "Behavioral Problems in Dementia," p 267. The use of pharmacologic treatments for behavioral problems is recommended only after nonpharmacologic ones prove ineffective, or when there is an emergent need such as extreme patient distress or risk of physical violence.

Nonpharmacologic Treatment

Cognitive Rehabilitation

Reality orientation, memory retraining, and cognitive training have all been proposed as possible techniques to perhaps improve cognitive function. A 2006 Cochrane review of cognitive training found no evidence of positive effects in patients with dementia (SOE=B). Given that new learning is a skill lost very early in the course of AD, an overemphasis on quizzing or retraining may lead to anxiety and self-depreciation. In general, a preferred approach is to provide support to accommodate for lost skills.

Supportive Therapy

Emotion-oriented psychotherapy, such as "pleasant events" and "reminiscence" therapy, and stimulation-oriented treatment, including art and other expressive recreational or social therapies, such as exercise or dance, are examples of psychosocial treatments that can minimize depressive symptoms and reduce behavioral symptoms. These interventions can be provided by professionals or informal caregivers who have been specifically trained. Support groups can provide meaningful support and education for both patients and caregivers. Early-onset dementia groups are especially helpful for patients with mild deficits and insight. Research has begun to demonstrate benefits of caregiver education and support in reducing behavioral symptoms and improving quality of life among patients and caregivers with dementia (SOE=C).

Other Therapies

There are some data supporting physical exercise as having effects on functional performance, cognitive function, and behavioral symptoms. Physical activity should be encouraged as part of the treatment plan. Early research also suggests a role for occupational therapy in providing caregiver education strategies and environmental modification.

Regular Appointments

One approach to ensuring optimal health care for patients with dementia is to schedule regular patient surveillance and health maintenance visits every 3–6 months. During such visits, the clinician should address and treat comorbid conditions, evaluate ongoing medications, and consider initiating medication-free periods. In addition, it is useful to check for sleep and behavioral disturbances and to provide guidance on proper sleep hygiene. Caregiver well-being should also be regularly assessed.

Family and Caregiver Education and Support

Research has demonstrated that caring for an individual with dementia is more difficult and more stressful than caring for someone with normal cognition. Working closely with family members and caregivers will help establish a therapeutic alliance. Education of family and caregivers about diagnosis, clinical course, treatment options, and management strategies is critical. Information about community resources as well as strategies for managing challenging behavioral symptoms can allow families to cope more effectively, reduce institutionalization, and improve quality of life. Relatives are often helpful sources of information about cognitive and behavioral changes, and generally they take the primary responsibility for implementing and monitoring treatment. Often, they are also responsible for medical and legal assistance. However, early identification of dementia can allow the affected individual to participate in treatment decisions and future planning. Subjects to pursue with family include medical and legal advance directives (also called advance care plans in some contexts). It is often best for a trusted relative to co-sign important financial transactions and attend to paying bills. See "Legal and Ethical Issues," p 26.

Community programs such as enrollment in adult daycare centers or respite programs can provide support to family caregivers, allowing the individual with dementia to remain at home longer. Patients also benefit from these programs through opportunities for socialization and structured activities. Although most care for dementia patients is provided in the home, many patients with dementia need admission to a long-term care facility at some point. Discussion about long-term care placement options should be started early rather than late, to provide the individual or family members time to complete arrangements and begin to adjust emotionally. Increasingly, hospice can be an alternative for end-stage dementia patients who wish to remain at home and have comfort as the goal for care. Caregivers often express concern about their own memory lapses, which should be addressed with counseling or neuropsychologic assessment. Caregiver distress is often reduced with support-group participation, which may relieve common feelings of anger, frustration, and guilt. Respite care is another community resource that offers caregivers relief. Caregiver support interventions involving individual and family counseling combined with regular participation in support groups have demonstrated improvement in caregiver well-being and delay in time to nursing-home placement. Use of support groups and counseling services by family caregivers has also been associated with a delay in nursing-home placement of ≥1 year (SOE=B).

Environmental Modification

Patients with dementia can be extremely sensitive to their environment; in general, a moderate level of stimulation is best. When they experience overstimulation, confusion or agitation can increase, whereas too little stimulation can cause boredom and withdrawal. As deficits change over time, this balance must be reevaluated and activities adjusted regularly. Familiar surroundings maximize existing cognitive functions, and predictability through daily routines is often reassuring. Other helpful orientation and memory measures in early stages include conspicuous displays of clocks, calendars, and to-do lists. Links to the outside world through newspapers, radio, and television can benefit some mildly impaired patients. Adaptive strategies for more impaired individuals can involve providing visual clues to assist patients (eg, picture of a toilet for the bathroom, or of food for the dining room) or to distract patients from exposure to unsafe situations (eg, STOP sign on door, covering elevator buttons). Attention to a simple and compassionate communication style can reduce behavioral symptoms in the patient and burden for the caregiver. Strategies such as using simple sentences, phrasing commands in a positive fashion, avoiding slang and pronouns, and speaking in a calm tone of voice can enhance communication.

Attention to Safety

In early stages, safety concerns may be minimal because the person with dementia is still able to make appropriate judgments about safety. However, the need for supervision usually increases as the disease progresses and the person becomes more forgetful and is no longer able to anticipate or avoid dangerous situations. Interventions should balance allowing as much independence as possible while ensuring safety, focusing initially on environmental strategies. Door locks or electronic guards prevent wandering, and many families benefit from registering with Safe Return through the Alzheimer's Association (www.alz.org). Patient name tags and medical-alert bracelets can assist in locating lost patients. Emerging technologies include watches and other devices that incorporate a global positioning system to monitor the individual's location.

Cognitive impairment affects driving skills, and the visuospatial and planning disabilities of even mildly demented patients can make them unsafe drivers. Discussions about driving are best started early in treatment. Patients with advanced dementia definitely should not drive, but clinicians disagree about whether mildly demented patients should drive. Referral for an independent driving assessment is recommended if there is any concern regarding safety. Certainly, when a patient has a history of traffic accidents or significant spatial and executive dysfunction, driving abilities should be carefully scrutinized. See also the older driver in "Assessment," p 48.

Pharmacologic Treatment

General Issues

Several factors should be considered when prescribing medications for older adults with dementia. Patients in the older age groups vary in their response, so treatments need to be individualized. In addition, age is associated with decreased renal clearance and hepatic metabolism. Older patients often take several medications simultaneously, so drug interactions and adverse events are likely. Medications with anticholinergic effects are a particular problem for patients with dementia because they can worsen cognitive impairment and lead to delirium. Another group of problem medications that can worsen cognition include those causing CNS sedation. Any nonessential medications with CNS adverse events should be considered carefully. The best strategy, in light of such factors, is to start with low dosages and increase dosing gradually ("start low and go slow"). The goal is to identify the lowest effective dosage, thus minimizing adverse events while avoiding subtherapeutic dosing. Before starting any treatment, a thorough medical examination should be conducted to identify and treat any underlying medical conditions that might impair cognition.

Cholinesterase Inhibitors (ChIs)

The primary medications available for stabilizing cognitive function in AD are ChIs. Currently, four ChIs approved by the FDA are available: tacrine (rarely prescribed because of hepatotoxicity), donepezil, rivastigmine, and galantamine. By slowing the breakdown of the neurotransmitter acetylcholine, these medications are thought to facilitate memory function because of the association of acetylcholine and memory.

In clinical trials, these medications demonstrate a modest delay in cognitive decline compared with placebo in patients with AD. Onset of behavioral problems and decline in ADLs is modestly delayed compared with treatment with placebo (SOE=A). In a Cochrane review of 10 randomized, double-blind, placebo-controlled trials, treatment for 6 months improved cognitive function on average –2.7 points (95% confidence interval, –3.0 to –2.3, $P < .00001$) on the 70-point Alzheimer's Disease Assessment Scale-Cognitive Subscale, as well as small improvement on measures of ADLs and behavior. Over the last decade, a large body of evidence has grown to support the modest clinical benefits of cholinesterase inhibitors in AD for both short- and long-term treatment. With the increase in focus on identifying a prodromal phase of AD, several clinical trials including a few randomized double-blind, placebo-controlled trials have sought to determine the efficacy of ChIs in MCI in preventing/delaying onset of AD, but to date no study has achieved its endpoint. However, some of the subanalysis suggests a positive response within specific populations toward prevention of progression to AD (ie, +*APOE* ϵ4 allele).

Results of studies of patients with dementing disorders other than AD are also becoming available. Widespread treatment in vascular dementia was not recommended in a meta-analysis because of the limited cognitive benefit and lack of sufficient data (SOE=B). Some studies suggest that ChIs may be helpful in managing attention and behavioral disturbances (eg, hallucinations) associated with dementia with Lewy bodies (SOE=B), and one ChI, rivastigmine, is approved by the FDA for mild to moderate dementia in Parkinson disease. There appears to be no role for ChIs in treating frontotemporal dementia, and in fact, evidence suggests they may worsen agitation (SOE=B). Because effects are modest in all disorders, patients and families should be counseled to have realistic expectations, and discontinuation of medication should be considered after a reasonable time period if decline continues at the rate expected without treatment. Clinical evaluation after 6 months of therapy is suggested. In the case of long-term therapy with initial positive responses to treatment but continued advancement of cognitive decline, the question of discontinuation effect on cognition ultimately arises. If cognitive decline persists despite maximal treatment with ChIs, the clinician should discuss the risks and benefits of therapy with the patient and caregivers. Tapering the medication over time may be considered. Abrupt discontinuation is not recommended.

All three commonly prescribed ChIs can be dosed once daily, either in oral form (donepezil and galantamine) or as a 24-hour patch (rivastigmine). Dosing adjustments should follow a slow titration curve to maximize the tolerable dosage while avoiding the emergence of adverse events, such as nausea, diarrhea, insomnia, headaches, dizziness, orthostasis, and nightmares. However, a lower initial dosage and/or an even slower titration curve can help further mitigate adverse events if they occur, especially GI adverse events. Increasing the dosage of donepezil to the recently approved dosage of 23 mg/d or rivastigmine patch to 13.3 mg/24 hours may offer some benefit in severe dementia, but is unlikely to affect overall global functioning and should only be used with caution given the observed increase in adverse events (SOE=A). The most serious adverse event associated with ChIs is the induction of bradycardia. Because of limited direct comparisons, there is currently no evidence for any difference in efficacy among the ChIs.

Memantine

Memantine, an N-methyl-D-aspartate antagonist, has been used worldwide for many years. It is thought to have neuroprotective effects by reducing glutamate-mediated excitotoxicity. Clinical trials in the United States support the efficacy of memantine in moderate to severe stages of AD (SOE=A). A Cochrane review of two 6-month studies showed modest beneficial effects on cognition, ADLs, and behavior. Memantine is approved by the FDA for treatment of moderate to severe AD. Research has not supported use in earlier stages of AD, and trials are ongoing to determine efficacy in other dementing diseases. A Cochrane review and a meta-analysis of memantine in vascular dementia found limited effect on cognition and no evidence to recommend widespread use (SOE=A). The recommended dosage of memantine in the management of Alzheimer-type dementia starts at 5 mg/d po, which may then be increased on a weekly basis in 5-mg increments to a target dosage of 20 mg/d dosed as 10 mg q12h after a 4-week titration period. For the extended-release formulation, the starting dosage of 7 mg/d can be increased to the maximum dosage of 28 mg/d over 3 weeks. The most common adverse events are constipation, dizziness, and headache. Memantine has been used safely as a single agent and in conjunction with ChIs for moderate to severe AD (SOE=B).

Other Cognitive Enhancers

Ongoing studies are assessing a variety of other agents in AD, including antioxidants and *Ginkgo biloba* extract. In a trial including >300 patients with moderately severe AD, treatment with vitamin E (α-tocopherol) or the selective monoamine oxidase B inhibitor selegiline (approved for treatment of Parkinson disease) lowered rates of functional decline but was not associated with evidence of cognitive improvement. However, this study involved patients with moderate to severe dementia, so effects on cognition earlier in the illness remain unknown. Results from a randomized placebo-controlled trial of vitamin E and donepezil in MCI showed some short-term benefit from donepezil in delaying conversion to AD but no effect of vitamin E. High-dose vitamin E supplementation was associated with increased mortality in a meta-analysis and is no longer recommended for the treatment of AD.

Extract from the leaf of the *Ginkgo* tree has been promoted primarily in Europe for peripheral vascular disease as well as for "cerebral insufficiency." Other studies in Europe and the United States have explored its use in AD. However, a recent large, multicenter, randomized, double-blind, placebo-controlled trial in normal individuals and individuals with MCI did not show any slowing of cognitive decline in either population over a median follow-up of 6.1 years.

Many patients also use OTC preparations for cognitive enhancement. A complete review of medications should always include questions about use of OTC medications.

Antidepressants

Antidepressant drug treatment is generally considered for AD patients with depressive symptoms, including depressed mood, appetite loss, insomnia, fatigue, irritability, and agitation. See "Depression and Other Mood Disorders," p 308. Anecdotal evidence exists that SSRIs can be helpful in managing the disinhibitions and compulsive behaviors associated with frontotemporal dementia. However, patients with dementia are at risk of falls, and the use of selective serotonin-reuptake inhibitors and selective norepinephrine-reuptake inhibitors can possibly exacerbate these risks, especially those with greater anticholinergic tone (eg, paroxetine).

Psychoactive Medications

Behavioral and psychologic symptoms of dementia such as paranoia, agitation, and irritability are best managed by nonpharmacologic strategies, such as reducing overstimulation, distraction, redirection, and physical activity. However, when medications are required, target symptoms should be identified and therapy selected accordingly. There is some limited evidence that first- and second-generation antipsychotics help control these symptoms, but recent trials have revealed that all antipsychotics increase the risk of "all-cause" mortality in the setting of dementia (SOE=A). Therefore, these medications must be used cautiously to manage delusions, hallucinations, and paranoia as well as some of the significant irritability associated with dementia. To help mitigate these risks, frequent attempts to taper off each medication should be undertaken (SOE=A). Medications such as carbamazepine^{OL} and valproic acid^{OL} are possible alternatives for managing irritability and agitation, but again both have limited evidence for effectiveness in dementia and can be associated with increased mortality risk as well (SOE=B). The use of benzodiazepines and medications with anticholinergic effects should be avoided. Finally, antidepressants with sedating effects such as mirtazapine and trazodone can be considered in the management of insomnia. For a complete discussion of nonpharmacologic and pharmacologic treatment of behavioral and psychologic symptoms, see "Behavioral Problems in Dementia," p 267.

Other Resources

Most primary care clinicians successfully treat and manage most patients with dementia, but referral to a specialist is sometimes necessary, especially for diagnosis. When the presentation or history is atypical or complex, particularly when the onset begins before age 60, consultation with a specialist in treating dementia patients (eg, geriatric psychiatrist, neurologist) can be useful.

Community support can be informal, in which neighbors or friends help out, or formal, through home-care or family service agencies, the aging or mental health networks, or adult daycare centers. Available specialized services include adult daycare and respite care, home-health agencies that can provide skilled nursing, help lines of the Alzheimer's Association, and outreach services offered by Area Agencies on Aging and Councils on Aging, which are mandated and funded under the federal Older Americans Act. Food services for the homebound are available from Meals-on-Wheels, and many senior citizens' centers and church and community groups, and hospitals offer transportation options.

For organizations providing information and referral for dementia patients and families, see the agencies and organizations section on the AGS Web site at www.americangeriatrics.org/health_care_professionals/directory_of_agencies.

REFERENCES

- Banerjee S, Wittenberg R. Clinical and cost effectiveness of services for early diagnosis and intervention in dementia. *Int J Geriatr Psychiatry*. 2009;24(7):748–754.

- Barnes DE, Yaffe, K. The projected effect of risk factor reduction on Alzheimer's disease prevalence. *Lancet Neurol*. 2011;10(9):819–828.

- Beerens HC, Zwakhalen SM, Verbeek H, et al. Factors associated with quality of life of people with dementia in long-term care facilities: A systematic review. *Int J Nurs Stud*. 2013;50(9):1259–1270.

- Farlow MR, Salloway S, Tariot PN, et al. Effectiveness and tolerability of high-dose (23 mg/d) verses standard-dose (10 mg/d) donepezil in moderate to severe Alzheimer's disease: A 24-week, randomized, double-blind study. *Clin Ther.* 2010:32(7):1234–1251.

CHAPTER 35—BEHAVIORAL PROBLEMS IN DEMENTIA

KEY POINTS

- Behavioral disturbances in dementia require evaluation of the specific symptoms, including the comfort of the patient, medical comorbidities, the environment of care, the needs of the caregiver, and the degree of distress of all those involved in the life of the demented adult.
- Delirium secondary to an underlying condition such as dehydration, urinary tract infection, or medication toxicity is a common cause of abrupt behavioral disturbances in patients with dementia.
- Nonpharmacologic interventions must be considered the first-line choice for all behavioral disturbances in dementia. These include caregiver education and support, patient-centered use of music, physical activity, support for activities of daily living, and cognitive stimulation programs.
- Pharmacologic treatment of behavioral disturbances in dementia is of limited efficacy and should be used only after environmental and nonpharmacologic interventions have been implemented.
- Increased mortality has been identified with the use of both first-generation antipsychotic agents such as haloperidol and perphenazine, as well as second-generation antipsychotic agents such as risperidone and olanzapine. All antipsychotic agents now carry an FDA warning regarding increased all-cause mortality in patients with dementia.
- Despite these FDA warnings, antipsychotic medications may be needed for treatment of distressing delusions and hallucinations, and antidepressants may be helpful if symptoms of depression are evident. There is limited evidence for considering mood stabilizers for symptoms such as impulsivity and aggression in patients who have a significant behavioral disturbance.

Most dementias are associated with a range of behavioral and psychologic disturbances, with as many as 80%–90% of patients developing at least one distressing symptom over the course of their illness. The development of behavioral disturbances or psychotic symptoms in dementia often precipitates early nursing-home placement and causes significant caregiver burden and distress. These disturbances are potentially treatable, and it is vital that they are anticipated and recognized early. As these symptoms emerge, it is essential to perform a thorough evaluation of contributing factors, identify the target symptoms of treatment, and implement appropriate interventions for the patient and caregiver.

Research that compares different treatment strategies for the behavioral and psychologic symptoms of dementia is growing in response to the great need for evidence-based treatment guidelines. Some conclusions can be drawn from randomized controlled trials of studies of medications for the treatment of depression and psychosis, but these results are limited by marginal efficacy and FDA warnings regarding increased mortality among patients with dementia who are treated with antipsychotc agents. Interventions using behavioral treatment modalities have also been studied, with more robust outcomes in the ability to delay the need for nursing-home placement (SOE=A) and improve quality of life among patients and caregivers (SOE=B). These studies have allowed for recommendations in many areas; however, many aspects of treatment must still draw on case reports and clinical experience.

CLINICAL FEATURES

Behavioral and psychologic symptoms are a common feature of all dementias. These include anxiety, apathy, depression, sleep disturbance, resistance to care, elation, irritability, disinhibition, wandering, hoarding, verbal disruptions, physical aggression, delusions, and hallucinations. Discrete psychiatric symptoms may develop that take on a variety of characteristics resembling mental disorders such as depression or mania; however, the course and features are more difficult to predict, and treatments are less reliably effective than when these disorders occur in younger adults without dementia. Depressive symptoms are common and often manifest as sadness, tearfulness, or a lack of interest in previously enjoyable activities. This depressive syndrome can also include a loss of interest in self-care, eating, or interacting with peers. A propensity for irritability and impulsivity can also occur. If these features become progressive, overt hostility or violence may ensue, and patients may be characterized as "agitated," reflecting a loss of the ability to modulate their behavior in a socially acceptable way. This behavior may involve verbal outbursts, physical aggression, resistance to bathing or other care needs, and restless motor activity such as pacing or rocking. Among the behavioral complications of dementia, the most severe disruptions in caregiving occur when patients develop physical behaviors such as hitting, scratching, or pushing, or when they develop paranoid delusions that lead to hostility and altercations with caregivers. This type of overlap across symptoms, in which some are associated with a well-described psychiatric disorder but others such as wandering and hoarding are considered atypical, often creates a significant challenge in diagnostic labeling. In this situation, the fairly nonspecific term *agitation* is commonly used to describe the patient, but it may best be accompanied by additional description as to whether the problem is accompanied by irritability, vocal or physical aggression, or motor disturbances. The term agitation is too broad and nonspecific to be clinically useful. Assessment of disruptive behavior must include a careful description of the nature of the symptom, when it occurs, where it develops, and if any precipitants or antecedents are identified. Treatment cannot be provided without adequate assessment of the behavioral disturbance.

In many cases, behavioral disruption can occur concomitantly with evidence of paranoia or delusional thinking, such as a fixed false belief that caregivers have stolen possessions or money, or are plotting against the patient. When delusions occur, the patient is then characterized as suffering from "psychotic" symptoms. Sensory experiences without stimuli such as hallucinations are another type of psychotic symptom that can accompany episodes of agitated behavior. Depending on the degree of communication deficits in a given patient, the ability to discern the presence of psychosis is variable, and in many cases disruptive behaviors can occur without clear evidence as to whether delusions or other psychoses may be precipitating the disturbance. Antipsychotic medications are commonly used in the management of disruptive behaviors, with the presumption that disturbed perceptions may be the underlying problem. There is little evidence to support this presumption, and there is increasing concern over both the lack of efficacy of antipsychotic agents for nonspecific symptoms of disruptive behavior in addition to risks of adverse events and mortality related to these medications in dementia.

Occasionally, a behavioral syndrome occurs that includes features of hyperactivity, mood lability, disinhibition, and grandiose beliefs that resemble a manic episode associated with bipolar affective disorder. The features of this "manic-like" syndrome are described below (p 271), and much like other mood symptoms in dementia, the features are similar but less predictable than those seen in younger adults and treatment strategies are more challenging. One key feature of the manic-like syndromes seen in dementia patients is the tendency to develop additional symptoms outside the typical course of a bipolar manic episode, such as resistance to care, stubbornness, wandering, and hoarding behaviors, as well as a significant degree of fluctuation in symptoms over the course of a single day.

The complaints from family caregivers and professional caregivers in a nursing home or assisted-living facility often arise from behavioral complications occurring during care that involve a resistance to bathing, dressing, feeding, or other routines. Environmental precipitants such as excessive stimuli or a change in the environment (eg, a new roommate, frequent changes in staff and caregivers) can induce behavioral problems. The presenting complaint may relate to internal cues such as pain, hunger, thirst, or other needs that the patient is not able to express. Family members may feel more overwhelmed than professional caregivers and may consequently attribute more overall distress to these episodes. Overt resistance to care is most often seen in later stages of dementia, but behavioral problems can also be a first sign of an incipient cognitive decline in earlier stages. Neuropsychiatric symptoms such as apathy, poor self-care, or paranoia may be the first indication of dementia before cognitive decline is recognized, such that an evaluation for dementia in any older adult who presents with new behavioral or emotional symptoms may reveal a previously undetected dementia syndrome.

Assessment and Differential Diagnosis

Comprehensive assessment includes a history both from the patient and from an informant or other source. The information should include a clear description of the behavior: temporal onset, course, associated circumstances, and its relationship to key environmental factors such as caregiver status and recent stressors. The problem behaviors and symptoms should then be considered in the context of the patient's family and personal, social, and medical history.

Rating scales are available for the behavioral and psychologic symptoms of dementia. Some of these include the Cohen-Mansfield Agitation Inventory (CMAI), the Neuropsychiatric Inventory (NPI), and the Behavioral Pathology in Alzheimer Disease Rating Scale (BEHAVE-AD). These allow the clinician to note and quantify the symptoms based on a caregiver interview.

A differential diagnosis of the disturbance should proceed based on findings of a comprehensive geriatric evaluation. The first step is to decide whether the disturbance is a symptom of a new condition, of a preexisting medical problem, or of an adverse drug event. Disturbances that are new, acute in onset, or evolving rapidly are most often due to a medical condition or medication toxicity. An isolated behavioral disturbance in a demented patient can be the *sole* presenting symptom for many acute conditions such as pneumonia, urinary tract infection, acute pain, angina, constipation, or poorly controlled diabetes mellitus. Additionally, the need to satisfy basic physical needs, such as hunger, sleepiness, thirst, boredom, or fatigue, which the patient cannot adequately communicate, can precipitate a behavioral disturbance. Medication intolerance or toxicity due to new or existing medications might also present as solely behavioral symptoms. Treatment or stabilization of the medical or physical cause is often sufficient to resolve the disturbance. Older adults with dementia may require several weeks longer to recover from routine medical problems than those who are cognitively intact.

The second step is to consider whether the behavioral disturbance is related to an environmental precipitant. These include disruptions in routine, time change (eg, with daylight savings time or travel across time zones), changes in the caregiving environment, new caregivers, a new roommate, or a life stressor (eg, death of a spouse or family member). Other common environmental precipitants include overstimulation (eg, too much noise, crowded rooms, close contact with too many people, too much time spent out of the familiar environment), understimulation (eg, relative absence of people, spending much time alone, use of television as a companion), and the disruptive behavior of other patients. For many disturbances, correcting an environmental precipitant or removing the stressor commonly improves the symptoms.

Another consideration is whether the disturbance results from stress in the patient-caregiver relationship. Caring for dementia patients is difficult and requires a degree of perseverance of which most caregivers are capable if proper guidance and support is provided. Inexperienced caregivers, domineering caregivers, or caregivers who themselves are impaired by medical or psychiatric disturbances can exacerbate or cause a behavioral disturbance. Caregiver burden can be a problem both in community settings and in nursing homes. Assessing the level of stress and burden on the caregiver is an important part of the evaluation of behavioral disturbances. Interventions to improve the patient-caregiver relationship and to provide caregiver education and support are a vital part of treatment of behavioral disturbances in dementia. Providing resources to caregivers such as referral to support groups and respite services is often very helpful. See also "Psychosocial Issues," p 18; and "Dementia," p 256; on family caregiver education and support.

After medical, environmental, and caregiving causes are excluded, it is often concluded that the behavioral problem is a manifestation of the dementia and may not be amenable to a pharmacologic intervention. Such disturbances that are closely linked to the dementia syndrome take on the form of a catastrophic reaction. A catastrophic reaction is an acute behavioral, physical, or verbal reaction to environmental stressors that results from an inability to make routine adjustments in daily life. The reaction might include anger, emotional lability, or aggression when patients are confronted with a deficit, such as the inability to find a word, or confusion about where they are or what they are supposed to do. Catastrophic reactions are best treated by identifying and avoiding their precipitants, by providing structured routines and activities, and by recognizing early signs of the impending catastrophic reaction so that the patient can be distracted and supported before reacting.

If the disturbance is not related to an identifiable cause or environmental precipitant, it may be a consequence of the brain deterioration that occurs during the course of dementia. Disturbances with a more insidious onset or that are persistent are more likely to be symptoms of the underlying disease. Epidemiologic and clinical studies suggest that such disturbances fall into three groups: mood symptoms, psychosis, and specific behavior problems that occur without significant specific psychiatric symptoms. The overlap in the symptoms of these groups can make treatment choices difficult. One approach is to decide whether the predominant symptom of a polysymptomatic disturbance is psychosis (delusions or hallucinations), mood symptoms (dysphoria, sadness, irritability, lability), aggression, or behavioral disruption, and then direct treatment toward the most distressing feature.

Behavioral disturbances can occur in all types of dementias, including Alzheimer type, vascular, and mixed. Frontotemporal dementia (ie, Pick disease) is a less common type of dementia often associated with prominent disinhibition, compulsive behaviors, and social impairment due to more advanced frontal lobe degeneration. In severe cases, a syndrome of hyperphagia, hyperactivity, and hypersexuality can occur that is related to bilateral temporal lobe atrophy. Another dementia associated with prominent psychiatric symptoms and behavioral disturbances is dementia with Lewy bodies. This form of dementia may be more common than previously thought. It is characterized by cognitive deterioration and parkinsonian features with prominent psychosis characterized by visual hallucinations. Affected older adults often suffer from distressing hallucinations and a fluctuating clinical course. These patients are extremely sensitive to the extrapyramidal adverse events of antipsychotic medications (eg, muscle rigidity and tremor) and often cannot tolerate even low dosages of second-generation antipsychotic medications.

TREATMENT APPROACH

The treatment of the psychiatric and behavioral disturbances in dementia is complex and may require several interventions as part of a comprehensive plan of care. Specialists should be consulted in refractory cases. In general, treatment begins with appropriate environmental and caregiver interventions. Caregiver education and support interventions have been useful in

Table 35.1—Behavioral Interventions for Dementia Care

- Evaluate and treat underlying medical conditions
- Correct sensory deficits; replace poorly fitting hearing aids, eyeglasses, and dentures
- Remove offending medications, particularly anticholinergic agents
- Keep the environment comfortable, calm, and homelike with use of familiar possessions
- Provide regular daily activities and structure; refer patient to adult day care programs, if needed
- Monitor for new medical problems
- Attend to patient's sleep and eating patterns; offer regular snacks and finger foods
- Install safety measures to prevent accidents
- Ensure that the caregiver has adequate respite
- Educate caregivers about practical aspects of dementia care and about behavioral disturbances
- Teach caregivers the skills of caregiving: communication skills, avoiding confrontational behavior management, techniques of ADL support, activities for dementia care
- Simplify bathing and dressing with the use of adaptive clothing and assistive devices if needed; offer toileting frequently and anticipate incontinence as dementia progresses
- Provide access to experienced professionals and community resources
- Refer family and patient to local Alzheimer's Association
- Consult with caregiving professionals, such as geriatric case managers

reducing distress and delaying the need for nursing home placement (SOE=A). Nonpharmacologic interventions should always be used as a first-line treatment in the management of disruptive, aggressive, or agitated behavior. For a list of key behavioral interventions that might ameliorate behavioral symptoms in patients with dementia, see Table 35.1. Having a daily routine and introducing meaningful activities is vital. Behavioral disturbances in patients with dementia may decrease with the use of music, particularly during meals and bathing, and with light physical exercise or walking (SOE=B). Massage, pet therapy, white noise, videotapes of family, and cognitive stimulation programs may also be helpful. If the disturbances persist despite best efforts, pharmacologic interventions for specific target symptoms are often necessary (see next section).

Treatments for Specific Disturbances

The core of treatment is identifying any possible underlying cause of the behavior change, recognizing that multiple causes may exist. Managing pain, dehydration, hunger, and thirst is paramount. The possibilities of positional discomforts or nausea secondary to medication effects should be considered because these are common possible culprits. Environmental modifications can improve patient orientation. Good lighting, one-on-one attention, supportive care, and attention to personal needs and wants are also important aspects of treatment. If there is sleep-wake cycle disturbance, efforts should be made to stabilize the sleep cycle by maintaining a consistent routine, using bright lights, or prescribing short-term use of medications (see the sleep disturbances section, below).

Mood Disturbances

In dementia patients experiencing mood symptoms, measures similar to those used in other behavior disturbances should be implemented, ie, the environment should be optimized by reducing adversive stimuli, and physical health should be assessed comprehensively. Recreational programs and activity therapies have shown positive results in improving mood in depressive symptoms in dementia. Criteria for the diagnosis of depression in Alzheimer dementia have been proposed that note common features of irritability and social isolation or withdrawal. The waxing and waning course of mood symptoms in dementia is attributed to the cognitive loss and reduced communication skills related to the dementia. In patients with depression that lasts ≥2 weeks and that results in significant distress, a trial of an antidepressant medication should be strongly considered. Similarly, if depressive symptoms last >2 months after behavioral interventions have been implemented, treatment with antidepressant medications is warranted.

First-line agents are the SSRIs, preferred for their favorable adverse-event profiles. Studies of depression in patients with dementia have demonstrated the efficacy of sertraline and citalopram versus placebo (SOE=B), but other studies using the same medications as well as paroxetine and fluoxetine have been inconclusive. For the antidepressants most commonly used to treat depressive symptoms in dementia, see Table 35.2.

The treatment of depression in dementia requires persistence. If a first agent has failed after administration of an adequate therapeutic dose for 8–12 weeks, an alternative agent should be tried. Venlafaxine, bupropion, mirtazapine, and the tricyclic agents desipramine and nortriptyline might be considered. Tricyclics should be avoided if a bundle-branch block or other significant cardiac conduction disturbance is present. For patients who have a partial response to an antidepressant, augmentation strategies might be considered. The addition of a stimulant such as methylphenidate[OL] (2.5–10 mg/d) may be helpful in some cases (SOE=C), but there is some risk of increasing psychotic symptoms if the patient tends to be suspicious or delusional. Also, the addition of stimulants such as methylphenidate to augment bupropion should be avoided, because bupropion already has stimulant effects. If the patient does not improve, the agents should be discontinued. If a patient continues to

Table 35.2—Medications to Treat Depressive Features of Behavioral Disturbances in Dementia

Medication	Daily Dosage	Uses	Precautions
Selective serotonin-reuptake inhibitors (SSRIs)			
Citalopram	10–20 mg	Depression, anxiety[OL]	GI upset, nausea, insomnia (common among all SSRIs)
Escitalopram	5–20 mg	Depression, anxiety	
Fluoxetine	10–40 mg	Depression, anxiety	Long half-life, greater inhibition of the cytochrome P-450 system
Paroxetine	10–40 mg	Depression, anxiety	Greater inhibition of cytochrome P-450 system, some anticholinergic effects
Sertraline	25–100 mg	Depression, anxiety	
Vilazodone	10–40 mg	Depression, anxiety	Take with food, dosage adjustment required in severe hepatic impairment, reduce dose to 20 mg if given with CYP3A4 inhibitors
Serotonin norepinephrine-reuptake inhibitors (SNRIs)			
Desvenlafaxine	25–50 mg	Depression, fibromyalgia	Nausea, hypertension, dry mouth, headaches, dizziness
Duloxetine	20–60 mg	Depression, diabetic neuropathy	Nausea, dry mouth, dizziness, hypertension
Mirtazapine	7.5–30 mg	Useful for depression with insomnia and weight loss	Sedation, hypotension
Venlafaxine	25–150 mg	Useful in severe depression, anxiety	Hypertension may be a problem, insomnia
Tricyclic antidepressants (TCAs)			
Desipramine	10–100 mg	Useful in severe depression, anxiety; high degree of efficacy	Anticholinergic effects, hypotension, sedation, cardiac arrhythmias (conduction delays)
Nortriptyline	10–75 mg	High efficacy for depression if adverse events are tolerable; therapeutic range 50–150 ng/mL	Anticholinergic effects, hypotension, sedation, cardiac arrhythmias (conduction delays)
Other			
Bupropion	75–225 mg	More activating, lack of cardiac effects	Irritability, insomnia
Trazodone	25–150 mg	When sedation is desirable	Sedation, falls, hypotension

be significantly depressed after several antidepressant trials and is in danger because of serious weight loss or suicidal ideas, electroconvulsive therapy might be considered. This is the most efficacious and rapidly effective treatment for severe major depression and has a favorable safety profile even in mild dementia (SOE=B).

Common adverse effects of antidepressants include sedation, insomnia, GI upset, falls, and for tricyclic agents cardiac adverse events. The serotoninergic-norepinephrine reuptake inhibitors venlafaxine, duloxetine, and desvenlafaxine may cause dose-related hypertension. Patients should be monitored for the development of *serotonin syndrome*, a potentially fatal result of multiple or high-dose agents that increase availability of serotonin (see Table 35.3).

Table 35.3— Clinical Signs and Symptoms of Serotonin Syndrome

- Use of medication(s) with serotonergic activity
- Cognitive and behavioral changes: agitation, hyperactivity, worsening confusion, restlessness
- Diaphoresis
- Diarrhea and GI upset
- Fever usually >100.5°F (38°C)
- Hyperreflexia with or without myoclonus
- Incoordination, ataxia, or new onset of falls
- Ocular clonus
- Rhabdomyolysis
- Shivering
- Seizures
- Tremor

Manic-like Behavioral Syndromes

Occasionally mood syndromes may develop in dementia patients that are characterized by pressured speech, disinhibition, elevated or irritable mood, intrusiveness, hyperactivity, impulsivity, and reduced sleep. These syndromes frequently bear a resemblance to the manic episodes observed in the context of bipolar affective disorder in younger adults, although they are generally considered to be secondary to the dementing disorder. The important distinction in the dementia patient is the frequent co-occurrence with confusional states and a tendency to have more of a fluctuating mood, ie, the patient's mood may be irritable or hostile as opposed

Table 35.4—Mood Stabilizers for Behavioral Disturbances in Dementia with Manic-like Features

Medication	Geriatric Dosage	Adverse Events	Comments
Carbamazepine[OLa,b]	200–1,000 mg/d (therapeutic level 4–12 mcg/mL)	Nausea, fatigue, ataxia, blurred vision, hyponatremia	Poor tolerability in older adults; monitor CBC, liver function tests, electrolytes every 2 weeks for first 2 months, then every 3 months
Lamotrigine[OLb]	25–200 mg/d	Skin rash, rare cases of Stevens-Johnson syndrome, dizziness, sedation, neutropenia, anemia	Increased adverse events and interactions when used with divalproex, slow-dose titration required
Lithium[OLa,b]	150–1,000 mg/d (therapeutic level 0.5–0.8 mEq/L)	Nausea, vomiting, tremor, confusion, leukocytosis	Poor tolerability in older adults; toxicity at low serum concentrations; monitor thyroid and renal function
Divalproex sodium[OLa,b]	250–2,000 mg/d (therapeutic level 50–100 mcg/mL)	Nausea, GI upset, ataxia, sedation, hyponatremia	Monitor CBC, platelets, liver function tests at baseline and every 6 months; better tolerated than other mood stabilizers in older adults

[a] Approved by FDA for treatment of bipolar disorder

[b] 2009 FDA warning regarding increase in suicidal thoughts and behaviors among all populations treated with anticonvulsant agents, including those used as mood stabilizers

to euphoric. The appearance of hypersexual behaviors may be observed in this clinical scenario, although sexual disinhibition frequently occurs with dementia as a consequence of reduced frontal-executive functioning and may not necessarily be part of a manic syndrome. Treatment of manic-like states, emotional lability, disinhibition, or irritability typically begins with the use of mood-stabilizing agents such as divalproex sodium[OL] (Table 35.4). The sustained-release preparation divalproex sodium is commonly recommended (SOE=C). In dementia patients, a typical starting dosage of divalproex is 125 mg q12h. The dosage should be titrated upward slowly while the patient is monitored for sedation, ataxia, and falls. Serum concentrations in the range of 50–100 mcg/mL have been shown to be effective, but individual variability in dosage and response is great. Because of the potential adverse effects on the liver and thrombocytopenia, transaminase levels and a CBC with platelets should be done before therapy is started, rechecked with each dosage increase, and repeated at least every 6 months while the patient remains on the medication. Alternatives to divalproex sodium are carbamazepine[OL], lamotrigine[OL], or lithium[OL]. Carbamazepine starting at 100 mg q12h (with monitoring of liver enzymes and CBC) is an acceptable alternative for manic-like states, mood lability, or irritability in dementia. Leukopenia is of concern with carbamazepine, and monitoring the CBC with every dosage increase and at least every 3 months while the patient remains on the medication is needed. Lamotrigine is approved by the FDA for the treatment of mania, but no trials have been conducted in older adults. Lithium is valuable as a mood stabilizer, but its use may be a problem in older adults because of enhanced sensitivity to adverse events. Increased lithium concentrations may occur in the context of reduced renal function and dehydration, resulting in ataxia, tremor, GI distress, and confusion.

Delusions and Hallucinations

Delusions (fixed false belief) or hallucinations (sensory experiences without stimuli), whether occurring independently or in association with mood syndromes, typically require specific pharmacologic treatment if the patient is disturbed by these experiences, or if the experiences lead to disruptions in the patient's environment that cannot otherwise be controlled. Clinical criteria for the diagnosis of Alzheimer dementia with psychosis specifies that the presence of delusions or hallucinations occur for at least 1 month, at least intermittently, and must cause distress for the patient. A sample of antipsychotic drugs is listed in Table 35.5, along with dosing information. The second-generation agents risperidone[OL], olanzapine[OL], quetiapine[OL], and aripiprazole[OL] are used more commonly than first-generation agents such as haloperidol[OL]. The first-generation agents are more likely to cause extrapyramidal adverse events, such as parkinsonism and tardive dyskinesia. Sedation, hypotension, and falls are common adverse events among all antipsychotic agents. As these medications are more widely used, differences in adverse-event profiles are emerging. The FDA has required that warnings regarding diabetes mellitus, hyperglycemia, ketoacidosis, and hyperosmolar states be included as a risk of therapy with all second-generation antipsychotic agents. Quetiapine is the most sedating of the second-generation agents. Clozapine[OL], the first of the second-generation agents to be introduced, is difficult to use because of the need for weekly CBC monitoring, adverse events of sedation and orthostatic hypotension, and the risk of agranulocytosis. Clozapine is still helpful in a small group of patients with psychosis associated with Parkinson dementia or dementia with Lewy bodies who are unable to tolerate the extrapyramidal adverse events of other agents;

Table 35.5—Antipsychotic Medications for the Treatment of Psychosis (Hallucinations and Delusions) in Dementia

Medication	Daily Dosage (mg)	Adverse Events*	Formulations	Comments
Aripiprazole[OL]	2–20	Mild sedation, mild hypotension	Tablet, rapidly dissolving tablet, IM injection, liquid concentrate	Give in AM
Asenapine[OL]	5–10	Sedation	Sublingual tablet	Only sublingual use
Clozapine[OL]	12.5–200	Sedation, hypotension, anticholinergic effects, agranulocytosis	Tablet, rapidly dissolving tablet	Weekly CBCs required; poorly tolerated by older adults; reserved for treatment of refractory cases
Haloperidol[OL]	0.5–3	Extrapyramidal symptoms, sedation	Tablet, liquid, IM injection, long-acting injection	First-generation agent
Iloperidone[OL]	1–12	Sedation, orthostatic hypotension	Tablet	Dosage reduction with use of CYP3A4 and CYP2D6 inhibitors
Lurasidone[OL]	40–80	Sedation	Tablet	Do not exceed 40 mg daily with CYP3A4 inhibitors
Olanzapine[OL]	2.5–15	Sedation, falls, gait disturbance	Tablet, rapidly dissolving tablet, IM injection	Weight gain, hyperglycemia
Paliperidone[OL]	1.5–12	Sedation, fatigue, GI upset, extrapyramidal symptoms	Sustained-release tablet, depot IM long-acting injection	Dosage reduction in renal impairment
Perphenazine[OL]	2–12	Extrapyramidal symptoms, sedation	Tablet	First-generation agent
Quetiapine[OL]	25–200	Sedation, hypotension	Tablet, sustained-released tablet	Ophthalmologic examination recommended every 6 months
Risperidone[OL]	0.5–2	Sedation, hypotension, extrapyramidal symptoms with dosages >1 mg/d	Tablet, rapidly dissolving tablet, depot IM long-acting injection, liquid concentrate	
Ziprasidone[OL]	40–160	Higher risk of QT_c prolongation	Capsule, IM injection	Warning about increased QT_c prolongation; little published information on use in older adults

*NOTE: All listed medications have warning about hyperglycemia, cerebrovascular events, and increase in all-cause mortality in patients with dementia.

quetiapine can also be used in this situation. Clinicians must be prepared to monitor for the emergence of adverse effects among all patients treated with antipsychotic agents and counsel caregivers regarding the possible adverse effects of these medications before treatment is started.

An increased risk of cerebrovascular events in patients with dementia was identified with use of second-generation agents in 2002. All such agents, including risperidone, olanzapine, aripiprazole, quetiapine, clozapine, ziprasidone, and paliperidone must carry this warning. It should be noted that most cerebrovascular events were not fatal.

The FDA required in 2005 that the manufacturers of aripiprazole[OL], olanzapine[OL], quetiapine[OL], risperidone[OL], clozapine[OL], and ziprasidone[OL] and all additional second-generation antipsychotic agents add a "black box" warning to their labeling describing an increased risk of mortality that has been observed in 17 placebo-controlled studies (SOE=A). In these studies, the rate of death for patients with dementia was approximately 1.6–1.7 times that of placebo. In most cases, the cause of death appeared to be heart related or from infections (eg, pneumonia). All new second-generation agents, including rapid-release clozapine and paliperidone, must carry this warning. Based on two observational studies, the FDA has required in 2008 that all first-generation antipsychotic agents also have a "black box" warning regarding an increase in all-cause mortality among patients with dementia who are treated with these agents (SOE=B). The mechanism of action of the increase in mortality is not understood, and the FDA has stated that it is not indicating that clinicians should never use these agents to treat patients with dementia and psychosis. It is strongly suggested that clinicians discuss the risks and benefits of treatment with these agents with families and

Table 35.6—Behavioral Management of Insomnia

- Establish a stable routine for going to bed and awakening
- Advise and educate caregivers regarding the natural fragmented sleep patterns associated with dementia
- Optimize sleep environment (attention to noise, light, temperature)
- Increase daytime activity, use of regular light exercise and exposure to natural sunlight
- Reduce or eliminate caffeine, nicotine, alcohol
- Reduce evening fluid consumption to minimize nocturia
- Give activating medications (eg, steroids) early in the day
- Control nighttime pain
- Limit daytime napping to periods of 20–30 min
- Use relaxation, stress management, breathing techniques to promote natural sleep
- Provide a safe environment for the patient to stay awake if unable to sleep

caregivers before starting therapy. More information on these warnings is available at www.fda.gov/.

Although antipsychotic agents have demonstrated efficacy in large controlled trials in the treatment of dementia with psychosis and aggression, overall positive effects have been relatively modest (SOE=B). Controlled studies of geriatric patients have had very high placebo responses. Although 45%–55% of patients improved on antipsychotic medications, the response to placebo ranged from 30% to 50% across studies. Studies of several antipsychotic agents show that risperidone and aripiprazole may be more effective than placebo for symptoms such as anger, aggression, and paranoid ideation when used for ≤12 weeks (SOE=B). However, use of antipsychotic agents did not appear to improve functional status, care needs, or quality of life. Antipsychotic agents clearly play an important role in the treatment of delusions, hallucinations, and aggression in dementia, but they must be part of a comprehensive treatment plan that includes frequent dosage evaluation, monitoring of adverse effects, and time-limited treatment.

There is some evidence that cholinomimetic agents such as donepezil or galantamine may reduce the onset of psychosis and behavioral disturbances of Alzheimer disease. Studies comparing these agents with placebo in patients with mild to moderate Alzheimer disease have suggested that they may reduce the rate of emergence of behavioral disturbances and psychosis (SOE=B). One area in which cholinesterase inhibitors may be likely to improve psychosis is in the case of dementia with Lewy bodies. Reduced visual hallucinations have been reported with cholinesterase inhibitor treatment (SOE=C). Galantamine^OL in dosages of 16–24 mg/d may be useful in the treatment of patients with Lewy body dementia, who are uniquely sensitive to the extrapyramidal adverse events of antipsychotic agents. More recent studies including patients with Alzheimer dementia and behavioral disturbances failed to demonstrate that agents such as donepezil or memantine were effective in reducing behavioral and psychologic disturbances once the symptoms were present.

Disturbances of Sleep

Treatment of insomnia and sleep-wake cycle disturbance should begin with improvement of sleep hygiene (Table 35.6). This consists of efforts to get the patient to go to sleep later every day, around 10:00 or 11:00 PM, while keeping the environment calm, comfortable, and conducive to sleep, into the next morning. If the sleep disturbance is associated with depression, suspiciousness, or delusions, those conditions should be treated.

For primary sleep disturbances when good sleep hygiene and increasing daytime activity level are not successful, trazodone^OL (25–50 mg at bedtime) or mirtazapine^OL (7.5–15 mg at bedtime) might be used (SOE=D). Benzodiazepines or antihistamines, such as diphenhydramine, should be avoided, because they carry a high risk of falls, hip fractures, disinhibition, and cognitive disturbance when prescribed for patients with dementia. See also "Sleep Problems," p 285.

Zolpidem^OL and zaleplon^OL are short-acting nonbenzodiazepine sedative hypnotics that may be helpful for sleep disturbances in older adults, although there have been no controlled trials for their use in sleep disturbances secondary to dementia. Zolpidem has been studied in older patients without dementia and appears to be effective in improving sleep onset, although it does not improve sleep duration because of its short half-life. The recommended dose of zolpidem in older adults is 5 mg, because an increased risk of adverse events appears to be dose related. Zaleplon has also been studied in older patients and appears to have similar properties.

Hypersexuality

If hypersexuality occurs in association with another recognizable syndrome such as a mania-like state, treatment of the specific syndrome, such as with mood stabilizers, should be undertaken. In men with dementia who are dangerously hypersexual or aggressive, clinical case reports have suggested that a trial of an antiandrogen might be attempted to reduce the sexual drive (SOE=D). Patients have been tried on oral progesterone^OL 5 mg/d at first. The dosage should be adjusted to suppress serum testosterone well below normal. If the patient responds well behaviorally, 10 mg of depot intramuscular progesterone may be given weekly to maintain reduced sexual drive. An alternative treatment to reduce sexual drive is leuprolide acetate^OL (5–10 mg IM every month), also an antiandrogen. The use of antipsychotic medications is often adopted clinically, given the seriousness of hypersexual behaviors in institutionalized settings such as nursing homes; however, there are no controlled studies supporting this use. Presumably, these medications may enhance the cognitive focus of the individual's perceptions by reducing any psychotic thinking that may in some way be contributing to hypersexual behavior. Studies of nonpharmacologic interventions are needed for this problem.

Intermittent Aggression or Agitation

When disruptive behavior occurs intermittently or episodically, such as once per week or less, behavioral interventions focusing on identifying the antecedents of the behavior and avoiding the triggers are often most useful. Behavior modification using positive reinforcement of desirable behavior has been shown to be helpful, and it also helps encourage the caregiver to focus on times when behavior is not a problem. Caregiver education and support, music therapy, and physical activity appear to show promise in reducing behavioral disturbances (SOE=B). Reminiscence; validation therapy; and environmental modifications of light, sound, and space may all help promote positive behavior. Distraction techniques, activity therapies, and aromatherapy also show promise in reducing troublesome behaviors (SOE=C).

Physical restraint in any form should be avoided if at all possible. If restraining measures are necessary, careful supportive care should be provided to the patient. Over time, it is usually possible to reduce or eliminate the amount of restraint. See also the section on quality issues in "Nursing-Home Care," p 153.

REFERENCES

- Ballard C, Corbett A. Management of neuropsychiatric symptoms in people with dementia. *CNS Drugs*. 2010;24(9):729–739.
- Olazaran J, Reisberg B, Clare L, et al. Nonpharmacological therapies in Alzheimer's disease: a systematic review of efficacy. *Dement Geriatr Cogn Disord*. 2010;30(2):161–178.
- Smith M, Schultz SK, Seydel LL, et al. Improving antipsychotic agent use in nursing homes: development of an algorithm for treating problem behaviors in dementia. *J Gerontol Nurs*. 2013;39(5):24–35.

CHAPTER 36—DELIRIUM

KEY POINTS

- The first key step in delirium management is accurate diagnosis, which involves administration of a brief mental status examination that includes testing attention and applying the Confusion Assessment Method diagnostic algorithm.
- All delirious patients require a thorough evaluation for reversible causes; all correctable contributing factors should be addressed.
- Patients who develop delirium are at increased risk of poor outcomes, including nursing-home placement, dementia, and death, and require an intensive interdisciplinary effort to maximize likelihood of a favorable outcome.
- Pharmacologic intervention should be reserved for key target symptoms; low-dosage, high-potency antipsychotics are usually the treatment of choice.
- Proactive, multifactorial interventions have reduced the incidence, severity, and duration of delirium.

Delirium remains under-recognized and often inappropriately evaluated and managed. Clinicians call delirium by many different names. *Acute confusional state* is the most common synonym. Other common synonyms include *acute mental status change*, *altered mental status*, *organic brain syndrome*, *reversible dementia*, and *toxic* or *metabolic encephalopathy*.

INCIDENCE AND PROGNOSIS

Delirium is common and associated with substantial morbidity and mortality. Approximately one-third of patients ≥70 years old admitted to a general medical service experience delirium: one-half of these are delirious on admission to the hospital, while the other half develop delirium in the hospital. Among those admitted to intensive care units, the prevalence of delirium is much higher, and when rates for delirium are combined with those for stupor and coma, prevalence rates exceed 75%. Up to one-third of older adults presenting to the emergency department are delirious. In postacute skilled-nursing facilities, 16% of new admissions meet criteria for delirium. The prevalence of delirium at the end of life is reported to be as high as 85%, while the overall prevalence in the community is reported to be 1%–2%, largely among older patients recently discharged from the hospital.

Although delirium is traditionally viewed as a transient phenomenon, there is growing evidence that it may persist for weeks to months in a substantial portion of affected individuals (SOE=A). A recent systematic review found that persistence rates for delirium at hospital discharge and at 1, 3, and 6 months after discharge were 45%, 33%, 26%, and 21%, respectively. Risk factors for delirium persistence predominantly relate to individual vulnerability, including advanced age, preexisting dementia, multiple comorbidities, and functional impairment, but also include severity of delirium and use of restraints. In some cases, persistent delirium never resolves, but there is no consensus as to the time frame when persistent delirium should be called dementia.

Evidence is mounting that delirium is strongly and independently associated with poor patient outcomes (SOE=A). A recently published meta-analysis that included almost 3,000 patients followed for a mean of 22.7 months demonstrated that delirium was independently associated with an increased risk of death (OR 2.0; 95% CI, 1.5–2.5), institutionalization (OR 2.4; 95% CI, 1.8–3.3), and dementia (OR 12.5; 95% CI, 11.9–84.2). Further, persistence of delirium may play an important role in its association with poor long-term outcomes. Rates of mortality, nursing-home placement, functional decline, and dementia are consistently higher in patients with persistent delirium than in patients whose delirium resolves more quickly.

DIAGNOSIS AND DIFFERENTIAL DIAGNOSIS

Under-recognition of delirium is a major problem. A recent systematic review recommended the Confusion Assessment Method (CAM) as the most useful bedside assessment tool for delirium. By judging the presence or absence of the four key CAM features (Table 36.1), clinicians can establish the diagnosis of delirium. Although the CAM can be completed by using observations from routine care, use of a formal mental status evaluation improves detection and reliability of the assessment. This assessment should evaluate level of consciousness, orientation, attention, and thought organization before using the CAM. In the absence of a formal evaluation or when there is doubt, any older adult with acute change in mental status should be considered delirious, and evaluated and managed as described below.

The Confusion Assessment Method for the Intensive Care Unit (CAM–ICU) (Table 36.1) is a variant of the CAM that is designed for ventilator-dependent patients or those unable to speak in the ICU and that

Table 36.1—Operationalizing the Confusion Assessment Method Diagnostic Algorithm

Confusion Assessment Method	Confusion Assessment Method–Intensive Care Unit Version
1. Acute change in mental status and fluctuating course	
Is there evidence of an acute change from the patient's baseline? Does the abnormal mental status or behavior fluctuate during the day (ie, come and go), or increase and decrease in severity? Suggest asking the patient if he or she has felt confused over the past 24 hours, using previous documented mental status examinations, and asking the nurse and/or family members about changes in mental status over the past 24 hours.	Is there an acute change from baseline? Did the abnormal behavior fluctuate over the past 24 hours? Suggest using Richmond Agitation and Sedation Scale (RASS) evaluations over the past 24 hours as well as collateral information from nurse and family.
2. Inattention	
Does the patient have difficulty focusing attention, eg, is easily distracted, or has difficulty keeping track of what is being said? Suggest tests of attention: ■ Recite a sequence of random numbers in forward or backward order ■ Recite days of week, months of year backward ■ Count backward from 20 to 1	Does the patient have difficulty focusing attention? Is there a reduced ability to maintain and shift attention? Suggest tests of attention: ■ Vigilance A letter test: HAVEAHAART ■ Picture recognition
3. Disorganized thinking	
Is the patient's thinking disorganized or incoherent? Examples: ■ Unclear/illogical flow of ideas ■ Rambling, incoherent speech ■ Severe disorientation ■ Perceptual disturbances or delusions with thought disorder	Was the patient's thinking disorganized or incoherent, such as rambling or irrelevant conversation, unclear or illogical flow of ideas, or unpredictable switching from subject to subject? Was the patient able to follow questions and commands throughout the assessment? Suggest asking the following questions: ■ Hold up this many fingers. (Examiner holds up 2 fingers.) Now do the same thing with the other hand. ■ Ask a series of simple yes/no questions: "Does one pound weigh more than two pounds?" "Will a stone float on water?"
4. Altered level of consciousness	
Is the patient's mental status anything other than alert? ■ Vigilant (hyperalert) ■ Lethargic (drowsy but easily aroused, unaware of some elements in the environment) ■ Stuporous (difficult to arouse, unaware of some or all elements in the environment) ■ Comatose (unarousable, unaware of all elements in the environment)	Any level of consciousness other than alert?
The diagnosis of delirium requires the presence of features 1 *and* 2 *and* either 3 or 4.	

SOURCE: Data from Inouye SK, van Dyck CH, Alessi CA, et al. Clarifying confusion: the Confusion Assessment Method: a new method for detection of delirium. *Ann Intern Med.* 1990;113(12):941–948; and Ely EW, Margolin R, Francis J, et al. Evaluation of delirium in critically ill patients: validation of the Confusion Assessment Method for the Intensive Care Unit (CAM-ICU). *Crit Care Med.* 2001;29(7):1370–1379.

does not require verbal responses from the patient. It includes the same four features as the CAM diagnostic algorithm but uses mental status testing that requires only yes/no answers, which can be indicated by a nod or raised finger. Attention is tested using the Attention Screening Examination, in which patients are required to immediately recall simple pictures. Disorganized thinking is tested by answers to a series of simple yes/no questions (eg, "Does 1 pound weigh more than 2 pounds?"). Recent evidence suggests that the sensitivity of the CAM-ICU may be lower than that of the standard CAM; therefore, for verbal patients, it is appropriate to use a verbal mental status evaluation before completing the CAM algorithm.

To improve recognition of delirium, medical centers are starting to use standardized screening of high-risk patients, such as those in the ICU, after major surgery, and very old patients. Such screening is particularly important for identifying cases of hypoactive delirium, which might otherwise go unnoticed by the care team. A brief but standardized screening assessment should be administered on a daily basis, or even more frequently in very high-risk patients, such as those in the ICU. Frequent standardized assessment and documentation of mental status is also important to allow detection of fluctuations, which are a key feature of delirium.

The differential diagnosis of delirium includes dementia, depression, and acute psychiatric syndromes.

Table 36.2—Mnemonic for Reversible Causes of Delirium

Drugs	Any new additions, increased dosages, or interactions Consider OTC drugs and alcohol Consider especially high-risk drugs (Table 36.5)
Electrolyte disturbances	Especially dehydration, sodium imbalance Thyroid abnormalities
Lack of drugs	Withdrawals from chronically used sedatives, including alcohol and sleeping pills Poorly controlled pain (lack of analgesia)
Infection	Especially urinary and respiratory tract infections
Reduced sensory input	Poor vision, poor hearing (lack of glasses, hearing aids in the hospital)
Intracranial	Infection, hemorrhage, stroke, tumor Rare; consider only if new focal neurologic findings, suggestive history, or diagnostic evaluation otherwise negative
Urinary, fecal	Urinary retention: "cystocerebral syndrome" Fecal impaction
Myocardial, pulmonary	Myocardial infarction, arrhythmia, exacerbation of heart failure, exacerbation of COPD, hypoxia

In many cases, it is not truly a "differential" diagnosis, because these syndromes can coexist and indeed are risk factors for one another. Instead, it is better thought of as a series of independent questions: Does this patient have delirium? Does he or she have dementia? Does he or she have depression? Does the patient have more than one disorder? The most common diagnostic issue is whether a newly presenting confused patient has dementia, delirium, or both. To make this determination, the clinician must ascertain the patient's baseline status. In the absence of prior knowledge or documentation of the patient's baseline, information from family members, caregivers, or others who know the patient is essential. An acute change in mental status from baseline is not consistent with dementia and suggests delirium. In addition, a rapidly fluctuating course (over minutes to hours) and an abnormal level of consciousness are also highly suggestive of delirium. Depression can also be confused with hypoactive delirium. Finally, certain acute psychiatric syndromes, such as mania, can present similarly to hyperactive delirium. Hyperactive patients are best initially evaluated and managed as if they have delirium rather than attributing the presentation to psychiatric disease and potentially missing a serious underlying medical disorder.

THE SPECTRUM AND NEUROPATHOPHYSIOLOGY OF DELIRIUM

The classic presentation of delirium is thought to be the extremely agitated patient. However, agitated or hyperactive delirium represents only 25% of cases. More common is hypoactive or "quiet" delirium, and delirium with mixed features. Evidence suggests that hypoactive delirium is associated with an equal or poorer prognosis than delirium with hyperactive or normal psychomotor features (SOE=B). Potentially, one of the reasons for this poorer prognosis is that hypoactive delirium is less frequently recognized. As described above, special case-finding efforts are necessary to detect quiet delirium among high-risk older patients. If agitation is present, behavioral control measures may be necessary (see below), but such measures alone are not adequate treatment for delirium, and in some cases they can exacerbate or prolong delirium.

RISK FACTORS

In the absence of a clear neuropathophysiologic basis for delirium, the cornerstone of its management focuses on the assessment and treatment of modifiable risk factors. Fortunately, several consistent risk factors for delirium have been identified. These risk factors are classified into two groups: baseline factors that predispose patients to delirium, and acute factors that precipitate delirium. Predisposing factors include advanced age, preexisting dementia, preexisting functional impairment in ADLs, and high medical comorbidity. Male gender, sensory impairment (poor vision and hearing), depressive symptoms, laboratory abnormalities, and history of alcohol abuse have also been reported in some studies. Acute precipitating factors include medications, especially those that are sedating or highly anticholinergic, surgery, uncontrolled pain, low hematocrit level, bed rest, and use of certain indwelling devices and restraints. A useful model suggests that delirium develops when the sum of predisposing and precipitating factors crosses a certain threshold. In such a model, the greater the predisposing factors, the fewer precipitating factors are needed for delirium to develop. This would explain why older, frail adults develop delirium in the face of stressors that are much less severe than stressors that can cause delirium in younger, healthy adults. For a mnemonic for reversible risk factors for delirium, see Table 36.2.

Delirium and Dementia

While dementia is an established risk factor for delirium, evidence is increasing that the relationship may be bidirectional. As described above, a recent meta-analysis demonstrated that nondemented patients who develop delirium are at increased risk of incident dementia over the next 1–5 years (SOE=B). Most of these studies did not involve detailed testing of neuropsychologic performance before the onset of delirium, so it remains unclear whether delirium was the herald of previously unrecognized cognitive impairment (or other brain vulnerability), or whether the delirium itself set forth a CNS process that initiated or accelerated onset of dementia. In either case, these findings suggest that previously intact patients who develop delirium need to be monitored closely, even if the acute symptoms of delirium resolve entirely. Complementing these studies in non-demented patients, a recent study demonstrated that patients with Alzheimer disease experienced accelerated cognitive decline after an episode of delirium. Further studies exploring the interrelationship of delirium with dementia should use serial cognitive testing performed both before and after the episode of delirium, to better define how delirium impacts cognitive trajectory.

Postoperative Delirium

Delirium may be the most common complication after surgery in older adults. The incidence is 15% after elective noncardiac surgery, and up to 50% after high-risk procedures such as hip fracture repair, aortic aneurysm repair, and coronary artery bypass grafting. In a prospectively validated clinical prediction rule for delirium after elective noncardiac surgery, seven risk factors were identified preoperatively: advanced age, cognitive impairment, physical functional impairment, history of alcohol abuse, markedly abnormal serum chemistries, intrathoracic surgery, and aortic aneurysm surgery. Patients with none of these risk factors had a 2% risk of delirium, those with one or two risk factors had a 10% risk, and those with three or more risk factors had a 50% risk. More recently, a clinical prediction rule for delirium after cardiac surgery has been validated. Four risk factors were identified: cognitive impairment, history of stroke or transient ischemic attack, depressive symptoms, and low or high albumin.

In addition to baseline risk factors, intraoperative and postoperative management plays an important role in the development of delirium. Multiple studies demonstrate that the type or route of intraoperative anesthesia, whether general, spinal, epidural, or combined, has little impact on the risk of delirium (SOE=A). However, the total dose of anesthetic agents may play an important role (SOE=B). A recent randomized trial used bispectral (BIS) monitoring to titrate the dosage of intraoperative sedative medications among hip-fracture patients undergoing surgical repair using spinal anesthesia. Patients in the low-dose arm had a markedly reduced rate of postoperative delirium relative to the high-dose arm (19% versus 40%, $P<.01$).

Postoperative medication management also plays an important role in delirium. Postoperative use of benzodiazepines and certain opioids, especially meperidine, is strongly associated with the development of delirium. Although pain medications can cause delirium, adequate pain management is also important, because high levels of postoperative pain have also been associated with delirium. Strategies to provide adequate analgesia with minimally effective doses of opioids should be used. These include the use of scheduled rather than as-needed dosing, patient-controlled analgesic pumps, regional analgesia, opioid-sparing analgesics, and nonpharmacologic approaches, such as ice packs. Low postoperative hematocrit level (<30%) has also been associated with postoperative delirium, although transfusions have not been shown to reduce delirium.

Evaluation and Management

All patients with newly diagnosed delirium require a careful history, physical examination, and targeted laboratory testing. Most treatable causes of delirium lie outside the CNS, and these should be investigated first. Moreover, multiple contributing factors are often present, so the diagnostic evaluation should not be terminated because a single "cause" is identified. For key steps in the evaluation and management of delirium, see Table 36.3.

The history should focus on the time course of the changes in mental status and their association with other symptoms or events (eg, fever, shortness of breath, medication change). Because medications are the most common and treatable cause of delirium, a careful medication history, using the nursing administration sheets in the hospital or a "brown-bag" review in the outpatient setting, is imperative. In the outpatient setting, it is also important to review the patient's use of OTC drugs, herbal or other supplements, and alcohol. The physical examination should include vital signs and oxygen saturation, a careful general medical examination, and a neurologic and mental status examination. The emphasis should be on identifying acute medical problems or exacerbations of chronic medical problems that might be contributing to delirium.

Laboratory tests and imaging studies should be selected on the basis of history and examination findings.

Table 36.3—Management of Delirium

Step	Key Issues	Proposed Treatment
Identify and treat reversible contributors	Medications	Reduce or eliminate offending medications, or substitute less psychoactive medications
	Infections	Treat common infections: urinary, respiratory, soft tissue
	Fluid balance disorders	Assess and treat dehydration, heart failure, electrolyte disorders
	Impaired CNS oxygenation	Treat severe anemia (transfusion), hypoxia, hypotension
	Severe pain	Assess and treat; use local measures and scheduled pain regimens that minimize opioids; avoid meperidine
	Sensory deprivation	Use eyeglasses, hearing aids, portable amplifier
	Elimination problems	Assess and treat urinary retention and fecal impaction
Maintain behavioral control	Behavioral interventions	Teach hospital staff appropriate interaction with delirious patients; encourage family visitation
	Pharmacologic interventions	If necessary, use low-dose high-potency antipsychotics (Table 36.5)
Anticipate and prevent or manage complications	Urinary incontinence	Implement scheduled toileting program
	Immobility and falls	Avoid physical restraints; mobilize with assistance; use physical therapy
	Pressure ulcers	Mobilize; reposition immobilized patient frequently and monitor pressure points
	Sleep disturbance	Implement a nonpharmacologic sleep hygiene program, including a nighttime sleep protocol; avoid sedatives
	Feeding disorders	Assist with feeding; use aspiration precautions; provide nutritional supplementation as necessary
Restore function in delirious patients	Hospital environment	Reduce clutter and noise (especially at night); provide adequate lighting; have familiar objects brought from home
	Cognitive reconditioning	Have staff reorient patient to time, place, person at least three times daily
	Ability to perform ADLs	As delirium clears, match performance to ability
	Family education, support, and participation	Provide education about delirium, its causes and reversibility, how to interact, and family's role in restoring function
	Discharge	Because delirium can persist, provide for increased ADL support; follow mental status changes as "barometer" of recovery

Most patients require at least a CBC, electrolytes, and kidney function tests. Urinalysis, urine toxicology for drugs of abuse, blood alcohol level, tests for liver function, serum medication levels, arterial blood gases, as well as chest radiographs, an ECG, and appropriate cultures are helpful in selected situations. Cerebral imaging is often performed but is rarely helpful, except in cases of head trauma or new focal neurologic findings. In the absence of seizure activity or signs of meningitis, electroencephalograms and cerebrospinal fluid analysis rarely yield helpful results.

Delirious hospitalized patients are particularly vulnerable to complications and poor outcomes. Special care is needed and requires an interdisciplinary effort by clinicians, nurses, family members, and others. A multifactorial approach is the most successful, because many factors contribute to delirium; thus, multiple interventions, even if individually small, can yield marked clinical improvement (Table 36.3). If delirium is not diagnosed and managed properly, costly and life-threatening complications and long-term loss of function can result.

Modifying the risk factors that contribute to delirium is critically important. Some factors, such as age and prior cognitive impairment, cannot be modified. However, some predisposing factors, such as sensory impairment, can be modified through proper use of eyeglasses and hearing aids. Newly admitted older adults should be screened for cognitive loss, severity of illness, sensory deficits, and markers of dehydration with a goal of addressing correctable risk factors proactively before the onset of delirium. Medications are the most common reversible causes of delirium. Anticholinergics, H_2-blockers, benzodiazepines, opioids, and antipsychotic medications should be replaced with medications that have no central effects. For example, H_2-blockers can be replaced by antacids or proton-pump inhibitors, and regular dosing of 650 mg of acetaminophen three to four times daily can reduce or eliminate the need for opioids in many patients (Table 36.4).

The delirious patient is susceptible to a wide range of iatrogenic complications, and careful surveillance is critical. Bowel and bladder function should be monitored closely, but urinary catheters should be avoided unless absolutely required for monitoring fluids or treating urinary retention. Bowel stimulants and fecal softeners can be used to prevent obstipation, particularly in those who are concomitantly using opioids. Complete bed rest

Table 36.4—Drugs to Reduce or Eliminate in the Management of Delirium

Agent	Adverse Events	Possible Substitutes	Comments
Alcohol	CNS sedation and withdrawal	If history of heavy intake, careful monitoring and benzodiazepines for withdrawal symptoms	Alcohol history is imperative
Anticholinergics (oxybutynin, benztropine)	Anticholinergic toxicity	Lower dosage, behavioral measures	Rare at low dosages
Anticonvulsants (especially primidone, phenobarbital, phenytoin)	CNS sedation and withdrawal	Alternative agent or none	Toxic reactions can occur despite "therapeutic" drug concentrations
Antidepressants, especially tertiary amine tricyclic agents (amitriptyline, imipramine, doxepin)	Anticholinergic toxicity	Secondary amine tricyclics (nortriptyline, desipramine), SSRIs, or other agents	Secondary amines as good as tertiary for adjuvant treatment of chronic pain
Antihistamines (eg, diphenhydramine)	Anticholinergic toxicity	Nonpharmacologic protocol for sleep, pseudoephedrine for colds	Must take OTC medication history
Antiparkinsonian agents (levodopa-carbidopa, dopamine agonists, amantadine)	Dopaminergic toxicity	Lower dosage; adjusted dosing schedule	Usually with end-stage disease and high dosages
Antipsychotics, especially low-potency anticholinergic agents and second-generation agents (clozapine)	Anticholinergic toxicity, CNS sedation	No agents or, if necessary, low-dosage high-potency agents	See note for Table 36.5 for warnings about second-generation antipsychotics
Barbiturates	CNS sedation, severe withdrawal syndrome	Gradual discontinuation or benzodiazepine substitution	In most cases, should no longer be prescribed; avoid inadvertent or abrupt discontinuation
Benzodiazepines, especially long-acting (eg, diazepam, flurazepam, chlordiazepoxide)	CNS sedation, potential for withdrawal	Nonpharmacologic sleep management, melatonin, intermediate agents (lorazepam, temazepam)	Associated with delirium in medical and surgical patients
Benzodiazepines: ultra short-acting (eg, triazolam, alprazolam)	CNS sedation and withdrawal	Nonpharmacologic sleep management, melatonin, intermediate agents (lorazepam, temazepam)	Associated with delirium in case reports and series
Chloral hydrate	CNS sedation	Nonpharmacologic sleep protocol, melatonin	No better for delirium than benzodiazepines
H_2-blocking agents	Possible anticholinergic toxicity	Lower dosage, antacids or proton-pump inhibitors	Most common with high-dosage intravenous infusions
Nonbenzodiazepine hypnotics (eg, zolpidem)	CNS sedation and withdrawal	Nonpharmacologic sleep protocol, melatonin	Like other sedatives, can cause delirium
Opioid analgesics (especially meperidine)	Anticholinergic toxicity, CNS sedation, fecal impaction	Local measures and nonpsychoactive pain medications around the clock, reserve opioids for breakthrough and severe pain	Higher risk in patients with renal insufficiency; must consider risks versus benefit
Almost any medication if time course is appropriate			**Consider risks and benefits of all medications in older adults**

should be avoided, because it can lead to increasing disability through disuse of muscles and the development of pressure ulcers and atelectasis in the lungs. Physical exercise and ambulation prevent the deconditioning often associated with hospitalization. Malnutrition can be avoided through the use of nutritional supplements and careful attention to intake of food and fluids. Some delirious patients may need assistance for eating.

Managing behavioral problems while ensuring both the comfort and safety of the patient can be challenging.

The patient should be placed in a room near the nursing station for close observation. Nonpharmacologic behavioral measures provide orientation and a feeling of safety. Orienting items such as clocks, calendars, and even a window view should be made available. Patients should be encouraged to wear their eyeglasses and hearing aids. Although use of physical restraints in the hospital has not been well studied, evidence from the long-term care setting suggests that such restraints probably do not decrease the rate of falls by confused ambulatory patients, and they may actually increase the risk of fall-related injury. Restraints, although objectionable, may be required because of violent behavior or to prevent the removal of important devices, such as endotracheal tubes, intra-arterial devices, and catheters. Whenever restraints are used, the indicators for use should be frequently reassessed, and the restraints should be removed as soon as possible.

Medications used as chemical restraints extract a costly toll in accidents, adverse events, and loss of mobility; they should be avoided if possible. Pharmacologic intervention may be necessary for symptoms such as delusions or hallucinations that are frightening to the patient when verbal comfort and reassurance are not successful. Some delirious patients display behavior that is dangerous to themselves or others and cannot be calmed by a family member or aide. Indications for pharmacologic intervention should be clearly identified, documented, and constantly reassessed.

Several recent meta-analyses have examined pharmacologic treatment of delirium. Relatively few studies met criteria for inclusion, with the largest having a sample size of 73 participants. One of these studies established the superiority of haloperidol to benzodiazepines. Most of the other studies demonstrated the equivalence of the second-generation antipsychotics with haloperidol. Until recently, none of the studies used a placebo control group. Based on this limited evidence (SOE=B), high-potency antipsychotics are the treatment of choice for agitation in delirium because of their low anticholinergic potency and minimal hypotensive effects. High-potency antipsychotics have substantial extrapyramidal symptoms and are contraindicated in patients with Parkinson disease, Lewy-body dementia, and a history of neuroleptic malignant syndrome. Moreover, they must be used cautiously in all patients, because they can actually prolong delirium and increase the risk of complications by converting a hyperactive, confused patient into a stuporous one whose risk of a fall or aspiration is increased. In older patients with mild delirium, low doses of haloperidol^{OL} (0.5–1 mg po or 0.25–0.5 mg parenterally) should be used initially, with careful reassessment before additional dosing. In more severe delirium, somewhat higher doses can be used initially (0.5–2 mg parenterally), with additional dosing every 60 min as required for symptom management. In patients with Parkinson disease and Lewy body disease, a second-generation antipsychotic with less extrapyramidal effects such as quetiapine^{OL} can be substituted. One must be careful to assess for akathisia (motor restlessness), which can be an adverse event of antipsychotic medications and can be confused with worsening delirium. The treatment for akathisia is less, not more, antipsychotic medication. As with physical restraints, in all cases in which pharmacologic restraint is used, the healthcare team must clearly identify the target symptoms necessitating use of the medications, frequently review the efficacy of these drugs in controlling the target symptoms, and assess the patient for adverse events and complications. For a summary of the pharmacologic management of agitated delirium, see Table 36.5.

Family Counseling

It is important to stress to family members that delirium is usually not a permanent condition, but rather that it improves over time. Unfortunately, as described above, persistence of delirium is common. Thus, when counseling families, it is important to point out that many cognitive deficits associated with the delirium syndrome can continue, abating weeks and even months after the illness. Advanced age (≥85 years old), preexisting cognitive impairment, and severe illness are risk factors for slow recovery of cognitive function. Careful monitoring of mental status and providing adequate functional supports during this period are necessary to give the patient the maximal chance of returning to his or her baseline level. Family members can play an important role in the hospital and postacute setting by providing appropriate orientation, support, and functional assistance. Hospitals are increasingly making provisions for family members to sleep overnight with relatives who are already delirious or at high risk of developing delirium. While symptoms of delirium may persist, acute exacerbation of cognitive dysfunction is not expected during the convalescent period and therefore likely heralds a new medical problem. Families should be counseled to seek prompt medical attention if a patient's mental status acutely worsens.

Models of Care

A growing body of literature has focused on the prevention and management of delirium. These studies can be best understood along a continuum, ranging from proactive interventions to prevent delirium or to reduce its severity and consequences, to reactive interventions designed to treat delirium after it has developed. The overall trend suggests that the more proactive, the more successful the intervention.

Table 36.5—Pharmacologic Therapy of Agitated Delirium

Agent	Mechanism of Action	Dosage	Benefits	Adverse Events	Comments
Haloperidol[OL]	Antipsychotic	0.25–1 mg po, IM, or IV q4h prn agitation	Relatively nonsedating; few hemodynamic effects	EPS, especially if >3 mg/d	Usually agent of choice[a]
Risperidone[OL]	Second-generation antipsychotic	0.25–1 mg po q4h prn agitation	Similar to haloperidol	Might have slightly fewer EPS than haloperidol	Small trials[b]
Olanzapine[OL]	Second-generation antipsychotic	2.5–5 mg po or IM q12h, max dosage 20 mg q24h (cannot be given by IV infusion)	Fewer EPS than haloperidol	More sedating than haloperidol	Small trials[b]; oral formulations less effective for acute management
Quetiapine[OL]	Second-generation antipsychotic	25–50 mg po q12h	Fewer EPS than haloperidol	More sedating than haloperidol; hypotension	Small trials[b]
Lorazepam[OL]	Benzodiazepine	0.25–1 mg po or IV q8h prn agitation	Use in sedative and alcohol withdrawal; history of neuroleptic malignant syndrome	More paradoxical excitation, respiratory depression than haloperidol	Second-line agent, except in specific cases noted

NOTE: EPS = extrapyramidal symptoms

Use of all these drugs for delirium is an off-label indication. Due to the small number and size of trials investigating the use of these agents in the treatment of agitation in delirium, the SOE=B.

[a] In a randomized trial comparing haloperidol, chlorpromazine, and lorazepam in the treatment of agitated delirium in young patients with AIDS, all were found to be equally effective, but haloperidol had the fewest adverse events.

[b] Second-generation antipsychotics have been tested primarily in small equivalency trials with haloperidol and recently in small placebo-controlled trials in the intensive care unit. The FDA requires a "black box" warning for all second-generation antipsychotics because of the increased risk of cerebrovascular events, stroke, and mortality in patients with dementia. First-generation antipsychotic agents also have an FDA "black box" warning regarding an increase in all-cause mortality among patients with dementia.

In a 1999 study, a unit-based proactive multifactorial intervention termed HELP (The Hospital Elder Life Program) reduced the incidence of delirium among hospitalized patients ≥70 years old by 40% (matched OR=0.60; 95% CI, 0.39, 0.92; number needed to treat [NNT] = 19.6) (SOE=A). Six intervention components were used selectively on the basis of patient-specific risk factors determined at an admission assessment: cognitive impairment, sleep deprivation, immobility, visual impairment, hearing impairment, and dehydration. Among these, the most successful component was a nonpharmacologic sleep protocol that involved trained volunteers offering patients warm milk, back rubs, and soothing music at bedtime; this intervention reduced the use of sedative-hypnotic medication. The HELP model was subsequently demonstrated to be cost-effective for hospitals in medium-risk patients, and for the healthcare system in all patients because of the large savings in postacute care.

Another approach with proven benefit for the prevention of delirium is proactive geriatrics consultation. Two randomized trials demonstrated that this model of care can reduce the incidence of delirium in older patients undergoing hip fracture repair. In most cases, consultation began preoperatively and continued throughout the duration of hospitalization. Daily recommendations were based on a structured protocol that covers key elements in delirium prevention, such as limitation of psychoactive medications. The geriatrics consultation group achieved a 30%–40% reduction in the incidence of delirium (NNT=5.6) (SOE=A).

Finally, several studies have examined treatment of delirium using multifactorial strategies similar to those used for delirium prevention. For the most part, these have not yielded as dramatic benefits as the prevention models (SOE=B), although some have demonstrated a reduction in delirium severity, duration, or faster cognitive recovery in the intervention group. A recent cluster randomized trial of a Delirium Abatement Program for postacute care showed improved detection of delirium among postacute care nurses at the intervention facilities but no reduction in delirium persistence. New trials are underway to test treatment interventions.

QUALITY MEASURES AND CONSENSUS GUIDELINES

The ACOVE guidelines include a single delirium quality indicator within its indicators for hospital care: If a diagnosis of delirium is suspected or definite in a hospitalized vulnerable older adult, then an evaluation for potentially precipitating factors should be undertaken, and identified causes treated. Medicare's

Table 36.6—Key Recommendations of the National Institute for Health and Clinical Excellence (NICE) Guideline for Delirium

Assess delirium risk factors when patients are admitted to the hospital.

Prevent delirium by addressing risk factors using a multicomponent intervention.

Screen for incident delirium by assessing recent changes or fluctuations in cognitive function, perception, physical function, and social behavior on admission and at least daily thereafter.

Diagnose delirium by performing a clinical assessment based on formal criteria conducted by a trained healthcare professional; document in medical record.

Manage delirium by:

- Identifying and managing possible underlying causes
- Ensuring effective communication, reorientation, and providing reassurance
- Considering the involvement of family, friends, and caregivers
- Providing care in a suitable environment

If a person with delirium is distressed or a risk to themselves or others:

- Use verbal and nonverbal deescalation techniques, such as quietly sitting at the bedside and engaging the patient in conversation, playing relaxing music.
- If these are not effective or inappropriate, consider short-term antipsychotics at the lowest clinically appropriate dosage and titrate cautiously according to symptoms.

SOURCE: Data from Young J, Murthy L, Westby M, et al. Diagnosis, prevention, and management of delirium: summary of NICE guidance. *BMJ*. 2010;341:247–249.

Nursing Home Compare Web site lists failure to resolve delirium within 14 days as a quality indicator for postacute care. The most recent, comprehensive consensus guideline for delirium was published in 2010 by the National Institute for Health and Clinical Excellence of the United Kingdom Health Service, based on "systematic reviews of the best available evidence and explicit considerations of cost-effectiveness" (Table 36.6) (SOE=C). Future guidelines will be strengthened by the growing literature on delirium recognition, prevention, and treatment.

REFERENCES

- Kolanowski AM, Hill N, Clare L, et al. Practical protocol for implementing cognitive stimulation in persons with delirium superimposed on dementia. *Nonpharmacol Ther Dement*. 2012;2(2):101–110.
- Marcantonio ER, Bergmann MA, Kiely DK, et al. Randomized trial of a delirium abatement program for post-acute skilled nursing facilities. *J Am Geriatr Soc*. 2010;58(6):1019–1026.
- Witlox J, Eurelings LS, de Jonghe JF, et al. Delirium in elderly patients and the risk of postdischarge mortality, institutionalization, and dementia: a meta-analysis. *JAMA*. 2010;304(4):443–451.
- Wong CL, Holroyd-Leduc J, Simel DL, et al. Does this patient have delirium? Value of beside instruments. *JAMA*. 2010;304(7):779–786.

CHAPTER 37—SLEEP PROBLEMS

KEY POINTS

- Comorbid psychiatric and/or medical conditions (rather than aging alone) are largely responsible for the increased prevalence of insomnia in older adults.
- Compared with younger adults, older adults generally take longer to fall asleep and have more nighttime wakefulness and more daytime napping. An earlier bedtime and earlier wake time are also common.
- Older adults also have less N3, or slow-wave, sleep (which is the deeper stage of sleep) than younger adults.
- The appropriate treatment of sleep problems must be guided by knowledge of likely causes and potential contributing factors.
- Several trials, meta-analyses, and guidelines recommend behavioral interventions (eg, cognitive-behavioral therapy for insomnia) as first-line treatment for chronic insomnia in older adults.

Sleep problems are common among older adults, particularly those with other psychiatric and medical conditions. More than two-thirds of older adults with multiple comorbidities have sleep problems. The most common sleep complaints among community-dwelling older adults are difficulty falling asleep (around 40%), nighttime awakening (30%), early morning awakening (20%), and daytime sleepiness (20%). At least one-half of community-dwelling older adults use OTC and/or prescription sleeping medications.

EPIDEMIOLOGY

Epidemiologic studies in older adults have demonstrated an association between sleep complaints and risk factors for sleep disturbance (eg, chronic illness, multiple medical problems, mood disturbance, less physical activity, physical disability) but little association with older age, suggesting that these risk factors, rather than aging per se, account for much of the increase in insomnia with age. However, certain sleep disorders do increase in prevalence with age, such as sleep-related breathing disorders (ie, sleep apnea), periodic limb movement disorder, restless legs syndrome, and circadian rhythm sleep disorders.

Insomnia is more common in women than in men across the life span (SOE=A). A meta-analysis of several epidemiologic studies from around the world found a risk ratio for insomnia in women compared with men that increased from young adulthood (risk ratio [RR]=1.28) to older age (RR=1.73). Self-reported sleeping difficulties are more common in older black Americans, particularly women and those with depression and chronic illness.

Late-life insomnia is often a chronic problem. In one British study, more than one-third of older adults with insomnia reported persistent severe symptoms at 4-year follow-up, and one-third of participants who reported use of prescription hypnotics were still using these agents 4 years later. Even among very old women (≥85 years old), there is evidence that more than 80% report sleeping difficulties, and many regularly use alcohol and/or OTC sleeping agents for sleep. Studies in the United States suggest that around 5% of older adults use sedative hypnotics on a daily basis. Insomnia has been reported as a predictor of death and nursing-home placement (particularly in older men). In addition, in several epidemiologic studies, subjective sleep disturbance was associated with worse health-related quality of life in older adults (SOE=B).

CHANGES IN SLEEP WITH AGING

In general, older adults have decreased sleep efficiency (time asleep divided by time spent awake in bed), stable or decreased total sleep time, and increased sleep latency (time to fall asleep) (Table 37.1). Older adults also report an earlier bedtime and earlier morning awakening, more awakenings during the night, more wakefulness during the night, and more daytime napping. Notable age-related changes in sleep structure as measured by polysomnography include changes in both nonrapid eye movement (NREM) and rapid eye movement (REM) sleep. Older adults have less N3, or slow-wave, sleep, which is the deeper stage of sleep, while the percentage of stage N1 and N2 sleep (the lighter stages of sleep) increases with age. The decline in slow-wave sleep begins in early adulthood and progresses throughout life, with a notable decline in middle age. Men have more decline in slow-wave sleep than women. Changes in REM sleep with age are less clear, but a decrease in REM sleep and an earlier onset of REM sleep in the night (ie, shorter REM latency) have been reported. Older adults also have a decrease in sleep spindles and K complexes on electroencephalography during sleep. In addition, older adults can have an advance in circadian rhythms of sleep and wake (ie, go to bed earlier, wake up earlier) and a reduced amplitude in circadian rhythms.

Most experts believe that the decreased sleep in older adults is due to a decreased *ability* to sleep, rather than a decreased *need* for sleep. However, after a period

Table 37.1–Age-Related Changes in Sleep

Sleep Characteristic	Age-Related Change*
Total sleep time	Decrease
Sleep latency (time to fall asleep)	Increase or no change
Sleep efficiency (time asleep over time in bed)	Decrease
Daytime napping	Increase
Stages N1 and N2	Increase
Slow-wave sleep (Stage N3)	Decrease
Percent rapid eye movement (REM)	Decrease
Wake after sleep onset	Increase

*Many seen by middle age

of sleep deprivation, older adults show less daytime sleepiness, less evidence of decline in performance measures, and a quicker recovery of normal sleep structure than younger people. Older adults have more sleep disturbance with jet lag and shift work, which may reflect physiologic changes in circadian rhythm with age. In studies comparing good sleepers with poor sleepers, poor sleepers were found to take more medications, make more clinician visits, and have poorer self-ratings of health. In addition, as noted above, among older adults chronologic age per se does not seem to correlate with higher prevalence of poor sleep.

EVALUATION OF SLEEP

Symptoms of sleep disturbance in older adults can be identified with simple screening questions, such as asking whether the person is satisfied with their sleep, whether sleep or fatigue interferes with daytime activities, and whether a bed partner or others complain of unusual behavior during sleep, such as snoring, interrupted breathing, or leg movements. Having the patient keep a sleep log for 1–2 weeks can be helpful in obtaining a careful description of the sleep complaint. Each morning, the patient should record the time they went to bed the prior night, the estimated amount of sleep, the number of awakenings, the time of morning awakening, when they got out of bed for the day, and any symptoms that occurred during the night. Any medications or other agents taken for sleep and time spent napping during the day should also be recorded. The patient's sleep log should be supplemented by information from a bed partner (if available) or from others who may have observed unusual symptoms during the night. Examples of sleep logs and validated sleep questionnaires are available in the literature. The focused physical examination depends on evidence from the history. For example, reports of painful joints should be followed by a careful examination of the affected areas. Reports of nocturia that disrupts sleep should be followed by evaluation for cardiac, renal, or prostatic disease, or diabetes mellitus. Mental status testing should also be considered, with a focus on memory and mood problems, particularly depression. The findings of the history and physical examination should guide laboratory testing.

Polysomnography is indicated when a sleep-related breathing disorder (sleep apnea) or narcolepsy is suspected, or when there are symptoms of violent or injurious behaviors during sleep (SOE=A). Polysomnography may be indicated when other unusual behaviors occur during sleep or if periodic limb movement disorder is suspected (SOE=B). Portable sleep monitoring systems for use in the home have been developed and are used primarily when sleep apnea is suspected. Wrist activity monitors (ie, wrist actigraphy) estimate sleep versus wakefulness based on wrist movement. Wrist actigraphy can be used in identifying circadian rhythm disorders (SOE=A) and in nursing-home residents, in whom traditional sleep monitoring can be difficult to obtain (SOE=B).

COMMON SLEEP PROBLEMS

Insomnia

Insomnia is defined as difficulty in falling or staying asleep, waking up too early, or experiencing sleep that is nonrestorative or poor in quality. To meet diagnostic criteria for insomnia, these symptoms must be associated with daytime impairment (such as fatigue, poor concentration, daytime sleepiness, or concerns about sleep). The prevalence of insomnia increases from about 10% in young adulthood to about 30% in those ≥65 years old. However, the prevalence of insomnia symptoms is even greater than the prevalence of insomnia using strict diagnostic criteria. Much of the increase in insomnia seen with older age seems to occur by middle age. In older adults in particular, insomnia is generally seen with other conditions, and older adults with insomnia are more likely to have medical and/or psychiatric illness than good sleepers. As mentioned previously, some evidence suggests that much of the increase in insomnia prevalence with older age is due to comorbid insomnia. Other risk factors for insomnia include female gender, social isolation, low socioeconomic status, and more medications.

Some studies report that an associated psychiatric disorder is present in 30%–60% of patients presenting with insomnia. Depression is the most common and the most strongly associated comorbid psychiatric illness with insomnia, and most patients with depression also have sleep complaints. Common sleep complaints with depression include early morning awakening, increased sleep latency, and more nighttime wakefulness. Chronic insomnia is a risk factor for development of major depressive disorder in older (and younger) adults, and studies suggest that insomnia symptoms commonly precede the onset of depressive symptoms. In depressed older adults with sleep disturbance, treatment of depression can improve sleep complaints. Conversely, lack of attention to sleep complaints in older depressed adults can make depression less likely to respond to treatment. See also "Depression and Other Mood Disorders," p 308. After depression, anxiety disorder is the psychiatric condition most commonly associated with insomnia symptoms, particularly difficulty falling asleep and early awakening. See also "Anxiety Disorders," p 319. Caregiving is also associated with insomnia, and older caregivers report more sleep complaints than do noncaregivers of similar age. In one study, nearly 40% of older women who were family caregivers of adults with dementia reported taking a sleeping medication in the past month. See also caregiving in "Psychosocial Issues," p 18; "Community-Based Care," p 166; and "Mistreatment of Older Adults," p 97.

Many medical problems are associated with insomnia in older adults. Epidemiologic studies in older adults suggest a greater prevalence of insomnia in those with conditions such as hypertension, heart disease, arthritis, lung disease, gastroesophageal reflux, stroke, neurodegenerative disorders (eg, dementia, Parkinson disease), and other comorbid conditions. Common symptoms of medical illness that can contribute to sleep disturbance (particularly nighttime awakening) include pain, paresthesias, cough, nocturnal dyspnea, gastroesophageal reflux, and nighttime urination. In older adults with sleeping difficulties who describe pain at night, the painful condition should be assessed and managed (see "Persistent Pain," p 119). Nighttime urination is common in both older men and women, and may be associated with insomnia and increased fatigue in the daytime.

Many medications can contribute to insomnia in older adults. Sleep can be impaired by diuretics or stimulating agents (eg, caffeine, sympathomimetics, bronchodilators, activating psychiatric medications) taken near bedtime. Some antidepressants, antiparkinson agents, antihypertensives (eg, propranolol), and cholinesterase inhibitors can induce nightmares and impair sleep. Required medications that are sedating (eg, sedating antidepressants) should be given at bedtime if possible. Chronic use of sedatives can cause light, fragmented sleep. For some sleeping medications, chronic use can lead to tolerance and the potential for increasing dosages. When chronic use of hypnotics is suddenly stopped, rebound insomnia can occur. Alcohol abuse is associated with lighter sleep of shorter duration. In addition, some older adults try to treat their sleeping difficulties with alcohol. Although nighttime alcohol causes an initial drowsiness, it can impair sleep later in the night. Finally, sedatives and alcohol can worsen sleep apnea; the use of these respiratory depressants should be avoided in older adults with documented or suspected untreated sleep apnea. See also "Addictions," p 336.

Sleep-Related Breathing Disorders

Sleep-related breathing disorders are characterized by disordered respiration during sleep. Central sleep apnea (CSA) syndromes are those in which respiratory effort is absent because of CNS or cardiac dysfunction. Obstructive sleep apnea (OSA) is characterized by an obstruction in the airway resulting in continued breathing effort but inadequate ventilation. In-laboratory polysomnography is the gold standard for diagnosis of these conditions (SOE=A). Portable devices that combine oximetry with additional measures (eg, heart rate, respiratory effort, nasal airflow) have shown some promise in diagnosing OSA in the home, but debate remains regarding the most appropriate use of these devices. These devices are less expensive, and monitoring can be performed more readily than in a sleep laboratory. The sensitivity of home testing is far lower than that of laboratory polysomnography (SOE=B).

In adults, CSA can be a primary disorder, secondary to neurodegenerative disease or stroke, or more commonly, the Cheynes-Stokes breathing pattern of heart failure. CSA is more common in older adults than in younger adults. Treatment of Cheynes-Stokes respiration focuses on management of the heart failure. The role of continuous positive-airway pressure (CPAP) in treatment of patients with CSA and heart failure is under debate, but evidence suggests that CPAP may improve survival if treatment is titrated to achieve improvement in the apnea–hypopnea index (AHI), but CPAP does not improve survival if AHI is not adequately treated (SOE=B). Nighttime oxygen supplementation can reduce the apnea and oxygen desaturation, but effects on important health outcomes are unclear (SOE=C).

OSA is common among older adults, but reported prevalence varies considerably. Patients with OSA usually present with excessive daytime sleepiness and may be unaware of their frequent arousals at night. Patients can have morning headache, personality changes, poor memory, confusion, and irritability. A bed partner may report loud snoring, cessation of breathing, and choking sounds during sleep. Patients are generally obese, but there is less association between obesity and OSA in older age. Other reported predictors identified in community-dwelling older adults include falling asleep at inappropriate times, male gender, and napping. OSA should be considered in patients with treatment-resistant hypertension. The classic sleep apnea patient is the obese, sleepy snorer with hypertension. However, obesity is less commonly associated with OSA in older adults, and many older OSA patients have a normal BMI. Large neck circumference has also been reported as a marker for sleep apnea in middle-aged adults but may not be a significant predictor of sleep apnea in older adults. Alcohol abuse and dependence is an important risk factor for sleep apnea, and sleep-disordered breathing is a significant contributor to sleep disturbance in men >40 years old with a history of alcoholism. Finally, there appears to be an association between sleep apnea and dementia. Of note, evidence suggests that OSA patients with mild-moderate dementia tolerate CPAP well, with acceptable adherence to treatment, improvement in OSA parameters, and some evidence of beneficial effects on cognition (SOE=B).

OSA is a treatable condition that is associated with cardiovascular disease, including hypertension, stroke, myocardial ischemia, arrhythmias, fatal and nonfatal cardiovascular events, and all-cause mortality (SOE=A). OSA is also associated with motor vehicle accidents (SOE=A), and there is mixed evidence for a relationship with cognitive impairment (SOE=B). The importance of mild degrees of sleep-disordered breathing in older adults is unclear. In one study, no association was found between mild or moderate sleep-disordered breathing and subjective sleep-wake disturbance. The long-term consequences of asymptomatic sleep-disordered breathing in older adults are also unclear.

Patients suspected of having OSA should be referred to a sleep laboratory for evaluation and, if the diagnosis is documented, treatment. As mentioned above, portable in-home monitoring devices are also available. CPAP reduces sleepiness and improves quality of life in people with moderate and severe OSA (SOE=A). Older adults are likely to tolerate CPAP as well as younger adults. Careful efforts to use devices (eg, variations in mask, humidification) that improve comfort can improve adherence with CPAP. Early successful adherence with CPAP can predict long-term adherence with CPAP treatment. Unfortunately, clinicians may not recommend CPAP in older adults, perhaps because they assume that the treatment will not be tolerated or successful in this population.

Other mechanical options are available as alternatives to CPAP, eg, bi-level PAP (biPAP), which reduces expiratory pressure in an effort to increase comfort). Evidence suggests that biPAP does not improve efficacy or adherence in the treatment of sleep apnea compared with CPAP (SOE=B), but these alternative devices can be appropriate in certain patients. Oral appliances are also available, but CPAP is more effective in improving OSA. Oral appliances are generally recommended only in patients with mild symptomatic OSA or in those unwilling or unable to tolerate CPAP (SOE=B). Several upper airway surgical approaches have also been used, but evidence of effectiveness from large trials is limited.

Periodic Limb Movements During Sleep and Restless Legs Syndrome

Periodic limb movements during sleep (PLMS) is a condition of repetitive, stereotypic leg movements that generally occur in non-REM sleep. PLMS increases in prevalence with age, but the significance of this is unclear, because many studies have found little relationship between PLMS and sleep disruption. In one study, evidence of PLMS was found in more than one-third of community-dwelling older adults. Some authors have suggested that the high prevalence of PLMS with age is associated with delayed motor and sensory latencies noted on nerve conduction testing. When PLMS is associated with clinical sleep disturbance or a complaint of daytime fatigue that is not better explained by another sleep disorder, this is termed periodic limb movement disorder (PLMD). Polysomnography is required to establish a diagnosis of PLMD.

Restless legs syndrome (RLS) is a condition of an uncontrollable urge to move one's legs at night, usually accompanied by an uncomfortable and unpleasant sensation of the legs that worsens with inactivity and improves with movement. The symptoms occur while the person is awake, and symptoms can also involve the arms. The diagnosis is based on the patient's description of the symptoms; polysomnography is not required to make the diagnosis. There may be a family history of the condition (particularly in patients with an earlier age onset of RLS) and, in some cases, an underlying medical disorder (eg, anemia, or renal or neurologic disease). RLS is 1.5 times more common in women than men, and evidence suggests that RLS prevalence increases with age. PLMS occurs in most (80%–90%) patients with RLS, but the presence of PLMS is not specific for RLS. RLS can also be seen in patients with dementia, in which the patient may not be able to adequately describe the symptoms. RLS should be considered in dementia patients who have symptoms such as rubbing or massaging of legs, increased motor activity (eg, pacing, wandering), and evidence of leg discomfort that occurs in the evening and/or with inactivity; and shows improvement with movement of the legs. Many medications can aggravate or induce RLS symptoms, such as antiemetics, antipsychotics, SSRIs, tricyclic antidepressants, and diphenhydramine. These and other medications should be addressed in patients with new or worsening RLS.

If pharmacologic treatment for PLMD or RLS is indicated (because of severity of symptoms or significant effects on quality of life), dopaminergic agents are the initial agent of choice. An evening dose of a dopamine agonist (eg, pramipexole or ropinirole, about 1–2 hours before bedtime) is effective in the treatment of RLS and PLMD (SOE=A). A nighttime dose of carbidopa-levodopa^{OL} may also be effective (SOE=A) and can be used for patients who need medication infrequently (ie, for as-needed use). However, some patients describe a shift of their symptoms to daytime hours with successful treatment of symptoms at night; this problem (termed augmentation) appears more frequently with use of carbidopa-levodopa as treatment for RLS. RLS can be associated with iron deficiency, in which case RLS symptoms can improve with iron replacement therapy (SOE=B). Patients with RLS should be screened for iron deficiency. Of course, the cause of the iron deficiency should also be addressed. Gabapentin^{OL} can also be effective (SOE=B), particularly in patients who cannot tolerate dopamine agonists. Benzodiazepines^{OL} and opioids^{OL} have also been used for RLS but likely have more adverse events than the dopaminergic agents in older adults.

Circadian Rhythm Sleep Disorders

Disturbances in circadian rhythms of the sleep-wake cycle may be more common with advanced age. In particular, older adults are more likely to have an advanced sleep phase (fall asleep early and awaken early) rather than a delayed sleep phase (fall asleep late and awaken late), but a delayed sleep phase can be seen in older adults. Some individuals have extremely irregular sleep-wake cycles, including some patients with dementia and nursing-home residents. Some common changes in sleep pattern seen in older adults (such as increased daytime napping and disrupted nighttime sleep) can be due to alterations in circadian rhythm. Dementia is associated with sleep-wake disturbance and frequent nighttime awakenings, nighttime wandering, and nighttime agitation.

A sleep log can help establish the presence of a circadian rhythm sleep disorder (SOE=B). Wrist actigraphy can also be useful for making a diagnosis (particularly in patients who are unable to complete a sleep log) and in monitoring treatment response in patients with a circadian rhythm sleep disorder (SOE=B), including older patients with dementia and nursing-home residents. Polysomnography is not routinely indicated in patients in whom a circadian rhythm sleep disorder is suspected, but referral to a sleep specialist may be indicated when symptoms do not respond to initial management, when the diagnosis is unclear, or when another sleep disorder is suspected (SOE=C). Treatment depends on the particular circadian rhythm sleep disorder. An advanced sleep phase may respond to appropriately timed (ie, evening) exposure to bright light (SOE=B) (see nonpharmacologic interventions, p 291). A delayed sleep phase may respond to appropriately timed morning bright light or evening melatonin, or both (SOE=B).

REM Sleep Behavior Disorder

REM sleep behavior disorder is characterized by excessive motor activities associated with dream enactment behavior during sleep and a pathologic absence of normal muscle atonia during REM sleep. The presenting symptoms are usually vigorous sleep behaviors associated with vivid dreams, and patients may first present because of injuries (to themselves or their bed partner). The condition can be acute or chronic, and it is much more common in older men (in some series, >85% of cases are older men). There may be a family predisposition. Transient REM sleep behavior disorder has been associated with toxic metabolic abnormalities, primarily drug or alcohol withdrawal or intoxication. The chronic form of the disorder can be idiopathic but is increasingly recognized as associated with neurodegenerative disorders such as Parkinson disease, Lewy body dementia, multisystem atrophy, and other conditions. Several psychiatric medications have been associated with REM sleep behavior disorder, including tricyclic antidepressants, monoamine oxidase inhibitors, fluoxetine, venlafaxine, cholinesterase inhibitors, and other agents. Polysomnography is indicated to establish the diagnosis. Removal of the offending agent is indicated for drug-induced REM sleep behavior disorder. Clonazepam^{OL} is reported to be effective for treatment of REM sleep behavior disorder, with little evidence of tolerance or abuse over long periods of treatment, but some patients (especially older adults) can experience adverse events from this agent. There is some evidence for the use of melatonin in the treatment of REM sleep behavior disorder in individuals with coexisting neurodegenerative disorders (eg, Parkinson disease, dementia with Lewy bodies) (SOE=C). Environmental safety interventions are also indicated, such as removing dangerous objects from the bedroom, putting cushions on the floor around the bed, protecting windows, and in some cases, putting the mattress on the floor.

CHANGES IN SLEEP WITH DEMENTIA

Older adults with dementia have more sleep disruption and arousals, lower sleep efficiency, a higher percentage of stage N1 sleep, and more sleep fragmentation than nondemented older adults. Circadian rhythm sleep disorders are more common with dementia, resulting in excessive daytime sleeping and nighttime wakefulness. Cholinesterase inhibitors (often used in treatment of the symptoms of dementia) can exacerbate insomnia and cause vivid dreams; changing dose timing to morning hours can help alleviate this problem. Sedative-hypnotic agents have not been adequately tested in patients with dementia. As mentioned above, evidence suggests that those with coexisting OSA and mild to moderate dementia can tolerate CPAP well, with improvement in OSA parameters and beneficial effects on cognition. Results of studies using melatonin for sleep disturbance in dementia have been mixed, but results of one large randomized controlled trial in patients with Alzheimer disease suggested melatonin was not effective for sleep disturbance in these individuals (SOE=B). Bright light therapy has also been used in dementia patients, with some beneficial effects on sleep and circadian rhythms (SOE=B), but the most appropriate timing of the light exposure is unclear.

Sleep Disturbances in the Hospital

Acute hospitalization can precipitate transient or short-term insomnia. This insomnia is likely multifactorial in origin and related to illness, medications, change from usual nighttime routines at home, and a sleep-disruptive hospital environment (eg, high noise levels at night). In one small uncontrolled study, nighttime melatonin levels increased in hospitalized older patients treated with daytime bright-light exposure. Another small study implemented "flexible medication times" that allowed inpatients to sleep longer in the morning, and their resulting in-hospital sleeping patterns were more similar to their at-home sleeping patterns. However, adherence with nonpharmacologic interventions can be difficult to achieve in the acute hospital. For example, one large clinical trial of nonpharmacologic interventions to prevent delirium in hospitalized older adults reported only a 10% adherence rate for the sleep protocol portion of the intervention. In a large study that tested the feasibility of a nonpharmacologic sleep protocol (consisting of a back rub, warm drink, and relaxation tapes) for hospitalized older adults administered by nurses, the use of sedative hypnotic medications was successfully reduced; the sleep protocol had a stronger association with improved quality of sleep than the sedative-hypnotic medications.

Sleeping medications are commonly prescribed in hospitalized older adults. A large Belgian study of consecutively admitted patients at a university hospital found that 45% of patients took a sleeping medication while in the hospital, with greater use among patients ≥60 years old. In this sample, >15% of patients who were newly prescribed a sleeping pill while in the hospital reported that they planned to use the medication after discharge to home. In another study of hospitalized older adults in India, among those prescribed a benzodiazepine for sleep during their acute hospitalization, over half were not taking a sleeping pill before their admission. Unfortunately, clear guidelines are not available to guide the choice of a sleeping medication for hospitalized older adults. Benzodiazepine receptor agonists are commonly used for insomnia in this setting, but prescribers should remember to try use of smaller dosages (than those used for younger adults) first, which are likely effective and safer in older adults. Sedating antihistamines (eg, diphenhydramine) should not be used as a sleep aid in hospitalized older adults because of possible complications related to anticholinergic adverse events (eg, delirium, urinary retention, constipation).

Sleep-related breathing disorders can be common in hospitalized adults, particularly among those with cardiac illness and stroke. In one study of older men on medicine wards in a Veterans Affairs hospital, survival among patients with heart failure and CSA was shorter than among heart failure patients without evidence of this disorder. Sleep apnea among stroke patients is associated with worse survival and less functional recovery. Sleep apnea patients should continue their use of CPAP when hospitalized, particularly when sedating and narcotic medications are used and in the peri- and postoperative period.

Sleep in the Nursing Home

Nursing-home residents often have marked sleep disruption, frequent nighttime awakening, and excessive daytime sleeping. In one study, up to 70% of caregivers reported that nighttime difficulties played a significant role in their decision to institutionalize the older adult, often because the sleep of the caregiver was being disrupted. Once in the nursing home, many residents nap on and off throughout the day and wake up frequently during the night. One study found that 65% of residents reported problems with their sleep and that the use of hypnotic medications was common, but no association was found between the use of sedative hypnotics and the presence, absence, or change in sleep complaints after 6 months of follow-up. In another study, the average duration of sleep episodes during the night in nursing-home residents was only 20 minutes. Nursing-home residents generally have little or no exposure to outdoor bright light, which likely exacerbates sleep-wake abnormalities. Other common conditions in nursing-home residents that can contribute to sleep disturbance include multiple physical illnesses, the use of psychoactive medications, debility and inactivity, increased prevalence of sleep disorders, and environmental factors (eg, nighttime noise, light, disruptive nursing care).

Recent evidence suggests that sleep disturbance is also common among older adults in assisted-living facilities. One prospective, observational cohort study found that sleep disturbance was common in this population, and subjective and/or objective evidence of sleep disturbance was associated with more symptoms of depression, decline in functional status, and worse health-related quality of life over 6 months of follow-up.

MANAGEMENT OF SLEEP PROBLEMS

Treatment of sleep problems in older adults must be guided by knowledge of likely causes and potential contributing factors. Sedative hypnotics have a documented association with falls, hip fracture, and daytime carryover symptoms of sedation in older adults. However, there is also some evidence that untreated insomnia symptoms are associated with increased risk of falls in older adults. If the initial history and physical examination do not suggest a serious underlying cause of the sleep problem, a trial of improved sleep habits (eg, sleep hygiene techniques) is usually the best first approach and may improve mild symptoms of insomnia (Table 37.2), but more intensive behavioral treatment (as described below) is indicated for the treatment of chronic insomnia. If the person takes daytime naps, it is important to determine whether these are needed rest periods or due to inactivity, boredom, or sedating medications. It is important to explain that daytime naps will decrease nighttime sleep.

Short-term hypnotic therapy may be appropriate in cases of transient, situational insomnia, particularly during bereavement, acute hospitalization, and other periods of temporary acute stress. Sedative-hypnotic medication treatment should not be withheld in situations when it is clearly indicated. People generally do not feel well if they do not sleep well. If a decision is reached to use a sedative-hypnotic in an older adult, the smallest dosage of the agent with the least risk of adverse events should be chosen. However, in older adults with chronic insomnia, sedative-hypnotic agents should be used cautiously because of the complications associated with their long-term use (see chronic hypnotic use, p 293). The chronic use of benzodiazepines can lead to dependence or cognitive impairment. The newer, nonbenzodiazepine hypnotics have been tested in healthy older adults and seem to have less risk of daytime carryover and tolerance to sedative effects. However, there has been little study of these (or other hypnotic) agents in older adults with significant medical comorbidity.

Table 37.2—Measures to Improve Sleep Hygiene

- Maintain regular rising time.
- Maintain regular bed time, but do not go to bed unless sleepy.
- Decrease or eliminate naps, unless necessary rest period.
- Exercise daily but not immediately before bedtime.
- Do not use bed for reading or watching television.
- Relax mentally before going to sleep; do not use bedtime as worry time.
- If hungry, have a light snack (except with symptoms of gastroesophageal reflux or medical contraindications), but avoid heavy meals at bedtime.
- Limit or eliminate alcohol, caffeine, and nicotine, especially before bedtime.
- Wind down before bedtime and maintain a routine period of preparation for bed (eg, washing up, going to the bathroom).
- Control the nighttime environment with comfortable temperature, quiet, and darkness.
- Try a familiar background noise (eg, a fan or other "white noise" machine).
- Wear comfortable bed clothing.
- If unable to fall asleep within 30 minutes, get out of bed and perform soothing activity such as listening to soft music or light reading (but avoid exposure to bright light).
- Get adequate exposure to sunlight or bright light during the day.

Behavioral and Nonpharmacologic Interventions

Behavioral treatment of insomnia is effective in older adults, including those with insomnia comorbid with other conditions (SOE=A). It is important not to confuse these effective insomnia behavioral interventions with simple sleep hygiene, because sleep hygiene (when used alone) is generally not effective for chronic insomnia. For a summary of such interventions, see Table 37.3. Several systematic reviews and meta-analyses of behavioral interventions for insomnia have been published; the strongest evidence currently supports cognitive-behavioral therapy for insomnia (which generally combines stimulus control, sleep restriction, and cognitive therapy) (SOE=A). These behavioral interventions produce reliable therapeutic benefits, including improved sleep efficiency, decreased nighttime wakefulness, and greater satisfaction with sleep; treatment is also helpful in reducing chronic hypnotic use. In at least two randomized trials of older adults with insomnia that compared cognitive-behavioral therapy with a prescription sedative-hypnotic agent, participants generally reported better improvement in their sleep patterns and more satisfaction with the cognitive-behavioral therapy (than with the sedative-hypnotic), and sleep improvements were better sustained over time with behavioral treatment.

Several small studies have also tested the effectiveness of exposure to bright light (either natural sunlight or with commercially available light boxes)

Table 37.3—Examples of Nonpharmacologic Interventions to Improve Sleep

Intervention	Goal	Brief Description
Stimulus control	To recondition maladaptive sleep-related behaviors	Patient is instructed to go to bed only when sleepy, not use the bed for eating or watching television, get out of bed if unable to fall asleep, return to bed only when sleepy, get up at the same time each morning, not take naps during the day.
Sleep restriction	To improve sleep efficiency (time asleep over time in bed) by limiting time in bed	Patient first keeps a sleep diary for 1–2 weeks to determine average total daily sleep time, then stays in bed only that amount of time plus 15 minutes, gets up at same time each morning, takes no naps in the daytime, gradually increases time allowed in bed as sleep efficiency improves.
Cognitive interventions	To change misunderstandings and false beliefs regarding sleep	Patient's dysfunctional beliefs and attitudes about sleep are identified; patient is educated to change these false beliefs and attitudes, including normal changes in sleep with increased age and changes that are pathologic.
Relaxation techniques	To recognize and relieve tension and anxiety	In progressive muscle relaxation, patient is taught to tense and relax each muscle group; in electromyographic biofeedback, the patient is given feedback regarding muscle tension and learns techniques to relieve it; meditation or imagery techniques are taught to relieve racing thoughts or anxiety.
Cognitive-behavioral therapy	Combines features of several behavioral interventions	Typically combines stimulus control, sleep restriction, and cognitive interventions, with or without relaxation techniques.
Bright light	To correct circadian rhythm causes of sleeping difficulty (ie, sleep-phase problems)	Patient is exposed to sunlight or a light box. For delayed sleep phase, 2 hours early morning light; for advanced sleep phase, 2 hours evening light; light intensity ≥2,500 lux. Appropriate timing of the light exposure is important. Shorter durations may be as effective. Routine eye examination is recommended before treatment; do not use light boxes with ultraviolet exposure.

on the sleep of older adults with insomnia (SOE=B). Variable results have been reported for insomnia, with better results seen for circadian rhythm disorders. As mentioned above, appropriately timed morning bright light may be useful in delayed sleep phase, and evening exposure may be useful in older adults with an advanced sleep phase. Even short durations of bright light may be useful. One study reported beneficial effects in older adults using a visor that provided 2,000 lux to each eye worn for only 30 minutes in the evening.

There is less evidence to support other nonpharmacologic interventions for insomnia, but some patients may find these methods useful. For example, bathing before sleep may enhance the quality of sleep in older adults, perhaps related to changes in body temperature with bathing. Moderate-intensity exercise also improves sleep in healthy, sedentary adults ≥50 years old who reported moderate sleep complaints at baseline. However, strenuous exercise should not be performed immediately before bedtime, because this can interfere with sleep. Studies have also suggested beneficial effects on sleep with Tai Chi (SOE=B).

Nonpharmacologic interventions have been studied in institutional settings. In a study of institutionalized demented residents with sleep and behavior problems, morning exposure to bright light was associated with better nighttime sleep and less daytime agitation. In a study of ambient bright light therapy (2,500 lux delivered in the morning, evening, or all-day compared with standard lighting) among older adults with dementia in a psychiatric hospital and a dementia-specific residential care facility, nighttime sleep increased significantly in participants exposed to morning and all-day light, with the increase most prominent in those with severe or very severe dementia. In another study of residents with dementia and behavioral problems, social interaction with nurses reduced behavioral problems and sleep-wake rhythm disorders in some residents. In another small trial in the nursing home, nighttime sleep increased and agitation decreased among residents randomized to receive a daytime physical activity program plus nighttime intervention to decrease noise and light disruption. In another trial that combined an enforced schedule of structured social and physical activity for 2 weeks in a small sample of assisted-living residents, treated residents had enhanced slow-wave sleep and improved performance in memory-oriented tasks. Two large multicomponent nonpharmacologic interventions on sleep in nursing-home residents had mixed results, with greatest effects on decreasing daytime sleeping but little effect on nighttime sleep (SOE=B).

Pharmacotherapy

Pharmacotherapy is generally considered in individuals with transient sleep problems, such as problems associated with an acute stressor, or in individuals with chronic insomnia that has not responded to behavioral therapy. As mentioned above, if a decision is made to use a sedative hypnotic in an older adult, the smallest dosage of an agent with the least risk of adverse events should be chosen and used for the shortest duration necessary. Short-acting sedative-hypnotic agents are recommended for patients with problems falling asleep, and intermediate-acting agents are recommended for patients with problems staying asleep (Table 37.4).

Benzodiazepines (eg, the intermediate-acting agents estazolam and temazepam) bind nonselectively to the gamma-aminobutyric-acid-benzodiazepine (GABA-BZ) receptor subunits. As a class, these agents have potential adverse events, including confusion, rebound insomnia, tolerance (to treatment effects), and withdrawal symptoms on discontinuation. Older adults can be more sensitive to the sedating effects of benzodiazepines, with greater risk of confusion and falls (SOE=B). Long-acting benzodiazepines (eg, flurazepam, quazepam), in particular, should not be used in older adults. Short-acting agents appear to have less association with falls and hip fractures, presumably due to less daytime carryover, but at least one study demonstrated an association of short-acting agents with falls at night (SOE=B). However, agents with rapid elimination in general also result in the most pronounced rebound and withdrawal syndromes after discontinuation. Rebound insomnia after discontinuation of short-acting agents is dose dependent and can be reduced by tapering the dosage before discontinuing the drug.

The nonbenzodiazepine-benzodiazepine receptor agonists (NBRAs [ie, nonbenzodiazepines such as eszopiclone, zolpidem, zaleplon]) are structurally unrelated to benzodiazepines but bind to the GABA-BZ receptor with relative selectivity for sedative and amnestic properties. These agents also have a relatively shorter duration of action than benzodiazepines with less risk of daytime carryover of sedating effects (SOE=B). Evidence suggests that NBRAs are relatively well tolerated in healthy older adults (SOE=B), but evidence is limited in older adults with significant comorbidity. Zolpidem is a nonbenzodiazepine imidazopyridine. In older adults, studies suggest that zolpidem does not result in rebound insomnia, agitation, or anxiety when discontinued; does not seem to result in impaired daytime performance on cognitive and psychomotor performance tests; and can have a therapeutic effect that outlasts the period of drug treatment. Zaleplon is a nonbenzodiazepine hypnotic from the pyrazolopyrimidine class, which has also been studied for short-term use in older adults with insomnia. Because of their rapid onset of action, zolpidem and zaleplon should be taken only immediately before bedtime or after the individual has gone to bed and has been unable to fall asleep. Eszopiclone is an s-isomer of the cyclopyrrolone zopiclone, and it has a longer duration of action than the other nonbenzodiazepines. In the United States, eszopiclone and extended-release zolpidem are approved for long-term use. Guidelines recommend that zolpidem (regular release) or zaleplon, like benzodiazepines, be used only short term (2–3 weeks) and that, if used longer, these agents be used no more than 2 or 3 nights per week. Concerns remain regarding the risks of confusion, falls, and fracture with chronic use of NBRAs in older adults (particularly those who are frail), and caution is warranted even with these newer agents.

The melatonin receptor agonist ramelteon does not act at GABA receptors; rather it is a selective MT1/MT2 receptor agonist. Ramelteon reduces sleep latency and increases total sleep time in older adults (SOE=B), without evidence of significant rebound or withdrawal effects with discontinuation.

The tricyclic antidepressant doxepin, which has been available for decades, is now available in a low-dose formulation (3–6 mg) that is approved for the treatment of insomnia characterized by problems with sleep maintenance (SOE=B). At low dosages, doxepin selectively antagonizes H_1 receptors, which is believed to promote the onset and maintenance of sleep. Low dosages of other sedating antidepressants such as trazodone^OL^ or mirtazapine^OL^ at bedtime have been used as sleeping aids for many years, but there is limited evidence to support this practice (SOE=D). Sedating antidepressants have been suggested for use at low dosages as a nighttime aid for sleep in depressed patients receiving another antidepressant at therapeutic dosages during the daytime. Other indications include patients with a history of psychoactive substance use problems, lack of response to other sleeping medications, suspected untreated sleep apnea (in which further respiratory depression is a concern), and fibromyalgia (when there is some evidence of antidepressant medication treatment effect). However, the adverse effects of sedating antidepressants may limit their usefulness.

Sedating antipsychotics should not be used in the routine management of insomnia in older adults without serious psychiatric illness. Sedating antipsychotics^OL^ are sometimes used for sleep complaints in patients with other serious psychiatric conditions that warrant treatment with an antipsychotic medication.

Chronic Hypnotic Use

In European studies, a relatively high prevalence of chronic sedative hypnotic use in older adults (5%–8% in older men, up to 25% in older women) has been reported. There is strong epidemiologic evidence for increased morbidity and mortality with chronic use of prescription sleeping pills; however, much of this literature is older and predates the availability of newer, nonbenzodiazepine hypnotics, so the relationship between the newer hypnotics and morbidity/mortality is not clear. In addition, after tolerance to hypnotics develops, long-term use of these agents can actually

Table 37.4—Prescription Medications Commonly Used for Insomnia in Older Adults

Class, Medication	Starting Dose (mg)	Usual Dose (mg)	Half-life (hours)	Comments
Intermediate-acting benzodiazepine				
Temazepam	7.5	7.5–30	8.8	Psychomotor impairment, increased risk of falls
Short-acting nonbenzodiazepines				
Eszopiclone	1	1–2	6	Reportedly effective for long-term use in selected individuals; may be associated with unpleasant taste, headache; avoid administration with high-fat meal
Zaleplon (a pyrazolopyrimidine)	5	5–10	1 (reportedly unchanged in older adults)	Reportedly little daytime carryover, tolerance, or rebound insomnia
Zolpidem (an imidazopyridine)	5	5	1.5–4.5 (3 in older adults, 10 in hepatic cirrhosis)	Reportedly little daytime carryover, tolerance, or rebound insomnia
Melatonin receptor agonist				
Ramelteon	8	8	1.5 (2.6 in older adults)	Dizziness, myalgia, headache, other adverse events reported; no significant rebound insomnia or withdrawal with discontinuation
Sedating antidepressants				
Doxepin	3	3–6	15.3 (doxepin); 31 (metabolite)	Somnolence/sedation, nausea, and upper respiratory tract infection reported; antagonizes central H_1 receptors (antihistamine); active metabolite; should not be taken within 3 hours of a meal
Mirtazapine^{OL}	7.5	7.5–45	31–39 in older adults; 13–34 in younger adults; mean = 21	Increased appetite, weight gain, headache, dizziness, daytime carryover; used for insomnia with depression
Trazodone^{OL}	25–50	25–150	Reportedly 6 ± 2; prolonged in older adults and obese individuals	Moderate orthostatic effects; administration after food minimizes sedation and postural hypotension; used for insomnia with depression

make sleep quality worse. Data reported from a longitudinal study of older adults in Germany indicated a higher rate of sleep-related complaints in those who took sleeping medications than in those who did not.

Several studies have shown that the bulk of prescription sleeping medication use occurs among chronic users, and not those with transient sleeping difficulties. In a study in Spain, long-term use was 2–3 times more common in older adults than in middle-aged respondents. In studies in Canada and France, sleep-promoting medications were prescribed for ≥1 year in more than two-thirds of people who were taking these agents. Studies in the United States have also demonstrated more benzodiazepine use by older adults and by women, with chronic use being more common in older adults.

Methods to help older chronic hypnotic users reduce or eliminate their use of these agents have been reported (SOE=B). In general, tapering of the hypnotic in chronic users is necessary to prevent rebound insomnia and other adverse withdrawal effects. One reported strategy involved decreasing the hypnotic dose by one-half for 2 weeks, followed by full withdrawal (perhaps with the use of a substitute pill at night), which was effective in eliminating hypnotic use without adverse events on nighttime sleep, depressive symptoms, or daytime sleepiness. In another small controlled trial in which benzodiazepine use was tapered to complete withdrawal over as many as 6 weeks, more success was seen in those participants randomized to receive a nightly dose of 2 mg of controlled-release melatonin rather than placebo. At follow-up 6 months later, nearly 80% of those who successfully discontinued benzodiazepines continued to report good sleep quality. Cognitive-behavioral therapy, when combined with gradual tapering of the hypnotic dose, has also been demonstrated to be helpful in reducing or eliminating chronic benzodiazepine use (SOE=B).

Nonprescription Sleeping Agents

Nearly half of older adults report using nonprescription OTC sleeping agents; however, there is little evidence to support this practice. Commonly used nonprescription agents include sedating antihistamines, acetaminophen, alcohol, melatonin, and herbal products. Sedating antihistamines (eg, diphenhydramine) are common ingredients in OTC sleeping agents as well as in combination analgesic-sleeping agents that are marketed for nighttime use. Diphenhydramine has potent anticholinergic effects, and tolerance to its sedating effects develops after several weeks, so it is not recommended for older adults. Individuals with mild nighttime discomfort and mild insomnia may have adequate relief with a simple pain reliever (eg, acetaminophen) at bedtime. Although alcohol causes some initial drowsiness, it can interfere with sleep later in the night and can actually worsen sleeping difficulties. Melatonin is available OTC. There is some evidence in older adults with insomnia that melatonin administration decreases sleep latency and wake time after sleep onset, and increases sleep efficiency (time asleep over time in bed), but results are mixed. However, there is evidence for effectiveness of melatonin in certain circadian rhythm sleep disorders. For example, blind people with abnormal circadian sleep-wake rhythms (eg, free-running rhythms not entrained to the external environment because of lack of light/dark perception) may correct with melatonin given at night (SOE=B). The melatonin dose in these studies has ranged from 0.5 to 10 mg, but lower doses may be most effective. Several weeks or months of treatment with nighttime melatonin may be required to correct the blind person's rhythm, and it is believed that melatonin treatment must be continued indefinitely, because the free-running rhythm will return if the melatonin is discontinued. Valerian is an herbal product with mild sedative action that has been marketed for insomnia. Its mechanism of action is uncertain, and it contains several potentially active compounds, with risk of adverse events. A systematic review found the existing evidence for efficacy of valerian to be inconclusive (SOE=C). Kava, another herbal product marketed for insomnia, has a significant risk of adverse events, including hepatotoxicity, and it is not recommended.

REFERENCES

- de Niet G, Tiemens B, Hutschemaekers G. Nursing care for sleep problems in psychiatry: is there a problem? *Br J Nurs.* 2009;18(7):429–433.
- Martin JL, Fiorentino L, Jouldjian S, et al. Sleep quality in residents of assisted living facilities: effect on quality of life, functional status, and depression. *J Am Geriatr Soc.* 2010;58(5):829–836.
- Rose KR, Beck C, Tsai PF, et al. Sleep disturbances and nocturnal agitation behaviors in older adults with dementia. *Sleep.* 2011;34(6):779–786.
- Yaffe K, Laffan AM, Harrison SL, et al. Sleep-disordered breathing, hypoxia, and risk of mild cognitive impairment and dementia in older women. *JAMA.* 2011;10;306(6):613–619.

CHAPTER 38—PRESSURE ULCERS AND WOUND CARE

KEY POINTS

- The normal wound-healing cascade comprises four phases: hemostasis, inflammatory, proliferative, and maturation.
- A pressure ulcer is defined as damage caused to skin and underlying soft tissue by unrelieved pressure when the tissue is compressed between a bony prominence and external surface over a prolonged period of time.
- Two main factors are believed to play a major role in pressure ulcer formation: pressure and shear forces. Intrinsic and extrinsic factors determine the tolerance of soft tissue to the adverse effects of pressure.
- Risk assessment and preventive strategies are required to decrease the incidence of pressure ulcers, although not all pressure ulcers are avoidable.
- The stage of an ulcer determines the appropriate treatment plan.

Wound healing is a complicated process, and it is important to understand the normal function of the wound-healing cascade regardless of the type of chronic wound (eg, pressure ulcers, venous stasis ulcers, diabetic foot ulcers, etc). Aging can affect the wound healing phases and thus delay or impede the healing process.

THE WOUND HEALING CASCADE

Hemostasis

Hemostasis is achieved when vasoconstriction of the blood vessels occurs and platelets arrive at the wound. Platelet degranulation provides the first signals that begin the wound-healing cascade. Alpha granules of the platelets contain the following growth factors: 1) platelet-derived growth factors (PDGF), 2) insulin-like growth factor-1, 3) epidermal growth factors, 4) fibroblast growth factor (FGF), and 5) transforming growth factor-β (TGF-β). These growth factors are released from platelets and leave the wound, migrating into the surrounding tissue and blood vessels. Growth factors release signals to inflammatory cells. Growth factors also stimulate production, movement, and delineation of wound cells that include epithelial cells, fibroblasts, and endothelial cells. This begins the inflammatory phase of wound healing, which is a catabolic process.

Inflammatory Phase

In the inflammatory phase, polymorphonuclear neutrophils begin the process of phagocytosis. Neutrophils release tumor necrosis factor-α (TNF-α) and the proinflammatory cytokines interleukins IL-2 and IL-4 at the site of injury. Neutrophils also release matrix metalloproteinase eight (MMP-8). MMP-8 removes the damaged extracellular matrix, which is replaced with new extracellular matrix.

Macrophages are the most important wound-healing cells, because they are involved in all phases of wound healing. Macrophages replace neutrophils in the wound and are responsible for several actions during the inflammatory phase. They initiate phagocytosis, are bactericidal, and promote angiogenesis. They also secrete more growth factors and signal for additional macrophages and monocytes to respond to the wound. They convert macromolecules into amino acids and sugars, nutrients that are necessary for wound healing. During this phase, mast cells, derived from the dermis, arrive at the site and stimulate local inflammation that increases the sensation of pain.

Proliferative Phase

Macrophages are the mediators for the start of the proliferative phase, which is initiated by the stimulation of the movement of fibroblasts, epithelial cells, and vascular endothelial cells to begin wound healing by the formation of granulation tissue. This phase is anabolic and can last for several weeks. Cell movement and production persist as a temporary matrix of fibrin and fibronectin is created. Granulation tissue provides a moist surface for cell migration and replaces the temporary matrix as it fills in the wound cavity. It contains fibroblasts, keratinocytes, macrophages, immature collagen, endothelial cells, and new blood vessels. It is very vascular and easily damaged.

The final step in the proliferative phase is the movement of keratinocytes from the epidermal layer of the wound edge into the wound to begin epithelialization. Keratinocytes form scar tissue as they travel and reproduce across the wound bed only in the presence of healthy granulation tissue. These cells synthesize TGF-β, TNF-α, and IL-1 B, all of which stimulate cell production, extracellular protein formation, and angiogenesis.

Endothelial cells promote development of new blood vessels quickly, which are necessary for nutrition for the new tissue. These cells stimulate fibrinolysis, breaking down the temporary matrix so that fibroblast movement and collagen synthesis can occur. The growth factors synthesized by endothelial cells are vascular endothelial growth factors, fibroblast growth factors, and PDGF.

Maturation Phase

The final phase of wound healing is the maturation phase or the remodeling phase. This phase can take months to years and is catabolic. Collagen fibers are the main substance in the wound, and fiber collection increases, creating a thick collagenous arrangement. Fibroblasts, matrix metalloproteinases (MMPs), tissue inhibitors of metalloproteinases (TIMPs), and TGF are vital to organizing, remodeling, and maturing of the collagen fibers. Fibroblasts stimulate production of collagen, elastin, proteoglycans, MMPs, and TIMPs. This action continues until the tensile strength of scar tissue is approximately 80% that of normal tissue. Apoptosis or programmed cell death decrease fibroblast and capillary density. The quality of scar tissue decreases, and the scar becomes less red and flat over time; this is known as remodeling of the scar.

As a person ages, wounds heal more slowly and can become chronic because of a delayed inflammatory phase when one or more chronic diseases are present. This can be attributed to changes within the wound-healing cascade, as well as to the influence of chronic disease and medications that affect tissue perfusion. Malnutrition and infection contribute to slower rates of wound healing in older adults.

The lack of tissue perfusion can significantly affect the rate of wound healing. Diagnoses such as anemia, diabetes, cardiovascular disease, hypotension, COPD, low blood protein levels, high temperature, and smoking can increase demand for oxygen and the metabolic rate. Microvascular changes in the circulatory system in diabetic patients also reduce tissue perfusion.

The use of corticosteroids can impede regeneration of the epidermis and collagen synthesis. Antibiotics, corticosteroids, and hormones can change the skin's protective barrier function. The inflammatory response is affected by other medications such as analgesics, antihistamines, and NSAIDs. Chemotherapeutic agents may interrupt the cell cycle and production of cells.

Pressure Ulcers

Pressure ulcers remain the most common chronic ulcer, affecting approximately 1 million adults in the United States. The Surgeon General's Healthy People 2010 document identified pressure ulcers as a national health issue for long-term care, and CMS has designated pressure ulcers as one of the three primary markers of quality of care in the long-term care setting. On October 1, 2008, CMS made the decision to stop paying for hospital-acquired Stage III and IV pressure ulcers. Pressure ulcers are monitored throughout the continuum of care. Thus, it is critical for clinicians to be aggressive in both pressure ulcer prevention and treatment programs.

Epidemiology

A pressure ulcer is defined by the National Pressure Ulcer Advisory Panel (NPUAP) as a localized injury to the skin and/or underlying tissue, usually over a bony prominence that results from pressure (including pressure associated with shear). A number of contributing or confounding factors are also associated with pressure ulcers; the significance of such factors is yet to be elucidated. Because pressure is the major physiologic factor that leads to soft-tissue destruction, the term pressure ulcer is most widely used and preferred over the terms decubitus ulcer or bedsore.

The true causes of pressure ulcers are still not fully understood. Most research into the causes of pressure ulcers has been in animal models. Two main factors are believed to play a major role in pressure ulcer formation: pressure and shear forces. It appears that the amount of pressure or shear force needed to create a pressure ulcer depends on the quality of tissue, the blood flow, and the amount of pressure applied. Hence, for patients with poor-quality tissue (ie, tissue with inadequate blood perfusion), it may take less sustained pressure over a shorter time to develop a pressure ulcer. Conversely, patients with good-quality tissue may be able to sustain more pressure over a longer time before an ulcer develops. Ulcers caused by shearing forces tend to develop deep in the fascia, whereas ulcers caused by friction tend to be quite superficial, starting in the epidermal and dermal layers. With aging, local blood supply to the skin decreases, epithelial layers flatten and thin, subcutaneous fat decreases, and collagen fibers lose elasticity. These changes in aging skin and the resultant lowered tolerance to hypoxia can predispose older adults to the development of pressure ulcers.

The incidence and prevalence of pressure ulcers vary greatly, depending on the setting. In long-term care, average incidence is 11%, with 50% reported as Stage II; in hospitals, average range of incidence was 7%–9% (higher rates are noted in intensive-care units, where patients are less mobile and have severe systemic illnesses) with a prevalence of 15%; and for those receiving home health care, incidence is 0%–17%.

The incidence of pressure ulcers differs not only by healthcare setting but also by stage of ulceration. The Stage I pressure ulcer (persistent erythema) is most common, accounting for 47% of all pressure ulcers. The Stage II pressure ulcers (partial thickness loss involving only the epidermal and dermal layers) are second, at 33%. Stage III (full-thickness skin loss involving subcutaneous tissue) and Stage IV (full thickness involving muscle or bone or supporting structures) pressure ulcers make up the remaining 20%. In 2007, the NPUAP introduced the diagnosis of deep-tissue injury. These pressure ulcers have been described by clinicians for many years with terms such as purple pressure ulcers, ulcers that are likely to deteriorate, and bruises on bony prominences. The incidence and prevalence of this specific ulcer remains unknown, because many were described as Stage I. The incidence of pressure ulcers among black Americans and white Americans differs, with blacks tending to have a higher incidence of Stage III and IV pressure ulcers. In fact, black Americans have higher incidence rates than white Americans in nursing homes. Whether this can be attributed to structural skin changes or to socioeconomic factors is unknown because of the paucity of pressure ulcer research among patients in U.S. minority groups.

Risk Factors and Risk-Assessment Scales

The literature abounds with lists of risk factors associated with pressure ulcer development. However, any disease process that renders an older adult immobile for an extended period of time increases the risk of pressure ulcer development. Both intrinsic and extrinsic factors determine the tolerance of soft tissue to the adverse effects of pressure. Intrinsic risk factors are physiologic factors or disease states that increase the risk of pressure ulcer development, eg, age, poor nutritional status, and decreased arteriolar blood pressure. Extrinsic factors are external factors that damage the skin, eg, friction and shear, moisture, and urinary or fecal incontinence (or both). Variables that appear to be predictors of pressure ulcer development include age ≥70 years old, impaired mobility, use of restraints, current smoking history, low BMI, altered mental status (eg, confusion), urinary and fecal incontinence, malnutrition, malignancy, diabetes mellitus, stroke, pneumonia, heart failure, fever, sepsis, hypotension, kidney failure, dry and scaly skin, history of pressure ulcers, anemia, lymphopenia, and hypoalbuminemia. Some physiologic risk factors (eg, diabetes mellitus, cerebrovascular accident) have been associated with microcirculatory impairment, thus leading to neural and endothelial compromise and increasing the risk of ulceration (SOE=C).

Because of the myriad risk factors associated with pressure ulcer development, various scales have been developed to quantify a person's risk by identifying the presence of factors in several categories. The Braden Scale (www.bradenscale.com [accessed Oct 2013]) and the Norton Scale are probably the most widely used tools for identifying older adults who are at risk of developing pressure ulcers. Both tools have been validated and are recommended by the Agency for Healthcare Research and Quality (AHRQ). The Braden Scale has a sensitivity of 83%–100% and a specificity of 64%–77%; the Norton Scale has a sensitivity of 73%–92% and a specificity of 61%–94%.

The AHRQ guidelines for preventing pressure ulcers recommend that bed- and chair-bound patients or those with impaired ability to reposition themselves should be assessed on admission to the hospital or the nursing home for additional factors that increase risk of developing pressure ulcers. Studies have demonstrated that incorporating systematic risk-assessment tools has significantly reduced the incidence of pressure ulcers (SOE=A). To date, the Braden Scale is the only tool to be validated in nonwhite populations (black, Asian, and Latino/Hispanic). The use of risk-assessment tools does not guarantee that all older adults at risk of pressure ulcers will be identified.

There is no agreement on how frequently risk assessment should be done. However, most clinical guidelines for pressure ulcers indicate that a risk assessment should be done on admission, at discharge, and whenever the patient's clinical condition changes (SOE=D). The appropriate interval for routine reassessment remains unclear. Studies by Bergstrom and Braden found that in a skilled-nursing facility, 80% of pressure ulcers develop within 2 weeks of admission and 96% develop within 3 weeks of admission. Moreover, the Institute for Healthcare Improvement has recently recommended that in hospitalized patients, risk assessment for pressure ulcers be done every 24 hours rather than the previous suggestion of every 48 hours.

Prevention

The AHRQ sponsored the development of recommendations for the prevention of pressure ulcers in adults. These clinical practice guidelines (*Pressure Ulcers in Adults: Prediction and Prevention,* published in May 1992) provide an excellent approach to evidenced-based pressure ulcer prevention. In 2009, the NPUAP and the European Pressure Ulcer Advisory Panel (EPUAP) published clinical guidelines on the prevention and treatment of pressure ulcers. It should be noted that the vast majority of recommendations remain expert opinion.

Skin Care

Evidence on the role of skin care in pressure ulcer prevention is limited. Most recommendations are based on expert opinions and clinical guidelines. Although experts believe that there is a relationship between skin care and pressure ulcer development, there is a dearth of supporting research. How the skin is cleansed may make a difference (SOE=D). In one study, the incidence of Stages I and II pressure ulcers was reduced by educating the staff and by using a body wash and skin protection products. Another study compared hyperoxygenated fatty acid compound in acute-care and long-term care patients and found reduced incidence of ulcers versus placebo compound (triisotearin). All experts do agree that once an older adult at risk of pressure ulcers has been identified, the goal of skin care is to maintain and improve tissue tolerance to pressure.

The frequency of skin assessment may serve as a deterrent to developing pressure ulcers. Hence, frequent assessment of the skin is essential to detect early signs of pressure damage (SOE=B). Thus, all older adults at risk should have a systematic skin inspection at least once a day, with emphasis on the bony prominences. Moreover, the skin should be observed for pressure damage caused by medical devices. The skin should be cleansed with warm water and a mild cleansing agent to minimize irritation and dryness of the skin. Every effort should be made to minimize environmental factors leading to skin drying, such as low humidity (<40%) and exposure to cold. Decreased skin hydration results in decreased pliability, and severely dry skin damages the stratum corneum. Dry skin should be treated with moisturizers (SOE=D).

Massaging over bony prominences should be avoided. Previously, it was believed that massaging the bony prominences promoted circulation. However, postmortem biopsies showed degenerated tissue in areas that were massaged but no degenerated tissue in areas not massaged. All efforts should be made to avoid exposing the skin to perspiration, wound drainage, or urine and fecal matter resulting from incontinence. When disposable briefs are used to manage incontinence, the patient must be checked and changed frequently, because perineal dermatitis can develop quickly. The use of disposable underpads to control excessive moisture and perspiration can help wick moisture away from skin. The use of moisturizers and moisture barriers should also be considered to protect the skin (SOE=D). Documenting all skin assessments, noting details of any pain that may possibly be related to pressure damage, is essential (SOE=C).

Nutrition

The literature remains unclear about protein-calorie malnutrition and its association with pressure ulcer development. The relationship between nutritional intake and pressure ulcer prevention is not always supported by randomized controlled trials. Some research supports the finding that undernourishment on admission to a healthcare facility increases a person's likelihood of developing a pressure ulcer. In one prospective study, high-risk patients who were undernourished on admission to the hospital were twice as likely to develop pressure ulcers as adequately nourished patients (17% and 9%, respectively). In another study, 59% of residents were undernourished and 7.3% were severely undernourished on admission to a long-term care facility. Pressure ulcers developed in 65% of the severely undernourished residents, but in none of the mild to moderately undernourished or well-nourished residents. However, all patients should be screened and assessed for nutritional status if they are at risk of pressure ulcers. Those patients that may be nutritionally compromised should be referred to a registered dietitian. An evidenced-based guideline for enteral nutrition and hydration should be followed for those patients who demonstrate nutritional risks (SOE=C).

Empirical evidence is lacking that the use of vitamin and mineral supplements (in the absence of deficiency) actually prevents pressure ulcers. Therefore, oversupplementing patients without protein, vitamin, or mineral deficiencies should be avoided. Before enteral or parental nutrition is used, a critical review of overall goals and wishes of the patient, family, and care team should be considered. Despite the lack of evidence regarding nutritional assessment and intervention, maintaining optimal nutrition continues to be part of national pressure ulcer prevention guidelines (SOE=D). The CMS guidelines on pressure ulcer care (F-Tag 314) for nursing homes suggest that a resident with a nutritional risk should have a minimum of 1.25–1.5 g/kg of protein per day.

Mechanical Loading

Minimizing friction and shear is important. This can be accomplished through proper repositioning, transferring, and turning techniques. The use of lubricants (eg, cornstarch and creams), protective films (eg, transparent film dressings and skin sealants), protective dressings (eg, hydrocolloids), and protective padding can be used to reduce the possibility of friction and shear. Older adults who are at risk of developing pressure ulcers should be repositioned at least every 2 hours. Research on optimal turning schedules is sparse. The first study—an observational study published in 1975—found that older adults turned every 2–3 hours had fewer ulcers. A more recent study suggests that depending on the support surface used, less frequent turning may be optimal to prevent pressure ulcers in a long-term care facility. Several nurse researchers investigated the effect of four different turning frequencies (every 2 hours on a standard mattress, every 3 hours on a standard mattress, every 4 hours on a viscoelastic foam mattress, and every 6 hours on a viscoelastic foam mattress). They found that the incidence of early pressure ulcers (Stage I) did not differ in the four groups. However, patients being turned every 4 hours on a viscoelastic foam mattress developed significantly less severe pressure ulcers (Stage II and

Table 38.1—Prevention of Heel Pressure Ulcers*

- Every day, assess the heels of patients at high risk of pressure ulcers.
- Use moisturizer on the heels twice a day; do not massage.
- Apply transparent film dressings to the heels of older adults prone to friction problems (eg, stroke patients).
- Apply hydrocolloid dressing (either single or extra thick) to the heels of patients with reactive hyperemia (pre-Stage I).
- Have patients wear socks to help prevent friction; remove at bedtime.
- Have patients in wheelchairs wear properly fitting padded sneakers or shoes.
- Place pillow vertically under the patient's legs (without hyperextending them) to support heels off the bed surface.
- Turn the patient every 2 hours, repositioning heels.

*SOE=D for all

higher) than the three other groups. Although the results of this study may indicate less turning may be appropriate when using a viscoelastic foam mattress, additional studies are needed to examine optimal turning schedules among different populations (SOE=C).

Bed-positioning devices such as pillows or foam wedges should be used to keep bony prominences from direct contact with one another. The head of the bed should be at the lowest degree of elevation consistent with medical conditions. The use of lifting devices, such as trapezes or bed linen, to move the patient in bed also decreases the potential for friction and shear forces. The heel is quite vulnerable to pressure ulcer development; studies suggest that approximately 20% of all pressure ulcer development is on the heels. This may be attributed to the limited amount of soft tissue over the heel. Specific clinical interventions to prevent heel pressure ulcers have been developed (Table 38.1) (SOE=D).

Patients seated in a chair should be assessed for good postural alignment, distribution of weight, and balance. They should be taught or reminded to shift weight every 15 minutes. The use of doughnuts as seating cushions is contraindicated, because they increase pressure over the area of contact and can actually cause pressure ulcers (SOE=C).

Mobility

Maintaining or improving mobility is one of the most effective ways to decrease pressure on bony prominences. For bedbound patients, there are benefits of both active and passive range-of-motion exercises. Patients not confined to bed should be encouraged to move from bed to chair to standing to ambulating to minimize the risk of developing pressure ulcers (SOE=C).

Support Surfaces

Any older adult identified as being at risk of developing pressure ulcers should be placed on a pressure redistribution device. The concept of pressure redistribution has been endorsed by the NPUAP. However, if pressure is reduced on one body part, this will result in increased pressure elsewhere on the body. Thus, the goal is to obtain the best pressure redistribution possible. In a systematic review of 49 randomized controlled trials that examined the role of support surfaces in preventing pressure ulcers, no one category of support surface was found to be superior to another; however, use of a support surface was more beneficial than a standard mattress (SOE=A). Two types of devices exist: static (foam, static air, gel or water, or a combination) and dynamic (alternating air, low air loss, or air fluidized). Most static devices are less expensive than dynamic surfaces. For the various types of support surfaces that can guide selection for particular situations, see Table 38.2. Most experts agree that the use of static devices is appropriate for pressure ulcer prevention (SOE=D). Two conditions warrant consideration of a dynamic surface:

- bottoming-out occurs (the static surface is compressed to <1 inch)
- the patient is at high risk of pressure ulcers, and reactive hyperemia is noted on a bony prominence despite the use of a static support surface

Although effective at reducing pressure, dynamic airflow beds have several potential adverse effects, including dehydration, sensory deprivation, loss of muscle strength, and difficulty with mobilization. The NPUAP has undertaken the task of trying to standardize support surfaces, because much confusion remains on which is the optimal support surface for any patient, depending on clinical characteristics (www.npuap.org/NPUAP_S3I_TD.pdf [accessed Oct 2013]).

Management

The AHRQ developed evidence-based guidelines on the management of pressure ulcers. This guideline, *Treatment of Pressure Ulcers*, published in December 1994, reviews the foundation for providing evidence-based pressure ulcer management. As noted previously, the NPUAP/EPUAP updated the guideline in 2009.

Assessment

A pressure ulcer will not heal unless underlying causes are identified and effective interventions implemented. When a pressure ulcer has developed, a systematic evaluation is necessary (SOE=D). For an approach to assessment and documentation when a pressure ulcer develops, see Table 38.3.

There is no universal agreement on a single system for classifying pressure ulcers. Most experts do agree

Table 38.2—Support Surfaces for Older Adults at Risk of Pressure Ulcers

Type	Examples	Support Area	Low Moisture Retention	Reduced Heat Accumulation	Shear Reduction	Pressure Reduction	Cost per Day
Static surfaces	Foam	yes	no	no	no	yes	low
	Standard mattress	no	no	no	no	no	low
	Static flotation—air or water	yes	no	no	yes	yes	low
Dynamic surfaces	Air fluidized	yes	yes	yes	yes	yes	high
	Low-air-loss	yes	yes	yes	?	yes	high
	Alternating air	yes	no	no	yes	yes	moderate

SOURCE: Adapted from Bergstrom N, Bennett MA, Carlson CE, et al. *Treatment of Pressure Ulcers. Clinical Practice Guideline No. 15.* Rockville, MD: US Department of Health and Human Services, Public Health Service, Agency for Health Care Policy and Research. December 1994:38. AHCPR Pub. No. 95-0652.

that the stage of an ulcer determines the appropriate treatment plan. However, staging alone does not determine the seriousness of the ulcer. Most systems use four stages to classify ulceration. Table 38.4 describes the most commonly used staging system by the NPUAP. This group has revised the staging system to include deep-tissue injury, an ulcer often described as a purple or maroon localized area of discolored intact skin or blood-filled blister due to damage of underlying soft tissue from pressure or shear, or both. The NPUAP also reclassified blisters and unstageable pressure ulcers. The new staging system has six stages: suspected deep tissue injury, Stage I, Stage II, Stage III, Stage IV, and unstageable. When eschar (thick brown or black devitalized tissue) is covering the ulcer, the ulcer cannot be accurately staged.

The challenge for most staging systems lies in the definition of the Stage I pressure ulcer. Attempts to classify the first stage of ulcer development are more variable than for any other stage. Most systems define the Stage I pressure ulcer as nonblanchable erythema of intact skin; both the AHRQ prediction and prevention guidelines and the Minimum Data Set (required by CMS for all patients in long-term care facilities) refer to Stage I pressure ulcer in these terms. However, it is difficult (at best) to blanch the skin of people with darkly pigmented skin. Thus, erythema can appear as a defined area of persistent redness in lightly pigmented skin, whereas in darker skin tones, the pressure ulcer can appear with persistent erythema, or blue or purple hues. In a recent study, black nursing-home residents were more likely to have pressure ulcers than their white counterparts. One explanation given for the variance was the inability to detect erythema as easily in darker tone skin.

Perhaps no other population is more vulnerable to heel ulcers than those patients admitted to intensive care units. They often are hemodynamically unstable, have multiple comorbid conditions, are on a poor plane of nutrition, and are immobile. An excellent 5-step universal heel pressure ulcer prevention algorithm has been developed as a quick and simple method to manage this challenging problem in the most vulnerable population. Following this universal guideline may decrease the development of heel ulcers (www.sageproducts.com/education/pdf/WCET%20April-June%202008%20reprint_low_res.pdf [accessed Oct 2013]).

Debridement

Debridement is necessary when the wound contains necrotic, devitalized tissue (SOE=C). Such tissue supports the growth of pathologic organisms and prevents healing. There are four major types of debridement methods used in the United States: mechanical, enzymatic, autolytic, and sharp (Table 38.5). Sharp/surgical debridement must be performed in the presence of advancing cellulitis, crepitus, fluctuance, and/or sepsis secondary to pressure ulcer-related infection (SOE=C). It should be noted that sharp debridement should be used cautiously on patients in the presence of immune incompetence, compromised vascular supply to the limb, or lack of antibacterial coverage in systemic sepsis. Biosurgery (ie, maggot or larva therapy), which is used widely in Europe, is another potential debridement option. The debridement method should be selected on the basis of the patient's health condition, the ulcer presentation, the presence or absence of infection, and the patient's ability to tolerate the procedure (Table 38.5).

Dressings

Numerous dressings are used in the healing of pressure ulcers. The use of wet-to-dry gauze has been discouraged by experts; it is actually a debriding technique that can damage the tissue matrix and prolong healing. Many experts advocate the use of hydrocolloid dressings (SOE=B). These dressings, when compared with gauze, have been found to significantly speed the healing process. This is most likely because hydrocolloids require fewer dressing changes (inflicting less trauma), block bacteria from penetrating the wound bed, and maintain a moist wound environment (facilitating increases in the growth factors needed in the healing process). Moreover, studies have demonstrated that the

Table 38.3—Detection, Assessment, and Management of Pressure Ulcers

Evaluate and Document	Consider These Strategies
Location	■ Examine high-risk sites. ■ Develop targeted pressure-relieving strategies (eg, positioning and repositioning, padding, seat cushions, heel elevation). ■ Limit shearing forces by special attention to positioning when the head of bed is elevated. ■ Lift rather than slide the patient. ■ Cleanse and dry regularly if wetted frequently.
Stage	■ Differentiate between minor Stage I lesions (nonblanchable erythema related to extravasation of RBCs into the interstitium) and deep-tissue injuries that can progress to full-thickness lesions. ■ Discuss with caregivers and families the possibility of significant pressure ulcer development when deep-tissue injury is identified.
Area	■ Record diameter of circular lesions. ■ Record lengths of largest perpendiculars for irregular lesions.
Depth	■ Measure depth from plane of skin. ■ Probe and measure extent of undermining or depth of sinus tracts.
Drainage	■ Estimate amount. ■ Identify degree of odor and purulence. ■ Monitor hematocrit if more than minor blood loss occurs with dressing changes. ■ Monitor serum albumin if volume of ulcer drainage is large.
Necrosis	■ Consider simple blunt debridement of small amounts of necrotic tissue. ■ Involve general or plastic surgeons for extensive debridement. ■ Monitor damage to healthy tissue whenever using blunt, enzymatic, or wet-to-dry dressings for debridement. ■ Monitor use of pressure dressings (which can cause necrosis) after blunt debridement. ■ Use silver-based dressings to decrease bacterial burden. ■ Use low-frequency nonthermal ultrasound to remove necrotic tissue.
Granulation	■ Identify granulation as an indication that wound healing is occurring. ■ Look for regression if other infections (eg, urinary tract infection or pneumonia) develop. ■ Develop strategies to protect and enhance growth of granulation tissue (eg, nourishment, vitamins, minerals; use of dressings to ensure moist wound surfaces). ■ Avoid damage with dressing changes.
Cellulitis	■ Differentiate from a thin rim of erythema surrounding most healing wounds. ■ Look for tenderness, warmth, and redness, particularly if there is progression. ■ Consider treatment with systemic antibiotics active against gram-positive cocci.
Nonhealing wound	■ Use negative-pressure wound therapy for excessive exudate. ■ Consider monochromatic infrared photo energy therapy.

use of hydrocolloids, when compared with the use of gauze, decreases direct and indirect institutional costs. It is essential to select an appropriate dressing, not on the basis of the stage of the pressure ulcer, but rather on the amount of wound exudate. For some of the most common dressings and the indications for their use, see Table 38.6. The most appropriate dressing should meet several criteria: absorptive, good wear time (dependent on goal), barrier to water and bacteria, conformable to body contours, non-sensitizing, effective skin adhesive, nonflammable, nontoxic, sterile, easy to use, and cost-effective.

Surgical Repair

Surgical repair remains a viable option for Stage III and IV pressure ulcers (SOE=D). However, because many Stage III and IV pressure ulcers eventually heal over a long period of time (if appropriately managed) and the rate of recurrence of surgically closed pressure ulcers is high, the benefits of surgery must be considered carefully. The most common types of surgical repairs are direct closure, skin grafting, skin flaps, musculocutaneous flaps, and free flaps.

Diet and Nutritional Supplements

The importance of diet and dietary supplements in a malnourished patient with a pressure ulcer is controversial. Per AHRQ treatment guidelines, nutritional support that achieves approximately 30–35 calories/kg/d and 1.25–1.5 g of protein/kg/d is recommended (SOE=C). Evidence to support the use of supplemental vitamins and minerals is limited. The use of amino acids such as arginine, glutamine, and cysteine has been noted to assist in ulcer healing.

Table 38.4—Staging System for Pressure Ulcers (National Pressure Ulcer Advisory Panel)

Stage	Definition	Comments
Suspected deep-tissue injury	Purple or maroon localized area of discolored intact skin or blood-filled blister due to damage of underlying soft tissue from pressure or shear, or both. The area may be preceded by tissue that is painful, firm, mushy, boggy, warmer, or cooler than adjacent tissue.	Deep-tissue injury can be difficult to detect in individuals with dark skin tones. Evolution can include a thin blister over a dark wound bed. The wound can further evolve and become covered by thin eschar. Evolution can be rapid and expose additional layers of tissue, even with optimal treatment.
Stage I	Intact skin with nonblanchable redness of a localized area usually over a bony prominence. Darkly pigmented skin may not have visible blanching; its color may differ from the surrounding area.	The area may be painful, firm, soft, and warmer or cooler than adjacent tissue. Stage I can be difficult to detect in individuals with dark skin tones.
Stage II	Partial-thickness loss of dermis presenting as a shallow open ulcer with a red-pink wound bed, without slough. Can also present as an intact or open/ruptured serum-filled blister.	Presents as a shiny or dry shallow ulcer without slough or bruising (the latter indicates suspected deep-tissue injury). This stage should not be used to describe skin tears, tape burns, perineal dermatitis, maceration, or excoriation.
Stage III	Full-thickness tissue loss. Subcutaneous fat can be visible but bone, tendon, or muscle is not exposed. Slough may be present but does not obscure the depth of tissue loss. Can include undermining and tunneling.	The depth of a Stage III pressure ulcer varies by anatomic location. The bridge of the nose, ear, occiput, and malleolus do not have subcutaneous tissue, and Stage III ulcers can be shallow. In contrast, areas of significant adiposity can develop extremely deep Stage III pressure ulcers. Bone/tendon is not visible or directly palpable.
Stage IV	Full-thickness tissue loss with exposed bone, tendon, or muscle. Slough or eschar can be present on some parts of wound bed. Often include undermining and tunneling.	The depth of a Stage IV pressure ulcer varies by anatomic location. The bridge of the nose, ear, occiput, and malleolus do not have subcutaneous tissue, and these ulcers can be shallow. Stage IV ulcers can extend into muscle or supporting structures, or both (eg, fascia, tendon, or joint capsule), making osteomyelitis possible. Exposed bone/tendon is visible or directly palpable.
Unstageable	Full-thickness tissue loss in which the base of the ulcer is covered by slough (yellow, tan, gray, green, or brown) or eschar (tan, brown, or black), or both, in the wound bed.	Until enough slough or eschar, or both, is removed to expose the base of the wound, the true depth (and therefore stage) cannot be determined. Stable (dry, adherent, intact without erythema or fluctuance) eschar on the heels serves as "the body's natural (biological) cover" and should not be removed.

SOURCE: Adapted with permission from the National Pressure Ulcer Advisory Panel, 2012 (www.npuap.org).

Table 38.5—Methods of Debridement

Type	Description	Advantages and Disadvantages
Mechanical	Use of physical forces to remove devitalized tissues; methods include wet-to-dry irrigation (using 19-gauge needle with 35-mL syringe), hydrotherapy, and dextranomer.	Can remove both devitalized and vitalized tissues; can cause pain.
Surgical, sharp	Use of scalpel, scissors, and forceps to remove devitalized tissue; laser debridement	Quick and effective if performed by skilled professional; should be used when infection is suspected; pain management is needed.
Enzymatic	Use of topical debriding agent to dissolve the devitalized tissue (chemical force)	Appropriate when there are no signs or symptoms of local infection; some agents can damage surrounding skin.
Autolytic	Use of synthetic dressings to allow the devitalized tissue to self-digest from the enzymes found in the ulcer fluids (natural force)	Recommended for those who cannot tolerate other forms of debridement and when infection is not suspected; may take a long time to be effective.
Biosurgery	Use of larvae to digest devitalized tissue	Quick and effective; good option for those who cannot tolerate surgical debridement.

SOURCE: Data from Bergstrom N, Bennett MA, Carlson CE, et al. *Treatment of Pressure Ulcers. Clinical Practice Guideline No. 15.* Rockville, MD: US Department of Health and Human Services, Public Health Service, Agency for Health Care Policy and Research. December 1994:47–49. AHCPR Pub. No. 95-0652.

New or Unproven Therapies

Throughout the years, a number of treatments have been advocated for the healing of pressure ulcers without sufficient data to support their various claims. Data on the therapeutic efficacy of hyperbaric oxygen, low-energy laser irradiation, and therapeutic ultrasound have not been established. However, areas of promise include the use of recombinant PDGF to stimulate healing and

Table 38.6—Common Dressings for Treating Pressure Ulcers

Dressing	Indications	Contraindications	Comments
Transparent film	Stage I, II Protection from friction Superficial scrape Autolytic debridement of slough	Draining ulcers Suspected skin infection or fungus	Apply skin prep to intact skin to protect from adhesive
Foam island	Stage II, III Low to moderate exudate Can apply as window to secure transparent film	Excessive exudates Dry, crusted wound	
Hydrocolloids	Stage II, III Low to moderate drainage Good periwound skin integrity Autolytic debridement of slough	Poor skin integrity Infected ulcers Wound needs packing	Leave in place 3–5 days Can apply as window to secure transparent film Can apply over alginate to control drainage Must control maceration Apply skin prep to intact skin to protect from adhesive
Alginate	Stage III, IV Excessive drainage	Dry or minimally draining wound Superficial wounds with maceration	Apply dressing within wound borders Requires secondary dressing Must use skin prep Must control maceration
Hydrogel			
(amorphous gels)	Stage II, III, IV	Macerated areas Wounds with excess exudate	Needs to be combined with gauze dressing Stays moist longer than saline gauze Changed 1–2 times/day Used as alternative to saline gauze for packing deep wounds with tunnels, undermining Reduces adherence of gauze to wound Must control maceration
(gel sheet)	Stage II	Macerated areas Wounds with moderate to heavy exudate	Needs to be held in place with topper dressing
Gauze packing (moistened with saline)	Stage III, IV	Wounds with depth, especially those with tunnels, undermining	Must be remoistened often to maintain moist wound environment
Silver dressings (silver with alginates, gels, charcoal)	Malodorous wounds High level of exudates	Systemic infection Cellulitis Signs of systemic adverse events, especially erythema multiforme Fungal proliferation Sensitivity of skin to sun Interstitial nephritis Leukopenia Skin necrosis Concurrent use with proteolytic enzymes	Wound highly suspicious for critical bacterial load Periwound with signs of inflammation Slow-healing wound

SOURCE: Copyright © 2012 by Rita Frantz. Adapted from Reuben DB, Herr K, Pacala JT, et al. *Geriatrics At Your Fingertips*, 15th ed. New York: American Geriatrics Society; 2013:274–275. Reprinted with permission.

skin equivalents that may prove to heal Stage III and IV pressure ulcers. Although the combined clinical evidence to support PDGF does suggest its ability to aid wound healing, the evidence is not sufficient to recommend this treatment for routine usage.

Electrical stimulation is the use of electrical current to stimulate a number of cellular processes important in pressure ulcer healing. It influences the migration of neutrophils, fibroblasts, and macrophages into the wound and increases the tensile strength of collagen. Electrical stimulation appears to be most effective on healing recalcitrant Stages III and IV pressure ulcers. In a meta-analysis of 15 studies evaluating the effects of electrical stimulation on the healing of chronic ulcers, the rate of healing per week was 22% for participants receiving electrical stimulation compared with 9% for controls. Thus, electrical stimulation should be considered for nonhealing pressure ulcers (SOE=B).

Negative-pressure wound therapy is widely used, although few randomized controlled trials have been published. This therapy promotes wound healing by applying controlled, localized, negative pressure to the wound bed. In one prospective study of 281 patients investigating the effects of using negative-pressure wound therapy to heal pressure ulcers, those patients using the adjunctive therapy had better healing outcomes than the cohort not using the therapy. Evidence is emerging that this therapy may be helpful in healing pressure ulcers (SOE=C).

The use of growth factors and skin equivalents in healing pressure ulcers remains under investigation, although the use of cytokine growth factors (eg, recombinant PDGF-BB), FGFs, and skin equivalents have been effective in diabetic and venous ulcers. In three small randomized controlled trials, growth factors had beneficial results with pressure ulcers, but the findings warrant further exploration. A greater understanding of the healing cascade may clarify the appropriate use of growth factors in pressure ulcer treatment.

In the past 5 years, there has been great interest in the use of phototherapy (laser, infrared, ultraviolet) and acoustic therapy (ultrasound). However, there remains a paucity of data to suggest that these therapies actually increase wound healing. Finally, the use of biological dressings for pressure ulcer treatment remains controversial. There is insufficient evidence to support the use of these dressings in the treatment of pressure ulcers. However, their use in diabetic foot ulcers is promising.

Monitoring Healing

Monitoring the healing of pressure ulcers can pose a challenge. The accurate measurements of a pressure ulcer can provide useful information about the effectiveness of ulcer treatment. However, results obtained using traditional measurements (ie, rulers and tracing paper) are highly variable among raters. In the past 8 years, two instruments to measure healing of pressure ulcers with some level of validity and reliability have been developed. The Pressure Sore Status Tool and the Pressure Ulcer Scale for Healing (www.npuap.org/PDF/push3.pdf [accessed Oct 2013]) are excellent tools for monitoring pressure ulcer healing. The use of high-frequency portable ultrasound to measure wound healing has been introduced. This technology, which can capture three-dimensional measurements, has been quite beneficial in objectively monitoring healing (SOE=C). Moreover, because ultrasound is "color blind," it can detect Stage I pressure ulcers in darkly pigmented skin.

Expert debate has been considerable regarding the use of reverse staging of pressure ulcers to monitor healing. Staging of pressure ulcers is appropriate only for defining the maximal anatomic depth of tissue damage. Because pressure ulcers heal to a progressively more shallow depth, they do not replace lost muscle, subcutaneous fat, or dermis before they reepithelialize. Instead, pressure ulcers fill with granulation (scar) tissue composed primarily of endothelial cells, fibroblasts, collagen, and extracellular matrix. A Stage IV pressure ulcer cannot become a Stage III, Stage II, and then Stage I; reverse staging does not accurately characterize the physiologic process during healing of the pressure ulcer. When a Stage IV pressure ulcer has healed, it should be classified as a healed Stage IV pressure ulcer, not as a Stage 0. The progress of healing can be documented only by describing ulcer characteristics or by measuring wound characteristics with a validated tool. It should be noted that CMS still requires reversed staging in long-term care, because the payment for pressure ulcers is based on its stage.

Ulcer care should be evaluated weekly for healing progress. There are no standard healing rates for pressure ulcers. Review of the literature suggests that most Stage I pressure ulcers heal within 1–7 days; Stage II, within 5 days to 3 months; Stage III, within 1–6 months; and Stage IV, within 6–12 months. Some full-thickness pressure ulcers may never heal, depending on comorbidity; however, no clear guidelines exist to determine when a pressure ulcer can be truly defined as recalcitrant or what characteristics must be present to predict that an ulcer will never heal.

Control of Infections

All pressure ulcers become colonized with both aerobic and anaerobic bacteria, and superficial swab cultures of the wounds have not been helpful in determining the organisms that may be causing the infection. Therefore, routine swab cultures are not recommended (SOE=B). The most common organisms isolated from pressure ulcers are *Proteus mirabilis*, group D streptococci, *Escherichia coli*, *Staphylococcus* spp, *Pseudomonas* spp, and *Corynebacterium* organisms. Patients with bacteremia are more likely to have *Bacteroides* spp in their pressure ulcers. However, some evidence suggests that quantitative tissue swab cultures can be used to determine the wound bioburden. Wound cleansing and dressing changes are two of the most important methods for minimizing the amount of bacterial colonization. Increasing the frequency of wound cleansing and dressing changes is an important first step when purulent or foul-smelling drainage is observed on the ulcer (SOE=C). When ulcers are not healing or have persistent exudate after 2 weeks of optimal cleansing and dressing changes, it is reasonable to consider the use of antimicrobials.

Topical antimicrobials have been shown to decrease the bioburden in pressure ulcers (SOE=B). The use of antimicrobials such as silver sulfadiazine and mupirocin ointment can be applied up to three times a day for 1–2 weeks, with careful monitoring for allergic reactions. Because prolonged use of these antimicrobials can result in resistant organisms, they should not be used indefinitely. In the past several years, the use of silver-impregnated dressings to decrease the bioburden has become quite popular. Although the exact mechanism of how silver kills the infecting organisms remains unknown, it is hypothesized that it stops the enzyme that feeds the proliferation of bacteria, viruses, and fungi. These dressings (eg, Aquacel Ag, Acticoat, Actisorb, Arglaes) control bacterial load and ideally control odor caused by the bacteria. The dressing selected determines how the silver is delivered, the length of treatment, the amount of exudate absorption, the incidence of maceration, the ease of dressing removal, and the pain intensity at dressing changes. Prolonged use of silver dressings should be avoided, and these dressing should be discontinued when the infection is controlled. The use of silver sulfadiazine in heavily contaminated or infected pressure ulcers until definitive debridement could be considered. It is important to select a dressing that meets the needs of the patient and the staff.

Because most topical antibiotics do not penetrate the wound bed, they are not effective for infection control. When ulcers fail to heal despite the treatments described above, it is reasonable to consider the possibility of cellulitis or osteomyelitis. These diagnoses can be established by biopsy of the ulcer for quantitative bacterial cultures or of the underlying bone. Cellulitis, osteomyelitis, bacteremia, and sepsis are all indications for use of systemic antibiotics.

Topical antiseptics (eg, povidone iodine, iodophor, sodium hypochlorite, hydrogen peroxide, acetic acid) reduce bacterial loads; however, most are cytotoxic to healthy granulation tissue needed for the wound to heal.

Bacteria from surrounding skin contaminate the wound within 24 hours. High levels of bacteria in wounds can delay or impede wound healing. An emerging area of interest in wound healing is the role of bacterial biofilms. Bacterial biofilms are bacteria that attach to wound surfaces and aggregate to form communities in a hydrated polymeric matrix of their own syntheses. Although wounds have been shown to have the characteristics that suggest the existence of bacterial biofilms, there remains a paucity of studies investigating the role of bacterial biofilms and wound healing. This is one of the most controversial areas of wound research.

Complications from Pressure Ulcers

The development of pressure ulcers can lead to several complications. Probably the most serious complication is sepsis. When a pressure ulcer is present and there is aerobic or anaerobic bacteremia, or both, the pressure ulcer is most often the primary source of the infection. Additional complications of pressure ulcers include localized infection, cellulitis, and osteomyelitis. Quite often, a nonhealing pressure ulcer indicates underlying osteomyelitis. Mortality can also be associated with pressure ulcer development. Several studies have noted the association of pressure ulcer development and mortality in both the hospital and nursing-home settings. In fact, the mortality rate has been as high as 60% for those older adults who develop a pressure ulcer within 1 year of hospital discharge.

Pressure ulcers can be painful. Thus, patients should be assessed for pain related to a pressure ulcer, its treatment, or both (SOE-B). A systematic review of the literature found that 1) pressure ulcers cause pain; 2) pain assessment was typically found to be self-reported using different versions of the McGill Pain Questionnaire, Faces Rating Scale, or Visual Analog Scale; 3) pain assessment instruments should be appropriate to the patient's cognitive level and medical challenges; 4) in some cases, topical medications can ease pain and although information on systemic medication is limited, pain medications have been found to negatively affect appetite; and 5) wound treatment is painful, particularly during dressing changes. Thus, the use of analgesics (especially during debridement), encouraging the patient to request a "time out" during any wound procedure, and use of dressings less likely to cause pain (eg, silicone-based dressings) should be encouraged.

Avoidable versus Unavoidable Pressure Ulcers

One of the most challenging decisions that are made in providing pressure ulcer care is to determine whether the ulcer was avoidable or unavoidable. CMS determines whether the ulcer was avoidable or not based on processes of care. Hence, if the process was consistently followed, the ulcer was unavoidable. Conversely, if consistent processes were not followed, then the ulcer was avoidable. In 2010, the NPUAP hosted a multidisciplinary conference to establish consensus on whether there are individuals in whom pressure ulcer development may be unavoidable and whether a difference exists between end-of-life skin changes and pressure ulcers.

Consensus was achieved for the following statements: most pressure ulcers are avoidable; not all pressure ulcers are avoidable; there are situations that render pressure ulcer development unavoidable, including hemodynamic instability that is worsened with physical movement and inability to maintain nutrition and hydration status and the presence of an advanced directive prohibiting artificial nutrition/hydration; pressure redistribution surfaces cannot replace turning and repositioning; and if enough pressure is removed from the external body, the skin cannot always survive.

REFERENCES

- National Pressure Ulcer Advisory Panel and European Pressure Ulcer Advisory Panel. *Pressure Ulcer Prevention and Treatment: Clinical Practice Guideline. 2009*. Washington DC: National Pressure Ulcer Advisory Panel.
- Reddy M, Gill SS, Kalkar SR, et al. Treatment of pressure ulcers: A systematic review. *JAMA*. 2008;300(22):2647–2662.
- Theisen S, Drabik A, Stock S. Pressure ulcers in older hospitalised patients and its impact on length of stay: a retrospective observational study. *J Clin Nurs*. 2012;21(3/4):380–387.

CHAPTER 39—DEPRESSION AND OTHER MOOD DISORDERS

KEY POINTS

- Treatment of depression may require up to 12 weeks before remission is complete, but an initial response to medication should be seen within the first 4 weeks.
- In a substantial minority of cases, trials of more than one antidepressant or combination therapy with two antidepressants may be required before remission is achieved.
- Executive cognitive dysfunction is easily assessed and when present predicts poor response to medication as well as the need for adapted psychotherapy.
- Exercise reduces depressive symptoms and should be prescribed for all depressed older adults who are capable of increasing their level of physical activity.
- Bipolar depression in older adults may be more common than previously thought and should be treated with a mood stabilizer rather than an antidepressant.

EPIDEMIOLOGY

Depression is a leading cause of disability-adjusted life years lost across the life span and projected to be more so within a generation. Mood disorders are implicated in 10% of all hospitalizations. However, prevalence studies of community residents demonstrate surprisingly low rates of depressive disorders among those ≥65 years old. Only 1%–2% of women and <1% of men interviewed with standardized instruments met diagnostic criteria for major depressive disorder (SOE=A). Both current and lifetime prevalence rates for older adults are lower than those for middle-aged adults; furthermore, these relatively low rates persist after accounting for possible premature death and institutionalization, both of which can be associated with depression. Similarly, the incidence of first-episode major depressive disorder decreases after age 65. Data demonstrating that older adults are less likely to recognize depression and to endorse depressed mood offer one explanation for the lower prevalence and incidence of depressive syndromes among older community residents.

However, the prevalence of depressive symptoms that do not meet the threshold for a *Diagnostic and Statistical Manual of Mental Disorders, 5th Edition, (DSM-5™)* clinical diagnosis is substantial in older adults, with most studies reporting rates in the range of 15%. These subsyndromal states are not inconsequential. "Minor" or "subsyndromal" depression, defined as the presence of depressed mood with from two to three additional symptoms of major depressive disorder has been associated with increased use of health services, excess disability, and poor health outcomes, including higher mortality.

The prevalence rates of both major and subsyndromal depression vary greatly by the setting in which older adults are seen and by methods used to identify cases. Increased rates of depression are found among older adults seen in healthcare facilities and inpatient settings. Major depressive disorder has been identified in 6%–10% of older adults in primary care clinics and in 12%–20% of nursing-home residents. More varied rates of 11%–45% have been reported among older adults requiring inpatient medical care. The reported prevalence rates of minor depression in outpatient medical settings have varied as well, with reported rates of 8% to >40%. In mental health settings, major depressive disorder is the most common diagnosis seen among older patients and accounts for >40% of outpatient caseloads and inpatient psychiatry admissions.

CLINICAL PRESENTATION AND DIAGNOSIS

The Geriatric Syndrome of Late-Life Depression

Although aging does not markedly affect the phenomenology of depression, older adults are more often preoccupied with somatic symptoms and less frequently report depressed mood and guilty preoccupations. Among those who do not acknowledge sustained sadness, a persistent loss of pleasure and interest in previously enjoyable activities (*anhedonia*) for at least 2 weeks is necessary for a diagnosis of major depressive disorder.

The diagnosis of depression in physically ill older adults is confounded by the overlap among symptoms of major depressive disorder and somatic illness. Patients with advanced physical illness may be preoccupied with thoughts about death or worthlessness because of marked disability, yet not meet criteria for a major depressive episode. The *DSM-5™* criteria require that the depressive symptoms are not a direct result of a general medical condition or medication used to treat it. The alternative diagnosis of mood disorder due to a general

Table 39.1—The 9-Item Patient Health Questionnaire (PHQ-9): Screening Questions and Complete Assessment

Two-question screening with the "PHQ-2"

Over the last 2 weeks, how often have you been bothered by the following problems?	**Not at all**	**Several days**	**More than half the days**	**Nearly every day**
A. Little interest or pleasure in doing things?	0	1	2	3
B. Feeling down, depressed, or hopeless?	0	1	2	3

If A + B = 3 or greater, ask the following:

Over the last 2 weeks, how often have you been bothered by the following problems?	**Not at all**	**Several days**	**More than half the days**	**Nearly every day**
Feeling tired or having little energy?	0	1	2	3
Poor appetite or overeating?	0	1	2	3
Trouble falling or staying asleep, or sleeping too much?	0	1	2	3
Feeling bad about yourself—or that you are a failure or have let yourself or your family down?	0	1	2	3
Trouble concentrating on things, such as reading the newspaper or watching television?	0	1	2	3
Moving or speaking so slowly that other people could have noticed? Or the opposite—being so fidgety or restless that you have been moving around a lot more than usual?	0	1	2	3
Thoughts that you would be better off dead or of hurting yourself?	0	1	2	3

SOURCE: Developed by Spitzer RL, Williams JBW, Kroenke K, et al., with an educational grant from Pfizer Inc. Copyright © Pfizer, Inc. All rights reserved.

Table 39.2—Indications to Start Antidepressant Therapy Based on Patient Health Questionnaire-9

PHQ-9 Score	Depression Severity	Clinician Response
1–4	None	None
5–9	Mild to moderate	If not currently treated, rescreen in 2 weeks. If currently treated, optimize antidepressant and rescreen in 2 weeks.
10–14	Major depressive disorder	Start antidepressant therapy.
≥15	Major depressive disorder	Start antidepressant therapy; obtain psychiatric consultation if suicidality or psychosis suspected.

medical condition should be used for patients with depression that appears to result directly from a specific medical condition (eg, hypothyroidism, pancreatic cancer, end-stage renal disease). In either case, when symptoms are disabling, treatment should be offered.

Screening

Simply screening for the presence of depressed mood and anhedonia identifies most medically ill patients who also meet diagnostic criteria for major depressive disorder. These symptoms are less likely to be confounded by those of a medical illness. When the clinician fears an older adult is minimizing distress or associated disability, it is helpful to obtain further information from involved family members or caregivers.

The nine items of the Patient Health Questionnaire (PHQ-9) cover the diagnostic criteria for major depressive disorder, and the initial two questions (the "PHQ-2") can be used for screening. In addition, serial administrations of the PHQ-9 can be used to reliably assess response to treatment.

For use of the PHQ-2 and PHQ-9, see Table 39.1. Patients scoring a total of ≥3 on the depressed mood plus anhedonia questions on the PHQ-2 should be assessed with the remaining seven questions of the PHQ-9. Patients scoring 3 on the anhedonia questions alone should also be fully assessed. A complaint of depression need not be present for a diagnosis of depressive disorder, provided the other symptoms significantly impair function and are not the direct result of somatic illness. For management based on PHQ-9 score, see Table 39.2.

At a score of ≥10, the PHQ-9 has good sensitivity and specificity for major depressive disorder among primary care patients versus a structured diagnostic interview conducted by a mental health professional. People scoring ≥15 and those with suicidal ideation may require psychiatric consultation. A change of 5 points is considered a minimal clinically important difference and evidence of response to treatment (Table 39.3). Remission is best defined as a total score of ≤5. When the score has changed by <5 points despite 4 weeks of treatment at recommended dosages, the medication should either be switched or combined with another antidepressant.

Another standardized instrument for evaluating depressive symptoms is the 15-item Geriatric

Table 39.3—Prescriber Response Guidelines at 4 Weeks Based on the Patient Health Questionnaire-9 and the Sequenced Treatment Alternatives to Relieve Depression (STAR*D) Studies

PHQ-9 Score or Change	Outcome	Clinician Response
No decrease or increase	Nonresponse	Switch medication
Decrease of 2–4 points	Partial response	Add medication
Decrease of ≥5 points	Response	Maintain medication
Score <5	Remission	Maintain medication

Depression Scale (GDS) (Table 39.4). Although it offers the convenience of a "yes/no" response, and it is virtually free of somatic and sleep queries, it does not query suicidal or death ideation and is not useful for assessing treatment response. Those who acknowledge thinking they would be "better off dead" or "hurting yourself" should be asked about the presence of a firearm in the home. Firearms are the leading means of suicide among older adults. The PHQ-9 and the GDS may be reliable when administered to people with mild to moderate dementia, but response to treatment with SSRI therapy in dementia with depression may be no better than with placebo (SOE=A).

Emerging evidence suggests that the diagnostic process for older patients should include an assessment of executive cognitive function. When present, executive dysfunction complicating depression predicts poor response to SSRI therapy and may be better addressed with psychotherapy (SOE=A).

Table 39.4—The Geriatric Depression Scale (GDS, 15-item)

Choose the best answer for how you felt over the past week.	
1. Are you basically satisfied with your life?	yes/**no**
2. Have you dropped many of your activities and interests?	**yes**/no
3. Do you feel that your life is empty?	**yes**/no
4. Do you often get bored?	**yes**/no
5. Are you in good spirits most of the time?	yes/**no**
6. Are you afraid that something bad is going to happen to you?	**yes**/no
7. Do you feel happy most of the time?	yes/**no**
8. Do you often feel helpless?	**yes**/no
9. Do you prefer to stay at home, rather than going out and doing new things?	**yes**/no
10. Do you feel you have more problems with memory than most?	**yes**/no
11. Do you think it is wonderful to be alive now?	yes/**no**
12. Do you feel pretty worthless the way you are now?	**yes**/no
13. Do you feel full of energy?	yes/**no**
14. Do you feel that your situation is hopeless?	**yes**/no
15. Do you think that most people are better off than you are?	**yes**/no

NOTE: Score one point for each bolded answer; 0–5 = normal, >5 suggests depression. For additional information on administration and scoring, refer to the following:

SOURCE: Courtesy of Jerome A. Yesavage, MD. http://www.stanford.edu/~yesavage/GDS.html; http://www.stanford.edu/~yesavage/GDS.english.short.score.html (accessed Oct 2013)

Bipolar Disorder

Although the prevalence of bipolar disorder is low, the increasing numbers of older adults means clinicians will encounter more patients with a bipolar disorder, particularly bipolar depression. Bipolar disorders do not "burn out" in old age. Indeed, few patients with bipolar disorder recover full function despite symptom remission. Among those with bipolar disorder, mania is a more frequent cause of hospitalization than depression, but depression accounts for more disability. Late-onset mania is seen equally among men and women. Age has little impact on the symptom profile except for less sexual preoccupation among older adults. Impaired cognitive processing, executive dysfunction, and changes in subcortical brain structures are common, further reducing the chances of return to full function.

The *DSM-5™* criteria for bipolar disorder type 1 (mania with or without depression) and type 2 (major depressive disorder without mania but with hypomania) are unchanged with age. The manic episode (prevalence 1 to 4 per 1000) often presents with confusion, disorientation, distractibility, and irritability rather than with elevated, positive mood. The clinical interview can be characterized by irrelevant content delivered with an argumentative, emotionally intense yet fluent quality. Grossly unrealistic ideas concerning finances, travel, or plans for the future are common. Inflated self-esteem, grandiosity, and contentious claims of certainty in the face of evidence to the contrary are also seen. The unsuspecting examiner may be puzzled or irritated by the difficulty of the clinical interaction until the diagnosis of mania is considered.

The presence of psychosis, sleep disturbance, and aggressiveness may lead to the mistaken diagnosis of dementia or depressive disorder rather than mania. Because mania in late life is genuinely less frequent than depression or dementia, these patients are often treated with antipsychotics, antidepressants, or benzodiazepines, which provide partial relief. Late-onset mania is more often secondary to or closely associated with other medical disorders, most commonly stroke, dementia, or hyperthyroidism, and also with medications, including antidepressants, steroids, stimulants, and other agents with known CNS properties. A search for treatable components that contribute acutely to the person's disability should be pursued. Risk factors for cerebrovascular disease, including excessive use of alcohol or tobacco, suboptimal control of hypertension, hyperlipidemia, and other cardiovascular risk factors, should be explored. Careful inquiry of the family may reveal repeated hypomanic episodes that did not seriously impair the individual but in retrospect are clear indications of earlier disease. The difficulty of recognizing the diagnosis, care for contributing conditions, age-related vulnerability to adverse events of medication, and the frequency with which structural brain changes are associated all make treatment more difficult.

Occurring in approximately 0.5% of the U.S. population, bipolar disorder type II is characterized by recurrent major depressive episodes interspersed with periods of hypomania. Because interpersonal difficulties can be minimal, and some symptoms can temporarily increase performance with tasks, past episodes of hypomania may be unrecognized by the patient and family. Major depressive episodes also occur in bipolar disorder I, in which the occurrence of one or more manic episodes is the distinguishing diagnostic feature. There are also mixed states in which criteria for both mania and major depressive disorder are present. As a result, the term "bipolar depression" spans the spectrum of bipolar disorders.

Psychotic Depression

The recognition of psychotic depression has particular relevance to primary care clinicians. Patients with psychotic depression have sustained fixed false beliefs (delusions) in association with depressed mood. These delusions are often plausible and focused on physical or medical preoccupations, such as the belief that one's bowels are "blocked with cancer" or "I know there's something there and the doctors are just not telling me." Psychotic depression may be suspected when the irrational belief focuses on somatic symptoms or around fears of a serious physical condition when no medical evidence can be identified to support the belief. Patients with somatic delusions often visit multiple specialists and obtain repeated testing to identify problems that they "know" exist rather than for the purpose of seeking relief from persistent somatic "worries." Nearly 25% of older adults with somatic delusions are not diagnosed, despite visits to other healthcare practitioners or specialists and multiple diagnostic tests and procedures. Recognition of the excess disability caused by somatic delusions will improve the rate of diagnosis and appropriate treatment of this type of depression.

TREATMENT

Overview

Although mood disorders are eminently treatable, effective treatment remains a goal not so easily attained. Only 50% of patients with major depressive disorder fully respond to an initial antidepressant treatment (SOE=A). An additional one-third recover when the antidepressant is switched to another agent or is combined with a second antidepressant or psychotherapy. For those who do recover, 40%–60% experience recurrence depending on the severity of the initial episode and persistence of symptoms. Although a substantial number of patients with "subclinical," "subsyndromal," or "minor" depression experience a remission of symptoms without intervention, each category is associated with as much as a 5-fold risk of a subsequent major depressive episode. Poor self-assessed health and perceived lack of social support may be the simplest and most reliable measures to predict a less benign course. The onset of macular degeneration, stroke, and myocardial infarction are reliable indicators of depression risk, especially in the context of a prior history of mood disorder. Although the need to prevent mood disorders is substantial, success to date has been limited to reducing the progression of minor to major depressive disorder and to preventing recurrent episodes of major depressive disorder.

The current approach to mood disorders in late life includes a more aggressive acute phase of treatment to bring about remission of the current episode, continuation treatment to prevent relapse, and maintenance treatment to prevent recurrence. Continuation treatment to stabilize the recovery involves ongoing treatment for an additional 6 months after symptom remission. Maintenance treatment (≥3 years) is provided to patients with bipolar disorders or a history of depression complicated by psychosis, suicidality, or recurrent episodes. The duration of maintenance therapy should be based on the frequency and severity of previous episodes and may need to be lifelong. Combined pharmacotherapy with psychotherapy is recommended for all patients with bipolar disorders and recurrent, severe psychotic or suicidal depression (SOE=B).

The First Weeks of Treatment

Substantial data indicate that 4 weeks is adequate to identify those patients who at 12 weeks will be nonresponders or partial responders (SOE=B). The sooner the response occurs, the sooner the remission is likely to be achieved. More severe depression at baseline is associated with slower response; higher self-esteem is associated with rapid response. At 4 weeks, one-third of medicated patients will be nonresponders, one-third will have responded fully, and one-third partially. As the duration of treatment extends, the response rate for both partial and nonresponders decelerates. The longer the patient remains symptomatic, the greater the indication that either the dosage or the medication should be changed. In addition, partial response predicts recurrence of a major episode of depression.

Pharmacotherapy of Single or Recurrent Episodes of Major Depression

Currently available antidepressants are thought to work through the enhancement of monoamine function either blocking the reuptake or stimulating receptors of serotonin, dopamine, or norepinephrine. For a summary of antidepressants and adverse effects in older adults, see Table 39.5. A series of reports from the Sequenced Treatment Alternatives to Relieve Depression (STAR*D) study team offer a genuine advance for older adults in primary care settings with a structured treatment protocol for use by clinicians. When the first SSRI in the STAR*D protocol (citalopram) did not achieve remission, augmentation with a non-SSRI (bupropion or buspirone) reliably achieved remission in one-third of patients. Stopping citalopram because of intolerability or lack of response and switching to bupropion, venlafaxine, or sertraline achieved remission in an additional one-fourth. Of those not well after the first and second trial of monotherapy or augmentation, subsequent augmentation with L-triiodothyronine[OL] (T_3) was superior to monotherapy with nortriptyline, mirtazapine, or tranylcypromine and to augmentation with lithium or the combination of venlafaxine plus mirtazapine. In summary, for patients who could tolerate citalopram but did not achieve remission, augmentation with bupropion or buspirone was superior to switching to another agent. However, patients who did not tolerate citalopram did as well with sertraline as with bupropion or venlafaxine.

When psychosis complicates major depressive disorder, the evidence directing choice of pharmacotherapy for older adults is evolving. Electroconvulsive therapy (ECT) is effective for depression complicated by psychosis and is often considered the treatment of choice for patients with severe depression accompanied by suicidal thoughts and for those who do not respond to augmentation therapies (SOE=B). Yet, few patients or their family members will consider ECT without having exhausted other alternatives. In the multisite Study of Pharmacotherapy of Psychotic Depression (STOP-PD), remission was achieved in >60% of the geriatric patients who received a combination of sertraline and olanzapine over 12 weeks. Remission rates with combination therapy were substantially better than with sertraline alone. The average end-of-study daily doses were nearly 150 mg of sertraline and more than 12 mg of olanzapine. Therefore, while ECT remains an effective treatment option for late-life psychotic depression, intensive antipsychotic and antidepressant pharmacotherapy can be an effective initial strategy.

Pharmacotherapy of Mania

For a summary of treatment of bipolar disorders in older adults, see Table 39.6. Expert opinion, guidelines, and the Systematic Treatment Enhancement Program for Bipolar Disorder (STEP-BD) reports are in agreement that anticonvulsants, called mood stabilizers in this context, are preferable both for acute treatment and for prevention of recurrence in late-life bipolar mania (SOE=A). The anticonvulsant divalproex is increasingly considered first choice for treatment and prevention of mania. A therapeutic blood level of 50–100 mcg/mL can be used to ensure safety as well as efficacy. When the level is subtherapeutic and the patient response inadequate, the dose should be increased. When the level is at or above the upper limit and there is little or no response after 2 weeks, the drug should be declared a failure. Partial response accompanied by a blood level within the therapeutic range indicates the need to increase the dosage or add an antipsychotic. Divalproex inhibits hepatic enzymes that metabolize medications frequently used by older adults. Patients taking β-blockers, type 1C antiarrhythmics (eg, flecainide, propafenone), benzodiazepines, or anticoagulants should be monitored more closely until the divalproex dosage has been stabilized. Laboratory tests (including CBC with platelets, AST, ALT, and amylase) to ensure safety are performed when treatment is started, when the dosage is increased, and at least every 6 months. Dosage reduction is indicated for tremor interfering with self-care, ataxia or unsteady gait, excess sedation, or heart rate <50 beats per minute. Divalproex should be held or discontinued if the following do not remit after dosage reduction or dosage withholding: platelet count <80,000/μL, or AST, ALT, or amylase 2-fold or more above upper limit of normal.

Response to divalproex requires at least a 3-week period, including titration to a therapeutic range. In the interim, individuals whose mania is exhausting or associated with overly aggressive behavior require an antipsychotic or benzodiazepine. A number of second-generation antipsychotics are approved by the FDA for the treatment of mania (Table 39.6). Meta-analyses indicate that these second-generation antipsychotics appear to be equally effective (SOE=A) such that the choice of an individual agent is based on adverse-event profile. However, the available data on the treatment of mania in these studies include few older adults.

Older adults who have had good results with lithium should not be switched to an alternative unless adverse events become disabling. Nonetheless, the use of lithium as initial treatment should be considered cautiously. Structural brain changes that may not be clinically apparent are associated with a higher risk of toxicity. Diabetes insipidus, hyperglycemia, thyroid abnormalities, severe tremor, confusion, heart failure, arrhythmia, and psoriasis are among the more frequent reasons for discontinuing lithium. Manifestations of lithium toxicity include GI complaints, ataxia, slurred speech, delirium, or coma. Toxicity in older adults can occur at plasma concentrations below the therapeutic threshold of 1 mEq/L. Mild tremor and nystagmus without functional consequences frequently accompany lithium treatment and should not be considered signs of toxicity. Dosage reduction is indicated for tremor interfering with self-care or resulting in ataxia or unsteady gait. The onset of diabetes insipidus can also be cause for discontinuing lithium.

Pharmacotherapy of Bipolar Depression

Similar to the treatment of mania, there is a relative consensus that mood stabilizers are preferable to antidepressants for acute treatment and prevention of recurrence of late-life bipolar depression (SOE=B). Indeed, antidepressants should be used with caution in bipolar depression because of the risk of a manic reaction as well as other adverse events and lack of efficacy.

Electroconvulsive Therapy

ECT is highly effective for the treatment of major depressive disorder and mania in older adults. ECT is the first-line treatment for patients at serious risk of suicide or life-threatening poor intake due to a major depressive disorder (SOE=B). Patients with delusional depression can demonstrate paranoia about their food or caregivers, precluding pharmacologic treatment because of unreliable oral intake. Also, delusional depression is less responsive to standard medication regimens. Therefore, ECT is generally the first-line treatment for these patients and is associated with response rates that approximate 80%.

The cognitive adverse events of ECT are the principal factor limiting its acceptance. Anterograde amnesia or the inability to learn new information can be pronounced initially, particularly during bilateral ECT, but improves rapidly after treatment is completed. Retrograde amnesia is more persistent, and the recall of events that immediately preceded ECT can be lost permanently. Although patients may complain that ECT has had a long-term effect on their memory, longitudinal studies have not demonstrated lasting cognitive effects; furthermore, improved memory, perhaps owing to recovery from depression, has been reported. There are few absolute medical contraindications other than the presence of increased intracranial pressure or unstable angina. Patients with coronary artery disease or cerebrovascular disease can be administered ECT safely by appropriate pharmacologic management of the autonomic responses that can occur during treatment. Nevertheless, a recent myocardial infarction or cerebrovascular event and unstable coronary artery disease increase the risk of complications. Right unilateral treatment produces fewer cognitive adverse events than bilateral treatment but is less effective unless doses markedly exceeding a patient's seizure threshold are used.

The selection of ECT over aggressive pharmacotherapy is generally made by weighing the risk of waiting for medication to work against the burden of hospital treatment, any medical conditions that can complicate general anesthesia, and fears of the patient and family. After a course of ECT, patients should be treated with continuation of pharmacotherapy after recovery. Patients not responding to intensive antidepressant treatment before receiving ECT have lower acute response rates and are more likely to relapse subsequently, even when antidepressant treatment is continued with a new medication. Although maintenance ECT is sometimes used to prevent relapse, the burden that maintenance ECT places on patients and their families may limit its usefulness for long-term management of late-life major depressive disorder. However, some patients who respond uniquely well to ECT can tolerate maintenance ECT performed on an outpatient basis.

Psychosocial Interventions

Although evidence-based psychosocial interventions are not accessible to all depressed older adults, many components of the interventions have common sense appeal and can be incorporated into the practices of geriatricians and primary care clinicians. For psychosocial interventions for older adults with mood disorders, see Table 39.7. Studies demonstrating the efficacy of psychotherapy for major depressive disorder in older adults have included problem-solving therapy (SOE=B), cognitive-behavioral therapy, and interpersonal psychotherapy. Problem-solving therapy involves working with the patient to identify practical life difficulties that are causing distress and providing guidance to help the patient identify solutions. The treatment is delivered generally in six to eight meetings

Table 39.5—Selected Antidepressants for Older Adults

Generic Name	Initial Dosage (mg)	Final Dosage (mg)	Amnesia, Arrhythmia Potential	Hypotensive Potential	Sedative Potential	Precautions	Comments
Monoamine Oxidase Inhibitors (MAOIs)							
Selegiline	6 q24h transdermal patch	12 q24h transdermal patch	Low	Moderate	Low	MAOI type B with life-threatening diet and drug interactions unlikely at prescribed dosage	Transdermal patch with less risk of adverse events or suicide
Tranylcypromine	10–20 qam	30–60 qam	Low	Moderate	Low	Life-threatening diet and drug interactions	When depression resistant to TCA/SSRI; stimulant, short half-life
SSRIs							
Citalopram	10 qam	20qam	Moderate	Low	Low	Arrhythmia risk, nausea, tremor; reduce dosage in renal insufficiency; serotonin syndrome	Fewer drug interactions, oral solution available
Escitalopram	10 qam	10–20 qam	Low	Low	Low	Nausea, tremor; reduce dosage in renal insufficiency; serotonin syndrome	Single enantiomere, FDA approved for GAD, oral solution available
Fluoxetine	10 qam; 90 once/week for delayed-release form	20–40 qam	Low	Low	Low	Prolonged half-life, nausea, tremor, insomnia, drug interactions, serotonin syndrome	Adverse events not life threatening; inhibits CYP1A2, -2B6, -2D6, -3A4; liquid preparation available; FDA approved for OCD, panic disorder
Paroxetine	10 qhs	20–40 qhs	Low	Low	Low	Nausea, tremor, drug interactions; reduce dosage in renal insufficiency; serotonin syndrome	Mild sedative effect; inhibits CYP1A2, -2B6, -2D6, -3A4; FDA approved for PTSD, OCD, panic disorder, GAD, social anxiety disorder
Sertraline	25 qam	100–200 qam	Low	Low	Low	Nausea, tremor, insomnia, serotonin syndrome	Fewer drug interactions; FDA approved for OCD, PTSD, social anxiety disorder
Selective Serotonergic and Noradrenergic Reuptake Inhibitors (SSRI/SNRI)							
Desvenlafaxine	50 qam	50-100 qam	Low	Low	Low	Headache, nausea, hypertension, dizziness; reduce dosage in renal insufficiency	Active metabolite of venlafaxine
Duloxetine	20 qam	30–60 qam	Low	Low	Low	Drug interactions (CYP1A2, -2D6 substrate); chronic liver disease, alcoholism, increased serum transaminase; reduce dosage in renal insufficiency or choose other agent; rare cases of liver toxicity	Equally SSRI and SNRI, narrow dosage range; FDA approved for neuropathic pain, GAD, maintenance treatment for major depressive disorder
Venlafaxine XR	37.5–75 qam	75–225 qam	Low	Low	Low	Mild hypertensive; headache, nausea, vomiting; do not stop abruptly; reduce dosage in renal insufficiency	SSRI and SNRI, fewer drug interactions: Specify XR for once daily dosing

Stimulants							
Methylphenidate[OL]	2.5 qam	20 qam	Low	Low	Low	Anorexia, insomnia, daytime use only	Quick results; for the frail and apathetic
Modafinil[OL]	100–200 qam	400 qam	Low	Low	Low	Few studies in older adults; potential for drug interactions	Once daily dosing
Tricyclic Antidepressants (TCAs)							
Desipramine	10–25 qhs	25–150 qhs	Moderate	Moderate	Low	Can be fatal in overdose; glaucoma, prostatic disease	Therapeutic level 125–300 ng/mL
Nortriptyline	10–25 qhs	25–100 qhs	Moderate	Moderate	Moderate	Lower final dosage, may be fatal in overdose; glaucoma, prostatic disease, diabetes	Therapeutic window 50–150 ng/mL
Others							
Bupropion	75 q12h 150 qam	150–300 300 extended release qam	Low	Low	Low	Dopaminergic, noradrenergic; agitation, insomnia, seizures; no anxiolytic properties	For apathetic depression, when TCA/SSRI are ineffective; available in immediate-release, sustained-release, and extended-release tablets
Buspirone[OL]	5 q12h	30 in divided doses	Low	Low	Low	Only for augmentation, not a benzodiazepine substitute	Antianxiety agent with no dependence
Hypericum perforatum (St. John's wort)[OL]	300 q12h	900 q8h	Low	Low	Low	Use standardized, freeze-dried extract 0.3% hypericin; drug interactions; little evidence of efficacy	Low adverse-event profile, OTC
Lamotrigine XR	25 q24h	200 q24h	Moderate	Low	Low	Prolonged half-life; can cause fine skin rash, also potential for Stevens-Johnson syndrome	Causes increase in valproate levels when used concurrently; FDA approved for bipolar depression; chewable and dissolvable dose formats available; specify XR for once daily dosing
Mirtazapine	7.5 qhs	15–45 qhs	Low	Low	Moderate	Prolonged half-life, dry mouth, weight gain; reduce dosage for renal insufficiency; potential for neutropenia	When depression resistant to TCA/SSRI; sedative, useful for insomnia
Trazodone	25–50 qhs	100–400 in divided doses	Low	High	High	Very sedating; rare cases of priapism with high dosages	Potentially useful for sleep disturbance
L-triiodothyronine[OL] (various T_3)	25 mcg qam	50 mcg qam	Moderate	Low	Low	Anorexia, arrhythmia, hypertension; only for augmentation	Rapid onset of action
Vilazodone	10 qam	40 qam	Low	Low	Low	Nausea, insomnia, no studies devoted to older adults	Metabolized by CYP3A4, FDA approved for major depressive disorder

NOTE: GAD=generalized anxiety disorder; PTSD=posttraumatic stress disorder; OCD=obsessive-compulsive disorder

Table 39.6—Medications Used to Stabilize Mood in Mania and Bipolar Depression

Generic Name	Initial Dosage (mg)	Final Dosage (mg)	Sedative Potential	Precautions	Indications
Anticonvulsants					
Carbamazepine	100 q12h 100 qhs	500 q12h 800 hs	Moderate	Delayed onset of action, drug interactions, dizziness, unsteady gait, anemia; CBC and serum chemistries at baseline, then q6mo; enhances cytochrome P450 activity and decreases other drug concentrations	FDA approved for acute manic and mixed bipolar I episodes; therapeutic concentration 4–12 mcg/mL
Divalproex sodium Extended-release Delayed-release	250 q12h 250 hs 250 hs	1000 q12h 1000 hs 500 hs	Moderate	Delayed onset of action, drug interactions, GI upset, tremor, weight gain, edema, thrombocytopenia, sedation; CBC and serum chemistries at baseline, then q6mo; inhibits hepatic enzymes and increases other drug concentrations; hepatotoxicity, pancreatitis; reduce dosage in renal insufficiency	FDA approved for acute manic and mixed bipolar I episodes; better tolerated than carbamazepine; therapeutic concentration 50–100 mcg/mL
Lamotrigine	25 hs	100 q12h	Low	Headaches; prolonged half-life; appearance of rash calls for immediate cessation; valproate reduces clearance of lamotrigine	FDA approved for bipolar I depression to prevent recurrence; does not alter cytochrome P450 activity
Antipsychotics					
Aripiprazole	5 qam	15 qam	Low	Prolonged half-life, may produce agitation at high dosages because of D_2 dopamine receptor agonist activity	FDA approved for acute manic and mixed bipolar I episodes and for adjunctive treatment of major depressive disorder
Olanzapine	2.5 qhs	15 qhs	Moderate	Slightly anticholinergic as dosage increases, weight gain, metabolic syndrome, diabetes	FDA approved for acute manic and mixed bipolar I episodes
Olanzapine/fluoxetine	6/25 qhs	12/25 qhs		Little data on use in older adults	FDA approved for bipolar depression
Quetiapine	25 qhs	750 in divided doses	Moderate	Sedation, weight gain, metabolic syndrome, diabetes, arrhythmia	FDA approved for acute manic and bipolar I and II depression; sedative; less extrapyramidal symptoms, tardive dyskinesia
Risperidone	0.25 qhs	6 in divided doses	Low	Extrapyramidal symptoms likely at doses >2 mg, weight gain, metabolic syndrome, diabetes	FDA approved for acute manic and mixed bipolar I episodes
Lithium compounds					
Lithium carbonate Controlled-release	300 q24h 450 q24h	300 q8h 450 q12h	Low	Renal clearance is sole route of elimination; toxicity may appear below therapeutic range; mild tremor is a benign universal adverse event but not when excessive or combined with ataxia; polyuria, polydipsia may be signs of diabetes insipidus; nausea, vomiting are signs of toxicity; risk of hypothyroidism, renal impairment	FDA approved for acute and maintenance therapy of mania in bipolar disorder, lowers risk of suicide; therapeutic level 0.6–1 mEq/L

Table 39.7—Types of Psychotherapy and Other Psychosocial Interventions for Depressed Older Adults

Therapy/Intervention	Distinguishing Attributes
Cognitive-behavioral therapy to prevent recurrent suicide attempts	Thoughts, feelings, images, beliefs leading up to the attempt are addressed, then reprised at end of treatment to assess benefit; flash cards and memory box used to remind oneself why life is worth living
Cognitive bibliotherapy	Self-help format using Burns' *Feeling Good* (1980) as a workbook to identify and challenge maladaptive cognitions; little contact with therapist
Interpersonal	Exploratory, present- rather than past-oriented; focused on interpersonal conflict, role changes, and role deficits
Brief psychodynamic	Problem-focused, transference not examined, identifies conflicts over dependency and independence, intrapsychic locus, insight-oriented
Life review, reminiscence	Recall of personal success and failure to master one's present and future; developed for older adults
Problem-solving	Focused on change, narrow and pragmatic; solutions elicited from patient not offered by therapist; can reduce executive dysfunction
Emotionally supportive	Meant to maintain present level of function or symptom control through expression of burdensome feelings without examination of the unconscious or search for insight
Dementia caregiver counseling	Focused on the caregiver role, combines elements of cognitive-behavioral and interpersonal therapy
Bereavement therapy	Restructuring the experience of the lost loved one and restoration of life goals
Complicated grief therapy	Uses retelling and imaging of the death scene; imaginary conversations with the deceased to decrease disbelief, longing, bitterness, and intrusive preoccupations
Behavioral	Educational with focus directed at reducing negative and increasing positive experiences
Social support intervention	Encourages social outreach, network development; counters thoughts that preclude formation of supportive relationships; enhances social communication and assertiveness skills
Control-relevant intervention	Adaptation of behavioral, problem-solving, and social support interventions to provide greater sense of autonomy to depressed nursing-home residents
Behavioral health management	Facilitates treatment of depression in primary care in a disease management model that encourages adherence without directly providing psychotherapy; often includes telephone contact with clinician and patient by a trained mental health counselor
Dialectical behavior therapy	Focus on acceptance of that which cannot be changed, nonjudgmental awareness, distress tolerance, impulse control, acting counter to depressive urges
Social rhythm therapy	Adjunct to interpersonal therapy with focus on maintaining regularity of daily routines and managing precipitants of rhythm disruption to sustain the emotional quality of roles and relationships
Treatment initiation program	Early intervention to address the older adult's attitudes about depression and treatment, including perceived need for care and stigma of illness and treatment
Family-focused therapy	Incorporates psychoeducation with enhancement of communication skills and behaviors along with relapse prevention planning
Depression care management	Promotes treatment of depression in primary care practices through the services of a depression care manager; use of treatment protocols, access to psychotherapy and follow-up regarding compliance with treatment and satisfaction with care
Problem adaptation therapy (PATH)	Using the framework of problem-solving therapy, PATH focuses on the patient, environment, and caregiver to reduce disability and depression among cognitively impaired, depressed, disabled older adults; distinguished from other psychotherapeutic interventions by in-home delivery

spaced 1–2 weeks apart. Cognitive and interpersonal psychotherapy are also time-limited but less highly structured. Psychotherapy for minor depression has been promising, with efficacy demonstrated particularly in individuals who have suffered a loss; the goal is prevention of progression to major depressive disorder. Also, caregivers of older adults can develop minor or major depressive syndromes that benefit from psychotherapy. Psychosocial interventions can be effective without psychotropic medication. However, psychotherapy combined with an antidepressant has been associated with a longer period of remission after recovery from the acute episode (SOE=A).

Aerobic exercise is also prescribed as a treatment for mild to moderate depression in older adults who are capable of increasing their level of physical activity. It incorporates the concept of behavioral activation central to cognitive-behavioral psychotherapy. Exercise performed with a partner also adds to the perception of social support. Exercise in combination with antidepressants can yield faster, more lasting results than either alone (SOE=B). Encouraging physical activity should be part of the prescription for all depressed older adults.

Originally developed with younger and middle-aged patients, evidenced-based psychosocial interventions for bipolar depression are applicable to older adults. Intensive psychosocial interventions improve recovery of function and prevent hospitalization associated with recurrence (SOE=B). Improvements in relationships and life satisfaction associated with the interventions exceed those expected from improvements in mood alone. The interventions include family-focused treatment, interpersonal and social rhythms therapy, and cognitive-behavioral therapy as indicated based on individual needs.

For patients with available family, family-focused treatment emphasizes shared planning to prevent relapses, improved listening and communication, and problem-solving skills. In interpersonal and social rhythms therapy, interpersonal problems and difficulties maintaining a physiologically stabilizing schedule of sleep, waking, and activity are examined to minimize destabilizing social and interpersonal situations. In individual cognitive-behavioral therapy, patients and therapists discuss problem solving, cognitive restructuring, and behavioral activation exercises to reverse negative self-attributions and increase rewarding habits. Enthusiasm for these interventions must be tempered by the frequency with which cognitive impairment accompanies bipolar disorder. Nonetheless, the major components of these interventions have a common sense quality and can be applied in primary care.

REFERENCES

- Alexopoulos GS, Raue PJ, Kiosses DN, et al. Problem solving therapy and supportive therapy in older adults with major depression and executive dysfunction: effect on disability. *Arch Gen Psychiatry*. 2011;68(1):33–41.
- Katon W, Lin E, Von Korff M, et al. Collaborative care for patients with depression and chronic illnesses. *N Engl J Med*. 2010;363(27):2611–2620.
- Rojas-Fernandez CH, Miller LJ, Sadowski CA. Considerations in the treatment of geriatric depression: Overview of pharmacotherapeutic and psychotherapeutic treatment interventions. *Res Gerontol Nurs*. 2010;3(3):176–186.

CHAPTER 40—ANXIETY DISORDERS

KEY POINTS

- Late-life anxiety is often seen with other medical illnesses or depression.
- Comorbid medical problems that commonly lead to anxiety include cardiovascular and pulmonary disorders.
- SSRIs, including citalopram and sertraline, are often used as first-line treatment for anxiety in late life.
- Nonpharmacologic therapies, particularly cognitive-behavioral therapy and other types of psychotherapies, are beneficial in older adults.

The term anxiety disorder encompasses a spectrum of psychiatric illnesses that includes panic disorder, phobias, obsessive-compulsive disorder, posttraumatic stress disorder, and generalized anxiety disorder. Older adults can suffer from the full spectrum of anxiety disorders. A thorough review of the *Diagnostic and Statistical Manual of Mental Disorders, 5th Edition, (DSM-5™)* should guide the clinician. Older adults can experience a subjective feeling of anxiety that can meet a level of clinical concern that warrants treatment but does not necessarily fulfill the full diagnostic criteria for an anxiety disorder. While such symptoms merit clinical attention, true anxiety disorders are the focus of this chapter.

Because the published literature on anxiety disorders in older adults is limited, some of the characterizations and treatment strategies described here are based on research conducted in younger populations. Such strategies have been modified to take into account the physiologic and psychologic differences between older and younger adults.

Numerous complexities are involved in a proper assessment of anxiety in older adults. Understanding the common issues faced in such an assessment will lead to a more accurate diagnosis and treatment plan. Examples of these complexities include differentiating anxiety disorders from symptoms related to medical conditions or medications, differentiating anxiety disorders from the appropriate ("normal") experience of anxiety associated with the stressors of late life, appropriately attributing the cause of anxiety to an adverse event of medication, and differentiating anxiety from depression. These common challenges are further complicated by the tendency of older adults to resist psychiatric evaluation because of stigma surrounding mental illness or frank denial of illness.

Assessment of anxiety in older adults generally begins with a clinical psychiatric interview to determine the course and nature of symptoms. The interview should include an evaluation of the patient's mental status, including appearance, stated mood, observed affect, and thought process. Consideration of the patient's social context and support systems is particularly relevant in the geriatric population. Assessment of any impairment in functioning related to the anxiety is an important part of the evaluation. A review of all medications, both prescription and OTC, should be done to exclude an alternative medical or pharmacologic explanation for what appears to be an anxiety disorder, or to identify an aggravating condition. Questioning should be done to explore substance use, because use of alcohol or other drugs can exacerbate anxiety symptoms, or may represent an attempt to self-medicate anxiety. Laboratory tests to check for common medical conditions such as renal, thyroid, or hematologic diseases are important. Urine toxicology should be considered in cases in which substance abuse or misuse is suspected.

Anxiety as a symptom and full-scale anxiety disorders are common problems. The ability to recognize and effectively treat anxiety in older adults is important, given the debilitating effects that an unhealthy level of anxiety can have in this population.

CLASSES OF ANXIETY DISORDERS

The types of anxiety disorders as currently defined in the *DSM-5™* are discussed in the following section.

Panic Disorder

Panic disorder is characterized by chronic, repeated, and unexpected panic attacks—spontaneous bouts of overwhelming and irrational fear, terror, or dread when there is no specific cause. During a panic attack, the person experiences a constellation of physical and cognitive symptoms that can include palpitations, sweating, trembling, shortness of breath, the feeling of choking, chest pain or discomfort, nausea or abdominal distress, dizziness or lightheadedness, feelings of derealization (ie, that one or others are unreal) or depersonalization (ie, feeling detached from oneself), paresthesias, chills or hot flashes, fear of losing control, "going crazy," or dying. A diagnosis of a true panic attack requires that at least four of the somatic symptoms listed above are experienced. Attacks are brief, lasting typically 10–30 minutes. In between panic attacks, individuals with panic *disorder* worry excessively about when and where the next attack may occur. A clinically significant degree of panic symptoms exists if the history reveals that recurrent and unpredictable panic attacks have occurred for at least 1 month and that time is being spent in worried anticipation of possible recurrence. Whether agoraphobia related to the panic attacks is present also needs to be considered. In such cases, agoraphobia involves the persistent fear of situations that might trigger a panic attack, such as fear of having an attack in the mall, and therefore remaining at home. Patients who experience one or more panic attacks may not necessarily warrant a diagnosis of panic disorder. Panic attacks in late life often present with limited symptoms often related to one or two organ systems, such as shortness of breath, nausea, and diarrhea; overwhelming feelings of pounding in the chest; or dizziness. These limited-symptom panic attacks are accompanied by feelings of doom, dread, or fears of dying. The literature suggests that the usual onset of panic disorder is between 15 and 40 years of age and that <1% will have a new-onset panic disorder after age 65, although a Canadian community health survey suggested that almost 25% of older adults with panic disorder in late life had onset after age 55. Panic attacks in older adults are commonly associated with other psychiatric diagnoses, including major depressive disorder, as well as with medical illnesses, including COPD, hyperthyroidism, and pheochromocytoma.

Specific Phobia

A specific phobia is defined as a marked, persistent, excessive, unreasonable fear in the presence of or in anticipation of a particular distinct trigger, such as a specific person, animal, place, object, event, or situation. Examples of simple phobias include fear of snakes, mice, dogs, elevators, flying, or heights. Commonly, the person's anxiety level increases instantly when the feared trigger is encountered. Interestingly, he or she is able to identify this fear as unrealistic and unsupported, even though the cognitive and physiologic responses persist. Specific phobias often involve a great amount of anticipatory anxiety (ie, thoughts of the *possibility* of encountering the feared stimulus), and avoidance behaviors are likely to be reported. The consequence is that the person experiences a variety of personal difficulties as a result of the anxiety. These behaviors interfere with work and daily routines, and they decrease the person's opportunities to experience pleasurable situations (for fear that a trigger might be present). They can also contribute to secondary symptoms, such as frustration, hopelessness, and a sense of lack of control in one's life. The level of anxiety or fear usually varies as a function of both the degree of proximity to the phobic stimuli and the degree to which escape is limited. Specific phobias may be seen with panic disorder, with or without agoraphobia. Among older adults, especially in urban settings, fear of crime seems to be particularly prevalent. Phobic disorders tend to be chronic and persist into old age. However, fear of falling is a specific phobia that is increasingly recognized to have an onset in later life. The prevalence of specific phobias in older adults is thought to be 3%–8%.

Obsessive-Compulsive Disorder (OCD)

OCD involves persistent thoughts (obsessions) and behaviors (compulsions) that are performed in an effort to decrease the anxiety experienced as a result of the obsessions. Obsessions are thoughts or ideas that come to a person's mind, often while completing a specific task or during a particular type of situation, that are generally experienced as intrusive. Compulsions are behaviors that are either clearly excessive or are not connected in any realistic way with the thought/obsession that they are designed to "neutralize." For example, a person may wash his or her hands repeatedly, for hours at a time, after shaking a stranger's hand; the unwanted thought is of possibly having been exposed to a disease. In this example, the act of washing is the compulsion. Other compulsive behaviors include turning lights on and off and checking locks on doors repeatedly. The obsessive-compulsive person may realize that this behavior is excessive but feels intense anxiety if he or she tries to control the compulsion. OCD is chronic and often disabling. Sufferers may spend many hours every day carrying out their compulsions. Depression and other symptoms of anxiety can also be comorbid illnesses in the older population.

In general, the prevalence of OCD is low, the 1-year prevalence being <1%. OCD first appearing in late life is unlikely. More commonly, symptoms of obsessions occur along with a depressive syndrome or early dementia. For example, obsessions about paying bills on time can occur in the context of difficulty in estimating time and planning.

Hoarding Disorder

Hoarding Disorder is now coded in the *DSM-5™*. It is a late-life disorder that previously was thought to be related to OCD. However, hoarding was minimally responsive to OCD treatments. Also known as senile squalor syndrome, it is characterized by extreme self-neglect. It usually manifests itself with compulsive hoarding and the pathologic collection and storage of objects, often including items collected from garbage cans and dumpsters that the individual believes have value and meaning.

Posttraumatic Stress Disorder (PTSD)

The distinctive feature of PTSD is that the person has experienced, either as a witness or a victim, a traumatic event to which he or she has reacted with fear and helplessness. Examples of such events include those that involve actual or threatened death or serious injury, other threats to personal integrity, witnessing an event that involves death or serious injury of another, or even hearing about death or serious injury of a family member or close associate. Commonly observed symptoms include the reexperiencing of the traumatic event, avoidance (both cognitively and behaviorally) of stimuli associated with the event, psychologic numbing, and increased physiologic arousal. Reexperiencing can take the form of recurrent, intrusive recollections or images, thoughts, or even physical perceptions of the traumatic event. Such experiences are commonly termed flashbacks. Symptoms of hyperarousal include difficulty falling or staying asleep, hypervigilance, and exaggerated startle response. Nightmares, or recurrent distressing dreams of the traumatic event, are evidence of both hyperarousal and reexperiencing. Disorders often seen with PTSD include depression, panic disorder, and substance-use disorders. Symptoms must be present for at least 1 month and cause clinically significant distress or impairment in social, occupational, or other important areas of functioning. Individuals who experience these symptoms after a recent trauma (from 2 days to 1 month) are diagnosed with acute stress disorder. PTSD must be considered if distress persists for >1 month, and is considered chronic PTSD if the symptoms last for <3 months.

While <50% of people exposed to a traumatic event go on to develop PTSD, those who experience symptoms of acute stress disorder are at higher risk than those who do not develop acute symptoms (SOE=B). In older adults, PTSD can have a delayed onset, eg, a new presentation of the disorder in a Holocaust survivor. It is postulated that lack of social supports in the context of new stressors in an older adult's life can contribute to such a presentation. PTSD symptoms have been suggested to be associated with increased cardiovascular events, as was seen in a prospective study from 2007.

Generalized Anxiety Disorder (GAD)

The distinctive symptoms of GAD include excessive anxiety and worry in addition to experiencing other symptoms, such as muscle tension, feeling easily fatigued, difficulty sleeping through the night, difficulty concentrating on a task, and feeling irritable or on edge. These symptoms need to have occurred for at least 6 months and must be accompanied by the sense that one cannot control the feelings of anxiety. In addition, these feelings of intense worry must be a result of more than one stressor. For example, intense worry over financial matters or a medical illness alone, even with all the associated symptoms, in and of itself does not indicate a diagnosis of GAD. Many older adults with GAD also have symptoms of depression. The clinician must try to distinguish between the two diagnoses. When these symptoms occur in the context of a major depressive disorder, it is the latter diagnosis that must be assigned, but it is not surprising that >25% of patients with major depressive disorder have symptoms that would qualify them for a diagnosis of GAD. Some studies suggest that GAD may be the most common anxiety disorder in older adults, with prevalence rates between 1.2% and 7.3%. That said, <1% of individuals >74 years old have new-onset GAD.

COMORBIDITY

Depression with Marked Anxiety

Anxiety can be a prominent symptom of depression in many older adults. In fact, anxiety can be the presenting symptom that belies an underlying diagnosis of major depressive disorder. It is commonly believed that the expression of anxiety is more culturally acceptable in this cohort of older adults than the expression of depression. Patients presenting with a chief complaint of anxiety should routinely be evaluated for a major depressive disorder. Patients suffering from a combination of depressive and anxious symptoms can have clinically significant levels of distress despite the fact that they do not meet the full criteria for a diagnosis of either disorder.

Anxiety and Medical Disorders

Comorbid anxiety and medical disorders are commonly present. In many cases, medical illness can mimic an anxiety disorder in its presentation. Medical illness can also exacerbate a concurrent anxiety disorder, or vice versa. Finally, adverse effects of medications can produce or contribute to anxiety symptoms.

COPD is a common medical illness that can mimic an anxiety disorder. The common cold or influenza can aggravate a concurrent anxiety disorder. Other common medical illnesses that can cause or contribute to an anxiety disorder include cardiovascular or pulmonary conditions and hyperthyroidism. Medical illnesses that can be exacerbated by high levels of anxiety include angina pectoris or myocardial infarction.

Adverse effects of medications include those commonly encountered with thyroid hormone replacements, antipsychotics, caffeine, and theophylline, and can also be the primary cause of anxiety symptoms. Given the complicated clinical picture that results when anxiety and medical disorders coexist, a thorough assessment, including a clinical history, review of both prescribed and OTC medications including herbal supplements (with an eye toward possible interactions), appropriate laboratory tests, and

Table 40.1—Treatment Strategies for Anxiety Disorders in Late Life

Disorder	First-Line Treatments	Second-Line Treatments or Adjunctive Therapies
Panic disorder with or without agoraphobia	SSRIs[a], SNRIs[a], CBT[a]	Benzodiazepines[b]
Social phobia	SSRIs[a] plus CBT[b]	Benzodiazepines[b]
Social phobia, specific type (eg, public speaking)	β-blockers[OL] plus CBT[b]	Buspirone[b]
Specific phobia (eg, rats, blood)	CBT[b] or benzodiazepines[b]	β-Blockers[b]
Obsessive-compulsive disorder	SSRIs[a], SNRIs[b], CBT[b]	Clomipramine[b]
Posttraumatic stress disorder	SSRIs[b], SNRIs[b]	CBT[b]
Generalized anxiety disorder	SSRIs[a], SNRIs[a], CBT[a]	Benzodiazepines[b]
Anxiety and medical disorders	Identify and treat underlying cause; use SSRIs[a] or SNRIs[a] in primary anxiety disorder.	Benzodiazepines[b]
Depression with severe anxiety	SSRIs[a], SNRIs[a],CBT[a]	Buspirone[b], benzodiazepines[b]

NOTE: SNRIs=serotonin-norepinephrine reuptake inhibitors; CBT=cognitive-behavioral therapy

[a]SOE=A in studies of the geriatric population

[b]SOE=A in studies of the general adult population; insufficient studies in the geriatric population

measurement of therapeutic medication concentrations when appropriate, is imperative before treatment begins. When medical illness and anxiety symptoms coexist, maximizing potential anxiolytic properties of a medical treatment should be considered. For instance, in the treatment of a patient with diabetic neuropathy and anxiety, it would be appropriate to consider maximizing the dosage of duloxetine to take full advantage of its anxiolytic effects.

PHARMACOLOGIC MANAGEMENT

Numerous drugs have been used over the years as anxiolytics: alcohol, barbiturates, antihistamines, benzodiazepines, antipsychotic medications, and β-blockers. Evidence to support the use of many of these agents is lacking. Although empirical studies of the use of medications in treating older adults were initially limited, the body of literature to support this practice is increasing, including several randomized controlled trials of the treatment of late-life anxiety disorders (most often GAD). For some disorders, the body of literature supporting the efficacy of these medications is gleaned from use in younger patients, modified by age considerations. For example, a study of time for treatment for an anxiety disorder suggested that, if a patient responds, continuing on medication for a year decreases risk of relapse. A brief description of the various classes of compounds currently favored as anxiolytics follows. For a summary of the treatment strategies for anxiety disorders in late life, see Table 40.1.

Antidepressants

Antidepressants have proved efficacious in the treatment of panic disorder, OCD, GAD, and PTSD in younger patients. Studies have demonstrated that SSRIs, particularly citalopram, are safe and efficacious in the specific treatment of late-life anxiety disorders. Given their relatively favorable adverse-event profile, the SSRIs should now be considered the medications of choice for these disorders (SOE=A). Further, SSRIs should also be considered treatments of choice for treating depression with severe anxiety symptoms. Compounds such as venlafaxine and duloxetine (serotonin-norepinephrine reuptake inhibitors) should be considered as alternatives for those patients who do not respond to SSRIs or who experience adverse events.

Benzodiazepines

Over the past several decades, benzodiazepines have been the most commonly prescribed anxiolytics for both younger and older patients, but their use is now discouraged. When needed because symptoms are severe, benzodiazepines with shorter half-lives and without active metabolites, such as lorazepam and oxazepam, are preferable for treating older adults because they are metabolized by direct conjugation, a process relatively unaffected by aging. However, the use of even short-acting benzodiazepines should be limited to <6 months because long-term use is fraught with complications, such as motor incoordination and falls, cognitive impairment, depression, and the potential for abuse and dependence.

Other Medications

Several studies have suggested that buspirone, an anxiolytic medication with some serotonin-agonist properties, is efficacious for treatment of GAD (SOE=A), although clinical experience is less positive. Buspirone appears to be a safer choice than benzodiazepines for patients taking several other medications or needing treatment for longer periods of time. One drawback of buspirone is the amount of time required to see a clinical response (approximately 4 weeks). At times, concomitant use of a short-acting benzodiazepine in the initial stage of treatment could be useful for some patients. Although antihistamines such as hydroxyzine^{OL} and diphenhydramine^{OL} are sometimes used to manage mild anxiety in younger patients, the anticholinergic properties of these agents can cause serious problems in older adults, in whom their use is not recommended. Second-generation antipsychotics, such as risperidone^{OL}, olanzapine^{OL}, and quetiapine^{OL}, are not recommended choices for treatment of a nonpsychotic older adult with an anxiety disorder.

Psychologic Management

Although pharmacotherapy is commonly the first-line treatment for late-life anxiety disorders, psychologic treatments are often efficacious, either alone or as adjuncts to medication (SOE=A). The psychotherapeutic remedies that have been most rigorously tested all fall under the rubric of cognitive-behavioral therapy. Techniques generally fall into three categories: 1) relaxation training used with music, visual imagery, aromatherapy, and instruction in relaxation techniques; 2) cognitive restructuring to help the patient identify triggers and stimuli that maintain anxiety, gain more control over the effect of such stimuli, and develop a range of coping strategies and tools; and 3) exposure with response prevention (ie, the individual is exposed to the feared stimuli and prevented from performing a compulsive action), which is used with and particularly effective for OCD. Graded desensitization, which is used in panic and phobias, relies on exposure to gradually more anxiety-producing stimuli, with techniques to manage and tolerate the resultant anxiety. Treatment of older adults typically includes a combination of these therapeutic approaches. Success depends on the appropriateness of the patient for psychotherapy; the patient's support system, intellectual functioning, and level of motivation; the degree of coordination of care with medical professionals; and the nature of the disorder. Consultation with a mental health professional can assist in determining the appropriateness of a referral.

References

- Baldwin D, Woods R, Lawson R, et al. Efficacy of drug treatments for generalised anxiety disorder: systematic review and meta-analysis. *BMJ*. 2011 Mar 11;342:d1199.
- Neville C, Teri L. Anxiety, anxiety symptoms, and associations among older people with dementia in assisted-living facilities. *Int J Ment Health Nurs*. 2011;20(3):195–201.
- Wolitzky-Taylor KB, Castriotta N, Lenze EJ, et al. Anxiety disorders in older adults: a comprehensive review. *Depress Anxiety*. 2010;27(2):190–211.

CHAPTER 41—PSYCHOTIC DISORDERS

KEY POINTS

- Hallucinations are perceptions without stimuli that can occur in any sensory modality (ie, visual, auditory, tactile, olfactory, gustatory). In late life, multimodal hallucinations are common.
- Delusions are abnormal beliefs that in late life are often paranoid or persecutory, such as a belief that one's safety is in jeopardy or that one's belongings are being stolen.
- Psychosis occurring for the first time in late life is often due to dementia or neurologic conditions such as Parkinson disease or stroke, as opposed to a primary psychotic disorder, such as schizophrenia.
- Dementia with Lewy bodies is associated with characteristically vivid visual hallucinations, often including people or animals.
- When psychotic symptoms arise in the context of depression, the symptoms are often "mood congruent," such as delusions that one is penniless or that one is already dead.

Psychotic symptoms are defined as either *hallucinations*, ie, perceptions without stimuli, or *delusions*, ie, fixed, false, idiosyncratic ideas. Hallucinations are abnormal perceptions without stimulus that can be in any of the five sensory modalities (auditory, visual, tactile, olfactory, gustatory). Delusions are fixed false beliefs or ideas that can be suspicious (paranoid), grandiose, somatic, self-blaming, or hopeless. This chapter focuses on conditions in which psychotic symptoms are prominent and central to making the diagnosis. It only briefly discusses other disorders, such as dementia, delirium, and the mood disorders, in which psychotic symptoms can occur but the defining features are in the cognitive or mood realms (discussed elsewhere; see "Dementia," p 256; "Delirium," p 276; and "Depression and Other Mood Disorders," p 308).

Hallucinations and delusions occur in a variety of disorders. The evaluation of an older adult with hallucinations and delusions should begin with evaluation for underlying sources such as delirium, dementia, stroke, or Parkinson disease. An acute onset of altered level of consciousness or inability to sustain attention suggests delirium. Next, a primary mood disorder should be considered. Only after other causes are excluded should the diagnosis of a schizophrenia-like state be made. Delirium, most often superimposed on an underlying dementia, is the most common cause of new-onset psychosis in late life.

SCHIZOPHRENIA AND SCHIZOPHRENIA-LIKE SYNDROMES

Schizophrenia is defined as a chronic psychiatric disorder characterized by positive symptoms (eg, hallucinations, delusions, and thought disorder) and negative symptoms (eg, social dilapidation and apathy). Mood disorder and cognitive disorder should be excluded before the diagnosis is made. In men, schizophrenia has a modal onset at age 18; onset after age 45 is uncommon. In women, modal age of onset is 28, and 20%–30% of cases begin after age 45. Approximately 85% of older adults with schizophrenia experienced onset of illness in early adult life. However, 10%–15% of cases of schizophrenia first come to clinical attention after patients are 45 years old. Schizophrenia with onset between the ages of 40 and 60 is called "late-onset schizophrenia," while patients with onset after age 60 are considered to have "very-late-onset schizophrenia-like psychosis."

In older adults, late-onset schizophrenia-like conditions are characterized by onset after age 44, prominent persecutory (paranoid) delusions, and multimodal hallucinations (SOE=C). For example, patients commonly complain that items are being stolen or report that they are being persecuted unjustly. Hallucinations often manifest in complaints, for example, that a neighbor is persistently banging on walls or the roof, that someone is pumping gas under the door, or that electrical sensations are being sent through the walls of the person's home and into his or her body. A schizophrenia-like psychosis can be diagnosed only when cognitive disorder, mood disorder, or other explanatory medical conditions such as delirium or focal brain pathology have been excluded.

The schizophrenia-like psychoses of late life differ from schizophrenia beginning in early life in two ways (SOE=C). First, thought disorder, a sign described as speech in which a series of thoughts are not connected to one another in a logical fashion, is much less common in older adults, comprising only 5% of cases. In early-onset schizophrenia, thought disorder is present in approximately 50% of cases. Thought disorder in schizophrenia occurs in the absence of an impaired sensorium (ie, delirium). When illogical speech occurs in late life, a delirium or dementia should be excluded. A second significant difference is the rarity of social deterioration and dilapidation among older adults. Thus, personality is often intact in late-onset cases. However, there is a dearth of long-term follow-up studies, so it is unknown whether social deterioration and personality changes occur after many years of symptoms.

Epidemiology and Clinical Characteristics

Late-onset schizophrenia is more common among women. The population-based incidence of late-onset schizophrenia is unknown, but the lifetime prevalence of schizophrenia is 1% among both men and women.

Late-onset schizophrenia-like psychoses affect predominantly women, with the female:male ratio ranging from 5:1 to 10:1. Many older adults with late-onset schizophrenia-like psychosis have been married at some time and have been able to hold responsible jobs and work efficiently, but premorbid isolation and "schizoid" (socially isolated personality) traits are common.

While many individuals with schizophrenia experience fewer hallucinations and delusions as they age, others remain significantly functionally impaired by psychotic symptoms. Moreover, older adults with schizophrenia have an increased risk of suicidal behavior compared with that of their peers without mental illness (SOE=C).

One condition that may be confused with late-onset schizophrenia is frontotemporal dementia, because it can involve features of socially inappropriate and odd behaviors as well as premorbidly odd or "schizoid" personality features. (See "Dementia," p 256.) While individuals with early-onset schizophrenia have more cognitive deficits than patients with late-onset schizophrenia, these cognitive changes remain relatively stable over time. Neither early-onset nor late-onset schizophrenia is considered a dementing illness, and rapid memory loss should prompt further evaluation for possible comorbid conditions, including dementia.

Treatment and Management

Nonpharmacologic

Because suspiciousness and paranoid delusions are commonly the most prominent symptoms, the clinician's first task in treating late-onset psychosis is often to establish a trusting therapeutic relationship with the patient. On occasion, the suspicious ideas are plausible (eg, the claim that the patient is being financially abused by a relative), but usually the delusions are bizarre and implausible. It is rarely effective to confront the patient with the unreality or implausibility of his or her ideas. The patient is more likely to respond positively if the clinician empathizes with the distress that the symptoms cause ("I can see how upset you are by all of this"). If patients ask whether the clinician "believes" them, a response such as, "I don't hear anything like that, but I appreciate the fact that you do" is both honest and empathetic. The symptoms are usually frightening and distressing to the patients and can lead to unusual behaviors. For example, patients who develop concerns that their food is being poisoned may exhibit unusual eating habits or food avoidance. Furthermore, suspiciousness can isolate the patient from friends and family. Therefore, encouraging patients to maintain important relationships and seeking their permission to discuss the source of symptoms with close family members or friends can help these patients maintain important, supportive relationships.

Pharmacologic

Clinical consensus and descriptive case series suggest that antipsychotic medications are as effective in late-onset schizophrenia as in early-onset cases (SOE=B). Most specialist clinicians recommend second-generation antipsychotic medications, because such agents are less likely to cause tardive dyskinesia (TD), an adverse event for which older age is a predisposing factor. Dosages should be increased at semiweekly or weekly intervals as needed. While dosages are being titrated, patients should be monitored for the emergence of extrapyramidal adverse events (eg, parkinsonian tremor, rigidity, dystonia) and other movement disorders. (See drug-induced movement disorders in "Neurologic Diseases and Disorders," p 480.) These should be treated by lowering the dosage and switching to an alternative antipsychotic if necessary. Polypharmacy should be avoided by reducing the dosage or switching the antipsychotic medication rather than by adding a medication for extrapyramidal symptoms. The more common adverse events with quetiapine are sedation and orthostatic hypotension; with risperidone, extrapyramidal symptoms; and with olanzapine, weight gain and sedation (Table 41.1).

No studies are available to guide the duration of treatment. Clinical experience suggests that patients who respond to antipsychotic medications should be continued on the minimal effective dosage for at least 6 months. Patients with early-onset schizophrenia and chronic stable symptoms may be able to tolerate a gradual reduction in dosage of antipsychotic medication. For all patients who relapse on treatment or when the dosage is lowered, maintenance over a longer term (at least 1–2 years) is recommended (SOE=D). Patients should be monitored for the emergence of TD, a syndrome characterized by repetitive involuntary movements of the oral and limb musculature. Rating scales for TD, such as the Abnormal Involuntary Movement Scale (AIMS) or the Dyskinesia Identification System Condensed User Scale (DISCUS), are clinically useful and easy to administer in the office or institutional setting. If TD develops, the dosage of the antipsychotic

Table 41.1— Dosing and Adverse Events of Commonly Used Antipsychotic Medications for Psychotic Disorders

Medication	Starting Daily Dosage (mg)	Maximal Daily Dosage (mg)	Adverse Events		
			EPS*	Drowsiness	Weight Gain
Aripiprazole	5	15	++ (akathisia)	+	+
Asenapine	5	10	+	+++	++
Clozapine	12.5	100	+	+++	+++
Haloperidol	0.5–1	5–10	+++	++	+
Iloperidone	1	12	+	++	+
Lurasidone	40	80	+	++	+
Olanzapine	2.5	10–15	+	++	+++
Paliperidone	1.5	12	++	++	+
Perphenazine	4	32	++	++	++
Quetiapine	25	200–300	+	+++	++
Risperidone	0.5–1	2–4	++	+	++
Ziprasidone	20	120	+	++	+

NOTE: + = uncommon, ++ = somewhat common, +++ = common

*EPS = extrapyramidal signs: rigidity, parkinsonian tremor, dystonia, akathisia

medication should be lowered if possible. Depending on the duration of exposure, TD may worsen or appear when the antipsychotic is discontinued or the dosage is lowered, or when switching from one antipsychotic to another. At the time antipsychotic medications are started or as soon as symptoms improve enough so that the patient can understand the risk, he or she should be informed of the risk of TD and the possibility that it can be irreversible.

Psychotic Symptoms

Delirium and Delusional Disorder

Hallucinations, particularly visual hallucinations, can be a symptom of delirium, even when it is mild. The onset of delirium is typically acute, and there is usually an identifiable metabolic, pharmacologic, or infectious cause. The mental status examination reveals multiple cognitive impairments and a diminished or waxing and waning level of consciousness. (See "Delirium," p 276.)

Some older patients present with long-standing chronic delusions without hallucinations. When these occur in patients with a normal mood and who do not have cognitive impairment, then a diagnosis of delusional disorder may be made. A recent study found that delusional disorder is more frequent among women and that men experience more severe symptoms. Most commonly, the delusions are persecutory or paranoid in nature, but delusions of jealousy or somatic delusions of bodily dysfunction are seen as well. Patients with somatic delusions may present to multiple health practitioners and request medical interventions. Management strategies include reassurance, amelioration of sensory deficits, and sometimes antipsychotic medication.

Mood Disorder

Delusions can be seen in major depressive disorder and in the manic phase of bipolar disorder. These delusions are described as "mood congruent." That is, in patients with depression, the delusional content usually reflects self-deprecation, self-blame, hopelessness, or the conviction of ill health. A patient may complain, for example, that he or she has no blood or that his or her intestines are not working; another patient may believe that he or she has caused a terrible wrong and deserves to be punished (a self-blaming delusion). Some patients become convinced that they are dying and that nothing can be done to help them when there is no physiologic evidence to support their concerns. Other common depressive delusions are the conviction that one has no insurance, no clothing, or no money when this is not true (delusion of poverty). Delusions congruent with mania are grandiose. Examples include the person's belief that he or she is infallible, can do impossible physical or intellectual activities, has skills and abilities that no other human being has, or is a special personage such as Jesus Christ. (See "Depression and Other Mood Disorders," p 308.)

Dementia

Patients with dementia experience both hallucinations and delusions. These are usually less complex than the delusions seen in schizophrenia or mood disorder. Common delusions in dementia are the belief that one's belongings have been stolen or moved, or the conviction that one is being persecuted. Delusions that one's spouse is unfaithful (delusions of infidelity) are also common. See "Dementia," p 256.

Management of psychosis in dementia is particularly challenging, because the use of antipsychotic medication warrants careful consideration of risks and adverse events. Nonpharmacologic interventions, such as redirection and reassurance, should be tried first. However, if the patient is physically aggressive or severely distressed by the psychotic symptoms, then a trial with low-dose antipsychotic medication is warranted (SOE=C). Both first- and second-generation antipsychotic medications are associated with numerous adverse events, including stroke and death, in patients with dementia (for a detailed discussion, see "Behavioral Problems in Dementia," p 267).

Second-generation antipsychotics have a class warning concerning the increased risk of developing hyperglycemia and diabetes in both younger and older patients with schizophrenia. The mechanism for these adverse events is unclear.

SYNDROMES OF ISOLATED HALLUCINATIONS

Charles Bonnet Syndrome

Between 10% and 13% of patients with significant visual impairment (bilateral acuity worse than 20/60) experience visual hallucinations. These can take the form of shapes such as diamonds or rectangles but more commonly consist of complex silent hallucinations such as small children, multiple animals, or a vivid scene such as one would see in a movie. This condition, first described more than 200 years ago, goes by the eponym Charles Bonnet syndrome. The criteria for this syndrome are as follows:

- silent visual hallucinations
- partially or fully intact insight (the patient is aware that the perceptions cannot be real but still reports that they appear absolutely real and vivid)
- visual impairment
- lack of evidence of brain disease or other psychiatric disorder

It has been suggested that this syndrome is a concomitant of the phantom limb syndrome caused by retinal lesions. However, visual hallucinations have also been reported in individuals with field defects caused by cortical lesions of the visual pathways.

The best treatment for the Charles Bonnet syndrome is education, reassurance, and support. Patients should be informed that the hallucinations are a sign of eye disease, not mental illness. An occasional patient has partial insight or loses insight and becomes very distressed by this symptom. When this distress is significant or leads to dangerous behavior, a cautious trial of low dosages of a second-generation antipsychotic medication is occasionally beneficial.

Psychotic Disorder Caused by a General Medical Condition

Patients with Parkinson disease, stroke, and other brain disorders may experience delusions and hallucinations without prominent cognitive impairment or other evidence of psychiatric disorder (SOE=C). Delirium caused by a superimposed condition should be excluded. In patients with Parkinson disease, psychotic symptoms are common and may be secondary to a prescribed dopaminergic agent, although some patients experience visual hallucinations before any medications are started. Education and support should be offered to all patients with these symptoms. Judicious discontinuation or dose reduction of nonessential antiparkinsonian medications often provides relief from psychotic symptoms. If patients experience significant emotional distress or if the symptoms lead to dangerous or upsetting behavior, cautious use of an antipsychotic medication is appropriate (SOE=B). Use of conventional or first-generation antipsychotic medications is usually avoided because of the potential for exacerbating parkinsonian symptoms (SOE=B). For patients with Parkinson disease and hallucinations or psychosis, quetiapine^{OL} 12.5–75 mg/d may be beneficial. Some patients require clozapine^{OL} 12.5–75 mg/d. However, patients taking clozapine should have a CBC with absolute neutrophil count done once a week for 6 months and then biweekly thereafter because of the risk of granulocytopenia.

Dementia associated with Lewy bodies is increasingly recognized as an important cause of hallucinations in late life. The clinical scenario typically involves cognitive decline accompanied by motor features of parkinsonism. However, prominent visual hallucinations are a key part of the diagnosis. These hallucinations are often vivid and troubling. See "Dementia," p 256.

Dementia associated with Lewy bodies presents a challenge similar to that of psychosis in Parkinson disease, because the medications in the class approved to treat psychosis (the antipsychotics) worsen the parkinsonian symptoms. At least two placebo-controlled clinical trials and multiple case studies report significant improvement through the use of cholinesterase inhibitors^{OL} (SOE=B). If an antipsychotic medication must be used, then the treatment strategies outlined above are appropriate if there is careful attention to the risk of extrapyramidal adverse events. Nonpharmacologic treatments include redirection, reassurance, and explanation.

References

- Collier E, Sorrell JM. Schizophrenia in older adults. *J Psychosoc Nurs Ment Health Serv*. 2011;49(11):17–21.
- Iglewicz A, Meeks TW, Jeste DV. New wine in old bottle: Late-life psychosis. *Psychiatr Clin North Am*. 2011:34(2):292–318.
- Schneider LS, Dagerman KS, Insel P. Risk of death with atypical antipsychotic drug treatment for dementia: meta-analysis of randomized placebo-controlled trials. *JAMA*. 2005;294(15):1934–1943.
- Weintraub D, Chen P, Ignacio RV, et al. Patterns and trends in antipsychotic prescribing for Parkinson disease psychosis. *Arch Neurol*. 2011:68(7):899–904.

CHAPTER 42—PERSONALITY AND SOMATIC SYMPTOM DISORDERS

KEY POINTS

- Personality disorders persist into late life and pose complex challenges in patients across various medical and psychiatric settings.
- Personality disorders can be more difficult to detect in late life because of age-associated changes in symptoms, comorbid psychopathology, and lack of age-adjusted diagnostic instruments.
- The goal of treatment of personality disorders in late life is not to cure the disorder but to decrease the frequency and intensity of symptoms. To this end, both psychotherapeutic and psychopharmacologic strategies are needed.
- Somatic symptom disorders represent the presence of physical symptoms without established underlying pathology and with strongly associated psychologic factors. Undifferentiated somatic symptom disorder and hypochondriasis are the most common forms seen in late life.
- Treatment of somatic symptom disorders must attend to the affected individual's distress and belief in the veracity of his or her symptoms. Repeated reassuring clinical visits help to build a therapeutic relationship. Both psychotherapy and pharmacotherapy can be helpful for some individuals.

PERSONALITY DISORDERS

Personality refers to the unique characteristics and qualities that define an individual's ability to form relationships, cope with life stress, and approach the tasks of daily living. Personality disorders are defined in the *Diagnostic and Statistical Manual of Mental Disorders, 5th Edition* (*DSM-5™*) by the presence of chronic and pervasive patterns of inflexible and maladaptive inner experiences and behaviors. These patterns lead to significant disruptions in several spheres of function, including cognitive perception and interpretation, affective expression, interpersonal relations, and impulse control. Individuals with personality disorders are often distinguished by repeated episodes of disruptive or noxious behaviors and, as a result, they often receive pejorative labels, depending on their form. Descriptive terms often applied to those with personality disorders include "difficult," "dramatic," and "strange," to name just a few. The developmental roots of personality disorders are believed to lie in childhood and adolescence, but their features can present clinically at any age in adulthood. Personality disorders are influenced by both genetic and environmental factors.

The *DSM-5™* describes ten personality disorders, grouped into three broad clusters that are based on common phenomenology; however, they are no longer documented on a separate axis. For late-life features of all ten personality disorders, see Table 42.1. Depressive and passive-aggressive personality disorders were two additional categories that were considered provisional in *DSM IV-TR*, but have not been included in *DSM-5™* because of a lack of empirical support. Some clinicians continue to see older adults who present with the symptom constellations of depressive and passive-aggressive personality disorders. Mixed diagnoses and those that do not fit into any existing category are labeled "personality disorder, not otherwise specified."

Many older adults with personality disorders can easily become overwhelmed by age-associated losses and stresses, largely because they lack appropriate coping skills and the personal, social, or financial resources to buffer their losses. In particular, admission to a hospital or long-term care setting poses a unique stress on all individuals with personality disorders in late life. The loss of a familiar environment, personal items, privacy, and the control over one's schedule can lead to a sense of disorganization and displacement. Conflict in an institutional setting begins when patients with personality disorders try to cope with the stresses from their new environment by exaggerating their maladaptive behaviors. An obsessive-compulsive person may attempt to maintain a sense of control by demanding rigid adherence to schedules and rules of hygiene. Dependent individuals may feel helpless and panicked without enough attention to their needs, responding with clinging behaviors and excessive questions or requests for assistance. Paranoid, antisocial, and borderline patients may refuse to cooperate with treatment plans or institutional rules.

Epidemiology

Prevalence rates of late-life personality disorders in the community range from 5% to 13%, which is a slightly lower range than the 10% to 20% prevalence estimates for individuals of all ages in the community. Prevalence rates in inpatient settings and with comorbid depression are much higher, ranging from 10% to >50%, depending on the method of diagnosis.

Table 42.1—Features of Personality Disorders

Cluster, Disorder	General Features*	Features Specific to Older Adults
Cluster A: Odd or Eccentric Behaviors		
Paranoid	Pervasive suspiciousness of the motives of others, which often leads to irritability and hostility	Episodes of paranoid psychosis, agitation, and assaultiveness
Schizoid	Disinterest in social relationships, coupled with isolative and sometimes odd behaviors	Poor, strained, or absent relationships with caregivers
Schizotypal	Characteristic appearance, behaviors, and beliefs that are strange, unusual, or inappropriate	Beliefs that can become delusional and lead to conflicts with others; relationships with caregivers can be strained or absent
Cluster B: Dramatic, Emotional, or Erratic Behaviors		
Antisocial	Poor regard for social norms and laws; lack of conscience and empathy for others; frequent reckless and criminal behaviors	Frequent remission of antisocial behaviors with less aggression and impulsivity
Borderline	Impaired control of emotional expression and impulses associated with unstable interpersonal relations, poor self-identity, and self-injurious behaviors	Persistent emotional lability and unstable relationships but less self-injurious and impulsive behaviors
Histrionic	Excessive emotionality and attention-seeking behaviors, sometimes appearing overly seductive or provocative	Behaviors that can become excessively disinhibited and disorganized, appearing manic
Narcissistic	Pervasive sense of entitlement, grandiosity, and arrogance, coupled with lack of empathy	Can present as hostile, enraged, paranoid, or depressed
Cluster C: Anxious or Fearful Behaviors		
Avoidant	Excessive sensitivity to rejection and social scrutiny; social demeanor that can be timid and inhibited	Social contacts that can be extremely limited, providing for inadequate support
Dependent	Excessive dependence on others to help make decisions and provide support	Commonly, comorbid depression; clinical appearance often with demanding or clinging behaviors if dependency needs not met
Obsessive-compulsive	Pervasive preoccupation with orderliness and cleanliness; a perfectionistic, rigid, and controlling approach that can become more inflexible and indecisive under stress	Obsessive-compulsive traits that can become exaggerated in efforts to maintain control over somatic and environmental changes

* Descriptions of the clusters and of the disorders in each cluster are based on the *Diagnostic and Statistical Manual of Mental Disorders. 5th ed.* Washington, DC: American Psychiatric Association; 2013. An alternative model of personality disorders is presented in the appendix of the *DSM-5™*, but it has not been officially adopted.

The most common personality disorders in late life are dependent, obsessive-compulsive, paranoid, and not otherwise specified. Although most research has demonstrated fewer diagnoses in older age groups, it is unclear whether this represents an actual difference in prevalence or merely reflects the fact that it is more difficult to make a diagnosis in late life. Some researchers have suggested that prevalence rates can be influenced by increased mortality among those with personality traits that are associated with higher rates of reckless, impulsive, and self-injurious behaviors. Other research exploring the neural substrates of emotion has demonstrated an attenuation of emotional reactivity in late life across a number of physiologic and behavioral parameters. These findings can partially explain the reduction in prevalence of the more impulsive and emotionally reactive personality features, such as those associated with borderline personality disorder.

Diagnostic Challenges

Establishing a diagnosis of personality disorder in older adults can be especially challenging because it requires a detailed, longitudinal psychiatric and psychosocial history. Older patients and their informants are not always able to provide sufficient history, especially when it may span ≥50 years. The history can be distorted by recall bias (the tendency to present more socially desirable traits) or memory impairment. Furthermore, schizotypal and paranoid individuals may be reluctant to engage in clinical interviews and share personal history, and antisocial and narcissistic individuals who lack insight into their problems may refuse to divulge relevant experiences. Records often do not provide sufficient information to determine prior personality dynamics. Remote diagnoses from previous decades cannot be easily correlated with current ones, because the diagnostic criteria for personality disorders have changed significantly in the past 50 years. As a result of all of these limitations, clinicians often are unable to make a diagnosis or end up making judgments based on insufficient information.

A further diagnostic challenge for clinicians is the need to isolate lifelong personality characteristics from a multitude of comorbid psychiatric and medical problems. Acute and chronic episodes of major depression, psychosis, and other major psychiatric disorders can considerably distort personality features. Even the current diagnostic nomenclature might serve to handicap late-life diagnosis because it is not age adjusted, and many criteria do not apply in late life. A final barrier to diagnosis can be present if the clinician erroneously considers all older patients to have disruptive personality features as a normal function of age.

Differential Diagnosis

In clinical settings, it is important to remember that not every older patient with prominent or troubling personality features has a personality disorder. Those who demonstrate rigid and maladaptive personality traits but without the pervasiveness or severity as represented by *DSM-5™* criteria are better described as suffering from certain personality traits or an adjustment disorder. An adjustment disorder might best characterize previously healthy and well-adjusted individuals who demonstrate acute changes in personality as a result of severe stresses. For example, physical pain and disability can lead to dependent or avoidant behaviors that resemble those seen in personality disorders, but without the pervasive pattern and degree of maladaptiveness. Often, the symptoms of major psychiatric disorders and those of personality disorders overlap considerably, and without longitudinal history it can be difficult to distinguish between them. For example, the odd thinking and unusual perceptual experiences seen in psychotic disorders can resemble behaviors seen in schizotypal personality disorder. The emotional lability of bipolar states can mimic behaviors of borderline and histrionic diagnoses, and depressive symptoms from dysthymic and depressive disorders can be almost indistinguishable from depressive personality traits. Diagnosis of a personality disorder becomes more certain when seemingly acute behaviors emerge as enduring and pervasive personality traits. This process depends on the opportunity to observe a person over time and in multiple settings or situations.

Personality disorders as described in *DSM-5™* must also be differentiated from the diagnosis of personality change due to a specific medical condition. When personality change is a direct result of brain damage, it has classically been described within the context of an "organic" personality disorder, although this term is no longer used in *DSM* nomenclature. Most often, personality changes with an "organic" source involve impairments in executive functioning, consisting of poor impulse control, poor planning, and greater vulnerability to irritability or agitation. Along these lines, Alzheimer disease and other dementias are often associated with personality changes, including apathy, egocentricity, and impulsivity. Frontal lobe injury can result in a disinhibited impulsive syndrome, or conversely, an apathetic, avolitional syndrome. Frontotemporal dementia has been associated with distinct personality changes characterized by odd social interactions and compulsive behaviors such as hoarding. (See "Dementia," p 256.) Temporal lobe epilepsy has been associated with personality change, including emotional deepening, verbosity, hypergraphia, hypersexuality, and preoccupation with religious, moral, and cosmic issues. Other disorders found in older adults that are associated with personality disorders include brain tumors, multiple sclerosis, and encephalopathies.

Long-Term Course

Personality disorders can follow one of four possible courses: persist unchanged, evolve into a different form or major psychiatric disorder (eg, depression), improve, or remit. Few disorders have actually been studied over time, and rarely into late life. Several studies have suggested that personality disorders can enter a period of relative quiescence in middle age, with fewer and less intense symptoms and increased adaptation (SOE=C). However, this period may precede their reemergence in late life. Other researchers have proposed that personality disorders characterized by emotional and behavioral lability, including antisocial, borderline, histrionic, narcissistic, and dependent disorders, tend to improve over time, although patients remain vulnerable to depression. Personality disorders characterized by an overcontrol of affect and impulses, including paranoid, schizoid, schizotypal, and obsessive-compulsive personality disorders, are thought either to remain stable or to worsen in late life.

Only antisocial and borderline personality disorders have been looked at longitudinally, and both have shown symptom improvement and even remittance into middle and later life for a significant percentage of patients (SOE=B). At the same time, there can be persistent psychopathology that is not recognized within the context of existing antisocial or borderline diagnostic criteria. In other words, chronic personality dynamics can manifest in new behaviors. For example, those with antisocial personality disorders demonstrate less aggressiveness, violence, and criminal acts as they age but can still have antisocial tendencies expressed through substance abuse, disregard for safety, and noncompliance with institutional rules. Older borderline patients display less impulsivity, self-mutilation, and risk taking but more aging-related symptoms, such as the use of multiple medications and nonadherence with treatment.

Treatment

The treatment of personality disorders in late life is complicated and often has limited success. Given the

Table 42.2—Therapeutic Strategies for Personality Disorders in Late Life*

Cluster A: Paranoid, Schizoid, Schizotypal Personality Disorders

- Always assess for and treat comorbid psychosis.
- Do not force social interactions, but offer support and problem-solving assistance in a professional and consistent manner.
- Do not challenge paranoid ideation; instead, solicit and empathize with emotional responses to inner turmoil and fear of paranoid states.

Cluster B: Antisocial, Borderline, Histrionic, and Narcissistic Personality Disorders

- Assess for and treat underlying mood lability, depression, anxiety, and substance abuse.
- Adopt a consistent, structured, and predictable approach with strict boundaries to contain disruptive behaviors.
- Adopt a team approach with all involved clinicians to devise a common plan; avoid staff splits between "supporters" and "detractors" of the patient.
- Use behavioral contracts and authority figures when necessary to address recurrent disruptive behaviors.
- Do not personalize belligerent behaviors directed toward staff members; instead, provide opportunities for staff to discuss frustration and negative thoughts and emotions with professional colleagues.

Cluster C: Avoidant, Dependent, and Obsessive-Compulsive Personality Disorders

- Assess for and treat underlying anxiety, panic, and depression.
- Provide regularly scheduled clinical contacts rather than on an as-needed basis.
- When possible, provide case managers to solicit the needs of avoidant patients and to provide extra reassurance and attention to the needs of dependent and obsessive-compulsive patients.

*SOE=D

chronic and pervasive nature of personality disorders, the overall goal of treatment in late life is not to cure the disorder but to decrease the frequency and intensity of disruptive behaviors. The first step should always be to clarify the diagnosis and then to identify recent stressors that may account for the current presentation. The resultant formulation can guide the selection of realistic target symptoms and therapeutic approaches, and allow a treatment team to anticipate future stressors. Treatment of personality disorders in late life uses the same basic approaches as with younger patients, but clinicians must incorporate a much broader understanding of the impact of age-related stressors and comorbid disorders. All forms of psychotherapy have been used to treat personality disorders in older adults, ranging from intensive and long-term insight-oriented approaches to equally intensive but more focused cognitive-behavioral models, such as dialectical behavior therapy. In late life, time and intensity of therapy may be more limited and, as a result, treatment must focus more on short-term approaches. Studies in adults generally find that comorbid personality disorders complicate the treatment of psychiatric illness, but that with consistent treatment, the prognosis is often favorable (SOE=B).

In outpatient settings, control over a patient's environment is limited, and clinicians must therefore rely on one-to-one interventions (if the patient is willing to cooperate with treatment). With some patients, it may be necessary to convey a basic formulation of their behaviors, along with suggested approaches, to caregivers and affiliated healthcare professionals, such as primary care providers, social workers, and visiting nurses. This communication is important when patients are vulnerable to self-harm or likely to cause significant disruptions in other settings when they are not understood and approached in a therapeutic manner. For some therapeutic approaches that can be used with various personality disorders, see Table 42.2.

Long-term care settings allow more opportunities for intervention. A staff meeting or case conference often provides the best forum to discuss disruptive patients and to coordinate a consistent treatment plan. Disruptive behaviors can sometimes be traced to particular activities or staff interactions, which can be adapted as part of an overall treatment strategy. Sometimes, disengagement from patients reduces the intensity of disruptive interactions. In other situations, the continuity of staffing and of daily schedules is critical. In all situations, a treatment plan should be well documented and conveyed to the patient, as well as to all involved staff and caregivers. All plans must provide appropriate limits to ensure the safety of patients and staff. A written contract, signed by all parties, may be needed with nonadherent patients to eliminate ambiguity. Although it is important to involve family members in the treatment plan, clinicians must recognize that patients with personality disorders often have conflictual relationships with them. Attention should also be given to individual staff members who must work with difficult patients. These staff members need opportunities to discuss feelings of anxiety and frustration, and to feel acknowledged and supported by administrative and other clinical staff.

There have been no studies looking specifically at pharmacologic strategies for personality disorders in late life, so extrapolation from guidelines used for younger people is needed. Psychotropic medications can be targeted at a particular personality disorder; specific symptoms or symptom clusters; or comorbid depression, anxiety, or psychosis. The goal is not to cure the disorder but to reduce the frequency and intensity of targeted symptoms. Antidepressant medication can be helpful for the target symptoms of depression and anxiety found in most personality disorders (SOE=B). Mood stabilizers (eg, lithium carbonate[OL] and divalproex sodium[OL]) and antipsychotic medications can reduce mood lability and impulsivity in borderline patients, and they can be useful with similar symptoms in antisocial personality disorder (SOE=B). Antianxiety agents are commonly used for transient agitation seen in borderline, antisocial, narcissistic, and paranoid disorders, and they may reduce social anxiety and panic in avoidant and dependent patients (SOE=C). Antidepressants are used commonly to treat impulsive aggression as well as obsessive-compulsive personality symptoms, although efficacy has not been established for the treatment of these symptoms (as it has been demonstrated for obsessive-compulsive disorder). Antipsychotic agents, both first- and second-generation, can treat the transient psychosis, agitation, and impulsivity seen in dramatic cluster and paranoid disorders, as well as the borderline psychosis and paranoia seen in cluster A disorders (SOE=B).

For personality disorders, psychotropic medications are best used as adjuncts to psychotherapy. In older adults, multiple medications should be avoided in general, and particularly when there is a history of nonadherence, confusion, or impulsivity. Attention must be given to potential interactions with multiple other medications used to treat medical disorders.

Finally, clinicians must recognize that in some cases it is best not to prescribe a psychotropic medication. Such cases include older adults with personality disorders and comorbid substance abuse, chronic nonadherence, or a history of or potential for abusive or self-injurious use of medications. Antisocial and borderline individuals often demonstrate such behaviors. Dependent patients often insist on medications as a means of fostering dependency on the clinician, and obsessive-compulsive patients can perpetuate a maladaptive relationship with the clinician through detailed and controlling discussions of medication management. In each example, medication management is corrupted by dysfunctional interpersonal behaviors that lie at the heart of personality disorders.

Somatic Symptom and Related Disorders

Somatic symptom and related disorders encompass a heterogeneous group of five diagnoses that have in common the presence of distressing physical symptoms, as well as abnormal thoughts, feelings, and behaviors in response to these physical symptoms. Previously, under *DSM IV-TR*, the somatic complaints occurred without objective organic causes; however, *DSM-5™* does not require that the somatic symptoms be medically unexplained. Instead, somatic symptom disorder can also accompany a diagnosed medical disorder as long as the somatic symptoms are associated with significant emotional distress and impairment. The *DSM IV-TR* diagnoses of somatization disorder, undifferentiated somatic symptom disorder, hypochondriasis, and some presentations of pain disorder are now included under the *DSM-5™* criteria as *somatic symptom disorder.* In somatic symptom disorder, the patient must have one or more distressing and/or disruptive somatic symptom(s) that is accompanied by at least one of the following: 1) concerns about the seriousness of the medical symptom that is out of proportion to what is typically experienced, 2) persistent high level of anxiety about the symptom, and/or 3) excessive time and energy are focused on the somatic symptom. The clinician can also specify if the somatic symptom disorder occurs with predominant pain.

Illness anxiety disorder is a preoccupation with being susceptible to or having an illness. Patients with illness anxiety disorder tend to have milder somatic symptoms but higher anxiety levels than those with somatic symptom disorder. Symptoms must be persistent for ≥6 months, and patient behaviors can be described as care seeking or care avoidant. *Conversion disorder* is defined by one or more symptoms of altered voluntary motor and/or sensory function that causes significant social and occupational impairment and is not explained by a neurologic disease. Motor symptoms of conversion disorders may include weakness, paralysis, and abnormal movements (eg, tremor) and gait disorders. Sensory symptoms include changes in vision or hearing, or skin sensation. *Psychological factors affecting medical conditions* are psychological or behavioral factors that have an adverse effect on a diagnosed medical condition. For example, a patient may exacerbate symptoms of chronic obstructive pulmonary disease because of anxiety, or a patient may manipulate insulin dosage in an attempt to lose weight. Finally, *factitious disorder*s are false symptoms associations with deception on the part of the patient. Patients with factitious disorder present as ill or injured without any obvious evidence of external reward or reinforcement. Distressing somatic symptoms that do not fit any of the above diagnoses are classified as *other or unspecified somatic symptom and related disorders.* Specific diagnostic criteria for these five conditions can be found in the *DSM-5™*.

These disorders are especially relevant to geriatric care because affected older adults are seen in all healthcare settings, and they tend to overuse medical services. Somatic symptom disorders in late life have not been well studied, and existing research has usually focused on select diagnoses, in limited or biased samples. Research also has looked at somatic symptom reporting rather than at specific diagnoses. Prevalence rates in middle and late life have been found to be <1%, except for one study, which found a prevalence rate of >36% for somatization disorder in women >55 years old seen in healthcare clinics. The presence of these disorders has not been found to be strongly associated with age. Increased somatic preoccupation and symptoms are, however, associated with depression in late life, and older age of onset for depression may be most predictive. In addition to depression, increased somatic preoccupation is associated with the presence of the personality trait of neuroticism, in which a person displays a tendency to experience more negative emotions. Somatic symptom disorders are found more commonly in women and in lower socioeconomic groups. Late onset of a somatic symptom disorder can suggest associated neurologic illness.

Clinical Characteristics and Causes

Somatic symptom disorders do not represent intentional, conscious attempts by older adults to present factitious physical symptoms. Somatic symptoms are experienced by the affected individual as real physical pain and discomfort, usually without insight into associated psychologic factors. Somatic symptom disorders do not represent delusional thinking as seen in psychotic states, and they are different from psychosomatic disorders, which are characterized by actual disease states with presumed psychologic triggers. They also differ from malingering, with its intentional and fully conscious goal of avoiding a specific responsibility such as work, and from factitious disorders (such as Munchausen syndrome), in which the patient's sole, semiconscious intent is to assume the sick role. Rather, somatic symptom disorders represent a complex interaction between mind and brain in which an affected person is unknowingly expressing psychologic stress or conflict through the body. It is not surprising, then, that depression and anxiety are associated with increased somatic expressions. In late life, somatic symptom disorders can be a way for a person to express anxiety and attempt to cope with accumulating fears and losses. These may include fears of abandonment by family and caregivers, loss of beauty and strength, financial setbacks, loss of independence, loss of social role (eg, through retirement, loss of spouse, occupational disability), and loneliness. The psychologic distress and anxiety over such losses can be less threatening and more controllable when shifted to somatic complaints or symptoms. In turn, the resultant state of debility might be reinforced by increased social contacts and support.

The causes of somatic symptom disorders are usually multifactorial and are often rooted in early developmental experiences and personality traits. Psychodynamic approaches suggest that these disorders result from unconscious conflict in which intolerable impulses or affects are expressed through more tolerable somatic symptoms or complaints.

Although psychodynamic explanations can apply across the life span, these conflicts often begin early in life, perhaps accounting for the relatively young age of onset for most somatic symptom disorders. In late life, psychologic conflict that results in significant depression and anxiety are, for the most part, the same conflicts that can lead to somatization. In addition, the presence of so many comorbid medical problems and the use of multiple medications can provide readily available somatic symptoms around which psychologic conflict can center. In long-term care, older adults are faced with many overwhelming losses, and their own bodies often serve as the last bastion of control. Somatic preoccupation thus serves as a means of coping with stress, even though it is maladaptive and can result in excessive and unnecessary disability.

Treatment

People with somatic symptom disorder do not usually present as such; by definition, they appear to have legitimate somatic complaints with an unknown physical cause. It is only after repeated but fruitless evaluations, multiple and persistent complaints and requests, and sometimes angry and inappropriate reactions to treatment that clinicians begin to suspect a somatic symptom disorder. In some cases, the manner of presentation and symptom complex is more immediately suggestive of a particular somatic symptom disorder. In any event, it is important for the clinician to remember that from the perspective of the patient, the symptoms and complaints are quite real and disturbing. It is never wise to challenge the patient or to suggest that the symptoms are "all in your mind," even after diagnostic evaluation has made it obvious that psychologic factors are involved. The typical response to such advice is for the patient to seek additional opinions and medical tests, which in turn can perpetuate a cycle of somatization that never addresses the underlying issues.

Instead, the clinician should attempt to foster an ongoing, supportive, consistent, and professional relationship with the affected patient. Such a relationship serves to provide reassurance as well as to protect the patient from excessive and unnecessary medical visits and procedures. The clinician should focus on responding to individual complaints, perhaps with periodic but regularly scheduled appointments, and to set limits on evaluation and treatment in a firm but empathetic manner. This can be difficult to do when patients become demanding and attempt to consume excessive amounts of time, but the clinician must endeavor to remain professional, without personalizing the situation or feel that he or she is failing the patient. Overall, the role of the clinician is to focus on reducing symptoms and rehabilitating the patient, and not attempting to force the patient to have insight into the potential psychologic nature of his or her symptoms. It would be hazardous to prematurely diagnose a somatic symptom disorder when there might actually be an underlying medical problem that has eluded diagnosis. For example, disorders such as multiple sclerosis, systemic lupus erythematosus, and acute intermittent porphyria commonly have complex presentations that elude initial diagnostic evaluation. Moreover, many somatic symptom disorders coexist with actual disease states, eg, many individuals with pseudoseizures also have an actual seizure disorder. At the same time, it is important for the clinician to set limits on what he or she can offer and to make appropriate referrals to specialists and mental health clinicians.

The mental health clinician should have an active role in addressing the somatic symptom disorder. Unfortunately, no particular treatment for any somatic symptom disorder has been found to have good efficacy, and most disorders tend to be lifelong. As a result, the goal of treatment is not to cure, but to control symptoms. The clinician first forms a therapeutic alliance based on empathetic listening and acknowledgment of physical discomfort, without trivializing the somatic complaints. Sometimes an offer to review all available medical records can be a tangible way of conveying one's seriousness to the patient. Underlying anxiety and depression must be identified and treated with psychotherapy and, when necessary, antidepressant or antianxiety medications, or both. Cognitive-behavioral therapy focuses on identifying distorted thought patterns and triggers of anxiety, and then replacing them with more realistic and adaptive strategies. A mental health professional can assist in determining whether cognitive-behavioral therapy may be of benefit. In many cases, however, the supportive nature of regular visits to a primary care provider may be sufficient to meet the needs of individuals with somatic symptom disorders.

References

- Balsis S, Woods CM, Gleason MEJ, et al. The over and underdiagnosis of personality disorders in older adults. *Am J Geriatr Psychiatry*. 2007;15(9):742–753.
- Hunt M. Borderline personality disorder across the lifespan. *J Women Aging*. 2007;19(1–2):173–191.
- Stevenson J, Datyner A, Boyce P, et al. The effect of age on prevalence, type and diagnosis of personality disorder in psychiatric inpatients. *Int J Geriatr Psychiatry*. 2011;26(9):981–987.

CHAPTER 43—ADDICTIONS

KEY POINTS

- Alcohol and other substance-abuse problems can remain undetected when screening questions are omitted during routine medical visits.
- Alcohol use can be an unrecognized cause of falls, cognitive decline, and medical problems (eg, anemia, increased liver function tests, hyponatremia thrombocytopenia).
- It is important to consider a diagnosis of alcohol or benzodiazepine withdrawal in older adults who develop delirium with hospitalization or facility placement.
- Cognitive impairment from chronic alcoholism in older adults can improve with sustained abstinence.
- Abuse of prescription drugs, including benzodiazepines and opioids, is often unrecognized.
- Smoking cessation efforts should persist throughout life.

The abuse and misuse of alcohol, psychoactive medications, illicit drugs, and nicotine have become significant public health concerns for the growing population of older adults. Substance abuse and dependence among older adults is common, and older adults are particularly vulnerable to the cognitive and physical effects of these substances. Clinicians and researchers therefore may need to change their thinking about the risks of use in this population. Typically, substance-use problems are thought to develop only in those who use substances in large quantities and at regular intervals. Among older adults, however, negative health consequences have been demonstrated at consumption amounts previously thought of as light to moderate, and certainly not in the amounts usually associated with a diagnosis of substance dependence. A growing number of effective treatments for these problems lead not only to reduced substance use but also to improved general health. Both the risks and the emergence of new treatments underscore the need to identify problems and provide appropriate treatment for older adults suffering from the effects of substance misuse.

DEFINITIONS OF SUBSTANCE ABUSE

Establishing valid criteria for determining which older adults would benefit from reducing or eliminating their substance use is the first step in successful intervention. *Substance dependence* has been defined as any use that imparts significant disability and warrants treatment. Many older adults are not recognized as having problems that are related to their substance use, partly because the diagnostic criteria are difficult to interpret and apply consistently to older adults. For instance, many older people drink at home by themselves; thus, they are less likely than younger drinkers to be arrested, get into arguments, or have difficulties in employment. Moreover, because many of the diseases caused or affected by substance misuse (eg, hypertension, stroke, and peptic ulcer disease) are common disorders in late life, the effects of substance use on older adults who have these disorders can be overlooked. The literature indicates that older problem drinkers are identified less often by clinicians and are less often referred for treatment than their younger counterparts.

Because of the difficulties in assessing older adults for substance dependence, many experts advocate screening to identify those who are at risk of problem behaviors or who have at-risk or problem use. *At-risk use* is defined as any use of a substance at a quantity or frequency greater than a recommended level. The level of use is often determined empirically based on association with significant disability. For instance, the recommended upper limit of alcohol consumption for older adults has been established as no more than an average of one standard drink per day and no more than two episodes of binge drinking (four or more drinks in a day) during a 3-month period. *Problem substance use* is defined as the consumption of any amount of an abusable substance that results in at least one problem related to this use. For example, the use of benzodiazepines by a patient who has a preexisting unsteady gait would be considered problem use.

On the other end of the spectrum, *abstinence* is defined as drinking no alcohol in the previous year. Approximately 60% of older adults are abstinent. If an older adult is abstinent, it can be useful to ascertain why alcohol is not used. Some individuals are abstinent because of a previous history of alcohol problems. For this reason, it is particularly important to obtain a history of both current and past use. Some older adults are abstinent because of recent illness; others have lifelong patterns of abstinence or low-risk use. Individuals who have a previous history of alcohol problems can require preventive monitoring to determine if any new stresses could exacerbate an old pattern. In addition, a previous history of at-risk drinking or alcohol dependence increases the risk of developing other mental health problems in late life, such as depressive disorders or cognitive problems, and can limit treatment response because of brain damage.

Low-risk or *moderate use* of alcohol is that which falls within the recommended guidelines for consumption and is not associated with problems. Older adults in this category not only consume amounts that fall within recommended drinking guidelines but also are able to reasonably limit their alcohol consumption, ie, they do not drink when driving a motor vehicle or boat, or when using contraindicated medications. However, a change in either physical health or prescription medications can increase even low-risk use to a problem level.

The most practical method for identifying individuals who could benefit from intervention is to determine the quantity and frequency of their use of abusable substances. This method has advantages over formal diagnostic interviews because of its brevity, easily interpretable results, and absence of stigmatizing language, such as "addiction," "alcoholism," "alcoholic," or "alcohol dependence." For more on screening, see the section below on identifying substance-use disorders, p 339.

MAGNITUDE OF THE PROBLEM

Drug Use

Little is known about the epidemiology of substance-use disorders among older adults other than alcoholism. The general belief is that older drug addicts are only younger addicts grown old and that few individuals initiate drug use in their later years. In the Epidemiologic Catchment Area study, lifetime prevalence rates of drug abuse and dependence were 0.12% for older men and 0.06% for older women, and lifetime history of illicit drug use was 2.88% for men and 0.66% for women. No active cases were reported in either gender. In contrast, a more recent study of an elder-specific drug program in a veteran population found that one-fourth had either a primary drug problem or concurrent drug and alcohol problems. This study may be a reflection of the growing number of older adults who used drugs during a time of expanded drug experimentation in the United States in the 1960s. Indeed, reports from the National Survey on Drug Use and Health suggest a rise in marijuana and cocaine use among individuals ≥50 years old, with the 1-year prevalence of marijuana use approaching 4% for the U.S. population aged 50–64 years, whereas use of illicit drugs has decreased in all younger age groups. Recent increases in hepatitis C among those ≥60 years old can reflect both a history of intravenous drug use, as well as increased risk of nosocomial infection with advanced age. Other studies to determine the prevalence and incidence of substance-use disorders (in later life) involving nicotine, caffeine, and benzodiazepines are needed.

Medication Use

An increasing problem with the older age group is the misuse or inappropriate use of prescription and OTC medications, with 2.1% of adults aged 50 in the National Survey on Drug Use and Health reporting using prescription-type drugs nonmedically, the most commonly used illicit class among those ≥65 years old. This problem includes the misuse of substances such as sedatives, hypnotics, narcotic and non-narcotic analgesics, diet aids, decongestants, and a wide variety of OTC medications. Community surveys have found that 60% of older adults are taking an analgesic, 22% are taking a CNS medication, and 11% are taking a benzodiazepine. Many medications used by older adults have the potential for inducing tolerance, withdrawal syndromes, and harmful medical consequences, such as cognitive changes, kidney disease, falls, and liver disease. A growing body of literature demonstrates a concerning increase in morbidity and mortality associated with the misuse of prescription and nonprescription medications, even though this is not considered as a disorder in the *Diagnostic and Statistical Manual of Mental Disorders, 4th Edition, Text Revision*.

Medication use by all older adults needs to be monitored carefully; prescribing potentially hazardous combinations of medications, medications with a high risk of adverse events, and ineffective or unnecessary medications should be avoided. See "Pharmacotherapy," p 81. A practical approach to monitoring psychoactive medications is to reevaluate the older patient's use every 3–6 months. Maintenance treatment should be continued only in those patients who have specific target symptoms and a documented response to the treatment. Patients who have no response or only a partial response should be reevaluated to consider the appropriate diagnosis and further care. In such cases, consultation with a geriatric mental health professional could be advantageous. See also "Depression and Other Mood Disorders," p 308; "Anxiety Disorders," p 319; "Psychotic Disorders," p 324; and "Personality and Somatic Symptom Disorders," p 329.

Alcohol Use

Community-based epidemiologic studies define the extent and nature of alcohol use in the older population by reporting percentages of abstainers, heavy drinkers, and daily drinkers. Abstention from alcohol ranges from 31% to 58%, and daily drinking ranges from 10% to 22% in samples of older adults. "Heavy" drinking, defined as a minimum of 12 to 21 drinks per week, is present in 3%–9% of the older population; alcohol abuse, as defined clinically, is present in approximately 2%–4%.

Cultural and Demographic Factors

The prevalence of alcohol use and alcohol-related problems among older adults is much higher for men than for women. Among younger adults, however, the ratio of male to female drinkers has changed over the past several decades, with the result that more women present for treatment. These changes are likely to continue to be reflected in the next generation of older women. Similar patterns by gender are seen with illicit drug use, except that benzodiazepines are much more commonly used by older women than by older men.

Conclusions are less clear from the few studies addressing differences among various ethnic groups. Depending on the study, older black Americans and older Hispanic Americans consume amounts of alcohol similar to or lower than the amounts consumed by older white Americans. The Epidemiologic Catchment Area data demonstrated significant differences in the 1-year diagnosis of alcohol abuse and dependence among black Americans (2.93% among men and 0.60% among women), white Americans (2.85% among men and 0.47% among women), and Hispanic Americans (6.57% among men and 0.0% among women). Increased leisure time and higher disposable income are more relevant risk factors for alcohol consumption among older adults than race or ethnicity.

Clinical Settings

Older adults constitute most admissions to acute-care facilities and are frequent users of outpatient medical services, including primary care. The prevalence rates for alcohol problems among hospital populations are substantially higher than those among community dwellers. High prevalence rates for problems related to drinking are also becoming more common in retirement communities. Data from a survey of a Veterans Affairs nursing home demonstrated that 35% of patients interviewed had a lifetime diagnosis of alcohol abuse. A significant number of patients seen in outpatient clinics also have active alcohol-use disorders. The high prevalence of alcohol-related problems in both hospital and outpatient populations underscores the need for thorough screening of older adults in medical settings.

Risks and Benefits of Substance Use

Benefits of Alcohol Consumption

Moderate alcohol consumption among otherwise healthy older adults has been promoted as having significant beneficial effects, especially with regard to cardiovascular disease. Findings from the cardiovascular literature have led to a host of articles in the popular press espousing the benefits of alcohol use.

Alcohol in moderate amounts can promote relaxation and reduce social anxiety. However, even though there are benefits of moderate drinking, the practice of recommending drinking to people who currently do not drink is not advocated. Many older adults do not drink because of past problems with drinking, family problems with drinking, the expense related to drinking, and the adverse effects of intoxication. There is no direct evidence to justify prescribing alcohol for individuals with heart disease or any other health condition.

Excess Physical Disability

Substance abuse has clear and profound effects on the health and well-being of older adults in all spheres of life. Older adults are particularly prone to the toxic effects of substances on many different organ systems because of both the physiological changes associated with aging and the changes associated with other illnesses common in late life. The social and economic impact is also tremendous. Substance abuse has adverse effects on self-esteem, coping skills, and interpersonal relationships, which may be compounded by losses that are common in the late stages of life.

Levels of alcohol consumption above seven drinks per week, so-called at-risk drinking, have been associated with a number of health problems, including an increased risk of stroke caused by bleeding, impaired driving skills, and an increased rate of injuries such as falls and fractures (SOE=A). The risk of breast cancer in women who consume three to nine drinks per week is approximately 50% higher than that of women who drink fewer than three drinks per week. Of particular importance to older adults are the potential harmful interactions between alcohol and both prescribed and OTC medications, especially psychoactive medications such as benzodiazepines and antidepressants. Alcohol also interferes with the metabolism of many medications, including warfarin.

Older adults who consume more than an average of four drinks per day or whose drinking has led to a diagnosis of alcohol dependence are at greatest risk of excess physical disability and physical illness related to drinking. The most common problems associated with alcohol dependence are alcoholic liver disease, COPD, peptic ulcer disease, and psoriasis. Moreover, unexplained multisystem disease should alert the clinician to probe more closely for alcohol use. With smoking, the risks are much clearer, including increased rates of pulmonary disease, especially cancer. Medications such as benzodiazepines are also associated with excess physical disability, increased rates of falls, and driving-related impairment. Research is beginning to demonstrate that the disability associated with these problems is also reversible with reduced substance use (SOE=B).

Mental Health Problems

Substance use can be a significant factor in the course and prognosis of nearly all mental health problems of late life. Use of alcohol, benzodiazepines, opioids, and cigarettes has been demonstrated to be related etiologically to mood disturbances, but these substances also complicate the treatment of concurrent mood disorders. Individuals with both alcoholism and depression have a more complicated clinical course of depression with an increased risk of suicide and more social dysfunction than nondepressed individuals with alcoholism. Overall, older adults with alcohol abuse or dependence are nearly three times more likely to have a lifetime diagnosis of another mental disorder. Alcoholism has been implicated in mood disorders, suicide, dementia, anxiety disorders, and sleep disturbances.

As might be expected, patients with alcohol-related dementia who become abstinent do not show a progression in cognitive impairment comparable to that of those with Alzheimer disease. The complex role of alcoholism in the development of Alzheimer disease is not fully understood, but alcoholism does lead independently to a syndrome of dementia. Interesting new hypotheses implicate glutamatergic toxicity, but overall, the mechanisms are not well understood. The criteria for alcohol-related dementia are as follows:

- clinically evident dementia at least 60 days after last alcohol use
- a history of significant use for at least 5 years, ie, at least 35 drinks per week for men and 28 per week for women
- the occurrence of this period of significant use within 3 years of the onset of cognitive deficits

Clinical features supporting the diagnosis include end-organ damage (eg, liver disease), cognitive stabilization or improvement after abstinence, and evidence of cerebellar atrophy in brain imaging. Further research is needed to understand the potential benefits of long-term abstinence in alcohol-related dementia. Similarly, those with comorbid depression and alcohol use are likely to have better depression outcomes if they become abstinent. Moderate alcohol use has also been demonstrated to have negative effects on the treatment of late-life depression, further underscoring the need for reducing moderate use in the context of chronic health problems in older adults.

Identifying Substance-Use Disorders

Although clinical examination remains the most valuable tool for identifying substance-use problems, screening instruments can help increase the sensitivity and efficiency of diagnosis. Several instruments have been developed for identifying alcohol-use disorders, including self-administered questionnaires and laboratory studies. Self-administered questionnaires provide a rapid, sensitive, and inexpensive method of screening for alcohol problems. Two questionnaires have been developed with these principles in mind: the Michigan Alcoholism Screening Test (MAST)—Geriatric Version, and the AUDIT C (Table 43.1). Both of these instruments have high sensitivity and specificity for identifying alcohol misuse in middle-aged and older adults. The CAGE is a brief clinician-administered screening test that may be useful to identify problem drinking (Table 43.2).

Treatment

Older adults with a substance-use problem often need a variety of treatments. It is therefore important to have an array of services available for older adults that can be tailored to their individual needs and that have the flexibility to adapt to changing needs over time. The most important aspect of treating an older adult who is misusing a substance is to engage the individual in the intervention. Older adults engaged in treatment have been shown to have robust improvement, especially compared with younger cohorts. The spectrum of interventions for alcohol abuse in older adults range from prevention and education for those who are abstinent or low-risk drinkers, to minimal advice or brief structured interventions for at-risk or problem drinkers, to formalized alcoholism treatment for drinkers who meet criteria for abuse or dependence. The array of formal treatment options available includes psychotherapy, education, rehabilitative and residential care, and psychopharmacologic agents. An example of the necessity to tailor care is the contrast between the at-risk drinker or benzodiazepine user and the severely dependent patient. The at-risk user will not likely need the intensity of services required for the severely dependent patient. Indeed, requiring the at-risk drinker to accept a set of rigorous services can be more detrimental than helpful.

Dependency on medications such as benzodiazepines is managed by placing the patient on a 24-hour equivalent of the dosage of the drug on which the patient is dependent; tapering the dosage by 10% every three half-lives; and providing supportive counseling via groups, psychosocial support, and 12-step programs. Symptoms of withdrawal from narcotics can be controlled when necessary with oral clonidine[OL]. Assuring that the patient enters a long-term treatment program increases the likelihood of long-term success. For smoking cessation, it is important to prepare the patient for quitting by discussing management strategies before quitting, setting a quit date, and implementing a monitoring plan for maintaining success.

Detoxification and Stabilization

The assessment of any substance abuser starts with a thorough history, physical examination, and laboratory tests. The patient's potential to suffer acute withdrawal should also be assessed. Severe withdrawal such as that from alcohol use can be life threatening and warrants careful attention. Patients with severe symptoms of dependency or withdrawal potential and patients with significant medical or psychiatric comorbidity can require inpatient hospitalization for acute stabilization before implementing an outpatient management strategy. Detoxification is achieved by placing the patient on the minimal amount of drug that suppresses withdrawal symptoms and then decreasing the dosage by 10% every three half-lives. In general, longer-acting formulations of the drug being abused are preferred to shorter-acting formulations, but many clinicians find that prescribing the specific drug that a patient was abusing makes the process more acceptable to the patient and minimizes the time needed to determine the initial dose.

For patients who are hospitalized for an elective surgery or condition unrelated to the substance problem, remaining vigilant for any evidence of withdrawal is extremely important. Unrecognized alcohol withdrawal can result in serious morbidity and mortality in older adults. Early symptoms include tachycardia, diaphoresis, tremulousness, and hypertension. These symptoms can progress to overt delirium, psychosis, and seizures. Intravenous lorazepam[OL] is the most expedient intervention in this scenario, followed by oral lorazepam, in tapering dosages.

Outpatient Management

Traditionally, outpatient substance-abuse treatment has been reserved for specialized clinics focused on substance abuse. However, it is becoming increasingly apparent that this model is inadequate in addressing the broader public health demand, and there is a need to involve a variety of clinicians and clinical settings to deliver substance-abuse treatment. This is particularly important for older adults, who frequently seek medical services but rarely seek specialized addiction services. The traditional addiction clinic is focused on supportive group psychotherapy and encouragement to attend regular self-help group meetings such as Alcoholics Anonymous, Alcoholics Victorious, Rational Recovery, or Narcotics Anonymous. For older adults, peer-specific group activities are considered superior to mixed-age group activities. Outpatient rehabilitation, in addition to focusing on active addiction issues, usually needs to address issues of time management. The management of this time, which is often the greater part of a patient's day, is critical to the prognosis.

Clinicians should be wary of focusing on abstinence as the only positive outcome of treatment and should commend patients for making progress in decreasing use as well as stopping. This can be particularly relevant for misuse of medications such as benzodiazepines, because eliminating the use may be more difficult. For benzodiazepines, the risk of adverse events such as falls is greater with higher dosages and with medications that have a longer half-life such as diazepam or clonazepam. Therefore, using medications with a half-life of 6–12 hours reduces the risks for that patient. If benzodiazepines seem to be indicated for an anxiety condition and treatment is started for the first time, shorter-acting agents that do not have active metabolites (eg, lorazepam) are preferred to long-acting preparations. However, for patients already receiving long-acting benzodiazepines (eg, diazepam at ≥50 mg/d), the risk of withdrawal complications is increased, and the dosage should be reduced very gradually. If the daily dose is greater than the equivalent of 100 mg of diazepam, then the patient should be hospitalized to start withdrawal. Ultimately, a transition to shorter-acting agents is ideal, but this should be done carefully and initially involve an equivalent dosage before any reductions are considered. The use of resources such as day programs and senior centers can be beneficial, especially for cognitively impaired patients. Supervised living arrangements, such as halfway houses, group homes, nursing homes, and residing with relatives, should also be considered.

Pharmacotherapy

The use of medications to support abstinence may be of benefit, but it is not well studied. For strength of evidence, see Table 43.3. Small-scale studies have demonstrated that naltrexone for alcohol abuse is well tolerated and efficacious in older adults. Naltrexone is available in both oral and long-acting injectable forms. Studies of antidepressants, including the SSRIs, do not support the widespread use of antidepressants as a treatment for alcohol misuse, although they can be effective in treating concurrent depression. Some of the general principles used in treating younger patients should be applied to older drinkers as well. For example, benzodiazepines are important in the treatment of alcohol detoxification,

Table 43.1—The AUDIT-C Questionnaire: The Alcohol Use Disorders Identification Test-Consumption Questions

The AUDIT-C is an alcohol screen that can help identify patients who are hazardous drinkers or who have active alcohol-use disorders (including alcohol abuse or dependence).

Read questions as written. Record answers carefully. Begin the AUDIT-C by saying, "Now I am going to ask you some questions about your use of alcoholic beverages during the past year." Explain that "alcoholic beverages" refers to beer, wine, vodka, etc. Code answers in terms of "standard drinks."

Question #1: How often did you have a drink containing alcohol in the past year?	
■ Never	0 points
■ Less than monthly	1 point
■ 2–4 times per month	2 points
■ 2–3 times per week	3 points
■ 4 or more times per week	4 points
Question #2: In the past year, how many drinks did you typically have when you drank?	
■ I did not drink in the past year	0 points
■ 1–2 drinks	0 points
■ 3–4 drinks	1 point
■ 5–6 drinks	2 points
■ 7–9 drinks	3 points
■ More than 10 drinks	4 points
Question #3: How often did you have 6 or more drinks on one occasion in the past year?	
■ Never	0 points
■ Less than monthly	1 point
■ Monthly	2 points
■ Weekly	3 points
■ Daily	4 points

The AUDIT-C is scored on a scale of 0 to 12 (scores of 0 reflect no alcohol use). In men, a score ≥4 is considered positive; in women, a score ≥3 is considered positive. Generally, the higher the AUDIT-C score, the more likely it is that the patient's drinking is affecting his or her health and safety.

References: Babor TF, Bohn MJ, Kranzler HR. The Alcohol Use Disorders Identification Test (AUDIT): validation of a screening instrument for use in medical settings. *J Stud Alcohol*. 1995;56:423–432 (www.queri.research.va.gov/tools/alcohol-misuse/alcohol-faqs.cfm).

Table 43.2—The CAGE Questionnaire

C	■ Have you ever tried to **C**ut down on your drinking?
A	■ Have you ever gotten **A**nnoyed at someone for criticizing your drinking?
G	■ Do you ever feel **G**uilty about your drinking?
E	■ Have you ever had an **E**ye-opener to steady your nerves or get rid of a hangover?

NOTE: A positive answer to one or more questions suggests problem drinking.

but they have no clinical place in maintaining long-term abstinence because of their potential for abuse and for fostering further alcohol or benzodiazepine abuse. Disulfiram can benefit some well-motivated patients, but cardiac and hepatic disease limits its use by older adults who abuse alcohol. Acamprosate has not been studied in older adults. Methadone maintenance has proven efficacy in opioid dependence. Older adults can be started and maintained on methadone, following the same principles of use as in younger patients. Comorbid medical and psychiatric disorders must be identified and properly treated, and they may necessitate the need for referral to, or consultation with, a psychiatrist with expertise in these areas. Buprenorphine, and buprenorphine with naloxone have been approved for outpatient treatment of opioid dependence. However, given the complexity of the treatment of opioid dependence, systematic training, practice, monitoring, regulation, and evaluation are necessary in a multidisciplinary treatment setting to optimize outcomes. Guidelines for developing treatment programs using buprenorphine are available on the Web site of the Substance Abuse and Mental Health Services Administration (http://buprenorphine.samhsa.gov/index.html [accessed Oct 2013]).

Tobacco Dependence

Tobacco dependence is a chronic disease that typically requires multiple attempts to quit with repeated interventions over the life span. Smoking cessation at any age slows the decline in lung function, and aggressive cessation efforts are appropriate even in the oldest-old patient. There is significant evidence to demonstrate that brief interventions performed at each

Table 43.3–Strength of Evidence for Research on Late-Life Addiction Treatment

Indication	Treatment Strategy	SOE	Comments	Limits
Detoxification				
Alcohol	Substitution with benzodiazepine	A	Prevents sequela such as seizures, severe withdrawal symptoms; should be driven by specific plan and measurement of effects	Few specific studies in older adults, who may be at greater risk of idiosyncratic responses
	Carbamazepine[OL] and other mood-stabilizing medications	C	Small-scale studies have shown promise, but these medications are somewhat more complicated to use.	Very limited evidence base for older adults
Benzodiazepines	Slow tapering	B	Effective in managing withdrawal	Limited evidence base for older adults; long-term outcomes not well correlated with success of detoxification
Opioids	Substitution/taper	B	Effective in managing withdrawal	Limited evidence base for older adults
Treatment Strategies				
Problem and at-risk drinking	Brief interventions	A	Randomized trials have showed efficacy in primary-care settings with less evidence in high-risk settings such as behavioral health, home care, and the emergency room.	Limited effect in those with alcohol dependence; limited dissemination
Alcohol dependence	Psychotherapy	C	Several naturalistic trials demonstrating increased adherence to treatment and generally better outcomes for older adults than for middle-aged adults. Individual therapy such as cognitive-behavioral therapy may be particularly effective.	Randomized trials designed to better understand age-dependent adherence and treatment outcomes are needed.
	Naltrexone	B	Well tolerated and showed some evidence of efficacy in post-hoc analyses.	
	Acamprosate	C	Inconsistent evidence base but approved for use	Very limited evidence base for older adults
	Disulfiram	C	Antabuse reaction can be particularly harmful for older adults with preexisting medical problems.	No age-specific studies or studies that have included significant numbers of older adults
	Other agents	D	Antidepressants and mood-stabilizing agents are all used clinically but with an inconsistent evidence base.	No age-specific studies or studies that have included significant numbers of older adults
Nicotine dependence	Nicotine replacement	B	Strong evidence base for use but limited evidence base specifically in older adults	
	Varenicline	B	Several evidence-based studies	Very limited evidence for older adults; case reports of depression and behavior disturbance
Opioid dependence	Methadone, buprenorphine	B	Strong evidence for decrease in use and improved function	Limited evidence base for older adults, many of whom have been on methadone for many years

office visit will promote smoking cessation (SOE=A). The basic elements of the approach are the "Five A's" from the Agency for Health Care Policy and Research:

- **A**sk patients about use of tobacco at every office visit.
- **A**ssess readiness to quit.
- **A**dvise patients to quit.
- **A**ssist patients in the quit attempt with aids such as a local cessation program and pharmacologic agents such as bupropion, nicotine replacement, or varenicline.
- **A**rrange both a quit date and a follow-up visit or contact to discuss the quit attempt.

Establishing abstinence from nicotine follows the same principles as that from other addicting substances. Initially, pharmacologic substitution with either nicotine gum or patch is followed by a gradual decrease in dosage. In several trials, antidepressant medications improved rates of continued abstinence, but only bupropion has been approved for this purpose by the FDA. Varenicline has not received specific attention in older adults and may be considered, because there is strong evidence for benefit in smoking cessation in younger adults (SOE=B). However, as of July 2009, the FDA requires a black box warning for varenicline because of neuropsychiatric symptoms such as depression and suicidality. As with other abstinence regimens, psychotherapy plus pharmacotherapy is better than pharmacotherapy alone.

Gambling

Gambling in late life is less prevalent than in young adulthood. However, older adults who have engaged in problematic and compulsive gambling behaviors earlier in life often continue this pattern of destructive behavior. Gambling in late life, both recreational and problematic, is associated with a higher prevalence of mental and physical health problems (SOE=B). Many older adults report that gambling is a means of coping with loneliness and boredom. While gambling activities can be a source of socialization, the clinician must be mindful of asking about problematic gambling when taking a history. These include symptoms such as preoccupation with gambling, restlessness or irritability when trying to quit, loss of control, need to bet more money with increasing frequency, "chasing" losses, and continuation of gambling despite negative social or occupational consequences. No medications have been helpful in reducing pathologic gambling behaviors. States that allow legalized gaming activities are required to post toll-free telephone numbers to access assistance with problematic gambling. Many 12-step programs are focused on problematic gambling. Older adults who engage in gambling activities should be screened for alcohol, smoking, and other substance-use disorders. Referrals to community resources and 12-step programs may be useful.

REFERENCES

- Blazer DG, Wu LT. The epidemiology of substance use and disorders among middle aged and elderly community adults: national survey on drug use and health. *Am J Geriatr Psychiatry*. 2009;17(3):237–245.
- Fiore MC, Jaen CR, Baker TB, et al. *Treating Tobacco Use and Dependence: 2008 Update*. Clinical Practice Guideline. Rockville, MD: U.S. Department of Health and Human Services. Public Health Service. May 2008.
- Gage S, Melillo KD. Substance abuse in older adults: policy issues. *J Gerontol Nurs*. 2011;37(12):8–11.

CHAPTER 44—INTELLECTUAL AND DEVELOPMENTAL DISABILITIES

KEY POINTS

- Individuals with intellectual disability surviving into adulthood and old age are increasing in numbers.
- Maladaptive and challenging behaviors, as well as difficulties learning and retaining new skills of coping and adaptation, are significant problems for adults with intellectual disability and, consequently, for their caregivers.
- Receptive and expressive communication impairments and coexisting cognitive limitations can contribute to diagnostic and treatment difficulties for medical, psychiatric, and behavioral problems.
- Physiologic changes related to age as well as disease states in individuals with intellectual disability can exacerbate or attenuate behaviors.
- Therapeutic interventions for maladaptive behaviors or psychiatric illnesses that coexist with intellectual disability can include medications and behavioral therapies.
- The term developmental disability can describe a variety of medical conditions that are not defined by intellectual disability. However, these conditions can contribute to challenging behaviors and impact an individual's quality of life.

Intellectual disability, as used in the *Diagnostic and Statistical Manual, 5th Edition,* is defined as an IQ of approximately 70 or below based on formal test results and impairment in adaptive functioning with onset before 18 years of age, the period of time defined for significant neural development. Unfortunately, differences over nomenclature for intellectual disability continue to exist based on historical, cultural, or geographic issues, or on perceptions of "correctness." Intellectual disability, or intellectual developmental disorder, must include a current intellectual and functional deficit with onset during the developmental period. All three of the criteria must be met.

A demographic issue to keep in mind is that not everyone with a developmental disability has intellectual disability. This chapter focuses on individuals with intellectual disability who may or may not have other comorbid conditions, such as cerebral palsy, epilepsy, and autism spectrum disorders.

PREVALENCE

The number of individuals with intellectual disability surviving into old age is increasing because of generally better health care overall, including earlier detection and treatment of some conditions. It is difficult to quantify the prevalence of older adults with intellectual disability because of methodologic considerations. It is even more problematic to consider the issues from the perspectives of other cultures and standards in areas other than Europe and North America. As reported in a 2003 Canadian study of Ontario, overall prevalence for intellectual disability was 7.18/1000 and 3.54/1000 for severe intellectual disability among teenagers (as would be expected). Also reported was an increase in the life expectancy for adults with intellectual disability and seniors with any type of developmental disability.

Life expectancy for individuals with intellectual disability has increased over time. In the 1930s, the average age at death for males suffering from intellectual disability was 15 years, and for females, 22 years. In 1932, for children 10 years old, only 28% were expected to survive to age 60. By the 1990s, that figure increased to >40% for institutionalized as well as for community-based individuals.

Published estimates of the number of people of all ages with intellectual disability have ranged from 1% to 2% in the United States, with 2% used in some more recent reports. Regardless of the number, it is proposed to double for individuals ≥60 years old by 2030. In general, longevity decreases with severity of intellectual impairment, certain comorbid conditions (eg, seizure disorders, Down syndrome), and the general health and wealth of the country or culture. In the same Canadian study, adults with Down syndrome who had a decreased life span had also increased their life expectancy to about 59 years of age.

Intellectual Disability and Mental Illness

The literature on older adults with intellectual disability and mental illness (other than dementia) has been relatively sparse over the last few decades. This makes it even more problematic to determine accurate numbers for a number of reasons: definitions have changed (ie, through various editions of the *DSM* and various versions of the *International Classification of Diseases [ICD]*), health care has improved, studies have been conducted in different countries or regions, standard methodologies are lacking, and the relative numbers of institutionalized versus community-based individuals have changed.

Over the last decades, several studies with diverse methodologies and equally uneven goals have been conducted, but there have been some common general conclusions, notably that the prevalence of psychiatric disorders among adults with intellectual disability is much greater than that of age-matched controls (SOE=B). Adults with intellectual disability have similar risk factors (biologic, psychologic, and social) for mental illnesses as their "normal" peers but may have additional risks depending on the cause of their mental disability. Older adults who were raised in institutions or who have not benefitted from modern medical care are also at greater risk.

There are many reports of greater than expected rates of certain mental illnesses or behavioral disorders associated with specific physical illnesses or genetic disorders. For example, older adults with autistic spectrum disorders exhibit higher rates of compulsive behaviors requiring psychiatric treatment.

There is general agreement that among all groups of older adults with intellectual disability, behavioral problems are more common, or at least more commonly diagnosed, than are major psychiatric disorders, such as major depressive disorders and psychotic disorders. Some terms, such as "challenging behaviors," are used to describe various behavioral symptoms of autism and fragile X syndrome, while other behaviors may have a relationship to brain abnormalities or to impaired acquisition of typically learned social behaviors. Additionally, some abnormal behaviors are learned and, in some situations perhaps, discovered maladaptive or problem behaviors become symptomatic. Learned problematic behaviors are likely to occur from years in an institutional setting.

There is nothing protective against a psychiatric disorder by virtue of having intellectual disability. The cloud of uncertainty is increased perhaps by lack of objective signs and an individual's ability to report their inner feelings. Some of life's stressors that are common for older adults may have a greater impact on those with intellectual disability. Loss of family or friends, income, residence, or vocational status may strain coping strategies as well as overwhelm caregivers or support systems, resulting in an overt decline in level of functioning or a worsening of symptoms.

Major psychiatric disorders are estimated to occur in about 10% of older adults with intellectual disability. Among the most common disorders is dementia. The presence of psychotic disorders increases with age as well. Some disorders are seen at a higher rate than in the general population, such as certain anxiety disorders. Mood disorders also continue into old age, and the management is complex if the individual's ability to participate in certain psychotherapies is limited. Some developmental disorders, such as Down syndrome, may increase the likelihood of some disorders such as obsessive-compulsive disorder, which may be three times more prevalent than in the general population. Again, the difference is in the presentation of symptoms in individuals with intellectual disability, and not in the possibility of psychiatric illness.

DIAGNOSTIC AND TREATMENT ISSUES

Clinicians face many diagnostic and treatment challenges when seeing patients with intellectual disability with or without comorbid issues of mental illness or challenging behaviors. The best treatment requires an accurate, or at least the most likely, diagnosis, and that requires obtaining the best history. Unfortunately, all too often the patient's history and his or her subjective reporting are limited or unavailable.

Barriers to communication can exist for both clinician and patient. Under these circumstances, the clinician should try to be as effective as possible by recognizing the limitations of the patient. For the purposes of this discussion, these limitations are grouped into three broad categories: self-awareness, communication abilities, and comorbid overshadowing.

For adult and older adult patients with intellectual disability, the clinician needs to estimate the degree to which the patient is aware of his or her problem, condition, or feelings. Barriers to that process of evaluation can come from the organic cause of intellectual disability or from the interviewer by asking questions that are too complex or by using vocabulary beyond the grasp of the patient.

The patient's receptive and expressive abilities need to be considered. These two abilities can be comparable in some individuals with intellectual disability or quite different in others with autism or fragile X syndrome. Differences in these abilities can be characteristic features for some conditions. The goal is to adapt the questions to fit the communication abilities of the patient. Collateral sources of information, such as family or caregivers who can provide histories, narratives, and other data, are critically important in both diagnostic and treatment considerations.

An enduring and important concept is that of diagnostic overshadowing, or the idea that the presence of intellectual disability itself makes the appropriate diagnosis and treatment of symptoms of mental illness or challenging behaviors more difficult. It exists as a barrier within the critical thinking of the clinician and, therefore, clinicians should remain aware when presented with a difficult situation.

Psychiatric and Mental Disorders in Aging Adults with Intellectual Disability

The prevalence of psychiatric disorders among adults with intellectual disability is about 5 times that of age-matched control groups. Depending on the exact population studied and the type of diagnoses included, rates range from 10% to 40%. It is, of course, more complicated because human aging and pathologic processes are neither simple nor linear. In older adults with intellectual disability, the occurrence and severity of psychiatric disturbances can vary by age and comorbid conditions. For example, in a study of individuals with Down syndrome who subsequently developed Alzheimer dementia, these individuals were far more likely to suffer from psychologic and behavioral symptoms with more rapid decline in functional status than those who did not develop dementia.

Some symptoms may improve as the patient ages or develops comorbid problems. In adults with Down syndrome, it is not uncommon to have complaints of significant obsessive and compulsive symptoms. This can be the primary focus of concern from young adulthood through the fifth or sixth decade of life or until symptoms of dementia become evident. As the dementia worsens, the anxieties of obsessions and compulsions can wane, and as memory function worsens, those symptoms are often lost or of little concern.

It is also true that some behaviors or conditions can worsen with age through various processes. Individuals with intellectual disability experience the same disorders of aging as others but possibly with reduced coping mechanisms. For example, they may be more affected by chronic pain conditions or by vision or hearing loss.

In lower-functioning individuals or in those with expressive communication disorders, a new behavioral concern can be a sentinel sign of a physical disorder. As a general rule, before determining that a new problem behavior should be the focus of a psychotropic medication or intervention, physical causes should be excluded. New-onset, self-injurious behavior in particular can be an important clue to occult illness. Self-injurious behavior to the ears can be a sign of otitis externa or media. Self-injurious behavior to the eyes can be a clue to vision loss or changes. Delaying attention for a treatable vision condition, eg, presbyopia, can cause permanent loss through self-injury, such as a detached retina or corneal scarring.

Dementias

Individuals with intellectual disability have a higher prevalence of dementias overall than age-matched controls in the general population; this is especially true for dementia associated with Down syndrome (SOE=A). The challenge is to diagnose the condition correctly given the individual's baseline cognitive impairment and diminished reporting skills. All causes of dementia are possible, but some are more likely than others. The dementia of alcoholism is considered relatively rare given the lower rates of alcohol dependence (and other substance use disorders) in this particular population. Similarly, so-called "pugilistic dementia" is higher than might be expected in this population because of repeated self-injuring blows to the head from coup/contra-coup effects.

For well over 100 years, it has been recognized that there is an association and a significantly increased risk of dementia and Down syndrome. Recent research has added imaging technology to the proof of common histologic pathology between Alzheimer dementia and Down syndrome. Adults with Down syndrome are at increased risk of the early onset of Alzheimer disease, with nearly 100% already having developed the characteristic histologic neuropathology of plaques and tangles by age 40. However, it is not typical for individuals with Down syndrome to develop overt dementia at that early an age. In an 1989 study, 49 of 96 patients with Down syndrome met criteria for dementia with an average age of onset of about 54 years ± 6 years. In general, the prevalence for dementia and Down syndrome is approximately 40% for those ≥50 years old and approximately 75% for those ≥60 years old (SOE=B).

The diagnosis of dementia among individuals with intellectual disability is made according to the same criteria as in the general population. The evaluation includes establishing presence of cognitive and adaptive deterioration; demonstration of deficits on examination (preferably with longitudinal follow-up showing progression of deficits); and exclusion of other possible causes of deterioration, such as medical or environmental factors, or other mental disorders, such as depression or delirium. See "Dementia," p 256.

Interest has been growing in attempting to demonstrate the efficacy of medications such as cholinesterase inhibitors (donepezil, rivastigmine, galantamine) and the glutamate antagonist memantine in individuals with intellectual disability. The body of evidence is increasing for modest palliative efficacy in this population. One randomized trial showed minimal benefit with the use of donepezil[OL] for patients with Down syndrome who developed progressive dementia (SOE=C). Another study failed to demonstrate any benefit from use of memantine in a placebo-controlled randomized trial of patients with dementia secondary to Down syndrome (SOE=A). It may be that Alzheimer dementia in Down syndrome is diagnosed relatively later in disease progression than in non-Down syndrome patients with Alzheimer dementia.

Adaptive Behavioral Difficulties

Adaptive behaviors are learned social and practical skills concerned with daily functions. Limitations in these skills have a negative impact on people's lives; however, these skill abilities are not fixed in place or easily assigned to a particular level of intellectual disability. In general, the greater the severity of intellectual disability, the lower the level of adaptive abilities. However, these abilities can be improved over time with behavioral supports.

Adaptive behavior skills can be conceptual, such as in language, reading, and writing; social such as rules, self-esteem, and sense of responsibility; and practical such as job skills, eating, dressing, using the phone, or taking medications. As in any group, aging adults with intellectual disability can lose or become less adept with some adaptive behavior skills, significantly impacting quality of life.

Behavioral Disorders

Maladaptive behaviors are observable phenomena that are counterproductive or disruptive for the individual. Various other terms are sometimes used to describe these acts, including target behaviors (behaviors targeted for extinction) or challenging behaviors. As many as 50%–60% of adults with intellectual disability have a maladaptive behavior (such as withdrawal, self-injury, stereotypy) that is severe or that occurs frequently, and follow-up studies show that these behaviors can persist for years. The proportion decreases with age for various reasons, except in Down syndrome, in which the proportion is higher and the incidence of behavioral problems increases with the degree of intellectual disability. Aggression is seen with similar frequency in all age groups and has an extremely variable presentation.

Diagnosis and Treatment

The diagnosis of a mental disorder in an older adult with intellectual disability is based on the same principles of history and examination that apply in the general population. However, as discussed above, the patient's presentation or reported symptoms can be different, and the perceptions of the clinician and the criteria used pose additional challenges.

Typically, it is difficult for patients to report their emotional or physical state because of impaired verbal skills or a limited awareness of their internal state. Often, mental disorders present as behavioral changes; therefore, the reports of family or other caregivers are extremely important. Their interpretation of an individual's behaviors or symptoms, as well as any physical or behavioral responses to therapeutic interventions, can be critically important.

It is important to not over-diagnose and therefore over-treat an individual's presentation. Because insight, judgment, and adaptive or coping skills are limited, individuals may be more likely to "act out," which may be incorrectly perceived as a serious symptom of illness when, in fact, it may just be frustration. Medication may not be called for in a situation in which supportive therapy and time could lead to resolution. Medication can be used, however, to create a window of opportunity to make behavioral supports or strategies more effective.

Changes in staff, residential or vocational settings, or family health should be reported and considered as precipitating factors for all behavioral changes. The concepts of applied behavioral analysis are important tools to use in determining cause and effect of problem behaviors.

Maladaptive behaviors, such as aggression, can be common in individuals with intellectual disability and can be either a learned response or an impulsive response to a stressor. An appropriate treatment or response, as mentioned earlier, might be instructional or behavioral. Preferred behavior programs reward desirable behavior using positive reinforcement.

Despite appropriate attempts to control physical aggression through behavioral methods, pharmacologic intervention may be necessary for the safety of the patient or those nearby. Very few medications are approved for the most common and challenging behaviors, and prescribing medications off-label is common. Medication management for symptoms of major mental illnesses in older adults with intellectual disability is not much different from that in the general population, keeping in mind the diagnostic caveats already mentioned. See "Dementia," p 256; "Behavioral Problems in Dementia," p 267; "Depression and Other Mood Disorders," p 308; "Anxiety Disorders," p 319; and "Psychotic Disorders," p 324.

It is beyond the scope of this chapter to discuss the various treatment options for such a diverse patient group. Autism spectrum disorders probably represent the largest diagnostic group among aging individuals for whom medication management is common and difficult. Self-injurious behaviors are certainly the most common reason medications are considered. Self-injurious behaviors include several potentially life-threatening behaviors that can cause damage to the brain, eyes, and ears, as well as the potential for systemic infections.

Table 44.1—Developmental Disabilities and Health Problems

System/Condition	Change with Developmental Disabilities	Management Strategies
Intellectual disability	Two-thirds of patients with developmental disabilities suffer from intellectual disability, many in the mild-to-moderate range.	Evaluation and referral to specialized services to maximize intellectual potential
Growth retardation	Usually found in patients with moderate to severe disabilities; it may present as short stature, inability to gain weight, lack of sexual development, or failure to thrive.	Medical evaluation for treatable causes
Sensory impairment	Nearly 90% of patients have impairments in hearing, vision, and speech. Strabismus is common, as is dysarthric speech.	Regular evaluation of hearing, vision, and speech; correction of deficits
Dental/oral conditions	Poor dentition and oral health are very common.	Oral hygiene and tooth brushing; regular dental visits
Thyroid	Thyroid problems can be a cause or a result of developmental disability.	Regular testing and treatment as indicated
Spinal deformities	Kyphosis, scoliosis, and lordosis are common among patients with muscle weakness and spasticity.	Monitoring of body habitus; physical therapy
Seizure disorders	Half of patients may suffer from some type of seizure disorder.	Diagnosis; anticonvulsant medications
Degenerative joint disease	Chronic muscle spasticity and mobility limitations often lead to osteoarthritis and joint disease. Strength and functional status may be prematurely impaired.	Physical therapy, occupational therapy, pain management
Osteopenia and osteoporosis	Lack of weight bearing leads to these chronic conditions in patients who are unable to ambulate.	Promotion of mobility (physical therapy); adequate calcium and vitamin D supplementation
Chronic pain syndromes	Muscle abnormalities and associated spinal deformities often result in chronic pain syndromes. Sensory abnormalities can result in the inability to describe the type, location, and source of the pain.	Regular monitoring of function and behavior to detect possible painful conditions; pain management
Functional decline	Aging patients with cerebral palsy and other similar conditions often develop fatigue, pain, weakness, and overuse syndromes that result in premature loss of function. This is referred to as *postimpairment syndrome* and often requires a reduction in work hours, increase in assistance or use of adaptive devices, and sometimes nursing-home placement.	Physical therapy, occupational therapy, pain management
Cardiac and pulmonary conditions	Patients with cerebral palsy and other similar physical disabilities typically require 3–5 times the energy level of unimpaired adults, predisposing patients to premature conditions of aging, such as hypertension, heart failure, and coronary artery disease.	Monitoring for hypertension, shortness of breath, angina; risk factor management
GI conditions	Gastroesophageal reflux disease and constipation common; constipation can be chronic and severe.	Monitoring; medications, fiber-rich diet, exercise
Incontinence	Many patients are incontinent of bowel and bladder from childhood, but others develop these problems with age.	Screening for treatable causes; identifying functional impairments that can limit toileting
Depression and mood disorders	Patients with cerebral palsy are 4 times more likely to develop depression than age-compared other adults. The stress associated with multiple disabilities is a risk factor, as is the premature decline in functional status associated with the disorder.	Regular screening; counseling and/or medications for those diagnosed with mood disorder

There are a few good guidelines. When two medication options exist, a risk-benefit analysis should be done to identify the best choice, ie, the option that poses the least potential for harm with the greatest potential for benefit. Changing only one medication at a time decreases the number of variables. New medications should be started at a low dosage, and results monitored ("start low and go slow"). If possible, dosages of all medications should be tapered, ultimately discontinuing pharmacotherapy. The use of antipsychotic medications should be avoided if possible. Second-generation antipsychotic medications should not be used for sleep or "anxiety."

MEDICAL DISORDERS

Adults with intellectual disability have more medical problems than age-matched individuals (approximately five medical conditions per person; those with more severe intellectual disability have more problems).

Approximately two-thirds of those in a community setting have chronic conditions or major physical disability. It is estimated that 50% of these medical conditions go undetected. Prompt detection and treatment is associated with better survival. Visual or hearing impairments are more common in individuals with intellectual disability; they increase with age and affect approximately 25%.

Life expectancy decreases with increasing severity of intellectual disability and with other morbidity, such as inability to ambulate, lack of feeding skills, and incontinence. Life expectancy for adults with intellectual disability is about 65 years, with the most common causes of death being cardiovascular and respiratory disorders, cancer, and dementia (particularly in Down syndrome).

Social Conditions

At least 80% of adults with intellectual disability live at home and are cared for by aging family members; 20% live in residential programs. It is estimated that about 40% of eligible individuals may not be served by the formal service system. This situation often leads to a crisis when the parent is no longer able to provide adequate care or is unable to manage a behavioral problem. It is estimated that about half of developmentally disabled adults with a behavior problem eventually need a different living arrangement. Typically, more than half of families have not made plans for the future care of adult relatives with intellectual disability. Clients in day programs or workshops do not typically have pensions or Social Security benefits to allow retirement. Not surprisingly, the degree of intellectual disability, physical health, and functional skills of the aging individual correlate with the degree of parental stress and burden, although maternal and family characteristics such as education and income are more correlated with overall life satisfaction and maternal well-being.

Developmental Disabilities and Comorbidity

Some developmental disabilities may not cause an intellectual disability but nonetheless can contribute to other morbidities and challenging behaviors, resulting in reduced quality of life. Among these disabilities are cerebral palsy, seizure disorders, and a host of genetic disorders too numerous to mention. Some genetic disorders have significant variability in their impact of cognitive functioning, such as William syndrome (a disorder of missing 25 genes). Some genetic disorders once thought to affect only a single generation or gender are now thought to have broader implications, such as fragile X syndrome.

Seizure disorders can negatively impact an individual both directly (if the seizures are uncontrollable) or indirectly (through the medications needed for seizure control). Pre- and postictal states can be times of distinct vulnerability for some individuals. Chronic pain conditions associated with some developmental disabilities, such as the contractures of cerebral palsy, can be a source of medical and psychiatric morbidity. Medical conditions that require frequent hospitalizations or surgeries can carry a great behavioral cost to the individual.

In general, as the degree of cognitive impairment increases, the risk of morbidity due to physical causes increases. For the approximate prevalence and severity of some common conditions found in individuals with developmental disabilities with and without intellectual disability, see Table 44.1.

References

- Bishop KM, Robinson LM, VanLare S. Healthy aging for older adults with intellectual and development disabilities. *J Psychosoc Nurs Ment Health Serv*. 2013;51(1):15–18.
- Chauhan U, Kontopantelis E, Campbell S, et al. Health checks in primary care for adults with intellectual disabilities: how extensive should they be? *J Intellect Disabil Res*. 2010;54(6):479–486.
- Livingston G, Strydom A. Improving Alzheimer's disease outcomes in Down's syndrome. *Lancet*. 2012;379(9815): 498–500.

Chapters

CHAPTER 45—DERMATOLOGIC DISEASES AND DISORDERS

KEY POINTS

- Photoaging increases the fragility of the skin and decreases the elasticity/tensile strength of the skin.
- Older adults are at risk of xerosis and neurodermatitis, or lichen simplex chronicus.
- Venous insufficiency can cause stasis dermatitis and chronic leg ulcers. Treatment should begin by controlling venous hypertension with compression therapy.
- Ultraviolet (UV) light exposure and age are associated with increased incidence of skin cancers, including squamous cell carcinomas, basal cell carcinomas, and melanomas.

AGING AND PHOTOAGING

The incidence and prevalence of skin disease increase with aging and sun exposure. Dermatologic care of older adults requires an awareness of cutaneous changes of aging and the effects of cumulative UV radiation exposure, as well as knowledge of the common tumors, inflammatory diseases, and infections seen in this population. The skin of older individuals is characterized by several changes, including increased fragility, graying of hairs, and increased wrinkles, particularly at rest. Each of the skin layers changes with aging. In normal young skin, the epidermis interdigitates with the dermis. With time, the epidermis becomes flattened with reduced keratinocyte turnover and melanocyte numbers, contributing in part to the decreased rate of wound healing. In the dermis, the fibroblasts are elongated and collapsed. Types I and III collagen and microfibrils of elastin all decrease, leading to the appearance of laxity and atrophy. Changes in hair include graying, which is caused by changes in follicular melanocytes, and a decrease in scalp hair density secondary to a shortened length of anagen (the growth phase of the hair cycle) and an increased proportion of hairs in telogen (the resting phase). In aging skin, the number of immune antigen-presenting cells, such as Langerhans cells, decrease, which may have consequences for cutaneous immune surveillance.

Aging of skin is a result of both intrinsic and extrinsic factors. The largest contributor is the cumulative exposure to UV light. This leads to the clinical appearance of lentigines, guttate hypomelanosis, poikiloderma, laxity, yellow hue, and leathery appearance. *Photoaging* refers to the effects of UV exposure on skin. UV light appears to activate signaling pathways that lead to increased matrix metalloproteinase activity and decreased collagen production. In a vicious cycle, the fibroblasts become elongated and collapsed and respond by decreasing collagen production. UV light also causes DNA injury in part via oxidative damage, which likely also contributes to the aging phenotype. Cutaneous malignancies are also more common in photodamaged skin because of photocarcinogenesis and UV light–mediated immunosuppression.

Prevention of photodamage involves using broad-spectrum sunscreens—sunscreens that protect against both UVA and UVB radiation—as well as avoiding direct sunlight and wearing protective clothing, including hats and sunglasses. Although there are claims that various topical agents decrease photodamage, only topical tretinoin has been shown to increase the thickness of the superficial skin layers, reduce pigmentary changes and roughness, and increase collagen synthesis (SOE=A). Topical and even oral antioxidants (particularly vitamins E and C) have been shown to have some photoprotective and chemoprotective capabilities. In addition, over 70 botanicals, including soy and green tea, are currently found in many cosmaceuticals, but pharmacokinetic, safety, and double-blinded efficacy studies are lacking.

INFLAMMATORY AND AUTOIMMUNE SKIN CONDITIONS

Seborrheic Dermatitis

Seborrheic dermatitis (Figure 45.1) is a chronic inflammatory dermatosis characterized by symmetric pink patches with overlying greasy bran-like scaling distributed in the areas where sebaceous glands are found, namely on the scalp, the face, and sometimes the presternal chest and intertriginous areas. On the face, the lesions are found on the forehead, medial portions of the eyebrows, upper eyelids, nasolabial folds and lateral aspects of the nose, retroauricular areas, and occasionally the occiput and neck. At times, the lesions may be arcuate or petaloid, resembling flower petals. Occasionally patients have features of both psoriasis and seborrheic dermatitis, particularly in the hairline and eyebrows, and this condition is therefore known as sebopsoriasis.

The pathogenesis of seborrheic dermatitis is unclear but may be related to the yeast colonies that normally colonize the skin, ie, *Malassezia furfur*. Seborrheic

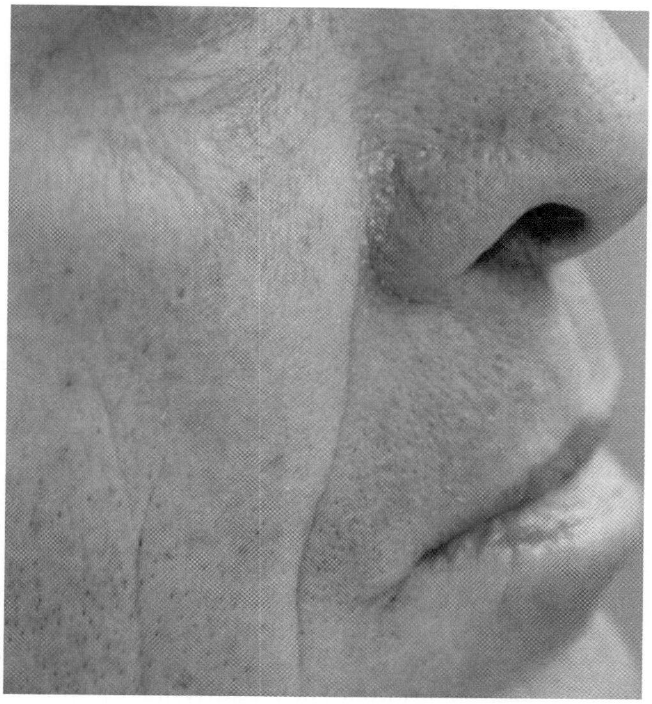

Figure 45.1—Seborrheic dermatitis. Erythema with greasy scaling noted along nasolabial folds.

dermatitis tends to be more prevalent in patients with Parkinson disease. Extensive and severe eruptions of seborrheic dermatitis often warrant an examination of HIV status. Rebound flares of seborrheic dermatitis can follow tapering of corticosteroid medications.

While seborrheic dermatitis can be treated, it cannot be cured or eliminated. Treatment can be in the form of creams (face and body) or shampoos (scalp). Medications that target yeast, including selenium sulfide, ketoconazole, and various tar shampoos, are effective. In an acute flare, patients can be treated with mild topical corticosteroids such as hydrocortisone 1%; if treatment is unsuccessful, a trial of topical calcineurin inhibitors can be tried. Aggressive topical or systemic therapy should be avoided because of risk of rebound.

Rosacea

Rosacea (Figure 45.2) is a common condition in fair-skinned people and has four subtypes with overlapping prevalence: erythematotelangiectatic rosacea has been reported in 96% of rosacea patients, papulopustular rosacea in 51%, phymatous rosacea in <5%, and ocular rosacea in 14%. In the erythematotelangiectatic subtype, there is persistent erythema of the central convex areas of the face (ie, nose, forehead, cheeks, and chin) with telangiectasias and flushing. In the papulopustular subtype, there are follicular and nonfollicular papules and pustules in addition to the persistent erythema. In the phymatous subtype, there is sebaceous hyperplasia and thickening of the skin, in part due to recurrent flushing and edema; in some cases, this leads to rhinophyma. In ocular rosacea, irritation and burning of the eye can present as conjunctival injection, blepharitis, episcleritis, chalazion, or hordeolum. Other variants of rosacea include granulomatous rosacea, periorificial dermatitis, and pyoderma faciale.

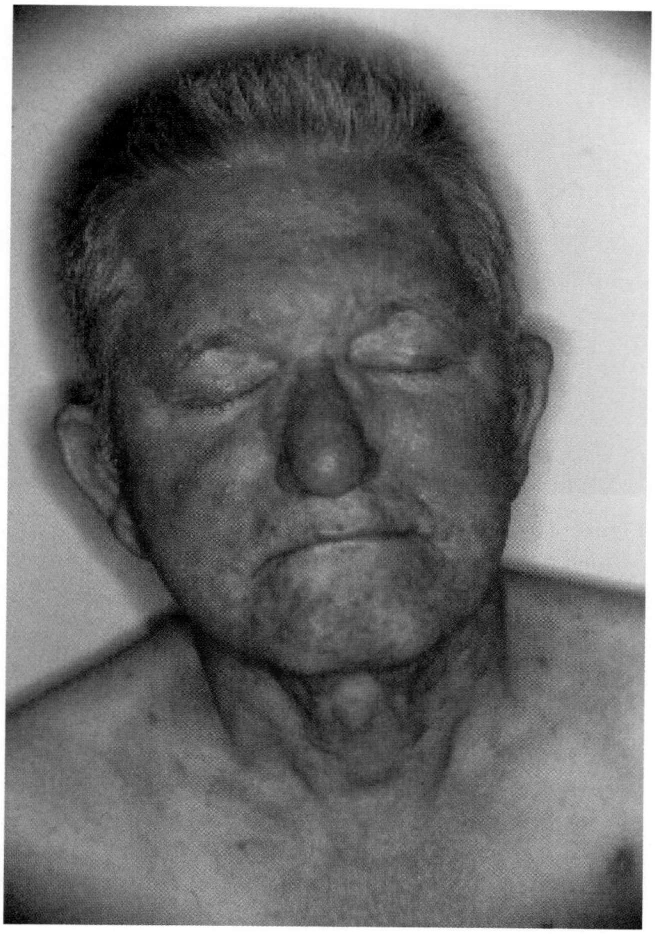

Figure 45.2—Rosacea. Diffuse erythema and erythematous papules and papulopustules are seen on the cheeks, forehead, and chin. The nose shows thickening of the skin and changes consistent with an early rhinophyma.

Incidence of rosacea peaks in the third and fourth decades, but the disease is seen in young and older adults as well. The cause of acne rosacea is likely multifactorial, including contributions from vasodilatation, *Demodex* mites, and propionobacterium. In addition, thermal stimuli, sunlight exposure, and a number of medications can contribute to rosacea, including oral niacin and topical steroids. Often, seborrheic dermatitis and rosacea are seen together.

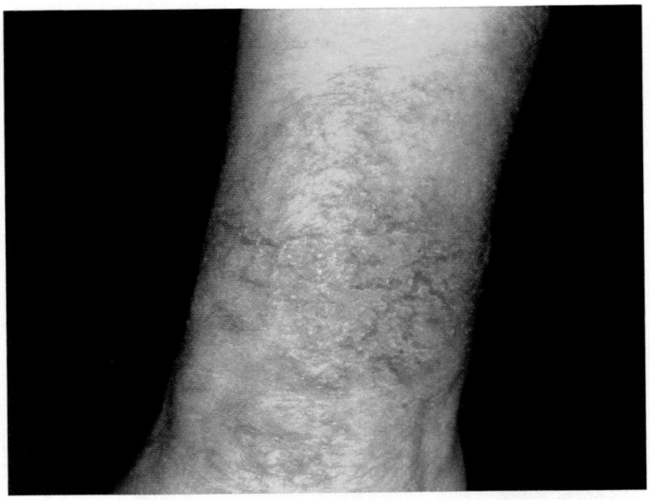

Figure 45.3—Eczema craquelé. Dry, erythematous, fissured, and cracked skin is seen on the lower legs of this patient.

The treatment of rosacea depends on the subtype and severity. Topical antibiotics such as benzoyl peroxide, erythromycin, and metronidazole can be used to treat papulopustular rosacea. Oral antibiotics such as tetracylines (eg, doxycycline, minocycline) and macrolides are used to treat moderate to severe cases. Alternative therapies include topical azelaic acid, topical tretinoin, and oral isotretinoin for severe cases. For the persistent erythema, nasal decongestants such as oxymetazoline hydrochloride have shown some promise in small case series. For treatment of the telangiectasias, lasers, such as the potassium-titanyl-phosphate laser, intense pulsed light, and the pulsed dye laser, can be used. Rhinophyma can be treated with surgical excision or electrosurgery.

Xerosis

Dryness of the skin, often a concern for older adults, is due to altered barrier function in the aging epidermis and a reduced ability to retain water. It is exacerbated by environmental factors such as decreased humidity; prolonged exposure to water, which can dilute out natural moisturizing factors; and use of harsh soaps, which can further damage the stratum corneum. This condition is often more pronounced on the legs. Depending on the severity of the dryness, xerosis can present as rough, itchy skin or as scales that give the skin a dry, cracked riverbed appearance known as *eczema craquelé* (Figure 45.3).

Treatment usually begins with avoiding the exacerbating factors mentioned above. Patients should be advised to take tepid showers and avoid using washcloths, sponges, or brushes to scrub the skin. Moisturizing agents, especially those containing lactic acid or α-hydroxy acids, can reduce roughness and scaliness. Moisturizing agents are often most helpful when applied immediately after a bath or shower. Home humidifiers may also be beneficial during seasons when home heating is being used. When irritation or inflammation is prominent, episodic use of mild topical corticosteroids for a short time provides relief.

Neurodermatitis

Neurodermatitis is a nonspecific term that is used to refer to chronic, pruritic conditions of unclear cause. Another commonly used term is *lichen simplex chronicus*. It is most common in adults >60 years old. The lesions show signs of chronic scratching, such as hyperpigmentation and lichenification (increased skin markings), along with redness and scaling. Scratching these lesions is often satisfying and leads to a vicious cycle of skin changes and more pruritus. Treatment consists of potent topical corticosteroids (often under occlusion), emollients, and behavior modification. Other causes of pruritus such as irritant or allergic contact dermatitis, drug allergy, or xerosis must be excluded.

Intertrigo

Intertrigo (Figure 45.4) is any infectious or noninfectious inflammatory condition of two closely opposed skin surfaces (intertriginous area). It is more common in older adults because of the increased skin folds secondary to decreased dermal elasticity. Additional contributory factors include decreased mobility, moisture, friction, and poor hygiene. Factors that increase moisture (eg, obesity) or decrease immunity (eg, diabetes or systemic corticosteroids) predispose patients to develop intertrigo. Commonly involved areas, such as the inframammary area, abdominal folds, groin, and axillae, appear erythematous, macerated, moist, and mildly malodorous. Differential diagnosis includes seborrheic dermatitis and inverse psoriasis. Intertrigo often is associated with superficial infection with bacteria or *Candida*. Successful treatment involves decreasing moisture with topical drying agents, such as corn starch and antifungal powder (eg, miconazole or nystatin powder). Physical means of keeping the area dry include bed sheets/handkerchiefs to separate skin folds and frequent airing, or careful use of a hairdryer. If candidal intertrigo is suspected, treatment involves the topical polyene and azole antifungals, such as topical nystatin or ketoconazole. Occasionally, a very mild topical corticosteroid such as 1%–2% hydrocortisone is needed for a short period to reduce inflammation and irritation (see also candidiasis, p 357).

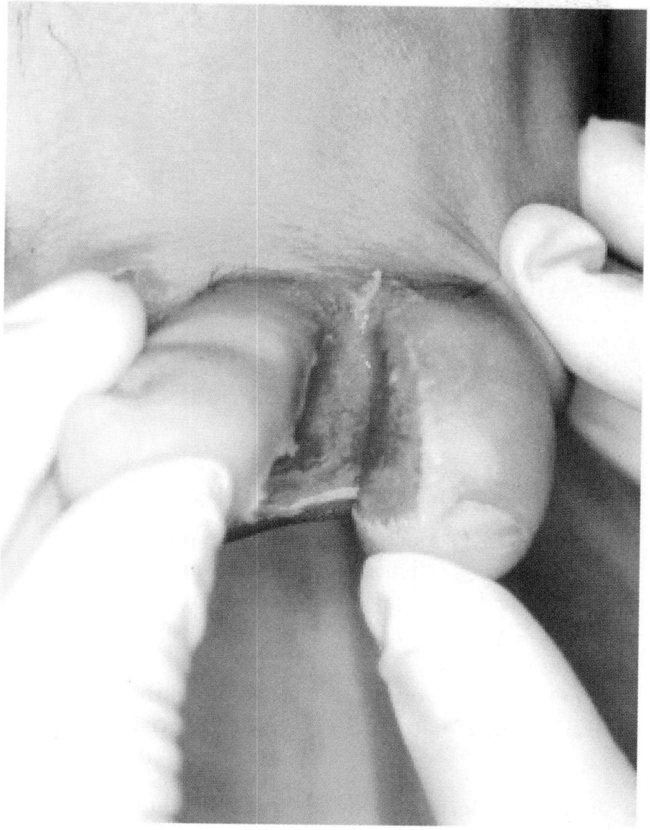

Figure 45.4—Intertrigo and candidiasis. This fungal infection is commonly found in the web space between the fourth and fifth toes. Moist erythema, maceration, and superficial erosion are apparent.

Bullous Pemphigoid

Bullous pemphigoid (Figure 45.5) is the most common autoimmune subepidermal blistering disease. It is a disease of older adults, with the age of onset commonly >60 years. Clinically, the disease has diverse manifestations. Typically, bullous pemphigoid presents as an extremely pruritic eruption with widespread blister formation. The blisters are typically tense, often filled with clear fluid. The distribution is symmetrical and widespread, although the flexural areas and lower trunk may be favored. Up to one-third of patients have mucous membrane involvement. The blisters often resolve without scarring. Early or atypical lesions may be nonbullous with primarily urticarial lesions (Figure 45.5).

Bullous pemphigoid is a prototypical organ-specific autoimmune disease with a humoral and cellular immune response targeted against two antigens in the hemidesmosome. With the help of autoreactive T cells, pathogenic B cells produce antibodies that target these two hemidesmosomal antigens. The antibodies trigger an inflammatory cascade of complement activation, the recruitment of neutrophils and eosinophils, and

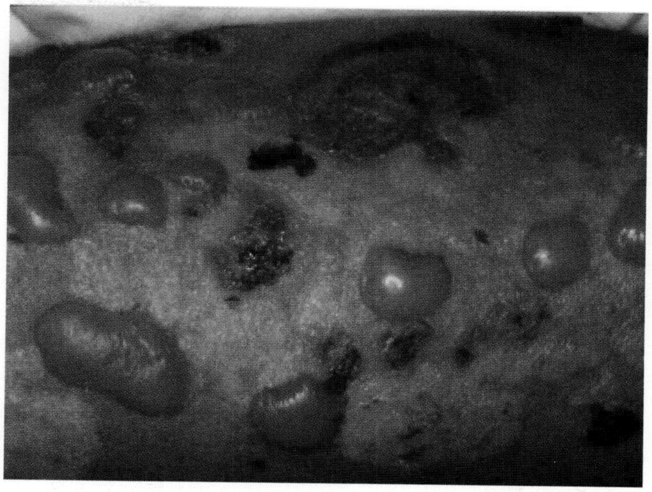

Figure 45.5—Bullous pemphigoid. Tense, fluid-filled, and hemorrhagic bullae on an erythematous base are seen on the trunk and extremities. Some of the bullae have ruptured and left a scab with crusting.

the elaboration of proteases. Bullous pemphigoid has been associated with medications, including diuretics, analgesics, antibiotics, and ACE inhibitors. Diagnosis is made by clinicopathologic correlation.

While the disease may last for months to years, it is often self-limited. Treatment should be commensurate to the severity of disease. Limited, localized disease can be treated with potent topical corticosteroids, topical calcineurin inhibitors, and nicotinamide with tetracycline. Systemic corticosteroids are the mainstay of more extensive treatment. Steroid-sparing agents (eg, azathioprine and cyclophosphamide) are often used to avoid the adverse events of corticosteroids.

Pruritus

Pruritus, a very common skin complaint, is associated with many cutaneous and systemic conditions. Severe pruritus can compromise quality of life. Pruritus can be idiopathic, related to a primary skin disease, or secondary to a systemic disease. In older adults, xerosis is the most common cause of chronic pruritus. However, evaluation must exclude other underlying pruritic dermatologic conditions, including infestations such as scabies; genetic or childhood diseases such as atopic dermatitis; and autoimmune blistering diseases, including bullous pemphigoid. Pruritus can be caused by medications (eg, dermal hypersensitivity reactions), related to chemical exposures (eg, irritant dermatitis or allergic contact dermatitis), or be a consequence of autosensitization to stasis dermatitis. Pruritus can be secondary to systemic diseases such as renal disease, cholestasis or chronic liver disease, thyroid disease, anemia, and occult malignancies. Finally, generalized pruritus can also be associated with generalized anxiety disorder, depression, and even psychosis, including delusions of parasitosis.

A thorough evaluation of pruritus in an older adult therefore includes a complete history and physical examination to exclude underlying and treatable skin disease. Distribution of the pruritus may help to determine the underlying cause. Involvement of flexural areas suggests atopic dermatitis or bullous pemphigoid, whereas primary involvement of the lower legs suggests an autosensitization to stasis dermatitis. Laboratory evaluation to exclude secondary causes includes a CBC and function tests of the liver, kidneys, and thyroid. It is also important to perform age-appropriate cancer screening, as warranted by the findings of above.

Treatment requires addressing the cause of the pruritus, if known, and relieving symptoms. If there is a primary dermatologic condition or a systemic disease, treatment should be tailored to the underlying disease. For example, prednisone may be warranted for bullous pemphigoid, and topical corticosteroids for atopic dermatitis. In addition, symptomatic relief often requires multiple modalities. Nonpharmacologic measures include open-wet dressings: in brief, a thin, white material such as a bed sheet can be moistened with lukewarm tap water and placed over the skin for 10–15 min; as the water evaporates, it can relieve pruritus. It is important to treat xerosis with frequent applications of emollients. Topical corticosteroids, such as 0.1% triamcinolone ointment, can also relieve xerosis and any underlying inflammation. Topical pramoxine, menthol in calamine preparations, and capsaicin[OL] cream can change the neurologic sensation of pruritus. These topical agents can also be used frequently with minimal adverse events in the short-term. Systemic therapy can include nonsedating oral antihistamines. Most trials investigating their use have used desloratadine in the treatment of chronic idiopathic urticaria. It has significantly improved patient-reported pruritus, sleep disruption, and interference with daily activities with a low incidence of adverse events (SOE=A). Cetirizine, fexofenadine, and levocetirizine are also used for this purpose. In severe, refractory cases, including cases secondary to systemic disease, patients can be referred to a dermatologist for UVB phototherapy or oral thalidomide.

Psoriasis

Psoriasis (Figure 45.6) is a chronic inflammatory skin disease characterized by well-demarcated plaques with overlying silvery scale. Chronic plaque psoriasis is the most common variant, and it characteristically involves the scalp, the gluteal cleft, and extensor surfaces. Hands and feet can be involved, as well as the nails, which may portend psoriatic arthritis. The other psoriatic subtypes are as follows:

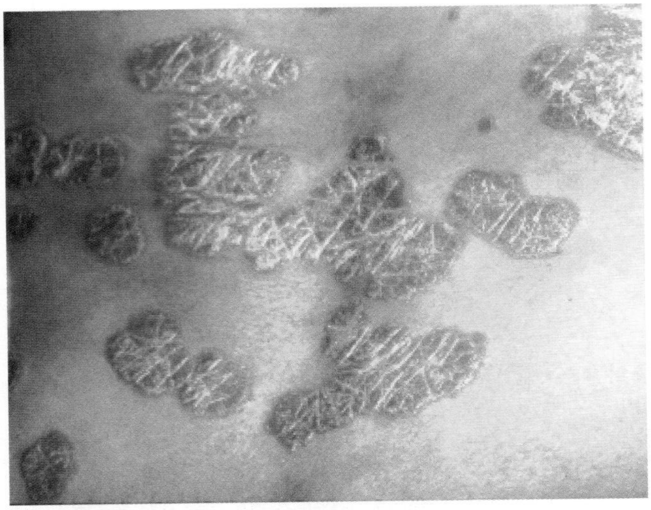

Figure 45.6—Psoriasis. Characteristic well-demarcated beefy red plaques with overlying silvery white scales are evident on the back of this patient.

- inverse pattern, in which lesions develop in skin folds, such as the neck, axillae, and genital area
- guttate, in which small papules (approximately 1 cm) appear over the upper trunk and proximal extremities, usually after a streptococcal or viral infection
- pustular, which is acute with generalized eruption of sterile pustules (2–3 mm) and fever
- palmoplantar pustulosis, in which sterile pustules are confined to the palms and soles
- erythrodermic psoriasis, in which the patient has generalized erythema

Psoriasis is common, affecting 2% of the population. The incidence is bimodal, first in the mid-20s and then at about 50–60 years of age. The cause is likely multifactorial. There is a strong genetic predisposition, with multigene mode of inheritance, as well as a role for environmental factors. Triggers that initiate or exacerbate disease include physical trauma (known as Koebner's phenomenon), infections (including streptococcal upper respiratory infections), stress, and medications (eg, oral corticosteroids, lithium, β-blockers, ACE inhibitors, NSAIDs). In psoriasis, the risk factors ultimately lead to the activation and recruitment of autoreactive Th1 and Th17 T cells to the skin. Cytokines such as tumor necrosis factor-alpha (TNF-α) and IL-23 likely lead to the activation of T cells, and IL-22 leads ultimately to increased keratinocyte proliferation.

Psoriatic arthritis, which is characterized by pain, swelling, and stiffness of affected joints, is also seen in 5%–35% of patients. Classically, psoriatic arthritis is an asymmetrical oligoarthritis of the small joints of the hands. Alternative patterns of presentation include inflammation restricted to the distal interphalangeal joints, symmetrical polyarthritis of the hands, and arthritis mutilans with telescoping of the involved digit. Also, some patients suffer from back pain in the form of spondylitis or sacroiliitis.

Because of the wide clinical spectrum of disease, treatment should be tailored to the individual, with special attention paid to the risks and benefits for the older patient. Therapies directed at the skin are appropriate for patients with limited disease. These include topical treatments such as topical corticosteroids, vitamin D derivatives (eg, calcipotriene), topical retinoids (eg, tazarotene), salicylic acid, and tar compounds. Long-term use of topical steroids is limited by the risk of cutaneous atrophy. In patients in whom topical therapy is unsuccessful and in those who have extensive disease, phototherapy can be of benefit. UV light therapy, including narrow-band UVB therapy and psoralen with UVA light (PUVA), can be used alone or in conjunction with topical therapies. Patients receiving UV light therapy must be able to stand for the duration of the treatment. Risks include increased incidence of skin cancer.

For those with widespread and recalcitrant disease, systemic agents are available. Oral immunosuppressive agents, including cyclosporine and methotrexate, are effective but require careful monitoring for adverse events. Toxicities of cyclosporine include hypertension and renal dysfunction. Toxicities of methotrexate include bone marrow suppression, liver fibrosis, and interstitial lung pneumonitis. Oral retinoids such as acitretin can be used in conjunction with other therapies such as UV light. Biologics can be effective in patients in whom traditional systemic therapies are either ineffective or contraindicated. These include agents that block the cytokine TNF, and T-cell surface molecules including adhesion molecules and co-stimulatory molecules. These agents have their own adverse events. In general, anti-TNF agents are contraindicated in those with a history of hepatitis C, multiple sclerosis, heart failure, and lymphoma. Antibodies targeting the common IL-12/IL-23 subunit (uztekinumab) have demonstrated remarkable efficacy and duration of response (up to 16 weeks from each treatment) in phase II and III studies. These antibodies are FDA approved, and many more new agents are under development.

Initiation of psoriasis involves both epithelial cells and immune cells, and as a result of this interaction, psoriatic skin lesions and/or joint issues may develop, as well as an underlying systemic inflammatory disease with potential cardiovascular implications and risks. Therefore patients with psoriasis should be counseled about diet, exercise, and weight control.

Stasis Dermatitis

Stasis dermatitis can be an early sign of chronic venous insufficiency of the legs. Chronic venous hypertension, caused mostly by incompetency of the venous valves, is the initial trigger for stasis dermatitis. Venous hypertension slows down the flow of blood in the microvasculature, damages the permeability barrier of the small vessels, and allows for the passage of fluid and plasma proteins into the tissue, leading to edema and extravasation of erythrocytes. These processes lead to decreased oxygen diffusion and metabolic exchange and to activation and attraction of inflammatory cells and mediators to the site. Stasis dermatitis typically develops in the medial supramalleolar areas. It is often associated with intense pruritus. Initially, pitting edema to the ankle is noted, which is often worse later in the day. Over time, these events lead to progressive induration and adherence of the skin and subcutaneous tissues. Venous ulcers can develop spontaneously or secondary to trauma, arising most often in the supramalleolar areas.

The goal of therapy is to control the venous hypertension by regularly using compression bandages or stockings and exercising the calf muscles to improve venous return. Topical treatment includes the judicious use of corticosteroids and emollients. Sensitization to ingredients in topical medications and emollients, including topical antibiotics, is common and frequently overlooked. Patch testing to exclude contact sensitization to these agents should be considered before use.

ULCERS

Venous and Arterial Ulcers

An ulcer is a wound with a loss of the epidermis. Ulcers of the lower leg are most often caused by vascular disease or neuropathy. Of leg ulcers caused by vascular disease, 72% are caused by venous disease, 22% have a mixed arterial and venous cause, and only 6% are caused by pure arterial disease. They have characteristic risk factors, morphologies, and distributions (Table 45.1).

Chronic leg ulcers are defined as open ulcers that fail to heal within a 6-week period. Treatment of the leg ulcers should be selected based on the cause of the ulceration. In addition to clinical criteria, ankle-brachial indices (ABI) can be used to determine the presence of underlying arterial disease; an ABI <0.8 is abnormal, and compression is contraindicated with an ABI <0.5.

Table 45.1—Characteristics of Venous and Arterial Ulcers

Characteristic	Venous Disease	Arterial Disease
Signs and symptoms	Limb heaviness, aching and swelling that is associated with standing and is worse at end of day, brawny skin changes	Claudication (pain in leg with walking), ankle-brachial index <0.9, loss of hair, cool extremities
Risk factors	Advanced age, obesity, history of deep-vein thrombosis or phlebitis	Age >40 years old, cigarette smoking, diabetes mellitus, hyperlipidemia, hypertension, male gender, sedentary lifestyle
Location of ulcers	Along the course of the long saphenous vein, between the lower medial calf to just below the medial malleolus	Over bony prominences

For venous ulcers, venous hypertension can be reversed by either elastic compression, ie, compression stockings, or by inelastic compression, ie, Unna boot. Debridement of necrotic and fibrinous debris is important for reepithelialization and can be achieved by mechanical or chemical methods, eg, collagenase treatment. Occlusive dressings can be used to help the wound heal; the type of dressing used depends on the ulcer type and amount of drainage (Table 38.6). Surgical options include pinch grafts, split-thickness skin grafts, and allografts. Pentoxifylline[OL] is a systemic agent with fibrinolytic and antithrombotic activities that has been reported to accelerate healing (SOE=C).

For arterial ulcers, the main goal is reestablishing the blood supply. Revascularization can be achieved with arterioplasty and bypass surgery. To preclude worsening of disease and development of new ulcers, patients should be encouraged to reduce their risk factors for arterial disease, including smoking, hyperlipidemia, hypertension, and diabetes mellitus. See peripheral arterial disease in "Cardiovascular Diseases and Disorders," p 378.

Pressure Ulcers

See "Pressure Ulcers and Wound Care," p 296.

INFECTIONS AND INFESTATIONS

Onychomycosis

See "Diseases and Disorders of the Foot," p 471.

Herpes Zoster

Herpes zoster represents reactivation of the varicella zoster virus (VZV), the virus that is responsible for varicella, ie, chickenpox. Classically, it is a disease of older adults, with more than two-thirds of cases in patients >50 years old. The lifetime risk of reactivation of VZV is 20% in healthy adults and 50% in immunocompromised individuals. During primary infection, ie, varicella, VZV establishes a latent infection in sensory ganglia. Partly because of the decline in the cellular immune response associated with age or immunosuppressive conditions (Table 60.1), the virus is reactivated and leads to painful ganglionitis. The infection spreads down the sensory nerve and is released around the sensory nerve endings in the skin, producing the characteristic lesions.

Usually, zoster begins with a prodrome of pain. In some people, the prodrome includes sensations of pruritus, tingling, tenderness, or hyperesthesia. The pain is followed by a painful eruption of grouped vesicles on an erythematous base, usually in a sensory distribution. In the localized form of zoster, the vesicles rarely cross midline (Figure 45.7). Rarely, prodromal pain is not followed by a cutaneous eruption, a condition called zoster sine herpete.

Herpes zoster infection has been associated with a number of complications, including post-herpetic neuralgia (PHN), scarring ophthalmic zoster, and Ramsay Hunt syndrome. The incidence and severity of PHN increase with increasing age and an immunocompromised state. In 7% of cases of herpes zoster, the ophthalmic branch of the trigeminal nerve is involved. Involvement of the nasociliary branch, which presents as vesicles on the tip of the nose (known as Hutchinson sign), requires careful ophthalmic examination to monitor for complications, such as neurotrophic keratitis and ulceration, scleritis, uveitis, and ultimately blindness. In the Ramsay Hunt syndrome, the geniculate ganglion is involved. In addition to producing vesicles in the pharynx and on the external ear or tympanic membrane, Ramsay Hunt is associated with facial palsy with or without tinnitus, vertigo, and deafness. Zoster is considered disseminated if it involves two noncontiguous dermatomes. In disseminated zoster, meningoencephalitis, hepatitis, and pneumonitis are also complications.

Although the symptoms of herpes zoster can be confused with a variety of conditions causing localized pain (ie, pleurisy, myocardial infarction, renal colic, cholecystitis, and glaucoma), the combination of the history and the characteristic physical examination (ie, the dermatomal distribution) facilitate the diagnosis. A Tzanck smear from the base of the vesicle can be performed to confirm the diagnosis. Detection of

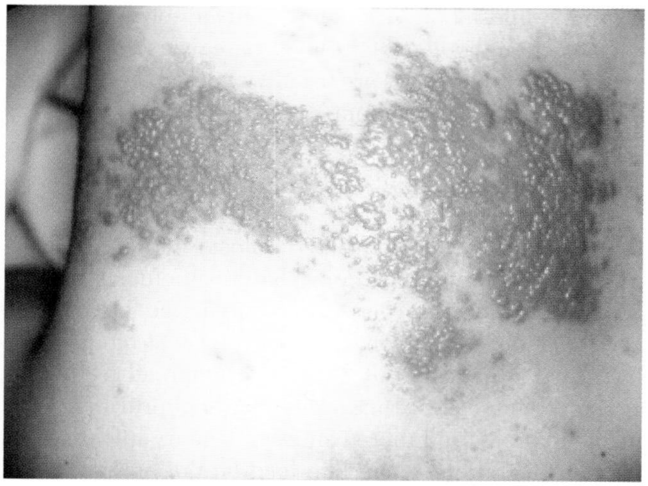

Figure 45.7—Herpes zoster. This patient has clusters of vesicles and pustules on an erythematous base involving a thoracic dermatome.

multinucleated giant cells suggests a herpes simplex or herpes zoster infection. Direct fluorescence antibody testing can be performed to confirm the presence of VZV. Polymerase chain reaction and viral cultures are the most sensitive means to confirm the diagnosis.

Early treatment with antiviral therapies, optimally within 72 hours of onset of rash, decreases disease duration and pain (SOE=A). FDA-approved therapies include acyclovir, famcyclovir, and valacyclovir, and their use should be monitored in patients who have reduced renal function. The addition of oral corticosteroids has not been shown to shorten the duration of complete recovery, although in one randomized controlled trial participants treated with a 3-week tapering dosage of prednisone had a greater chance of being pain-free 1 month after the onset of the lesions (SOE=B). Intravenous antiviral therapy is reserved for immunocompromised individuals and for those who demonstrate signs of disseminated disease or complications. Most cases of acute herpes zoster are self-limited, but the probability of developing PHN increases with advanced age. PHN occurs in approximately 20% of zoster patients ≥70 years old and is difficult to treat. Acute herpetic neuralgia refers to pain preceding or accompanying the eruption of rash that persists up to 30 days from its onset. Subacute herpetic neuralgia refers to pain that persists beyond healing of the rash but that resolves within 4 months of onset. PHN refers to pain persisting beyond 4 months from the initial onset of the rash. Prevention of PHN can be attempted by vaccinating to decrease the incidence of acute zoster and PHN, by treating the acute zoster infection itself, or by treating acute zoster very early with preventive pain medications such as tricyclic antidepressants or anticonvulsants. Anticholinergic adverse events of tricyclics are common and may limit their use in older adults.

Treatment of PHN can be challenging. Systematic reviews of randomized controlled trials of treatments of PHN with evaluation periods of >24-hour duration found no single best treatment. Tricyclic antidepressants[OL], opioids, topical capsaicin, gabapentin, topical lidocaine, pregabalin, and tramadol can alleviate the pain of PHN, but the long-term benefits of most therapies are not known and adverse events are common. Intrathecal methylprednisolone may relieve pain in patients refractory to the oral and topical measures discussed above.

Because of the high incidence and high morbidity associated with herpes zoster, prophylaxis by zoster vaccination is recommended for patients >60 years old. Vaccination is associated with a statistically significant decrease in zoster incidence and incidence of PHN (SOE=A). The vaccine is more effective in preventing zoster infection in patients 60–69 years old than in those ≥70 years old. However, it appears to prevent PHN to a greater extent in older research participants than in those 60–69 years old. In a large community-based study of participants ≥60 years old, herpes zoster vaccination was associated with a 55% reduced risk of herpes zoster in those who had received the vaccine compared with those who had not.

Candidiasis

Candidiasis has a wide spectrum of presentation. Cutaneous candidiasis is often seen in intertriginous areas; it can be superimposed on intertrigo caused by psoriasis or seborrheic dermatitis (see intertrigo, p 352). *Candida* pustules can also develop on the backs of bedridden patients and on other areas prone to moisture and occlusion. In these areas, candidiasis is characterized by red patches, sometimes with erosions. Often, there are peripheral satellite pustules. Candidiasis can also affect the scrotum, the nails, the genital area, and corners of the lips, causing perleche. Oral thrush is an example of mucocutaneous candidiasis, observed most commonly in patients on corticosteroid inhalers, antibiotics, or immunosuppressive medications; or with concomitant systemic illnesses, such as diabetes mellitus. A potassium hydroxide preparation of skin scrapings of the involved site can confirm the diagnosis. The presence of spores and pseudohyphae is consistent with candidiasis.

Topical treatments are generally effective; topical medications should be applied beyond the margins of the lesion. Most commonly used are topical polyenes such as nystatin, and topical azoles such as miconazole, clotrimazole, ketoconazole, and econazole. Other topical agents that are effective are terbinafine, butenafine, and ciclopirox. Topical therapies can be used twice a day until symptoms resolve and subsequently twice a week for prophylaxis as necessary. In the event of pruritus, pain, and burning, a low-dose topical corticosteroid can sometimes be used in conjunction with topical antifungal therapy, but these symptoms generally resolve with use of topical antifungal medications. In patients with widespread candidiasis, oral therapy with an azole has a response rate of 80%–100%. Effective eradication of candidiasis generally also requires treating the underlying intertrigo by keeping the moist areas dry with drying agents and physical barriers to keep the skin folds separated (eg, bed sheets).

Scabies

Human scabies is a pruritic eruption caused by the mite *Sarcoptes scabiei* var *hominis*. The entire 30-day life cycle is confined to the human epidermis. After fertilization, adult female mites lay eggs, which mature over 10 days. For first-time infestations, sensitization can take 2–6 weeks; therefore, symptoms may not be seen until a month after infestation, making it difficult to make a diagnosis before disease spread. Scabies is spread primarily by person-to-person contact and is common in institutionalized older adults.

Scabies is characterized by intense pruritus, worse at night, and a symmetrically distributed cutaneous eruption. The eruption is most often characterized by small erythematous papules, sometimes accompanied by linear excoriations. The pathognomic sign is a burrow that is characterized by a wavy, threadlike lesion about 1–10 mm long. The lesions are distributed over the interdigital webs, the flexural wrists, the umbilicus, the wrists, the ankles, and the feet. In men, lesions are also seen on the scrotum and penis. In women, the areolae, nipples, and genital areas are commonly affected. Immunocompromised patients can get crusted scabies, characterized by thousands of mites per gram of epidermis. Other manifestations include vesicles and indurated nodules. The lesions may be nonspecific, and the diagnosis should be considered in anyone with intense pruritus.

Diagnosis can be confirmed by microscopic examination of skin scrapings in mineral oil. This allows direct visualization of the adult mites, nymphs, eggs, or fecal matter (scybala). Occasionally, diagnosis can also be made by skin biopsy. Treatment includes topical creams such as 5% permethrin cream applied head to toe and left on for 8–14 hours, or systemic medications such as ivermectin (200 mcg/kg). Therapies are generally not effective against the eggs; therefore, patients require retreatment in 1–2 weeks after the eggs mature. Clothes, linens, and towels should be either washed in hot water and dried in high heat or left in a closed bag for 10 days to prevent reinfestation by fomites. In the absence of human contact, the mite cannot survive. Caregivers should also be treated because they are usually exposed, even though they may not have symptoms.

Louse Infestations

Lice can infest the body (pediculosis corporis), scalp (pediculosis capitis), or pubic hair (pediculosis pubis). With pediculosis corporis or capitis, lice are spread from person to person through physical contact or fomites. Pediculosis pubis is usually spread by sexual contact. In all cases, patients complain of pruritus of the involved areas, and there can be secondary infection. In pediculosis corporis, the lice feed on the body but live on clothing, where they lay eggs, often near the seams. In pediculosis capitis, the lice lay eggs on the proximal part of the hair shaft. The eggs (or nits) are visible as white specks cemented to the hair at an oblique angle. Patients with pediculosis pubis also have nits on the pubic hair and commonly have more organisms.

Treatment involves eradicating the lice and larvae, treating close contacts, and treating the secondary infection. Pyrethrin or its derivatives (permethrin) are ovicidal and can be used as a single 10-minute topical treatment. People who come into contact with the patient, including caregivers and those who share bedding, should be evaluated for lice and treated. Combs, brushes, hats, clothing, bedding, and towels must be washed with hot water.

BENIGN GROWTHS

Seborrheic Keratoses

Seborrheic keratoses (Figure 45.8) are benign growths that are extremely common in adults >40 years old. They are tan, gray, or black waxy or warty papules and plaques. They often have a stuck-on appearance with follicular prominence. They can be found anywhere on the body except on mucous membranes, palms, and soles. Occasionally, some lesions are darkly pigmented, and differentiation from a melanoma can be difficult without a biopsy. These growths can be removed for cosmetic purposes with cryosurgery or shave excision if necessary.

Cherry Angiomas

Cherry angiomas are the most common acquired cutaneous vascular proliferations. They usually appear in people in their 20s and increase in number over time. They are round to oval, bright red, dome-shaped or polypoid papules ranging in size from <1 mm to several millimeters. Cherry angiomas are benign, consisting of dilated, congested capillaries and postcapillary venules. However, they can bleed when traumatized. These

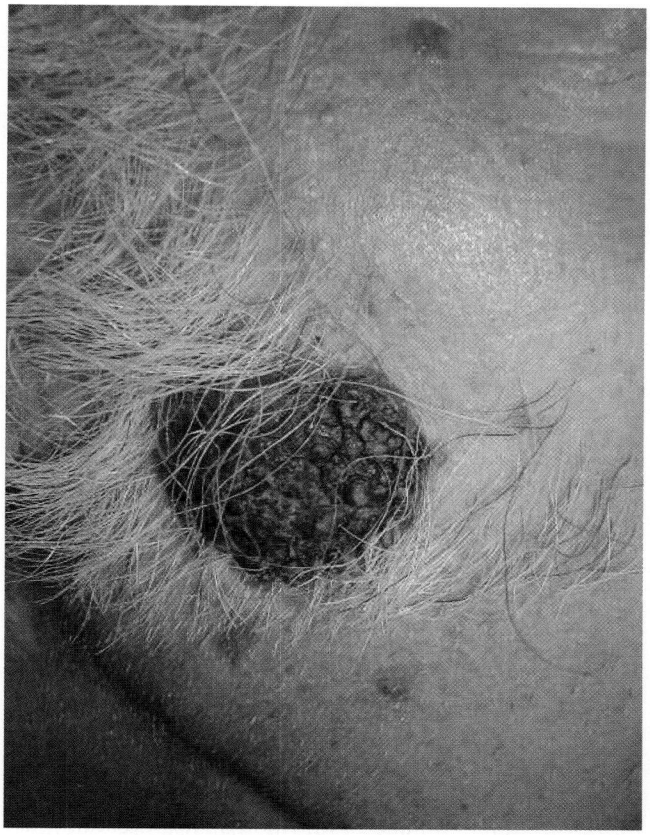

Figure 45.8—Seborrheic keratoses. These lesions present as waxy, warty stuck-on papules in a variety of colors.

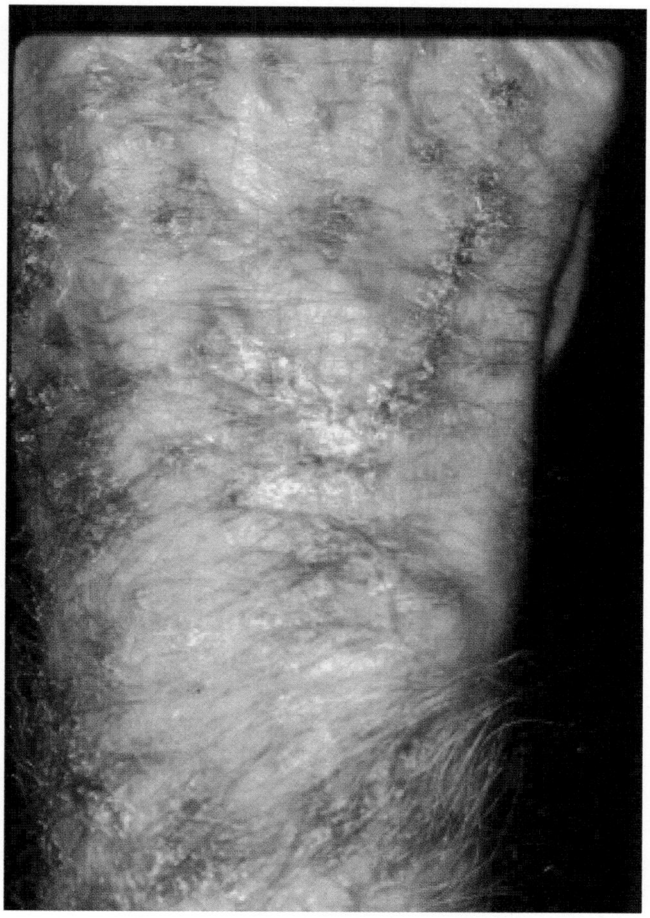

Figure 45.9—Actinic keratoses. These rough, scaly, red-brown macules on sun-exposed skin are premalignant.

lesions can be removed with excision, electrodessication, or laser ablation.

Actinic Keratoses

Actinic keratoses (Figure 45.9) are precancerous lesions caused by chronic UV radiation. They are seen in fair-skinned people and characterized by occasionally tender, rough, poorly circumscribed, erythematous papules with white or yellow scaling. They appear most often in areas with prolonged sun exposure, including the face, neck, ears, arms, and the dorsum of the hands. The scalp of alopecic men is commonly affected. Clinical variants include hypertrophic, pigmented, and lichenoid types. Some may have an overlying thick, hard, raised crust known as a *cutaneous horn*. Actinic keratosis or actinic damage of the lips is called *actinic cheilitis*.

Actinic keratoses are considered premalignant growths, precursors of squamous cell carcinoma. It is unclear how many progress to squamous cell carcinoma; reports vary from 0.24% to 20%. Actinic keratoses are treated to prevent progression to squamous cell carcinoma. They may respond to medical and surgical management. They can be easily treated in the office setting with cryotherapy (liquid nitrogen) or photodynamic therapy. Alternatively, they can respond to topical chemotherapeutic agents such as 5-fluorouracil, and immunomodulators such as imiquimod[OL]. When lesions are numerous, topical treatment with 5-fluorouracil or imiquimod is preferred over cryotherapy (SOE=B). These topical therapies are associated with a transient reaction characterized by bright erythema and discomfort.

SKIN CANCER

Basal Cell Carcinoma

Basal cell carcinoma (Figure 45.10) is the most common cancer in the United States. While the tumors may be locally invasive, the risk of metastasis is low. There are many clinical subtypes, including nodular, superficial, and pigmented (which can be confused for melanoma). The three major clinical subtypes are the following:

- nodular—the most common variant; appears as a waxy, translucent papule with overlying telangiectasias, often with central ulceration

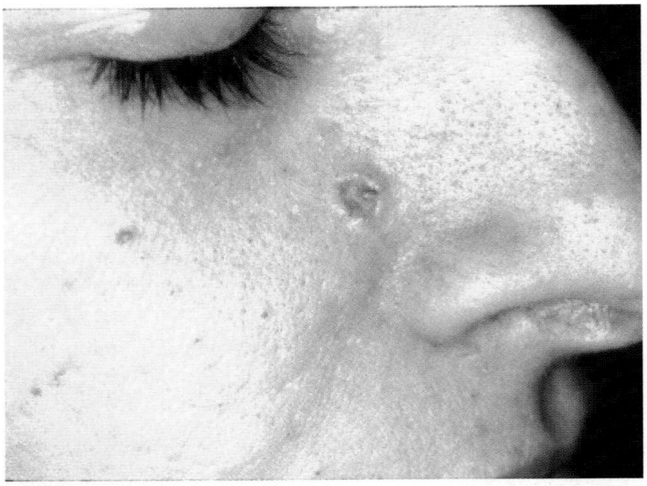

Figure 45.10—Basal cell carcinoma. This is a pearly, fleshy papule but is ulcerated in the center and has a characteristic rolled border.

- morpheaform—has a scar-like appearance and can look atrophic
- superficial—appears as an erythematous macule or papule with fine scale or superficial erosion often surrounded by telangiectasia

Risk factors for basal cell carcinoma include age, UV exposure, immunosuppression, genetic syndromes, and chemical exposures. Definitive treatment of basal cell carcinoma is surgical excision. Because of its higher cure rate, Mohs micrographic surgery is warranted for basal cell carcinomas that have indistinct borders, are >2 cm in diameter, are recurrent, or have high-risk histologic features (ie, morpheaform). An additional benefit of Mohs micrographic surgery is that it spares tissues and therefore can provide additional cosmetic benefits. Basal cell carcinomas that develop in poor surgical candidates can also be treated with ablative methods such as cryosurgery and radiation. Superficial basal cell carcinomas can be treated with less invasive techniques such as curettage with electrodessication and topical imiquimod therapy.

Squamous Cell Carcinoma

Squamous cell carcinoma is the second most common form of skin cancer. It generally presents as an occasionally tender, erythematous papule, plaque, or nodule with keratotic scale. The lesions can develop scaling and crusting. Squamous cell carcinomas are locally invasive and can cause subsequent tissue destruction. The risk of metastasis is low but higher than that of basal cell carcinomas. The risk of metastases increases with size of the tumor, high-risk histologic features (eg, poor differentiation, perineural invasion), depth of invasion, and location. Squamous cell carcinomas on the lip and ear can behave more aggressively. Squamous cell carcinomas also have a propensity to develop in longstanding, nonhealing wounds and in burn and radiation scars; these lesions are known as Marjolin's ulcers and are associated with a higher risk of metastasis.

Like other nonmelanoma skin cancers, squamous cell carcinomas are associated with cumulative sun exposure and age. They tend to be found on sites chronically exposed to the sun, such as the face, the dorsum of hands, and arms. Additional risk factors include exposure to arsenic, ionizing radiation, and immunosuppression. Definitive treatment consists of surgical excision. In anatomically sensitive areas or with high-risk tumors, Mohs micrographic surgery is indicated. If surgery is contraindicated, palliative measures with lower cure rates (such as ionizing radiation) can be used.

Melanoma

Melanomas are malignant tumors of melanocytes. They have a higher risk of metastasis than basal cell carcinomas and squamous cell carcinomas. In addition to spreading locally, they are associated with distant metastases to the skin, brain, lung, liver, and small intestine. The tumors present usually as atypical pigmented lesions. There are four clinical types:

- lentigo maligna—an irregularly shaped tan or brown macule that has been enlarging slowly; the type seen most commonly on atrophic, sun-damaged skin of older adults
- superficial spreading—an irregularly shaped macule, papule, or plaque with great variation in color (Figure 45.11) and that can occur anywhere but most commonly on the trunk or proximal extremities
- nodular—a papule or nodule, often brown, black or gray, that has been growing rapidly; can be red or amelanotic
- acral lentiginous—a dark brown or black patch found on the palms, soles, or nail beds with a pigmented streak of the cuticle known as Hutchinson sign (Figure 45.12) found in all skin types; incidence is highest in adults ≥65 years old

The incidence of melanoma continues to increase. Mortality due to melanoma has also increased but at a lower rate, in part because of earlier detection. Risk factors for melanoma include family history, fair skin type, red hair, history of dysplastic or numerous nevi, and sunlight exposure, particularly intermittent blistering sunburns in childhood.

Melanomas are usually asymptomatic. If detected early, they can be associated with a high rate of

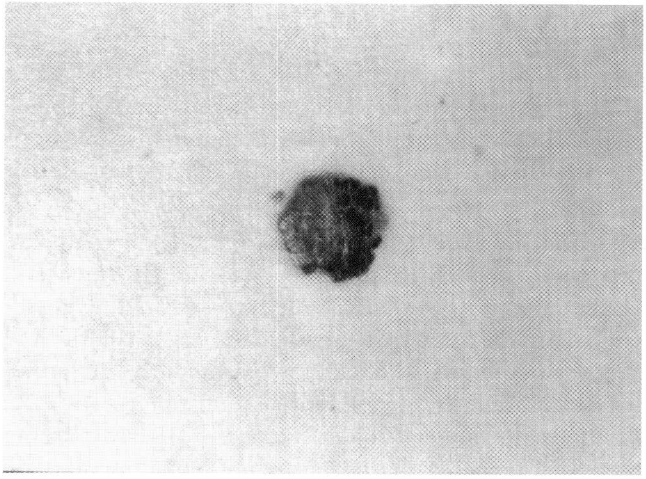

Figure 45.11—Melanoma. This lesion has irregular variegation in pigment (shades of brown and blue-black) as well as irregular borders, suggesting melanoma.

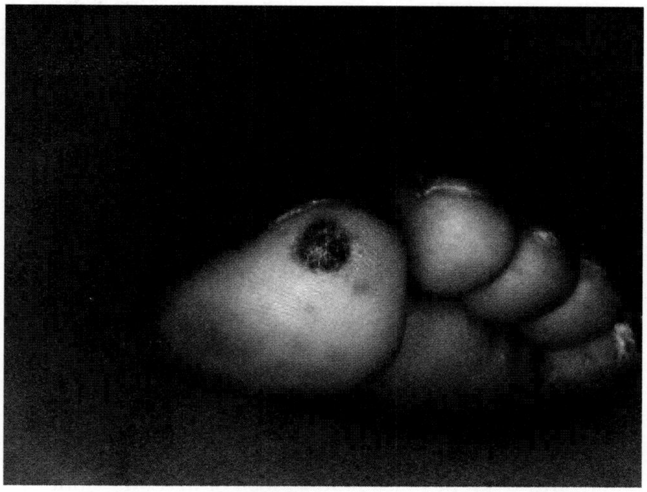

Figure 45.12—Acral lentiginous melanoma. This type of melanoma presents as a dark macular growth with irregular borders on volar surfaces of palms and soles (as in this case) and nails.

cure. Therefore, regular skin examinations and early recognition are important. A new pigmented skin lesion or a change in the color, size, surface, or borders of a preexisting mole should be biopsied. A useful mnemonic when examining skin for melanoma or atypical moles is ABCD: **a**symmetry, **b**orders, **c**olor, **d**iameter >6 mm.

Risk factors for metastases and mortality due to melanoma are depth of invasion, ulceration, and number of mitoses. Treatment is tailored to the perceived aggressiveness of the tumor. If caught early with a Breslow depth <1 mm, definitive treatment is surgical excision. If Breslow depth is ≥1 mm, standard treatment is wide excision, and sentinel node biopsy may be indicated. Adjuvant therapy such as interferon is sometimes used in cases with lymph node involvement. If there is evidence of distant metastases, treatment options include immunotherapy such as interleukin-2, pegylated interferon alpha-2b and/or chemotherapy.

Until recently, 95% of patients with stage IV melanoma died within 5 years. In 2010–2011, two breakthroughs in the treatment of metastatic melanoma have engendered tremendous excitement. The first was FDA approval of ipilimumab, a monoclonal antibody that binds to cytotoxic T lymphocyte–associated antigen 4, which functions as a negative feedback mechanism within the immune system. Ipilimumab blocks this negative feedback and allows the T cells of the immune system to attack the melanoma cells. The second breakthrough was approval of vemurafenib, a drug that can inhibit mutated BRAF protein, which has been identified in >50% of melanomas. Melanoma cells with this mutation depend on activated signaling through the mitogen-activated kinase pathway. Vemurafenib is a potent inhibitor of melanoma cells with the BRAF V600E mutation and thus inhibits the kinase pathway, subsequently blocking proliferation of the melanoma cells.

References

- Askew DA, Mickan SM, Soyer HP, et al. Effectiveness of 5-fluorouracil treatment for actinic keratosis: a systematic review of randomized controlled trials. *Int J Dermatol.* 2009;48(5):453–463.
- Cadogan MP. Herpes zoster in older adults. *J Gerontol Nurs.* 2010;36(3):10–14.
- Currie BJ, McCarthy JS. Permethrin and ivermectin for scabies. *N Engl J Med.* 2010;362(8):717–725.
- Derby R, Rohal P, Jackson C, et al. Novel treatment of onychomycosis using over-the-counter mentholated ointment: a clinical case series. *J Am Board Fam Med.* 2011;24(1):69–74.
- Garcia-Albea V, Limaye K. The clinical conundrum of pruritus. *J Dermatology Nurses Assoc.* 2012;4(2):87–105.
- Naldi L, Rebora A. Seborrheic dermatitis. *N Engl J Med.* 2009;360(4):387–396.
- Nestle FO, Kaplan DH, Barker J. Psoriasis. *N Engl J Med.* 2009;361(5):496–509.

CHAPTER 46—ORAL DISEASES AND DISORDERS

KEY POINTS

- Because teeth become less sensitive with age, it is not uncommon to observe profound yet asymptomatic untreated dental disease in older adults. This justifies the need for regular dental evaluations every 6–12 months and even more frequently if an individual's salivary flow is diminished as an adverse event of medication.
- Periodontitis caused by plaque formation within the gingival sulcus (that should be controlled with regular oral hygiene) can lead to loss of alveolar bone height, decreased support around the tooth, malposition, loosening, and eventual loss of the tooth. There is a growing body of evidence that bacteremia and circulating inflammatory factors due to periodontal infection are cofactors in multiple serious cardiovascular diseases.
- Dentures usually aid in speech and restore diminished facial contours, but improved ability to masticate is unpredictable and improved oral intake is a less likely outcome. Dental implants diminish patient's insecurity with their prosthetics but do not enhance eating ability or improve patients' dietary quality.
- Oral cancer screening can detect oral cancer early, potentially translating into improved outcomes and better survival rates.
- Antibiotic prophylactic coverage before invasive dental procedures to avoid infective bacterial endocarditis or infection of implanted prostheses (eg, prosthetic joints) is indicated only for specific high-risk situations. Patients at increased risk of these orally seeded infections should be counseled to maintain excellent oral hygiene to minimize incidence and severity of orally seeded bacteremia.
- Pulmonary pathogens responsible for institution-acquired pneumonia have been repeatedly documented as colonizing dental plaque on teeth and on pharyngeal mucosa. Daily oral hygiene in institutional health settings, such as hospitals (especially intensive care units) and nursing homes, is therefore an essential preventive measure that should be taught to direct care staff and its daily practice, whether by the patient or provided or assisted by staff, monitored as part of infection control.
- Osteonecrosis of the jaw has been reported in up to 5% of patients who have received extended intravenous treatment with bisphosphonates for management of bony metastases. This complication does not seem to affect those receiving bisphosphonates for osteoporosis to a greater extent than those not receiving bisphosphonates.

The oral cavity is involved in initiating food intake, producing speech, and protecting the GI tract and upper airway. Dysfunction and disease in the mouth can therefore profoundly affect overall health and social functioning and can be particularly important for older adults who are frail or nutritionally at risk. Findings prevalent in older adults (eg, decay, missing teeth, periodontal disease, salivary hypofunction) do not represent normal aging, and individuals with such conditions should be urged, and assisted in their efforts, to obtain preventive and therapeutic care.

AGING OF THE TEETH

Most age-related changes in teeth are subtle (Table 46.1) but become significant in the presence of environmental factors or disease. For a combination of reasons, the teeth of older adults are typically less sensitive or wholly insensitive to temperature changes and, importantly, to the sensations that commonly herald dental disease in younger adults. It is not uncommon to observe profound yet asymptomatic untreated dental disease in older adults.

DENTAL DECAY

Dental *caries*, or decay, is a bacterially caused demineralization and cavitation that can attack teeth throughout life. *Recurrent caries* refers to decay at the interface between a dental restoration (such as a filling or crown) and the tooth. For the anatomy of the tooth, see Figure 46.1. Older adults have more restored teeth (and usually the restorations are older and more extensive) and thus are more likely to have recurrent

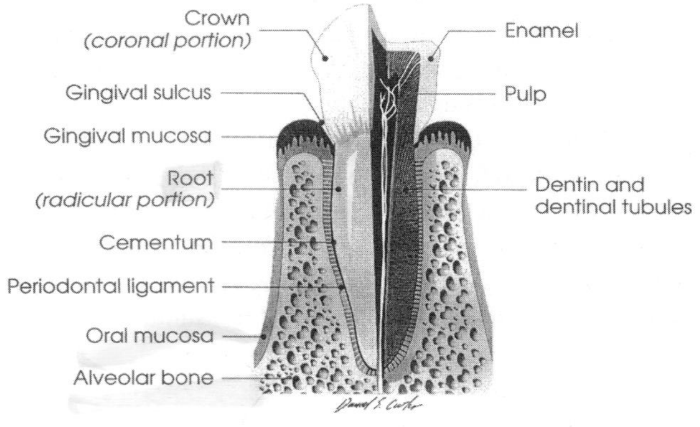

Figure 46.1—Dental and periodontal anatomy

Table 46.1—Clinical Significance of Selected Age-Related Changes in Oral Tissues

Tissue Affected	Nature of Change	Clinical Significance
Tooth dentin	Increased thickness	Diminished pulp space
	Diminished permeability resulting from sclerosis of dentinal tubules	Diminished sensitivity of dentin; diminished susceptibility to effects of bacterial metabolites; increased tooth brittleness
Dental pulp	Diminished volume	Diminished reparative capacity; diminished sensitivity and change in nature of sensitivity
	Shift in proportion of nervous, vascular, and connective tissues	Diminished reparative capacity; diminished sensitivity and change in nature of sensitivity
Salivary glands	Fatty replacement of acini	Possibly less physiologic reserve

caries. The teeth of older adults can have more caries of the root surfaces than are typically seen in younger adults because prior periodontal disease exposes the root surface, thereby predisposing it to demineralization and an increased risk of decay. Both recurrent and root caries are generally asymptomatic and can become advanced before discovery, often resulting in destruction of much or all of the tooth.

Untreated, advanced caries commonly results in necrosis of the remaining pulp, which usually leads to an acute or chronic dental abscess. These infections may not present with pain but they should not be ignored, because severe metastatic infections of dental and oral origin have been reported in virtually every organ system. In particular, α-hemolytic (viridans) streptococci of the oral cavity have long been implicated in close to one-third of the cases of bacterial endocarditis reported annually in the United States, and bacteria associated with dental abscesses (eg, *Staphylococcus aureus)* have been cultured from aspirates of infected hip arthroplasties.

The risk factors for dental caries are the same at any age, but many of the risk factors increase in prevalence with age. A primary risk factor is poor oral hygiene, which often occurs in older adults when visual acuity, manual dexterity, or arm flexibility is impaired, or when salivary flow is diminished. Another risk factor is frequent ingestion of sticky foods with a high content of sucrose, such as cake, candy, and cookies. Other risk factors include infrequent dental visits because of financial, access, or educational barriers; the presence of permanent or removable artificial teeth (more common with increasing age); and limited lifetime exposure to fluoride, widely used in the United States only in the past 50 years. White older Americans have a higher incidence of root caries than either black or Hispanic older Americans, but they are more likely to have received dental treatment for the lesions. Recurrent caries are also more common in white older Americans because of the greater likelihood that they have received prior dental treatment.

The prevention of caries involves daily oral hygiene with fluoride toothpaste, limitation of sugar intake, and regular dental examinations. The treatment of dental caries includes topical high-potency fluoride for remineralization, removal of demineralized tooth structure ("drilling"), and replacement of removed tooth structure with fillings or crowns. When caries involves the dental pulp, root canal treatment or tooth extraction becomes necessary.

Diseases of the Periodontium

The investing tissues of the teeth, termed the *periodontium*, consist of the gingiva, the alveolar bone, and a collagenous sleeve (termed the *periodontal ligament*) located between the tooth root and the surrounding bone. Periodontal disease occurs when microorganic colonies (*plaque*) form on the teeth near the gingiva and between the gingiva and the root surface within the gingival sulcus. The most common form of periodontal disease is gingivitis, in which the inflammatory reaction to plaque is limited to the gingiva. Gingivitis develops more rapidly in older adults than in younger ones, but in both groups the changes—including gingival edema and light bleeding on brushing—rapidly resolve after plaque removal. If the inflammatory process extends to the periodontal ligament and alveolar bone, the process is termed *periodontitis*. In periodontitis, there is destruction of the hard and soft tissues of the periodontium due to immune-regulated osteolytic and proteolytic host defenses. In most adults, the process of periodontitis is marked by long periods of disease quiescence punctuated by bursts of localized destructive inflammation. The prevalence of active periodontitis is 20%–40% of dentate adults. By their 50s, more than 90% of Americans with teeth show ≥2 mm of lost alveolar bone height, the primary marker of prior periodontal disease activity. In advanced cases of periodontitis, the decreased support around a tooth leads to its malposition, loosening, and eventual loss.

Epidemiologic data and clinical observation support the concept that those who reach advanced age without significant periodontal bone loss will not likely experience a worsening of the disease in senescence. In contrast, other adults who have experienced a more rapid rate of bone loss commonly will have lost teeth in their 40s and 50s. In addition to age, risk factors for periodontitis include smoking and poor oral hygiene. Black and Hispanic Americans have a significantly higher prevalence of advanced periodontitis than white Americans. Preventing gingivitis and periodontitis is largely a matter of oral hygiene and regular dental examinations and cleanings. Managing periodontal disease involves debriding the roots below the gingiva, which may require surgical access. Adjunctive therapy with topical antibiotics such as chlorhexidine oral rinse (SOE=B) or systemic antibiotics such as minocycline (SOE=B) or metronidazole (SOE=C) can also be useful in periodontal therapy.

Periodontitis has long been reported to be worse in patients with poorly controlled diabetes mellitus. Investigations also support the contention that periodontitis, as a cause of chronic inflammation, impedes effective diabetes control. Periodontal disease can be rapidly destructive in a patient whose immune system is impaired by disease or immunosuppressive therapy. Epidemiologic data also correlate osteoporosis and tooth loss due to periodontitis. Periodontal disease and the pathogens responsible for it have been linked epidemiologically and immunologically with coronary artery disease, peripheral vascular disease, cerebrovascular disease, and pneumonia. There is also epidemiologic association between gram-negative pneumonia, gram-negative periodontal pathogens, salivary hypofunction, and impaired swallowing (SOE=C). Numerous reports in the dental, infectious disease, and critical care literature demonstrate increasing prevalence of pulmonary pathogens from dental and oral plaque with increasing length of stay (SOE=B). Several studies have demonstrated significantly reduced incidence of institution-acquired pneumonia, reduced mortality, and reduced length of hospital stay in patients on ventilators (SOE=B) and those in nursing homes (SOE=C) when a program of daily oral hygiene is instituted.

The prevention and control of periodontal disease revolve around daily oral care, ie, tooth brushing and flossing to remove bacterial plaque on the teeth, particularly within the gingival sulcus. Properly used, electronic toothbrushes can facilitate oral hygiene for people with impaired manual dexterity and make plaque removal by caregivers easier and more effective as well. Regular dental evaluation, every 6–12 months, is important to ensure that the periodontium is healthy or to provide early intervention if it is not.

TOOTHLESSNESS

Advanced age was once considered synonymous with the need for false teeth, but that stereotype is fading. In the early 1960s, more than 70% of adult Americans ≥75 years old were edentulous. By the 1990s, fewer than 40% of this group were edentulous, most likely because of some level of preventive and restorative dental care in childhood or early adulthood.

Nevertheless, removal of one or more teeth in an older adult may be necessitated by various combinations of physiologic and behavioral factors. The leading cause is inability or unwillingness to access and pay for restorative dental treatment in the face of a symptomatic dental disease, usually stemming from dental caries. A second common cause is loosening of teeth as a consequence of periodontal disease, to the point that mastication becomes painful or ineffective. A third common cause is removal of otherwise healthy teeth that, because of the absence or loss of other teeth for the preceding or other reasons, would hinder the fabrication or function of a dental prosthesis to replace missing teeth.

Nearly 50% of Americans ≥85 years old have no natural teeth. There are unique problems associated with the edentulous state. Functionally, the teeth aid in mastication and enunciation. Aesthetically, the teeth support the lips and cheeks and keep the nose and chin a fixed distance apart. When a person has lost all teeth and there are no prosthetic replacements, the facial appearance is dramatically changed because of the lack of tissue support and the diminished vertical height of the lower half of the face. Chewing ability is severely compromised, yet the impact on nutritional intake is difficult to characterize. Several longitudinal studies have demonstrated correlation between loss of teeth and increased intake of carbohydrates, and decreased intake of protein and selected micronutrients.

Removable dentures can aid in speech and restore diminished facial contours, but they are less predictably successful in restoring the ability to masticate. Edentulous people with dentures can generally eat a wider range of foods than edentulous people without dentures. Yet dentures restore, on average, only about 15% of the chewing ability of the natural dentition. The range of foods regularly eaten by denture wearers is significantly restricted in comparison with the dietary range of people with natural teeth. Denture wearers also have to chew more times before they swallow food, and they swallow their food in larger particles. Older patients and their clinicians who hope that dentures will restore oral intake in cases of malnutrition or unexplained weight loss are usually disappointed, whereas those who hope for a more socially acceptable appearance, clearer speech, and modest improvement in chewing comfort and range of dietary choices are more likely to be satisfied.

Dentures often are a considerable source of discomfort, dysfunction, and embarrassment for older adults. This is because the alveolar processes that originally held the natural teeth continually remodel and diminish in volume once the natural teeth are gone. For most patients, dentures require frequent professional adjustment and periodic replacement. Alveolar ridge resorption is most severe in the oldest patients who have had the longest time without natural teeth; this effect is more pronounced in those with osteoporosis.

For health of the oral mucosa, dentures should be kept clean by removing them and cleaning them after meals and by soaking them in a commercial disinfectant several times each week. Dentures should remain out of the mouth for several hours each day; most people choose to leave their dentures out during sleep. Fractured or broken dentures, as well as denture looseness or soreness, should be brought to a dentist's attention without delay. However, because neither dental services nor dentures are currently covered by Medicare and <10% of older Americans have private dental insurance, many older adults continue to use inadequate or even damaging dentures.

For the past 30 years, the dental profession has refined the placement and restoration of a variety of implanted devices that integrate with bone of the jaws and can more effectively anchor oral prostheses. Dentures that are retained in this manner are preferred by patients in comparison with mucosal-borne prostheses, but studies have not demonstrated enhanced chewing ability or significant improvements in dietary intake or quality. Rehabilitation with implants costs from 3 to 20 times as much as traditional dentures and is therefore financially out of reach for many patients.

SALIVARY FUNCTION IN AGING

Saliva is critical for protecting the tissues of the oral cavity and maintaining their function in speech, mastication, swallowing, and taste perception. Saliva buffers the intraoral pH, contains a wide spectrum of antimicrobial factors, remineralizes and lubricates the oral surfaces, and keeps the taste pores patent. In the absence of disease, the major salivary glands undergo regressive histologic changes with age. Yet data from the Baltimore Longitudinal Study on Aging and the Veterans Affairs Dental Longitudinal Study have demonstrated that with healthy aging, flow from the parotid glands under both resting and stimulated conditions remains essentially unchanged. In both studies, flow from the submandibular glands did not change with age; in data from other centers, there has been a measurable but clinically minor decrease. It has been suggested that the major salivary glands demonstrate "organ reserve," in which the capacity of youthful glands exceeds ordinary demands, but that with age-related changes, functional reserves dwindle. By extreme old age, healthy glands function adequately under normal conditions but are more susceptible to factors that impede function, such as dehydration or drug-induced hypofunction.

Complaints of dry mouth are very common among older adults. The leading causes are medications that have this as an adverse event. Commonly implicated are medications with anticholinergic effects, including tricyclic antidepressants, opioids, antihistamines, antihypertensives (including diuretics, ACE inhibitors, calcium channel blockers, and both α- and β-blockers), and antiarrhythmic agents. Separate studies have found that 72% of institutionalized older adults received at least one (and some as many as five) potentially xerostomic medications daily and that 55% of >4,000 rural community-dwelling older adults took at least one potentially xerostomic medication daily. Dry mouth can also be due to local disease, such as salivary gland tumors and blocked ducts, or to systemic disease. Sjögren syndrome affects approximately 3 million Americans, predominantly women, ≥50 years old. Cevimeline (30 mg q8h), a cholinergic agent, is approved for dry mouth in patients with Sjögren syndrome. Depression has been reported to diminish saliva flow, as have poorly controlled diabetes mellitus and hypothyroidism.

Dry mouth is also an adverse consequence of therapeutic irradiation of the head and neck. In the total dosage range administered for oral and oropharyngeal squamous cell carcinoma, salivary flow is commonly obliterated as a consequence of short-term direct effects on the glands and long-term fibrosis of their vascular supply. As a result, patients who have undergone radiation of the head can experience rapidly destructive dental caries and painful oral mucositis, which can affect nutritional status.

Treatment of older adults with dry mouth requires attention to both diagnosis and prevention. Diminished oral secretions increase the risk of serious oral disease. Medications that reduce salivary flow should be decreased, discontinued, or substituted for, if possible. Systemic causes, as well as a history of irradiation of the head and neck, should be excluded. Patients who have had irradiation should be considered for a 3-month course of oral pilocarpine (5–10 mg q8h), which may restore some salivary function. Saliva substitutes and oral lubricants, available without prescription and used as needed, can provide transient relief but replenish none of the protective properties of saliva. Patients should be counseled on the greatly increased risk of oral disease and educated on the need to limit dietary sugar, optimize daily oral hygiene practices, and have more frequent dental examinations.

COMMON ORAL LESIONS

Squamous cell carcinoma accounts for 96% of oral and oropharyngeal malignancies. Of the 28,000 new cases of

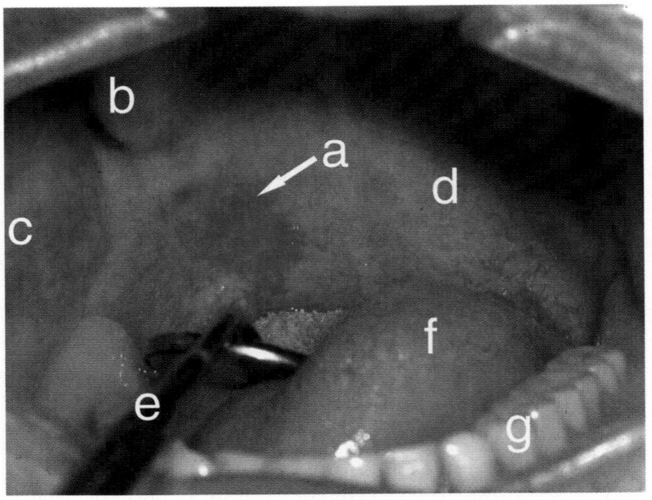

Figure 46.2—Erythroplakia in a 72-year-old man with a history of cigar smoking and alcohol abuse. Lesion confirmed by biopsy to be invasive squamous cell carcinoma, poorly differentiated.

Key: a = erythroplakia; b = right posterior maxillary alveolar ridge; c = inner aspect of right cheek; d = soft palate; e = tongue retractor; f = tongue dorsum; g = mandibular denture

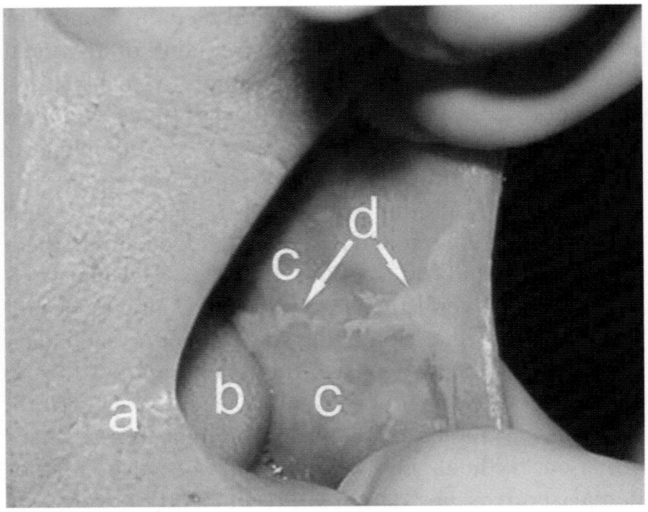

Figure 46.3—Leukoplakia in a 66-year-old man with a history of smoking. Lesion confirmed by biopsy to be carcinoma in situ.

Key: a = right lip commissure; b = tongue; c = inner aspect of left cheek; d = leukoplakia

oral cancer reported in the United States annually, ≥95% occur in people ≥40 years old; age is the primary risk factor identified in epidemiologic analyses. The 5-year survival rate for white Americans is approximately 55% and for black Americans, 34%. Carcinoma of the lip, tongue, and floor of the mouth represents >65% of all oropharyngeal cases. Lip cancer affects men eight times more frequently than women; most other sites affect men at a ratio slightly below 2:1. Oral cancer is strongly linked with the use of tobacco, particularly cigarettes (SOE=A). Lip cancer is strongly correlated with pipe and cigar smoking (SOE=A). Alcohol is a potent cofactor that enhances the effects of tobacco. Other potential risk factors—dentures, poor oral care, oral viral disease (particularly human papilloma virus), oral lichen planus, and candidiasis—have been suggested, but none has shown the unambiguous associations of age, smoking, and alcohol use.

Oral malignancies appear clinically as painless red, white, or mixed red and white areas of the oral mucosa that may be ulcerated or indurated. Red and mixed lesions (termed *erythroplakia*) (Figure 46.2) display cellular atypia in as many as 93% of cases and should be biopsied immediately. White lesions (*leukoplakia*) (Figure 46.3) are malignant or premalignant <10% of the time and merit close monitoring; biopsy is indicated if a lesion does not resolve in 14 days or is increasing in size. Less invasive diagnostic tools can be used for determining whether a white or red lesion in the mouth merits biopsy, such as scraping (exfoliative cytology) and in situ staining. Early identification markedly improves outcome: 5-year survival without nodal involvement in white Americans is 80% and in black Americans is 69%, but survival rates decline with nodal involvement (41% and 30%, respectively) and with distant metastases (18% and 12%). A thorough oral cancer screening, which can be completed in <2 minutes, consists of a head and neck nodal assessment followed by inspection of the oral cavity using gauze to retract the tongue and tongue blades to enhance visualization of the cheeks, lips, and vestibules. Although oral cancer screening is easy to learn, straightforward to perform, requires minimal instrumentation, and causes no discomfort to the patient, few older smokers receive oral evaluations as part of the routine physical examination.

The treatment of localized oral squamous cell carcinoma is generally surgical, although large but localized tumors can be managed with radioactive implants. More extensive disease necessitates surgery followed by beam irradiation. Concern over the deleterious adverse effects of irradiation (described in the preceding section) has led to the development of techniques that seek to limit destruction of healthy tissues surrounding a tumor. Radiation alone has been used to shrink inoperable tumors. Newer protocols combine surgery and chemotherapy with the goal of a cure.

Certainly not every oral lesion is malignant, but because most clinicians have not been trained to distinguish among different oral lesions or even normal oral anatomic structures, a brief overview is provided. Exostoses can form on either or both sides of the palatal suture at the crest of the roof of the mouth in about 20% of the population. Termed "torus" (plural

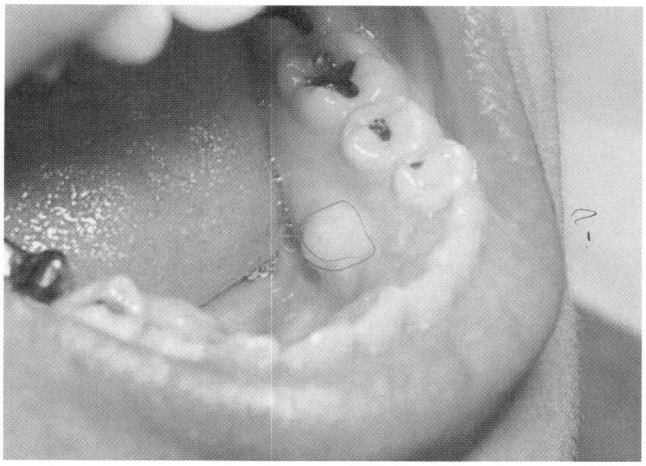

Figure 46.4—Mandibular torus

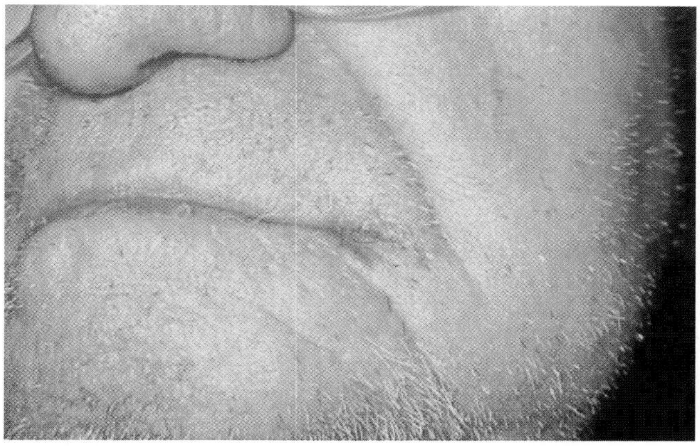

Figure 46.5—Angular cheilitis

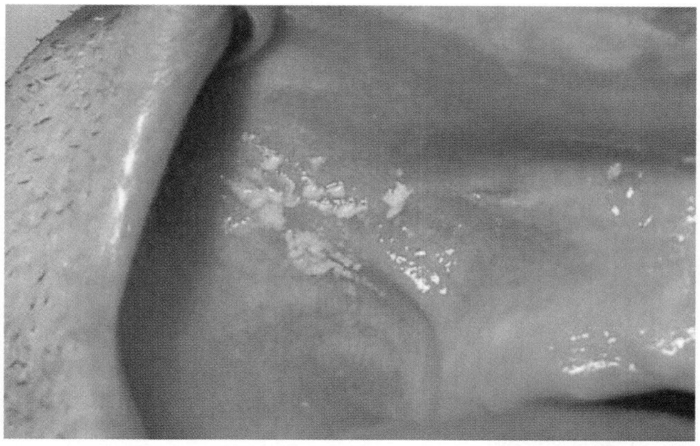

Figure 46.6—Thrush

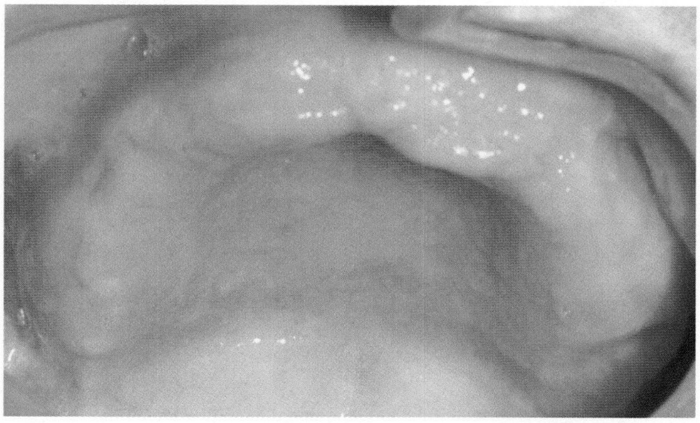

Figure 46.7—Denture stomatitis due to a maxillary complete (ie, replacing all the teeth of the upper jaw) denture

"tori"), these also are commonly found on the medial aspects of the mandible as well (Figure 46.4). Tori can grow slowly throughout adulthood and sometimes reach dimensions that can predispose to trauma from food and impede swallowing.

The parotid ducts enter the mouth under small flaps of tissue termed Stenson's papillae, which are located lateral to the maxillary second molars. These can be distinguished from pathologic polypoid structures by applying gentle pressure to the preauricular area—saliva will be excreted only if the structure is Stenson's papilla.

The dorsum of the tongue in some individuals displays irregular patterns of hyperkeratotic and denuded reddened areas lacking lingual papillae. This presentation is variously termed geographic tongue (because the pattern looks map-like) and migratory glossitis (because the patterns change over time) and is no basis for concern.

Candidiasis presents as diffusely erythematous mucositis, cracking at the corners of the mouth (angular cheilitis [Figure 46.5]), curd-like white patches (thrush [Figure 46.6]), or erythema in denture-bearing areas (denture stomatitis [Figure 46.7]); it can be wholly asymptomatic or result in taste dysfunction, burning, itching, and pain. Older adults are particularly susceptible to candidiasis because of denture use, salivary hypofunction, the prevalence of diabetes mellitus, and the use of antibiotics for pulmonary and urologic diseases. Use of inhaled corticosteroids places oropharyngeal structures in the path of the spray, increasing their risk of localized candidal colonization. Management of candidiasis involves first excluding any immunopathologic cause for the disease, followed by administering topical or systemic antifungal agents and optimizing oral and denture hygiene.

Herpes simplex is a virus that resides preferentially in the trigeminal ganglion and periodically causes intraoral outbreaks. These outbreaks are limited to the hyperkeratotic areas of the palate (Figure 46.8), the gingiva, and the extraoral aspects of the lips. They begin as clusters of small, circular, red-rimmed yellowish blisters that burst and coalesce into irregular denuded lesions. They are highly contagious until healed. Herpes can be readily distinguished from another episodic, painful oral outbreak, aphthous ulcer (Figure 46.9), in that the latter tend to appear as

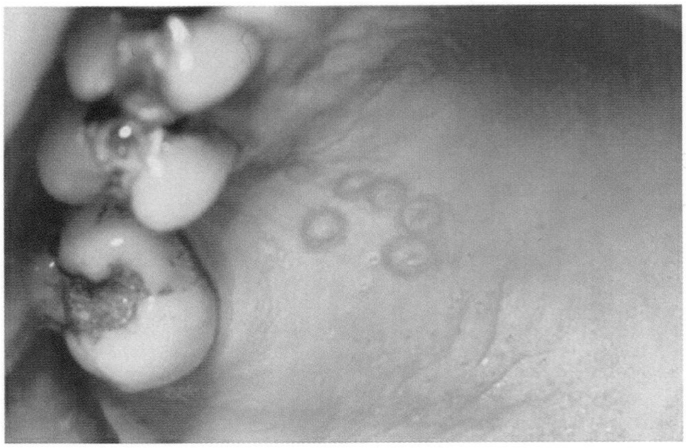

Figure 46.8—Early lesions of herpes simplex, right palate

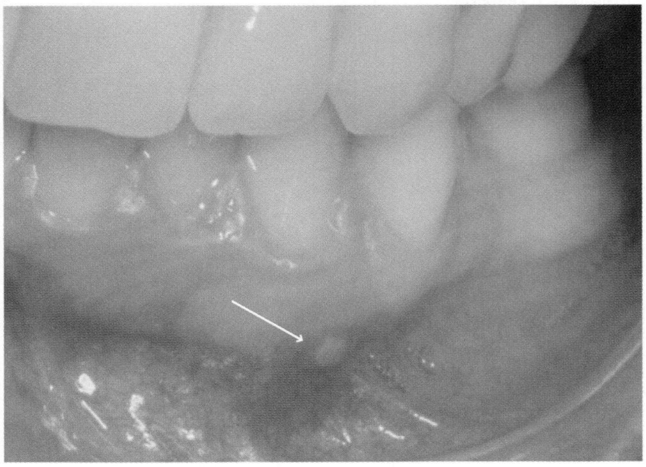

Figure 46.9—Aphthous ulcer

isolated lesions and form only on the parakeratinized tissues of the mouth (ie, inner aspects of the cheeks and lips, floor of the mouth, and lateral border of the tongue). Aphthous ulcerations are not known to be contagious.

An idiopathic disruption of the desquamation of tongue filiform papillae (normally about 1 mm long), which seems to become more prevalent with advancing age, results in elongation of the papillae (to ≥3 mm) and the appearance of a "hairy tongue." This condition is prone to staining from a variety of foods (eg, tea, coffee), from tobacco use, and from medications (eg, bismuth). "Hairy tongue" can also serve as a substrate for bacterial and/or fungal growth. Any of these, all of which are exacerbated by salivary hypofunction, can confer on the tongue notable colorations (eg, "black hairy tongue" [Figure 46.10]), but none is associated with symptoms.

Burning mouth syndrome is a chronic orofacial pain disorder usually without other clinical signs. It typically affects women ≥50 years old, particularly in Asian Americans and Native Americans. The pain most

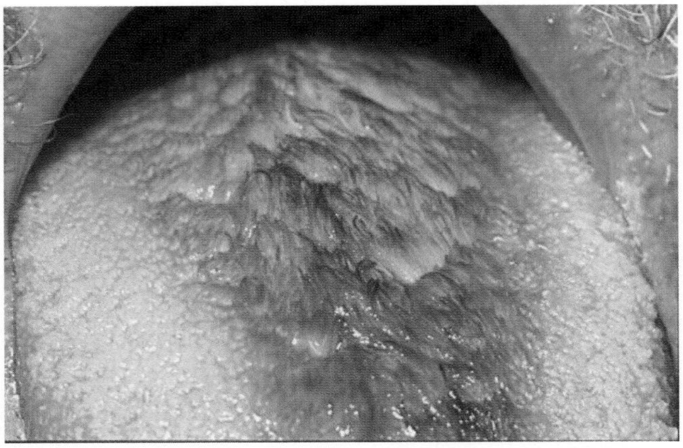

Figure 46.10—Black hairy tongue

commonly affects the lips, tongue, and palate. Multiple causes have been suggested, including xerostomia, denture use, candidiasis, nutritional deficiencies, and psychiatric disorders. Treatment is symptomatic and empirical.

CHEMOSENSORY PERCEPTION

Olfactory function declines with age. A decreased ability to identify odors and to rank their intensities affects both older men (to the greater extent) and women. Several medications have been implicated in olfactory dysfunction, as has Alzheimer disease, among other disorders common among older adults. Impaired olfaction in older adults has been anecdotally implicated as a risk factor for eating spoiled food or failing to notice gas leaks or domestic fires.

Taste perception changes with aging. The subjective perception of saltiness and sweetness blunts with advancing age. This change potentially has clinical significance, possibly playing a role in a person's tendency to oversalt foods or crave sweets.

Complaints of taste and smell dysfunction are common among older adults. Often the complaint derives from medication use, but other causes are possible (Table 46.2 and Table 46.3). Some medications may have no primary effect on taste but reduce saliva flow and lead to impaired taste perception. The sense of "taste" can actually be more accurately termed "flavor," ie, the full range of sensations that accompany eating, including temperature, texture, sound, and smell in addition to the perception of sweet, salt, sour, and bitter. Older adults are prone to impaired flavor perception because of changes in olfaction and oral stereognosis, salivary hypofunction, and the presence of dentures, which present physical and thermal barriers. Flavor enhancement strategies have had positive effects on both food preference and caloric intake among frail older adults.

Table 46.2—Medications That Interfere With Gustation (Taste) and Olfaction (Smell)

	Gustation[a]	
Acyclovir	Enalapril	Pentoxifylline
Allopurinol	Ethacrynic acid	Phenytoin
Amiloride	Ethambutol	Procainamide
Amitriptyline	Fenoprofen	Prochlorperazine
Amphotericin B	Gemfibrozil	Promethazine
Ampicillin	Hydrochlorothiazide	Propafenone
Baclofen	Imipramine	Propranolol
Buspirone	Labetalol	Ritonavir
Captopril	Levamisole	Saquinavir
Chlorpheniramine	Lomefloxacin	Sulfamethoxazole
Desipramine	Mexiletine	Sulindac
Dexamethasone	Nabumetone	Terfenadine
Diclofenac	Nelfinavir	Tetracyclines
Dicyclomine	Nifedipine	Trifluoperazine
Diltiazem	Ofloxacin	Zidovudine
Doxepin	Pentamidine	
	Olfaction[b]	
Amitriptyline	Dexamethasone	Morphine
Amphetamine	Enalapril	Pentamidine
Beclomethasone dipropionate	Flunisolide	Pirbuterol
	Flurbiprofen	Propafenone
Cocaine	Hydromorphone	Tocainide
Codeine	Levamisole	Zalcitabine

[a] Gustation: source lists >250 agents reported to disturb the sense of taste; agents listed are limited to those for which taste disturbance was determined objectively through threshold or intensity scaling or both, using one or more standardized solutions.

[b] Olfaction: source lists >40 agents reported to disturb the sense of smell; agents listed are limited to those for which olfactory disturbance was determined objectively through experiment or clinical trial.

SOURCE: Data from Schiffman SS, Zervakis J. Taste and smell perception in the elderly: effect of medications and disease. *Adv Food Nutr Res.* 2002;44:247–346.

Table 46.3—Nonpharmacologic Causes of Taste and Smell Dysfunction in Older Adults

Gustatory dysfunction

Oral causes:

Burning mouth syndrome
Candidiasis
Laceration
Malignancy
Salivary hypofunction
Therapeutic irradiation of head
Thermal or chemical burn

Other causes:

Alzheimer disease, other neurodegenerative disorders
CNS tumor
Endocrinopathies (eg, diabetes mellitus, Cushing syndrome, adrenocortical insufficiency, hypothyroidism)
Head trauma
Nutritional deficiencies (vitamin B_{12}, zinc)
Psychiatric disorders
Stroke

Olfactory dysfunction

Upper aerodigestive and respiratory causes:

Dental infection
Periodontal disease
Poor oral hygiene, including poor denture hygiene
Sinusitis
Tobacco smoking or use of nasal snuff
Tumor of airway or sinus
Upper respiratory infection (bacterial or viral)

Other causes:

Alzheimer disease, other neurodegenerative disorders
CNS tumor
Exposure to volatile or particulate toxins
Head trauma
Nutritional deficiencies (niacin, zinc)
Psychiatric disorders
Stroke

COMMON MEDICAL CONSIDERATIONS IN DENTAL TREATMENT OF OLDER ADULTS

The mouth contains about 10^{11}–10^{13} microorganisms, and the rich vascular supply beneath the relatively delicate mucosal covering predisposes to episodes of orally seeded bacteremia. Approximately one-third of the reported cases of infective endocarditis are caused by organisms normally found only in the mouth. Case reports of prosthetic implants infected by organisms originating in infected oral tissues have for years compelled clinicians to administer antibiotics prophylactically before invasive dental care for patients with such history. However, the recommendations from the American Heart Association in 2007 reflect that tooth brushing and eating in the presence of gingival inflammation are recognized to present, over time, as much as or a greater source of bacteremia than dental care, and that there is growing concern that widespread, short-term antibiotic treatment promotes the emergence of drug-resistant strains of microorganisms. Prophylactic coverage is now recommended only in specific high-risk situations. While those recommendations are directed at preventing infective endocarditis, bacteremia-induced infections of prosthetic implants (such as joint arthroplasties, stents, vascular patches, and shunts) are less common than endocarditis, and the link between their occurrence and dental disease far more tenuous. As such, the case for antibiotic coverage in such situations is also less robust and should be the exception rather than the rule.

Correlation between length of stay in nursing homes, hospitals, and intensive care units, and colonization of dental and oral mucosal plaque with known pulmonary pathogens (SOE=B), is compelling justification for ensuring daily oral care is a required nursing task. Direct care staff should receive training, and the daily practice of such care carefully monitored as a component of infection control (SOE=B).

Because of the rich vascular supply of the head and neck, invasive dental treatment of a patient on anticoagulants presents particular risk of prolonged bleeding. Generally, if the INR is ≤3.5, the risk of uncontrolled oral hemorrhage is minimal and outweighed by the protective effects of anticoagulation (SOE=B).

The risk of precipitating a hypertensive episode or an ischemic cardiac event in a susceptible patient due to accidental intravascular injection of epinephrine as a part of dental care is quite remote and should not in general be of concern. The common forms of injectable local anesthetic solutions used by dentists do contain some vasoconstricting agent to prolong the anesthetic effect. In general, the amount of endogenous epinephrine that might be secreted in response to pain induced by dental treatment (due to inadequate anesthesia) is likely far greater than would be introduced by dental personnel.

REFERENCES

- Jensen SB, Pedersen AM, Vissink A, et al. A systematic review of salivary gland hypofunction and xerostomia induced by cancer therapies: management strategies and economic impact. *Support Care Cancer*. 2010;18(8):1061–1079.
- Silverman SL, Landesberg R. Osteonecrosis of the jaw and the role of bisphosphonates: a critical review. *Am J Med*. 2009;122(2 Suppl):S33–S45.
- Weening-Verbree L, Huismand-de Waal G, van Dusseldorp L, et al. Oral health care in older people in long term care facilities: A systematic review of implementation strategies. *Int J Nurs Stud*. 2013;50(4):569–582.

CHAPTER 47—RESPIRATORY DISEASES AND DISORDERS

KEY POINTS

- With age, forced vital capacity (FVC), forced expiratory volume in 1 second (FEV_1), and Pao_2 all decrease, while the A-a gradient increases.
- Clinically significant dyspnea is often under-reported and unrecognized in older adults.
- 5%–10% of people ≥65 years old meet the criteria for asthma.
- COPD is the fourth leading cause of death in older adults. Pharmacologic treatment of COPD chiefly consists of inhaled bronchodilators and steroids.
- Smoking cessation will slow the decline in lung function at any age.

AGE-RELATED PULMONARY CHANGES

Studies of age-specific changes in pulmonary function are limited by common, important comorbidities experienced by older adults, which include smoking-related diseases, occupational and industrial exposures, and other significant organ dysfunction such as heart failure or deconditioning. These limitations notwithstanding, decrements in various aspects of pulmonary function occur with aging.

Because of changes in connective tissue, the size of the airways is reduced and the alveolar sacs become shallow. Chest wall compliance is reduced as a consequence of kyphoscoliosis, calcification of the costal cartilage, and arthritic changes in the costovertebral joints. Sarcopenia results in intercostal muscle atrophy, and diaphragmatic strength is reduced by 25%. These processes result in a decline of FVC and FEV_1 of 25–30 mL/year in nonsmokers and approximately double that (60–70 mL/year) in smokers ≥65 years old. The normal alveolar-arterial gradient (A-a gradient) increases with age and can be approximated by the following formula: (age/4) + 4 (in mmHg). The Pao_2 decreases with age and can be approximated by the following equation: $Pao_2 = 110 - (0.4 \times \text{age})$.

COMMON RESPIRATORY SYMPTOMS AND COMPLAINTS

There is a common misperception that older adults tend to overestimate or exaggerate respiratory symptoms; however, the opposite is more often true. For example, many older adults and their clinicians tend to underestimate the importance of dyspnea, which may go undiagnosed until disease is advanced. This is partly because dyspnea is blamed on deconditioning and age. Older adults often adjust their activity level to compensate for the often insidious decline in lung function and resultant disabling dyspnea. Such changes in lifestyle often go unnoticed by family, the clinician, and even the patient. Pulmonary or cardiac disorders, or both, may underlie such modifications in lifestyle, and testing (eg, pulmonary function tests, chest radiography, or cardiac echocardiography) can reveal major abnormalities such as asthma, emphysema, or pulmonary fibrosis. Another complicating feature of symptom recognition is that older adults often have more than one explanation for their problems. A patient may have overlapping symptoms of dyspnea, cough, and wheezing because of a combination of diseases such as asthma or emphysema, obstructive sleep apnea, heart failure, and gastroesophageal reflux. This may also be physically deconditioned, adding to symptom presentation.

Rhinosinusitis

There are no data to determine if either acute or chronic rhinosinusitis manifests itself any differently in older than in younger adults, so guidelines from the American Academy of Otolaryngology–Head and Neck Surgery do not advise different approaches to diagnosis or treatment based on age. Acute (<4 weeks in duration), subacute (4–12 weeks in duration), and chronic (>12 weeks in duration) rhinosinusitis are further subclassified as uncomplicated when inflammation is restricted to the nasal cavity and sinuses or complicated when inflammation extends beyond these areas (eg, soft-tissue or neurologic involvement). Bacterial rhinosinusitis is associated with purulent nasal discharge and facial pain or pressure. Treatment may focus on pain relief with simple analgesics, as well as on relief of nasal obstruction by saline irrigation. Antibiotics are generally not prescribed for patients who have mild illness but are advised if symptoms persist another 7 days, or if the symptoms worsen at any time. Early treatment with antibiotics in patients with mild disease has been shown to be harmful (SOE=B). In patients with clear nasal discharge, the cause of the rhinosinusitis is likely viral, and treatment should be symptomatic only. Although topical α-adrenergic decongestants may be

80
.4
32.0

effective, their use should be restricted in older adults, particularly those with hypertension or voiding symptoms from prostate disease. Chronic rhinosinusitis is treated with a variety of topical agents. A Cochrane review demonstrated that saline irrigation is more effective than placebo and offers a safe approach for many older patients. Topical nasal steroids are more effective than saline irrigation but can cause more epistaxis and local irritation. Allergic causes of rhinosinusitis are best treated by avoidance of the inciting allergens if possible, although topical nasal steroids are often required. Anti-allergy medications may also have a role in treatment of allergic rhinosinusitis in older patients but should be used judiciously, especially antihistamine formulations that also have anticholinergic effects.

Dyspnea

Dyspnea becomes prominent in end-stage lung diseases such as COPD and idiopathic pulmonary fibrosis. Importantly, the level of dyspnea is the best predictor of quality of life, yet it does not correlate with either oxygenation or pulmonary function test results. A thorough history and physical examination can help tailor both testing and empirical treatment choices. For example, in older adults presenting with dyspnea and associated nocturnal cough, common diseases such as asthma, emphysema, allergic rhinitis with postnasal drip, and gastroesophageal reflux disease should be considered first. Minimal testing (eg, pulmonary function tests only) followed by an empiric trial directed toward the most likely cause would be a reasonable approach. In the same patient, the presence of significant weight loss or constitutional symptoms (eg, fever, night sweats) could suggest other disease, such as malignancy or tuberculosis. At times, the particular language the patient chooses to describe the dyspnea can be revealing, such as "heavy" for cardiac dysfunction or deconditioning or "tight" for angina or asthma. The common causes of dyspnea to consider in older adults include COPD, cardiac disease, asthma, interstitial lung disease, and deconditioning.

Chronic Cough

Fortunately, most patients can be reassured that chronic cough, although particularly annoying, usually has a benign cause in individuals without a history of chronic lung disease or smoking. By far, the most common causes of chronic cough are postnasal drip, asthma, and gastroesophageal reflux. These three diagnoses account for >90% of the causes identified in most series, so a reasonable approach to the treatment of chronic cough is empiric treatment for these conditions (SOE=C). Not infrequently, a combination of these conditions may contribute, and treatment for multiple causes may be warranted when single therapies are ineffective. In older adults, the possibility of silent aspiration needs to be considered, especially in patients with frequent pneumonias or neurologic deficits or who are residents in extended-care facilities. In these cases, a modified barium swallow can evaluate oropharyngeal and esophageal aspiration. Less common yet important differential diagnostic considerations of cough in older adults include medication effects (eg, ACE inhibitors), heart failure, laryngeal dysfunction, *Bordetella pertussis* infection, chronic cough after viral upper respiratory tract infection or secondary bacterial infection, recurrent aspiration, or respiratory tract abnormalities such as bronchiectasis or central airway tumors. A careful history and physical examination should help direct the diagnostic evaluation or empiric treatment of cough.

Wheezing

Wheezing w/
cough w/ or dyspnea → asthma
if no — not asthma

Although asthma is a common cause of wheezing in all age groups, it is not the principal cause in older adults, particularly if the wheezing is not associated with cough or dyspnea. Wheezing in older adults is most commonly caused by COPD or heart failure—called "cardiac asthma." Rates of heart failure rise in the older age groups, and associated pulmonary edema may present as cardiac asthma. Other common causes of wheezing to consider include postnasal drip, and chronic bronchitis in older adults with a history of cough, sputum production, and tobacco use. Uncontrolled gastroesophageal reflux disease can also contribute to wheezing and asthma symptoms in older adults.

MAJOR PULMONARY DISEASES

Asthma

After childhood, the prevalence of asthma has a second peak after the age of 65 years; 5%–10% of older adults meet criteria for obstruction and bronchial hyperreactivity, particularly in nonsmokers. Asthma deaths in older adults account for >50% of asthma fatalities annually. This is likely due to reduced awareness of bronchial constriction on the part of the patient (with attendant delays in seeking medical attention), as well as under-recognition and undertreatment on the part of clinicians. In addition to accounting for most asthma deaths, older adults with asthma also suffer significant negative consequences to their health-related quality of life. Methacholine challenge testing is a safe, effective method to identify asthma in older adults. Population studies of asthma in older adults have shown that unlike younger adults, who may need only symptomatic treatment, most older adults require continual treatment programs to control

Table 47.1—Example of an Asthma Action Plan

Green zone: Doing well No cough, wheeze, chest tightness, or shortness of breath during day or night Can do usual activities *Peak flow:* ≥80% of my best peak flow	Take these long-term medications as prescribed: Medicine 1: how much, when to take it Medicine 2: how much, when to take it
Yellow zone: Getting worse Cough, wheeze, chest tightness, or shortness of breath, *or* Waking at night due to asthma, *or* Can do some, but not all, usual activities *Peak flow:* 50%–79% of my best peak flow	Keep taking your Green zone medications and add quick-relief medication (a short-acting β_2-agonist). If your symptoms return to Green zone after 1 hour of above treatment, continue monitoring. If your symptoms do *not* return to Green zone after 1 hour of treatment, take another dose of the short-acting β_2-agonist and add oral steroid.
Red zone: Medical alert Very short of breath, *or* Quick-relief medications have not helped, *or* Cannot do usual activities, *or* Symptoms are the same or get worse after 24 hours in the Yellow zone *Peak flow:* <50% of my best peak flow	Take a short-acting β_2-agonist and oral steroid. Then call your doctor *now*. Go to the hospital or call an ambulance if you are still in the Red zone after 15 min *and* you have not reached your doctor.

their disease (SOE=B). Overall asthma management does not differ between older and younger people. Inhaled corticosteroids (or other controller drugs such as leukotriene-receptor antagonists) are the mainstay of therapy in both older and younger patients, with use of the lowest effective dosage and counsel regarding rinsing of the oropharynx to avoid thrush. Oral corticosteroids are discussed in COPD, below. The bronchodilator response to inhaled β-agonists declines with age, but β-agonists are still the mainstay as-needed reliever medication for asthma treatment. The potential for adverse events of β-agonists—eg, hypokalemia or possible QT prolongation in cardiac patients on digoxin or other medications—warrants adequate controller use in older asthmatic patients to minimize their overreliance on the β-agonist. Use of long-acting β-agonists is helpful for long-term maintenance therapy and nocturnal symptoms. In older adults, theophylline is fraught with adverse events and drug interactions, and it should be considered a third-line medication to be used only once daily in the evening for severe asthma or COPD, targeting a serum level of 5–15 mg/L if tolerated. In addition to pharmacologic treatment, asthma "action plans" should be addressed in the event of worsening pulmonary symptoms. See Table 47.1 for an example of an asthma action plan, which provides patient instruction as a function of how he or she is feeling. Patients should keep a copy of such a plan in a convenient location for easy reference.

Chronic Obstructive Pulmonary Disease

COPD affects approximately 15 million people in the United States and is the fourth most common cause of death after heart disease, cancer, and stroke. The prevalence of COPD in patients ≥65 years old is at least 10% and is increasing along with COPD mortality rates, especially in older adults. Episodes of acute respiratory failure that require mechanical ventilation are associated with mortality rates ranging from 11% to 46%. The National Lung Health Education Program Executive Committee has noted that the morbidity and mortality from COPD accounts for more than $15 billion per year in U.S. medical care expenditures. COPD is a leading cause of hospitalization in the United States and accounts for 19.9% of the total hospitalizations for patients 65–75 years old and 18.2% for patients >75 years old. In one study, patients >65 years old who were admitted to an intensive care unit with COPD had a hospital mortality of 30% and a 1-year mortality of 59%. See also "Palliative Care," p 111.

The diagnosis of airflow limitation is challenging in that no single item or combination of items from the history and clinical examination excludes airflow limitation. For criteria often used to make the diagnosis of COPD, see Table 47.2. FEV_1/FVC decreases with age, so using a fixed $FEV_1:FVC$ ratio to separate normal from obstructive creates a risk of overdiagnosis of COPD in older adults. Up to one-fifth of current smokers and one-seventh of individuals >50 years old who have never smoked can be misidentified as abnormal when a fixed cut-off is used. Current guidelines recommend against screening asymptomatic older adults for COPD. In smokers, chronic cough is the most commonly reported symptom associated with COPD diagnosis. Wheezing noted on physical examination is the most potent predictor of airflow limitation; individuals with obstructive airflow limitation are 36 times more likely to have wheezing than those without this problem. Other findings associated with an increased likelihood

Table 47.2—GOLD[a] Guidelines for COPD

Key Factors for Considering a Diagnosis of COPD	
Dyspnea	Progressive or worsens over time Worse with exercise Persistent (present daily) Described as "increased effort to breathe," "heaviness," "air hunger," "gasping"
Chronic cough	May be intermittent and nonproductive
Sputum production	Any pattern of chronic sputum production can indicate COPD
Risk factors	Tobacco smoke Occupational dusts and chemicals Smoke from home cooking and heating fuel Family history, genetic variant (α-1 antitrypsin deficiency)
Spirometric Classification of COPD	
FEV_1/FVC <70%[b] applies to each category	
Mild	FEV_1 ≥80% predicted
Moderate	50% ≤ FEV_1 <80% predicted
Severe	30% ≤ FEV_1 <50% predicted
Very severe	FEV_1 <30% predicted or FEV_1 <50% predicted and chronic respiratory failure

NOTE: FEV_1 = forced expiratory volume in 1 sec; FVC = forced vital capacity

[a] GOLD=Global Initiative for Chronic Obstructive Lung Disease

[b] Using the criteria FEV_1/FVC <70% may overdiagnose COPD in older, nonsmoking adults; some experts recommend using FEV_1/FVC <65% after the age of 70, because the changes seen may be related to structural changes that occur in the airways with increasing age.

of airflow limitation include a barrel-shaped chest, hyperresonance on percussion, and a forced expiratory time of >9 seconds measured during the clinical bedside examination.

Smoking cessation at any age slows the decline in lung function, and aggressive cessation efforts are appropriate even in the oldest-old patient. For a commonly used approach for addressing smoking cessation with patients (The "Five A's" method), see "Addictions," p 336.

The chief components of daily medication therapy in COPD consist of a β-agonist, ipratropium bromide or tiotropium, or both in combination (Table 47.3 and Table 47.4). For more severe disease, the use of long-acting β-agonists such as salmeterol, along with a combined albuterol and ipratropium bromide metered-dose inhaler as needed, or the long-acting anticholinergic tiotropium with albuterol-only rescue inhalers, can achieve improved adherence and long-term control by reducing the number of inhalers by one. Concern has been raised over risk of cardiovascular events associated with anticholinergic medications, although in a randomized controlled trial of 6,000 patients with COPD, tiotropium use was associated with decreased cardiovascular mortality. Use of inhaled corticosteroids has been associated with some improvement in lung function, airway reactivity, frequency of exacerbations, and respiratory symptoms, but they have not been shown to impact the rate of decline in lung function (SOE=A). Combination therapy with inhaled corticosteroids and a long-acting β-agonist has been associated with better lung function and symptom control but without survival benefit. A landmark investigation documented that use of systemic corticosteroids (intravenous followed by oral) reduces the duration and recurrence of acute exacerbations of COPD for up to 6 months (SOE=A). Importantly, there is no benefit to a course of systemic steroids for >14 days for acute exacerbation of COPD. For the few patients (5%–10%) who chronically use systemic corticosteroids, the risks of peptic ulcer disease, hypertension, cataracts, diabetes mellitus, osteoporosis, psychosis, seizures, poor wound healing, infections, and aseptic necrosis of the hip must be carefully considered. Appropriate preventive measures should also be taken in circumstances of prolonged use, such as monitoring for signs of osteopenia or osteoporosis; using the lowest possible dosage of corticosteroids; and using supplemental vitamin D, calcium, and perhaps a bisphosphonate for those at risk of osteoporosis.

Long-term oxygen therapy benefits patients who have a resting Pao_2 of ≤55 mmHg on room air (SOE=A). Use of oxygen for at least 15 hours per day improves survival, exercise tolerance, sleep, and cognitive function. Other possible beneficial interventions in older adults with COPD include pulmonary rehabilitation via exercise training and respiratory therapy and education. Home-based, self-administered exercise and strength-building programs may also have a role in pulmonary rehabilitation of older patients with COPD. Both major depressive disorder and anxiety are present in up to 40% of patients with COPD; these diagnoses should be screened for and treated appropriately. In older adults, anxiety is associated with the level of physical functioning and disability and is a major predictor of emergency department visits and hospitalization.

Paramount to the care of older adults with asthma or COPD is adequate instruction in the proper use of peak expiratory flow meters and inhalers. Neurologic, muscular, and arthritic diseases in older adults can lead to suboptimal timing and lack of coordination in the actuation of the inhaler device. Only 60% of older adults have been reported to have adequate technique with a metered-dose inhaler; this number decreases to 36% when objective criteria are used. While the use of spacers improves technique, 85% of older adults do not use the spacer when it is prescribed. Breath-activated dry-powder inhalers require less coordination but do require a certain minimal negative peak inspiratory flow for adequate drug delivery. The clinician should observe the patient actually using the inhaler. Cost is another additional barrier to adherence in over one-quarter of patients with COPD, particularly when out-of-pocket costs exceed $20.

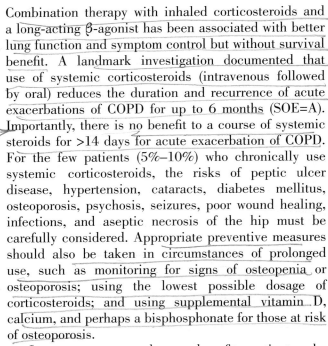

Table 47.3—Inhaled Bronchodilators and Corticosteroids for COPD

Class	Medication	Duration (hours)	Dosage
Short-acting			
β_2-Agonist	Albuterol sulfate	4–6	2 puffs q6h
β_2-Agonist	Levalbuterol	4–6	2 puffs q6h
β_2-Agonist	Pirbuterol	4–6	2 puffs q6h
Anticholinergic	Ipratropium bromide	4–6	2 puffs q6h
Inhaled corticosteroid (ICS)	Triamcinolone acetonide	4–6	1 or 2 puffs q6-8h
Long-acting			
β_2-Agonist	Formoterol fumarate	8–12	1 puff q12h
β_2-Agonist	Salmeterol xinafoate	8–12	1 puff q12h
β_2-Agonist	Arformoterol	8–12	15 mcg nebulized q12h
Anticholinergic	Tiotropium bromide	>24	1 puff q24h
Anticholinergic	Aclidinium	12	1 puff q12h
ICS	Beclomethasone diproprionate	12	1 or 2 puffs q12h
ICS	Budesonide	12	1 or 2 puffs q12h or nebulized
ICS	Fluticasone	12	1 puff q12 h
ICS	Mometasone furoate	24	1 or 2 puffs q24h

Table 47.4—COPD Therapy[a]

Class	Treatment
Mild COPD $FEV_1 \geq 80\%$	Short-acting β_2-agonist when needed
Moderate COPD $50\% \leq FEV_1 < 80\%$	Long-acting bronchodilator if needed for added benefit or if ≥2 exacerbations per year Rehabilitation
Severe COPD $30\% \leq FEV_1 < 50\%$	Regular treatment with one or more bronchodilators[b] Inhaled steroids[c] or if significant symptoms and lung function response or if ≥2 exacerbations per year Rehabilitation
Very severe COPD $FEV_1 < 30\%$ ***or*** $FEV_1 < 50\%$ plus chronic respiratory failure	Regular treatment with one or more bronchodilators[b] Inhaled steroids[c] or if significant symptoms and lung function response or if repeated exacerbations Treatment of complications Long-term oxygen therapy if respiratory failure
COPD exacerbation (increased breathlessness, wheezing, cough, and sputum of acute onset and beyond normal day-to-day variation)	Increased dosage and/or frequency of β_2-agonists with or without anticholinergics. Add steroid (eg, methylprednisolone 30–40 mg/d po for 7–10 d). Add antibiotics if increased sputum with increased purulence or increased dyspnea (cover *Streptococcus pneumoniae, Heamophilus influenzae, Moraxella catarrhalis).* CBC, chest radiograph, ECG, arterial blood gas; titrate oxygen to 90% sat and recheck arterial blood gas. If two or more of severe dyspnea, respiratory rate ≥25, or P_{CO_2} 45–60, then noninvasive positive-pressure ventilation reduces risk of ventilator use and mortality and length of hospital stay.

[a] $FEV_1/FVC < 70\%$ for all levels of severity

[b] β_2-agonists, ipratropium, slow-release theophylline (caution in older adults with other conditions and taking other medications)

[c] Consider osteoporosis prophylaxis.

SOURCE: Data from *Global Initiative for Chronic Obstructive Lung Disease (GOLD)*; 2007. www.goldcopd.org (accessed Oct 2013).

Obstructive Sleep Apnea

Sleep-related breathing disorders are very common in older adults, obstructive sleep apnea (OSA) being the most frequent. As in younger patients, OSA in older patients is more common in men. The estimated prevalence of OSA in older men ranges from 13% to 28% and in women from 4% to 20%. Age-related changes of respiratory anatomy and physiology, such as increased upper airway adipose tissue deposition and pharyngeal bony changes, may predispose older adults to sleep apnea. Body habitus as a risk factor for apnea is less important in older patients than in younger patients. In the Heart Health Study, prevalence of OSA did not differ by racial group. Black women are significantly younger than white women at the time of diagnosis of OSA. Black patients with OSA are more obese and have higher rates of hypertension than whites with OSA. Medications, alcohol consumption, and abnormal upper airway configuration are additional risk factors for OSA. OSA has been associated with cerebrovascular accidents, myocardial infarctions, and a 3-fold increase in mortality (SOE=B). Untreated OSA is associated with significant cognitive impairment, including executive function impairment and depression in older patients. Most patients with OSA remain undiagnosed and therefore without treatment of this life-threatening, yet potentially treatable disease. Clinicians should consider the diagnosis of OSA in patients who have complaints of daytime somnolence, frequent daytime napping, or drowsiness while driving. A history of snoring or witnessed apneas or hypopneas by a bed partner should also prompt further evaluation. Treatment options include addressing upper-airway obstruction via weight loss, avoiding alcohol and sedatives, sleeping on one's side or upright, correcting metabolic disorders such as hypothyroidism, and using continuous positive-airway pressure (CPAP) via a nasal mask. To increase adherence to the use of CPAP, the treatment can be ordered with "nasal pillows" to increase comfort and "ramping technique" to give a delayed rise in the applied pressure after the individual has fallen asleep. Diagnosis and treatment issues are generally the same for both young and old, and the major consideration for the clinician is a high index of suspicion and clinical recognition of this disease. See "Sleep Problems," p 285.

Idiopathic Pulmonary Fibrosis (IPF)

There are >100 causes of interstitial lung diseases; however, IPF is the most common among older adults. It has a mean age of onset of 55 years and is increasing in prevalence with the aging population. IPF is extremely frustrating because of its relentless progression. The median survival is 3–5 years. Survival is even worse in patients with IPF and pulmonary hypertension. The presentation is normally one of insidious dyspnea (often unrecognized because of a decrease in the activity level on the part of the patient) and cough with dry inspiratory rales on examination. Clubbing is often a prominent finding on physical examination in IPF (40%–70%), as opposed to emphysema, which rarely causes clubbing (prompting a search for another disease such as occult lung cancer). Older adults often present with advanced disease because of the insidious onset of symptoms. IPF should be considered in older adults with a restrictive ventilatory defect or a reduced diffusing capacity on pulmonary function testing, or both. Chest radiographs often show reticular opacities in the mid and lower lung zones. High resolution CT scans show characteristic areas of subpleural reticulation and honeycombing. The diagnosis can often be made by experienced pulmonologists and radiologists, based on clinical and radiographic findings.

There is no known effective or curative therapy for IPF. Oral corticosteroids (0.5 mg/kg/d) for 3–6 months is the most common initial therapy, yet only 10%–20% of patients respond and adverse events are often prominent. Combination therapy with oral corticosteroids, azathioprine, and N-acetylcysteine may reduce decline of lung function, but further studies are needed to determine efficacy of this regimen. Lung transplantation is the only treatment for end-stage IPF. However, risks associated with lung transplant need to be carefully considered, especially in patients ≥65 years old whose survival after transplant is lower than that of younger patients. Although the current treatment options are limited, early referral to a subspecialist experienced in fibrotic lung diseases is warranted if the patient wishes to consider further therapeutic attempts or to enroll in a randomized controlled trial of newer pharmacologic agents. The primary care provider may initiate the evaluation by obtaining a history and searching for evidence of chemical exposure, smoking, asbestosis, connective tissue syndromes, chronic aspiration, or a family history of lung diseases. Chest CT and pulmonary function tests are helpful in guiding subsequent management decisions. Patients with advanced disease may benefit from a palliative care approach (see "Palliative Care," p 111).

Pulmonary Thromboembolism

The incidence of pulmonary thromboembolism triples between the ages of 65 and 90 years and has a reported 10% recurrence rate within 1 year. Age >70 years has been independently associated with missed antemortem diagnosis. Importantly, 10%–20% of patients with documented pulmonary embolism have an entirely normal blood-gas profile (ie, normal $Pa{O_2}$ and normal A-a gradient for age). Age-specific risk factors for pulmonary thromboembolism include hypercoagulability due to increases in fibrinogen, activated protein-C resistance due to factor-V Leiden gene mutation, malignancy, stasis (decreased mobility due to stroke, heart failure, or arthritis), or vessel injury (due to trauma or varicosities). The diagnostic evaluation is not different for young and older patients. Anticoagulants are central to therapy, and their use is generally guided by the same principles in patients of any age. Because of lessened cardiopulmonary reserve in older patients, achieving therapeutic levels of heparin quickly may be even more important to avoid major adverse hemodynamic or oxygenation defects.

The trend toward increased use of low-molecular-weight heparin preparations for outpatients, while achieving anticoagulation with warfarin, is supported by large, well-designed randomized controlled trials (SOE=A). There should be an overlap of approximately 1–3 days between heparinization and adequate warfarin therapy with an INR target of 2–3. Long-term anticoagulation (≥6 months) is preferred to shorter term (eg, 3 months) unless there are increased risks of bleeding. Indeed, patients with multiple ongoing risk factors for pulmonary thromboembolic disease are to be considered for anticoagulation therapy for up to 2 years or longer. Recurrent pulmonary thromboembolism is usually treated with lifelong anticoagulation therapy.

INTENSIVE CARE OF THE CRITICALLY ILL

See "Hospital Care," p 130.

REFERENCES

- Akgün KM, Crothers K, Pisani M. Epidemiology and management of common pulmonary diseases in older persons. *J Gerontol A Biol Sci Med Sci.* 2012;67(3):276–291.
- Engbers MJ, van Hylckama Vlieg A, Rosendaal FR. Venous thrombosis in the elderly: incidence, risk factors and risk groups. *J Thromb Haemost.* 2010;8(10):2105–2112.
- Managing coexistent asthma and chronic obstructive pulmonary disease in older populations is challenging. *Drugs & Therapy Perspectives.* 2013;29(5):141–144.
- Monteiro MB, Berton DC, Moreira MA, et al. Effects of expiratory positive airway pressure on dynamic hyperinflation during exercise in patients with COPD. *Respiratory Care.* 2012;57(9):1405–1412.

CHAPTER 48—CARDIOVASCULAR DISEASES AND DISORDERS

KEY POINTS

- Increasing age is associated with extensive changes throughout the cardiovascular system that lead to a progressive decline in cardiovascular reserve capacity and to substantive alterations in the clinical presentation, response to therapy, and prognosis of cardiovascular disease in older adults.
- Older adults account for the majority of patients hospitalized with acute coronary syndromes (ACS), and >80% of deaths attributable to ACS occur in patients ≥65 years old. Although the benefits of current treatments for ACS are generally similar in older and younger patients, older patients are at increased risk of major complications from therapeutic interventions.
- Atrial fibrillation (AF), the most common sustained dysrhythmia in clinical practice, increases in prevalence with age, and >50% of all patients with AF are ≥75 years old. Most older patients with AF respond to rate-control medications in conjunction with antithrombotic therapy, but some patients require antiarrhythmic drug therapy to maintain sinus rhythm and alleviate symptoms.
- The prevalence of peripheral arterial disease (PAD) increases progressively with age, and the presence of PAD is often predictive of concomitant coronary artery and cerebrovascular disease. Management of patients with PAD should therefore include appropriate treatment of hypertension, dyslipidemia, diabetes, and tobacco abuse in accordance with existing practice guidelines.

EPIDEMIOLOGY

The prevalence of cardiovascular disease (CVD) increases progressively with age, exceeding 80% in both men and women >80 years old (Table 48.1). Similarly, the annual incidence of CVD increases from 1.0% in men 45–54 years old to 7.4% in men 85–94 years old, and from 0.4% in women 45–54 years old to 6.5% in women 85–94 years old. Because of the high prevalence of CVD in older age, adults ≥65 years old account for 61% of hospitalizations for CVD in the United States, including over 50% of percutaneous and surgical coronary revascularization procedures, 59% of defibrillator implantations, 73% of arterial endarterectomies, and 80% of permanent pacemaker insertions. In addition, women comprise an increasing proportion of cardiovascular hospitalizations and procedures with increasing age.

Over the past 50 years, lifestyle changes and medical advances have led to a progressive decline in age-adjusted mortality rates from CVD. Nevertheless, CVD remains the leading cause of death in the United States, accounting for approximately one-third of all deaths in 2007. Notably, cancer is the leading cause of death among adults up to age 75, and it is only after age 75 that CVD becomes the dominant cause of death. Thus, among 814,000 deaths in the United States from cardiac and cerebrovascular diseases in 2007, more than 80% occurred in adults ≥65 years old and 67% occurred in the 6.1% of the population ≥75 years old. Mortality rates from CVD are higher in men than in women at all ages, but women account for more than 50% of CVD deaths among adults 65 years or older. CVD mortality rates are highest in black Americans and then decrease in order among non-Hispanic whites, Hispanic Americans, Native Americans, and Asians/Pacific Islanders. With the aging of the population, it may be anticipated that the absolute number of cardiovascular deaths in older adults will increase markedly over the next several decades.

EFFECTS OF AGING ON CARDIOVASCULAR FUNCTION

Normal aging is associated with diverse changes throughout the cardiovascular system (Table 48.2), and these changes are accentuated by common comorbid conditions, particularly hypertension, diabetes, obesity, and atherosclerosis.

These age-related changes in numerous organ systems intersect with the cardiovascular system to substantially alter the clinical features, response to therapy, and prognosis of older adults with prevalent cardiovascular diseases.

Table 48.1—Prevalence (percent of population) of Cardiovascular Disease in Americans by Age and Sex

Age Cohort	Men	Women
20–40 years old	14.2	9.7
40–60 years old	39.3	37.2
60–80 years old	72.6	71.9
>80 years old	80.1	86.7

SOURCE: Data from NHANES 2005–2008.

Table 48.2—Principal Effects of Aging on the Cardiovascular System

Age Effect	Clinical Implication
↑ Arterial stiffness	↑ Afterload and systolic blood pressure
↓ Myocardial relaxation and compliance	↑ Risk of diastolic heart failure and atrial fibrillation
Impaired responsiveness to β-adrenergic stimulation	↓ Maximum cardiac output; impaired thermoregulation
↓ Sinus node function and conduction velocity in the atrioventricular node and infranodal conduction system	↑ Risk of sick sinus syndrome, atrioventricular block, left anterior fascicular block, and bundle-branch block
Impaired endothelium-dependent vasodilation	↑ Demand ischemia and risk of coronary artery disease and peripheral arterial disease
↓ Baroreceptor responsiveness	↑ Risk of orthostatic hypotension
↓ Exercise response (↓ maximal heart rate, maximal cardiac output, $\mathrm{Vo_2}$ max, coronary blood flow, peripheral vasodilation)	↓ Exercise capacity and ↑ cardiac complications (ischemia, heart failure, shock, arrhythmias, death) with illness

Cardiovascular Risk Factors

Major Risk Factors

In general, the 4 major risk factors for cardiovascular disease—hypertension, diabetes mellitus, dyslipidemia, and smoking—continue to exert significant influence on cardiovascular risk in older adults. In addition, because the incidence and prevalence of cardiovascular diseases are higher in older than in younger individuals, the absolute number of cases attributable to a given risk factor tends to increase with age. Moreover, because the prevalence of hypertension, diabetes mellitus, and dyslipidemia all increase with age, older adults are more likely to have multiple risk factors that act in concert with age-related cardiovascular changes to promote the development and progression of heart and vascular disorders.

Hypertension

Pulse pressure (the difference between systolic and diastolic blood pressure) increases with age, and isolated systolic hypertension becomes the dominant form of hypertension in older adults, especially women. In the Framingham Heart Study and other epidemiologic studies, increased systolic blood pressure was identified as the strongest risk factor for incident cardiovascular disease in older adults, including those >80 years old (SOE=A). In some but not all studies, pulse pressure was equivalent or stronger than systolic blood pressure as a marker for cardiovascular risk. In addition, although the prevalence of diastolic hypertension declines with age, its presence confers increased cardiovascular risk independent of the systolic blood pressure, particularly in men. See "Hypertension," p 402.

Diabetes Mellitus

The prevalence of diabetes mellitus increases with age, at least up to age 80, and approximately half of all patients with diabetes in the United States are ≥65 years old. As in younger individuals, the impact of diabetes on cardiovascular risk is greater in older women than in older men. In the Framingham Heart Study, for example, the adjusted risk for incident coronary heart disease was 2.1 in older women with diabetes compared with 1.4 in older men with diabetes. Notably, the excess risk associated with diabetes was greater in both men and women >65 years old than in younger individuals.

Dyslipidemia

Population mean total serum cholesterol levels increase in men until approximately age 70 and then level off. In women, total cholesterol levels tend to rise rapidly after menopause and average 15–20 mg/dL higher than in men after age 60. Low-density lipoprotein (LDL) cholesterol levels track with total cholesterol levels in men and women, while high-density lipoprotein (HDL) cholesterol levels average about 10 mg/dL higher in women than in men throughout adult life. The strength of association between total cholesterol and LDL-cholesterol levels and incident CAD declines with age, especially after age 80, in part because of the confounding effects of comorbid conditions and nutritional factors. Nevertheless, low HDL-cholesterol levels (<40 mg/dL in men, <50 mg/dL in women) and high total cholesterol to HDL-cholesterol ratios (≥5.5 in men, ≥5 in women) remain independently associated with coronary events even among adults >80 years old (SOE=A). In addition, clinical trials have demonstrated beneficial effects from lipid-lowering therapy with statins in moderate- and high-risk patients, ie, those with established coronary heart disease, diabetes, or multiple other risk factors (cerebrovascular or peripheral vascular disease, smoking, hypertension) up to 85 years of age (SOE=A). Conversely, the value of lipid-lowering therapy for primary prevention of cardiovascular disease in older adults, especially those >80–85 years old, remains uncertain.

Smoking

Unlike other risk factors, the prevalence of smoking declines with age, in part due to successful smoking cessation and in part because of premature deaths attributable to smoking. In 2006, approximately 12.6% of men and 8.3% of women ≥65 years old in the United States were active smokers, declining to <5% among individuals >85 years old. In most but not all studies, smoking remains a strong and independent risk factor for fatal and nonfatal cardiovascular disease events among older adults. In addition, several large observational studies have shown that among older smokers, smoking cessation is associated with substantial reductions in cardiovascular risk within 2–6 years relative to continued smoking.

Other Risk Factors

Obesity is associated with increased cardiovascular risk in young and middle-aged people, in part because of its association with hypertension, diabetes mellitus, and dyslipidemia. The importance of obesity as a cardiovascular risk factor among older adults, especially those >80 years old, is less clear. Indeed, among older adults with CAD, heart failure, or renal insufficiency, there is evidence that being overweight or mildly obese (ie, BMI 25–35 kg/m^2) exerts a favorable effect on prognosis, while being underweight (BMI <20 kg/m^2) confers the highest mortality risk (SOE=B).

Increased levels of the inflammatory marker C-reactive protein (CRP) are associated with increased risk of incident CAD events and cardiovascular death in older adults, but the clinical utility of CRP in guiding management is undefined, and routine measurement of CRP is not currently recommended. Similarly, although increased levels of fibrinogen, D-dimer, and plasmin-antiplasmin complex have been associated with increased risk of myocardial infarction in older adults, use of these markers to identify patients at increased risk is not recommended.

The value of quantitation of coronary artery calcium content by CT scanning is controversial. Coronary artery calcium scores increase with age, while the correlation of calcium scores with the severity of clinically significant coronary artery stenoses declines with age. Nonetheless, calcium scores ≥100 (Agatston method) are associated with increased risk of incident coronary events in older adults, and higher scores are associated with progressively higher risk. Despite this, the value of routine CT scans to screen for CAD, even in patients with multiple risk factors, remains to be defined.

In the Cardiovascular Health Study, several subclinical markers of cardiovascular disease were found to identify individuals at increased risk of subsequent cardiovascular events. These included increased carotid artery intima-media thickness assessed by carotid ultrasonography, increased left ventricular mass by echocardiography, borderline or decreased left ventricular ejection fraction, and decreased ankle-brachial index. As with CT scanning, the clinical use and cost-effectiveness of these measures require further study, but in patients with diabetes or multiple other risk factors, the presence of any of these markers may identify patients likely to benefit from more aggressive management (SOE=C).

Coronary Artery Disease

Epidemiology

Autopsy studies indicate that up to 70% of adults ≥70 years old have significant CAD, defined as ≥50% obstruction of one or more coronary arteries. The prevalence of clinical CAD increases with age in both men and women, while the incidence of angina pectoris peaks between the ages of 65 and 84 and decreases modestly thereafter. Of an estimated 1.2 million fatal and nonfatal myocardial infarctions (MIs) occurring annually in the United States (excluding silent MIs), two-thirds are in adults ≥65 years old, including 44% in those ≥75 years old. In addition, the proportion of MIs occurring in women increases from 26% among those 45–64 years old, to 35% in those 65–74 years old, and to 55% in those ≥75 years old. Mortality after acute MI increases exponentially with age, with >80% of MI deaths occurring in adults ≥65 years old, and approximately 60% occurring among those ≥75 years old.

Acute Coronary Syndromes

The acute coronary syndromes (ACS) comprise unstable angina, non-ST-elevation MI (NSTEMI), and ST-elevation MI (STEMI). Unstable angina and NSTEMI are often considered together because they are pathophysiologically similar and clinically difficult to distinguish at the time of presentation, pending analysis of cardiac biomarker proteins (ie, troponin or creatine phosphokinase).

Presentation

The proportion of patients with ACS who present with chest pain declines with age, especially after age 80, and shortness of breath is the most common initial symptom in patients >80–85 years old. In addition, older ACS patients are more likely than younger patients to present with altered mental status, confusion, dizziness, or syncope, and the prevalence of these symptoms approaches 20% among patients ≥85 years old. The time from onset of symptoms to initial presentation at a medical facility also tends to be longer in older patients, in part due to the decreased prevalence of chest pain, although other factors likely contribute to delays in presentation.

The initial ECG is more likely to be nondiagnostic of ACS in older than in younger patients due to the higher prevalence of prior MI, conduction abnormalities (especially left bundle-branch block), left ventricular hypertrophy, and paced rhythm. In addition, the proportion of ACS associated with ST elevation declines with age, further reducing the diagnostic accuracy of the ECG. Importantly, the combination of presentation delays, altered symptomatology, and nondiagnostic ECGs often results in substantial delays to initiation of treatment, thereby limiting the potential benefits of current therapies and contributing to higher complication rates and worse outcomes.

Therapy

All patients with suspected ACS should immediately receive aspirin 160–325 mg, regardless of age (SOE=A). Oxygen should be administered to maintain an arterial oxygen saturation of at least 92% (SOE=B), but routine use of oxygen in patients with arterial oxygen saturations >92% is of unproven value and may be harmful (SOE=C). Patients with ongoing chest discomfort should receive intravenous nitroglycerin initially, followed by intravenous morphine if nitroglycerin is ineffective. Patients with STEMI should also receive oral metoprolol or atenolol in the absence of contraindications (ie, heart rate <45–50 beats per minute, systolic blood pressure <100 mmHg, advanced heart block, moderate or severe heart failure, active bronchospasm). An ACE inhibitor should be administered to hemodynamically stable patients with adequate renal function (estimated creatinine clearance ≥30 mL/min), especially those with left ventricular (LV) systolic dysfunction or clinical heart failure, or both (SOE=A). An angiotensin-receptor blocker (ARB) may be substituted in patients with known intolerance to ACE inhibitors due to cough. Early administration of high-dose statin therapy (eg, atorvastatin 80 mg) has been associated with improved outcomes in some but not all studies, and some experts recommend its routine use; data in patients >75–80 years old are, however, very limited (SOE=C).

The role of adjunctive antithrombotic therapy (ie, in addition to aspirin) in patients with ACS continues to evolve. In general, low-molecular-weight heparins (enoxaparin, dalteparin) have been associated with more favorable outcomes than intravenous unfractionated heparin (SOE=B), including in older adults, but appropriate dosage adjustment for renal function is essential to minimize the risk of bleeding. Fondaparinux, a factor Xa inhibitor, and bivalirudin, a direct thrombin inhibitor, have been associated with improved clinical outcomes and fewer major bleeding complications than either unfractionated or low-molecular-weight heparin, with similar benefits in younger and older patients (SOE=A). Fondaparinux is not currently approved for treatment of ACS in the United States, and it is contraindicated in patients with creatinine clearance <30 mL/min and in those weighing <50 kg. Dosage reduction is also required in patients >75 years old because of reduced clearance. Bivalirudin is currently approved only for treatment of patients undergoing percutaneous coronary intervention. Dosage reduction is required in patients with impaired renal function. A loading dose of clopidogrel 300–600 mg should be given to patients undergoing early coronary angiography in whom percutaneous coronary intervention (PCI) is anticipated, but it is prudent to withhold clopidogrel in patients who may be candidates for coronary bypass surgery rather than PCI, because perioperative bleeding risks are increased for up to 5 days after even a single dose of clopidogrel. Prasugrel at a loading dose of 60 mg is an alternative to clopidogrel in patients <75 years old. Glycoprotein IIb/IIIa inhibitors (eptifibatide, tirofiban, abciximab) reduce the risk of ischemic complications in selected patients with ACS, but the value of routine use of these agents in older adults receiving aspirin, clopidogrel (or prasugrel), and heparin is uncertain, while the risk of bleeding is increased; therefore, judicious use of these agents is warranted.

Reperfusion therapy with a fibrinolytic agent or PCI is indicated in patients presenting within 6–12 hours of onset of STEMI (or MI associated with new left bundle-branch block). Fibrinolytic therapy reduces mortality in STEMI patients <75 years old, as well as in carefully selected patients ≥75 years old. The risk of intracranial hemorrhage after administration of a fibrinolytic agent increases with age, especially after age 75, and is higher with fibrin-selective agents, such as tissue plasminogen activator or reteplase, than with the nonselective agent streptokinase. PCI has been associated with superior outcomes relative to fibrinolysis in patients up to 85 years old, provided the procedure can be performed within 90–120 minutes of the patient's arrival at the hospital.

In the setting of non-ST-elevation ACS, early PCI has been associated with improved outcomes in high-risk patients, including older adults, especially those with ongoing ischemia, extensive ECG changes, decreased LV systolic function, or hemodynamic instability (hypotension, tachycardia, heart failure) (SOE=A). In hemodynamically stable patients without active chest pain or major ECG abnormalities, an initial strategy of optimal medical therapy is appropriate.

Routine use of antiarrhythmic agents, including lidocaine and amiodarone, is not recommended in patients with ACS. Similarly, intravenous magnesium and the combination of glucose-insulin-potassium have not been shown to be beneficial. Dihydropyridine calcium channel blockers are contraindicated in patients with acute MI (SOE=A), and the use of diltiazem and verapamil should be limited to the treatment of supraventricular tachyarrhythmias (including atrial fibrillation and atrial flutter) in patients unresponsive to or intolerant of β-blockers. Digoxin is not indicated for patients with ACS, including those with heart failure, and it also has limited efficacy in the treatment of atrial fibrillation.

After documented ACS, patients should be maintained on aspirin, a β-blocker, an ACE inhibitor (or ARB), and a statin in the absence of contraindications (SOE=A). Clopidogrel 75 mg (or prasugrel 10 mg for patients <75 years old) is recommended for at least 3–12 months for all ACS patients undergoing PCI (3 months for patients receiving bare metal stents, 6–12 months for patients receiving drug-eluting stents), as well as for those with non-ST-elevation ACS in whom PCI is not performed. Patients with large anterior MIs associated with apical wall motion abnormalities should receive warfarin for 3–6 months to maintain an INR of 2–3 to reduce the risk of mural thrombus formation and embolization. In addition, aggressive interventions should be undertaken to control all treatable cardiovascular risk factors, and appropriate recommendations about diet, exercise, and sexual activity should be conveyed before hospital discharge. Whenever feasible, patients should be referred to a structured cardiac rehabilitation program, because such programs have been associated with improved functional, emotional, behavioral, and clinical outcomes, including 25%–30% reduction in mortality, and the beneficial effects are at least as great in older as in younger patients (SOE=A).

Chronic Coronary Artery Disease

Presentation and Diagnosis

As is the case with ACS, older patients with chronic CAD are more likely than younger patients to present with exertional fatigue or shortness of breath rather than classical angina pectoris. In addition, older patients tend to present later in the course of disease, in part because more sedentary lifestyles result in delays in symptom onset or reduced symptom severity. Coronary angiographic studies and autopsy series indicate that older patients tend to have more severe and diffuse CAD, including more triple-vessel and left main CAD, as well as higher prevalence of prior MI and associated LV dysfunction.

The diagnosis of CAD is similar in older and younger adults, except that older adults have, on average, a higher pretest likelihood of having significant coronary obstructions. As a result, false-positive rates on stress tests tend to be lower in older adults, while false-negative rates tend to be higher. Diminished exercise capacity can also contribute to higher false-negative rates on exercise stress tests (but not pharmacologic stress tests) in older patients.

In most patients with stable symptoms thought likely to be due to coronary ischemia, a stress test is the initial diagnostic test of choice. When feasible, an exercise test is preferable to a pharmacologic test because it is more physiologic and provides additional information about exercise tolerance and the hemodynamic response to exercise not afforded by pharmacologic testing. In patients unable to exercise because of poor physical conditioning or comorbid illness (especially orthopedic or neurologic disorders), pharmacologic stress tests such as dobutamine echocardiography or adenosine (or regadenoson) thallium (or sestamibi) provide equivalent diagnostic sensitivity and specificity relative to exercise tests.

In patients with accelerating symptoms or a markedly abnormal stress test in whom coronary revascularization may be a suitable therapeutic option, coronary angiography provides definitive information about the precise location and severity of coronary stenoses. Although the risks of coronary angiography increase slightly with age, in experienced centers the procedure can be performed with very low risk of major complications (<2% combined risk of all major complications, including death), even in patients of very advanced age (ie, nonagenarians and beyond).

Alternative approaches to the diagnosis of CAD include coronary artery calcium scores, CT coronary angiography, MRI scans, contrast echocardiography, and ambulatory ST-segment monitors. Although some of these techniques hold considerable promise and may eventually supplant stress testing or coronary angiography, or both, in selected situations, none is presently recommended for routine use.

Medical Therapy

Control of risk factors is the foundation for reducing CAD progression in patients of all ages. Diabetes, hypertension, and lipid abnormalities should be treated in accordance with published guidelines. For current recommendations for management of hypertension in older adults, see "Hypertension," p 402. The target LDL-cholesterol level in all patients with established CAD is <100 mg/dL, and a goal of <70 mg/dL is a reasonable option in very high-risk patients, especially those with concomitant diabetes (SOE=A). Individuals who smoke should be strongly encouraged to discontinue use of all tobacco products, and behavioral or pharmacologic support, or both, should be routinely offered to all patients who indicate an interest in smoking cessation (see "Addictions," p 336). A diet low in saturated fat and cholesterol but high in fruits, vegetables, and whole-grain products should be prescribed, and patients should be encouraged to engage in at least 30 minutes of aerobic exercise, such as walking, at least 5 days per week. Modest weight reduction is advisable in patients who are markedly overweight (BMI ≥35 kg/m^2), but as noted above, the value of weight loss in older patients with lesser degrees of obesity has not been established.

All patients with chronic CAD should receive aspirin 75–325 mg/d (SOE=A). Lower dosages are associated with decreased incidence of GI intolerance and bleeding complications but somewhat higher risk of aspirin resistance. Therefore, the optimal dose of aspirin may vary, but 75–160 mg is appropriate in most patients. In the small percentage of patients with true aspirin allergy or intolerance, clopidogrel 75 mg/d is a reasonable alternative. Although the combination of aspirin with either clopidogrel or warfarin is somewhat more effective than aspirin alone in reducing the risk of ACS in patients with CAD, the additional expense and higher risk of major hemorrhage makes combination therapy less desirable in the absence of specific indications (eg, clopidogrel after PCI or warfarin for atrial fibrillation).

Statin therapy is indicated for all patients with CAD, even in those with untreated LDL-cholesterol levels within the desirable range, because statins have been shown to reduce mortality and major cardiac events regardless of the pretreatment LDL-cholesterol level (SOE=A). Statin dosages should be sufficient to reduce the LDL-cholesterol level by 30%–40% and to ensure that the target LDL-cholesterol level is achieved. Statins have been shown to improve clinical outcomes in trials involving patients up to 85 years old, and observational studies support the use of statins for secondary prevention in older patients as well. Although altered hepatic metabolism and the use of multiple medications may place older patients at increased risk of statin-related adverse events, studies have not consistently shown an increased incidence of major statin toxicity in older adults. There is some evidence, however, that statin-associated myalgias may be more common in older adults. In addition, recent studies suggest that long-term statin use may be associated with an increased risk of incident diabetes and cognitive impairment in a small percentage of patients.

ACE inhibitors have been shown to reduce mortality and cardiovascular morbidity in patients up to 85 years old with CAD, peripheral arterial disease, or diabetes. Routine use of ACE inhibitors is recommended for most patients with established CAD in the absence of contraindications (SOE=A). ARBs are an acceptable alternative in patients unable to tolerate ACE inhibitors because of cough. Both classes of agents should be used cautiously, if at all, in patients with estimated creatinine clearance <30 mL/min (unless receiving dialysis). Renal function and serum potassium levels should be monitored closely when starting or titrating ACE inhibitors or ARBs.

All patients with prior MI should be treated with a β-blocker in the absence of contraindications or limiting adverse effects (SOE=A). In addition, β-blockers are indicated for all patients with an LV ejection fraction ≤40%, regardless of cause. β-Blockers are also the most effective anti-ischemic agents and should be considered the medications of first choice for treatment of angina pectoris or other ischemic symptoms. The dosage of β-blocker should be titrated to maintain a resting heart rate of 50 to no more than 70 beats per minute. Up to 20%–30% of patients are unable to tolerate β-blockers because of adverse events, but there is no convincing evidence that older patients experience more adverse events than younger patients.

Calcium channel blockers are effective anti-ischemic agents, either as first-line therapy in patients unable to take β-blockers, or in combination with either β-blockers or long-acting nitrates. Calcium channel blockers are relatively contraindicated in patients with heart failure or an LV ejection fraction <40%. Leg edema due to venodilation is a common adverse effect of dihydropyridine calcium channel blockers, whereas constipation occurs more commonly with the nondihydropyridines, especially verapamil; both problems appear to be more common in older patients.

Long-acting nitrate preparations, such as isosorbide mononitrate, are less effective anti-ischemic agents than β-blockers or calcium channel blockers, in part because of the high rate of tolerance that develops during long-term use and the need for a daily nitrate-free interval of at least several hours. These agents are therefore best used as adjunctive therapy in patients with persistent symptoms despite treatment with a β-blocker or calcium channel blocker, or both. Headache is the most common adverse effect associated with nitrates, but most cases resolve with continued use. Occasionally patients develop hypotension, dizziness, falls, or syncope, most commonly on initiation of nitrate therapy.

Ranolazine, alone or in combination with conventional antianginal medications, reduces angina and improves exercise tolerance in patients with symptomatic CAD. In addition, the benefits of ranolazine are similar in older and younger patients. Ranolazine is generally well tolerated, although adverse events, including constipation and dizziness, tend to be more common in patients >70 years old than in younger patients. Ranolazine increases the

QT interval slightly, but a significant proarrhythmic effect has not been reported.

Revascularization

Adults >65 years old currently account for over half of all PCIs and coronary bypass operations performed in the United States, and both of these procedures are now routinely performed in octogenarians. In patients with chronic CAD, the principal indication for coronary revascularization is relief of symptoms to improve quality of life. In patients <70 years old, clinical trials conducted more than 20 years ago demonstrated that coronary bypass surgery decreased mortality relative to medical therapy in patients with stenosis of the left main coronary artery, in patients with severe multivessel CAD and LV systolic dysfunction, and in other patient subgroups. The applicability of these findings to the current population of older patients is unclear, especially in light of the availability of more effective medical treatments. In addition, neither coronary bypass surgery nor PCI has been shown to reduce the risk of MI in patients with stable CAD. Conversely, complication rates, including mortality, increase with age after both PCI and coronary bypass surgery, especially among patients >80 years old. However, despite the failure of revascularization procedures to reduce mortality or major coronary event rates in most patients with stable CAD, some trials of these interventions have demonstrated improved symptoms and quality of life in older patients in whom aggressive medical therapy did not elicit an adequate response (SOE=A). Therefore, it is appropriate to offer revascularization on an individualized basis to older patients with persistent symptoms and impaired quality of life attributable to coronary ischemia.

Several trials have compared PCI and coronary bypass surgery in patients who are suitable candidates for either procedure. In general, long-term outcomes are similar with either approach. Short-term mortality, major complication rates (including cognitive dysfunction), hospital length of stay, and convalescence time are all increased with surgery relative to PCI, but the need for subsequent revascularization procedures and late mortality are higher after PCI. PCI is also somewhat less effective in relieving symptoms (SOE=A). Some studies suggest that in selected patients with diabetes, surgery may be associated with better outcomes than either PCI or medical therapy. Overall, in choosing between revascularization procedures, factors favoring PCI include severe CAD that is amenable to complete revascularization by PCI, increased risk of perioperative complications (eg, multiple comorbid conditions, renal insufficiency, frailty), and personal preference to avoid a major operation. Factors favoring bypass surgery include more severe CAD (especially if complete revascularization by PCI is unlikely), high-risk coronary anatomy (eg, left main disease or high-grade stenosis of the proximal left anterior descending artery not suitable for PCI), personal preference to minimize the need for subsequent revascularization procedures, and possibly diabetes. In all cases, the benefits and risks of all major therapeutic options—continued medical therapy, PCI, or bypass surgery—should be discussed in detail with the patient and family before deciding the best course of treatment.

An additional important consideration in assessing the risk of bypass surgery is the potential for postoperative cognitive impairment and functional decline. Up to 50% of older patients undergoing bypass surgery using extracorporeal circulation experience measurable cognitive impairment after surgery (SOE=B). Although complete recovery occurs in most patients within 3–6 months, a small percentage has persistent cognitive dysfunction. Bypass surgery performed without extracorporeal circulation (so-called "off pump" surgery) has been associated with a lower incidence of postoperative cognitive dysfunction in some but not all studies and should be considered when technically feasible. Functional decline is also common after major cardiac surgery, and return to the preoperative functional status often takes several months, with some patients experiencing persistent irreversible functional loss. To minimize functional deficits, rehabilitation should be started in the hospital as soon as possible after surgery, and patients should be referred to a structured cardiac rehabilitation program after hospital discharge whenever possible.

Valvular Heart Disease

Valvular heart diseases include aortic stenosis (AS), aortic regurgitation (AR), mitral stenosis (MS), and mitral regurgitation (MR).

Epidemiology

The prevalence of AS increases with age, approaching 15% in octogenarians, and AS is the most common valvular abnormality requiring surgery in older adults. AS in patients >70 years old is usually due to fibrosis and calcification of a previously normal trileaflet aortic valve, rather than to a congenitally bicuspid valve or rheumatic disease, which are the most common causes of AS in middle-aged adults.

AR may be acute or chronic, and the incidence of both increases with age. Although up to 30% of older adults have some degree of AR detectable by echocardiography, in most cases it is mild or moderate in severity, and only rarely is it severe enough to require surgical intervention. The most common causes of acute AR in older adults include infective endocarditis, dissection of the ascending aorta, malfunction of a previously implanted prosthetic valve (eg, dehiscence or thrombosis), and chest trauma. Chronic AR may be due to pathology of the valvular apparatus (eg, calcific or rheumatic valve disease, prior endocarditis, chronic malfunction of a valve prosthesis) or to dilatation of the aortic root resulting in poor coaptation of the valve leaflets (from, eg, ascending aortic root aneurysm, sinus of Valsalva aneurysm, chronic ascending aortic dissection).

Rheumatic MS is uncommon in older adults in the United States, but occasionally patients in their 70s or 80s will present with symptoms attributable to previously undiagnosed rheumatic disease. Alternatively, the diagnosis may be established incidentally when a patient undergoes echocardiography for another reason (eg, new-onset atrial fibrillation). More commonly, MS in older adults is due to nonrheumatic calcification of the mitral valve annulus and subvalvular apparatus, leading to a narrowed orifice and decreased excursion of the valve leaflets.

MR of at least mild severity is present in up to one-third of older adults, but only a small proportion require surgical intervention. As with AR, MR may be acute or chronic. Causes of acute MR include papillary muscle dysfunction or rupture due to acute myocardial infarction, rupture of a chordae tendinae related to myxomatous degeneration (ie, mitral valve prolapse), and destruction of the valvular apparatus due to infective endocarditis. Chronic MR may be due to myxomatous degeneration, annular dilatation associated with ischemic or nonischemic dilated cardiomyopathy, mitral annular calcification, rheumatic mitral valve disease, or prior endocarditis.

Diagnosis

The echocardiogram is the study of choice for diagnosing valvular disorders. For AS, it is essential for assessing disease severity, evaluating left ventricular function, and determining the presence of associated valvular lesions. Moderate AS is indicated by an aortic jet velocity (AJV) of 3–4 meters/second or an aortic valve area (AVA) of 1–1.5 cm^2; severe AS is indicated by an AJV >4 meters/second or AVA <1 cm^2. Occasionally, technical considerations or the presence of severe LV dysfunction preclude accurate echocardiographic assessment of AS severity; in these cases, right- and left-heart catheterization is definitive.

In patients with acute severe AR, echocardiography demonstrates a short duration AR jet with rapid deceleration and premature closure of the mitral valve. In patients with severe chronic AR, the AR jet is typically more prominent and of longer duration, often persisting throughout diastole. The left ventricle is usually dilated, and there are signs of LV diastolic volume overload. In advanced cases, there may be evidence of LV systolic dysfunction, as evidenced by a reduced ejection fraction. Echocardiography is the definitive test for diagnosing MS, quantifying disease severity, and evaluating for the presence of other valvular lesions, especially MR. Severe MS is indicated by a mitral valve area <1 cm^2.

Echocardiography with Doppler assesses the cause and severity of either acute or chronic MR. Echocardiography also provides important information about left ventricular size and function, left atrial size, pulmonary artery pressure, and the presence and severity of other valvular lesions.

Clinical Features and Treatment

See Table 48.3.

Infective Endocarditis

See Infective Endocarditis in "Infectious Diseases," p 501.

HEART FAILURE

See "Heart Failure," p 395.

CARDIAC ARRHYTHMIAS

Epidemiology

Age-related changes in the cardiac conduction system, coupled with the increasing prevalence of cardiovascular diseases at older age, lead to a progressive increase in the incidence and prevalence of conduction abnormalities and heart rhythm disturbances in older adults. In a cohort of 1,372 healthy adults ≥65 years old participating in the Baltimore Longitudinal Study on Aging (BLSA), >90% of men and women demonstrated supraventricular ectopic activity and >75% demonstrated ventricular ectopic activity on 24-hour ambulatory electrocardiographic recordings. In addition, almost 50% of men and women exhibited short runs of supraventricular tachycardia, while 13% of men and 4% of women had three or more consecutive ventricular premature depolarizations. In contrast, <0.5% of men and women in this cohort had runs of five or more beats of ventricular tachycardia. In a related study, approximately 4% of women >60 years old developed supraventricular tachycardia (SVT) during an exercise test, whereas the proportion of men developing SVT with exercise was found to increase with age, approaching 15% in those ≥80 years old.

Table 48.3—Cardiac Valvular Conditions

Condition	Symptoms	Findings	Treatment
Aortic stenosis (AS)	Angina, DOE, heart failure, light-headedness, presyncope/syncope	*Physical examination*: mid/late systolic ejection murmur radiating to carotids, S4 gallop, left ventricular heave *ECG*: LVH	*Medical*: no effective therapy *Percutaneous*: transcatheter aortic valve implantation in selected patients at high surgical risk *Surgical*: AVR[a] indicated for severe AS with symptoms, bioprosthetic valves preferred in older patients
Aortic regurgitation (AR)	Can be acute or chronic; asymptomatic or minimally symptomatic in mild/moderate AR; DOE, heart failure, angina in severe AR	*Physical examination*: ↑ pulse pressure, bounding/collapsing pulses, diastolic decrescendo murmur, systolic ejection murmur *ECG*: LVH (severe chronic AR), tachycardia (acute AR) *Chest radiograph*: cardiomegaly (severe chronic AR), pulmonary congestion (acute AR)	*Medical* (less severe cases): control of hypertension and other cardiac risk factors; vasodilator therapy with nifedipine, hydralazine, or ACE inhibitor as alternative to AVR in severe chronic AR (SOE=D) *Surgical*: AVR[a] indicated for acute severe AR complicated by heart failure or hemodynamic instability, and for chronic AR with onset of heart failure, LVEF <50%, or left ventricular end-systolic dimension ≥5.5 cm
Mitral stenosis (MS)	Gradually worsening DOE early, orthopnea and leg edema late, progressive decline in exercise capacity	*Physical examination*: early diastolic opening snap, low-pitched ("rumbling") diastolic murmur at apex, pulmonary hypertension, right heart failure	*Medical*: diuretics for volume overload and β-blockers for decreased exercise tolerance *Percutaneous*: balloon valvuloplasty safe and effective, but most older adults are not good candidates because of extensive calcification and commissural fusion or concomitant mitral regurgitation *Surgical*: MVR[a] effective but with 5%–15% operative mortality in older patients
Mitral regurgitation (MR)	Can be acute or chronic; marked shortness of breath, orthopnea in acute severe MR; progressive DOE in chronic MR	*Physical examination*: pulmonary rales, tachycardia, narrow pulse pressure, S3, and short harsh systolic murmur in acute severe MR; holosystolic murmur radiating to axilla, S3, pulmonary hypertension, right heart failure in chronic severe MR	*Medical*: afterload reduction and aggressive control of hypertension *Percutaneous*: transcatheter mitral valve repair in selected patients *Surgical*: mitral valve repair preferred over MVR[a] (and for MVR bioprosthetic valves[b] are preferred over mechanical in older patients); all effective but with 5%–15% operative mortality in older patients. Surgical intervention is indicated: ■ Urgently for acute severe MR with heart failure ■ At onset of symptoms or with LVEF of <60% or left ventricular end-systolic dimension ≥4 cm for chronic severe MR (SOE=B) ■ When mitral valve repair is deemed likely to be successful in asymptomatic patients with chronic severe MR and an LVEF ≥60% (SOE=B) ■ With increased pulmonary artery pressure or new-onset atrial fibrillation in patients with chronic severe MR and an LVEF ≥60% (SOE=C)

NOTE: DOE = dyspnea on exertion; LVH = left ventricular hypertrophy; LVEF = left ventricular ejection fraction; AVR = aortic valve replacement; MVR = mitral valve replacement

[a] Older adults being considered for AVR and MVR should have coronary angiography first because significant coronary artery disease is present in >50% of patients.

[b] After MVR with bioprosthetic valve, anticoagulation to maintain INR of 2–3 is recommended for 3 months, followed by maintenance therapy with aspirin 75–100 mg/d in the absence of risk factors for thromboembolism (SOE=C).

In the absence of structural heart disease, the presence of supraventricular and ventricular arrhythmias had no effect on mortality or the incidence of cardiac events in BLSA participants, except that exercise-induced SVT was associated with an increased risk of developing atrial fibrillation during follow-up. Conversely, in patients with prevalent cardiovascular disease, increased ventricular (but not supraventricular) ectopy was associated with an increased risk of cardiovascular mortality. In addition, although patients with preexisting atrial fibrillation were excluded from the BLSA ambulatory monitoring study, atrial fibrillation, whether paroxysmal or persistent, has been shown to be an independent predictor of increased mortality in both men and women (SOE=A).

Age-related degenerative changes in and around the sinoatrial and atrioventricular (AV) nodes lead to an increase in bradyarrhythmias with advancing age. Although resting heart rate is unaffected by age in healthy individuals, the incidence and prevalence of sinus node dysfunction ("sick sinus syndrome") and AV-nodal block increase progressively with age. As a result, >75% of permanent pacemakers are implanted in patients ≥65 years old, and approximately half are in patients ≥75 years old. The prevalence of infranodal conduction disorders, including left anterior fascicular block and left and right bundle-branch block, also increases with age.

Atrial Fibrillation

Atrial fibrillation (AF) is the most common sustained arrhythmia encountered in clinical practice. The incidence and prevalence of AF increase exponentially with age, such that the prevalence of AF in octogenarians is approximately 10%. Among older patients with valvular heart disease or HF, the prevalence of AF is even higher, approaching 30%. The prevalence of AF is higher in men than in women, and higher in whites than in other racial and ethnic subgroups. Currently, >50% of patients with AF are ≥75 years old, and it is projected that by 2050 half of all adults with AF will be ≥80 years old. As noted above, AF is an independent predictor of increased mortality in older adults, conferring relative risks of 1.10–1.15 in men and 1.20–1.25 in women. The proportion of strokes attributable to AF also increases exponentially with age: AF accounts for about 1.5% of strokes in patients 50–59 years old but 23.5% of strokes in patients 80–89 years old. In addition, women with AF are at increased risk of stroke relative to men, especially after age 75, and the relative risk of stroke in women compared with that in men is approximately 1.8 (ie, an 80% greater risk) in this age group.

Clinical Features

Symptoms related to AF are highly variable. Most commonly, patients experience palpitations, shortness of breath, or impaired exercise tolerance. However, some patients are entirely asymptomatic, while others present with acute pulmonary edema. Less commonly, stroke, transient ischemic attack, or an acute coronary syndrome may be the initial manifestation. Physical examination reveals an irregularly irregular rhythm with heart rates ranging from <60 beats per minute (eg, in patients with sinoatrial dysfunction and in those taking a β-blocker) to >150 beats per minute. Increased systolic blood pressure is a common but nonspecific finding. Pulmonary crackles may be present in patients with acute HF, while a heart murmur may be heard in patients with valvular heart disease. Rarely, an enlarged or nodular thyroid may be detected, or signs of deep venous thrombosis may be evident, because hyperthyroidism and venous thromboembolism predispose to this dysrhythmia.

Diagnosis

In patients with ongoing AF, the standard 12-lead electrocardiogram is diagnostic. Additional laboratory studies should include evaluation of serum electrolytes (especially potassium and magnesium) and an assessment of thyroid function. A transthoracic echocardiogram is indicated in all patients with new-onset AF to evaluate LV size and function, left atrial size, pulmonary artery pressure, and the cardiac valves. Further evaluation in selected cases might include a chest radiograph, serial cardiac biomarker proteins to exclude acute MI, a brain natriuretic peptide level, a D-dimer level, lower-extremity venous Dopplers, and an evaluation for pulmonary embolism.

Management

The objectives of therapy for AF include relieving symptoms and minimizing the risk of thromboembolic events, particularly stroke. The principal strategies for relieving symptoms are control of heart rate and maintenance of normal sinus rhythm. Several clinical trials comparing "rate control" with "rhythm control" have consistently demonstrated that in patients who are asymptomatic or minimally symptomatic, therapy directed at controlling the heart rate with AV-nodal blocking agents such as a β-blocker, diltiazem, verapamil, or digoxin, alone or in combination, is associated with fewer hospitalizations and favorable trends in stroke and mortality rates relative to therapy directed at maintaining sinus rhythm through the use of antiarrhythmic medications (SOE=A). Based on these findings, rate control in conjunction with systemic anticoagulation is the preferred treatment for AF patients with minimal or no symptoms. In general, β-blockers are the most effective agents for rate control, followed by diltiazem and verapamil. Digoxin is not recommended as first-line therapy but may be a useful adjunct in patients with persistently increased heart rates despite β-blockers or rate-lowering calcium channel blockers. Recently, the Rate Control Efficacy (RACE-II) trial found that lenient heart rate control (resting heart rate <110 beats per minute) was noninferior to strict heart rate control (resting heart rate <80 beats per minute) with respect to major clinical outcomes in patients with chronic AF (mean age 68 years). Based on these findings, guidelines have been modified to reflect the safety and efficacy of lenient rate control.

Patients who experience significant shortness of breath, fatigue, or exercise intolerance attributable to AF may be best managed with antiarrhythmic drug therapy aimed at maintaining sinus rhythm. Selection of an antiarrhythmic agent is challenging. Amiodarone is the most effective medication available, but it is associated with multiple adverse events (eg, thyroid dysfunction, neurologic disorders, pulmonary toxicity, ophthalmologic disturbances, liver function abnormalities), some potentially serious, as well as numerous drug interactions. Dronedarone, a newer agent, is less effective than amiodarone but has fewer adverse events. However, dronedarone is contraindicated in patients with advanced heart failure, and recent data indicate that dronedarone may be associated with increased mortality, stroke, and hospitalizations for heart failure in older patients with chronic (permanent) AF. Sotalol is less effective than amiodarone and is contraindicated in patients with significant renal insufficiency. Flecainide and propafenone are contraindicated in patients with CAD or heart failure. Quinidine and procainamide have limited efficacy and are accompanied by relatively frequent adverse events, while disopyramide is generally contraindicated in older adults because of its anticholinergic effects. Alternatives to antiarrhythmic drug therapy for maintenance of sinus rhythm include catheter ablation of the arrhythmogenic foci, usually through pulmonary vein isolation, and the surgical maze procedure. Pulmonary vein isolation has been associated with "cure" rates of >80% in younger patients with paroxysmal AF, but experience is limited with this procedure in older patients with persistent AF. Nonetheless, catheter ablation may be considered in older patients with refractory symptoms attributable to AF who have failed treatment with at least two antiarrhythmic drugs and who have normal or only mildly increased left atrial size. The surgical maze procedure results in long-term maintenance of sinus rhythm in >90% of cases but requires an open heart procedure; it is, however, a reasonable option in older patients with AF undergoing open heart surgery for other indications if a surgeon with expertise in performing the procedure is available.

All older patients with paroxysmal or persistent AF require stroke prophylaxis, regardless of whether a rate-control or rhythm-control strategy is adopted. Until recently, the two main options for stroke prophylaxis were warfarin titrated to maintain an INR of 2–3 and aspirin 75–325 mg/d, alone or in combination with clopidogrel. In patients with nonvalvular AF, numerous trials have shown that warfarin reduces the relative risk of stroke by 65%–70%, whereas aspirin reduces the relative risk of stroke by 20%–25% (SOE=A). Conversely, warfarin is associated with a higher risk of hemorrhagic complications, and older patients may have additional risk factors for major bleeding, such as colonic polyps or GI arteriovenous malformations. In patients 65–74 years old who are not considered candidates for warfarin, the addition of clopidogrel to aspirin reduces the risk of stroke but increases the risk of bleeding. In patients ≥75 years old, the value of aspirin, alone or in combination with clopidogrel, for reducing the risk of thromboembolic events is uncertain. For these reasons, the choice of warfarin versus aspirin (with or without clopidogrel) for stroke prophylaxis in older adults is often challenging. To aid in the decision-making process, it is helpful to stratify AF patients according to stroke risk, for which the $CHADS_2$ score is currently the most widely used risk-stratification scheme. $CHADS_2$ assigns 1 point for chronic heart failure, hypertension, age ≥75 years, and diabetes, and 2 points for prior stroke or transient ischemic attack. Annual stroke risk increases from about 2% in patients with a $CHADS_2$ score of 0 to about 18% in patients with a $CHADS_2$ score of 6. In general, patients with a $CHADS_2$ score of 0 are at low risk of stroke, and the risks of warfarin outweigh the benefits; therefore, aspirin therapy is appropriate in these patients. Patients with a $CHADS_2$ score of ≥2 are at significant risk of stroke, and in most cases the beneficial effects of warfarin outweigh the potential for adverse events. In patients with a $CHADS_2$ score of 1, either warfarin or aspirin is acceptable, but warfarin is preferred in older patients in the absence of contraindications. Note that all patients ≥75 years old have a $CHADS_2$ score of at least 1, and the vast majority will have a score of ≥2 (given the high prevalence of hypertension, diabetes, and heart failure in this age group), so that warfarin is the recommended therapy for stroke prevention in most older AF patients.

More recently, an updated risk stratification scheme, CHA2DS2-VASc, has been shown to be more accurate than the $CHADS_2$ score in identifying patients at low risk of stroke. CHA2DS2-VASc assigns 2 points for age ≥75 years, 1 point for age 65–74 years, 1 point for vascular disease (coronary, peripheral, or aortic), and 1 point for female sex. Using CHA2DS2-VASc, all women ≥65 years old and all men ≥75 years old have a score of at least 2 and are therefore candidates for systemic anticoagulation.

One of the most common reasons for not prescribing warfarin in older patients with AF is concern about the risk of falls and the potential for serious bleeding complications, particularly intracranial hemorrhage. However, in older patients with a $CHADS_2$ score of ≥2, the risk of thromboembolic stroke greatly exceeds the risk of fall-related intracranial bleeding, and it has been estimated that a patient would have to fall almost 300 times in 1 year for the risk of intracranial hemorrhage to outweigh the benefit of stroke prevention. Therefore, in most cases the perception of high fall risk alone is insufficient justification for withholding warfarin.

Three newer oral antithrombotic agents have been investigated for use in stroke prophylaxis in patients with AF: dabigatran, rivaroxaban, and apixaban. Dabigatran is a direct thrombin inhibitor that is more effective than warfarin for reducing stroke risk and is also associated with a lower risk of intracranial hemorrhage. After oral administration, dabigatran has a predictable anticoagulant effect. As a result, it can be given as a fixed dose without laboratory monitoring. In addition, drug-drug and drug-food interactions are substantially less frequent than with warfarin. Disadvantages of dabigatran include twice-daily dosing, relatively short duration of action (ie, missing doses may lead to subtherapeutic anticoagulation), inability to routinely monitor level of anticoagulation (the INR is unreliable and not recommended), lack of reversibility in case of bleeding or other adverse events, requirement for dosage adjustment in patients with renal impairment (see below), and higher cost than warfarin. The most common adverse events with dabigatran are bleeding and dyspepsia, and recent reports have raised concern that older adults may be at increased risk of serious bleeding with dabigatran. The recommended dosage of dabigatran for patients with relatively preserved renal function (creatinine clearance ≥30 mL/min) is 150 mg q12h. For patients with creatinine clearances of 15–30 mL/min, the recommended dosage is 75 mg q12h. Dabigatran is not recommended for patients with more severe renal insufficiency. In summary, although dabigatran offers several advantages over warfarin, its role in the management of older patients with AF remains uncertain, and additional experience with this agent is needed, particularly in patients >75–80 years old.

Rivaroxaban and apixaban are orally active reversible inhibitors of coagulation factor Xa. In a large randomized trial comparing rivaroxaban with warfarin in over 14,000 patients with AF, of whom 77% were 65 years or older and 38% were 75 years or older, rivaroxaban was found to be noninferior to warfarin with respect to both prevention of thromboembolic events and bleeding complications. Results were similar in older and younger patients. Although bleeding risk was higher in older patients, the net benefit was similar across the age spectrum. The recommended dosage of rivaroxaban is 20 mg/d for patients with a creatinine clearance ≥50 mL/min and 15 mg/d for patients with a creatinine clearance of 15–50 mL/min; rivaroxaban is not recommended for patients with more severe renal impairment. More recently, a large randomized trial involving more than 18,000 patients with AF (median age 70 years, 31% were ≥75 years old) compared apixaban with warfarin. Overall, apixaban was superior to warfarin with respect to thromboembolic events, major bleeding complications, and mortality. Results were consistent across age groups, and there was a clear advantage of apixaban both in patients 65–74 years old and in those ≥75 years old. The dose of apixaban in this study was 5 mg twice daily (2.5 mg twice daily in patients with 2 or more of the following: age ≥80 years old, weight ≤60 kg, and creatinine ≥1.5 mg/dL). At the time of this writing, apixaban has not been approved for use in the United States. As with other antithrombotic agents, the main adverse events associated with rivaroxaban and apixaban are bleeding complications. Other adverse events appear to be relatively infrequent, although additional experience is needed in a broader range of older patients with higher comorbidity burden than those enrolled in the clinical trials. Costs of these agents are also likely to be substantially higher than generic warfarin. Despite these cautions, it seems likely that newer antithrombotic agents will play an increasingly important role in the management of older patients with AF over the next several years.

Other Supraventricular Arrhythmias

Atrial flutter most often occurs in older patients with concomitant AF, and for this reason management is similar to that for AF as discussed above. Occasionally, patients have incessant atrial flutter without evidence of AF. Patients with symptomatic persistent atrial flutter in whom response to medical therapy is not satisfactory should be considered for catheter ablation of the atrial flutter focus. This procedure is successful in alleviating atrial flutter in >70% of cases, although some patients subsequently develop atrial fibrillation.

Atrial tachycardia, AV-nodal reentrant tachycardia, accessory pathway-mediated SVT, and multifocal atrial tachycardia are less common than AF and atrial flutter in older patients, especially after age 75. Management is similar for older and younger patients with these arrhythmias and generally involves treatment of the underlying condition and pharmacotherapy aimed at rate control or arrhythmia suppression. In selected patients with recurrent symptomatic episodes, antiarrhythmic medications or catheter ablation may be considered.

Ventricular Arrhythmias

In general, frequent ventricular premature beats, ventricular couplets, and short runs of nonsustained ventricular tachycardia require no specific therapy unless highly symptomatic, in which case β-blockers are the medications of first choice. Patients with longer episodes of ventricular tachycardia associated with dizziness or syncope should be referred to a cardiologist or electrophysiologist for consideration of antiarrhythmic drug therapy or an implantable cardiac defibrillator. In addition, patients with New York Heart Association class II–III heart failure, an LV ejection fraction of ≤35%, and a remaining life expectancy of at least 1 year may be considered for an implantable cardiac defibrillator (see "Heart Failure," p 395), regardless of whether ventricular arrhythmias are clinically manifest.

Bradyarrhythmias

Increasing age is associated with a progressive increase in the incidence and prevalence of bradyarrhythmias. Patients with mild bradycardia (resting heart rate 50–60 beats per minute) are often asymptomatic; indeed, bradycardia may protect against the development of angina pectoris in patients with CAD. Patients with more marked bradycardia (resting heart rate 40–50 beats per minute) may experience fatigue, lightheadedness (especially on standing), or reduced exercise tolerance. Presyncope or syncope may occur in patients with profound bradycardia, manifested by a heart rate of <40 beats per minute or asystolic pauses of ≥3 seconds, whether due to sinus node dysfunction or heart block within the AV node or infranodal conduction system.

Diagnostic evaluation of patients with suspected symptomatic bradycardia should start with exclusion of significant electrolyte abnormalities, measurement of the thyrotropin level to exclude hypothyroidism, and a review of the patient's medications (including OTC medications and dietary supplements). The most commonly used medications associated with bradycardia in older adults are β-blockers (including eye drops), diltiazem, verapamil, clonidine, amiodarone and other antiarrhythmic agents, and cholinesterase inhibitors. In patients with orthostatic hypotension, presyncope, or syncope, blood pressure should be measured in the supine, sitting, and standing positions. Detection of significant orthostatic hypotension should prompt a search for potentially treatable causes, including adverse events of medication(s), dehydration, or autonomic dysfunction (eg, due to diabetes, amyloidosis, parkinsonism, or other neurologic disorders). Patients with presyncope or syncope should undergo carotid sinus massage to evaluate for carotid hypersensitivity. An abnormal response to carotid massage is defined as unequivocal reproduction of the patient's symptoms (eg, syncope), asystole ≥3 seconds, or a decrease in systolic blood pressure ≥50 mmHg in the absence of symptoms or ≥30 mmHg in association with symptoms (eg, dizziness, presyncope).

In patients with intermittent symptoms, it is essential to establish a correlation between symptoms and bradyarrhythmias before considering pacemaker implantation. If symptoms occur daily or almost every day, a 24–48 hour ambulatory monitor may be helpful for confirming or excluding bradycardia (or other heart rhythm disorder) as the proximate cause. In patients whose symptoms occur at least once a month (but not daily), a 30-day event monitor may provide a definitive diagnosis. In patients with rare (ie, less than monthly) but recurrent symptoms of a serious nature (eg, syncope with injury), an implantable loop recorder may be considered. These devices, which may be left in place for a year or longer, have increased diagnostic yield in patients with infrequent syncopal events. Head-up tilt testing may be useful in diagnosing vasovagal (neurocardiogenic) syncope in younger patients, but it is of limited use in older adults because of low specificity and a high prevalence of "false-positive" tests (see "Syncope," p 204).

Invasive electrophysiologic (EP) testing is not usually indicated for the diagnosis of syncope or bradyarrhythmias. However, in patients with recurrent unexplained syncope and a nondiagnostic noninvasive evaluation, EP testing may be helpful, especially in patients with CAD, cardiomyopathy, or with evidence of infranodal conduction system disease (eg, right or left bundle-branch block). In such cases, EP testing may distinguish syncope due to bradycardia (eg, high-grade infranodal AV block) from that due to a tachyarrhythmia (eg, sustained monomorphic ventricular tachycardia), thus facilitating appropriate therapy.

Management of bradycardia includes correction of any treatable causes (eg, hypothyroidism) and elimination of potentially offending medications, if possible. In patients with confirmed symptomatic bradycardia not amenable to conservative management, permanent pacemaker implantation is warranted. Class I indications for permanent pacing are listed in Table 48.4. In patients with sinus rhythm and preserved atrioventricular conduction (ie, normal PR interval and narrow QRS complex), atrial pacing is the preferred pacing mode. Patients with sinus rhythm but impaired atrioventricular conduction are often best served by dual-chamber (ie, atrial and ventricular) pacing, whereas patients with bradycardia in the context of atrial fibrillation or atrial flutter should receive a single-chamber ventricular pacemaker. Dual-chamber pacemakers (often referred to as DDD or DVI pacemakers in accordance with the universal pacemaker code) have been associated with reduced incidence of atrial fibrillation and heart failure relative to single-chamber ventricular pacemakers (VVI), but beneficial effects on mortality and stroke have not been demonstrated.

Tachy-Brady Syndrome

The tachy-brady syndrome is a common variant of "sick sinus syndrome," in which patients manifest both tachyarrhythmias (most commonly SVT or atrial fibrillation) and bradyarrhythmias, either or both of which can result in symptoms. Treatment of the tachyarrhythmias with AV-nodal blocking agents or antiarrhythmic medications often exacerbates symptoms related to bradycardia, for which pacemaker implantation may be required.

PERIPHERAL ARTERIAL DISEASE

Peripheral arterial disease (PAD) encompasses disorders of the abdominal aorta, renal and mesenteric arteries, and the iliofemoral-popliteal arterial tree. The prevalence of PAD increases with age and is higher in men than in women. In one study, the prevalence of PAD increased from 5.6% in adults 38–59 years old, to 15.9% in adults 60–69 years old, and to 33.8% in adults 70–82 years old. In another study, the prevalence of symptomatic PAD in nursing-home residents with a mean age of 81 years was 32% in men and 26% in women. In addition to age, risk factors for PAD include hypertension, diabetes, cigarette smoking, and to a lesser extent in older adults, family history.

Abdominal aortic aneurysms (AAA) are usually asymptomatic in the early stages. As the aneurysm enlarges, patients may notice abdominal pulsations or experience back pain or abdominal discomfort. Symptoms of leg PAD include claudication with exertion and skin changes related to chronically impaired circulation. In advanced cases, rest pain, ulcers, or dry gangrene may develop. Physical findings associated with PAD may include a pulsatile abdominal mass, bruits over the renal or femoral arteries (or both), diminished or absent peripheral pulses, and skin changes ranging from hair loss and hyperpigmentation to ulcers and gangrene.

Diagnosis

It is estimated that at least 50% of patients with PAD are either asymptomatic or attribute their symptoms to another disorder (eg, arthritis); this proportion is likely even higher in older adults because of a more sedentary lifestyle. Diagnosis of PAD therefore requires a high index of suspicion and a proactive approach. Current guidelines recommend a formal history and physical examination to screen for symptoms and signs of PAD in all adults 50–69 years old with risk factors for atherosclerosis, as well as in all individuals ≥70 years old with or without risk factors (SOE=C). Men ≥60 years old with a family history of AAA and men 65–75 years old who have ever smoked should undergo an abdominal ultrasound to screen for the presence of AAA (SOE=B).

Individuals with symptoms or physical findings suggestive of PAD should undergo assessment of the ankle-brachial index (ABI), the ratio of the systolic blood pressure obtained at the ankle to the blood pressure obtained over the ipsilateral brachial artery. A normal ABI is 1.0–1.4, and an ABI <0.9 has been reported to be 95% sensitive and 99% specific for leg PAD. An ABI of 0.91–0.99 is considered borderline low, while an ABI >1.4 is usually associated with stiff, noncompressible arteries, which are commonly seen in older patients with atherosclerosis or long-standing hypertension. An ABI <0.40 is generally associated with critical PAD and severely impaired perfusion of the distal limb.

Patients with moderate or severe symptoms and an abnormal ABI should undergo additional evaluation if percutaneous or surgical revascularization is being contemplated. Imaging procedures that may be useful in selected cases include Doppler flow velocity measurements, ultrasonic duplex scanning, magnetic resonance angiography, and CT angiography. If revascularization is indicated based on symptoms and the results of noninvasive testing, contrast angiography is usually required before performing the revascularization procedure.

Table 48.4—Arrhythmic or Conduction Disturbance Indications for Permanent Pacemaker Implantation

- Symptomatic bradycardia due to sinus node dysfunction (SOE=C), second-degree atrioventricular (AV) block (SOE=B), or third-degree AV block (SOE=C)
- Asystole ≥3 sec or any escape rate <40 beats per minute in awake patients with advanced second- or third-degree AV block, whether symptomatic or asymptomatic (SOE=C)
- Type II second-degree AV block (SOE=B), intermittent third-degree AV block (SOE=B), or alternating bundle-branch block (SOE=C) in patients with chronic bifascicular or trifascicular block
- Recurrent syncope caused by carotid sinus stimulation associated with asystole ≥3 sec in the absence of medications that depress the sinus node or AV conduction (SOE=C)
- Symptomatic chronotropic incompetence (inability to increase heart rate commensurate with increased activity level) (SOE=C)
- Transient or persistent second- or third-degree infranodal block associated with bundle-branch block after acute myocardial infarction (SOE=B)
- Third-degree AV block after catheter ablation of the AV junction (SOE=C)
- Conditions requiring medications that result in symptomatic bradycardia (SOE=C)

Treatment

PAD is considered a CAD risk-equivalent, indicating that patients with PAD have a ≥20% risk of experiencing a new coronary event within 10 years (SOE=A); in patients with comorbid diabetes or established CAD, the risk is even higher. Indeed, most deaths in patients with PAD are attributable to CAD or its complications (eg, heart failure, arrhythmias) rather than to PAD per se. The importance of PAD as a risk marker for CAD provides the rationale for the proactive approach to diagnosis described above, as well as for the aggressive treatment of prevalent cardiovascular risk factors. Thus, the target LDL-cholesterol level in patients with PAD is <100 mg/dL, and blood pressure should be treated in accordance with current guidelines (see "Hypertension," p 402). Smoking cessation should be strongly encouraged, and patients who indicate an interest in quitting should be offered counseling in combination with drug therapy (see "Addictions," p 336).

In addition to risk factor management, patients with significant leg PAD should engage in a regular exercise program, preferably under supervision (SOE=A). Exercise should include walking for at least 30–45 minutes at least 3 times a week for a minimum of 12 weeks (SOE=A). Data from multiple randomized trials and at least one large meta-analysis indicate that the beneficial effects of exercise on maximal walking capacity exceed those of available pharmacotherapies. In addition, the greatest improvements in walking ability occur in individuals who exercise to near maximal pain threshold for a period of at least 6 months.

Pharmacotherapy for PAD includes aspirin 75–325 mg/d to reduce the risk of MI, stroke, or vascular death (SOE=A). Clopidogrel 75 mg/d is more effective than aspirin in reducing cardiovascular risk in patients with PAD, but it is also considerably more expensive. There is no evidence that the combination of aspirin and clopidogrel is superior to either agent alone. For these reasons, clopidogrel is recommended as a reasonable alternative to aspirin in selected patients (SOE=B). In addition to antiplatelet therapy, routine treatment with an ACE inhibitor or ARB for the prevention of cardiovascular events is reasonable in patients with symptomatic PAD (SOE=B).

Currently, the only pharmacologic agent that has been shown to improve symptoms and walking distance in patients with claudication is the phosphodiesterase inhibitor (type III) cilostazol. At dosages of 100 mg q12h, cilostazol increases maximal walking distance by 40%–60%, and a therapeutic trial of this agent is recommended for all patients with lifestyle-limiting claudication (SOE=A). Although cilostazol is generally well tolerated, it is not recommended in patients with heart failure. Pentoxifylline is another agent approved for use in patients with symptomatic PAD, but the clinical effectiveness of this drug is marginal and not well established (SOE=C).

Revascularization is indicated for patients with severe symptoms attributable to PAD that have not responded to a reasonable trial of aggressive risk factor modification, exercise, and pharmacotherapy. Revascularization is also indicated for patients with critical-limb ischemia, defined as rest pain, ulceration, or gangrene; in this context, revascularization has been shown not only to improve symptoms but also to reduce the likelihood of subsequent amputation. The choice of revascularization procedure, ie, percutaneous transluminal angioplasty with or without stenting versus surgical revascularization, depends on lesion location and severity, likelihood of success, risk of major complications, and experience and technical expertise of the interventionalist and surgeon. Importantly, these two therapeutic approaches should be viewed as complementary rather than competing strategies, and the choice of revascularization procedure should be tailored to individual patient circumstances and preferences.

Indications for AAA repair include development of symptoms, rapid aneurysmal dilatation detected during serial assessments (≥1 cm in 1 year), and aneurysms ≥5.5 cm in diameter. Patients with asymptomatic AAAs 4–5.4 cm in diameter should undergo repeat evaluations at intervals of 6–12 months. The choice of open or endovascular surgical repair of AAAs is based on location of the lesion and patient comorbidities and prognosis. Open repair is favored for suprarenal AAAs and for patients with fewer comorbidities and a remaining life expectancy of >10 years, because this procedure has reduced rates of long-term leakage and rupture (SOE=B). Endovascular repair is suitable for patients with infrarenal AAAs and for those who have a higher surgical risk or shorter remaining life expectancy, because it is associated with lower perioperative complications and mortality (SOE=B).

VENOUS THROMBOEMBOLIC DISEASE

Older adults are at markedly increased risk of developing venous thromboembolic disease (VTED), including deep venous thrombosis (DVT) and pulmonary embolism (PE), because of age-related changes in the hemostatic system that predispose to thrombosis; venous stasis related to illness, injuries (eg, hip fracture), and immobility (especially hospitalization and residence in long-term care); incompetency of the superficial and deep veins, including failure of the venous valves; and the high prevalence of systemic illnesses associated with thrombogenesis (eg, heart failure, cancer, neurologic diseases). As a result, the incidence and prevalence of both DVT and PE increase exponentially with age.

Screening and Prophylaxis

In long-term care settings, screening for VTED risk is recommended every 5–7 days. VTED risk factors include age >60 years old, active cancer, acute infection, indwelling central venous catheter, chronic lung disease, dehydration, history of VTED, having a first-degree relative with VTED, heart failure, hypercoagulable state, immobility, inflammatory bowel disease, obesity, rheumatoid arthritis, and treatment with an aromatase inhibitor, hormone therapy, megestrol acetate, selective estrogen-receptor modulator, or erythroid-stimulating agent to a hemoglobin concentration >12 g/dL. Immobility is defined as the presence of ≥1 of the following: being bedridden or bedridden except for bathroom privileges, unable to walk at least 10 feet, recent reduction in ability to walk at least 10 feet for at least 72 hours, and having a lower limb cast. For some risk factors (eg, fractures), VTED prophylaxis is recommended for 35 days. If the individual has ≥2 risk factors and is immobile, prophylaxis for 10 days or until the immobility resolves is recommended. If there is immobility but only a single risk factor, consideration should be given to pneumatic compression with ongoing risk assessment.

VTED prophylaxis with subcutaneous unfractionated or low-molecular-weight heparin, fondaparinux, or intermittent pneumatic compression of the calves is indicated in all hospitalized older adults who are not fully ambulatory, as well as in transitional care and long-term care residents at increased risk of VTED, as outlined above. For VTED prophylaxis in the perioperative setting, see Perioperative Care, Table 14.3.

Diagnosis

Symptoms and signs of VTED are similar in older and younger patients, but it is important to recognize that most patients with DVT or PE, or both, are asymptomatic; therefore, a high index of suspicion for these conditions must be maintained, particularly in hospitalized patients and in residents of transitional-care facilities and nursing homes. The utility of most routine tests, including blood tests, arterial blood gases, chest radiographs, and ECGs, for diagnosing VTED is quite low, and the presence of "normal" findings on each of these tests does not exclude a diagnosis of DVT or PE. The plasma D-dimer level, when performed using ELISA, has a high sensitivity for VTED but very low specificity in older adults; therefore, a normal D-dimer level in an older patient with low to intermediate clinical suspicion for VTED essentially excludes the diagnosis. Noninvasive tests for DVT include leg venous Dopplers, impedance plethysmography, and CT of the legs; rarely, contrast venography may be required to establish the diagnosis. When positive, noninvasive tests provide presumptive evidence for DVT, but negative tests do not exclude DVT or PE, especially in patients for whom the clinical suspicion is high. Similarly, ventilation/perfusion lung scanning and spiral CT of the chest are useful when the findings are unequivocally normal or abnormal. However, indeterminant ventilation/perfusion scans are common in older patients, and 10%–20% of patients with PE have false-negative spiral CT scans. Therefore, in patients with high clinical suspicion for PE but negative noninvasive evaluations, pulmonary angiography should be performed as the definitive diagnostic procedure. Although clinicians are often reluctant to recommend pulmonary angiography, data from the PIOPED study indicate that this procedure is generally well tolerated by older adults, and that the risks of the procedure are lower than those of either empiric anticoagulation in patients without PE, or not anticoagulating patients with PE.

Management

Treatment of acute DVT or PE includes intravenous unfractionated heparin to maintain the activated partial thromboplastin time in the range of 50–70 seconds (1.5–2 times the control value), full-dose low-molecular-weight heparin adjusted for weight and renal function, or subcutaneous fondaparinux adjusted for weight and renal function (all SOE=A). Warfarin should be started and heparin or fondaparinux continued until the INR is 2–3 with at least 24-hour overlap. Patients who are not candidates for anticoagulation should be considered for an inferior vena caval filter, recognizing that although such devices reduce the risk of PE, the risk of recurrent DVT and postphlebotic syndrome may be increased. The duration of warfarin therapy depends on the risk of recurrent VTED. In patients with a first episode of DVT or PE due to a reversible factor (eg, immobilization in the hospital), warfarin should be continued for 3 months. In patients who develop DVT or PE in the absence of an identifiable or reversible cause, warfarin therapy should be continued for at least 6–12 months (SOE=B), and possibly indefinitely (SOE=C). Ultrasonography can be used to document recanalization of the vein after a limited course of anticoagulation; if no recanalization is observed, a longer course of anticoagulation should be strongly considered. Because the efficacy of warfarin for the prevention of recurrent VTED is reduced in patients with cancer, low-molecular-weight heparin is recommended for the first 3–6 months of therapy, followed by warfarin indefinitely (or until the cancer is resolved). In patients with recurrent VTED, long-term treatment with warfarin is recommended, and placement of an inferior vena caval filter should be considered in patients with recurrent VTED despite therapeutic anticoagulation. In addition to the above measures, regular exercise, such as walking, is recommended to reduce the risk of recurrent DVT, and elastic compression stockings are recommended for up to 2 years after an episode of DVT to reduce the risk of postphlebitic syndrome.

REFERENCES

- Dumont C J, Keeling AW, Bourguignon C, et al. Predictors of vascular complications post diagnostic cardiac catheterization and percutaneous coronary interventions. *Dimens Crit Care Nurs.* 2006;25(3):137–142.

- Fuster V, Ryden LE, Cannom DS, et al. 2011 ACCF/AHA/HRS focused updates incorporated into the ACC/AHA/ESC 2006 Guidelines for the management of patients with atrial fibrillation. *J Am Coll Cardiol.* 2011;57(11):e101–e198.

- Rooke TW, Hirsch AT, Misra S, et al. 2011 ACCF/AHA focused update of the guideline for the management of patients with peripheral artery disease (updating the 2005 guideline). *J Am Coll Cardiol.* 2011;58(19):2020–2045.

- Somes J. Syndromes of "holiday heart." *J Emerg Nurs.* 2011;37(6);577–579.

- Zipes DP, Camm AJ, Borggrefe M, et al. ACC/AHA/ESC 2006 Guidelines for the management of patients with ventricular arrhythmias and the prevention of sudden cardiac death. *Circulation.* 2006;114(10):e385–484.

CHAPTER 49—HEART FAILURE

Chapters

KEY POINTS

- Heart failure (HF) is the leading cause of hospitalization in older adults and a major source of chronic disability.
- Compared with younger patients, older patients with HF are more likely to be women and more likely to have preserved left ventricular systolic function.
- ACE inhibitors, angiotensin-receptor blockers, β-blockers, and aldosterone antagonists reduce morbidity and mortality from HF with reduced ejection fraction (systolic HF). Optimal medical therapy for HF with preserved ejection fraction (diastolic HF) is undefined.
- Optimal management of HF in older patients often requires a multidisciplinary approach.

EPIDEMIOLOGY

Heart failure (HF) affects more than 5.5 million Americans, and >650,000 new cases are diagnosed each year. The incidence and prevalence of HF increase progressively with age, and HF is the leading cause of hospitalization and rehospitalization in older adults. The median age of patients hospitalized with HF is 75 years, and approximately two-thirds of deaths attributable to HF occur in patients ≥75 years old. In addition, HF is a major cause of chronic disability and impaired quality of life in older adults, and it is a common factor contributing to loss of independence and admission to a long-term care facility. Although the incidence of HF is somewhat higher in men, women comprise slightly over half of prevalent HF cases.

ETIOLOGY AND PATHOPHYSIOLOGY

HF in older adults is often multifactorial in origin. Hypertension is the most common antecedent cardiovascular condition in both men and women with HF, and it is the principal cause of HF in 60%–70% of women. In men, 30%–40% of HF is attributable to hypertension, and a similar proportion is attributable to coronary artery disease (CAD). Other common causes of HF in older adults include valvular heart disease and nonischemic dilated cardiomyopathy. Less common causes include hypertrophic cardiomyopathy, restrictive cardiomyopathy (eg, amyloidosis), and pericardial disease.

The rising prevalence of HF with increasing age reflects the combination of age-related changes in cardiovascular structure and function that serve to diminish cardiovascular reserve, in conjunction with the rising prevalence of cardiovascular diseases with increasing age (especially hypertension and CAD) that predispose to HF. While up to 90% of HF patients <65 years old have low left ventricular (LV) ejection fraction (LVEF; ie, HF with reduced ejection fraction, henceforth referred to as systolic HF), approximately 40% of men and two-thirds of women >65 years old with HF have an LVEF ≥50% (ie, HF with preserved ejection fraction, henceforth referred to as diastolic HF). The rising prevalence of diastolic HF in older patients is due to age-associated changes in LV diastolic function, coupled with the increasing importance of hypertension as the etiologic mechanism for HF in older adults, particularly women.

Although this chapter uses the traditional nomenclature of "systolic" and "diastolic" heart failure, many experts prefer the terms "heart failure with reduced ejection fraction" and "heart failure with preserved ejection fraction," respectively. This preference reflects concerns about misleading connotations of the traditional labels. Virtually all patients with "systolic" HF also have diastolic dysfunction, and most patients with "diastolic" HF have systolic functional impairment as well.

CLINICAL FEATURES

As in younger patients, exertional shortness of breath, fatigue, orthopnea, and leg edema are the most common symptoms of HF in older adults. However, exertional symptoms may be less prominent in older adults because of a more sedentary lifestyle. Conversely, the prevalence of atypical symptoms increases with age, and older HF patients may present with decreased mental acuity, confusion, lethargy, irritability, anorexia, abdominal discomfort, or altered bowel function.

Classical physical findings of HF in younger patients include tachycardia, narrowed pulse pressure, increased jugular venous pressure, hepatojugular reflux, an S3 gallop, moist pulmonary crackles, diminished breath sounds at the lung bases (due to pleural effusions), and pitting edema of the legs. However, many or even all of these findings may be absent in older HF patients, especially those with diastolic HF, in whom an S3 gallop and signs of right-heart failure are not usually present. In addition, pulmonary crackles in older patients may be due to comorbid chronic lung disease or atelectasis, and peripheral edema may be due to hepatic or renal disease, venous insufficiency, hypoalbuminemia, or medications (especially calcium channel blockers).

In summary, the symptoms and signs of HF in older adults are often atypical and nonspecific, and it is therefore important for the clinician to maintain both a high index of suspicion and a healthy measure of skepticism when evaluating an older patient for possible HF.

DIAGNOSIS

The diagnosis of HF can usually be established on clinical grounds in patients who present with a constellation of classical symptoms and signs. Often, however, the diagnosis is uncertain, and additional supporting evidence is required.

The standard chest radiograph remains the most useful initial test for determining the presence of pulmonary congestion and pleural effusions, as well as for excluding pneumonia as a cause of shortness of breath in older adults. However, the chest radiograph may be difficult to interpret in older adults with chronic lung disease, kyphoscoliosis, or poor inspiratory effort, and the absence of pulmonary congestion on chest radiograph does not exclude a diagnosis of HF.

The ECG may show LV hypertrophy, acute ischemia or prior myocardial infarction, left atrial enlargement, or atrial fibrillation—all of which predispose to the development of HF—but the ECG is not usually helpful in establishing a diagnosis of either acute or chronic HF. Similarly, although it is appropriate to obtain a CBC, routine chemistry panel, thyroid studies, a urinalysis, and in selected cases, cardiac biomarker proteins (ie, troponin, creatine kinase) in patients with suspected HF, in most cases these tests are insufficient for confirming the diagnosis.

In recent years, B-type natriuretic peptide (BNP) and its precursor N-terminal pro-BNP (NT-proBNP) have proved to be of value in establishing the presence of HF and, in particular, in distinguishing shortness of breath due to HF from that attributable to noncardiac causes. However, BNP and NT-proBNP levels increase with age, especially in women, as well as with decreasing renal function. As a result, the specificity of increased levels of these peptides decreases with age, and the clinical significance of an isolated increased BNP or NT-proBNP level in an older adult may be difficult to interpret. Despite these caveats, a BNP level <100 pg/mL in an older adult with suspected acute HF makes the diagnosis very unlikely (likelihood ratio negative approximately 0.1), whereas a BNP level ≥500 pg/mL is consistent with active HF (likelihood ratio positive approximately 6).

Once a diagnosis of HF has been established, it is important to determine the cause and to assess LV function, because these factors often affect management. In most patients with recently diagnosed HF, an echocardiogram with Doppler is indicated for the assessment of left and right ventricular size, systolic and diastolic function, atrial size, left and right ventricular wall thicknesses, valve function, pulmonary artery pressure, and the pericardium. In patients with suspected CAD who are suitable candidates for revascularization, a stress test should be performed, followed by coronary angiography if the stress test indicates severe CAD, especially in a multivessel distribution.

MANAGEMENT

The goals of HF management are to decrease symptoms, improve quality of life, reduce acute exacerbations requiring hospitalization, and increase survival. Hypertension, hyperlipidemia, and diabetes should be treated in accordance with current guidelines. Smoking cessation should be strongly encouraged and supported if indicated, and alcohol intake should be limited to no more than 2 drinks/day in men and 1 drink/day in women. NSAIDs should be avoided because they promote water and sodium retention, and they antagonize the effects of diuretics and renin-angiotensin system inhibitors. CAD should be treated with anti-ischemic medications and, if indicated, percutaneous or surgical revascularization. Similarly, valvular lesions should be managed in accordance with established practice guidelines. Patients should be screened for anemia and thyroid dysfunction, and appropriate therapy should be initiated.

Nonpharmacologic Therapy

Patients should be counseled to restrict dietary sodium intake to no more than 2 g/d (SOE=C). Fluid restriction is not usually necessary except in patients with advanced HF or hyponatremia, but patients should be advised to avoid excess fluid intake (ie, the oft-quoted dictum to drink 8–10 glasses of water every day does not apply to individuals with HF, renal insufficiency, or other fluid-retaining states). Most patients with HF should also be advised to engage in regular exercise such as walking, stationary cycling, swimming, or water aerobics. Exercise duration and intensity should be adjusted to the individual patient's level of conditioning, severity of HF, and comorbidities, but should be gradually increased over time, if possible, to achieve 30–60 minutes of aerobic exercise most days of the week. These activities should be complemented

Table 49.1—Recommended Dosages of ACE Inhibitors, Angiotensin II Receptor Blockers, and β-Blockers in Patients with Heart Failure

Agent	Starting Dosage	Target Dosage
ACE Inhibitors		
Benazepril[a]	2.5 mg/d	40 mg/d
Captopril	6.25 mg q8h	50 mg q8h
Enalapril	2.5 mg/d	10–20 mg q12h
Fosinopril	5–10 mg/d	40 mg/d
Lisinopril	2.5–5 mg/d	20–40 mg/d
Moexipril[a]	3.75 mg/d	15 mg/d
Perindopril[a]	2 mg/d	8–16 mg/d
Quinapril	5 mg q12h	10–20 mg q12h
Ramipril	1.25–2.5 mg/d	10 mg/d
Trandolapril	1 mg/d	4 mg/d
Angiotensin II Receptor Blockers		
Azilsartan[a]	20–40 mg/d	80 mg/d
Candesartan	4 mg/d	32 mg/d
Eprosartan[a]	400 mg/d	400 mg q12h
Irbesartan[a]	75 mg/d	150–300 mg/d
Losartan[a]	25 mg/d	50–100 mg/d
Olmesartan[a]	20 mg/d	40 mg/d
Telmisartan[a]	20 mg/d	80 mg/d
Valsartan	40 mg q12h	160 mg q12h
β-Blockers		
Bisoprolol[b]	1.25 mg/d	10 mg/d
Carvedilol	3.125 mg q12h	25–50 mg q12h
Carvedilol ER	10 mg/d	80 mg/d
Metoprolol XL	12.5–25 mg/d	200 mg/d

[a] Not approved for heart failure by the FDA

[b] Not approved for heart failure by the FDA but has been shown to be effective in heart failure

by stretching and strengthening exercises, as well as by gait and balance exercises if indicated.

Patients should be instructed to keep an ongoing record of their daily weight. Weights should be obtained in the morning without clothes after going to the bathroom but before eating. A "dry weight" should be established (based on the home scale, not the office scale), and the patient should be instructed to contact the clinician if the weight varies by more than 2–3 pounds above or below the dry weight. Alternatively, selected patients may be provided with detailed instructions for self-adjustment of diuretic dosages based on daily weights.

Older patients with moderate or advanced HF, multiple comorbidities, or a recent HF exacerbation requiring hospitalization may benefit from participation in a structured HF disease management program. Such programs offer enhanced education and follow-up, usually by an HF nurse specialist or multidisciplinary team, in some cases supplemented by telemonitoring devices. They have been shown to reduce hospitalizations and inpatient costs, as well as to improve quality of life in older HF patients (SOE=A).

Pharmacotherapy of Systolic HF

ACE inhibitors, angiotensin-receptor blockers (ARBs), and β-blockers have been shown to improve outcomes and reduce mortality in multiple large prospective trials involving a broad range of HF patients with decreased LV systolic function (SOE=A), and these agents are now considered the cornerstone of therapy for systolic HF. Although older patients, especially those with multiple comorbid conditions, have been markedly under-represented in these trials, the available evidence indicates that the beneficial effects of these agents likely extend to older patients.

For ACE inhibitors approved for the treatment of HF, along with recommended initial and maintenance dosages, see Table 49.1. In general, treatment of older HF patients should be started at the lowest dosage and gradually titrated to the maintenance dosage as tolerated. Contraindications to ACE inhibitors include known intolerance to these agents, hyperkalemia (serum potassium ≥5.5 mEq/L), and severe renal insufficiency (estimated creatinine clearance <30 mL/min) in patients not currently undergoing dialysis. Common adverse events include cough in 5%–10% of patients during long-term treatment, mild worsening of renal function (often transient), hyperkalemia, hypotension, and GI distress. Renal function and potassium concentrations should be monitored at least weekly during initiation and titration of ACE inhibitor therapy.

ARBs are indicated as an alternative to ACE inhibitors in HF patients unable to tolerate the latter class of medications because of cough, allergic reactions, or GI disturbances. Contraindications and adverse events associated with these agents are otherwise similar to those of ACE inhibitors. In particular, the incidence of renal insufficiency, hyperkalemia, and hypotension are comparable with equivalent dosages of ACE inhibitors and ARBs. Combination therapy with an ACE inhibitor and ARB is not currently recommended because of an increased incidence of adverse events in the absence of a clear clinical benefit.

β-Blockers counteract the deleterious effects of chronic activation of the adrenergic nervous system in HF patients, and β-blockers have been shown to improve ventricular function and symptoms while reducing the risk of both sudden and nonsudden cardiac death (SOE=A). As with ACE inhibitors and ARBs, treatment should be started at the lowest available dosage and gradually titrated to the maintenance dosage over several weeks (Table 49.1). Contraindications to starting β-blocker therapy include severe decompensated HF, active bronchospastic lung disease, marked bradycardia (heart rate <45–50 beats per minute), relative hypotension (systolic blood pressure <90–100 mmHg), significant atrioventricular nodal block (PR interval

≥240 msec, or higher degrees of block), and known intolerance to β-blockers. Occasionally, HF symptoms will worsen on initiation or titration of a β-blocker (and patients should be warned about this possibility), but in most cases this is a transient phenomenon and the vast majority of HF patients (>80%) are able to tolerate long-term β-blocker therapy when judiciously initiated and titrated.

Diuretics are an essential component of HF therapy in most patients, and they remain the most effective agents for relief of congestion and edema. In general, the diuretic dosage should be adjusted to maintain euvolemia, manifested by the absence of pulmonary rales, an S_3 gallop, increased jugular venous pressure, hepatojugular reflux, and peripheral edema. Some clinicians recommend obtaining serial BNPs as a means of assessing volume status, with a BNP level <100–200 pg/mL indicative of optimal intravascular volume. Some patients with mild HF respond satisfactorily to a thiazide diuretic, but most require maintenance therapy with a loop diuretic, such as furosemide, bumetanide, or torsemide. Patients with advanced HF or concomitant renal insufficiency, or both, may be resistant to conventional dosages of loop diuretics; in these patients, the addition of metolazone at 2.5–10 mg/d is often effective, but careful monitoring of electrolytes is required. The principal adverse events associated with diuretic therapy are electrolyte disturbances, including hypokalemia, hyponatremia, and hypomagnesemia; close monitoring of these electrolytes, as well as renal function, is therefore warranted. Thiamine deficiency may occur during long-term treatment with loop diuretics and can contribute to apparent diuretic resistance. Although routine monitoring of thiamine levels is not currently recommended, supplemental thiamine in the form of a multivitamin is reasonable in older patients requiring long-term therapy with a loop diuretic (SOE=D). Older patients are also at increased risk of dehydration during diuretic treatment due to attenuation of the thirst response and diminished oral fluid intake, especially during periods of illness. Therefore, clinicians should remain vigilant for possible signs of dehydration, including excess weight loss during daily weight monitoring.

The aldosterone antagonist spironolactone has been shown to reduce mortality and hospitalizations in patients with New York Heart Association (NYHA) class III–IV HF (Table 49.2) and an LVEF <30% (SOE=A), with similar benefits in older and younger patients. Similarly, the selective aldosterone antagonist eplerenone has been associated with improved outcomes in patients with recent myocardial infarction complicated by HF or an LVEF <40% (SOE=A), and, more recently, in patients with NYHA class II HF and an LVEF ≤35% (SOE=A). Based on these studies, spironolactone 12.5–25 mg/d or eplerenone 25-50 mg/d is recommended in patients with moderate to severe LV dysfunction and persistent NYHA class II–IV HF symptoms despite triple-drug therapy with an ACE inhibitor (or ARB), β-blocker, and diuretic. Spironolactone and eplerenone are contraindicated in patients with serum creatinine ≥2.5 mg/dL or serum potassium ≥5 mEq/L. Older adults are at increased risk of worsening renal function and hyperkalemia during aldosterone antagonist therapy, and frequent monitoring of electrolytes and creatinine is necessary. Up to 10% of patients develop painful gynecomastia during long-term treatment with spironolactone; this adverse event is much less frequent with eplerenone.

Table 49.2—New York Heart Association Functional Class

Class	Symptoms
I	*No symptoms and no limitation in ordinary physical activity* Walking, climbing stairs, or doing household chores does not cause undue shortness of breath, palpitations, chest discomfort, or fatigue.
II	*Slight limitation of physical activity* Ordinary physical activity causes shortness of breath, palpitations, chest discomfort, or fatigue; able to walk >2 blocks and climb 2 flights of stairs.
III	*Marked limitation of physical activity* Less than ordinary physical activity (eg, walking <2 blocks) causes shortness of breath, palpitations, chest discomfort, or fatigue; no symptoms at rest.
IV	*Severe activity limitation* Unable to carry out any physical activity (eg, walking in the house, dressing, bathing, toileting) without shortness of breath, palpitations, chest discomfort, or fatigue; symptoms may be present at rest.

Digoxin improves symptoms and reduces HF hospitalizations in patients with chronic systolic HF but does not decrease mortality. Digoxin nevertheless remains a reasonable therapeutic option in patients with persistent limiting symptoms or recurrent hospitalizations, or both, who have not had a satisfactory response to the measures discussed above. Retrospective analyses based on a large randomized trial suggest that the optimal digoxin concentration for improving clinical outcomes is 0.5–0.9 ng/mL, which is substantially lower than the "therapeutic range" previously reported by most clinical laboratories. Therefore, digoxin should be dosed to maintain the digoxin concentration <1 ng/mL, and a dosage of 0.125 mg/d is likely to be sufficient in most older patients with relatively preserved renal function, while a lower dosage might be required in patients with moderate or severe renal insufficiency. Adverse effects of digoxin include nausea, visual disturbances, and cardiac arrhythmias (bradyarrhythmias as well as supraventricular and ventricular tachyarrhythmias). However, with appropriate monitoring of the serum digoxin concentration, serious digoxin toxicity is infrequent, and there is no convincing evidence that older patients are at increased risk of life-threatening digitalis intoxication. Amiodarone, quinidine, and verapamil, as well as several other medications, are associated with up to a 2-fold increase in serum digoxin concentrations when used concurrently, and the dosage of digoxin should be reduced by 50% in patients receiving these medications.

The combination of hydralazine-nitrates is recommended for HF patients with contraindications to ACE inhibitors and ARBs (eg, severe renal insufficiency), and in black Americans with advanced HF as an adjunct to ACE-inhibitor and β-blocker therapy. The starting dosage of hydralazine is 25–50 mg q8h, titrating to a maximal dosage of 100 mg q8h. The starting dosage of isosorbide dinitrate is 10 mg q8h titrating to a maximal dosage of 30–40 mg q8h. Common adverse events associated with hydralazine include palpitations, nausea, and dizziness; rarely, a drug-lupus syndrome may occur during prolonged therapy at high dosage (≥300 mg/d). The most common adverse event from isosorbide dinitrate is headache; this usually resolves with continued use.

In summary, optimal treatment of systolic HF usually requires a minimum of three medications and, in some cases, up to seven. In addition, because HF in older patients almost never occurs as an isolated disease process, almost all patients are taking one or more additional medications for other coexisting illnesses. Thus, pharmacotherapy of the older HF patient is problematic from the perspective of adherence, high potential for drug interactions and adverse events, and cost. Therefore, it is essential that therapy be individualized, taking into consideration the multiple and often competing factors that influence quality of life and other desirable clinical outcomes in older adults with multiple chronic illnesses and limited life expectancy.

Pharmacotherapy of Diastolic HF

In contrast to systolic HF, few clinical trials have been directed at treatment of diastolic HF, and to date no trials have demonstrated a beneficial effect on mortality with any intervention in patients with this condition. However, several agents have been shown to reduce hospitalizations due to diastolic HF, including the ARB candesartan (SOE=A), the ACE inhibitor perindopril (SOE=B), and the β-blocker nebivolol (SOE=B). Digoxin also reduces hospitalizations due to HF in patients with HF and preserved LV systolic function, but at the expense of increased hospitalizations for unstable angina (SOE=B). The I-PRESERVE trial, completed in 2008, showed no effect of the ARB irbesartan on mortality, hospitalizations, or other cardiac outcomes in older adults with diastolic HF. Results of the NHLBI-sponsored TOPCAT trial, which is comparing spironolactone to placebo in patients with diastolic HF, are anticipated in 2013 or 2014. Based on the available evidence, optimal therapy for diastolic HF remains undefined. Current recommendations include aggressive treatment of hypertension and other risk factors, appropriate management of comorbid CAD, and maintenance of sinus rhythm or effective rate control in patients with atrial fibrillation (SOE=D). Diuretics should be used judiciously to maintain euvolemia while avoiding overdiuresis, because patients with diastolic HF are often "volume-sensitive." The addition of an ACE inhibitor or ARB, and possibly a β-blocker (especially in patients with CAD), is appropriate to reduce the risk of hospitalization, recognizing that the impact of these agents on other clinically relevant outcomes is unproved.

Device Therapy, Mechanical Circulatory Support, and Heart Transplantation

The implantable cardioverter-defibrillator (ICD) has been shown to reduce mortality from sudden cardiac death in patients with systolic HF and an LVEF of ≤35%, including patients with either ischemic or nonischemic HF (SOE=A). However, few older patients were enrolled in the ICD randomized trials, and a recent meta-analysis suggested that the benefit of ICDs in reducing mortality is lower in older than in younger patients, most likely due to competing risks (SOE=A). In addition, major complications related to ICD implantation are 2-fold greater in patients ≥80 years old than in younger patients (SOE=B). Nonetheless 40%–45% of ICDs in the United States are implanted in patients ≥70 years old. Importantly, ICDs have not been shown to improve survival in patients with NYHA class I or IV HF, and there is no survival benefit within the first 12–18 months after implantation. Also, quality of life is impaired in patients who receive one or more ICD shocks, and up to 20% of shocks are inappropriate, ie, occurring in the absence of a life-threatening tachyarrhythmia. Older patients appear to be at increased risk of inappropriate ICD discharges due to the higher incidence of atrial fibrillation with rapid ventricular response in patients >75 years old.

Based on available evidence, prophylactic ICD placement is recommended in patients with NYHA class II or III HF, an LVEF ≤35%, and a remaining life expectancy of at least 1 year. ICD implantation should be deferred for at least 40 days after acute myocardial infarction and for at least 90 days after a new diagnosis of dilated cardiomyopathy, in the latter case because LV function often improves after initiation of β-blocker and ACE inhibitor therapy.

Given that HF patients >75–80 years old have limited remaining life expectancy, especially if they have multiple comorbid illnesses or frailty, and that ICDs may not reduce mortality in this age group, the selection of older patients for ICD therapy must be individualized. Patients should be advised about the potential benefits and risks of ICD implantation, including the possibility of an adverse effect on quality of life. Although many older patients elect to forego ICD implantation after an informed discussion, those who choose to undergo the procedure should not be denied solely on the basis of age, assuming that appropriate indications for ICD therapy are present. In these patients, it is, however, appropriate to discuss circumstances under which the patient would want to have the device disabled, especially at end of life due to progressive HF or other terminal illness.

Cardiac resynchronization therapy (CRT) has been shown to improve symptoms, exercise tolerance, quality of life, and survival in selected patients with advanced systolic HF and persistent severe symptoms (NYHA class III or IV) despite conventional medical therapy (SOE=A). CRT involves placement of a biventricular pacemaker with one lead in the right ventricle and a second lead inserted retrograde into the coronary sinus to stimulate the left ventricle. CRT is indicated in patients with dyssynchronous LV contraction, most commonly related to left bundle-branch block, which is present in up to 30% of patients with systolic HF. The basis for CRT, as the name implies, is to "resynchronize" LV contraction, thereby increasing myocardial efficiency, stroke work, ejection fraction, and cardiac output. Although few older patients have been enrolled in the CRT trials, observational studies indicate that appropriately selected older patients derive significant benefit from CRT (SOE=B). Therefore, because the main objective of CRT is to improve symptoms and quality of life, and because the risk of CRT is modest, it seems reasonable to offer CRT to older patients with severe LV dysfunction, advanced HF symptoms, and evidence of LV dyssynchrony (eg, left bundle-branch block or QRS duration ≥150 msec).

A recent technological advance in the management of HF patients who remain highly symptomatic despite optimal medical and device therapy is the development of implantable mechanical left ventricular assist devices (LVADs). LVADs have been shown to reduce symptoms, increase exercise tolerance, and improve quality of life and survival in selected patients with severe systolic HF, including adults in their 70s and 80s. Although originally reserved for use as a "bridge" to heart transplantation, LVADs are now often implanted to alleviate symptoms and improve quality of life in patients who are not candidates for heart transplantation (ie, as "destination therapy"). As a result, an increasing number of older adults are receiving LVADs, and this trend is likely to accelerate as the safety and efficacy of these devices continue to improve. In addition, many centers have extended the upper age limit for heart transplantation to 70–75 years, so that a small number of older patients with end-stage HF and limited comorbidities may be considered candidates for this procedure.

Recurrent Hospitalization

Multiple studies indicate that up to 50% of patients with HF are readmitted within 3–6 months after an initial hospitalization for HF. The most common cause of readmission is nonadherence to the medication regimen or to dietary sodium and fluid recommendations, or both. Other causes include inadequate follow-up, poor social support, and failure to seek medical attention promptly when symptoms worsen. Intercurrent cardiac events, such as an acute coronary syndrome or recurrent atrial fibrillation, are less common causes of repetitive hospitalizations.

Patients who experience recurrent HF hospitalization within 3–6 months after an index admission should be questioned carefully about adherence to the medication regimen, use of OTC medications (especially NSAIDs and "dietary supplements"), recent dietary choices, and daily fluid intake. Patients should also be asked if they have been monitoring their weight and if there have been any recent changes. In patients who acknowledge nonadherence to the medication regimen or sodium restriction, reasons for nonadherence should be explored; in the case of medications, these often include concerns about adverse events, cost, efficacy, and excess number of pills. Nonadherence to sodium restriction often involves lack of knowledge about the salt content of foods, inability to acquire low-sodium foods, frequent eating out, and poor sense of taste. If possible, strategies should be developed to overcome these barriers, and the importance of future adherence as a means to prevent subsequent admissions emphasized. A multidisciplinary team approach, including the physician, an HF nurse specialist (if available), dietitian, social worker, pharmacist (preferably with expertise in geriatric drug prescribing), and home-health representative, is most likely to result in significant changes in health behavior, thereby fostering improved adherence and self-efficacy, ultimately leading to decreased risk of early readmission (SOE=A). When feasible, the patient's partner and family should be actively engaged in the evaluation and teaching process.

Prognosis

The prognosis of older patients with HF is poor, with median survival rates of 2–3 years. However, the prognosis is also heterogeneous, with 25%–30% of patients dying within 1 year after initial diagnosis, 50% surviving 1–5 years, and 20%–25% surviving >5 years. Increasing age plays a critical role in prognosis; eg, in a study of Medicare beneficiaries hospitalized with HF in 2008, 1-year mortality rates in patients 65–74, 75–84, and ≥85 years of age were 22.0%, 30.3%, and 42.7%, respectively. Women and patients with diastolic HF have somewhat better survival rates than men and patients with systolic HF, respectively, but other outcomes, including hospitalization rates, functional status, and quality of life, do not differ significantly among these subgroups. Other factors that adversely affect prognosis include more severe symptoms (eg, higher NYHA functional class), lower systolic blood pressure, the presence of CAD (an important factor contributing to worse outcomes in men), diabetes (especially in women), peripheral arterial or cerebrovascular disease, cognitive impairment or dementia, renal insufficiency, anemia, and hyponatremia. Patients with higher BNP also have a worse prognosis, especially if the BNP remains substantially increased despite aggressive therapy.

End-of-Life Care

In light of the poor prognosis of older HF patients, it is appropriate to initiate discussions about end-of-life care early in the course of treatment, and to readdress these issues as clinical circumstances evolve. See "Palliative Care," p 111. Patients should be counseled to prepare an advance directive, which may include the appointment of a surrogate decision maker and the delineation of interventions desired in the event of clinical worsening and approaching death. Patients with ICDs should be asked to indicate under what conditions they would want the ICD turned off to avoid repetitive painful shocks at the end of life. For patients with particularly poor prognosis and remaining life expectancy of <6 months (eg, NYHA class IV symptoms despite appropriate medical therapy), clinicians should offer the option of a transition to palliative care and hospice as part of a candid discussion of prognosis and care goals.

References

- Hjelm C. The influence of heart failure on longitudinal changes in cognition among individuals 80 years of age and older. *J Clin Nurs*. 2012;21(7-8):994–1003.
- Lindenfeld J, Albert NM, Boehmer JP, et al. Executive Summary: HFSA 2010 Comprehensive Heart Failure Practice Guideline. *J Card Fail*. 2010;16(6):475–539.
- Lowery J, Hopp F, Subramanian U, et al. Evaluation of a nurse practitioner disease management model for chronic heart failure: a multi-site implementation study. *Congest Heart Fail*. 2012;18(1):64–71.
- Santangeli P, Di Biase L, Dello Russo A, et al. Meta-analysis: age and effectiveness of prophylactic cardioverter-defibrillators. *Ann Intern Med*. 2010;153(9):592–599.

CHAPTER 50—HYPERTENSION

KEY POINTS

- Age-related changes in blood-pressure regulation lead to greater variability in blood pressure and greater postural changes. Multiple blood-pressure readings, including postural measurements, are needed to accurately and safely diagnose and manage hypertension.
- Treating hypertension is beneficial, independent of age, and reduces stroke, heart failure, and cardiovascular and overall mortality.
- Choice of initial antihypertensive drug therapy should be individualized according to the patient's comorbidities. Thiazide diuretics are the preferred first-line agents unless there are contraindications or other compelling reason for other agents.
- Caution is needed in treating frail, older adults with antihypertensives. "Start low and go slow." Monitoring for falls, decrease in orthostatic blood pressure, and other adverse drug events is essential.

Table 50.1—Classification of Blood-Pressure Levels

Category	Systolic (mmHg)		Diastolic (mmHg)
Normal	<120	*and*	<80
Prehypertension	120–139	*or*	80–89
Hypertension			
Stage 1	140–159	*or*	90–99
Stage 2	>160	*or*	> 100

NOTE: Diagnoses should be based on the average of two or more readings taken at each of two or more visits after an initial screening.

SOURCE: Data from *JNC 7 Express: The Seventh Report of the Joint National Committee on Prevention, Detection, Evaluation, and Treatment of High Blood Pressure*. Bethesda, MD: National High Blood Pressure Education Program, National Heart, Lung and Blood Institute, National Institutes of Health, US Department of Health and Human Services; May 2003:3 (Table 1).

EPIDEMIOLOGY AND PHYSIOLOGY

Systolic blood pressure progressively increases with age, whereas diastolic blood pressure plateaus in the fifth to sixth decade. According to the National Health and Nutrition Examination Survey (NHANES) 1999–2004, 67% of the noninstitutionalized adults ≥60 years old had hypertension, which was significantly higher than the 58% reported in NHANES III (1988–1994). Although hypertension prevalence increased in all age groups, in both sexes, and in non-Hispanic whites and non-Hispanic blacks, the increase was greatest among older black Americans, especially women (SOE=A). Many observational studies have documented that the risk associated with hypertension does not decrease with age, although the association between hypertension and mortality is weaker in the very old. Current criteria defining hypertension, eg, the Seventh Report of the *Joint National Committee on Prevention, Detection, Evaluation, and Treatment of High Blood Pressure* (*JNC 7*; see references at end of chapter and Table 50.1), do not adjust for age. Over the last few decades, awareness and control rates of hypertension have improved significantly. Nevertheless, these rates are the lowest in older adults versus their younger counterparts. Based on NHANES 1999–2004, 26% of hypertensive older adults were unaware of their disease, 33% were untreated, and 57% of the treated were uncontrolled. Many factors contribute to poor rates of blood-pressure control, including lack of awareness of having hypertension and misinformation on desired normal blood-pressure goals; these issues appear to be particular barriers among older black and Hispanic women. Factors related to healthcare providers' practices and concepts about hypertension in older adults also contribute to the age-related disparities in control rates.

Vascular structural changes and neurohumoral alterations contribute to the progressive increase in blood pressure with aging. Large vessels become less distensible with age. This is related to structural changes in the media (elastin fracture, collagen deposition, and calcification), atherosclerosis, and endothelial dysfunction. These changes lead to increased peripheral vascular resistance and decreased vascular compliance, the physiologic hallmark of hypertension in older adults. Decreased sensitivity of the baroreflex, perhaps related to decreased arterial distensibility, contributes to an increase in blood-pressure variability and sympathetic nervous system activity. The dynamic regulation of vascular tone is affected by impairments in vasodilator systems (eg, production of nitric oxide by vascular endothelial cells and vasodilation mediated by β-adrenergic receptors) and by heightened vasoconstriction mediated by α-adrenergic receptors. Changes in kidney function as well as in systems that are involved in sodium balance, such as the renin-angiotensin system, lead to an increase in salt sensitivity and the blood-pressure response to dietary sodium. Approximately two-thirds of older hypertensive adults have salt-sensitive hypertension.

In addition to the increase in blood-pressure level, blood-pressure dysregulation in aging renders older adults at increased risk of orthostatic and postprandial hypotension. Maintaining normal blood pressure and cerebrovascular and coronary perfusion in the face of hypotensive stimuli related to postural challenge, meals, or medications requires the integrated coordination of multiple compensatory mechanisms both centrally and peripherally. The age-associated decline in baroreflex sensitivity and changes in sympathetic nervous system function impair the dynamic regulation of blood pressure. Because of the blunted sensitivity of the baroreflex, a greater decrease in blood pressure occurs before the increase in heart rate and other compensatory mechanisms are activated. Other pathophysiologic changes that impair blood-pressure regulation include arterial and cardiac stiffness and a decrease in early diastolic filling. Finally, changes in the circadian control of blood pressure predisposes older adults to higher relative night-time blood pressure and greater early morning blood-pressure rise, both leading to increased risk of stroke and myocardial infarction.

CLINICAL EVALUATION

Accurate measurement of blood pressure is the most critical aspect of the diagnosis of hypertension in older adults. Because variability in blood pressure increases with age, the diagnosis of hypertension requires at least 3 blood-pressure readings taken on 2 separate visits. Ambulatory (home) blood-pressure monitoring is recommended for patients with extreme blood-pressure variability or possible "white-coat" hypertension. Ambulatory (home) blood-pressure monitoring is also recommended for the evaluation of resistant hypertension and when there is concern regarding hypotensive episodes, including postural hypotension. Additional clinically useful information derived from ambulatory blood-pressure monitoring is the mean blood pressure over a 24-hour period and the diurnal blood-pressure rhythm. A diminished nocturnal fall in blood pressure (<10% of waking values)—the non-dipping pattern—has been associated with higher cardiovascular risk.

Indirect or cuff blood pressures correlate very well with direct, intra-arterial measures in most older adults. In rare individuals, extreme rigidity of the peripheral arteries may prevent complete compression of the brachial artery when the cuff is inflated, resulting in a falsely high blood-pressure measurement. This is referred to as pseudohypertension and should be considered in cases of what appears to be resistant hypertension or when there are marked adverse events—especially hypotension—when antihypertensive therapy is started. Clinicians should also be aware of an auscultatory gap, which can lead to underestimation of the true systolic blood pressure and can indicate arterial stiffness. This can be avoided by inflating the blood-pressure cuff 40 mmHg higher than the pressure required to occlude the brachial pulse.

Once hypertension has been diagnosed, the remainder of the clinical evaluation centers on excluding secondary forms of hypertension and risk stratification by identifying target-organ damage, other cardiovascular risk factors, and the presence of comorbid conditions. Although most older patients have essential hypertension, secondary forms of hypertension should be suspected in the presence of malignant hypertension, a sudden increase in diastolic blood pressure, new worsening level of blood-pressure control, or resistant hypertension (poorly controlled blood pressure on a regimen of 3 antihypertensive medications, including a diuretic). Renovascular disease is the most common secondary form of hypertension among older adults (see "Kidney Diseases and Disorders," p 420). Hyperaldosteronism, obstructive sleep apnea, and use of NSAIDs are other causes of secondary hypertension that can be reversed. Treatment decisions are based on both risk stratification and overall evaluation of the patient's life-expectancy and functional status. Higher risk strata are those with target-organ damage (eg, left ventricular hypertrophy) or comorbid illnesses such as diabetes mellitus and hyperlipidemia, renal disease, or congestive heart failure. In older adults, risk stratification should also include an overall evaluation of functional abilities, life expectancy, and personal healthcare wishes. Those who have a short life expectancy or are extremely frail should be counseled and monitored closely for adverse events to medications. Final decisions regarding treatment or target blood pressure should be based on goals of care and patient/family preferences.

Hypertensive older adults should always be counseled about lifestyle modification because doing so may lower the need for antihypertensive medications. Obtaining a lifestyle history, including smoking history, dietary intake of sodium and fat, alcohol intake, and the level of usual physical activity is essential and should be a part of hypertension evaluation. Contrary to common belief, older adults are able and willing to change their lifestyle but require specific education and monitoring.

TREATMENT

Treatment of hypertension in older adults is safe and effective. Meta-analyses of more than 40 randomized clinical trials of antihypertensive therapy have provided compelling evidence that treatment is effective in reducing cardiovascular (eg, chronic heart failure) and cerebrovascular (eg, stroke) morbidity and mortality (SOE=A). In a meta-analysis of outcome trials in systolic hypertension among older adults, treatment was associated with significant reductions in overall mortality, cardiovascular events, and stroke (SOE=A). The treatment effect was largest in men, in those

≥70 years old, and in those who had greater pulse pressures.

In those ≥80 years old, the evidence is not as robust. Until the Hypertension in the Very Elderly Trial (HYVET) study was completed in 2007, few participants in randomized controlled trials of hypertension treatment were >80 years old and almost none were >85 years old. This randomized controlled trial of 3,845 participants >80 years old ended early when its data safety monitoring board identified a significant 21% reduction in total mortality (10.1% versus 12.2%, ARR 2.2%, NNT 45 over a median of 1.8 years) in the intervention (extended-release indapamide plus perindopril if needed to achieve a goal systolic blood pressure of 150 mmHg) relative to the placebo control group (RR 0.76; CI 95%, 0.62–0.93; *P*=.007). The treatment group also demonstrated improvements in fatal and nonfatal stroke (RR 0.59; CI 95%, 0.40–0.88; *P*=.009) and heart failure and reported fewer adverse events. It is important to note that the participants in this trial were generally healthy, community-living older adults—those with dementia, living in nursing homes, or an inability to walk were excluded. The study design also required participants to have a standing blood pressure >140 mmHg at entry into the trial. For these reasons, the HYVET study results cannot be generalized to apply to frail, very old individuals. A HYVET substudy that assessed cognitive function and the rate of dementia developing in study participants, HYVET-COG, identified similar rates of incident dementia in the treatment and control groups.

As with treatment of other chronic conditions in older adults, it is important to balance the recognized beneficial effects of treatment for hypertension with the potential impact on the individual's functional status and quality of life. A treatment approach that is least likely to result in adverse events and that targets a reduction in systolic blood pressure to <140 mmHg and diastolic blood pressure to <90 mmHg should be developed. For individuals with type 2 diabetes, the JNC-7 guidelines recommend a systolic blood-pressure goal of <130 mmHg. However, the benefit of achieving this target has not been confirmed in clinical trials and cannot be generalized to older adults. For patients with markedly increased systolic blood pressure, an intermediate target, such as <160 mmHg, may be an appropriate initial goal in the absence of target-organ damage.

Although it is clear that any increase in blood pressure above normal (>115/80 mmHg) is positively and linearly associated with morbidity and mortality, some studies have shown increased mortality with blood-pressure reduction—especially diastolic blood pressure (<70 mmHg)—below a certain threshold, creating a J-shaped curve in relation to mortality (SOE=B). The significance of these concerns remains controversial. This relationship has been evaluated in older participants enrolled in the Systolic Hypertension in the Elderly Trial. This post hoc analysis suggested that an on-treatment diastolic blood pressure <70 mmHg was associated with more cardiovascular events only in those with a history of underlying coronary heart disease. While cardiovascular mortality was not increased as a function of lower diastolic pressures to as low as 55 mmHg, hazard ratios were higher for noncardiovascular mortality. It therefore seems reasonable to attempt to avoid excessive reductions in diastolic blood pressure (eg, diastolic levels <70 mmHg), especially in individuals with coronary heart disease.

Treatment should focus on systolic blood pressure because among older hypertensive adults, it is a stronger predictor of adverse outcomes than diastolic blood pressure. The systolic blood pressure alone correctly classifies the blood-pressure stage of >99% of older hypertensive adults. In addition, analysis of data from the Systolic Hypertension in the Elderly Trial demonstrates a significant relationship between pulse pressure and the risk of stroke and overall mortality that is independent of the level of mean arterial pressure.

Lifestyle Modification

Nonpharmacologic therapy is an important adjunct to drug treatment in all patients because of synergistic effects with antihypertensive drugs and the benefits realized through the reduction in other cardiovascular risk factors. Lifestyle modifications that target the typical characteristics of the older hypertensive adult—overweight, sedentary, and salt-sensitive—are likely to be effective. The randomized Trial of Nonpharmacologic Interventions in Elderly study, which evaluated the effects of dietary sodium restriction and weight loss in older adults, demonstrated that relatively modest reductions in dietary sodium intake (1.8 g/d) and in body weight (4 kg) are accompanied by a 30% decrease in the need to reinitiate pharmacologic treatment. A meta-analysis of randomized trials assessing the effects of dietary sodium restriction demonstrated a significant reduction in systolic (a mean decrease of 3.7 mmHg for each decrease of 2.4 g/d of sodium) but not in diastolic blood pressure (SOE=A). This differential reduction in systolic pressure is particularly well suited for the older hypertensive patient. Stress-reduction techniques and increasing potassium intake in the form of fruits and vegetables also lower blood pressure. Increasing physical activity is particularly critical because the benefit of exercise may surpass lowering blood pressure to affect other domains such as balance and cognitive function (SOE=C). Those with significantly higher blood

Table 50.2—General Treatment Recommendations for Hypertension

- Begin with a nonpharmacologic approach.
- Base drug selection or combination therapies on individual patient characteristics.
- Use a low-dose diuretic as the first choice for initial pharmacologic therapy in patients with uncomplicated hypertension unless there is a compelling reason for an alternative choice.
- When starting drug therapy, begin at half the usual dosage, increase dosage slowly, and continue nonpharmacologic therapies.
- Treatment goals should be gauged by systolic blood pressure and based on the patient's comorbidity profile.
- Avoid excessive reduction in diastolic blood pressure (<50 mmHg).

pressure (eg, >160 mmHg in systolic blood pressure) may be considered for concomitant pharmacologic therapy.

Pharmacologic Treatment

The general approach to pharmacologic management of older hypertensive adults is similar to that presented in the JNC-7. General principles regarding drug selection are reviewed here and summarized in Table 50.2. Initial drug choice is influenced by the presence or absence of comorbid conditions (eg, diabetes mellitus, coronary artery disease or history of myocardial infarction, heart failure, prostatism), cost, and compliance. A once-a-day regimen with long-acting medications is more likely to be successful. Medications should be started at the lowest dosage and cautiously increased during follow-up visits (every 4–6 weeks). If the response is inadequate or there is evidence of adverse events, a drug from a different class can be substituted. However, before adding new drugs, the following should be considered: polypharmacy, nonadherence, and drug interactions.

Thiazide diuretics, calcium channel blockers, and ACE inhibitors are all effective as initial treatment (SOA=A). Centrally acting agents (eg, clonidine, methyldopa) and α-blockers are not recommended as first choice. β-Blockers in noncardiac patients are also not recommended for first choice. Many patients will not reach their systolic blood pressure goal on a single medication; JNC-7 recommends starting patients on two medications if their initial blood pressure is >20 mmHg above the target level. However, adding two medications simultaneously may lead to a precipitous drop in blood pressure that may be tolerated less well in older patients than in younger patients. Therefore, caution should be exercised if two medications are to be started.

Diuretics

Therapy with low-dose thiazide-type diuretics (eg, hydrochlorothiazide ≤25 mg/d, or the equivalent) has demonstrated significant benefits in mortality, stroke, and coronary events in randomized clinical trials in older hypertensive adults (SOE=A). The adverse-event profile includes hypokalemia, hyperuricemia, hypomagnesemia, hyponatremia, and possible glucose intolerance. Adverse events are more likely to occur with higher dosages, so lower dosages are recommended. Adequate potassium replacement during diuretic-based treatment decreases the risk of arrhythmias and glucose intolerance. Thiazide diuretics are also well suited for use in combination therapies because of synergistic effects with other classes of antihypertensive medications. Loop diuretics may be used for hypertension but are usually reserved for those with heart failure or chronic kidney disease. Their adverse-event profile includes increasing glucose concentration, headaches, ototoxicity, and electrolyte disturbances. Aldosterone antagonists (spironolactone, eplerenone) are also useful in hypertension and may be used in those who are prone to hypokalemia.

ACE Inhibitors

ACE inhibitors block the production of angiotensin II and are effective in lowering blood pressure in older hypertensive adults. They lower peripheral vascular resistance through their humoral and structural effects on the vasculature without causing reflex tachycardia as seen with direct vasodilators. They are also effective in slowing the progression of hypertension nephrosclerosis and are particularly advantageous in those with concomitant diabetes or heart failure (SOE=A). Their use in African Americans has been questioned, but data from the African American Study of Kidney Disease and Hypertension (AASK) trial showed a significant beneficial effect in African Americans (SOE=A). Their adverse-event profile includes cough, hyperkalemia, angioedema, renal insufficiency (especially in those with renal artery stenosis), and in rare instances neutropenia and agranulocytosis. Black Americans are at greater risk of cough and angioedema than white Americans.

Angiotensin-Receptor Blockers

Angiotensin-receptor blockers (ARBs) block the effect of angiotensin II on the type 1 angiotensin receptor. ARB therapy may be considered as first line or as an alternative to an ACE inhibitor, especially in those with diabetes, heart failure, or microalbuminuria. ARBs are excellent choices for those who cannot tolerate ACE inhibitors (SOE=A).

Renin Inhibitors

Renin inhibitors (eg, aliskiren) are approved for hypertension treatment. They are as effective as ACE inhibitors or ARBs in their blood-pressure lowering effects, with the advantage of no dose-related increases in adverse events in older adults (SOE=B). However, no outcome data are available for older adults, and renin inhibitors are significantly more expensive than other antihypertensives. They are associated with diarrhea, and there are no data on safety in those with a GFR <30 mL/min/1.73 m^2.

Calcium-Channel Antagonists

Therapy with long-acting dihydropyridine calcium-channel antagonists (CCAs) (nifedipine-like) is effective in reducing stroke risk in older hypertensive patients (SOE=A). CCAs in combination with ACE inhibitors have been shown to be superior to the diuretic–ACE inhibitor combination in patients with multiple vascular risk factors. Because of age-related changes in the pharmacokinetics of CCAs, lower dosages should be used. Adverse events are related to vasodilator mechanisms and include ankle edema, headaches, and postural hypotension. CCAs are also associated with constipation. Non-dihydropyridine CCAs can suppress left ventricular function and may precipitate heart block in older adults with conduction defects. Unless there is a strong indication for their use, they should be avoided as first choice for hypertension management. Short-acting CCAs should not be used to treat hypertension.

β-Receptor Antagonists

Several meta-analyses have questioned the efficacy of β-blockers in treating uncomplicated hypertension. Compared with placebo, β-blockers, especially atenolol, provide no reduction in all-cause mortality and myocardial infarction, and only modest reduction in stroke, which is smaller than the risk reduction seen with other antihypertensives (SOE=A). Based on available evidence, β-blockers are not preferred as first-line agents, unless there is a strong indication, such as heart failure, prior myocardial infarction, acute coronary syndrome, stable angina, prevention of perioperative cardiac complications, or hypertrophic obstructive cardiomyopathy. Because of their effectiveness in the management of symptomatic coronary artery disease, in secondary prevention after myocardial infarction, and in management of heart failure, β-receptor antagonists should be considered for older adults whose hypertension is complicated by these comorbid conditions (SOE=A).

α-Receptor Antagonists

α-Receptor antagonists are not appropriate for first-line therapy of hypertension. The treatment arm that included participants randomized to therapy with the α-receptor antagonist doxazosin in the ALLHAT study was stopped early because of a higher rate of cardiovascular complications, including a 2-fold greater likelihood of being hospitalized for heart failure. α-Receptor antagonist therapy might be considered as part of a multidrug regimen, especially in those with prostatism because these drugs have been shown to be efficacious in improving obstructive urinary symptoms.

Other Classes

Direct vasodilators (hydralazine and minoxidil) are considered last-line therapy because of their toxic adverse-event profile, which includes tachycardia, arrhythmia, and fluid retention. Centrally acting agents (eg, clonidine) are also poorly tolerated in older adults and can be associated with sedation, bradycardia, and reflex hypertension, as well as tachycardia if abruptly stopped. Alpha-beta blockers have an antihypertensive effect, but their tolerability is an issue in older adults. Labetalol is useful in hypertensive urgencies and carvedilol in congestive heart failure. Their adverse events include weakness and significant orthostatic hypotension.

Follow-Up Visits

Attempts to reduce blood pressure to target levels too rapidly are unnecessary and likely deleterious. For most patients, an interval of 4–6 weeks between visits is appropriate to determine the need for dosage adjustment. At all follow-up visits, it is imperative to determine both supine and standing blood pressure measurements. It is good practice to adjust antihypertensive drug dosages to achieve the target (seated) blood pressure only after determining whether postural hypotension is present.

Blood-pressure monitoring while outside the clinic setting may be essential, especially in those who cannot tolerate even small doses of antihypertensives. Home blood-pressure monitoring may also aid in promoting adherence to therapy (SOE=B). If available, an interdisciplinary geriatric team is well suited to provide a well-rounded approach to hypertension management (eg, nurses to provide feedback on the degree of blood-pressure control, dietitians to review dietary information and adherence, pharmacists to promote adherence to the medical regimen, and social workers to review the financial burden associated with medical therapy).

When a patient's blood pressure has not been successfully reduced to the target level, cautiously increasing the dosage, adding another medication (particularly a thiazide diuretic if the patient is not already taking one), or switching to another class of medication should be considered. Patients should also be counseled to continue their lifestyle modifications. Achieving the target blood-pressure goal may take many months. When this goal is not attained despite adherence to a three-drug regimen, an evaluation for refractory or resistant hypertension (especially renovascular disease, hyperaldosteronism, and sleep apnea) should be considered. After more than a year of appropriate stable blood-pressure control, step-down treatment may be considered; dosages may be decreased cautiously, with close blood-pressure monitoring. Patients who have successfully modified their lifestyle (eg, weight loss) are most likely to be able to reduce their dosage or eliminate antihypertensive medications.

SPECIAL CONSIDERATIONS

Hypertensive Emergencies and Urgencies

Increased blood pressure per se in the absence of signs or symptoms of target-organ damage does not constitute a hypertensive emergency. Rapidly and too aggressively decreasing blood pressure in a patient with incidentally discovered increased blood pressure is potentially harmful and can cause complications, such as coronary or cerebral hypoperfusion syndromes (SOE=B).

Examples of true hypertensive emergencies in older adults include hypertensive encephalopathy, acute heart failure with pulmonary edema, dissecting aortic aneurysm, and unstable angina. These patients present with symptoms and signs of vascular compromise of affected organs. Management of these emergencies requires an acute hospital setting, with the parenteral administration of a short-acting antihypertensive agent and continuous blood-pressure monitoring to immediately reduce blood pressure, although not initially to a normal target level. Blood pressure should not be lowered emergently more than 25% within the first 2 hours, with a goal of achieving 160/100 mmHg gradually over the first 6 hours of therapy (SOE=D).

Hypertension in the Long-Term Care Setting

Approximately one-third to two-thirds of residents in long-term care facilities have hypertension. Special considerations are warranted in the care of residents with respect to making the correct diagnosis and defining the goals of therapy and its effects on quality of life. Blood-pressure measurements in long-term care settings may not be accurate because of measurement errors and the temporal variability in blood pressure, particularly in relation to meals. Blood pressure appears to be highest in the morning before breakfast. Postprandial hypotension is common among long-term care residents, affecting about one-third of this population. It has been associated with otherwise unexplained syncope and found to be a significant independent risk factor for falls, syncope, stroke, and overall mortality.

Several factors should be considered in the management of hypertension in this setting. First, the advanced average age and comorbidity of residents in long-term care facilities raises controversy surrounding the question of whether the benefits of antihypertensive therapy extend to this population. If the beneficial effects of treatment are less evident, the potential adverse events and risks of therapy should be weighed more heavily in defining the goals of therapy. Even an intervention as seemingly innocuous as a sodium-restricted diet needs to be evaluated in the context of the high prevalence of protein-energy malnutrition among nursing-home residents. Second, the average resident in long-term care takes 9 to 10 medications, and most have 3 or more comorbid conditions. The addition of an antihypertensive medication increases the possibility of an adverse event in this frail, at-risk group. Third, several studies have identified the use of antihypertensive medications, particularly vasodilators, as a risk factor for falls in this high-risk population, experiencing an average of 2 falls each year (SOE=B). It is therefore important to assess both postural and postprandial blood pressure in this population. Randomized controlled trials that could provide clear risk-benefit evidence to support an approach to antihypertensive .management in the long-term care population have not yet been conducted. Available data suggest that diuretic therapy is effective in controlling systolic blood-pressure increases and that blood-pressure reduction with diuretics lowers the prevalence of postural hypotension.

REFERENCES

- Aronow WS, Fleg JL, Pepine CJ, et al. ACCF/AHA 2011 Expert Consensus Document on Hypertension in the elderly: a report of the American College of Cardiology Foundation Task Force on Clinical Expert Consensus documents developed in collaboration with the American Academy of Neurology, American Geriatrics Society, American Society for Preventive Cardiology, American Society of Hypertension, American Society of Nephrology, Association of Black Cardiologists, and European Society of Hypertension. *J Am Coll Cardiol.* 2011;57(20):2037–2114.
- Klymko KW, Artinian NT, Price JE, et al. Self-care production experiences in elderly African Americans with hypertension and cognitive difficulty. *J Am Acad Nurse Pract.* 2011;23(4):200–208.
- National Institute for Health and Clinical Excellence. Hypertension: clinical management of primary hypertension in adults. CG127.2011. http://guidance.nice.org.uk/CG127/Guidance/pdf/English (accessed Oct 2013).
- Ritchie LD, Campbell NC, Murchie P. New NICE guidelines for hypertension. *BMJ.* 2011;343:d5644.

CHAPTER 51—GASTROINTESTINAL DISEASES AND DISORDERS

KEY POINTS

- Although physiologic changes of aging can affect GI function, most GI symptoms and signs are due to pathologic conditions.
- Medications used to treat many of the illnesses affecting older adults can cause GI symptoms and disorders.
- Colon cancer is a common and often preventable cause of death.

The structure and function of the GI tract are affected both by physiologic changes of aging and by the effects of accumulating disorders involving many body systems. In association with advancing age, changes in connective tissue can limit the elasticity of the gut, and changes in the nerves and muscles can impair motility. Disturbances of epithelial, muscle, or neural function may all result from age-related enteric neurodegeneration and loss of excitatory enteric neurons. Accumulating disorders and diseases are often associated with increased use of medications by older adults, many of which have direct effects on intestinal mucosa and motility. Some disease states, such as atherosclerosis and diabetes mellitus, can adversely influence GI function and lead to symptoms and complications. GI problems can quickly compromise the older adult's ability to maintain adequate nutrition and lead to fatigue and weight loss.

ESOPHAGUS

Dysphagia

Dysphagia implies either the inability to initiate a swallow, or a sensation that solids or liquids do not pass easily from the mouth into the stomach; it is a common problem, affecting up to 40% of adults ≥65 years old and more than 60% of institutionalized older adults. Patients with oropharyngeal dysphagia complain of foods getting stuck shortly after they swallow, inability to initiate a swallow, impaired ability to transfer food from the mouth to the esophagus, nasal regurgitation, and coughing. Cerebrovascular accidents, Parkinson disease and other neuromuscular disorders such as myasthenia gravis and amyotrophic lateral sclerosis, Zenker's diverticulum, oropharyngeal tumors, and prominent cervical osteophytes are the most common causes of oropharyngeal dysphagia in older adults. As patients with advanced dementia progress, increased oropharyngeal apraxia, with pouching, "cheeking" of food, and refusal to swallow occur; in patients with Parkinson disease, tremor of the tongue causes hesitancy and defects in swallowing.

In contrast, patients with esophageal dysphagia usually point to the sternum when asked to localize the site. Dysphagia for both solids and liquids from the onset usually implies a motility disorder of the esophagus. In contrast, dysphagia for solids that progresses later to involve liquids suggests mechanical obstruction. Progressive dysphagia results from either cancer or peptic stricture, whereas intermittent dysphagia is most often related to a lower esophageal ring or esophageal dysmotility, such as achalasia or diffuse esophageal spasm. It is particularly important to obtain a detailed review of medications because anticholinergics, antihistamines, and diuretics may reduce salivary flow. Slurred speech can indicate weakness or incoordination of muscles involved in articulation and swallowing. Dysarthria and nasal regurgitation of food suggest weakness of the soft palate or pharyngeal constrictors. Food regurgitation, halitosis, a sensation of fullness in the neck, or a history of pneumonia accompanying dysphagia may be the result of a pharyngoesophageal (or Zenker's) diverticulum, which may be associated with a poorly relaxing or hypertensive upper esophageal sphincter. Painful swallowing (odynophagia) typically results from infection due to fungi or viruses, drug-induced esophagitis, or malignancy. Esophagitis (gastroesophageal reflux disease [GERD]) causes heartburn but not odynophagia, which results from viruses, medications, or cancer. While common in AIDS patients, esophageal candidiasis occurs in debilitated older adults on broad-spectrum antibiotics, immunosuppressive medications, and both oral and inhaled corticosteroids, and among those with hematologic malignancies. This disorder may or may not be accompanied by oropharyngeal candidiasis.

Endoscopy is the best first test to evaluate dysphagia; it allows biopsies and therapeutic interventions, such as dilation. However, lower esophageal rings or extrinsic esophageal compression can be overlooked during endoscopy (SOE=C). In such cases, radiologic evaluation with a 13-mm barium tablet or a solid bolus with barium, such as a marshmallow or bread, can identify the level and nature of obstruction. If results of these tests are normal, an esophageal motility study should be performed. For patients with oropharyngeal dysphagia, videofluoroscopy allows detailed analysis of swallowing mechanics, identifies whether aspiration is present, and evaluates the effects of different barium consistencies.

Nasopharyngolaryngoscopy is a bedside procedure that evaluates the oropharynx, vallecula, piriform recesses, larynx, and perilaryngeal regions for pooled secretions or retained food; its utility is uncertain.

The treatment of dysphagia depends on its underlying cause. Esophageal cancer requires resection, chemotherapy, or radiation therapy. For patients who are poor surgical candidates, palliative endoscopic techniques, such as endoscopic mucosal resection for early esophageal cancer, radiofrequency or photodynamic therapy for high-grade dysplasia in Barrett's esophagus, and stent placement in obstructing esophageal cancer, may be considered. After stroke or head or neck surgery, or in degenerative neurologic diseases, swallowing rehabilitation and dietary modifications to facilitate oral intake are required. In some cases, feeding with a cup, straw, or spoon may improve swallowing. Endoscopic dilation is performed in patients with esophageal webs or strictures.

Gastroesophageal Reflux Disease

GERD is defined as chronic symptoms or mucosal damage produced by the abnormal reflux of gastric contents into the esophagus. Highly specific symptoms of GERD include heartburn, regurgitation, or both, which occur often after meals and are aggravated by recumbency and relieved by antacids. Among adults ≥65 years old, symptoms of heartburn or acid regurgitation occur at least weekly in 20% of the population and at least monthly in 59%, rates similar to those observed in younger adults. Because of degradation of the gastroesophageal junction, reduced visceral sensitivity, and impaired esophageal clearance, age is associated with an increase in esophageal acid exposure and reduced severity of reflux symptoms.

In >80% of patients, GERD is caused by transient inappropriate lower esophageal sphincter relaxations that lead to acid reflux into the esophagus. Some patients may have reduced lower esophageal sphincter tone, which permits reflux when intra-abdominal pressure rises. Sliding hiatal hernias occur in about 30% of patients ≥50 years old and may contribute to acid reflux and regurgitation. Poor esophageal peristalsis leads to delayed clearance of the refluxate and increased acid exposure time. In patients receiving anticholinergic medications, reduced salivary secretion decreases the buffering capacity of the esophagus against refluxed acid and can aggravate mucosal injury.

Patients with uncomplicated heartburn or regurgitation should be treated empirically with acid-suppressing medications after excluding possibly harmful medications, elevating the head of the bed, and waiting 2 hours before going to bed. If such therapy is unsuccessful, or if there are symptoms suggesting complicated disease, an upper endoscopy should be performed. Individuals, particularly white men, who have longstanding symptoms or who require continuous therapy for reflux, need endoscopic screening for Barrett's esophagus, a premalignant condition to esophageal adenocarcinoma. The frequency and severity of reflux symptoms are poorly predictive of the presence of Barrett's esophagus, particularly in patients ≥65 years old.

The presence of anemia, dysphagia, GI bleeding, recurrent vomiting, and weight loss suggests complicated GERD. Patients with these signs and symptoms should be considered for endoscopy. This is the procedure of choice to evaluate mucosal integrity and confirm the diagnosis of dysplasia or cancer in cases of Barrett's esophagus (SOE=B). However, many patients with reflux symptoms do not have esophagitis. In such cases, 24-hour ambulatory esophageal pH testing helps to confirm the diagnosis. This noninvasive test is also useful for patients with noncardiac chest pain or reflux-associated pulmonary and upper respiratory symptoms or to monitor the esophageal acid exposure in patients with refractory symptoms. Esophageal manometry is used to document the presence of effective esophageal peristalsis in patients in whom antireflux surgery is being considered and to exclude an underlying esophageal motility disorder, such as achalasia, as the cause of the symptoms. In patients with resistant reflux symptoms, a recently introduced technology, ambulatory esophageal pH-impedance monitoring, allows for measurement and quantification of both acid and nonacid reflux.

Proton-pump inhibitors (PPIs) are the treatment of choice for patients with GERD, but they are expensive; some of them, such as omeprazole and lansoprazole, are available OTC. PPIs heal esophagitis in 85% of cases and eradicate heartburn and regurgitation in 80%. In comparison, H_2 antagonists ameliorate symptoms and heal esophagitis in only 60% of cases. For dysphagic older adults, various formulations of PPIs, such as orally disintegrating tablets, are available. Regardless, therapy should be maintained for at least 8 weeks. After acute medical therapy alleviates symptoms, the patient should be given a trial off medication. Endoscopy, esophageal motility, and ambulatory 24-hour pH monitoring should be performed if the most potent medical therapy still results in a poor response. A wireless pH recording device is a convenient method for ambulatory pH monitoring (SOE=B). Recurrence of symptoms is common after therapy is stopped, and lifelong therapy may be needed. Intermittent therapy with an H_2 antagonist or PPI may be successful in some patients with mild to moderate symptoms without severe esophagitis if behavioral maneuvers are not helpful. Depending on the initial therapy rendered, the medical schedule is adjusted in a step-up or step-down fashion to the most cost-effective regimen. The need for maintenance medical therapy is determined by the rapidity of recurrence. Among patients whose symptoms recur <3 months after stopping therapy, their disease may best be managed with continual drug therapy. Patients whose symptoms recur ≥3 months after stopping treatment may be adequately managed with intermittent use of medication and behavioral maneuvers. The induction of hypergastrinemia and gastric carcinoid tumors in rats treated with omeprazole has raised safety concerns about the long-term safety of PPIs. However, although patients treated with omeprazole for up to 5 years have shown gastritis and gastric atrophy, no neoplastic changes have been seen. Because gastric acidity normally protects against ingested pathogens, another concern with gastric-acid inhibition is an increased risk of enteric infections, particularly *Clostridium difficile*. In a similar fashion, acid-suppressive therapy also allows pathogen colonization of the upper GI tract with an increased risk of community-acquired pneumonia. The long-term use of medications that suppress gastric acid production may also produce malabsorption of dietary protein-bound vitamin B_{12}. While a single case-control study suggested that chronic PPI use may slightly increase the risk of hip fractures (possibly via decreased absorption of calcium) in patients >50 years old, a 2008 update by the American Gastroenterological Association Institute found the current evidence insufficient to support recommendations regarding bone density measurements and calcium replacement in long-term PPI users (SOE=B). Calcium citrates should be used in patients on PPIs, because its absorption does not require acid. PPIs can cause arthralgias, myalgias, and progressive weakness due to myopathy that may be mistakenly attributed to other diseases or medications in older adults. Care of patients with GERD must weigh benefits and risks of PPI use.

Older adults with large hiatal hernias, with persistent regurgitation despite PPI therapy, or who do not wish to take PPIs long term, should be considered for antireflux surgery. This can be performed laparoscopically, with success rates of >90%.

Drug-Induced Esophageal Injury

Decreased esophageal peristaltic clearance, which is common among older adults, may be associated with pill retention. Esophageal injury can then occur as a result of prolonged contact of the caustic contents of the medication with the esophageal mucosa. The site of injury is commonly at the level of the aortic arch, of an enlarged left atrium, or of the esophagogastric junction. Because salivation and swallowing are markedly reduced during sleep, pill intake immediately before lying down and without adequate fluid bolus leads to pill retention and injury. Taking medications with at least 8 ounces of water or other fluid helps dissolve tablets or capsules and can also reduce the risk of injury or GI complaints. Patients with medication-induced esophageal injury may present with sudden and severe odynophagia in which even swallowing saliva is difficult. A classic example is the older patient in a nursing home given a number of medications with a small amount of water while recumbent before sleep.

Tetracyclines, particularly doxycycline, are the most common antibiotics that induce esophagitis. Aspirin and all of the NSAIDs can also damage the esophagus. Other offenders include potassium chloride, quinidine, iron, and bisphosphonates. Because of this, bisphosphonates should be used cautiously in patients with esophageal dysfunction and taken with at least 8 ounces of water to minimize the risk of the tablet getting stuck in the esophagus and causing damage. In addition, patients should stand or sit upright for at least 30 minutes and should not eat during this interval. Intravenous formulations of bisphosphonates (eg, zoledronic acid) are now available and provide an alternative in very high-risk patients.

Upper endoscopy, the most sensitive diagnostic tool, may reveal a discrete ulcer of variable size with normal surrounding mucosa. These lesions typically heal spontaneously within a few days, and it is unclear whether therapy is needed. Sucralfate suspension provides a protective coat on the esophageal mucosa and promotes healing. (Sucralfate is approved only for treating duodenal ulcers; its use for treating stomach or esophageal ulcers is off-label.) Strictures may be noted in those who use NSAIDs. Endoscopic dilation may be needed if a stricture is found. If possible, potentially caustic oral medications should be discontinued or a liquid preparation substituted.

Esophageal Cancer and Endoscopic Palliation

Esophageal cancer is commonly diagnosed at an advanced, incurable stage in older patients who are not candidates for tumor resection. These patients are plagued by symptoms of esophageal obstruction or fistula formation, dysphagia, aspiration, and weight loss. In such instances, endoscopic palliation can be achieved with either laser therapy or a single, permanent, metal stent placement. Photodynamic therapy uses a photosensitizing agent in combination with endoscopic laser exposure.

Stenting with self-expanding metal stents is preferable therapy for patients with a malignant stricture or an esophagobronchial fistula, because it relieves dysphagia and aspiration in up to 95% of patients and has a low complication rate (SOE=B). The disadvantages of stents include their high cost, tumor ingrowth, and stent migration.

STOMACH

Dyspepsia

Dyspepsia implies chronic or recurrent pain or discomfort in the upper abdomen. The major causes of dyspepsia are gastric or duodenal ulcer, gastroesophageal reflux, and gastric cancer. Because symptom pattern is inadequate for accurate diagnosis, endoscopy is the test of choice. Endoscopy is normal in up to 60% of patients, who are then classified as having functional dyspepsia. It is unclear whether *Helicobacter pylori* gastritis causes symptoms of dyspepsia.

Because the incidence of gastric cancer increases with age, upper endoscopy should be considered in older adults presenting with new onset of dyspepsia. *Helicobacter pylori* testing should be performed using a 13C-urea breath test or fecal antigen test. Treatment is then targeted at the underlying diagnosis. For patients with ulcer and documented *H pylori* infection, a trial of *H pylori* therapy should heal the ulcer and abolish the ulcer diathesis. For most patients with functional (or nonulcer) dyspepsia, reassurance and a course of antisecretory therapy using either H_2-receptor antagonists or PPIs is recommended.

Treatment of *H pylori* can lead to or possibly exacerbate reflux esophagitis. One possibility is that ammonia production by *H pylori* buffers acid. Alternatively, reversal of *H pylori*–induced gastritis (and associated hypochlorhydria) can increase gastric acid secretion and precipitate previously asymptomatic reflux. Despite this association, eradication of *H pylori* should not be avoided solely to prevent the development or exacerbation of reflux esophagitis.

Those who are *H pylori* negative should be given a 2-month empirical trial of a PPI. Such empirical PPI therapy is also the most cost-effective approach in populations with a prevalence of *H pylori* infection of <10% (SOE=A).

NSAID-Induced Gastric Complications

NSAID-induced injury results from both local effects and systemic prostaglandin inhibition. The risk of ulcers and their complications is three times greater in those who use NSAIDs than in those who do not. Most of these ulcers are asymptomatic and uncomplicated. For those ≥60 years old, the relative risk increases even more, to 5-fold. Older patients, particularly women, are 2–4 times more likely than younger patients to be hospitalized with peptic ulcer disease. Older adults with a prior history of bleeding ulcer are at increased risk of recurrent ulcer and complications. NSAIDs also have been implicated as an important factor in nonhealing ulcers. The presence of *H pylori* infection can have a synergistic effect on NSAID-induced ulcer disease. Older adults with NSAID-induced ulcers tend to present with anemia, bleeding, or perforation without the warning symptoms of dyspepsia or abdominal pain. In addition, older NSAID users commonly require emergency surgery for serious complications and have higher rebleeding rates, greater transfusion requirements, longer hospital stays, and higher mortality rates than do younger patients. When NSAIDs are used in older patients, the concomitant use of misoprostol or a PPI may reduce the risk of gastric bleeding by approximately 50% (SOE=A). In one trial, more patients remained in remission during maintenance treatment with omeprazole (61%) than with misoprostol (48%, P=.001), and with either drug than with placebo (27%, P<.001; absolute risk reduction [ARR] 12.7%). High-risk patients, particularly those who have experienced a GI complication, such as ulcer bleeding or perforation, should be placed on long-term PPI therapy; this approach reduces the risk of further bleeding (ARR approximately 9% over 13 months of treatment) (SOE=B).

Peptic Ulcer Disease

In the United States, *H pylori* infection is responsible for about 80% of duodenal ulcers and 60% of gastric ulcers. Most older adults with ulcers complain of dyspepsia, although bleeding, anemia, and acute abdominal pain can also occur. Typically, the diagnosis of peptic ulcer is made by upper GI radiography or endoscopy. Endoscopy is more sensitive and specific than double-contrast barium study (92% versus 54%, and 100% versus 91%, respectively). It is important to differentiate benign gastric ulcers from gastric cancer by obtaining multiple endoscopic biopsies and by repeating the endoscopic examination 2 months after therapy to verify complete ulcer healing.

The goal in evaluating an older patient with upper GI symptoms is to quickly establish a definitive diagnosis, avoiding costly and risky diagnostic procedures. Medications that can cause dyspepsia, especially NSAIDs, should be eliminated when possible. If early satiety, weight loss, occult GI bleeding, or otherwise unexplained anemia is present, an endoscopy should be performed to exclude malignancy.

Among patients with dyspepsia who test positive for *H pylori*, antibiotic therapy may be beneficial for up to 30% of those with underlying peptic ulcer, but those with nonulcer (functional) dyspepsia will have a variable response. *H pylori* testing should not be performed in asymptomatic people. All PPIs are effective in inducing ulcer healing with rates of 80%–100% at 8 weeks.

Biliary Disease

Gallstones primarily form in the gallbladder and can obstruct the cystic or common bile duct, causing biliary pain, cholecystitis, and cholangitis. When stones obstruct the ampulla, pancreatitis may occur. Biliary pain is acute, severe upper abdominal pain, usually in the epigastrium or right upper quadrant, and it may last for >1 hour. The pain may radiate to the back or scapula and is often associated with restlessness, nausea, or vomiting. Older patients with complicated cholelithiasis may not have fever or leukocytosis; their pain may be nonspecific rather than in the right upper quadrant, or they may experience only vomiting with no pain. Older patients with cholecystitis may present with acute change in mental status. Episodes are typically separated by several weeks. Postprandial epigastric fullness, fatty food intolerance, and regurgitation are nonspecific symptoms and are not related to gallstones. If biliary disease is suspected in older patients, ultrasonography should be the initial imaging modality. Abdominal CT scanning may be used if common bile duct stones or ductal obstruction are suspected. Magnetic resonance cholangiography and endoscopic ultrasonography are two very accurate imaging modalities to detect common bile duct pathology, including gall stones. However, for patients with obstructive jaundice, cholangitis, or suspected biliary pancreatitis in whom the probability of common bile duct stones is high, therapeutic endoscopic retrograde cholangiopancreatography is preferred.

Gallstones can be found in 35% of women and 20% of men by 70 years of age because of an age-related increase in the lithogenicity of bile. While many older adults with cholelithiasis are asymptomatic, biliary disease is the predominant indication for urgent abdominal operations in this population; in adults >80 years old, hepatobiliary disease accounts for 20% of all abdominal surgeries. An isolated increase in alkaline phosphatase without jaundice may be a presenting manifestation of biliary obstruction in older patients and should always be evaluated. If cholelithiasis is detected in patients with biliary pain, laparoscopic cholecystectomy is the procedure of choice. However, this procedure is not indicated in patients with gallstones without biliary pain or complications. In the rare older patient who is unable to undergo surgery, treatment with ursodeoxycholic acid or lithotripsy, or both, may be attempted. In patients with common bile duct obstruction due to gallstones, endoscopic sphincterotomy and bile ductal drainage is adequate in preventing recurrent cholangitis, and the gallbladder may be left *in situ*. In any older patient with gall stones, the possibility of gallbladder cancer should be considered. In older adults presenting with biliary pain who have had a cholecystectomy, a retained common bile duct stone should be suspected and evaluated by endoscopic retrograde cholangiopancreatography, magnetic resonance cholangiography, or endoscopic ultrasonography. In patients with abnormal liver function tests, right upper quadrant pain, and an increased common bile duct diameter, biliary manometry should also be considered. If sphincter of Oddi dysfunction is confirmed, endoscopic sphincterotomy should be performed. For patients with malignant jaundice, treatments are mostly palliative, with either surgery or percutaneous or endoscopic stenting. Such drainage improves quality of life, decreases pruritus, and improves nutritional state, but it does not improve survival.

COLON

Constipation

Chronic constipation affects about 30% of adults ≥65 years old, more commonly women. Common causes include low-fiber diet and inadequate fluid intake, inactivity, and medication, but it may result from metabolic causes, pelvic floor relaxation, or neurodegenerative conditions resulting from loss of excitatory (eg, cholinergic) enteric neurons and interstitial cells of Cajal. Evaluation of constipation depends foremost on the history and physical examination. Understanding the patient's usual pattern of bowel movement and fecal consistency provides useful clues to the cause and a better understanding of the patient's treatment goals. Abdominal and pelvic examination is a necessary first step in the evaluation, and sometimes a plain film of the abdomen is useful for detecting fecal impaction. Colonic obstruction should be excluded when clinically indicated.

Constipation has been defined as a fecal frequency of <3 times per week. However, some individuals may complain of straining at defecation or a sense of incomplete defecation despite a daily bowel movement. A more objective diagnosis of constipation is based on colonic transit times. Estimation of the colonic transit time is accomplished by having the patient ingest a gelatin capsule containing radiopaque markers, followed by a plain abdominal film 5 days later. Normally, all markers should have passed by that time point. If not, their distribution on the plain film may suggest either colonic inertia or pelvic floor dyssynergia (outlet delay), or both.

Table 51.1—Management of Chronic Constipation

Step 1	Stop all constipating medications, when possible.
Step 2	Increase dietary fiber to 6–25 g/d, increase fluid intake to ≥1,500 mL/d, and increase physical activity; or add bulk laxative provided fluid intake is ≥1,500 mL/d. If fiber exacerbates symptoms or is not tolerated, or patient has limited mobility, go to Step 3.
Step 3	Add an osmotic (eg, 70% sorbitol solution, polyethylene glycol [Miralax]).
Step 4	Add stimulant laxative (eg, senna, bisacodyl), 2 or 3 times per week. (Alternative: saline laxative, but avoid if creatinine clearance <30 mL/min.)
Step 5	Use tap water enema or saline enema 2 times per week.
Step 6	Use oil-retention enema for refractory constipation.

Patients with irritable bowel syndrome often complain of constipation that alternates with periods of diarrhea or normal bowel evacuation. Such patients have normal colonic transit times. Lumbosacral spinal disease can lead to colonic hypomotility (inertia) and dilation, decreased rectal tone and sensation, and impaired defecation. Older adults with Parkinson disease may have constipation worsened by physical inactivity or medication use. In middle-aged and older women, the pelvic floor muscles may acquire laxity that contributes to problems with fecal incontinence.

Most patients with prolonged colonic transit have colonic inertia, defined as the delayed passage of radiopaque markers through the proximal colon. Outlet delay is a form of idiopathic constipation in which markers move normally through the colon but stagnate in the rectum. This is typically seen in older women with fecal impaction and megarectum, and in women with pelvic floor dyssynergia who demonstrate abnormal responses of the pelvic floor muscles during defecation. Older patients with megacolon or megarectum have chronic fecal retention, increased rectal compliance and elasticity, and blunted rectal sensation, all leading to fecal impaction and soiling.

Defecography is a technique in which thick barium simulating feces is introduced into the rectum, and evacuation is monitored by fluoroscopy while the patient sits on a commode. Assessment of the anorectal structure and function is then made at rest and during barium expulsion. Anorectal manometry evaluates rectal sensation and compliance, reflex relaxation of the internal anal sphincter, and the competence of the anal sphincters.

For most patients with constipation and normal colonic transit time, fluids, dietary fiber, and bulk laxatives, such as psyllium seed or calcium polycarbophil, are effective in increasing the frequency and softening the consistency of feces with a minimum of adverse events. Patients who respond poorly or who do not tolerate fiber may require laxatives. Use of stimulant laxatives such as bisacodyl and senna 2–3 times a week is generally safe. Fecal softeners, such as docusate sodium, have few adverse events but are less effective than laxatives (SOE=C). Constipation among patients with dementia is common, especially if psychotropic medications are being used. Because the patient cannot be relied on to describe symptoms, a proactive approach is needed (Table 51.1 and Table 51.2).

Management of slow-transit constipation, which is the most common type in frail older adults, requires daily osmotic laxatives, such as sorbitol, lactulose, or a polyethylene glycol solution. Severe intractable colonic inertia with megacolon may require subtotal colectomy and ileorectostomy. Pelvic floor dysfunction requires biofeedback, relaxation exercises, and the use of suppositories.

Patients with fecal impaction should first have their colon evacuated with enemas or polyethylene glycol electrolyte solution until cleansing is complete. Recurrence of fecal impaction is then prevented with a fiber-restricted diet, together with cleansing enemas twice weekly or daily oral intake of 12–16 fluid ounces of polyethylene glycol solution.

Fecal Incontinence

Fecal incontinence, defined as the recurrent uncontrolled passage of fecal material for at least 1 month, is a disturbing disability because it affects quality of life and can lead to social isolation. Fecal incontinence may be minor, with inadvertent passage of flatus or soiling of underwear with liquid feces, or it may be major, with involuntary leakage of feces. Fecal incontinence affects 2%–7% of adults, mostly older adults in poor general health.

Fecal continence depends on many factors, such as physical and mental function, fecal consistency, colonic transit, rectal compliance, internal and external anal sphincter function, and anorectal sensation and reflexes. Normal defecation is a complex sequential process that starts with the entry of feces into the rectum, leading to reflex relaxation of the internal anal sphincter. If defecation is desired, the anorectal angle is voluntarily straightened, and abdominal pressure is increased by straining. This results in descent of the pelvic floor, contraction of the rectum, and inhibition of the external

Table 51.2—Medications that May Relieve Constipation

Medication	Onset of Action	Starting Dosage	Site and Mechanism of Action
Bulk laxatives—not useful in managing opioid-induced constipation			
Methylcellulose[a] (Citrucel[a])	12–24 h (up to 72 h)	2 to 4 caplets or 1 heaping tablespoon with 8 oz water q8–24h	Small and large intestine; holds water in feces; mechanical distention
Psyllium[a] (Metamucil[a, b])	12–24 h (up to 72 h)	1 or 2 capsules, packets, or teaspoons with 8 oz water or juice q8–24h	Small and large intestine; holds water in feces; mechanical distention
Polycarbophil[a] (FiberCon[a], others)	12–24 h (up to 72 h)	1,250 mg q6–24h	Small and large intestine; holds water in feces; mechanical distention
Chloride channel activator			
Lubiprostone *(*Amitiza*)*		24 mcg q12h with food	Enhances chloride-ion intestinal fluid secretion; does not affect serum sodium or potassium concentrations; for idiopathic chronic constipation
Opioid antagonists			
Alvimopan (Entereg)		Initial: 12 mg po 30 min to 5 h before surgery Maintenance: 12 mg po q12h the day after surgery × 7 days max	Hospital use only; for accelerating time to recovery after partial large- or small-bowel resection with primary anastomosis; contraindicated if >7 consecutive days of therapeutic opioids
Methylnaltrexone (Relistor)	30–60 min	Weight-based dosing: <38 kg: 0.15 mg/kg 38 to <62 kg: 8 mg 62–114 kg: 12 mg >114 kg: 0.15 mg/kg (all SC q48h); if CrCl <30 mL/min, decrease dosage 50%	Peripheral-acting opioid antagonist for the treatment of opioid-induced constipation in palliative care patients who have not responded to conventional laxatives
Osmotic laxatives			
Lactulose[a] (Chronulac)	24–48 h	15–30 mL q12–24h	Colon; osmotic effect
Polyethylene glycol[a] (Miralax[a])	48–96 h	17 g powder q24h (approximately 1 tablespoon) dissolved in 8 oz water	GI tract; osmotic effect
Sorbitol 70%[a]	24–48 h	15–30 mL q12–24h; max 150 mL/d	Colon; delivers osmotically active molecules to colon
Saline laxatives			*Class effect:* potential hyperphosphatemia in patients with renal insufficiency
Magnesium citrate[a] (Citroma[a])	30 min–3 h	120–240 mL × 1; 10 oz q24h or 5 oz q12h followed by 8 oz water × ≤5 d	Small and large intestine; attracts, retains water in intestinal lumen
Magnesium hydroxide[a] (Milk of Magnesia[a])	30 min–3 h	30 mL q12–24h	Osmotic effect and increased peristalsis in colon
Sodium phosphate/ biphosphate emollient enema[a] (Fleet[a])	2–15 min	14.5-oz enema × 1, repeat prn	Colon; osmotic effect
Stimulant laxatives			
Bisacodyl tablet[a] (Dulcolax[a])	6–10 h	5–15 mg × 1	Colon; increases peristalsis
Bisacodyl suppository[a] (Dulcolax[a])	15 min–1 h	10 mg × 1	Colon; increases peristalsis
Senna[a] (Senokot[a])	6–10 h	2 tablets or 1 teaspoon qhs	Colon; direct action on intestine; stimulates myenteric plexus; alters water and electrolyte secretion
Surfactant laxative (fecal softener)			
Docusate[a] (Colace[a])	24–72 h	100 mg q12–24h	Small and large intestine; detergent activity; facilitates admixture of fat and water to soften feces (effectiveness questionable); does not increase frequency of bowel movements

[a] Available OTC

[b] Psyllium caplets and packets contain ≥3 g dietary fiber and 2–3 g soluble fiber each. A teaspoonful contains approximately 3.8 g dietary fiber and 3 g soluble fiber.

SOURCE: Reuben DB, Herr KA, Pacala JT, et al. *Geriatrics At Your Fingertips,* 15th ed. New York, NY: American Geriatrics Society; 2013:129–130. Reprinted with permission.

anal sphincter, which causes evacuation of the rectal contents.

Decreased anal sphincter tone can result from trauma (eg, anal surgery) or neurologic disorders (eg, spinal cord injury or a secondary effect of diabetes mellitus). Vaginal delivery associated with anal sphincter tears or trauma to the pudendal nerve can result in fecal incontinence immediately or after many years. Decreased rectal compliance resulting from ulcerative or radiation proctitis leads to increased fecal frequency and urgency. Impaction is a common cause of fecal incontinence in older adults because it inhibits the internal anal sphincter tone, permitting leakage of liquid feces. Idiopathic fecal incontinence caused by denervation of the pelvic floor musculature occurs most commonly in constipated middle-aged and older women.

The history and physical examination often provide clues to the cause of fecal incontinence. A flexible sigmoidoscopy may be considered to exclude inflammation or tumor. The next step is anorectal manometry, which measures resting anal sphincter tone, the squeeze pressure, the rectoanal inhibitory reflex, rectal sensation, and rectal compliance. Abnormalities of the anal sphincters, the rectal wall, and the puborectalis muscle can be further evaluated by use of endorectal ultrasound. Typically, a defect in the internal anal sphincter is associated with low resting sphincter pressure, whereas defects in the external sphincter are associated with lower anal squeeze pressure.

Medical therapy is aimed at reducing fecal frequency when symptoms are not associated with constipation and at improving fecal consistency. The former is achieved with antidiarrheal drugs (eg, loperamide), the latter by supplementing the diet with a bulking agent (eg, methylcellulose). Older adults with incontinence related to cognitive impairment or physical debility may benefit from a regular defecation program. Biofeedback therapy is a painless, noninvasive method of retraining the pelvic floor and the abdominal wall musculature, and is recommended for patients with fecal incontinence associated with a structurally intact sphincter (SOE=A). Surgery may involve sphincter repair or implantation of an artificial sphincter. Colostomy may be needed for patients with intractable symptoms in whom other treatments have failed. A synthetic sphincter device, consisting of an inflatable cuff with a valve that allows the cuff to deflate for defecation, can maintain continence (SOE=C).

Chronic Diarrhea

Chronic diarrhea, defined as a decrease in fecal consistency lasting for >4 weeks, not only may decrease the quality of life in older adults but also may lead to significant morbidity and mortality given its impact on fluid and electrolyte balance. Many disorders and medications are associated with chronic diarrhea, and they all need to be considered; their relative prevalence varies with the clinical setting. Common causes of chronic diarrhea are irritable bowel syndrome, inflammatory bowel disease (Crohn disease, ulcerative colitis, and microscopic colitis), malabsorption syndromes (such as lactose intolerance, small intestinal bacterial overgrowth, chronic pancreatitis, and gluten-sensitive enteropathy), and chronic infections. A thorough medical history is essential to define fecal consistency, volume and frequency, and the presence of urgency or fecal soiling. Fecal incontinence is frequently confused with diarrhea in older adults. Malodorous feces and weight loss may suggest fat malabsorption, while visible blood suggests inflammatory bowel disease. If the diarrhea occurs during fasting or at night, a secretory etiology (eg, neuroendocrine tumor) needs to be considered. Large-volume watery diarrhea is more likely to be due to a small-intestinal disorder or microscopic colitis, whereas small-volume frequent diarrhea with tenesmus reflects distal colonic inflammation. All medications (particularly laxatives and OTC products) and diet, including possible use of sorbitol-containing products and use of alcohol, need to be reviewed. Depending on the initial history and physical examination, the diagnostic approach to chronic diarrhea is complex and multifaceted, involving fecal analyses, exclusion of infectious causes, structural evaluation by colonoscopy, biopsies, small-bowel radiography, and abdominal CT imaging. Recent guidelines for the diagnosis and management of diarrhea have been published (www.gastro.org/practice/medical-position-statements) [accessed Oct 2013]). Treatment of chronic diarrhea depends on the underlying diagnosis and may require referral to a specialist.

Diverticular Disease

The prevalence of diverticular disease is age dependent, increasing to 30% by age 60 and to 65% by age 85. Although most patients remain asymptomatic, 20% develop diverticulitis, and 10% may develop diverticular bleeding. Therefore, the mere presence of diverticulosis does not require specific therapy. A diet high in fiber appears to be associated with a reduced risk of developing diverticular disease and may reduce the risk of subsequent complications.

Uncomplicated diverticulosis is often an incidental finding on screening sigmoidoscopy, colonoscopy, or barium enema. Some patients may complain of nonspecific abdominal cramping, bloating, flatulence, and irregular bowel habits. Diverticular bleeding is usually painless and self-limited, and it rarely coexists with acute diverticulitis. Diverticulitis usually presents with left lower quadrant pain, although nausea, vomiting, constipation, diarrhea, and dysuria or frequency may occur. The physical examination usually reveals left lower quadrant tenderness, a tender mass, and abdominal distention. Generalized tenderness suggests perforation and peritonitis. Low-grade fever and leukocytosis are common, but their absence in older adults does not exclude the diagnosis. Urinalysis may reveal sterile pyuria induced by adjacent colonic inflammation; the presence of mixed colonic flora on urine culture suggests a colovesical fistula. Other potential complications include perforation, obstruction, and abscess formation.

CT scanning is the optimal imaging method in acute diverticulitis. CT features of acute diverticulitis include increased density of soft tissue within pericolic fat and colonic diverticula, thickening of the bowel wall, soft-tissue masses (phlegmon), and pericolic fluid collections (abscess formation). CT can also identify peritonitis; obstruction; and fistula to the bladder, vagina, and abdominal wall. However, in approximately 10% of patients, diverticulitis cannot be distinguished from colon cancer, because both may show focal thickening of the bowel wall. In such cases, on resolution of the acute inflammation, a colonoscopy is indicated. In older adults, CT-guided percutaneous drainage of localized abscesses may obviate emergent surgery and eventually permit single-stage elective surgical resection.

Most (85%) patients with simple diverticulitis respond to medical therapy. In contrast, all patients with complicated diverticulitis require surgery. Indications for emergency surgery are free perforation with peritonitis, obstruction, clinical deterioration or lack of improvement with conservative management, and an abscess that cannot be drained percutaneously. Indications for elective surgical intervention are recurrent or intractable symptoms, persistent mass, obstruction, and fistula or abscess formation.

Mild diverticulitis with left lower quadrant pain, low-grade fever, and minimal physical findings is often treated on an outpatient basis, with clear liquids and oral antibiotics, such as ciprofloxacin 500 mg q12h or metronidazole 500 mg q8h, or both. Hospitalization is needed only if no improvement is seen. Once the episode resolves, solid food is reintroduced and the colon is evaluated, preferably by colonoscopy. For patients with moderate to severe symptoms, treatment with bowel rest, fluids, and intravenous antibiotics is initiated, with the aim to avoid urgent surgery. Antibiotics should be active against gram-negative rods and anaerobes. If there is no improvement, either the diagnosis is incorrect or an abscess, peritonitis, fistula, or obstruction is present. Older immunosuppressed patients with multiple underlying medical conditions may present with minimal symptoms or signs even with frank peritonitis, and the diagnosis is commonly delayed. In such cases, early surgical intervention should be considered. Diffuse peritonitis requires fluid resuscitation, broad-spectrum antibiotics, and emergency laparotomy.

After successful medical therapy of the first episode of diverticulitis, one-third of patients will remain asymptomatic, another third will have episodic abdominal cramps (painful diverticulosis), and the remaining will proceed to a second attack of diverticulitis. Therefore, elective surgery is not necessary for all patients with diverticulitis who respond to medical therapy. If surgery is performed, progression of diverticulitis in the remaining colon occurs in only 15%, and the need for further surgery is reduced to <10%.

Irritable Bowel Syndrome

Irritable bowel syndrome (IBS) is a functional GI disorder with remissions and exacerbations, characterized by abdominal pain, bloating, and either constipation or diarrhea, or both. IBS results from altered bowel motility, visceral hypersensitivity, and enhanced perception by the brain of many visceral stimuli. A common mediator for all these abnormalities is serotonin, and serotonin-receptor agonists and antagonists are used in the management of IBS. Although psychosocial factors are commonly involved in IBS, they are not known to have a causative role.

Because the clinical symptoms characteristic of IBS are not specific, it is important to be mindful of features that are not consistent with IBS. These include weight loss, first onset of symptoms after age 50, nocturnal diarrhea, family history of cancer or inflammatory bowel disease, rectal bleeding or obstruction, and laboratory abnormalities (eg, anemia, leukocytosis, abnormal chemistries, positive fecal cultures, or the presence of parasites in the feces). In older patients, the diagnosis should be made only after other conditions (ie, ischemia, diverticulosis, colon cancer, or inflammatory bowel disease) have been carefully excluded. An appropriate evaluation of an older adult with symptoms consistent with IBS should include a colonoscopy to exclude structural abnormalities of the colon. A CT scan of the abdomen and a small-bowel series may also be useful. If the history, physical examination, and laboratory or imaging studies are negative, the diagnosis of IBS can then be made and subcategorized as IBS with constipation, IBS with diarrhea, or IBS with alternating constipation and diarrhea.

Depending on the IBS subtype, treatment includes reassurance, antispasmodics, antidiarrheals, fiber supplements, and serotonin-receptor agents, such as alosetron. Although quite effective, the latter medications may precipitate intestinal ischemia and should be used with caution, particularly in older patients. It is important to establish a definitive diagnosis of IBS, avoid repetitive investigations, and clarify that although IBS is not life threatening, it can certainly negatively impact quality of life. It is also important that clinicians listen actively to patients' symptoms, validate their feelings, provide empathy, set realistic shared goals, negotiate treatment strategies instead of issuing directives, help patients take responsibility for treatment decisions, establish limits on the duration and frequency of visits and phone calls, and maintain a continuing relationship as part of chronic disease management.

Occult Gastrointestinal Bleeding

Older patients are commonly noted to have a positive fecal occult blood test or are diagnosed with unexplained iron-deficiency anemia, or both. Although colorectal cancer is a leading concern in such patients, other causes (of which there are many) include esophagitis, peptic ulcers, esophageal and gastric malignancies, intestinal or colonic angiodysplasia, benign colon polyps, inflammatory bowel disease, or hemorrhoids. A positive fecal occult blood test should not be attributed to esophageal varices or colonic diverticula, because it is rare for such lesions to bleed in an occult fashion. The presence of fecal occult blood should not be attributed to aspirin or warfarin use or to alcohol ingestion.

Detection of fecal occult blood has a low sensitivity and a high rate of false-positive results, leading to more invasive and expensive tests. Despite these limitations, annual fecal occult blood testing is currently recommended as one method of screening for colon cancer and has been associated with up to a 33% reduction in mortality from colon cancer (SOE=A). Because of the high prevalence of colorectal cancer and adenomatous polyps in older adults with a positive fecal occult blood test, colonoscopy is performed and, if negative, is followed by an upper endoscopy. If symptoms of upper GI disease are present, there is a high likelihood for a positive endoscopy. However, in older patients at risk of colon cancer, the presence of a proximal lesion should not preclude evaluation of the colon. Patients with normal upper and lower tract may require evaluation for a small-bowel source using video capsule endoscopy, followed if necessary by balloon enteroscopy. The most common cause of bleeding from the small bowel is angiodysplasia, followed by tumors or ulcers that are commonly caused by NSAIDs. Unrecognized gluten-sensitive enteropathy can result in iron-deficiency anemia, because iron is absorbed in the proximal small bowel, and multiple biopsies should always be taken from the duodenum to confirm this diagnosis histologically.

In one prospective study in which patients with iron-deficiency anemia were evaluated with colonoscopy, endoscopy, and if these tests were negative, radiographic examination of the small intestine, a source of bleeding was identified in 62% of cases. A lesion was seen on colonoscopy in 25%, on upper endoscopy in 36%, and on both in 1% of patients. Peptic ulcer disease was the primary abnormality in the upper GI tract, but cancer was detected on colonoscopy in 11% of patients. In cases in which the source is not found, video capsule endoscopy, simple and noninvasive and with a higher diagnostic yield than radiography, should be considered.

Colonic Angiodysplasia

The terms *angiodysplasia*, *arteriovenous malformation*, and *vascular ectasia* have been used interchangeably. Angiodysplasias occur most often in the cecum and ascending colon, where they may cause bleeding, particularly in patients ≥60 years old. However, angiodysplasias occur throughout the GI tract and may be multiple or coexist in several different regions of the GI tract. They may be asymptomatic or cause occult or clinically overt GI bleeding.

Angiodysplasias are dilated, thin-walled vessels in the mucosa and submucosa that are lined by endothelium or by smooth muscle. Although they are mostly tortuous veins, arteriovenous communications or enlarged arteries may be present, leading to brisk bleeding. The pathogenesis of angiodysplasias is not well understood. They may result from local ischemia associated with cardiac, vascular, or pulmonary disease. More recently, increased expression of angiogenic factors, ie, basic fibroblast growth factor and vascular endothelial growth factor, has been detected in segments of colon with angiodysplasia.

Angiodysplasias are usually diagnosed during endoscopy or colonoscopy, appearing as 5- to 10-mm cherry-red, ectatic blood vessels radiating from a central vascular core. Angiodysplasias can also be diagnosed by angiography. If they are serendipitously detected during routine endoscopy or colonoscopy, angiodysplasias should not be treated. However, an actively bleeding angiodysplasia should be treated. Whether angiodysplasias were the cause of bleeding in patients who have stopped bleeding and, in particular, in patients who are found to have both angiodysplasias and diverticula is a more difficult problem. In such cases, bleeding from angiodysplasias is almost always from the cecum or ascending colon.

Colonic Ischemia

Ischemic colitis is typically encountered in patients ≥65 years old who have atherosclerosis or atrial fibrillation or who have had surgical bypass or vascular grafting procedures. The main symptoms at presentation are abdominal pain and lower GI bleeding. Colonoscopy reveals segmental edema, hemorrhages, gray-black pseudomembrane formation, and focal ulcers, mostly in the region of the splenic flexure and typically sparing the rectum. Treatment is mostly supportive, but even with treatment, colonic strictures can ensue. The development of peritoneal signs calls for surgical intervention with colonic resection of the involved segment.

Clostridium difficile Infection and Pseudomembranous Colitis

Clostridium difficile infection is becoming increasingly recognized among hospitalized patients and is the source of epidemics in hospitals and long-term care facilities for older adults. A hypervirulent strain, NAP1/BI/027, has been implicated as the responsible pathogen in selected *C difficile* outbreaks and is capable of enhanced production of toxins A and B. The infection is often precipitated by the use of antibiotics, such as cephalosporins, penicillins, or clindamycin. Clinically the disease presents with watery diarrhea, crampy abdominal pain, fever, abdominal tenderness and distention, and an increased WBC count. Serious complications, such as ileus with dehydration and electrolyte abnormalities, toxic megacolon, perforation, and death, may occur. *Clostridium difficile* infection should be considered when acute abdominal distention occurs in older hospitalized adults without diarrhea but with associated severe leukocytosis; it carries high mortality. *Clostridium difficile* infection can be recognized endoscopically by the appearance of diffuse or segmental pseudomembranes coating an edematous mucosa, but the diagnosis is often made by the detection of *C difficile* cytotoxins in the feces either by cytotoxin tissue culture assay, latex agglutination, or enzyme-linked immunoassays. Metronidazole 250 mg po q6h is effective in 85% of cases, and it may be given intravenously in severe cases of ileus or megacolon. Vancomycin (125 mg q6h) is also highly effective but only if given orally. Antibiotic treatment for *C difficile* colitis should be for 10–14 days to reduce the risk of relapse. Relapses may occur in up to 20% of cases and require repeat treatment with metronidazole, vancomycin, or a combination of vancomycin and rifampin (SOE=D). To prevent the disease in predisposed individuals and to avoid relapses, restitution of the colonic flora with lactobacilli or *Saccharomyces boulardii* has been used (SOE=D).

Acute Colonic Pseudo-Obstruction

Acute colonic pseudo-obstruction is manifested by acute massive dilation of the colon without evidence of mechanical obstruction. In older adults, it is often related to neurologic disease, such as Parkinson or cerebrovascular disease, trauma, recent orthopedic surgery, or use of narcotics. Infections, particularly *C difficile*, and colonic ischemia need to be excluded. Urgent colonoscopy not only can assist with the diagnosis but also allows placement of a decompression colonic tube. Parenteral fluids and supportive measures, discontinuation of narcotics, and the use of neostigmine intravenously often lead to rapid resolution.

Colonic Polyps and Colon Cancer

Polyps do not usually cause symptoms, but they may bleed or predispose the patient to cancer. Colonic polyps are usually classified as neoplastic (adenomas) or non-neoplastic (hyperplastic). Approximately 40% of the U.S. population ≥50 years old has one or more adenomas. Detection and removal of adenomas significantly decrease the morbidity and mortality associated with colorectal cancer. Old age and male gender are major risk factors. First-degree relatives of patients with adenomas are also at increased risk of colorectal cancer and should undergo screening. Adenomas are most often detected by colon cancer screening tests, primarily sigmoidoscopy. Because adenomas do not typically bleed, the fecal occult blood test is an insensitive screening method. Older age, villous histology, and size >1 cm are independent risk factors for malignancy within an adenoma. The risk of colon cancer also increases with the number of high-risk adenomas that are present.

Colorectal cancer is the third leading cause of cancer in the United States and the second leading cause of cancer death. The risk of colorectal cancer increases dramatically with age, with >90% of cases occurring in people >50 years old. Women are more likely than men to harbor right-sided colonic adenomas. The risk of colorectal cancer in patients with rectal bleeding is age related and may reach 25% in patients ≥80 years old. Up to 40% of colorectal cancer arises proximal to the splenic flexure, and <10% is within the reach of the digital rectal examination. Because it is impossible to identify the source of bleeding by clinical criteria, a colonoscopy should be performed in all cases of hematochezia, occult GI bleeding, iron-deficiency anemia, or even melena after a negative upper endoscopy (SOE=C). Other symptoms, such as abdominal pain, altered bowel habits, or pencil-thin feces are less predictive of colorectal cancer but do require thorough investigation, starting with a colonoscopy. Typically, right-sided cancers present with iron-deficiency anemia and occult GI bleeding, whereas left-sided cancers lead to obstructive symptoms, changes in bowel habits, and overt hematochezia.

A 3-year interval for surveillance colonoscopy is safe and cost-effective for most patients with adenomas. If only a small tubular adenoma is found, the interval may be extended to 5 years; in contrast, after removal of a large villous adenoma, a 1-year follow-up is recommended. After a negative screening or surveillance colonoscopy, an examination interval of 5 years appears to be safe. Patients with colorectal cancer should also have regular colonoscopic surveillance for adenomas starting 1 year after surgery, because these patients have adenoma or cancer recurrence rates of 25%–30% at 3 years.

References

- Atassi K. Strategies to increase colorectal cancer screening. *Nurse Pract*. 2012;37(7):21–26.
- Friedlander EA, Pallentino J, Van Beauge SS. *J Am Acad Nurs Pract*. 2012;22(12):674-683.
- Rofes L, Arreola V, Almirall J, et al. Diagnosis and management of oropharyngeal dysphagia and its nutritional and respiratory complications in the elderly. *Gastroenterol Res Pract*. 2011; Vol 2011; Article ID:818979.
- Williams JJ, Beck PL, Andrews CN, et al. Microscopic colitis—a common cause of diarrhea in older adults. *Age Ageing*. 2010;39(2):162–168.

CHAPTER 52—KIDNEY DISEASES AND DISORDERS

KEY POINTS

- As the kidney ages, it is less able to maintain homeostasis in response to physiologic stress.
- Serum creatinine is a poor marker of kidney function. Kidney function is best measured by the glomerular filtration rate (GFR).
- Prerenal azotemia causing acute intrinsic renal damage is more common in older adults than in younger ones.
- Chronic kidney disease (CKD) is very common in the older population and is classified into five stages based on GFR. Preventing progression of CKD is important at any age.
- Referral to a nephrologist for patients with advanced (Stage 4) CKD is helpful for assisting with management and for discussing the options and likely outcomes of dialysis or a kidney transplant.

Age-related anatomic, hemodynamic, and hormonal changes in the kidneys affect crucial functions that maintain homeostasis of fluids, electrolytes, volume, and acid-base balance. Under normal conditions, the aging kidney is able to maintain homeostasis; however, under stress, the adaptive response of the kidney to maintain homeostasis is impaired. For some of the changes seen in renal tubular functioning with aging, see Table 52.1.

MONITORING KIDNEY FUNCTION

The most important indicator of kidney function to be monitored with aging is the GFR. Cross-sectional studies have shown a progressive decline in GFR after the age of 30–40 years in both men and women. Traditionally, BUN and serum creatinine have been monitored to assess kidney function. However, these are notoriously insensitive indicators of loss of renal function, typically not increasing until 75% of function has been lost. Muscle mass, the main source of serum creatinine, declines with age, especially in frail older adults. Because the decline in muscle mass tends to parallel the decline in kidney function, most older adults maintain a stable serum creatinine, frequently leading to overestimation of kidney functioning through creatinine measurement. Kidney function can be profoundly impaired even though serum creatinine concentration is normal. For example, an 80-year-old woman with a serum creatinine of 1 mg/dL can have an estimated GFR of around 30 mL/min, a level at which almost all medications need significant dosing adjustment.

Because direct measurement of GFR is both expensive and time consuming, formulas for estimating GFR have been developed. These formulas predict GFR far more accurately than measures of serum creatinine, but they tend to become less accurate in the oldest and frailest patients. The most commonly used and practical method for estimating GFR is to calculate creatinine clearance by using the Cockcroft-Gault equation:

$$\text{Creatinine clearance} = \frac{(140 - \text{age})(\text{weight in kg})(0.85 \text{ if female})}{(72)(\text{stable serum creatinine in mg/dL})}$$

Many clinical laboratories now provide estimates of GFR based on the Modified Diet in Renal Disease (MDRD) formula, and this information can be requested when submitting samples for a basic or comprehensive metabolic panel. However, the MDRD formula is unreliable in acute illness and at extreme weights and extreme age. Research studies are typically using the CKD Epidemiology Collaboration of MDRD. Determining the actual GFR by performing a 24-hour creatinine clearance can be useful for sensitive medication dosing, such as antibiotics and chemotherapy, and for assessing the risk of ischemic, toxic, or metabolic events in the aging kidney.

ELECTROLYTE DISORDERS

Older adults are vulnerable to dehydration and/or volume overload. For age-related changes that predispose older adults to osmolar abnormalities, see Table 52.1. Precipitants of osmolar disturbances include the following:

- Decreased thirst sensation in older adults, especially with concomitant cognitive impairment
- Impaired access to fluids and/or sodium, especially in institutionalized patients
- Fluid and/or sodium loss from diarrhea, vomiting, or diaphoresis
- Volume and pressure changes related to surgery
- Increased fluid intake, especially from injudicious administration of intravenous fluids
- Medications, especially diuretics (particularly thiazides) and NSAIDs
- Conditions and medications that cause syndrome of inappropriate antidiuretic hormone secretion (SIADH), such as pulmonary malignancies, infections, and antidepressant medications
- Comorbidities, especially cardiac and hepatic dysfunction

Table 52.1–Declines in Kidney Function with Aging

Function	Mechanisms	Clinical Significance
Glomerular filtration rate (GFR)	Numerous	Increased susceptibility to acute and chronic kidney disease
Sodium conservation	Decrease in distal tubular sodium reabsorption, renin levels and activity, and aldosterone levels	Increased susceptibility to hyponatremia from salt loss caused by excessive diaphoresis, GI losses, etc
Sodium excretion	Decrease in GFR and response to atrial natriuretic peptide	Increased percentage of nocturnal sodium load excretion contributing to nocturia and susceptibility to hypernatremia
Renal concentrating capacity	Decrease in tubular water transport in response to arginine vasopressin release	Decreased response to hyperosmolar and volume-deprived conditions
Renal diluting capacity	Unclear; may be due to decrease in GFR	Decreased response to hypo-osmolar and volume-overloaded conditions
Acid and ammonium excretion	Decrease in GFR and renal mass	Increased susceptibility to metabolic acidosis

Disorders of Sodium Balance

Serum sodium concentrations are abnormal in >25% of older adults presenting acutely to the hospital. Increasing age is a strong independent risk factor for both hyponatremia and hypernatremia.

Hyponatremia

Hyponatremia has been reported to occur in 11.3% of hospitalized geriatric patients and in up to 22.5% of older adults in long-term care facilities. Enhanced osmotic release of antidiuretic hormone (ADH) and impaired diluting ability predispose older adults to a higher incidence of hyponatremia. Thiazide diuretics have also been implicated in up to 30% of cases in older adults. When administered with other medications such as sulfonylureas, SSRIs, or NSAIDs, thiazides potentiate the peripheral action of ADH and impair free water excretion.

Patients with hyponatremia are generally asymptomatic until the serum sodium concentration falls below 125 mEq/L. The osmotic shift of water from the extracellular to the intracellular space with hyponatremia can cause brain edema, leading to symptoms of apathy, disorientation, lethargy, muscle cramps, anorexia, nausea, agitation, headache, and seizures. If hyponatremia develops rapidly, muscular twitches, irritability, and convulsions can occur. The only manifestations of chronic hyponatremia may be lethargy, confusion, and malaise. Recognizing hyponatremia, discerning its primary cause, and instituting therapy are important to avoid severe neurologic sequelae, including central pontine demyelinolysis. Urgent or emergent treatment of hyponatremia is indicated with the appearance of the above symptoms or with acute severe hyponatremia (serum sodium concentration <120 mEq/L).

Hyponatremia can develop when plasma osmolality is increased (hypertonic hyponatremia usually caused by hyperglycemia), normal (isotonic hyponatremia usually presenting as pseudohyponatremia in hyperlipidemic or hyperproteinemic states), or most commonly, decreased (hypotonic hyponatremia). Hypotonic hyponatremia results from three major causes related to extracellular fluid (ECF) volume status:

- Contracted ECF volume (primary salt depletion)
- Expanded ECF volume (dilutional hyponatremia)
- Normal ECF volume (SIADH)

Hypotonic Hyponatremia with Contracted ECF Volume (Primary Salt Depletion)

Older adults who have lost both salt and water caused by concurrent illness are frequently hypovolemic and hyponatremic because of excess (sodium) losses and oral replacement with water only. A urine sodium concentration of <10 mEq/L indicates extrarenal salt depletion; possible causes include the following:

- Decreased salt intake
- Excessive sweating and replacement with hypotonic fluid
- Excess GI losses
- Third spacing

A urine sodium concentration of >20 mEq/L indicates renal salt loss; possible causes include the following:

- Use of diuretics, particularly thiazides or ACE inhibitors, or both
- Adrenal insufficiency
- Pituitary insufficiency
- Intrinsic renal disease with salt wasting

In older adults with hyponatremia and ECF volume depletion, the urgency for correction of serum sodium depends on the magnitude and rate of development of hyponatremia (see treatment of hyponatremia, below).

Hypotonic Hyponatremia with Expanded ECF Volume (Dilutional Hyponatremia)

In this condition, both free water and sodium excretion are impaired. Common conditions include heart failure, hepatic cirrhosis, and renal disease, including nephrotic syndrome. In these conditions, a decrease in effective arterial volume stimulates the renin-angiotensin-aldosterone axis, thus promoting salt and water retention. The urine sodium concentration is typically <10 mEq/L.

Hypotonic Hyponatremia with Normal ECF Volume (SIADH)

In this condition, ADH is released inappropriately when neither serum hyperosmolality nor volume depletion is present. Urine sodium concentration is usually >40 mEq/L, and serum uric acid can be <4 mg/dL. Pulmonary pathology, including infections and malignancy, is prominent among many conditions associated with SIADH. In addition, several agents potentiate the action of ADH, including angiotensin, nicotine, vincristine, morphine, cyclophosphamide, histamine, and sulfonylureas. Centrally acting drugs such as SSRIs and anticonvulsant medications can also cause SIADH.

Treatment of Hyponatremia

Treatment depends on the pathogenesis of the hyponatremia and the severity of symptoms. Asymptomatic patients with hypovolemic hyponatremia and those with hypotension are best treated by the administration of isotonic saline to replenish the intravascular volume. Water restriction is indicated in asymptomatic patients with hypervolemic hyponatremia or SIADH. The addition of loop diuretics can be effective in prompting both salt and water excretion in hypervolemic states.

Symptomatic hyponatremia warrants treatment with intravenous hypertonic saline. Patients treated with either isotonic or hypertonic saline should be reassessed frequently for adequacy of volume repletion by monitoring skin turgor, jugular venous pressure, and urine sodium concentration. Care must also be taken not to induce fluid overload and pulmonary vascular congestion. The administration of normal saline at 75 mL/h should raise serum sodium concentration by approximately 0.3–0.4 mEq/h. If there are concerns about heart disease, a slower rate of 50 mL/h is advisable. The serum sodium concentration should be determined as necessary and regulated as dictated by the clinical situation.

The amount of sodium required to increase the plasma sodium concentration to a desired value can be more carefully determined using the following formula:

Sodium deficit = lean body weight in kg × (desired Na – measured Na) × 0.6 [in men] or 0.5 [in women]

In patients with serum sodium concentrations <120 mEq/L or in those with neurologic symptoms, the sodium deficit to increase plasma sodium concentration to 120 mEq/L is calculated and administered as 3% hypertonic saline. As an example: a 60-kg woman started on a thiazide diuretic presents 5 days later with lethargy, confusion, and a serum sodium of 110 mEq/L. The amount of sodium required to increase the plasma sodium concentration to a safe level of 120 mEq/L is:

Sodium deficit = 60 × (120–110) × 0.5 = 300 mEq

Because 3% hypertonic saline contains 513 mEq/L of sodium, 600 mL of this solution will provide the required amount of sodium.

The rate of administration should be adjusted to provide enough sodium to raise the plasma sodium concentration by 0.3–0.4 mEq/h (7–10 mEq/24 h), because correction at a rate >0.5 mEq/h has been associated with severe neurologic complications, including osmotic demyelinating syndrome. For the example noted above, 600 mL of hypertonic saline administered at a rate of 25 mL/h over 24 hours should raise plasma sodium from 110 mEq/L to 120 mEq/L. Once a safe serum sodium concentration is reached (120 mEq/L), the sodium and volume deficit can be corrected with isotonic saline.

Conivaptan and tolvaptan are nonselective ADH-receptor antagonists that have been approved by the FDA for use as an intravenous infusion for inpatient treatment of euvolemic or hypervolemic hyponatremia. In initial studies, conivaptan effectively raised plasma sodium concentration up to 9 mEq/L in the acute setting over 4 days, but plasma sodium concentrations were not maintained at the higher level over several additional days. While nonselective ADH-receptor antagonists look promising, their role remains unclear for treatment of hyponatremia in older adults.

Hypernatremia

Serum sodium concentration can increase from either a net loss of water or a gain of sodium from ingestion. The impaired ability of the aging kidney to concentrate urine thus results in excess free water loss, and conserved sodium can predispose older adults to hypernatremia. Further risks of hypernatremia in older adults stem from impaired thirst and decreased fluid consumption. Patients with a depressed level of consciousness or immobility with decreased ability to obtain access to free water are at greatest risk of hypernatremia; mortality can be as high as 70%.

Older adults with systemic illnesses, infections, fever, dementia, and neurologic disorders are at significant risk of dehydration and hypernatremia. Medications that inhibit the action of ADH (eg, lithium, demeclocycline) should be avoided in older adults. In addition, medications that can cloud the sensorium, osmotic diuretic agents, tube feedings containing high protein and glucose, and bowel cathartics should be used carefully in older adults to minimize risk of hypernatremia.

Cellular dehydration can lead to severe neurologic sequelae, including obtundation, stupor, coma, and death. Free water deficits should be corrected by administering intravenous dextrose solution or enteral free water. Free water deficit should be replaced over 72 hours and can be calculated as follows:

Free water deficit (L) = (serum sodium/140 – 1) × weight in kg × 0.6 [in men] or 0.5 [in women]

Ongoing losses should also be included in the replacement.

Disorders of Potassium Balance

Hypokalemia in older adults generally results from renal loss of potassium through the use of diuretics and GI loss from vomiting, diarrhea, fistula drainage, and the use of enemas. Inadequate intake of potassium can also contribute to the development of hypokalemia. Treatment is most commonly accomplished by administration of oral potassium.

Several factors contribute to the increased risk of hyperkalemia in older adults, including the following:

- An age-related decline in aldosterone levels, leading to decreased potassium excretion in the distal tubule
- A defect in distal renal acidification, possibly leading to increased incidence of type 4 renal tubular acidosis or hyporeninemic hypoaldosteronism
- Medications that interfere with the renin-angiotensin-aldosterone axis, including ACE inhibitors, angiotensin-receptor blockers (ARBs), potassium-sparing diuretics, eplerenone, heparin, NSAIDs, and β-blockers. The concomitant use of sodium channel blocking drugs (eg, trimethoprim, pentamidine) has similar effects.

Hyperkalemia is most commonly seen in the setting of CKD. It is also seen in acute conditions causing acidosis. It is advisable to repeat potassium measurements when hyperkalemia is found, because potassium concentrations can be falsely increased from acidosis being produced by repeated fist clenching and unclenching during a blood draw. The urgency of treatment of hyperkalemia in older adults varies with the cause, duration, and the presence of signs of cardiac toxicity. In cases of mild hyperkalemia, restricting potassium-rich foods, discontinuing medications that cause hyperkalemia (see above), and using loop diuretics are effective. In patients with CKD and metabolic acidosis, the administration of sodium bicarbonate is a practical way of minimizing increases in serum potassium concentration. Ensuring that the patient is also on diuretic therapy may allow for ACE inhibitors to be restarted at a lower dosage if needed.

Adding sodium polystyrene sulfonate orally is useful for moderate hyperkalemia (eg, potassium concentration <7.0 mEq/L). Rapidly acting transient therapy with agents such as insulin with glucose, calcium, and nebulized β-agonists is indicated for signs of cardiac toxicity or severe increases in serum potassium concentration. The use of sodium polystyrene sulfonate in older adults must be weighed against its potential adverse events, which include osmotic diarrhea when used in combination with a cathartic agent. Chronic oral administration can lead to sodium retention and edema and to significant mucosal injury in the upper and lower GI tracts.

NEPHROTIC SYNDROME

Nephrotic syndrome consists of urinary excretion of >3 g of protein per day, with associated hypoalbuminemia, hyperlipidemia, edema, and a hypercoagulable state. Hypertension and renal failure are also seen in about one-third of cases in older adults. Nephrotic syndrome can result from primary glomerular disease or from secondary glomerular disease caused by infection, malignancy, exposure to allergens or medications, or multisystem disease.

The histologic lesions of nephrotic syndrome in order of approximate frequency in the older population (based on cumulative data from several studies) are as follows:

- Membranous nephropathy, 54%
- Minimal change, 19%
- Amyloidosis, up to 10%
- Mesangial and membranoproliferative glomerulonephritis, 9% each
- Focal segmental glomerulosclerosis, 7%

The histopathology of nephrotic syndrome is unpredictable based on only clinical data; therefore, renal biopsy is essential for early diagnosis and appropriate therapy.

Renovascular Disease

Renovascular disease is primarily an illness of the older population. Most risk factors for renovascular disease increase with age and include smoking, atherosclerosis, thromboembolic disease, hypertension, hyperlipidemia, diabetes mellitus, dissecting aortic aneurysms, vasculitis, and neurofibromatosis. Renovascular disease is closely associated with other vascular disease and is present in 24% of those undergoing coronary angiography (SOE=A). In patients with renovascular disease, mortality is typically related to cardiovascular events rather than to renal impairment. Stenosis of the renal artery needs to be >70%–80% of the luminal area to cause changes in pressure and blood flow. These changes in turn activate the renin-angiotensin system in an attempt to restore renal perfusion.

Renal artery stenosis should be suspected in cases of new-onset diastolic hypertension, inability to control hypertension despite therapy with maximal doses of three antihypertensive agents, abruptly worsening hypertension that was previously stable, azotemia induced by treatment with an ACE inhibitor or an ARB, or hypertension accompanied by widespread vascular disease. Diagnostic test options include renal angiography (the "gold standard"), magnetic resonance angiography (which is 95% sensitive and specific), CT angiography (90%), and captopril renogram (70%).

Atherosclerosis is a progressive disorder, and management of renovascular disease needs to address the underlying process as well as the stenotic lesion. Therapy is based on aggressive management of the above risk factors. Antihypertensive regimens should include angiotensin blockade. Although 2%–6% of patients treated with an ACE inhibitor or an ARB may have an increased serum creatinine concentration as an expected complication of therapy, modest increases in creatinine should not deter prescribing these medications, which reduce morbidity and mortality in patients with hypertension and vascular disease (SOE=A for ACE inhibitors, SOE=B for ARBs).

Renovascular angioplasty, with or without stenting, carries significant risks, particularly in patients with abdominal aortic atherosclerosis. Renal function declines abruptly in about 25% of patients after revascularization. Numerous case series of angioplasty with stenting show complication rates of 0–8% for embolization, 0–3% for dialysis, 0–4% for death, and 11%–26% for restenosis over an average of 10 months, while hypertension was significantly improved or cured in an average of 57% of cases (SOE=B). Invasive procedures should be limited to those in whom medical management has been unable to satisfactorily control blood pressure, those who develop heart failure, and those with progressive decline in renal function.

Acute Kidney Injury (AKI)

More than half of patients with AKI are >60 years old. Changes in renal function with aging (Table 52.1) create a progressive decline in renal reserve and compromise the kidney's ability to respond to sudden excesses or deficits of salt or water. Older adults are thus particularly vulnerable to superimposed renal complications during acute illnesses. Chronic conditions such as hypertension accelerate this age-related loss of renal reserve, and increased vulnerability to AKI in these patients should be anticipated.

Predisposing factors for AKI are more common with aging and include the following:

- Reduced renal blood flow and GFR
- Volume contraction
- Medications, especially NSAIDs, ACE inhibitors, ARBs, and diuretics
- Surgery
- Arrhythmias
- Sepsis
- Toxins, including intravenous contrast dyes
- Thromboembolic disease
- Urinary obstruction

AKI has three primary causes: prerenal azotemia, intrinsic renal damage, and postrenal AKI. The BUN-to-creatinine ratio is useful in determining the cause but may not always be applicable in older adults. In prerenal and postrenal failure, the BUN-to-creatinine ratio is generally greater than 20:1, but in intrinsic renal damage, the ratio remains close to normal at 10:1. Hypovolemic prerenal azotemia, acute tubular necrosis, obstructive uropathy, and renal embolic syndromes are much more common in older patients than in younger ones.

Even though older adults may be at higher risk of developing AKI and renal recovery can take longer, age is not an important determinant of survival in patients with AKI. Therefore, age should not be used as a discriminating factor in making therapeutic decisions. Most patients respond well to treatment of AKI with dialysis. Therefore, prompt therapy with dialysis should be started to treat uremic symptoms and to prevent complications, including infection, heart failure, and bleeding.

Prerenal Azotemia

Prerenal azotemia is due to hypoperfusion of the kidney. The aged kidney's impaired ability to retain sodium and concentrate urine, along with age-related impairment of thirst and declines in renal plasma flow, GFR, and autoregulation of renal plasma flow can render the kidney more susceptible to prerenal failure.

Several clinical conditions can cause renal hypoperfusion. Hypovolemia, frequently from dehydration, excessive diuresis, or GI fluid loss, is a major cause of prerenal failure in older adults. The use of ACE inhibitors, ARBs, NSAIDS, and α-adrenergic blockers can further exacerbate prerenal azotemia by compromising renal blood flow due to increased vascular resistance. Reduced cardiac output, most commonly from exacerbations of heart failure, is another common cause of hypoperfusion.

Prompt identification of prerenal AKI and treatment of its underlying causes are critical, because restoration of perfusion often results in recovery of renal function. If uncorrected, prerenal AKI can result in intrinsic renal disease, namely acute tubular necrosis, which has a prerenal cause in >50% of older patients.

Intrinsic Renal Disease

Intrinsic renal disease results from three pathologic processes: acute tubular necrosis, acute interstitial nephritis, and acute glomerulonephritis.

Acute Tubular Necrosis (ATN)

Ischemia is the most common cause of ATN in older adults. Evolution of prerenal azotemia to frank ATN is more common in older patients with AKI (23%) than in younger ones (15%). Renal hypoperfusion leading to ATN is generally due to systemic hypotension in which the normal autoregulation of renal blood flow and GFR are interfered with by therapeutic interventions or by preexisting renovascular disease in situations such as:

- Complications of surgery, accounting for about 30% of cases
- Vasodilation and hypotension from infection and sepsis, accounting for about 30% of cases
- Antibiotic use for treatment of sepsis, particularly aminoglycosides and vancomycin
- Radiocontrast agents
- Atheroembolic renal disease as a complication of arterial cannulation

The differentiation between prerenal azotemia and established ATN generally depends on the analysis of urinary electrolytes, urine osmolality, and careful inspection of urinary sediment for the presence of granular "muddy brown" casts. Typically in prerenal azotemia, the fractional excretion of sodium (FE_{Na}) is <1%, the urinary sodium concentration (U_{Na}) is <20 mEq/L, the urine osmolality is >500 mOsm/kg, and muddy brown casts are absent. In ATN, usual values are FE_{Na} >3%, U_{Na} >20 mEq/L, and urine osmolality <300 mOsm/kg, and muddy brown casts are more likely to be present.

Treatment of patients with ATN is generally supportive. Early management of patients with established ATN should include investigating the cause, assessing volume status and systemic hemodynamics, and instituting appropriate therapeutic measures designed to prevent or reduce worsening kidney function. Interventions should include maintaining adequate hemodynamic status to ensure renal perfusion and avoiding further injury by removing or decreasing the effect of any nephrotoxins. Medication dosing needs to be adjusted to the level of renal function to prevent toxicity and further renal injury. Careful attention should be paid to nutritional status and correction of fluid and electrolyte abnormalities. When required, older patients respond well to treatment with dialysis to alleviate uremic symptoms and complications of AKI such as volume overload, bleeding, disorientation, catabolic state, and electrolyte disturbances.

Acute Interstitial Nephritis

Acute interstitial nephritis induced by medication is becoming increasingly common in older adults. Diagnosis is made by seeing eosinophils in the urine or doing a renal biopsy. Medications such as NSAIDs and ACE inhibitors can cause interstitial inflammation and acute interstitial nephritis. In addition, >40 other commonly used medications have been implicated in causing acute interstitial nephritis. Commonly implicated antibiotics include β-lactam antibiotics, particularly methicillin, and fluoroquinolones, particularly ciprofloxacin. Therapy consists of discontinuing the offending agent. Rarely, a short trial of oral corticosteroids may be necessary when the interstitial inflammation is severe with persisting increased creatinine after the offending agent has been stopped.

Acute Glomerulonephritis

The clinical features of hematuria, proteinuria, sodium and fluid retention, decreased renal function, and hypertension seen in acute glomerulonephritis are seen in all age groups. The diagnosis may be delayed in older adults because of incorrectly attributing symptoms to preexisting conditions, to common conditions found in older adults (particularly heart failure), or to "normal" aging.

Rapidly progressive glomerulonephritis is the most common form of acute glomerulonephritis in older adults. Many patients have systemic vasculitis, a group of disorders characterized by inflammation and necrotizing lesions of the blood vessel walls, including Wegener granulomatosis and polyarteritis nodosa. Rapidly progressive glomerulonephritis should be considered in patients with AKI and fever, weight loss, arthritis, abdominal pain, myopathy, cardiac disease, or CNS dysfunction. Clinically, renal function declines rapidly and is accompanied by hematuria, pyuria, moderate to severe proteinuria, and RBC casts in the urine sediment. Histologic examination reveals severe crescentic involvement, commonly affecting more than half of the glomeruli. A pauci-immune crescentic glomerulonephritis is frequently diagnosed on immunofluorescence, but antiglomerular basement membrane disease has also been reported. Often, these patients have sera that are antineutrophil cytoplasmic antibody (ANCA)-positive but no immune deposits on renal biopsy. Therapy for rapidly progressive glomerulonephritis includes pulse steroids, cyclophosphamide, and plasmapheresis. While successful treatment has been reported in small, uncontrolled case series, the overall prognosis for older adults with rapidly progressive glomerulonephritis is poor.

Diffuse poststreptococcal acute glomerulonephritis is associated with streptococcal infection of the throat and skin in older adults, with an incidence as high as 22.6% in patients >55 years old. The prognosis is generally favorable.

Postrenal Acute Renal Failure

Postrenal obstruction is a common and often treatable cause of AKI in older adults. Symptomatic obstructive uropathy with rising BUN and creatinine concentrations is often seen in older men with prostatic hypertrophy. Ureteric obstruction in women can arise from pelvic tumors of the ovary, uterus, or cervix. In addition, other retroperitoneal malignancies, such as lymphoma, bladder carcinoma, and rectal tumors can also present with AKI in the geriatric population. The typical symptoms of urinary tract obstruction, such as urinary frequency and voiding difficulties, may not be readily apparent in older adults. Careful review of medications, particularly anticholinergic agents, can be useful. Measurement of postvoid residual urine volumes as well as renal ultrasonography may be necessary to establish the diagnosis. Prompt urologic evaluation is warranted in cases of documented urinary tract obstruction.

CHRONIC KIDNEY DISEASE

Kidney function as measured by GFR declines 10% per decade after age 40 in 70% of the population. Glomerulosclerosis (fibrosis of the kidney) increases with age, leading to CKD. CKD has many causes in older adults, including glomerulopathies (especially diabetic nephropathy), tubulointerstitial nephritis (often medication-induced), obstructive nephropathies, and renovascular disease. Progression of medical illnesses, especially chronic hypertension, often leads to development of CKD late in life. Clinical progression of CKD in older adults frequently manifests as a decompensation of preexisting medical illness such as heart failure, diabetes mellitus, hypertension, or dementia.

NHANES III data suggest that 6.6 million people >60 years old have CKD. The incidence varies between ethnic and racial groups. Diabetes and hypertension, both important causes of CKD, are more common in black, Hispanic, and some Native American populations. Black Americans with diabetes or hypertension are more than twice as likely to develop kidney failure than other ethnic or racial groups, and the odds increase for individuals with a first-degree relative on dialysis for any reason.

Chronic Kidney Disease Classification

In 2002, The National Kidney Foundation (NKF) issued clinical practice guidelines and established the current classification nomenclature for chronic renal disorders. Chronic renal insufficiency, the term that had been used traditionally, was renamed chronic kidney disease, classified into five stages based on GFR regardless of underlying diagnosis. CKD is defined as either kidney damage or decreased kidney function for ≥3 months. CKD progresses from Stage 1, kidney damage with preserved GFR, to Stage 5, kidney failure defined as a GFR of <15 mL/min/1.73 m^2 or the need to start renal replacement therapy. Stage 3 CKD has more recently been subdivided into 3A and 3B. Patients with eGFR close to 60 mL/min/1.73 m^2 are unlikely to have significant complications from CKD, while those closer to 30 mL/min/1.73 m^2 typically have complications such as anemia and need more aggressive management. Estimates of eGFR should always be done with the patient in stable health.

Management

Emphasis in older adults should be on preserving residual renal function using the same approaches as in younger people. Basic treatment principles include correcting reversible causes; controlling blood pressure; using ACE inhibitors, ARBs, and aldosterone antagonists; optimally controlling blood glucose; treating hyperlipidemia; minimizing proteinuria; aggressively managing phosphorous concentration; and moderately restricting dietary protein. Detailed clinical guidelines are available on the NKF Web site at www.kidney.org. Clinicians should expect a minor bump in serum creatinine when starting patients on an ACE or

ARB. This is to be expected and will typically stabilize at the new level within 3 weeks. This does not indicate a true decline in renal function but rather a change in intraglomerular pressure.

Declines in GFR are accompanied by a broad range of complications, including hypertension, anemia, malnutrition, metabolic bone disease, neuropathy, depression, impaired functional status, and increased cardiovascular morbidity and mortality. Early recognition of impaired kidney function allows screening for and managing these complications, thus preventing comorbidities and reduced quality of life. Guidelines of the NKF recommend referral to a nephrologist when a patient reaches Stage 4 CKD for management of the complications of impaired function such as acidosis, phosphorous retention, and anemia. Preparation for renal replacement therapy should also begin during Stage 4, so referral should be made to a nephrologist when the GFR falls to <30 mL/min/1.73 m^2.

Medication Use in Chronic Kidney Disease

Prescribing medications in the CKD population is complicated by age-associated changes in pharmacokinetics and pharmacodynamics (see "Pharmacotherapy," p 81) and compounded by diminished renal clearance. Most medications or their metabolites are renally excreted. Adjustments in dosage or dosing frequency may be needed once the estimated GFR falls to <50 mL/min/1.73 m^2. Almost all dosages need to be adjusted after the GFR falls to <30 mL/min/1.73 m^2.

Management of Anemia

Screening for anemia should start when patients reach Stage 3B CKD. The anemia is typically normochromic and normocytic and is primarily caused by reduced production of erythropoietin by the kidneys. It is important to exclude other causes before treatment is started. In older adults, vitamin $B_{12,}$ folate, thyrotropin, and iron studies (including transferrin saturation) should be checked. In case of iron deficiency, a bowel evaluation should be performed.

Approximately 50% of patients who reach end-stage kidney disease are iron deficient for dietary reasons (a result of poor appetite and animal protein restriction) by the time renal replacement therapy is needed. Iron should be replaced before starting other therapy for anemia. The goal is to raise the transferrin saturation to >20%. Giving erythropoietin to replace lost RBC mass requires adequate iron stores to support accelerated erythropoiesis. Most patients can tolerate oral iron, and stores can be replenished over a period of time. If the patient has severe or symptomatic anemia, iron can be given intravenously using iron sucrose, which is better tolerated than older iron preparations and much less likely to cause flu-like symptoms.

Once iron deficiency is corrected, treatment with human recombinant erythropoietin can be started. This medication is expensive, and Medicare requires the physician to certify that the anemia is due to kidney failure and that iron stores are adequate. Current Medicare guidelines require a hemoglobin concentration of <9 g/dL to qualify for erythropoietin therapy. Two large randomized control trials, CREATE and CHOIR, demonstrated that normalization of hemoglobin with erythropoietin increased vascular events. Some controversy still exists over the goal of replacement hemoglobin; further analysis of data on erythropoietin treatment supports a target hemoglobin concentration of 9.5–10.5 g/dL.

Calcium, Phosphorus, and Renal Bone Disease

Abnormalities of calcium, phosphorus, and parathyroid hormone (PTH) are common in patients whose GFR is <60 mL/min/1.73 m^2. All patients with impaired renal function should be screened regularly for these abnormalities. Phosphorous retention begins early in CKD, with serum phosphorous concentrations often remaining normal, while PTH will increase. Restriction of dietary phosphorus should start if the PTH is increased, even if serum phosphorus remains normal. Phosphorous concentrations should be maintained between 2.7 and 4.6 mg/dL in patients with Stage 3 or 4 CKD. Phosphorous binders should be used as soon as the PTH concentration starts to increase. Hyperphosphatemia leads to secondary hyperparathyroidism and consequent ectopic calcification and renal osteodystrophy. The PTH values will help to distinguish between high turn-over bone disease and adynamic bone disease. Some patients also need supplementation with vitamin D, but care needs to be taken if serum calcium concentration starts to increase. Calcium and phosphorous concentrations need to be carefully monitored when vitamin D supplementation is prescribed; a nephrologist can be very helpful in this area.

In the older population, renal osteodystrophy is often complicated by osteoporosis. CKD is one of many risk factors for osteoporosis. The incidence of fractures in patients with kidney failure is 4 times that of age-matched controls. Dual-energy x-ray absorptiometry (DEXA) scanning can be used to diagnose osteoporosis. Although data on their use in the CKD population are sparse, bisphosphonates are the recommended treatment of choice for osteoporosis in the early stages of renal impairment. Small studies have shown measurable increases in bone mineral density and reductions in fractures in the dialysis population (SOE=C). Bisphosphonates are also efficacious in the transplant population. They are contraindicated in adynamic bone disease, because they inhibit osteoclastic bone resorption. Calcitonin is probably safe in patients with adynamic bone disease, but no efficacy data are available (SOE=D). No safety or efficacy data are available on the use of estrogens and their derivatives in CKD.

Depression

Depression is very common in any population suffering from chronic disease, but it has been under-recognized in the CKD population, especially those on dialysis. In one study, 13% of dialysis patients had been diagnosed with depression, while 43% tested positive on a randomly administered depression screening test, suggesting that the true rate of depression is 3 times that of the recognized rate. Therefore, screening for depression in patients with CKD and in those on dialysis is warranted. Depression can be difficult to diagnose in the dialysis population, because the vegetative symptoms can be similar to those of uremia or insufficient dialysis. Functional and cognitive decline are particularly common presenting symptoms in older adults with kidney disease.

Most depression screening instruments have been validated in the kidney failure population. Very low doses of SSRIs can safely be used for treatment. Long-acting medications such as fluoxetine and paroxetine should be avoided, while the shorter-acting sertraline and citalopram are safer in this population. See "Depression and Other Mood Disorders," p 308.

Nutrition

Dietary requirements for patients with CKD are complex. Intake of protein, phosphorus, and potassium all need to be controlled while maintaining adequate energy intake. Once a patient reaches Stage 4 CKD, an experienced renal dietitian should be involved in the patient's nutritional management. The recommended protein intake for patients with Stage 4 CKD is 0.6 g/kg/day. This diet is unpalatable to most people, and a goal of 0.75 g/kg/d is frequently prescribed to increase compliance. Adequate dietary energy intake is easier to achieve at this level of protein restriction. Protein restriction also helps with control of phosphorus and reduces metabolic acidosis. Dietary phosphorus should be limited to 800–1,000 mg/d. Benefits of severe dietary restrictions in frail or institutionalized older adults have not been proved.

Adequate nutrition and dietary therapy in older adults with advanced kidney disease is complicated by many common age-related factors. Lack of transportation, lower income, and loss of social/family support can compromise access to therapeutic food choices. Loss of teeth, impaired sensory function, and medications that reduce appetite or cause nausea can also impede adequate nutritional intake. Comorbid conditions such as depression, cognitive deficits, mobility impairment, or loss of function from stroke, arthritis, or Parkinson disease pose obstacles to appropriate food preparation.

Table 52.2—Remaining Life Expectancy (years) on Dialysis in the United States

Age (years)	Dialysis Population	General Population
40–44	6.7–9.2	30.1–40.8
50–54	5.1–6.9	22.5–31.5
60–64	3.7–5.1	16.0–22.8
70–74	2.7–3.5	10.8–15.2
80–84	2.0–2.4	6.9–8.8

END-STAGE KIDNEY DISEASE

Epidemiology

End-stage kidney disease, requiring dialysis or transplant for survival, is primarily a disease of the older population. The mean age at the start of renal replacement therapy is 62.3 years for men and 63.4 years for women. The incidence of treated end-stage kidney disease in the age group 70–79 years old is 1,673 per million person-years and peaks at 80–85 years of age at 1,931 per million population and is increasing. More than 55% of end-stage kidney disease patients are >60 years old. Increases in renal replacement therapy for the older population likely indicate a greater willingness to offer treatment to older adults as well as lengthening life expectancy with attendant progression of CKD.

Renal Replacement Therapy

Advanced renal failure with no identifiable reversible cause necessitates renal replacement therapy, ie, dialysis or renal transplant, before uremic symptoms develop. Older patients become symptomatic at lower concentrations of serum creatinine. Increasing numbers of older patients are being accepted for renal replacement therapy. Age should not be the sole exclusion criterion from dialysis.

Most older patients with established end-stage kidney disease are treated with hemodialysis. Hemodialysis does not provide normal life expectancy, but it can provide meaningful extension of life (Table 52.2). The median survival time for octogenarians on hemodialysis is about 24 months. The overall mortality in older adults on hemodialysis is influenced by several factors, including comorbid vascular disease, infection, malnutrition, malignancy, and voluntary withdrawal from dialysis. Although older adults are more likely to suffer hypotension and silent ischemia during hemodialysis treatments, many older patients can be rehabilitated and have a quality of life that is comparable to that of their age-matched counterparts without end-stage kidney disease.

Guidelines of the NKF call for referral to a nephrologist when a patient develops Stage 4 CKD. Early referral ensures adequate time for discussing options for renal replacement therapy and for creating adequate access to dialysis. For patients opting for hemodialysis, creation of a native arteriovenous fistula, the optimal dialysis access, can require up to 6 months before use.

Hemodialysis and continuous ambulatory peritoneal dialysis appear to be about equally effective in older adults. Therefore, the mode of renal replacement therapy should be individualized in older patients, especially with regard to underlying medical conditions and psychosocial factors. Hemodialysis can be appropriate for debilitated older patients because less self-care is involved. In-center hemodialysis can also have a social benefit for those who are living alone or depressed. Patients with severe cardiovascular disease and blood pressure that is difficult to control might benefit from continuous ambulatory peritoneal dialysis. Outside of the United States, mainly in Canada and Europe, home-assisted peritoneal dialysis is available and provided by visiting nurse services in those countries. This makes it a more attractive option in older patients who might not be able to manage on their own.

Offering dialysis to patients with dementia is controversial. Sometimes, distinguishing between cognitive impairment related to uremia and progressing dementia can be difficult. It is certainly reasonable to offer a trial of dialysis for 4–6 weeks to see if cognition improves with correction of the electrolyte abnormalities. It should be made clear that the decision to continue dialysis is contingent on improvement in cognition, and families should be helped to prepare for withdrawal of dialysis if that should be the ultimate course.

The use of dialysis in nursing-home patients is also controversial. Patients who can no longer manage to live alone and who require 24-hour care because of functional limitations are not good candidates for dialysis. Studies using MDS (minimum data set) from nursing-home patients have shown that patients undergo a steady and sustained functional decline after initiation of dialysis and that the 1-year mortality in this group is >50%.

Kidney Transplantation: Older Donors, Older Recipients

About 60,000 patients are currently on the kidney transplant wait list, and the list grows every year with an average wait time of 5 years. Older patients are increasingly considered for transplantation. As in younger patients, mortality rates in older patients with transplants are considerably less than in those maintained on dialysis. Remaining life expectancy doubles for a dialysis patient once moved from the wait list to transplantation. Transplantation is routinely considered for patients in their seventies, who generally do well with suitable donors. Living donor transplants are growing at about 4% per year, eliminating the need to be on the wait list for a deceased donor kidney. Older patients and their families should be encouraged to explore the option of transplantation as soon as the need for renal replacement therapy arises.

Older patients undergo the same transplantation evaluation process as younger patients. However, older patients are more likely than younger patients to have vascular contraindications to transplantation, as well as other contraindications such as metastatic cancer and dementia. Older renal transplant recipients demonstrate lower acute rejection rates, lower incidence of chronic rejection, and higher risk of infection and sepsis than younger recipients, and they have greater survival probability than patients remaining on dialysis even when corrected for levels of comorbidity (SOE=A). Both donor and recipient age are independent additive risk factors for chronic allograft failure. Immunosuppressive therapy should be adjusted in older recipients. Older recipients who do not have a suitable living donor may be offered expanded criteria deceased donor organs as a way to reduce wait times on the transplant list. Several studies have shown poorer outcomes with these kidneys than with regular criteria donor kidneys or living transplants.

Hospice

Most people who choose to withdraw from dialysis are >65 years old. The decision to withdraw can be precipitated by a catastrophic insult such as a major stroke or myocardial infarction, but in almost half of cases, failure to thrive is the driving reason. About 20% of the dialysis cohort withdraws from dialysis in any given year. Of the patients who do choose to withdraw from dialysis, less than half use hospice. Patients enrolled in hospice are far more likely to die at home; in a 2006 study, only 22.9% of patients enrolled in hospice who withdrew from dialysis died in the hospital versus 69% of non-hospice patients. Once a patient on chronic dialysis withdraws, death within 7–14 days is almost certain. End-of-life symptoms are of a nature that makes a home death very manageable. There are well-defined cultural difference in the willingness of patients and their families to consider withdrawal from dialysis and end-of-life planning. The patient's primary clinician has a unique role in educating nephrologists and patients about the value of hospice and the opportunity to end life outside the hospital.

REFERENCES

- Adler SM, Verbalis JG. Disorders of body water homeostasis in critical illness. *Endocrinol Metab Clin North Am.* 2006;35(4):873–894.
- Bond TC, Spaulding AC, Krisher J, et al. Mortality of dialysis patients according to influenza and pneumococcal vaccination status. *Am J Kidney Dis.* 2012;60(6):959–965.
- Chan M, Kelly J, Batterham M, et al. Malnutrition (subjective global assessment) scores and serum albumin levels, but not body mass index values, at initiation of dialysis are independent predictors of mortality: a 10-year clinical cohort study. *J Ren Nutr.* 2012;22(6):547–557.
- Klassen S, Krepinsky JC, Prebtani AP. Pantoprazole-induced acute interstitial nephritis. *CMAJ.* 2013;185(1):56–59.
- Levey AS, de Jong PE, Coresh J, et al. The definition, classification, and prognosis of chronic kidney disease: a KDIGO Controversies Conference report. *Kidney Int.* 2011;80(1):17–28.

CHAPTER 53—GYNECOLOGIC DISEASES AND DISORDERS

KEY POINTS

- Many older women do not spontaneously discuss gynecologic problems, many of which are treatable, with their healthcare providers.
- Symptomatic urogenital atrophy is common in postmenopausal women and is readily reversed with the administration of local estrogen.
- Half of all cases of invasive cancer of the vulva are in women >70 years old.
- Pessaries can improve comfort and bladder function in some older women with pelvic organ prolapse.
- Any genital bleeding in a postmenopausal woman should be evaluated.

Most older women do not seek regular gynecologic care, perhaps in part because they are reticent about discussing personal gynecologic problems and they believe these are normal aging changes. Consequently, important and treatable disorders often go undiagnosed until they become severely disabling. For example, although urinary incontinence affects 16 million adults in the United States, the average time between onset and reporting to a clinician is 8.5 years; gynecologic problems such as genital prolapse and atrophic vaginitis often exacerbate urinary incontinence. Full gynecologic examination should be a routine part of a complete history and physical examination for all older women who are amenable to screening.

HISTORY AND PHYSICAL EXAMINATION

The American College of Obstetrics and Gynecology recommendations for primary care of women ≥65 years old include inquiring not only about routine gynecologic issues but also about involuntary loss of urine or feces, sexual behavior patterns and potential exposure to sexually transmitted diseases, and use of alternative medical treatments.

Nongynecologic medical problems that can have significant gynecologic effects should be noted in the history. For example, breast cancer therapy typically leads to severe urogenital atrophy. Obesity can result in hyperestrogenic states due to peripheral conversion of androgens to estrogen. Osteoporotic lordosis causes increased intra-abdominal pressure and resultant predisposition to genital prolapse. Previous obstetrical events can cause neuromuscular damage to the pelvic floor and eventual development of urinary incontinence and genital prolapse.

If a woman is on hormone therapy (HT), the regimen should be reviewed annually to ensure adherence, need for continued therapy, and absence of adverse events. If the uterus is present, estrogen must be combined with a progestin to prevent development of endometrial intraepithelial neoplasia (formerly referred to as endometrial hyperplasia) (see estrogen therapy in “Endocrine and Metabolic Disorders,” p 506). The history should also include inquiry about abdominal distention, early satiety, new-onset pelvic pain, as well as abnormal vaginal discharge or bleeding (signs of gynecologic malignancies). The pelvic examination also presents an opportunity to discuss sexual function with the patient. Although the lack of available, sexually capable men may limit an older woman’s sexual activities, many older women are interested in maintaining sexual relationships. Issues related to sexual activity such as atrophy-related dyspareunia, postcoital bleeding, and sexually transmitted diseases should be addressed. Many women require reassurance that enjoyable sexual activity is possible and normal at their age. Also, women who maintain regular sexual activity are less likely to have significant vaginal atrophy. See “Disorders of Sexual Function,” p 446.

Most ambulatory older women can assume the lithotomy position for a pelvic examination. The dorsal position, in stirrups for a pelvic examination, requires flexion and external rotation of the hips. Patients with osteoarthritis who find the lithotomy position uncomfortable or impossible to assume will need to use an alternative position. The left lateral decubitus position is one alternative. The patient lies on her left side, with knees flexed. The upper hip (right) is flexed to a greater degree and the right leg is elevated, exposing the perineum. An adequate speculum and bimanual examination can usually be done in this position. A bedbound patient can be examined by positioning an inverted bedpan under the sacrum to elevate the pelvis. Because the vaginal introitus can be small and stenotic, smaller speculums may be needed. Water-based lubricants facilitate the examination and can be used if a Pap smear is to be performed.

The pelvic examination of older women should include the following:

- examination of the vulva for abnormal pigmentation, erythema, or raised lesions

- examination for signs of urogenital atrophy, including urethral caruncle, vaginal dryness, pale vaginal mucosa, loss of rugae, and reduced vaginal caliber and depth
- Valsalva maneuver performed by the patient to evaluate for pelvic organ prolapse and urinary incontinence
- careful palpation for pelvic masses or ovarian enlargement on bimanual examination
- a Pap smear if indicated (see cervical cancer in "Prevention," p 70)

Bimanual examination and perineal inspection performed annually can detect vulvar, vaginal, or ovarian pathology. A rectal examination can also be performed at the same time to identify masses, detect occult bleeding, and evaluate the anal sphincter.

Ovaries become smaller with aging, and any palpable adnexal tissue should prompt consideration of malignancy. Although uterine fibroids are common, any increase in uterus size should be investigated. An ovarian or uterine mass could be evaluated by abdominal or pelvic ultrasound (using a vaginal probe) to determine location and character. Additional investigation with the use of MRI as well as serum tumor markers can be useful. When the nature (benign or malignant) of the mass cannot be determined, further evaluation with laparoscopy ultimately depends on clinical judgment.

Treatment of Menopausal Symptoms

Estrogen is labeled by the FDA for treatment of menopausal vasomotor symptoms and urogenital atrophy and for prevention of osteoporosis, but HT has historically been used for other reasons as well.

Menopause on average occurs at age 51 in the United States, and the average American woman is postmenopausal for one-third of her life. In light of the risks and benefits of HT found in the Women's Health Initiative Trial, many women and their clinicians choose to treat or prevent the sequelae of estrogen deficiency in menopause. Individualization of therapy is essential. Strategies for risk reduction include considerations of the following:

- route of administration of estrogen
- dosage
- duration of use
- selection of the progestational agent (when the uterus is intact)

Vasomotor symptoms or hot flushes are the most common symptom of the climacteric, occurring in up to 80% of perimenopausal women. Symptoms persist for >5 years in 25% of women and are lifelong in a small minority. Although the cause of the vasomotor response remains unknown, vasomotor symptoms are usually relieved within the first cycle of HT (SOE=A). Low-dose therapy can be started, and estrogen dosages titrated until symptoms improve. When estrogen is contraindicated or not acceptable, SSRIs^{OL} or progestins are considered the second most effective therapies (SOE=B). The anticonvulsant gabapentin also has been shown to have efficacy in treatment of vasomotor symptoms. Clonidine^{OL}, methyldopa^{OL}, vitamin E, or herbal remedies such as yams and black cohosh have also been tried, although evidence to support their use is inconsistent (SOE=C). Recently, the FDA has warned the compounding pharmaceutical industry against making claims that "bio-identical compounded" hormone preparations are more effective and/or safer than traditional FDA-approved hormone products because of lack of head-to-head comparison trials. See also estrogen therapy in "Endocrine and Metabolic Disorders," p 506; and HT and osteoporosis prevention in "Osteoporosis," p 243.

Urogenital Atrophy

The lower genital tract is exquisitely sensitive to estrogen. Urogenital atrophy occurs in all postmenopausal women. Proliferation and maturation of the vaginal epithelium depends on adequate estrogen stimulation. With reduced estrogen production, genital blood flow decreases, leading to further decline in delivery of estrogen to those tissues. This reduction in microvascularity leads to vaginal dryness, mucosal pallor, decreased rugation, mucosal thinning, inflammation with discharge, and ultimately decreased vaginal caliber and depth. With progressive atrophy, the vaginal Pap smear–maturation index shows atrophic changes with a decrease in mucosal superficial cells and an increase in intermediate and basal cells. Vaginal pH can be measured using pH paper; a reading >5.0–5.5 usually denotes significant atrophy. Many women experience dyspareunia, burning, and even vaginal bleeding in some cases.

These changes are readily reversed by administration of local estrogen (SOE=A). The intravaginal use of estrogen cream, one-quarter to one-half an applicator (1 g) as infrequently as two nights per week, allows topical estrogen therapy with minimal (if any) absorption into the circulation, endometrial proliferation, or other systemic effects. The available prescription estrogen creams appear to be therapeutically equivalent. Women complaining of irritation and burning from these creams may better tolerate compounded estradiol or estriol in a hypoallergenic medium. The estrogen ring can be used for 3 months per ring, and vaginal tablets are available for use twice a week. Estrogen cream is also an excellent lubricant for use during pessary insertion. (See also "Disorders of Sexual Function," p 446.) In women concerned about systemic absorption of locally administered estrogen, serum estradiol levels can be monitored at baseline and 6–8 weeks after initiation of therapy; dosage can be reduced if any significant increase in levels is noted.

VULVOVAGINAL INFECTION AND INFLAMMATION

Postmenopausal women are susceptible to a broad range of vulvovaginal infections. Candidal infection, common in diabetic and obese patients who are plagued with moisture and irritation, can be treated with oral, intravaginal, and topical antifungal agents. Women should be questioned about their ability to insert a vaginal applicator before beginning therapy. Topical corticosteroids can be used to hasten relief of symptoms of vulvar irritation. Combination therapy with a steroid and antifungal cream may be necessary, because older women commonly have more chronic, untreated candidal infections that spread from the vulva to the inguinal areas. Other vaginal infections such as *Trichomonas* and *Gardnerella* vaginosis that are common in women of reproductive age are less common in older women, likely because of the higher vaginal pH. A wet preparation revealing sheets of inflammatory cells without bacterial forms can represent advanced atrophy rather than an infectious cause. In women with inflammatory atrophy, the vagina will look inflamed (ie, petechia) with serous exudate, rather than thin, pale, and dry as is typical in advanced atrophy. Local estrogen cream may thus need to be considered as well. A clinician should not be hesitant to inquire about sexual practices when a woman presents with recurrent vaginal infections, vesicular lesions, or other changes suggestive of a sexually transmitted disease.

DISORDERS OF THE VULVA

With aging, the skin of the vulva loses elasticity, and the underlying fat and connective tissues undergo degeneration, with loss of collagen and thinning of the epithelial layer. Consequently, postmenopausal women not on estrogen are predisposed to a variety of dermatologic disorders. The assessment of vulvar complaints must include direct examination. Any pigmented lesion that does not respond to topical corticosteroid or estrogen treatment should be promptly biopsied if consistent with individual treatment goals of the patient.

Vulvar skin irritation can result from a variety of agents and causes burning, itching, and edema. Hygienic products used for urinary or fecal incontinence can lead to chemical dermatitis, as can urine or feces themselves. Treatment of incontinence is important to solve this problem. Vulvar burning or pain is rarely caused by estrogen deficiency, and this complaint should be investigated rather than treated with ever-increasing dosages of estrogen.

Vulvodynia, a chronic vulvar pain syndrome, is seen in both pre- and postmenopausal women. The International Society for the Study of Vulvovaginal Diseases (ISSVD) categorizes vulvodynia as either generalized or localized. The condition is further divided into provoked (sexual, nonsexual), unprovoked, or mixed. Treatment of vulvodynia can be challenging and should be approached in a comprehensive manner that includes local anesthetic agents, antidepressant therapy and/or other pain-modulating agents, as well as pelvic floor rehabilitation. Additionally, the expertise of sexual counselors, mental healthcare providers, and pain management specialists should be sought as part of the patient's treatment plan, because a team approach yields better outcomes.

Vulvar excoriation can result from scratching an inflamed vulva. Local corticosteroids such as hydrocortisone 1% ointment applied daily, sitz baths, or use of a bidet can help alleviate vulvar irritation. Any chronically irritated area should be biopsied to exclude malignancy.

Nonneoplastic Vulvar Lesions

Lichen sclerosus causes over one-third of all vulvar dermatoses and can extend beyond the vulva to the perirectal areas. Squamous cell carcinoma of the vulva can arise in 4%–5% of patients with untreated lichen sclerosus. There is epithelial thinning with edema and fibrosis of the dermis. It can progress to shrinkage and adherence of the labia minora with reduction in introital caliber. Lesions are typically shiny, white or pink, and parchment-like; they can be asymptomatic or cause itching, vaginal soreness, and dyspareunia. Diagnosis is confirmed on biopsy of the involved vulvar areas. Recommended treatment involves application of clobetasol propionate 0.05% twice per day. Treatment should be continued for at least 3 months and geared toward normalization or improvement of the skin. Once improvements are noted, reduction in the dosage or frequency of application can be considered. Periodic visits to assess compliance, exclude new lesions, and monitor for skin thinning are important. Further measures include wearing cotton underwear and avoiding irritant soaps. Topical emollient agents, including lanolin, can be helpful.

Table 53.1—Classification of Pelvic Organ Prolapse

Class	Description
1st degree	Extension to the mid-vagina
2nd degree	Approaching the hymenal ring
3rd degree	At the hymenal ring
4th degree	Beyond the hymenal ring

SOURCE: Data from American College of Obstetricians and Gynecologists. *Pelvic Organ Prolapse*. Washington, DC: American College of Obstetricians and Gynecologists. Technical Bulletin No. 214; 1995.

Lichen simplex chronicus, sometimes described as the end of the itch-scratch cycle has been previously described by many other terms, including neurodermatitis and squamous hyperplasia. Lichen simplex chronicus is a localized type of atopic dermatitis that can arise from either extrinsic or intrinsic insults. It can present as hyperplastic, elevated, white keratinized lesions that can be difficult to distinguish clinically from vaginal intraepithelial neoplasia (VIN) or condylomata. Biopsy should precede treatment. Topical mid-potency corticosteroids such as triamcinolone 0.1% twice daily for a few weeks (or longer with thick lesions) typically resolve the lesions; intermittent therapy may be necessary. It is essential not only to remove all irritants or allergens but also to control itching with the cautious use of antihistamines to allow for healing of the involved skin.

Other problematic vulvar lesions include lichen planus, which presents as erosive, ulcerative lesions of the vulva or vagina that can result in significant discomfort and scarring. Ultra-potency corticosteroids applied topically, estrogen cream applied locally, and hydrocortisone applied intravaginally are recommended. Compromised coital ability due to involvement of the vagina is often addressed through surgery or vaginal dilation. Although lichen planus and lichen sclerosus may be difficult to distinguish clinically, the hallmark distinction is that lichen sclerosus does not involve the vagina and extragenital lesions are rare, while lichen planus frequently involves the vagina and extragenital sites such as the oral cavity.

Vulvar Neoplasia

The classification system used by the ISVVD revised the nomenclature of vulva intraepithelial neoplasia (VIN) in 2004. The older terms VIN 1, 2, or 3 have been replaced by VIN usual type versus VIN well differentiated. VIN usual type appears to be related to the human papilloma virus, occurs in younger women, and tends to be multifocal. It includes warty, baseloid, and mixed types, VIN well differentiated does not appear to be related to human papilloma virus, most commonly presents as a unifocal lesion, and is seen primarily in postmenopausal women.

Because benign, premalignant, or malignant vulvar lesions may have similar clinical appearances, all suspicious, unusual, or symptomatic vulvar lesions should be biopsied. The prognosis of VIN differentiated type as well as its progression to squamous cell carcinoma is variable. The gold standard for treatment of unifocal VIN differentiated type is surgical incision with a margin of 0.5–1.0 cm. Surveillance for recurrence is recommended.

Invasive cancer of the vulva is an age-related malignancy; half of all cases occur after age 70. The vast majority are squamous cell carcinomas. Malignant melanoma, sarcoma, basal cell carcinoma, and adenocarcinoma account for <20% of cases. Treatment involves surgery (radical vulvectomy), occasionally accompanied by radiation.

Disorders of Pelvic Floor Support

Childbearing and other activities that increase intra-abdominal pressure cause progressive weakening of the connective tissue and muscular supports of the genital organs and can lead to genital prolapse. Constipation, chronic coughing, and heavy lifting commonly increase intra-abdominal pressure. Common symptoms of prolapse include pelvic pressure, lower back pain, urinary or fecal incontinence, difficulty with rectal emptying, or a palpable mass. Traditional classification of vaginal prolapse includes differentiated protrusion of the posterior vaginal wall (enterocele or rectocele), descent of the anterior vaginal wall (cystocele), and prolapse of the vaginal apex or uterus. These conditions are demonstrated by having the patient bear down or cough while in the dorsal lithotomy position, but the full extent of prolapse is better appreciated with a standing Valsalva maneuver. Vaginal prolapse is a pelvic organ hernia through the vaginal hiatus.

For the 1995 American College of Obstetrics and Gynecology classification of pelvic organ prolapse, see Table 53.1. The International Continence Society and the American Urogynecologic Association adopted a subsequent, rather complex prolapse classification system (Pelvic Organ Prolapse Quantification) that is based on measurement of the distance between vaginal anatomic sites and the hymenal ring, as well as on vaginal length and perineal dimensions. The purpose of this classification, which is used by specialty societies, is to more objectively and reproducibly describe the degree of prolapse.

Progression of mild prolapse (first- or second-degree [Table 53.1]) can be addressed with adequate estrogenization and Kegel exercises to strengthen the pelvic floor musculature (SOE=C). Genital prolapse does not always lead to bladder dysfunction and should not be assumed to be the cause of incontinence (see "Urinary Incontinence," p 220). Correcting advanced prolapse can cause or exacerbate urinary incontinence by "unkinking" the urethra or bladder neck. However, large cystoceles or rectoceles can result in urinary retention, and reducing the cystocele can restore normal bladder function.

Pessaries

Pessaries are commonly used in an effort to delay or avoid surgery. Their use in older women may be indicated to provide comfort and restore bladder function when comorbid illness makes surgery undesirable (SOE=C). Such women may elect long-term pessary use with ongoing oversight by their primary health care provider or gynecologist. Available pessaries are made from rubber, plastic, or silicone. A variety of shapes and sizes are available: donuts, rings, cubes, inflatable balls, and foldable models.

The choice of pessary is influenced by the degree of prolapse, presence of incontinence, type of accompanying tissue relaxation, and ease of care. Patients with prolapse and no incontinence require only space-occupying types (eg, donut). Those with stress incontinence benefit from a foldable lever-type, which restores bladder neck support. Ring pessaries are easier to insert and remove and may be preferred by older women, especially those who used a contraceptive diaphragm in their youth. For those with advanced degrees of apical or anterior wall prolapse, a more rigid pessary (eg, Gellhorn) may be needed. Although more difficult to insert and remove, this pessary type is very popular because of its high degree of efficacy. Self-care can be more challenging. Cube pessaries should be used with caution, because they can adhere to the vaginal walls because of the suction effect and result in mucosal ulcerations when removed.

Pessary selection often proceeds by trial and error and may require multiple office visits; the optimal pessary fits snugly but comfortably and allows voiding and defecating without difficulty. After pessary selection and insertion, clinical follow-up within a few days is essential to ascertain satisfactory usage. After initial fitting and recheck, pessaries should be removed, cleaned, and the vaginal walls inspected.

Pessary care requirements often influence the selection of a device and the amount of follow-up required. If an older woman's mobility or manual dexterity permits, she should remove the pessary two nights per week, wash it with soap and water, and reinsert it with a water-soluble lubricant after arising in the morning. She should use 1 g vaginal estrogen cream the two nights the pessary is out. Women who cannot perform this level of self-care should be assisted at periodic office or home visits if needed (eg, every 6–12 weeks) by a nurse practitioner. All women with pessaries should be instructed to report any unusual discharge, bleeding, or discomfort, and any changes in bladder or bowel function, and all should have a pelvic examination once or twice a year. If discomfort is present or the device becomes uncomfortable, a different size or type should be tried. Pessaries do not work as well with marked vaginal outlet relaxation. If a pessary is left in place for long periods without monitoring, fistulation can develop, or fibrous tissue can form around the pessary, and removal under anesthesia may be necessary.

Surgery for Prolapse

Surgical treatment of vaginal prolapse can be classified as either reconstructive or obliterative. Reconstructive procedures are designed to restore normal anatomy, whereas obliterative procedures result in total or partial closure of the vaginal canal. Vaginal reconstructive procedures include sacrospinous fixation (for apical prolapse), anterior repairs (for a cystocele), and posterior repairs (for a rectocele). These can safely be done under regional anesthesia, which minimizes anesthetic risks. Abdominal reconstructive procedures include sacrocolpopexy (for apical prolapse) and paravaginal repairs (for a cystocele); they typically require general anesthesia. Urinary and fecal incontinence procedures can also be performed at the time of the prolapse surgery. See also "Urinary Incontinence," p 220.

Age, in itself, is not a contraindication to surgery for genital prolapse. When a proven protocol for perioperative care, including preoperative medical clearance, regional anesthesia, infection prophylaxis, and deep-vein thrombosis prophylaxis, is followed, vaginal surgery offers a safe alternative to pessary use for older women with symptomatic genital prolapse. See also "Perioperative Care," p 102.

POSTMENOPAUSAL VAGINAL BLEEDING

Postmenopausal bleeding (defined as bleeding after 1 year of amenorrhea) occurs in a significant number of older women. A referral to gynecology is needed to establish this diagnosis. The challenge is not only to exclude gynecologic malignancies but also to alleviate the symptoms and eliminate the cause of benign conditions. Causes of bleeding can be grouped according to anatomic areas and endocrine dysfunction (Table 53.2). Not all complaints of postmenopausal bleeding are related to the reproductive organs; patients may be confused as to the origin of the bleeding. Proper evaluation involves complete pelvic examination

Table 53.2—Causes of Postmenopausal Vaginal Bleeding

Cervical	■ Carcinoma Cervicitis Polyp
Endocrinologic	■ Exogenous hormones Perimenopausal ovarian function
Ovarian	■ Functioning ovarian tumor
Uterine	■ Endometrial atrophy Hyperplasia Neoplasia Polyp Submucosal leiomyoma
Vaginal	■ Atrophy Inflammation Tumor Ulceration
Vulvar	■ Carcinoma Laceration or ulceration Urethral caruncle
Other	■ Coagulation disorder Rectal lesion Urinary tract infection

looking for any vaginal, cervical, or uterine source and directed diagnostic studies. Endometrial hyperplasia and cancer can be evaluated by taking an endometrial biopsy or by measuring the endometrial thickness on vaginal probe ultrasound. Although neither ultrasound nor biopsy is 100% specific, an endometrial thickness of <5 mm on transvaginal ultrasound essentially excludes endometrial intraepithelial hyperplasia and malignancy, although recurrent postmenopausal bleeding warrants endometrial sampling. The use of saline hysterosonography is helpful in evaluating the endometrial cavity and determining if there is global thickening or a focal lesion. Global thickening is amenable to in-office endometrial biopsy, while focal lesions are best evaluated and biopsied under direct visualization. Hysteroscopy with dilation and curettage is best used for these situations or for cases in which tissue cannot otherwise be adequately sampled or when bleeding persists. New techniques to destroy the endometrial lining (ablation) by heat, cold, radiotherapy, or excision can be helpful in women whose bleeding is proved to be due to nonmalignant conditions, but it is generally not used in postmenopausal women.

Exogenous hormone replacement is a common cause of postmenopausal bleeding. Megestrol used for appetite stimulation can also cause postmenopausal vaginal bleeding. Women on continuous combined estrogen–progesterone replacement who continue to have bleeding after 1 year should be evaluated. Some specialists recommend biopsy if bleeding persists beyond 6 months. Women on cyclic hormone therapy who bleed at an unexpected time during the cycle should also be evaluated. See also estrogen therapy in "Endocrine and Metabolic Disorders," p 506.

References

- Abernethy K. Managing vaginal dryness in menopause. *Practice Nursing*. 2013;24(5):230–234.
- Kingsberg SA, Wysocki S, Magnus L, et al. Vulvar and vaginal atrophy in postmenopausal women: Findings from the REVIVE (REal Women's VIews of Treatment Options for Menopausal Vaginal Changes) Survey. *J Sex Med*. 2013 May 16.
- Kuncharapu I, Majeroni BA, Johnson DW. Pelvic organ prolapse. *Am Fam Physician*. 2010; 81(9):1111–1117.
- Mold JW, Holtzclaw BJ, McCarthy L. Night sweats: a systematic review of the literature. *J Am Board Fam Med*. 2012;25(6):878–893.
- Stewart KM. Clinical care of vulvar pruritus, with emphasis on one common cause, lichen simplex chronicus. *Dermatol Clin*. 2010;28(4):669–680.

CHAPTER 54—PROSTATE DISEASE

KEY POINTS

- A number of treatment options exist for benign prostatic hyperplasia (BPH), including watchful waiting, medications, minimally invasive procedures, and more extensive operations. The choice is influenced by the extent of symptoms, the presence of complications from outflow obstruction, and patient preferences.
- The use of 5α-reductase inhibitors for BPH is especially indicated when the prostate gland is large.
- Two trials of prostate cancer screening using serial prostate-specific antigen (PSA) measurement in men 55–74 years old indicate that screening leads to significant overdiagnosis and overtreatment of clinically insignificant tumors. The trials show somewhat conflicting results on mortality after a decade of screening, one showing no mortality benefit and the other observing a very modest benefit. Men should be well informed about the risks and benefits of PSA screening before making a decision whether or not to be screened.
- Several treatment options exist for men with localized prostate cancer, including watchful waiting, resection of the gland and seminal vesicles, and radiation therapy. How the patient balances the potential benefits and burdens of the various options will influence the choice of therapy.
- For patients with chronic prostatitis, efforts should be made to identify the causative organism, and even with a prolonged course of appropriate antibiotics, a cure can be expected in fewer than half the patients.

With advancing age, the prevalence of prostate diseases increases dramatically. The three most common conditions are BPH, prostate cancer, and prostatitis. Self-reported prostate disease affects about 3 million American men. BPH develops in over half of men ≥65 years old and affects the overwhelming majority of men >85 years old. Prostate cancer is the second leading cause of cancer death in men, and many men have asymptomatic or low-grade tumors that cause few or no health problems. The prevalence of prostatitis is similar to that of ischemic heart disease or diabetes mellitus.

BENIGN PROSTATIC HYPERPLASIA

Epidemiology

BPH is a noncancerous enlargement of the epithelial and fibromuscular components of the prostate gland. The epithelial component normally makes up 20%–30% of prostate volume and contributes to the seminal fluid. The fibromuscular component comprises 70%–80% of the prostate and is responsible for expressing prostatic fluid during ejaculation. Age and long-term androgen stimulation induce development of BPH. Microscopic appearance of BPH can be seen as early as age 30, is present in 50% of men by age 60, and is present in 90% of men by age 85. In half of these cases, microscopic BPH develops into palpable macroscopic BPH. Of those with macroscopic BPH, only half develop clinically significant disease that is brought to medical attention. BPH is one of the most common conditions in aging men; in the United States annually it accounts for more than 1.7 million office visits and 250,000 surgical procedures.

Prostatism, or Lower Urinary Tract Symptoms

The symptoms of BPH are nonspecific; other diseases can result in identical symptoms. The pathophysiology of BPH symptoms is not completely understood, but presumably it involves the periurethral zone of the prostate gland, which results in obstructed urine flow and compensatory responses of the bladder, such as hypertrophy and decreased capacity. The urethral obstruction has both mechanical (obstructing mass) and dynamic (smooth muscle contractions) components. The resulting lower urinary tract symptoms are divided into irritative (eg, frequency, urgency, nocturia) and obstructive (eg, hesitancy, intermittency, weak stream, incomplete emptying) manifestations. These 7 lower urinary tract symptoms compose a quantitative symptom index for severity assessment and treatment response monitoring, which was developed by the American Urological Association and adopted by the World Health Organization, known as the International Prostate Symptom Score. Although tracking symptom severity is useful in the longitudinal management of patients, symptom severity has not been found to correlate with prostate size, urine flow rates, or postvoid residual volume. BPH primarily affects quality of life, although complications such as recurrent urinary tract infection, bladder stones, urinary retention, chronic renal insufficiency, and hematuria can develop.

Table 54.1—Management Options for Benign Prostatic Hyperplasia

Category	Interventions	Rationale	Comments
Lifestyle modification	Reduce nighttime fluids to manage nocturia; eliminate bladder irritants (eg, caffeine, alcohol, nicotine)	Factors outside the urinary tract contribute to urinary symptoms	Often sufficient management for mild symptoms; complements management for moderate to severe symptoms
Pharmacologic management	α-Adrenergic antagonists Selective α_1: prazosin[OL] Long-acting selective α_1: terazosin, doxazosin Long-acting selective α_{1a} subtype selective: tamsulosin, silodosin, alfuzosin	Relaxation of smooth muscle in hyperplastic prostate tissue, prostate capsule, and bladder neck decreases resistance to urinary flow	Adverse events: dizziness, mild asthenia, headaches, postural hypotension (reduced with careful dosage titration, not present with selective α_{1a} subtypes), abnormal ejaculation, rhinitis
	5α-Reductase inhibitors: finasteride, dutasteride	Reduced tissue levels of dihydrotestosterone result in prostate gland size reduction	Most effective for men with larger prostates (>40 g); results may not be evident for up to 6 months
Surgery	Transurethral resection of the prostate; transurethral incision of the prostate; open prostatectomy; transurethral vaporization of the prostate; stent placement	Removal or expansion of periurethral prostate tissue reduces obstruction to urinary flow	Indicated for recurrent urinary tract infection induced by benign prostatic hypertrophy, recurrent or persistent gross hematuria, bladder stones, renal insufficiency

Diagnosis

Differential diagnosis of lower urinary tract symptoms includes endocrine disorders (especially diabetes mellitus), neurologic disorders, urinary tract infections, sexually transmitted diseases, kidney or bladder stones, and medications (especially medications with anticholinergic and diuretic effects). Digital rectal examination (DRE) can be unremarkable or reveal an enlarged, smooth, rubbery, symmetrical gland. Urinalysis is routinely performed to evaluate for urinary tract infection, hematuria, and glycosuria. A baseline serum creatinine measurement assesses kidney function and the possibility of obstructive uropathy or intrinsic renal disease, or both. Additional optional tests include postvoid residual urine volume (often done by office or bedside bladder scan), urine flow rates, and pressure flow studies. These tests can be considered when the diagnosis is uncertain or an invasive treatment is being planned.

Treatment Approaches

BPH therapy depends on the patient and is driven by the impact of symptoms on the patient's quality of life (Table 54.1). All patients should be educated regarding lifestyle modification by adjusting fluid intake (eg, avoiding caffeine) and avoiding medications (especially anticholinergics) that aggravate symptoms. Men with mild to moderate symptoms may be satisfied with lifestyle modification only. Both medical and surgical treatments are also available, with medication the usual first approach. Indications for surgical treatment include patient preference, dissatisfaction with medication, and refractory urinary retention, as well as renal dysfunction, bladder stones, recurrent urinary tract infections, or hematuria if these are clearly due to prostatic obstruction.

Medical Treatment

The two main pharmacologic approaches are α-adrenergic antagonist and 5α-reductase inhibitor therapy (SOE=A).

α-Adrenergic antagonists, or α-blockers, are directed at the dynamic component of urethral obstruction. Smooth muscle of the prostate and bladder neck has a resting tone mediated by α-adrenergic innervation. α-Blockers relax the smooth muscle in the hyperplastic prostate tissue, prostate capsule, and bladder neck, thus decreasing resistance to urinary flow. Of the two major α-adrenergic receptors, α_1 receptors predominate in the prostate, with the α_{1a} subtype comprising 70% of these receptors. α-Blockade development for BPH therapy has progressed from selective α_1 agents (eg, prazosin, alfuzosin) to long-acting selective α_1 agents (terazosin, doxazosin) and then to long-acting α_{1a} subtype selective agents (tamsulosin, silodosin). The most common adverse events of α_1 agents are dizziness, mild asthenia (fatigue or weakness), and headaches. Postural hypotension occurs infrequently and can be minimized by careful dosage titration. For patients undergoing cataract surgery, intraoperative floppy iris syndrome (IFIS), characterized by sudden intraoperative iris prolapse and pupil constriction, is a potential risk of all α-blockers with the greatest frequency and severity of IFIS among those using tamsulosin (SOE=B).

The enzyme 5α-reductase is required for the conversion of testosterone to the more active dihydrotestosterone. Finasteride and dutasteride are inhibitors of 5α-reductase and reduce tissue levels of dihydrotestosterone, thus reducing prostate gland size. Improvements in symptom scores and urine flow rates may not be evident for up to 6 months. The 5α-reductase inhibitors are most effective in men with larger prostates

(>40 g, about the size of a plum) (SOE=A). Because 5α-reductase inhibitors reduce serum PSA levels by an average of 50%, after 6 months of therapy, men receiving prostate cancer surveillance will need a new baseline serum PSA determination.

When used together over years, the combination of α-adrenergic antagonists with 5α-reductase inhibitors has been shown to be safe and to reduce clinical progression of BPH better than either agent alone (SOE=A). In particular, a lower risk of urinary retention, urinary incontinence, renal insufficiency, and recurrent bladder infections is associated with combination therapy. Trials of BPH therapy with the herbal preparation *Serenoa repens,* or saw palmetto, show conflicting results. Limited data from smaller studies suggested that it improves urinary symptoms and flow measures in men with BPH. However, a recent Cochrane review found that compared with placebo, *S repens* monotherapy does not improve urinary symptoms or maximal urinary flow rate even at double and triple the usual dosage. See also "Complementary and Alternative Medicine," p 90.

Surgical Treatment

Surgical management includes transurethral resection of the prostate (TURP), transurethral incision of the prostate (TUIP), open prostatectomy, transurethral vaporization of the prostate, and device insertion such as stent placement. Surgical approaches offer the best chance for symptom improvement but also have the highest rates of complications. The benefits of various surgical treatments are generally considered equivalent, but complication rates differ. TURP is the standard of care to which other BPH treatments are compared, and it has an 80% likelihood of successful outcome in properly selected patients (SOE=A). Usually performed under spinal anesthesia, TURP involves passage of an endoscope through the urethra to surgically remove the inner portion of the prostate. Long-term complications can include retrograde ejaculation, urethral stricture, bladder neck contracture, incontinence, and impotence. TUIP is an endoscopic procedure via the urethra to make one or two cuts in the prostate and prostate capsule, relieving urethral constriction. Limited to use in small prostate glands (<30 g), TUIP offers lower rates of retrograde ejaculation, bleeding, and contractures. Open prostatectomy involves removal of the inner portion of the prostate through a retropubic or suprapubic incision. It is best used for patients with larger prostates or with complicating conditions such as bladder stones or urethral strictures. Open prostatectomy is associated with incisional morbidity, longer hospitalization, and greater risk of impotence. Transurethral vaporization of the prostate uses a high-energy electrode inserted via the urethra to vaporize the prostate. This approach has little bleeding but creates more prolonged irritative voiding. Prostatic stents are used to maintain expansion of the prostatic urethra and have both temporary and permanent uses.

PROSTATE CANCER

Incidence and Epidemiology

Prostate cancer is the most common noncutaneous cancer and the second leading cause of cancer deaths among men in the United States. Since 2010, it has been estimated that over 200,000 men would be diagnosed with and over 30,000 men would die annually from prostate cancer. Incidence increases with age; prostate cancer is rare in men <40 years old. A prevalence study of 340 healthy men scheduled for organ donation, reported in 2008, found the prevalence of prostate cancer was 0.5% in men <50 years old, 23.4% in men 50–59 years old, 35% in men 60–69 years old, and 45.5% in men >70 years old. Earlier autopsy studies that included debilitated men have found prevalence rates as high as 80% in men >80 years old. The incidence of disease varies according to race, with black Americans having the highest risk in the world. Among black men, prostate cancer occurs at an earlier age, has a higher mortality rate, and tends to be at a more advanced stage at diagnosis. Family history is a contributing factor. Men with one first-degree relative affected have more than a 2-fold increased risk (SOE=B). Androgens are necessary for prostate cancer pathogenesis; the disease does not occur in men castrated before puberty. History of sexually transmitted disease can be associated with an increased risk of prostate cancer (SOE=B). The association between prostate cancer and omega-3 fatty acid intake, alcohol intake, or vasectomy is inconclusive.

Symptoms

Cancer usually arises in the peripheral zone of the prostate. Most men, especially those with early-stage, potentially curable disease, are asymptomatic. Prostate cancer spreads by three routes: direct extension, the lymphatics, and the bloodstream. Direct invasion of the urethra and bladder can lead to irritative voiding symptoms, urinary incontinence, and hematuria. Extension of disease to adjacent nerves can cause impotence and pelvic pain. Nodal metastasis can cause extrinsic ureteral obstruction. Leg edema can develop from lymphatic obstruction. Hematogenous metastasis to bone can cause severe local pain, normochromic normocytic anemia, pathologic fractures, and spinal cord compression. Less commonly, hematogenous metastasis involves viscera, namely the lung, liver, and adrenal glands.

Screening Controversy

The benefit of early detection and the best approach to treatment of prostate cancer are controversial. There is a large reservoir of prostate cancer that does not need to be diagnosed because most men with prostate cancer die with the disease, not from it. However, the well-recognized burden of progressive prostate cancer is a potential impetus for early detection and management.

Results of two prospective, randomized controlled trials of prostate cancer screening report somewhat conflicting findings. The Prostate, Lung, Colorectal, and Ovarian Cancer Screening Trial found no significant difference in prostate cancer mortality between screened and unscreened groups after 7–10 years of follow-up. The European Randomized Study of Screening for Prostate Cancer, which was actually a collection of smaller trials in different European countries, found a 20% decrease in prostate cancer mortality in the screened subgroup aged 50–64 years over a mean of 9 years of follow-up; the absolute risk difference associated with screening was 0.071%, meaning that 1,410 men would need to be screened and 48 additional cases of prostate cancer would be treated for every prostate cancer death prevented. Both trials documented significantly increased prostate cancer incidence associated with screening. Men who were >74 years old at baseline were not enrolled in either trial. The two trials had significant methodologic differences, particularly for inclusion criteria, enrollment size, frequency and mode of screening, definition of a positive PSA level, and follow-up.

Screening for prostate cancer remains a controversial topic with different recommendations and guidelines from various task forces and specialty societies. In 2012, the U.S. Preventive Services Task Force issued updated recommendations giving routine screening for prostate cancer a "D" rating, meaning that "there is moderate or high certainty that the service has no benefit or that the harms outweigh the benefits." The U.S. Preventive Services Task Force noted that "The reduction in prostate cancer mortality 10 to 14 years after PSA-based screening is, at most, very small, even for men in the optimal age range of 55 to 69 years." The American Cancer Society's 2011 guideline recommends that men discuss screening with their doctor to make an informed decision, starting at age 50, or younger if risk factors are present. Other societies, including the American Urological Association, have recommended offering PSA measurement and DRE to well-informed men with at least a 10-year remaining life expectancy, starting at age 40–50. Many of these societies are in the process of updating their guidelines. Because screening for prostate cancer may lead to harm, including psychologic stress and adverse effects of further diagnostic testing, or adverse effects of treatment if prostate cancer is detected, clinicians should carefully discuss options and consequences with patients before proceeding with screening in asymptomatic men.

Screening and Diagnostic Tests

DRE allows palpation of the posterior surfaces of the lateral lobes of the prostate, where cancer most often begins. Cancer characteristically is hard, nodular, and irregular. Although DRE is less sensitive than PSA in detecting prostate cancer, it can sometimes detect cancers in men who have a normal PSA level. Its use as a single screening test is greatly limited, however, because parts of the prostate gland cannot be palpated. About half of the cancers thought to be limited to the prostate on the basis of DRE are found during surgery to have already spread. DRE has many false-positive results; only about one-third of men with positive DRE tests have prostate cancer on biopsy. Local extension of prostate cancer into the seminal vesicles can often be detected by DRE, which may be valuable in staging of disease. Thus, despite its limitations, DRE has a role in prostate cancer staging and in screening asymptomatic patients who choose to be screened.

The serum PSA test is not specific for prostate cancer. PSA increases in benign conditions of the prostate, namely, hypertrophy and prostatitis, and in transient response to conditions such as ejaculation and prostatic massage. The sensitivity of the PSA test is also imperfect. Decreased PSA values have been associated with acute hospitalization and use of medications such as 5α-reductase inhibitors and saw palmetto. PSA levels are normal in 30%–40% of men with cancer confined to the prostate (ie, false-negative tests). The reported positive predictive value of PSA in screening studies is 28%–35%: about one-third of men with increased PSA levels have prostate cancer demonstrated by fine-needle biopsy.

Several approaches to improve the accuracy of PSA testing have been developed. PSA density is derived from the PSA concentration divided by the volume of the prostate gland (measured by ultrasound). Prostate cancer results in higher PSA levels per unit volume than BPH and should therefore yield a higher PSA density. The PSA rate of change or velocity is more specific for prostate cancer than a single PSA measurement. Using a PSA velocity value of ≥0.75 ng/mL/year achieves 90% specificity, whereas using a single PSA level >4 ng/mL achieves 60% specificity. This high specificity for PSA velocity is realized even in normal-range serum PSA levels (<4 ng/mL). Another approach involves age-adjusted PSA reference ranges because PSA values increase with age. Finally, the ratio of free to complexed

Table 54.2—Staging Systems for Prostate Cancer

TNM Stage	Jewett-Whitmore Stage	Description
T_1	A1, A2	Tumor is an incidental finding.
T_{1c}		Tumor is identified by needle biopsy as a follow-up to screening that detected increased PSA.
T_2	B1, B2	Tumor is palpable, confined to prostate.
T_3	C1, C2	Tumor extends beyond the prostate capsule, may involve seminal vesicles.
T_4	C2	Tumor invades adjacent structures (eg, bladder neck, rectum, pelvic wall).
N	D1	Lymph node metastasis present.
M	D2	Distant metastasis present.

NOTE: TNM = tumor, regional node, metastasis

SOURCE: For further details, see AUA Prostate Cancer Clinical Guidelines Panel. *Report on the Management of Clinically Localized Prostate Cancer.* Baltimore, MD: American Urological Association; 1995.

PSA can be measured, recognizing that PSA bound to α_1-antichymotrypsin accounts for a larger proportion of total PSA with prostate cancer than with BPH.

Abnormal DRE or PSA tests lead to transrectal ultrasound-guided biopsy of the prostate for pathologic diagnosis. Cancer can appear as a hypoechoic density, but ultrasonography is not specific enough to be used as a screening tool. Any suspicious areas (by DRE or ultrasound) are biopsied. In addition to, or in the absence of suspicious areas, spring-loaded core needle biopsies are routinely taken from the base, middle, and apex of each lobe (six samples total, termed sextant biopsy). Sextant biopsy can be enhanced by extended biopsy schemes that sample more gland areas, particularly the lateral aspects. In a systematic review, prostate biopsy schemes that consist of 12 cores (standard sextant biopsy plus laterally directed cores) achieved a reasonable balance between cancer detection rates and adverse events.

Grading

The Gleason grading system is the most commonly used system that is based on the histologic appearance of prostate cancer. The Gleason grade ranges from 1, or well differentiated, to 5, or poorly differentiated. The Gleason score is the sum of the most common Gleason grade observed plus the next most common Gleason grade seen. The Gleason score ranges from 2 to 10. Gleason scores are sometimes grouped as 2–4, well differentiated; 5–7, moderately differentiated; 8–10, poorly differentiated. Well-differentiated tumors have a favorable prognosis; poorly differentiated tumors, an unfavorable prognosis (SOE=A). Most clinically detected tumors are moderately differentiated.

Staging

Staging of prostate cancer is necessary for planning disease management. Two classification systems are used: the tumor, regional node, metastasis (TNM) system and the Jewett-Whitmore (ABCD) system (Table 54.2). Usually detected by transurethral resection of the prostate, incidentally discovered cancers are staged according to the amount of tissue involved (T_1 or A). Stage T_{1c} reflects the growing number of tumors detected because of an increased PSA level. Tumors detectable by DRE and confined to the prostate (T_2 or B) are subdivided on the basis of the amount of tumor that is palpable. Staging is also based on the degree of extension and invasion of surrounding structures in tumors that extend beyond the prostatic capsule (T_3 to T_4 or C), and on presence of metastasis (M_1 or D).

The initial staging evaluation includes PSA level, DRE findings, transrectal ultrasonography results, and Gleason score. Bone scans may be performed on patients with PSA values >10 ng/mL, Gleason scores >6, or complaints of bone pain (SOE=D). For patients electing active treatment, surgical assessment of lymph node involvement (pelvic lymphadenectomy) is performed by itself or in conjunction with prostate surgery or implantation of radioactive seeds. CT scans are often used for active treatment planning.

In the past, CT scans, MRI scans, pedal lymphangiography, and pelvic lymph node dissection were routinely used in various combinations to evaluate the extent of prostate cancer. In the initial staging evaluation of patients with prostate cancer, these tests should be eliminated because they have been associated with unacceptably high false-negative and false-positive results. A subset of patients appears to benefit from CT scans combined with fine-needle aspiration. Patients who have a PSA >25 ng/mL, a Gleason score >6, and a palpable abnormality on DRE are recommended to undergo a CT scan with fine-needle aspiration if a lymph node >6 mm is present (SOE=D). Many of these patients will be diagnosed with nodal metastasis and are thus spared the need for bilateral pelvic lymph-node dissection and its associated morbidity.

The serum PSA level should be used to eliminate the staging radionuclide bone scan (SOE=C). In the asymptomatic, newly diagnosed, previously untreated prostate cancer patient, a PSA concentration ≤10 ng/mL has been associated with rare (0%–0.8%) findings of skeletal metastases. Adopting recommendations to eliminate the staging radionuclide bone scan in this population will substantially reduce testing, because 50%–60% of men with newly diagnosed prostate cancer have a serum PSA concentration in this range.

Table 54.3—Management Approaches for Prostate Cancer

Management	Description	Comments	Selected Adverse Effects
Localized			
Watchful waiting	Prostate cancer is not treated until symptoms develop	Offered to men with <10 years of remaining life expectancy; significant medical comorbidities; small, well-differentiated tumors; or unwillingness to bear treatment burdens Awaiting symptoms sacrifices opportunity for cure	Anxiety
Radical prostatectomy	Surgical removal of the entire prostate gland and seminal vesicles	Offered to men who have no surgical contraindications Adverse effects realized immediately	Erectile dysfunction, urinary incontinence
External beam radiation therapy	Standard regimen delivers 6,000–7,000 rads of pelvic radiation over 5- to 8-week period	Radiation reaches tissues outside the prostate, including pelvic lymph nodes Adverse effects occur initially from radiation-induced inflammation, then develop over time as scar tissue develops	*Acute:* proctitis, urethritis *Chronic:* erectile dysfunction, urinary incontinence, bowel dysfunction
Brachytherapy	Radioactive seeds (eg, iridium, palladium) are implanted into the prostate gland using CT scan guidance	Improvements in prostate imaging allow uniform distribution of seed, overcoming past limitations Adverse effects occur initially from radiation-induced inflammation, then develop over time as scar tissue develops	*Acute:* prostatitis, urinary retention, hematuria *Chronic:* erectile dysfunction, urinary incontinence, bowel dysfunction
Locally Advanced			
Radiation therapy	See external beam radiation (above)	Offered to men with prostate cancer extending beyond capsule or into seminal vesicles Asymptomatic cancer period may be prolonged	See external beam radiation (above)
Androgen deprivation	Hormone therapy can be combined with radiation therapy	Neoadjuvant androgen deprivation provides additional benefit toward increased survival and freedom from metastases; because of adverse effects, controversy exists regarding early versus delayed use of androgen deprivation	Erectile dysfunction, loss of libido, loss of stamina, increased fatigue, hot flashes, diminished muscle mass, premature osteoporosis
Advanced/Metastatic			
Complete androgen ablation	Combined approach of reducing androgens to castration levels and inhibiting binding of androgen to its receptor	Includes orchiectomy or LHRH agonists with antiandrogens	Erectile dysfunction, loss of libido, loss of stamina, increased fatigue, hot flashes, diminished muscle mass, premature osteoporosis
Orchiectomy	Surgical castration	Oldest, safest, least expensive approach; rejected by half of American men	Erectile dysfunction, loss of libido, loss of stamina, increased fatigue, hot flashes, diminished muscle mass, premature osteoporosis
LHRH agonists	Chemical castration	Alternative to surgical castration, equally effective Causes initial increase in serum testosterone levels	Erectile dysfunction, loss of libido, hot flashes, gynecomastia, insomnia, GI upset, dizziness
Antiandrogens	Inhibit binding of androgen to its receptor	Used at initiation of LHRH-agonist therapy to block effect of increased testosterone levels Used after castration to block effect of residual small amount of androgen being produced by adrenal glands	Erectile dysfunction, loss of libido, gynecomastia, insomnia, GI upset, dizziness
Other	Symptom-specific approaches are used as indicated	For example, focal radiation therapy can be provided to the site of a bony metastasis to reduce both pain and risk of fracture	Intervention specific

NOTE: LHRH = luteinizing hormone-releasing hormone

Management of Localized Disease

Localized cancer lends itself to cure, but the prevalence of men dying with prostate cancer (often asymptomatic) but not from the disease questions the necessity of treatment. There remains a lack of evidence that treatment prolongs life when treatment is compared with watchful waiting. Thus, three approaches to localized prostate cancer are routinely advocated: watchful waiting, radical prostatectomy, and radiation therapy (Table 54.3).

Watchful waiting (also called *expectant* or *conservative management; surveillance)* is the approach offered most commonly to men with <10 years of remaining life expectancy, who have significant medical comorbidities, or whose tumor is small and well to moderately differentiated. Conservative management studies have shown that 10-year disease-specific survival is 89%–96% for men with Gleason score 2–5 tumors, 70%–82% for men with Gleason score 6 tumors, 30%–58% for men with Gleason score 7 tumors, and 13%–40% for men with Gleason score 8–10 tumors. Because most men with prostate cancer are asymptomatic, watchful waiting attempts to spare men the burden of unnecessary treatment. However, waiting for symptoms in men with prostate cancer before starting treatment means sacrificing the opportunity for cure. Patients are offered palliation if and when symptoms develop. A newer approach, active surveillance, combines the concept of expectant management with the option for deferred curative intent treatment. The optimal selection criteria and surveillance strategy for active surveillance have not been defined. Active surveillance selection criteria include cases detected by PSA screening with Gleason scores <7 and small volume involvement (<3 of 6 biopsy cores, <50% malignant involvement within each core). The National Comprehensive Cancer Network guidelines for active surveillance suggest serum PSA measurement as often as every 3 months, DRE as often as every 6 months, and repeat prostate biopsy as often as every 12 months (SOE=C).

Radical prostatectomy involves the surgical removal of the entire prostate gland and the seminal vesicles. It can be performed through a perineal (incision near the rectum) or retropubic (lower abdominal incision) approach. The perineal approach allows an easier vesicourethral anastomosis and less bleeding, whereas the retropubic approach allows access to the pelvic lymph nodes and spares the neurovascular supply to the corpora cavernosa (with improved potency). The major complications of radical prostatectomy are urinary incontinence and erectile dysfunction. Surgery is thought to have the highest incidence of posttreatment sexual dysfunction. In a population-based study of 1,291 men undergoing radical prostatectomy for clinically localized prostate cancer, 59.9% reported erections not firm enough for sexual intercourse and 8.4% were incontinent 18 months later (SOE=C). After radical prostatectomy, men are more likely to experience stress incontinence, with symptoms ranging from occasional leakage to no urinary control. Bladder neck contractures also occur, resulting in obstructive voiding symptoms and urinary retention. The relationship between these symptoms and sense of bother is not direct; for example, those with the most leakage may have little bother while those with minimal leakage may report substantial bother.

Data regarding the benefits of radical prostatectomy are still lacking. Two randomized controlled trials have compared radical prostatectomy with watchful waiting. In one study of 695 men with 10-year follow up, prostatectomy compared with watchful waiting reduced both death from prostate cancer (10% versus 15%) and distant metastases (15.2% versus 25.4%). In the second study of 142 men, no statistically significant differences in survival were found; however, the study lacked sufficient power to detect moderate treatment differences. Both studies were conducted before prostate cancer detection with PSA testing was available. Two surgical improvements currently under investigation to reduce morbidity include the laparoscopic approach and robotic assistance. The laparoscopic approach has raised concerns of poorer results related to positive surgical margins, return of continence, and preservation of potency. Robotic approaches have not shown advantage in hospital length of stay, postoperative pain, or blood replacement (SOE=C). Long-term outcomes are not yet known for either the laparoscopic or robotic approach. Thus, radical prostatectomy can be offered to men with locally confined disease, with >10 years of remaining life expectancy, and without contraindications to undergoing surgery (SOE=B).

Radiation therapy is provided through external beam radiation or through implantation of radioactive sources (known as *brachytherapy*). The standard regimen of external beam radiation delivers a total of about 6,000–7,000 rads over 5–8 weeks. Hypofractionated schemes use higher doses per fraction that achieve biologically similar doses over 4–5 weeks. Pelvic lymph nodes can be radiated as well. Proctitis and urethritis are common acute adverse events. Chronic complications include erectile dysfunction, urinary incontinence, and chronic proctitis. The incidence of urinary stress incontinence after radiation therapy is significantly less than with surgery but that of irritative voiding dysfunction is greater. Bowel dysfunction, uncommon after surgery, affects more than half of patients after radiation. Bowel symptoms include diarrhea, rectal urgency, and fecal soiling. Most patients classify these bowel symptoms as minor with little to no effect on quality of life.

Conformal radiation therapy is a mode of high-precision external-beam radiation that uses high-resolution CT scan data and advanced computer technology to conform the radiation dose to the three-dimensional configuration of the tumor. This newer technology shows promise in reducing complications and adverse events. Local control and cancer survival rates appear to be comparable to those of radical prostatectomy, at least for the first 5–8 years (SOE=C). Comparisons between treatments are difficult because men undergoing radiation treatment tend to be older, less medically fit, and usually have not been pathologically staged.

Brachytherapy involves retropubic or perineal implantation of radioactive seeds, usually iridium or palladium. Improvements in three-dimensional imaging of the prostate through CT scan or ultrasound guidance have allowed more uniform distribution of seeds throughout the prostate and overcome many of the past limitations of brachytherapy. Potency is better preserved with seed implants. Urinary symptoms include frequency, dysuria, and urge incontinence. Bowel symptoms include rectal urgency and rectal bleeding. The morbidity of seed implants appears to improve over time after the initial seed placement and associated prostate inflammation and swelling. In retrospective series, it appears that brachytherapy is comparable to radical prostatectomy and external beam radiation for low-risk disease. However, brachytherapy outcomes appear less favorable for tumors with higher Gleason score or higher pretreatment PSA levels (SOE=C).

Management of Locally Advanced Prostate Cancer

Locally advanced prostate cancer extends beyond the capsule or invades the seminal vesicle, without evidence of distant or nodal metastasis. Radiation therapy is the recommended treatment, and neoadjuvant androgen deprivation provides additional benefit toward increased survival and freedom from metastases (SOE=B). However, controversy exists as to when androgen deprivation should be started. Patients may have a prolonged asymptomatic cancer period, while significant negative quality-of-life changes from long-term androgen deprivation occur, including loss of stamina, increased fatigue, hot flashes, diminished muscle mass, and premature osteoporosis. While radiation therapy with neoadjuvant androgen deprivation is a standard approach for locally advanced disease, some advocate that patients should be given the choice of early versus delayed androgen deprivation.

Management of Advanced Disease

Advanced disease is treated with androgen ablation and symptom-specific approaches, such as focal radiation therapy to painful bone metastasis. Androgen ablation aims to eliminate prostate cancer growth stimulation and includes orchiectomy or luteinizing hormone-releasing hormone (LHRH) agonists with antiandrogens. Orchiectomy and LHRH agonists are equally effective at reducing androgens to castration levels. Orchiectomy is the oldest, safest, least expensive approach but is rejected by nearly half of American men. LHRH agonists such as leuprolide and goserelin result in castration levels about 1 month after an initial increase in serum testosterone levels. Antiandrogens (eg, flutamide) are often given before starting LHRH agonists to blunt the effects of the initial testosterone increase. Antiandrogens inhibit the binding of androgen to its receptor. After castration, a small amount of adrenal androgen exists and may allow continued stimulation of prostate cancer growth. Antiandrogens can be combined with chemical or surgical castration, a practice called *complete androgen ablation*. Survival rates for antiandrogens alone are inferior to those for chemical or surgical castration alone; complete androgen ablation offers slight improvement in survival over that offered by castration only (SOE=B).

Radiation therapy is useful for relieving the pain of isolated bone metastasis and reducing the risk of fracture of bones with significant destruction. Diffuse bone metastases require alternative approaches. Bone-seeking radiopharmaceuticals such as strontium or radium can be beneficial for pain control (SOE=B). Androgen deprivation decreases bone pain in two-thirds of symptomatic patients (SOE=B). Bisphosphonates also decrease bone pain (SOE=B).

PROSTATITIS

Etiology

Prostatitis is an inflammatory condition of the prostate that can result from acute bacterial, chronic bacterial, or nonbacterial causes. The most common sources of acute or chronic infection are ascending urethral infection or reflux of infected urine into the prostatic ducts, or both. Direct extension or lymphatic spread from the rectum or hematogenous spread also occurs. Acute prostatitis is an infectious process that is more common in younger men than in older men. Pathogens in men ≤35 years old often include *Neisseria gonorrhea* and *Chlamydia trachomatis*. In older men, acute prostatitis is associated with indwelling urethral catheter use, and coliforms are the suspected bacterial cause. In >80% of patients with prostatitis, no infectious agent is identified.

Diagnosis

Acute bacterial prostatitis is characterized by fever, chills, dysuria, and a tense or boggy, extremely tender prostate. Because bacteremia can result from manipulation of the inflamed gland, minimal rectal examination is indicated. Gram's stain and culture of the urine can identify the causative agent.

Chronic bacterial prostatitis presents classically as recurrent bacteriuria caused by the same organism, although most patients do not have this presentation. Patients have varying degrees of obstructive or irritative voiding symptoms and perineal pain. The prostate often feels normal. First-void or midstream urine is compared with expressed prostatic secretion or urine collected after prostatic massage. The expressed sample should reveal leukocytosis and the causative agent. Sterile expressant with leukocytosis suggests nonbacterial prostatitis.

Treatment

Acute bacterial prostatitis is treated with antibiotics and can require hospitalization. The severe inflammation allows antibiotics to penetrate the prostate, and prompt response to empiric therapy is expected. CT or MRI should be considered to evaluate for an abscess if recovery is delayed. Antibiotic selection should be based initially on results of a urine Gram's stain, with subsequent consideration of sensitivity profiles. Fluoroquinolones are highly effective in most cases.

Antibiotics are less effective for chronic bacterial prostatitis because of their poor penetration of the prostate. Prolonged therapy (6–16 weeks) offers a cure rate of 30%–40%. Continuous low-dose antibiotic suppression therapy can be offered for those with frequent symptomatic relapse. Total prostatectomy offers cure but at a high risk-to-benefit ratio. Transurethral resection of the prostate is safer but cures only one-third of patients.

Nonbacterial prostatitis is treated symptomatically. A small percentage of cases can involve occult infections, and empiric antibiotic therapy is often used. Efforts to reduce pain and discomfort include anti-inflammatory agents, sitz baths, fluid adjustments (avoid caffeine), anticholinergic agents, and α-adrenergic antagonists.

References

- Moyer VA. Screening for Prostate Cancer: U.S. Preventive Services Task Force Recommendation Statement. *Ann Intern Med.* 2012;157:120–134.
- Nazarko L. Urinary incontinence: Providing respectful, dignified care. *Br J Community Nurs.* 2013;18(2):58–67.
- Paolone DR. Benign prostatic hyperplasia. *Clin Geriatr Med.* 2010;26(2):223–229.
- Sharp VJ, Takacs EB. Prostatitis: diagnosis and treatment. *Am Fam Physician.* 2010;82(4):397–406.

CHAPTER 55—DISORDERS OF SEXUAL FUNCTION

KEY POINTS

- Normal age-associated changes lead to decreased sexual interest and ability; however, complete sexual dysfunction is not a part of healthy aging.
- Physiologic changes in sexual response occur in both men and women. It is important to distinguish between normal age-associated changes and pathologic conditions that can be related to medications or medical disorders.
- Many older women have sexual dysfunction but do not report it to their primary care providers unless asked.
- Multiple options are available to treat male and female sexual dysfunction.
- Sexuality is an important part of quality of life for many older adults; treatment of sexual dysfunction can lead to improvements in quality of life.

Our understanding of sexual function and dysfunction in older men has increased significantly in recent years. There is less scientific information on the sexuality of older women, possibly because of the difficulty of measuring the female sexual response. However, the 2007 National Social Life, Health, and Aging Project (NSHAP) provided insights into the sexual activity, behavior, and problems of older men and women in America.

FEMALE SEXUALITY

Age-Associated Changes

Many factors play an important role in the sexual response of older women, including changes that occur with menopause, cultural expectations, relationship problems, previous sexual experiences, chronic illnesses, and depression. American women live about 29 years after menopause and outlive their spouses an average of 8 years. Although the frequency of intercourse decreases with aging, sexuality remains important for older women. Among 513 women 75–85 years old in the NSHAP, 37.2% were married, 1.2% were living with a partner other than the spouse, and 16.7% reported sexual activity with their spouse or other partner in the previous year. Of those who were sexually active with their spouse or other partner, 54.1% reported sexual activity at least 2 or 3 times per month. Among those women who had a spouse or other partner but had been sexually inactive in the previous 3 months, 64.8% attributed the inactivity to the partner's physical health problems or limitations and 24.8% to their own health problems.

The female sexual response cycle changes with aging. During the excitement phase, the clitoris may require longer direct stimulation, and genital engorgement is decreased. Vaginal lubrication is reduced, although with increased foreplay and gentle stimulation, lubrication is usually adequate for intercourse. During the plateau phase, there is less expansion and vasocongestion of the vagina. During orgasm, fewer and weaker contractions occur, although older women can still achieve multiple orgasms. Occasionally during orgasm, older women experience spastic and painful contractions of the uterine musculature. During the resolution phase, vasocongestion is lost more rapidly. Most of these changes are thought to be due to a decline in serum estrogen concentration after menopause, but a vasculogenic component can contribute to postmenopausal sexual dysfunction.

Female Sexual Dysfunction

For the most part, menopause is accompanied by decreased sexual function, with decreased sexual interest, responsiveness, and coital frequency. In addition, there is an increase in urogenital symptoms, often not discussed with the clinician. For example, in the NSHAP, among women 75–85 years old who were sexually active, the most common sexual problem was lack of interest (49.3%), followed by difficulty with lubrication (43.6%), inability to climax (38.2%), lack of pleasure during sex (24.9%), and pain during intercourse (11.8%).

Dyspareunia, defined as pain with intercourse, can be due to organic or psychologic factors, or a combination. For example, a woman can experience an episode of dyspareunia because of postmenopausal vaginal atrophy. With each subsequent sexual encounter, she anticipates pain, causing inadequate arousal with decreased lubrication. Because of this cycle, the woman continues to experience dyspareunia, even after the vaginal atrophy has been treated. The most common organic cause of dyspareunia is atrophic vaginitis due to estrogen deficiency. Other causes include inadequate lubrication, localized vaginal infections, cystitis, Bartholin cyst, retroverted uterus, marked uterine prolapse, endometriosis, pelvic tumors, excessive penile thrusting, or vaginismus (involuntary muscle spasms).

Systemic or local estrogen therapy can improve symptoms of vulvovaginal atrophy, but it has little effect on libido or sexual satisfaction (SOE=B). Libido is thought to depend on testosterone (even in women), rather than on estrogen. The ovaries and adrenals are the main sources of androgens in women. The effects of female androgen deficiency were originally identified in women treated for advanced breast cancer with oophorectomy and adrenalectomy. When deprived of androgens, these women reported loss of libido. Hypoactive sexual desire disorder (HSDD) is defined as decreased libido that causes personal distress and is not due to a psychiatric or medical illness or a substance (such as medication). HSDD is thought to be due to low testosterone. Because there are no normative data on plasma total and free testosterone in women and no well-defined clinical syndrome of androgen deficiency, the Endocrine Society has not recommended making a diagnosis of androgen deficiency in women.

Older women commonly have multiple medical conditions, some of which affect sexuality. However, scientific studies on the effect of chronic diseases and medications on the sexuality of older women are limited. Women with diabetes mellitus are less likely to be sexually active, and report decreased libido and lubrication and longer time to reach orgasm. Rheumatic diseases affect sexuality via functional disability. After mastectomy for breast cancer, 20%–40% of women experience sexual dysfunction, possibly because of disruption of body image, marital and family problems, spousal reaction, adjuvant therapy, or the psychologic impact of a breast cancer diagnosis. Several drugs can adversely affect sexual function, including antidepressants (with higher rates for SSRIs and lower rates for bupropion), antihypertensives, antipsychotics, antiestrogens, antiandrogens, anticholinergic drugs, narcotics, alcohol, and illicit/recreational drugs. Psychosocial factors also have an important role in sexual dysfunction. Women commonly marry men older than themselves and live longer than men. Consequently, heterosexual older women are likely to spend the last years of their lives alone. Even when a partner is available, he might have erectile dysfunction (ED). Finally, lack of privacy can be a problem when an older couple lives with their children or in a nursing home.

Evaluation and Treatment

The history is the most important part of the evaluation of sexual function. Careful and sensitive questioning can detect problems that a woman might not otherwise volunteer. Clinicians should ask about dyspareunia, lack of vaginal lubrication, and previous negative experiences, such as rape, child abuse, or domestic violence. Medications should be carefully reviewed. A woman with dyspareunia should undergo a pelvic examination to exclude organic causes.

Decreased lubrication, vaginal discomfort, itching, and dyspareunia due to atrophic vaginitis respond well to topical estrogen therapy (SOE=A). Improvement of symptoms and of the vaginal maturation index can be expected within 2–4 weeks of starting treatment. The low-dose vaginal estradiol ring (releases estradiol at 7.5 mcg/d, to be replaced every 90 days) or vaginal tablet (1 tablet [10 mcg/d] for 2 weeks, then 1 tablet twice a week) deliver low-dose estradiol locally with lower systemic absorption and risks of systemic adverse events than conjugated estrogen cream. The estradiol ring and tablet are also better tolerated than topical estrogen creams because of ease of use and comfort. If the patient is not a candidate for or does not want to use topical estrogen, water-soluble vaginal lubricants (eg, Astroglide, K-Y Jelly, Replens) are beneficial. Vaginal lubricants are also first-line treatment for women with hormone-sensitive cancers. Local estrogens should be prescribed only with the approval of the patient's oncologist, because safety data in this population are limited. Importantly, local stimulation through regular intercourse helps maintain a healthy vaginal mucosa. Longer foreplay allows more time for vaginal lubrication, just as older men often need longer and more direct stimulation to achieve an adequate erection.

Decreased libido without identifiable cause may respond to testosterone, but no androgen preparation is approved by the FDA for hypoactive sexual desire disorder in women. Several placebo-controlled, randomized trials showed that low-dose testosterone patch delivering 300 mcg/d dosed twice weekly or daily improves sexual desire in women with natural or surgical menopause and on systemic estrogens (SOE=A). Androgenic adverse events such as acne and hirsutism were uncommon, and concentrations of high-density lipoprotein cholesterol did not decrease as in studies with oral methyltestosterone.

More recent studies, including the ADORE study (see references), demonstrated that the testosterone patch is also effective in women with natural or surgically induced menopause who have decreased libido and are not taking estrogens. Although the testosterone patch seems effective (SOE=A), there are only limited data on the long-term safety of the testosterone patch in women.

Finally, older women should receive education about male sexual aging in addition to female sexual aging. Otherwise, an older woman might mistakenly attribute her partner's diminished erection and need for more genital stimulation to her own inability to arouse her partner. Other psychologic issues, including depression, history of sexual abuse, and relationship problems, should be addressed and treated with antidepressants, psychotherapy, and marital therapy, as necessary (SOE=C). A sex therapist can be identified on the Web site of the American Association of Sex Educators, Counselors, and Therapists (www.aasect.org). For a summary of treatments for female sexual dysfunction, see Table 55.1.

Table 55.1—Treatment Options for Sexual Dysfunction in Older Women

Symptom	Possible Cause	Therapy
Decreased desire	Low testosterone from natural or surgical menopause Chronic illness Depression Relationship problems Medications	Testosterone[OL] is not recommended by the Endocrine Society Treatment of underlying illness Antidepressant medication Marital therapy Review of drugs ingested
Decreased lubrication	Vaginal dryness or atrophy from postmenopausal status Antiestrogens and anticholinergic medications	Longer foreplay, regular intercourse, lubricants, topical estrogens Review of medications, including OTC drugs
Delayed or absent orgasm	Neurologic disorders, diabetes Psychologic problems	Treatment of underlying illness Cognitive-behavioral therapy, masturbation, Kegel exercises
Pain with intercourse	Organic cause Vaginal dryness, atrophy Vaginismus (involuntary vaginal contractions)	Treatment of underlying physical condition Longer foreplay, regular intercourse, lubricants, topical estrogens Psychotherapy, cognitive-behavioral therapy

MALE SEXUALITY

Age-Associated Changes

As men age, their sexuality changes. The frequency of sexual intercourse and the prevalence of engaging in any sexual activity decrease. Young men report having intercourse 3 to 4 times per week, whereas only 7% of men 60–69 years old and 2% of those ≥70 years old report the same frequency. Among men 60–70 years old, 50%–80% engage in any sexual activity, a prevalence rate that declines to 15%–25% among men ≥80 years old (SOE=A). However, sexual interest often persists despite decreased activity. The man's level of sexual activity, interest, and enjoyment in his younger years often determines his sexual behavior with aging. Factors contributing to a man's decreased sexual activity include poor health, social issues, partner availability, decreased libido, and ED. Although men 75–85 years old continue to prefer vaginal intercourse, approximately 50% report difficulty with erectile function.

Aging is associated not only with changes in sexual behavior but also with changes in the stages of sexual response. During the excitement phase, there is a delay in erection, decreased tensing of the scrotal sac, and loss of testicular elevation. The duration of the plateau stage is prolonged, and pre-ejaculatory secretion is decreased. Orgasm is diminished in duration and intensity, with decreased quantity and force of seminal emission. During the resolution phase, detumescence and testicular descent are rapid. The refractory period between erections is also longer. However, erectile failure is not a part of healthy aging but rather is frequently caused by age-associated disease or its treatment (eg, radical prostatectomy for prostate cancer) (SOE=B).

Erectile Physiology and Dysfunction

Penile rigidity results from a complex interaction between the brain, spinal cord, testosterone, neurotransmitters, arterial inflow, and venous outflow. In brief, testosterone, mental health, and an attractive partner typically stimulate sexual interest (libido). Fantasy, visual, tactile, or other erotic stimuli (eg, erotic scents or sounds) trigger neural impulses from the brain or spinal cord to the penis. Neural impulses cause release or synthesis of various neurotransmitters (eg, nitric oxide, cGMP), which induce arterial vasodilation and increased penile arterial inflow. Increasing arterial inflow impedes venous outflow, which results in penile tumescence. As the intrapenile (ie, intracavernosal) pressure equilibrates to mean arterial pressure, the penis becomes rigid. Thus, there are many steps along the path that can be broken and result in ED.

ED, the inability to achieve or maintain an erection adequate for sexual intercourse, is the most common sexual problem of older men. The prevalence of ED increases with age; by 70 years of age, 67% of men have ED. This high prevalence is important; in a study comparing affected and unaffected men, men with sexual dysfunction reported impaired quality of life. For a summary of the causes of sexual dysfunction in men, see Table 55.2.

The most common cause (30%–50%) of ED in older men is vascular disease (SOE=A). Risk of vascular ED increases with traditional vascular risk factors, eg, diabetes mellitus, hypertension, hyperlipidemia, and smoking. In fact, ED is a predictor of future major atherosclerotic vascular disease (ie, myocardial infarction and stroke).

Obstruction from atherosclerotic arterial occlusive disease likely impedes the intracavernosal blood flow and pressure needed to achieve a rigid erection. In addition, atherosclerotic disease can cause ischemia of trabecular smooth muscle and result in fibrotic changes leading to failure of venous closure mechanisms. Venous leakage leading to vascular ED can also result from Peyronie disease, arteriovenous fistula,

Table 55.2—Causes of Sexual Dysfunction in Older Men

Causes (in order of prevalence)	Characteristics
Vascular disease	■ Gradual onset Vascular risk factors: diabetes mellitus, hypertension, hyperlipidemia, tobacco use
Neurologic disease, eg, radiation therapy, spinal cord injury, autonomic dysfunction, surgical procedures	■ Gradual onset Neurologic risk factors: diabetes mellitus; history of pelvic injury, surgery, or irradiation; spinal injury or surgery; Parkinson disease; multiple sclerosis; alcoholism Loss of bulbocavernosus reflex
Medications, eg, anticholinergics, antihypertensives, cimetidine, antidepressants	■ Sudden onset Lack of sleep-associated erections or lack of erections with masturbation Temporal association with a new medication
Psychogenic, eg, relationship conflicts, performance anxiety, childhood sexual abuse, fear of sexually transmitted diseases, "widower's syndrome"	■ Sudden onset Sleep-associated erections or erections with masturbation are preserved
Hypogonadism	■ Gradual onset Decreased libido more than erectile dysfunction Small testes, gynecomastia Low serum testosterone concentration
Endocrine, eg, hypothyroidism, hyperthyroidism, hyperprolactinemia	■ Rare, <5% of cases of erectile dysfunction

or trauma-induced communication between the glans and the corpora. In anxious men who have excessive adrenergic-constrictor tone and in men with injured parasympathetic dilator nerves, ED can result from insufficient relaxation of trabecular smooth muscle.

The second most common cause of ED in older men is neurologic disease (17%–37%). Disorders that affect the parasympathetic sacral spinal cord or the peripheral efferent autonomic fibers to the penis impair penile smooth muscle relaxation and prevent the vasodilation necessary for erection. In patients with prostate cancer, all forms of (curative) treatment frequently cause neurogenic erectile failure (brachytherapy or external radiation, 50%; radical prostatectomy with nerve sparing, 45%–80%) and pain on orgasm (SOE=B). Common health problems such as diabetes mellitus, stroke, and Parkinson disease can cause autonomic dysfunction that results in erectile failure. Finally, surgical procedures such as cystectomy and proctocolectomy commonly disrupt the autonomic nerve supply to the penis, resulting in postoperative ED.

Numerous commonly used medications have been associated with ED for which the mechanism, for the most part, is unknown. In approximately 5% of men with ED, the ED is drug-induced. Those medications with anticholinergic effects, such as antidepressants, antipsychotics, and antihistamines, can cause ED by blocking parasympathetic-mediated penile artery vasodilatation and trabecular smooth muscle relaxation. Almost all antihypertensive agents have been associated with ED; of these, clonidine and thiazide diuretics have higher incidence rates, whereas ACE inhibitors and angiotensin-receptor blockers have lower incidence rates (SOE=B). One mechanism by which antihypertensives can cause ED is lowering blood pressure below the threshold needed to maintain sufficient blood flow for penile erection, especially in those men who already have penile arterial disease. OTC medications such as cimetidine and ranitidine can also cause ED. Cimetidine, an H_2-receptor antagonist, acts as an antiandrogen and increases prolactin secretion; thus, it has been associated with loss of libido and erectile failure. Ranitidine can also increase prolactin secretion, although less commonly than does cimetidine.

The prevalence of psychogenic ED correlates inversely with age. In approximately 9% of men ≥65 years old with ED, the ED is psychogenic. Psychogenic ED can develop via increased sympathetic stimuli to the sacral cord, inhibiting the parasympathetic dilator nerves and thus inhibiting erection. Common causes of psychogenic ED include relationship conflicts, performance anxiety, childhood sexual abuse, and fear of sexually transmitted diseases. Older men may have "widower's syndrome," in which the man involved in a new relationship feels guilt as a defense against subconscious unfaithfulness to his deceased spouse.

Hyperthyroidism, hypothyroidism, and hyperprolactinemia have been associated with ED. However, <5% of ED is caused by endocrine abnormalities. Thus, endocrine evaluation of men with ED but intact libido is of limited value (SOE=B).

The role of androgens in erection is becoming clearer. Hypogonadism is moderately common in older men. Hypogonadal men show smaller and slower developing erections in response to fantasy, which is improved with androgen replacement. However, even men with castrate levels of testosterone can attain erections in response to direct penile stimulation. It may be that erection from direct penile stimulation is less androgen dependent, whereas erection from fantasy is more androgen dependent. Nevertheless, testosterone is necessary for intracavernosal nitric oxide synthesis. Thus, testosterone plays a large role in libido and a smaller role in erectile function. For example, hypogonadal men do respond better to phosphodiesterase inhibitors after testosterone replacement therapy.

Evaluation of Erectile Dysfunction

The initial step is to obtain a sexual, medical, and psychosocial history. Sexual history should clarify whether the problem consists of inadequate erections, decreased libido, or orgasmic failure. The onset and duration of ED, the presence or absence of sleep-associated erections, and the associated decline in libido are clues to the likely cause.

Sudden onset (in the absence of pelvic surgery) suggests psychogenic or drug-induced ED. A psychogenic cause is likely if there is a sudden onset but retention of sleep-associated erections or if erections with masturbation or a different partner are intact (SOE=A). If sudden-onset erectile failure is accompanied by lack of sleep-associated erections and lack of erection with masturbation, temporal association with new medication should be investigated. A gradual onset of ED associated with loss of libido suggests hypogonadism. Gradual onset associated with intact libido (most common presentation) suggests vascular, neurogenic, or other organic causes.

Medical history is directed at discerning those factors likely to be contributing to ED. Vascular risk factors include diabetes mellitus, hypertension, coronary artery disease, peripheral arterial disease, hyperlipidemia, and smoking. Neurogenic risk factors include diabetes mellitus; history of pelvic injury, surgery, or radiation; spinal injury or surgery; Parkinson disease; multiple sclerosis; or alcoholism. An extensive medication review, including OTC medications, is essential. Finally, the psychosocial history should assess the patient's relationship with the sexual partner, the partner's health and attitude toward sex, economic or social stresses, living situation, alcohol use, and affective disorders.

On physical examination, attention should be paid to signs of vascular or neurologic diseases. Peripheral pulses should be palpated. Signs of autonomic neuropathy (eg, orthostatic hypotension and absent heart rate response to standing) and loss of the bulbocavernosus reflex suggest neurologic dysfunction. The genital examination includes palpating the penis for Peyronie plaques and assessing for testicular atrophy. A femoral bruit and diminished (or absent) pedal pulses suggests arterial insufficiency. An absent bulbocavernosus reflex suggests penile neuropathy. A loss of secondary sexual characteristics, small testes, and gynecomastia suggest hypogonadism or hyperprolactinemia.

Appropriate laboratory evaluations are those that target relevant comorbid conditions such as diabetes mellitus and vascular disease or that evaluate neurologic disorders if suggested by the physical examination. The measurement of serum testosterone should be considered in the setting of other symptoms of androgen deficiency. For specific recommendations regarding testing, see "Endocrine and Metabolic Disorders," p 506.

An at-home therapeutic trial of a phosphodiesterase inhibitor (sildenafil or vardenafil) is considered first-line evaluation and treatment. The initial dose should be low (sildenafil 25–50 mg or vardenafil 5–10 mg) in men suspected of having neurogenic ED. A poor response suggests vasculogenic ED. Further therapeutic trial with sildenafil at 100 mg or vardenafil at 20 mg may prove to be effective. An at-home therapeutic trial using tadalafil (5–10 mg) can be considered, but the long half-life complicates matters if an adverse event occurs with the first dose.

More extensive diagnostic tools are available but not commonly used. Nocturnal penile tumescence testing is of little value, except to confirm a psychogenic cause. The penile-brachial pressure index can be helpful in assessing arteriogenic ED. This index measures the loss of systolic pressure between the arm and the penis. When measured before and after exercise, it can be used to assess for a pelvic steal syndrome, which is the loss of erection associated with initiation of active pelvic thrusting, presumably due to the transfer of blood flow from the penis to the pelvic musculature. More invasive and expensive tests such as Doppler ultrasound to assess penile arterial function, dynamic infusion cavernosometry to assess venous leakage syndrome, and penile arteriography are generally reserved for research or penile vascular surgery candidates.

Treatment of Erectile Dysfunction

Multiple effective therapeutic options are available for the treatment of ED. Treatment should be individualized and based on cause, personal preference, partner issues, cost, and practicality (Table 55.3).

Oral therapy for ED with sildenafil, vardenafil, tadalafil, or avanafil has revolutionized treatment of male sexual dysfunction. Sildenafil is a type-5 phosphodiesterase inhibitor that potentiates the penile response to sexual stimulation. It improves the rigidity and duration of erection. It is taken 1 hour before sexual activity and has no effect until sexual stimulation occurs. Because absorption is attenuated when sildenafil is ingested with a fatty meal, patients need to be educated about this issue. Vardenafil is a more potent and specific phosphodiesterase inhibitor.

Table 55.3—Treatment Options for Erectile Dysfunction

Treatment	Route/ Administration	Applicable Conditions	Onset	Duration of Action	Dosage	Selected Adverse Events
Sildenafil	Oral	N, A?, V?	60 min	4 h	25–100 mg	Headache, flushing, rhinitis, dyspepsia, transient color blindness; contraindicated with nitrate use and α-blockers
Vardenafil	Oral	N, A?, V?	45 min	4 h	5–20 mg	Headache, flushing, rhinitis, dyspepsia; contraindicated with nitrate use and α-blockers
Tadalafil	Oral	N, A?, V?	45–60 min	24–36 h	5–20 mg	Headache, dyspepsia, flushing, rhinitis; contraindicated with nitrate use and α-blockers
Avanafil	Oral	N, A?, V?	30 min		100 mg	Headache, flushing, prolonged erection; contraindicated with nitrate use and α-blockers
Vacuum device	External	P, N, V, A?	<5 min	30 min	—	Petechiae, bruising, painful ejaculation
Papaverine^OL	Intracavernosal	N, A?, V?	10 min	30–60 min	15–60 mg	Prolonged erection, fibrosis, ecchymosis
Alprostadil	Intracavernosal	N, A?, V?	10 min	40–60 min	5–20 mcg	Prolonged erection, pain, fibrosis
Phentolamine^OL	Intracavernosal	N, A?, V?	10 min	30–60 min	0.5–1 mg	Prolonged erection, fibrosis, headache, facial flushing
Medicated urethral system for erection (MUSE)	Intraurethral	N, A?, V?	10–15 min	60–80 min	250–1,000 mcg	Penile pain or burning, hypotension
Penile prosthesis	Surgical	N, A, V		replacement in 5–10 years	—	Infection, erosion, mechanical failure
Sex therapy	Counseling	P	weeks	years	weekly	Anxiety

NOTE: A = arteriogenic; N = neurogenic; P = psychogenic; V = venogenic; ? = possibly

A lower effective dose and better adverse-event profile (no effect on color vision) make vardenafil a reasonable option. Tadalafil is a longer-acting phosphodiesterase inhibitor with an adverse-event profile similar to that of vardenafil but with the added potential problem of muscle pain. Avanafil is a more recently approved phosphodiesterase inhibitor; it is taken 30 minutes before sexual activity. All four of these agents are contraindicated for concomitant use with nitrate medications, because the combination can produce profound and fatal hypotension. In addition, combined use of α-blockers with phosphodiesterase inhibitors should be done with caution, starting with the lowest dose of either. Choosing among these phosphodiesterase inhibitors should likely be based on price and patient preference. All phosphodiesterase inhibitors result in sufficient penile rigidity for an approximately 50% success rate at vaginal intercourse. Because of the longer duration of action of tadalafil, men tend to select it when given the choice (SOE=B).

Vacuum tumescence devices are another option. The apparatus consists of a plastic cylinder with an open end into which the penis is inserted. A vacuum device attached to the cylinder creates negative pressure within the cylinder, and blood flows into the penis to produce penile rigidity. A penile constriction ring placed at the base of the penis then traps the blood in the corpora cavernosa to maintain an erection for about 30 minutes. The vacuum device is effective for psychogenic, neurogenic, and venogenic ED, but it requires a lot of manual dexterity. Local pain, swelling, bruising, coolness of penile tip, and painful ejaculation are potential adverse events. It is important to remove the constriction ring after 30 minutes.

Intracavernous injection of vasoactive drugs such as papaverine, phentolamine, and alprostadil are effective in producing erections adequate for sexual activity (SOE=A) but are used much less frequently since oral therapy has become available. Alprostadil, which is the only agent approved by the FDA for intracavernosal injection, produces erections that last 40–60 minutes. Phentolamine^OL is mainly used in combination therapy with papaverine^OL or alprostadil, or both. Potential adverse events are bruising, ecchymoses or hematoma, local pain, fibrosis from repeated injections, and priapism. Alprostadil appears to cause less scarring and priapism than papaverine. If an erection lasts >4 hours, detumescence is necessary by aspiration of blood from the corpora cavernosa or injection of phenylephrine because of the potential for intracavernosal hypoxia and fibrosis of trabecular smooth muscle, which can prevent future erections. In general, intracavernosal therapy should probably be reserved for patients in whom oral therapy with a phosphodiesterase inhibitor is not effective. Alprostadil can also be administered intraurethrally using medicated urethral system for erection (MUSE). This system contains a small pellet of alprostadil that is placed within the urethra and is rapidly absorbed through the urethral mucosa to produce an erection within 10–15 minutes. Possible adverse events are penile pain, urethral burning, and a throbbing sensation in the perineum. The sexual partner may also experience burning or irritation if the intraurethral alprostadil is expelled during sexual activity.

Testosterone supplementation increases libido and can improve ED in men with true hypogonadism (SOE=B). It is available as an intramuscular injection (testosterone enanthate or cypionate) or topical transdermal patch and gel. Possible adverse events associated with testosterone include polycythemia, prostate enlargement, gynecomastia, and fluid retention. It is important to perform a digital rectal examination to assess the prostate and obtain a baseline prostate-specific antigen level before beginning therapy. If prostate-specific antigen or hematocrit increases with testosterone therapy, it usually does so within 6 months. Therefore, these levels should be checked every 3 months during the first year of therapy, then every 12 months thereafter.

Surgical implantation of a penile prosthesis is another therapeutic option. Mechanical failure, infection, device erosion, and fibrosis are possible complications. However, since the availability of alprostadil and, more recently, phosphodiesterase inhibitors, surgical implantation of a penile prosthesis is rarely done (ie, men with severe arterial occlusive disease). Nevertheless, long-term patient satisfaction with penile prosthesis is actually higher than with oral therapy (SOE=B). Penile revascularization surgery has limited success.

Men with psychogenic ED should be referred to a mental health or other professional specializing in treatment of sexual disorders for further evaluation and treatment.

REFERENCES

- Katz A. Sex, health and aging. *Nurs Womens Health.* 2011;15(6):519–521.
- Penay N, Al-Azzawi F, Bouchard C, et al. Testosterone treatment of hypoactive sexual desire disorder (HSDD) in naturally menopausal women: the ADORE study. *Climateric.* 2010;13(2):121–131.
- Qaseem A, Snow V, Denberg TD, et al. Hormonal testing and pharmacologic treatment of erectile dysfunction: a clinical practice guideline from the American College of Physicians. *Ann Intern Med.* 2009;151(9):639–649.
- Wierman ME, Basson R, Davis SR, et al. Androgen therapy in women: an Endocrine Society Clinical Practice Guideline. *J Clin Endocrinol Metab.* 2006;91(10):3697–3710.

CHAPTER 56—MUSCULOSKELETAL DISEASES AND DISORDERS

KEY POINTS

- In addition to arthritis, musculoskeletal complaints in older adults can result from other disorders, including derangement of tendons, bursae, muscles, connective tissue, and nerves.
- Imaging and laboratory studies should be used to confirm clinical impressions rather than to search for a diagnosis. Older adults often exhibit incidental abnormalities on imaging and laboratory testing that may lack immediate clinical relevance.
- Comorbid medical conditions and treatments should be considered, and potential toxicities weighed against potential treatment benefits.
- Exercise and other nonpharmacologic treatments should be considered in the management of all articular and regional musculoskeletal problems.

DIAGNOSTIC APPROACH TO MUSCULOSKELETAL COMPLAINTS IN OLDER ADULTS

The following three questions yield information critical to the diagnosis of musculoskeletal complaints:

1. Do the symptoms arise from the joint or elsewhere?
2. Is the process inflammatory?
3. How many joints are involved?

Do the symptoms arise from the joint or elsewhere? Arthritis symptoms or pain and stiffness are usually accompanied by physical findings of warmth, swelling, tenderness at the joint line, and painful passive motion (with the patient relaxed). Pain on active but not passive motion, and tenderness elicited on palpation of structures around the joint suggest a periarticular source and resulting bursitis, tendinitis, etc, rather than arthritis.

Arthritis—reproducible on active and passive joint range of motion; joint line is painful or tender on palpation; range of motion may or may not be limited. Inflammatory signs, including warmth, erythema, swelling, or effusion, may be present.

Tendinitis—reproducible on active but not passive range of motion; inflammatory signs may be present. Range of motion is preserved unless limited because of contracture. Maneuvers that are specific to the region are helpful when pain is elicited (eg, forced supination against resistance results in anterior shoulder pain due to bicipital tendinitis).

Bursitis—tenderness on palpation over the bursa. Active range of motion may be painful, but passive range of motion is neither painful nor limited unless there is an underlying arthritis. Inflammatory findings may be present.

Bone—present and not reproducible with range of motion. Localized tenderness may be present, and the source may be distinct from the joint.

Is the process inflammatory? Older adults with arthritis should be assessed for inflammatory signs and symptoms. Stiffness that is present on awakening and that persists for hours is a prominent feature of inflammatory arthritis; this stiffness often recurs after periods of inactivity. In contrast, noninflammatory stiffness generally resolves within an hour after awakening or recurs during use of the affected joint. Unintentional weight loss, fever, loss of appetite, or a general feeling of poor health are features of a systemic illness and can accompany an inflammatory arthritis. The presence of rash, fever, stomatitis, dysphagia, Raynaud phenomenon, or true muscle weakness suggests an autoimmune rheumatologic disorder. Inflammatory features of arthritis should also be sought out during the physical examination. Joints that are palpably warmer than surrounding tissues, visibly red, or swollen are inflamed. Effusions may be palpated.

How many joints are involved? Identifying the number of involved joints can often be helpful in guiding diagnosis (Table 56.1). A monoarthritis can be infectious (eg, bacterial, fungal), crystal-mediated, traumatic, or degenerative. Arthrocentesis should be performed to evaluate the cause of an undiagnosed monoarthritis to exclude an infection and to evaluate for crystals. Arthritis involving 2 or 3 joints (pauci-articular or oligo-articular arthritis) can also be crystal mediated or degenerative, but it can also be due to reactive arthritis (Reiter syndrome), spondyloarthritis, or related to inflammatory bowel disease. Finally, the differential diagnosis of arthritis involving ≥4 joints (polyarticular arthritis) includes crystal-mediated arthritis, degenerative arthritis, rheumatoid arthritis, systemic lupus erythematosus, and viral arthritis (eg, hepatitis, parvovirus B19, etc).

Diagnostic Testing

Laboratory testing should be pursued with the caveat that many tests are neither sensitive nor specific, but they can play a confirmatory role when interpreted

Table 56.1— Differential Diagnosis of Arthritis According to Number of Affected Joints

Monoarthritis (1 joint)	Pauci-arthritis (2 or 3 joints)	Polyarthritis (≥4 joints)
Infection (eg, bacterial, fungal, tuberculosis, Lyme disease)	Crystal-mediated	Crystal-mediated
Crystal-mediated	Enteropathic (eg, inflammatory bowel disease)	Immune complex (eg, lupus, serum sickness, hypersensitivity drug reaction)
Trauma	Infection (eg, Lyme disease, rheumatic fever, endocarditis)	Infection (eg, Lyme disease, viral arthritis, rheumatic fever, endocarditis)
Hemarthrosis	Psoriatic arthritis	Psoriatic arthritis
Osteoarthritis	Reactive (Reiter syndrome)	Reactive (Reiter syndrome)
	Sarcoidosis (knees, ankles)	Rheumatoid arthritis
	Ankylosing spondylitis	Osteoarthritis
	Osteoarthritis	
	Amyloid (shoulder)	

in the appropriate clinical context. The Westergren erythrocyte sedimentation rate (ESR), rheumatoid factor, and antinuclear antibodies are three laboratory tests frequently used to evaluate rheumatic disease. Although these laboratory studies are of great value to confirm a diagnosis in older adults with clinically apparent disease, the abnormal values should be interpreted cautiously because of reduced specificity of these tests with aging, ie, the tests may be abnormal in healthy older adults.

The ESR can be increased in older adults even in the absence of identifiable illness; it increases normally with aging according to the following formula: men: 17.3 + 0.18 (age); women: 22.1 + 0.18 (age). The ESR is useful in evaluating patients with headache, fever of unknown origin, or unintentional weight loss if giant cell arteritis is suspected; however, diagnosis requires biopsy of the temporal artery. ESR increases can also accompany nonrheumatic systemic illness and therefore cannot distinguish, based on the laboratory result alone, giant cell arteritis from systemic infection, myeloma, or other advanced malignancy.

Rheumatoid factor is an antibody (usually IgM) that reacts with the Fc portion of IgG. It can be detected in 70%–80% of patients with rheumatoid arthritis but is not specific to this disease. It can also be detected in up to 30% of apparently healthy older adults, but when present is usually at a titer of 1:80 or less. This test may be most useful in evaluation of older adults with symmetric inflammatory polyarthritis that is characteristic of rheumatoid arthritis. More recent studies suggest that using anti-cyclic citrullinated peptide antibodies (anti-CCP) together with the rheumatoid factor latex assay enhances specificity in the diagnosis of rheumatoid arthritis. Neither test should be used to evaluate older adults with diffuse and vague musculoskeletal complaints in the absence of symmetric inflammatory small-joint findings on examination.

Antinuclear antibodies (ANAs) are immunoglobulins directed against DNA, RNA, and other nuclear or cytoplasmic proteins. Both the pattern of immunofluorescence (rim, speckled, nucleolar, or diffuse) and titer provide useful clinical information. ANAs can be found in healthy older adults but usually are in a diffuse pattern, and at a low titer, in the absence of rheumatic disease. The ANA test is highly sensitive for systemic lupus erythematosus in that a negative test essentially excludes a diagnosis of lupus. ANAs can be present in high titers in older adults with systemic or medication-induced lupus, inflammatory muscle disease, or scleroderma.

Arthrocentesis should be performed when infection or crystalline-mediated inflammatory joint disease is suspected. Fluid should be sent for cell count, Gram stain, culture, and crystal analysis. Bloody effusions may be due to joint trauma and may signal a coagulopathy or periarticular fracture.

Radiographs

Radiographs should be obtained to confirm a diagnosis of arthritis and distinguish inflammatory (eg, rheumatoid arthritis) or destructive (eg, septic, psoriatic) arthritis from noninflammatory (eg, osteoarthritis) forms of arthritis. Inflammatory joint findings are symmetric joint space narrowing, juxta-articular or generalized osteopenia, and erosions at or next to the joint. In contrast, degenerative arthritis or osteoarthritis is characterized by asymmetric joint space narrowing, osteophytes, sclerosis, and subchondral cysts. Presence of radiographic osteoarthritis does not exclude the possibility that a periarticular or inflammatory condition coexists. Radiographs can also help distinguish arthritis from a periarticular or bony process (eg, osteomyelitis, periostitis, fracture, tumor).

MRI provides high-resolution imaging of articular (cartilage, synovium, meniscus, ligaments) and periarticular structures (bone, tendon, bursae) and should be performed when joint instability is suspected (eg, internal derangement of the knee after trauma, cervical spine in rheumatoid arthritis before elective surgery). MRI is also the imaging modality of choice to evaluate back pain with neurologic deficits and to assess spinal cord integrity at any level. MRI can detect intraosseous processes, including infection, occult fracture, and avascular necrosis. It is significantly more expensive than plain radiographs; the incremental cost should be weighed against the gain in clinically relevant information that MRI imaging will yield.

Despite the high level of resolution achieved with MRI, CT scanning remains the imaging modality of choice to evaluate cortical abnormalities of axial bone (eg, spine, sacroiliac joint) and of intermediate to large joints.

EVALUATION OF REGIONAL MUSCULOSKELETAL COMPLAINTS

The Painful Shoulder

Shoulder pain is a common problem in older adults. Pain in the shoulder can be referred (from the cervical spine, heart, or subdiaphragm), occur as a local manifestation of a systemic process (eg, rheumatoid arthritis, polymyalgia rheumatica, or amyloidosis), or arise from the shoulder itself (eg, bursitis, tendinitis, capsulitis, and arthritis).

Subacromial bursitis causes a dull ache that precludes sleeping on the affected side with tenderness to palpation diffusely along the shoulder. Bicipital tendinitis causes pain in the anterior-lateral aspect of the humeral head. Forced supination of the forearm against resistance with the elbow flexed at 90 degrees reproduces the pain (Yergason sign). In contrast, rotator cuff tendinitis results in shoulder pain that is worse between 60 and 120 degrees of abduction. Patients may have mild to no symptoms on passive abduction but often "drop" their arm when asked to abduct against gravity. This is difficult to distinguish clinically from an incomplete tear of the rotator cuff. However, patients with a complete rotator cuff tear are unable to sustain the weight of their arm against gravity at all. Older adults are susceptible to rotator cuff injuries with even minor trauma (eg, lifting groceries, catching their fall). Adhesive capsulitis (ie, "frozen" shoulder) is a painful loss of range of motion in all directions; it can result from stroke, trauma, untreated arthritis, or relatively minor injury. Patients with diabetes can develop adhesive capsulitis without any inciting event. Osteoarthritis, rheumatoid arthritis, and calcium pyrophosphate dihydrate deposition disease (CPPD) can all contribute to shoulder pain, as can calcium hydroxyapatite (Milwaukee shoulder). Plain radiographs are most useful in assessing the shoulder for evidence of joint degeneration and can demonstrate calcification of the tendons (calcific supraspinatus tendinitis) or superior migration of the humeral head in the case of a complete rotator cuff tear. Shoulder pain often responds to local steroid injections administered in conjunction with physical therapy. Surgical intervention is rarely pursued for these conditions in older adults.

The Painful Elbow

Bursitis and arthritis most commonly cause elbow pain, although tendinitis can contribute in overuse syndromes; the latter circumstance may result in medial or lateral epicondylitis. Olecranon bursitis, with swelling of the bursa and pain only at the extremes of range of movement, is commonly associated with rheumatoid arthritis and gout, both of which also result in palpable nodules or tophi. Olecranon bursitis can be managed conservatively by using padding and avoiding pressure on the elbow. Excessive redness, warmth, or exquisite tenderness prompts evaluation for infection. Unlike bursitis, arthritis results in painful passive motion (supination or flexion) and tenderness on palpation over the joint line. Arthritis of the elbow can be part of an inflammatory arthritis (eg, rheumatoid arthritis, spondyloarthropathy, gout) but should be evaluated for an infectious cause if it presents as a monoarthritis. Overlying cellulitis does not preclude joint aspiration for culture and cell count, but empiric antibiotic coverage is warranted.

The Painful Wrist

Few conditions cause wrist pain. Arthritis of the wrist results in painful passive motion that is usually accompanied by fullness and tenderness on palpation that can be due to either synovial tissue inflammation or joint effusion. Inflammatory arthropathies that affect the wrist may also result in other involved joints that can be appreciated on examination (rheumatoid arthritis, gout, CPPD). Monoarthritis should be evaluated for the possibility of septic arthritis, gout, or pseudogout. Radiographs are useful in distinguishing between these different types of arthritis. MRI should be pursued in patients with tenderness over the ulnar styloid process to detect impending extension tendon rupture that requires tendon transfer surgery. Occasionally, wrist pain can be a manifestation of periostitis. Examination reveals tenderness on compression of the distal radius or ulna that can be confirmed on radiograph or bone scan.

In carpal tunnel syndrome, the impingement of the median nerve causes pain and paresthesia of the hand that are prominent at night. Carpal tunnel syndrome can be the result of overuse or arthritis of the wrist joint, or a manifestation of a systemic disease (eg, diabetes, hypothyroidism, amyloidosis). The diagnosis is confirmed by electrodiagnostic evaluation, demonstrating nerve conduction delay at the wrist. Older adults with cervical spine arthritis can manifest a "double crush" phenomenon (compression of the median nerve of the wrist and compression of the sixth and seventh cervical nerves) that can be detected on electrodiagnostic testing. Management options include the consistent use of neutral wrist splints (SOE=B) and judicious glucocorticoid injections (SOE=B) into the carpal tunnel, taking care not to inject the median nerve. Surgical decompression should be pursued if conservative measures fail or if thumb apposition weakness or thenar muscle atrophy is apparent.

The Painful Hip

Hip pain in older adults can be referred from the spine, retroperitoneal area, or knee, or can arise in the joint and surrounding area. Trochanteric bursitis results in pain that is localized over the lateral proximal thigh and that can be reproduced on palpation over the greater trochanter. Patients often complain of difficulty sleeping on the affected side. Response is good to localized glucocorticoid injection to the affected tissue. Iliotibial band syndrome also causes lateral thigh pain that is worse with walking and can be reproduced by having the patient bend forward at the waist while crossing the legs. Although responsive to steroid injection, iliotibial band syndrome should also be managed with stretching exercises and massage. Arthritis is suggested by hip pain that is reproduced on passive motion, often accompanied by reduced range of motion, especially internal rotation. Weakness of the hip muscles may be notable with a positive Trendelenburg sign or lurch during walking. Pain that is diffuse and bilateral and accompanied by prolonged morning stiffness should raise the possibility of polymyalgia rheumatica. Plain radiographs are useful to evaluate for osteoarthritis, rheumatoid arthritis, Paget disease of the bone, and fractures, while avascular necrosis is best demonstrated by MRI. Patients with hemoglobinopathy, traumatic injury to the hip, or malignancy, and those who are receiving chronic steroid therapy and who report hip pain that is not reproduced on passive motion, should be evaluated with a radiograph or MRI for avascular necrosis, osteomyelitis, or bone metastasis. Therapies are aimed at the underlying cause but usually include devices to reduce weightbearing on the affected hip (eg, cane, orthotics), weight loss and exercise, medications, and surgery.

The Painful Knee

According to data from the third National Health and Nutrition Examination Survey (NHANES III), knee pain affects >20% of adults ≥60 years old, with an incidence approaching 30% for those ≥80 years old.

The anserine bursa is located inferomedially to the knee joint, and when inflamed causes knee pain that is most notable at night. There is exquisite tenderness to palpation over the area, with occasional swelling and erythema. Injection with a small amount of glucocorticoid mixed with anesthetic can be both diagnostic and therapeutic (SOE=C). In contrast, knee pain with visible fluid or swelling at the superior aspect of the knee is more consistent with suprapatellar bursitis. This is commonly exacerbated by frequent kneeling and is common in gardeners and painters. Because mechanical irritation with prolonged kneeling aggravates the suprapatellar bursa, avoidance of kneeling is recommended rather than injections or NSAIDs. Adequate padding between the knees while sleeping (for anserine bursitis) and thick padding while kneeling (for suprapatellar bursitis) can alleviate symptoms as well as prevent recurrence (SOE=C).

Degenerative arthritis or osteoarthritis should be suspected with a history of knee pain that is aggravated by activity (eg, bending, stooping, walking) and alleviated with rest. The skin may or may not be warm. Passive motion and palpation of the joint line reproduces the pain. Usually there is no joint effusion, but occasionally there may be a small effusion. Patients with posterior knee pain should be examined for a popliteal cyst. Inspection of both popliteal fossae with the patient standing can reveal asymmetric fullness on one side and can be confirmed by ultrasound. The knee should be assessed for ligamentous instability (medial and lateral collateral and cruciate ligaments) by gently stressing the joint in all directions. Patients should be asked about symptoms of locking or instability. Rotational extension can elicit pain localized to the site of meniscal disease, and MRI is needed to assess the extent of damage. Other causes of knee pain include crystalline-mediated (gout, CPPD), rheumatoid, psoriatic, and reactive arthritis, as well as avascular necrosis of the femur or tibia, referred pain from hip disease, and septic arthritis.

The Patient with Diffuse Pain

Patients complaining of pain that is diffuse and does not respect articular boundaries, or of persistent symptoms despite maximal medical and adjunctive therapy should be evaluated further. Persistent pain with diffuse tenderness of periarticular regions warrants evaluation for metabolic disturbances that affect bone such as vitamin D deficiency, hyperparathyroidism, or hypothyroidism. Systemic infection of any source can manifest with diffuse pain. Chronic somatic pain can be a manifestation of depression as well.

Fibromyalgia is a chronic disorder characterized by chronic, widespread muscle pain and tenderness that is associated with nonrestorative sleep and fatigue. It is frequently accompanied by fatigue, insomnia, depression, and anxiety. Although the average age of fibromyalgia patients is reported to be in the 40s, older adults are not spared from the development or persistence of this condition. The precise cause of fibromyalgia is not known, but research suggests it is related to impairment with the processing of pain in the CNS. No clinical laboratory tests or imaging studies are available to confirm a diagnosis. Commonly requested laboratory (eg, thyroid, vitamin D, antinuclear antibody, sedimentation rate, C-reactive protein, Lyme serology) and imaging studies are usually negative or normal.

Aerobic exercise and stretching, as well as Tai Chi, are recommended for all but should be started slowly, and progressed patiently, to avoid overuse and strain injuries. Tricyclic antidepressants[OL] can be helpful (SOE=B) but should be started at low dosages and increased slowly with caution because of anticholinergic adverse events. Duloxetine, pregabalin, and gabapentin[OL] have been studied in treatment of fibromyalgia and may have modest benefit for some patients (SOE=B).

For an approach to complaints of back or neck pain, see "Back and Neck Pain," p 465.

GENERAL MANAGEMENT STRATEGIES

Comorbid Conditions

Thorough assessment of comorbid illnesses is a necessary part of caring for older adults with musculoskeletal disorders. Diseases and their treatments often compete and complicate medical management, while increasing risk of functional limitations. In addition, specific diseases in combination are of clinical importance. For example, comorbid heart disease with rheumatoid arthritis can present a significant clinical challenge, due to potential effects of anti-inflammatory therapy or joint replacement on risk of significant cardiovascular complications.

Arthritis and pain contribute to functional limitations in late life, and the accompanying muscle weakness increases risk of further functional decline and disability. Being overweight or obese contributes to mobility limitations that are compounded by arthritis of weight-bearing joints. Rehabilitative interventions targeting muscle weakness and obesity are recommended for maintaining function despite the ongoing presence of articular and nonarticular diseases. See "Frailty," p 177; and "Malnutrition," p 209.

Older adults with arthritis of weight-bearing joints are at increased risk of injurious falls and fracture, attributed in part to proprioceptive deficits. Studies suggest that pain may increase the propensity to trip on an obstacle. These factors suggest that alleviating painful symptoms along with muscle and proprioception training should be implemented along with other strategies for falls prevention. See "Falls," p 234.

Nonpharmacologic Strategies

As with any chronic disease treatment, patient education should be considered the first step in management of musculoskeletal disorders. Involvement of family and other caregivers can be helpful and is a priority. Educational groups or classes have been shown to reduce pain severity, clinician office visits, and reliance on medications, while improving self-efficacy and promoting physical activity (SOE=B).

Several well-designed studies have demonstrated the integral value of exercise in managing rheumatoid arthritis, osteoarthritis, polymyositis, and systemic lupus erythematosus (SOE=A). Exercise and even modest weight reduction (eg, 15 lbs) can substantially decrease knee pain due to osteoarthritis (SOE=A). Patients should be provided with an exercise "prescription" that details warm-up activities, followed by instructions for the type of exercise (eg, strengthening, flexibility, and endurance), intensity, duration, and frequency during a given week. Patients should be advised to watch for signs of excessive joint strain, including swelling, fatigue, weakness, pain during activity, or pain that lasts >1–2 hours after exercise.

Therapeutic ultrasound is widely prescribed for pain and loss of function due to osteoarthritis. Ultrasound uses high-frequency (0.8–1 MHz) sound waves to reduce painful symptoms by pulsed delivery for acute pain and inflammation, or by continuous delivery for patients with chronic symptoms that have resulted in joint limitations (SOE=C).

Cold and heat are useful adjuncts that can decrease both pain and muscle spasms (SOE=C). Use of ice or cold packs should be limited to 20 minutes or when the area becomes numb. Cautious use of heat can reduce pain and muscle spasm but should be limited to 20-minute intervals using a heating modality that is unlikely to cause skin injury. Contrast therapy, which alternates between hot and cold treatment modalities, can provide additional therapeutic benefits than either alone (SOE=C).

Massage can alleviate painful symptoms. Acupuncture has been included as a potentially useful adjunct for patients with back pain and for knee osteoarthritis. Transcutaneous electrical nerve stimulation (TENS) is yet another alternative that delivers electrical stimulation that can be combined with acupuncture (SOE=B). Finally, neuromuscular electrical stimulation (NMES) delivers low-voltage electrical impulses through surface electrodes placed over motor points of the targeted muscle, inducing muscle contraction. NMES may be an alternative for patients who are unable to participate in exercise because of severe pain or contraindications (SOE=D).

Occupational and physical therapists can recommend devices that serve to alleviate painful symptoms, stabilize lax joints, lessen joint strain, improve gait mechanics and stability, and lessen risk of falling (SOE=C). Involvement of therapy services early in the management plan is highly advisable.

Pharmacologic Therapies for Pain

Selection of medications requires particularly careful attention to potential for adverse drug events in the geriatric population. Medications generally are indicated only for significant symptoms or when nonpharmacologic approaches have failed. Topical balms and creams, applied 2 or 3 times daily, can help control arthritis symptoms in small and intermediate joints (SOE=C). Capsaicin cream is effective for osteoarthritis of the hand(s) and knees but must be used carefully to avoid contact with mucous membranes, particularly to the eyes (SOE=B).

Acetaminophen (500–1,000 mg q8h) remains the preferred simple analgesic for older adults (SOE=A). The risk of nephropathy from acetaminophen remains low when it is used in modest dosages in patients without preexisting kidney disease and with cautious supervision in patients with renal insufficiency. However, excessive dosages can result in hepatotoxicity.

NSAIDs can be prescribed at either analgesic (lower) or anti-inflammatory dosages, but because of their toxicity in older adults, they are recommended only in suitable candidates for short periods. Analgesic medications include choline magnesium trisalicylate (750 mg q8h) and ibuprofen (200–800 mg q8h). Nonacetylated salicylates such as salsalate or magnesium choline salicylate and COX-2 agents are thought to have lower GI toxicity when used short term, but equivalent GI toxicity may result when used long term; they are far more expensive than generic ibuprofen. All agents in this class are equally effective at their recommended dosages. Patients with a high risk of GI bleeding and ulceration should either avoid NSAIDs or be given prophylaxis concurrent with NSAID use (ie, prostaglandin analogs or proton-pump inhibitors). Patients prescribed NSAIDs should be monitored for renal insufficiency and fluid retention, which can be particularly severe in patients who have heart failure or are taking ACE inhibitors. Delirium is common in older adults with NSAID use. COX-2 inhibitors have been associated with higher rates of stroke and myocardial infarction, leading to the withdrawal of rofecoxib from the market, followed by manufacturers' withdrawal of valdecoxib. Some relatively selective COX-2 inhibitors remain available (ie, celecoxib, nabumetone, and meloxicam).

Because of their adverse events, prednisone and other glucocorticoids should be used judiciously. Consultation with a rheumatologist can be helpful when considering immunosuppressive treatments. Dosages used depend on the particular disease being treated, with benefits usually realized within 5–10 days. Toxicities of glucocorticoids include cataracts, poor wound healing, gastric ulcers, mental status change, hyperglycemia, hypertension, osteoporosis, and immunosuppression. Full recovery of the hypothalamic-pituitary axis can require up to a year after chronic steroid use. Individuals on chronic steroid therapy should also receive therapy to prevent osteoporosis, usually with calcium, vitamin D, and bisphosphonates.

Finally, narcotic medications, started in low dosages and titrated slowly, are often useful in managing acute or chronic musculoskeletal pain that is unresponsive to exercise, use of assistive devices, hot and cold therapies, or acetaminophen. See also "Persistent Pain," p 119.

APPROACH TO SPECIFIC RHEUMATOLOGIC DISEASES

Osteoarthritis

Depending on the source of data and which joint is involved, osteoarthritis (OA) is present in 50%–90% of older adults. It is the major cause of knee, hip, and back pain in older adults, and it will increase in both incidence and prevalence with the aging of the population and increasing rates of obesity. Yet, caution needs to be exercised to avoid the reflexive conclusion that joint pain in the geriatric age group is necessarily the result of underlying OA.

Cartilage degeneration is the hallmark of OA, with fibrillation and ulceration that begins superficially and eventually extends into deeper layers. However, evidence indicates that OA is not a purely degenerative disease restricted to the cartilage; subchondral bone abnormalities and focal synovial inflammation have also been seen in pathologic specimens. These pathologic characteristics are thought to arise as a result of repetitive cycles of degradation and repair responses that eventually become inadequate to maintain joint health. Inflammatory cytokines, matrix-degrading metalloproteinase enzymes, and chondrocyte apoptosis are likely contributors to this process.

OA commonly affects the hands, knees, hips, and cervical and lumbar spine, but it can develop in any joint that has suffered injury or other disease. On examination, bony enlargement and crepitus suggest OA. In the fingers, this enlargement is called Heberden nodes when it occurs in the distal interphalangeal joints and Bouchard nodes in the proximal interphalangeal joints. Joint tenderness and warmth may appear, but intense inflammation suggests an alternative or concomitant diagnosis. Osteophytes are the radiographic counterpart of this enlargement, and asymmetric joint space narrowing is common (Figure 56.1). MRI can help evaluate back and neck symptoms that may require surgical intervention.

The objectives of OA management are to alleviate painful symptoms, prevent disease progression,

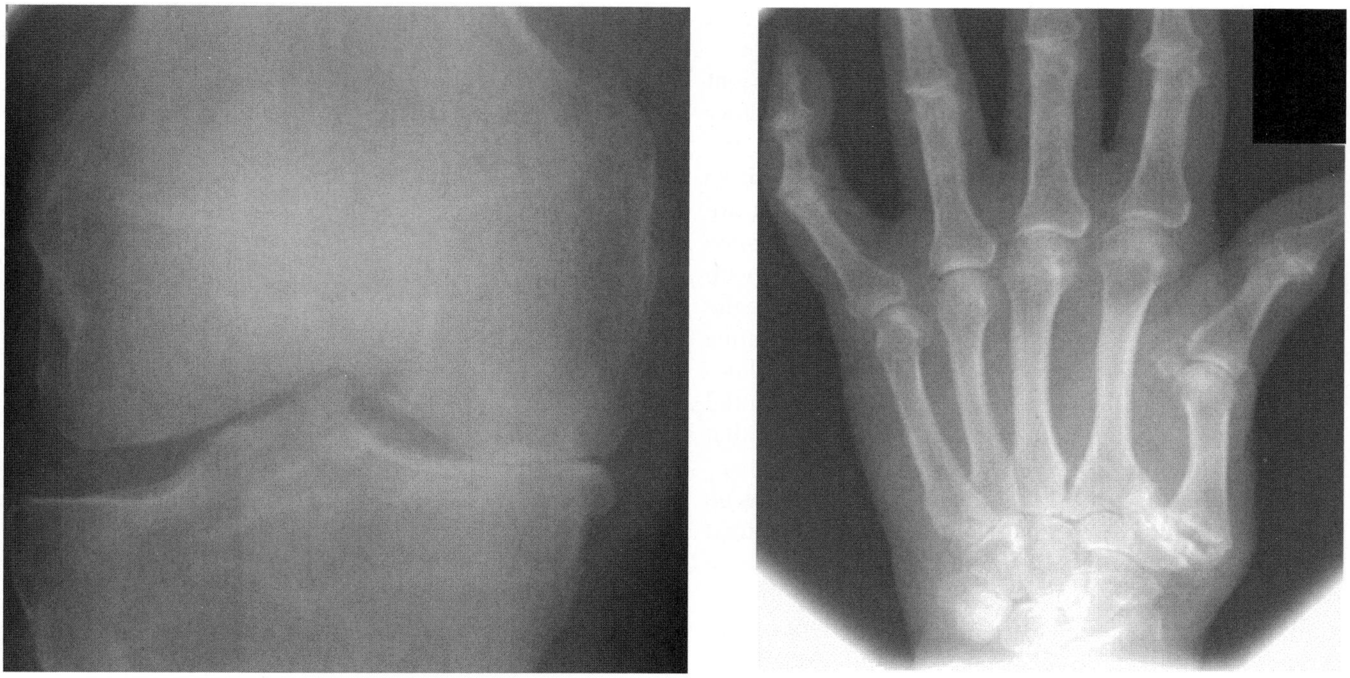

Figure 56.1—*Left:* Radiographic osteoarthritis of the knee with medial compartment osteophytes, joint space narrowing, and sclerosis. *Right:* Radiographic osteoarthritis of the hand with osteophytes, asymmetric joint space narrowing, and sclerosis of varying degrees of the thumb base (carpometacarpal joint) and proximal interphalangeal joints

maximize function, and minimize disease-related complications. Weight reduction can help reduce pain and improve function in patients with OA of the knee, hip, or spine. In knee OA, neoprene braces can alleviate patellofemoral symptoms by improving patellar tracking and can provide a greater sense of joint stability by improving joint proprioception. Specific orthoses designed to reduce medial knee pain by unloading the medial compartment of the knee include a valgus unloader brace and a lateral wedge insole. A simpler investment in a well-designed running shoe can also lessen pain and damage by decreasing the impact transmitted during ambulation. Finally, a properly fitted and used cane can provide stability as well as unloading the symptomatic knee or hip.

Topical therapies (eg, analgesic balms, capsaicin, topical NSAIDs) can be useful in hand or knee OA (SOE=C). Regular and consistently prescribed acetaminophen is the initial pharmacologic recommendation (SOE=A), followed by low-dose narcotic medications, or in cases of narcotic intolerance, NSAIDs. Studies evaluating glucosamine and chondroitin sulfate for pain have conflicting results, with more recent higher quality studies showing no superiority over placebo for patients with knee OA (SOE=A).

Glucocorticoid injections can be used for knee pain, although whether they are more effective than placebo injection is unclear (SOE=B). Hyaluronic acid and hyaluronan polymers given in a series of weekly injections in the knee are approved for intra-articular viscosupplementation therapy. The benefits of these preparations vary substantially between patients but last longer than benefits of corticosteroid injections in those who respond (SOE=B).

Several surgical procedures and joint replacement can be considered for patients with advanced large-joint OA. Arthroscopic debridement for knee OA is usually reserved for patients who report mechanical symptoms (eg, locking, "giveway" weakness), but effectiveness has not been proved (SOE=C). Joint-"sparing" high tibial osteotomy can realign the knee but requires considerable rehabilitation. Unicompartment joint replacement can be performed in patients whose disease is limited to one compartment (eg, isolated medial, lateral, or patellofemoral knee OA) (SOE=B). Total joint arthroplasty can be considered in patients with more extensive, disabling disease of the knee or hip. Although surgery remains the definitive intervention, it should be performed when the patient is likely to be able to withstand both the surgery and the ensuing rehabilitation and is debilitated enough from the OA that the benefits of surgery outweigh its risks.

Rheumatoid Arthritis

Although significantly less prevalent than osteoarthritis, rheumatoid arthritis (RA) is an important disease of older adults. Up to 40% of patients with RA are

>60 years old; some of these individuals have aged with the disease, while 20%–55% develop RA late in life.

Older adults with late-onset RA may present similarly to young adults with acute inflammatory polyarthritis that involves the small joints of the hands and feet and that is accompanied by a positive rheumatoid factor. Seronegative presentations that are unique to older adults include the "RS3PE" syndrome of remitting seronegative symmetrical synovitis with pitting edema, and an inflammatory arthritis of the shoulder and hips similar to polymyalgia rheumatica (PMR). In fact, descriptive studies suggest that late-onset RA should be considered in the differential diagnosis of PMR and vice versa. Other diseases that mimic RA include CPPD and carcinoma polyarthritis.

As with young adults, the diagnosis of RA relies on clinical, radiologic, and laboratory criteria. In contrast to young adults with RA, older adults with RA are more likely to have a higher initial ESR.

Descriptive studies suggest that patients with seropositive RA, even if of late onset, should be managed aggressively, including use of disease-modifying anti-inflammatory drugs (DMARDs) (SOE=B). Methotrexate is well tolerated, but older adults may require a lower dose; it should be given with daily folic acid supplementation. Cases of lymphoproliferative disease have been reported with long-term methotrexate treatment. Hydroxychloroquine is well tolerated, but patients must be monitored for retinal toxicity. Leflunomide has been demonstrated to prevent radiographic progression in younger adults, but experience is minimal in older adults (SOE=B). It has a relatively fast onset of action (about 4 weeks) compared with other DMARDs. Older agents, such as penicillamine, sulfasalazine, gold, and cyclophosphamide, are less well tolerated by older adults, and are rarely used.

Several biologic agents for RA are available, but experience with these agents in older adults is limited, so their use is generally limited to those in whom conventional DMARD therapy has not been effective. These agents work by inhibiting tumor necrosis factor α (etanercept, infliximab, adalimumab, golimumab, and certolizumab), antagonizing the interleukin-1 receptor (anakinra), serving as a fusion protein co-stimulation modulator via inhibition of CD28 (abatacept), or binding the CD20 antigen on B-lymphocytes (rituximab); they are given via injection or infusion. Infliximab, adalimumab, and rituximab all increase the risk of granulomatous infections with organisms such as *Mycobacterium tuberculosis*, atypical mycobacteria, yeast, *Listeria,* and *Nocardia.* Infliximab can also cause postinfusion fever, chills, headache, chest pain, and dyspnea. Anakinra is associated with bacterial respiratory tract infections.

Low-dose prednisone (10–20 mg/d) may be used as the primary treatment for seronegative PMR-like disease and the "RS3PE" syndrome. However, in contrast to classic PMR, late-onset RA may not respond promptly to low-dose prednisone. Prednisone alone is often not sufficient in managing seropositive RA but may be useful as an adjunctive agent. Its use is associated with increased risk of infectious complications, fluid retention, and osteoporosis.

Gout

Gout can cause both severe pain and debility. Women generally do not develop gout until menopause, at which time the rate in women approaches that in men. Diuretic use is an important predisposing factor. The clinical characteristics of gout can differ appreciably in older adults. Gout can present as a subacute smoldering oligoarthritis rather than as an acute, monarticular, and incapacitating attack, as in classic podagra affecting the first metatarsophalangeal joint. Tophaceous deposits in the distal and proximal interphalangeal joints can be mistaken for, or coexist with, osteoarthritis. Similarly, tophi at the extensor surfaces can be confused with rheumatoid nodules. Acute attacks can be precipitated by trauma, acute nonarticular illness requiring hospitalization, dehydration (acute gout is particularly common after surgery), and abrupt changes in uric acid concentration.

For a diagnosis of gout to be established, the presence of sodium urate crystals from synovial fluid or an aspirate of a tophus must be demonstrated. Sodium urate crystals are strongly negatively birefringent and needle-shaped and can be demonstrated in synovial fluid obtained in the intercritical phase, as well as during an acute flare. Radiographs show juxta-articular erosions of the involved joints. An overhanging edge (ie, Martel sign) can be seen and is helpful in distinguishing gout from rheumatoid arthritis. With rare exception, asymptomatic hyperuricemia precedes the development of gouty arthritis. However, hyperuricemia is not uniformly present at the time of an acute gout attack, and the presence of hyperuricemia neither confirms a diagnosis of gout nor necessitates starting urate-lowering medication.

An acute gout attack is best managed with a short-acting NSAID in those who can tolerate it, although narcotic medications or oral, intramuscular, or intra-articular glucocorticoids can be used. Intramuscular or short-term oral glucocorticoids (prednisone 30 mg/d for 5 days, or methylprednisolone beginning at 24 mg/d and tapering over 6 days) are preferred in managing a polyarticular gouty flare. Colchicine can also be used to treat an acute gouty attack. The approved dose of colchicine for an acute attack is 1.2 mg orally at the onset of the attack and then 0.6 mg 1 hour later (total dose 1.8 mg).

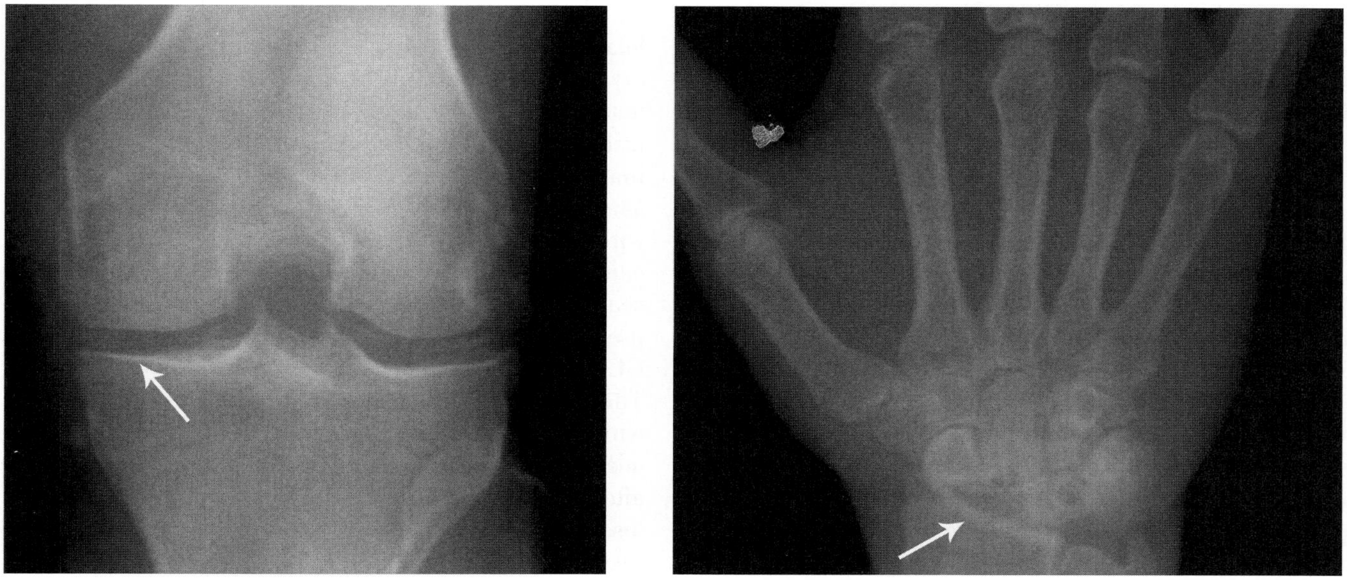

Figure 56.2—*Left:* Chondrocalcinosis of the meniscus. *Right:* Chondrocalcinosis of the triangular fibrocartilage of the wrist distal to the ulna

For patients who have recurrent episodes of gout, colchicine can be added prophylactically to reduce the frequency of recurrent gouty attacks. Conventional dosing is 0.6 mg orally q12h; the dosage should be reduced to 0.6 mg/d to three times weekly in patients with renal insufficiency; colchicine dosage adjustment is warranted among patients with hepatic insufficiency. Medications such as allopurinol, febuxostat, or probenecid, which can acutely lower uric acid levels, should not be used in the management of acute gout, because premature lowering of uric acid level paradoxically intensifies and prolongs an acute gout attack. Probenecid works as a uricosuric agent but is ineffective if creatinine clearance is <30–40 mL/min. Allopurinol and febuxostat lower serum uric acid via inhibition of xanthine oxidase and are beneficial in management of chronic gout, particularly for those with tophi, renal stones, or for whom colchicine is ineffective; the dosage should be adjusted in patients with renal or hepatic impairment.

Calcium Pyrophosphate Dihydrate Deposition Disease

CPPD, also known as "pseudogout," has many manifestations. Depending on the joint affected, it can mimic rheumatoid arthritis, inflammatory osteoarthritis, gout, or septic arthritis. It is most commonly diagnosed by finding chondrocalcinosis on plain radiographs (Figure 56.2). CPPD is associated with disorders of calcium metabolism (eg, hypomagnesemia, hypophosphatemia, hyperparathyroidism), hypothyroidism, and hemochromatosis. CPPD of the wrist can mimic rheumatoid arthritis but can be distinguished by prominent synovitis and chondrocalcinosis of the wrist and metacarpophalangeal joints; it is rheumatoid factor and anti-CCP antibody negative. CPPD can also mimic inflammatory osteoarthritis but with rapid joint destruction of the wrist, patellofemoral knee compartment, and hip joint.

CPPD can also cause an acute, intermittently inflammatory arthritis of the knee, hip, wrist, and metacarpophalangeal joints, with elbow, shoulder, and ankle involvement less common. CPPD can mimic an acute gout attack with sudden onset of pain and swelling that coincide with or immediately follow an acute illness or traumatic event such as surgery. When fever is present, distinguishing CPPD from septic arthritis is imperative yet can be challenging.

Arthrocentesis with crystal analysis is diagnostic and useful to distinguish CPPD from gout and infection. CPPD crystals are weakly positively birefringent rhomboids or squares. Chondrocalcinosis is apparent on plain radiographs (Figure 56.2), appearing as a stippled or linear calcification of the articular cartilage of the knee, wrist, hip, shoulder, and symphysis pubis.

Arthrocentesis with intra-articular steroid injection can result in significant relief of painful symptoms with CPPD. Short-acting NSAIDs and steroidal agents are also useful in management of CPPD in patients who can tolerate them (SOE=C). Intra-articular and parenteral corticosteroids are recommended for patients who cannot tolerate NSAIDs. Given once and possibly repeated in 1–2 days, triamcinolone acetonide (60 mg IM), betamethasone (7 mg IM), or methylprednisolone (125 mg IV) are all effective. Use of oral colchicine to prevent future acute episodes of CPPD has not been substantiated in clinical trials but is a conventional approach.

Polymyalgia Rheumatica

Polymyalgia rheumatica (PMR) is a condition unique to older adults. Approximately 53 new cases develop per 100,000 persons per year, with an estimated prevalence of 600 cases per 100,000 and higher prevalence with increasing age.

PMR should be suspected in adults ≥50 years old with persistent pain or stiffness of the upper arms, shoulders, hips, or thighs that is accompanied by constitutional symptoms of fatigue, low-grade fever, anorexia, and weight loss. Patients frequently lack physical evidence of an inflammatory arthritis of the small hand joints, distinguishing PMR from rheumatoid arthritis, and they also have normal muscle bulk and strength.

Diagnostic criteria include limb-girdle stiffness, an ESR often >50 mm/h, and normal levels of muscle enzymes. Recent studies of PMR have confirmed the presence of synovitis identical to that seen in rheumatoid arthritis, with synovial thickening, effusions, and lymphocytic synovial infiltration.

Mild symptoms of PMR can respond to NSAIDs. However, most patients require prednisone (10–20 mg/d as a single dose given in the early morning) (SOE=B). Symptoms should dramatically abate within 7 days, if not sooner. Dosage reduction should be gradual, with monitoring for symptom recurrence and laboratory studies (C-reactive protein, ESR) suggesting reactivation. Short-acting NSAIDs can be added to assist with controlling symptoms during the taper. Concomitant giant cell arteritis or an alternative diagnosis of rheumatoid arthritis should be considered in patients whose response to therapy is incomplete or not sustained. The duration of treatment required varies considerably, from 3 months to several years. Osteoporosis prophylaxis is recommended for all patients on systemic steroids for >2 months.

Giant Cell Arteritis

Giant cell arteritis (GCA) is a granulomatous vasculitis that involves large and medium-sized arteries. The overlap between GCA and polymyalgia rheumatica (PMR) is notable. Approximately 10%–20% of patients with PMR will also have GCA, and 50%–66% of patients with GCA have PMR symptoms. Therefore, all patients with PMR with any symptoms above the neck should have a temporal artery biopsy to evaluate for GCA.

Head and neck manifestations of GCA include headache, jaw, and tongue claudication with tenderness, erythema, or nodularity occasionally palpable along the temporal artery. Optic nerve pallor or swelling portends ischemia with impending blindness that warrants immediate glucocorticoid therapy. GCA can also appear as sudden blindness with no prior systemic illness or with claudication in the arms. Other manifestations can include stroke, ischemic necrosis of tongue or scalp, or rarely myocardial infarction. Aortic aneurysm, predominantly thoracic, is a late manifestation of GCA even when previously appropriately treated. The incidence of aneurysm in GCA is about 10%, with discovery of thoracic and abdominal aneurysm occurring at a median of 5.8 and 2.5 years, respectively, after GCA diagnosis. Constitutional symptoms of weight loss, malaise, fever, and depression may be the only manifestations of GCA.

Temporal artery biopsy is the gold standard for diagnosis; a specimen several centimeters in length should be obtained from the symptomatic side and immediately processed by frozen-section staining of multiple cross- and longitudinal sections; a section of the contralateral side can be obtained if the initial specimens are negative. Evidence of vasculitis without giant cells suggests other diagnoses (eg, polyarteritis nodosa) that may require cytotoxic therapy. Ultrasound, angiography, MRI with gadolinium, and positron emission tomography have been investigated as diagnostic modalities for demonstrating vascular inflammation; however, none has replaced biopsy as the gold standard diagnostic test.

Patients suspected of having GCA should begin prednisone treatment while awaiting biopsy to reduce the risk of sudden blindness. Fortunately for diagnostic purposes, pathologic evidence of GCA persists for up to 2 weeks after prednisone therapy has been started. Prednisone is given at a dosage of 40–60 mg/d and should be maintained for at least 1 month before considering dosage reduction. Intravenous glucocorticoids (prednisolone or methylprednisolone 80–100 mg) are occasionally recommended for patients at high risk of blindness or impending ischemic events of other organs. Treatment should continue for approximately 1–2 years. Long-term glucocorticoid therapy warrants prophylaxis for osteoporosis. Published studies of methotrexate as a steroid-sparing agent have not consistently demonstrated a benefit. In addition, concomitant administration of low-dose aspirin may decrease the risk of cranial ischemic complications. Monitoring for return of symptoms of PMR or temporal arteritis, increase of inflammatory markers, and radiographic screening for aortic aneurysms should continue lifelong after ceasing immunosuppressive therapy.

Systemic Lupus Erythematosus

Systemic lupus erythematosus is an autoimmune multisystemic disease that most commonly affects women of child-bearing age, yet up to 20% of cases are seen in older adults. When onset is after 50 years of age, the condition is referred to as "elderly onset lupus."

Elderly onset lupus should be considered in the differential diagnosis of rash (need not be malar in distribution), nonerosive arthritis, serositis (pleuritis, pericarditis), cytopenias (leukopenia, hemolytic anemia, or thrombocytopenia), neuropsychiatric symptoms (cognitive, seizures), symptoms of sicca (in the absence of medication-induced dry mouth), and Raynaud phenomenon. Renal involvement (eg, urinary casts, proteinuria) is less common in older lupus patients than in younger lupus patients. Additional physical findings can include periungual or palmar erythema, asymptomatic oral or nasal ulcers, and livedo reticularis—when present, these should raise suspicion of anticardiolipin antibody syndrome (venous or arterial thromboembolic phenomena). Vague manifestations for which lupus should be considered include fever, Raynaud phenomenon, and thromboembolic phenomena (including stroke).

The diagnosis rests on a constellation of clinical criteria along with serologic evidence of autoimmunity (positive antinuclear antibody, anti-double-stranded DNA, anti-Sm, or false-positive test for syphilis). Rheumatoid factor, anti-Ro/Sjögren syndrome (SS) A, and anti-La/SSB antibodies are more often positive in patients with elderly onset lupus.

Distinguishing elderly onset lupus from drug-induced lupus erythematosis is often clinically difficult. Both have a positive antinuclear antibody test, although drug-induced lupus erythematosis is associated with a speckled pattern with antihistone antibodies. Anti-double-stranded DNA and hypocomplementemia, both useful in monitoring disease activity in younger patients, are less frequently found in older patients. Renal biopsy should be pursued to evaluate patients with proteinuria or who have an active urine sediment to determine the underlying histopathology before starting treatment. Serologic evaluation for thromboembolic phenomena includes IgG and IgM anticardiolipin antibody levels and lupus anticoagulant testing, with mixing studies for a circulating anticoagulant, to explain prolonged partial thromboplastin times.

Treatment recommendations are based entirely on extrapolation from younger adults; no studies of these therapies have been done in older adults with lupus (SOE=D). Short-acting NSAIDs can be used to treat arthritis and serositis in older adults who can tolerate them. Hydroxychloroquine is effective in managing skin and joint manifestations (begun at 200 mg/d for a week, then increased to 400 mg/d). However, older adults should be evaluated for age-associated macular degeneration and monitored for visual field deficits possibly related to drug-induced retinopathy while receiving hydroxychloroquine treatment. Patients who are cardiolipin and lupus anticoagulant positive should receive preventive anticoagulant therapy. Intravenous methylprednisolone and monthly intravenous pulse cyclophosphamide is reserved for severe or renal (with an active urine sediment) or CNS disease. Methotrexate[OL], azathioprine[OL], mycophenolate mofetil[OL], or cyclosporine[OL] can be of benefit as corticosteroid-sparing agents.

Polymyositis and Dermatomyositis

Inflammatory muscle diseases, including polymyositis and dermatomyositis, form a heterogeneous and uncommon group of skeletal muscle diseases. Incidence of these diseases peaks in adults in their 50s, but they can occur at any age.

Muscle weakness is the central feature of myositis, and it is most prominent in the proximal muscle groups. Patients report difficulty with tasks such as standing from a chair, ascending stairs, or lifting a light package above the head. Muscle tenderness is usually not a manifestation and should raise suspicion of other conditions. Arthritis, when present, is inflammatory and occasionally erosive, suggesting overlap with rheumatoid arthritis. Esophageal dysmotility can cause dysphagia, hoarseness, and aspiration. Arrhythmia, symptoms of congestive heart disease, dyspnea on exertion, or persistent cough can also be present and suggest cardiac muscle involvement or coexistent interstitial lung disease. Raynaud phenomenon or Sjögren syndrome can also be present. Dermatomyositis is characterized by a facial rash that can involve the eyelids (heliotrope) or the nose and malar areas, or be more generalized. Rash can also be apparent over the neck and upper torso in sun-exposed areas. Gottron papules (skin thickening over the metacarpophalangeal and interphalangeal joints) can also be seen.

Initial diagnostic efforts should focus on excluding conditions that can result in muscle weakness, such as medication (eg, steroids, HMG-CoA reductase inhibitors), and metabolic derangements (eg, thyroid disorders, diabetes, vitamin D deficiency, electrolyte abnormalities) before muscle biopsy is pursued. Serum levels of muscle enzymes (creatine kinase, aldolase) are usually markedly increased. Electromyographic testing is used to exclude neuropathy and to identify the presence of an irritable myopathy. MRI using fat-suppression sequences can help to select which muscle to biopsy. Muscle biopsy remains the gold standard to confirm the diagnosis and also to distinguish among the subtypes of myositis. A diagnosis of polymyositis warrants an evaluation for cardiac and pulmonary disease; a diagnosis of dermatomyositis, and less so with polymyositis, warrants a search for an underlying malignancy. Associations with colon, lung, breast, prostate, ovarian, and uterine tumors are prominent, as is remission of polymyositis and dermatomyositis after treatment of the underlying malignancy.

Glucocorticoids are the initial therapy for polymyositis and dermatomyositis. Oral prednisone at 1 mg/kg/d is a typical starting dosage; for severe disease, an initial dose of methylprednisolone 1,000 mg IV is often used over 3 consecutive days. Prednisone can be tapered after an initial phase of improved muscle strength and normalized muscle enzyme concentrations. However, prolonged glucocorticoid use at high dosages can result in a myopathy with resultant proximal muscle weakness. Therefore, tapering the total dose by 10%–20% per month should be attempted. Methotrexate[OL], given orally or parenterally, in a weekly pulse regimen can be combined with corticosteroids and can also have a steroid-sparing effect in long-term therapy. Weekly oral methotrexate[OL] or mycophenolate mofetil[OL] may be effective in managing refractory skin manifestations of dermatomyositis.

Supervised exercise over 6-week and 6-month study periods has proved beneficial in polymyositis (SOE=B), improving function without aggravating underlying disease.

Sjögren Syndrome

Sjögren disease is a systemic, multiorgan chronic disease with lymphocytic infiltration of exocrine glands. Sicca symptoms (dry mouth and dry eyes) are common but are frequently caused by medications and other underlying connective tissue syndromes. Sjögren disease should be considered in patients with interstitial lung disease; malabsorption; CNS disease that mimics multiple sclerosis; unexplained renal, liver, or thyroid disease; or rash. The presence of palpable purpura and C4 hypocomplemententemia are recognized predictors for the development of lymphoma.

Sugar-free candies and artificial saliva can alleviate symptoms of xerostomia. Early and regular dental care should be ensured. Symptomatic treatment of xerophthalmia consists of lubricating ointments and artificial tears. Treatment of an underlying inflammatory disease (eg, rheumatoid arthritis, systemic lupus erythematosus, myositis, or scleroderma) can improve symptoms as well.

References

- Dasgupta B, Cimmino MB, Maradit-Kremers H, et al. 2012 Provisional classification criteria for polymyalgia: a European League Against Rheumatism/American College of Rheumatology collaborative initiative. *Arthritis Rheum*. 2012;65(4):943–954.
- Huizinga TW, Pincus T. In the clinic: Rheumatoid arthritis. *Ann Intern Med*. 2010;153(1):ITC1-1-ITC1-15.
- Khanna D, Khanna PP, Fitzgerald JB, et al. 2012 American College of Rheumatology Guidelines for Management of Gout. Part 1: *Arthritis Care Res*. 2012;64(10):1431–1446.
- Shelton LR. A closer look at osteoarthritis. *Nurse Pract*. 2013;38(7):30–36.
- Tsokos GC. Systemic lupus erythematosus. *N Engl J Med* 2011;365(22):2110–2121.
- Zhang W, Nuki G, Moskowitz RW, et al. OARSI recommendations for the management of hip and knee osteoarthritis: part III: Changes in evidence following systematic cumulative update of research published through January 2009. *Osteoarthritis Cartilage*. 2010;18(4):476–499.

CHAPTER 57—BACK AND NECK PAIN

KEY POINTS

- Back problems are the third most common reason for physician visits by older adults.
- Most episodes of back pain in older adults resolve within 4 weeks.
- The history and physical examination of the back, hips, and legs are the most important tools in assessing back pain. Clinical syndromes and diagnostic imaging tests are often poorly correlated. These tests should be used sparingly and interpreted in the context of the patient's clinical features.
- Pain that is insidious in onset, progressive in its course, and nonpositional; that is associated with night pain and systemic symptoms or signs; and that persists for >1 month should raise concerns about tumor or infection. Nonsystemic causes of pain are characterized by intermittent, often positional pain that is worse at onset and usually improves with time.
- Neck pain is most often due to mechanical disease of the cervical spine and is best diagnosed on physical examination.

BACK PAIN

Back problems are the third most common reason for physician visits by older adults. In the Framingham study, 22% of patients ≥68 years old had back pain on most days. Until recently, we knew little about the natural history of back pain in older adults. A recent 10-year study of 550 community-dwelling adults ≥70 years old documented 1,528 episodes of low back pain severe enough to restrict activity. Of these episodes, 80% lasted ≤1 month; only 6.4% lasted >3 months.

Several specific causes for pain in older adults are rarely seen in younger individuals. These include lumbar spinal stenosis, osteoporotic vertebral compression fractures, and osteoporotic sacral fractures. Systemic conditions such as tumors and infections, although a rare cause of back pain, are more common in older adults. Diagnostic imaging studies can complicate the evaluation of pain in older adults, because the prevalence of anatomic abnormalities unrelated to back pain is very high.

A systematic approach to the diagnosis of lower back pain in older adults requires knowledge of the typical presentation of common back conditions of older adults, an understanding of the anatomy of the lumbar spine, the identification of physical findings associated with common abnormalities, and the judicious use of diagnostic imaging studies (Table 57.1). The lack of specificity of diagnostic imaging tests heightens the importance of the history and physical examination in evaluation.

SYSTEMIC CAUSES

The history and physical examination can usually distinguish systemic from mechanical causes of back pain. Systemic conditions such as tumors or infections of the spine generally have an insidious onset of pain that becomes more and more persistent over time. This pain is usually nonpositional, can occur at night, and can be associated with systemic symptoms and signs. The pain of mechanical disease is usually intermittent, positional, and often worse at onset. The absence of the typical physical examination findings of motor weakness of the L4- through S1-innervated muscles of the hip and foot may also indicate systemic disease. The likelihood of cancer as a cause of back pain increases in adults ≥50 years old, those with a previous history of cancer, and those with pain that persists >1 month.

Fever, discrete local vertebral tenderness, upper lumbar or thoracic pain, and nonpositional pain can indicate vertebral infection. Approximately 10% of older adults with endocarditis have back pain. Infection can produce back pain in individuals at risk of endovascular infections, such as those on hemodialysis, with chronic indwelling venous access catheters, with a history of recent or chronic urinary tract infections, or with a history of intravenous drug abuse.

A number of visceral problems, such as abdominal aortic aneurysms, bladder distention secondary to urinary retention, large uterine fibroids, and intra-abdominal infections or tumors, can present with back pain. Referred pain from these conditions should be suggested by the historical pattern of the pain, the absence of positional changes, and a normal physical examination of the lumbosacral spine.

NONSYSTEMIC CAUSES

Lumbar Spinal Stenosis

Lumbar spinal stenosis results from a narrowing of either the central or lateral aspect of the lumbar spine canal. The characteristic symptom of lumbar spinal stenosis is pain in the back radiating into the buttock or leg that is worse on standing and walking and relieved with sitting. The anatomic features of lumbar spinal stenosis on diagnostic imaging studies are often found in asymptomatic older adults. The clinician must

Table 57.1—Conditions Causing Back Pain in Older Adults

Condition	History	Examination	Laboratory Tests, Imaging
Tumor	Persistent, progressive pain at rest; systemic symptoms	No focal abnormalities	Anemia, increased ESR, abnormal bone scan or MRI
Infection	Persistent pain, fever; at-risk patient (eg, indwelling catheter)	Tender spine	Increased ESR, WBC count; positive bone scan or MRI
Unstable lumbar spine	Recurring episodes of pain on change of position	Pain going from flexed to extended position	MRI or CT showing one disc space narrowed and sclerotic spondylolisthesis
Lumbar spinal stenosis	Pain on standing and walking relieved by sitting and lying	Immobile spine; L4, L5, S1 weakness	MRI or CT scan showing stenosis
Sciatica	Pain in the posterior aspect of leg; may be incomplete	Often positive straight leg raise; L4, L5, S1 weakness	Variable diagnostic imaging findings
Vertebral compression fracture	Sudden onset of severe pain; resolves in 4–6 weeks	Pain on any movement of spine; no neurologic deficits	Vertebral end-plate collapse; compression fracture seen on plain film
Osteoporotic sacral fracture	Sudden lower back, buttock, or hip pain	Sacral tenderness	H-shaped uptake on bone scan

NOTE: ESR = erythrocyte sedimentation rate

Table 57.2—Innervation of Lower Extremities

Function	Muscle	Peripheral Nerve	Nerve Root
Great toe dorsiflexion	Extensor hallucis longus	Deep peroneal	L5
Ankle dorsiflexion	Tibialis anterior	Deep peroneal	L4, L5
Ankle eversion	Peroneus longus, brevis	Superficial peroneal	L5, S1
Ankle plantar flexion	Gastrocnemius, soleus	Tibial	S1, S2
Knee extension	Quadriceps	Femoral	L3, L4
Hip flexion	Iliopsoas	Femoral	L2, L3
Hip adduction	Adductor magnus, brevis, longus	Obturator	L3, L4
Hip abduction	Gluteus medius	Superior gluteal	L4, L5
Hip extension	Gluteus maximus	Inferior gluteal	L5, S1

ensure that the patient has the appropriate historical and physical findings of this condition before making the diagnosis of lumbar spinal stenosis.

Flexion of the lumbar spine results in an increase in spinal canal volume and a decrease in nerve root bulk. Extension of the lumbar spine results in a decrease in spinal canal volume and an increase in nerve root bulk. Therefore, positions that flex the spine, such as sitting, bending forward, walking uphill, and lying in a flexed position, all relieve symptoms, while positions that extend the lumbar spine, such as prolonged standing, walking, and walking downhill, all exacerbate symptoms.

Pain in the calf when walking can mimic the claudication of arterial insufficiency and is referred to as *pseudoclaudication*. Continued walking after this point can result in paresthesia, numbness, and weakness in one or both legs. Other clues that a patient has lumbar stenosis are that walking uphill is easier than walking downhill, and walking with an assistive device, such as a shopping cart, which allows some flexion of the lumbar spine, is usually better tolerated. These symptoms are usually progressive and consistent, not intermittent. There is often subtle weakness in the muscles innervated by the L4, L5, and S1 nerve roots. (See Table 57.2 and the assessment section, below.)

Sciatica

In addition to the pseudoclaudication syndrome, which produces pain in all or part of the distribution of a sciatic nerve, older adults can develop an acute sciatic syndrome similar to that seen in younger individuals.

Acute sciatica usually occurs spontaneously, with no clear causal event. Pain can be felt in any position and is usually not relieved with sitting. The clinical course varies. In one study, 50% of patients were significantly improved in 10 days, while in another study, 80% of patients had remission of symptoms within 8 weeks. Although there are no studies that have specifically evaluated sciatica in older adults, most clinicians find that older patients with this syndrome follow the favorable clinical course of younger ones.

Osteoporotic Vertebral Compression Fractures

Although only one-third of vertebral compression fractures are symptomatic, the symptoms can be

Table 57.3—Assessment of Lower Back Pain in Older Adults

Symptoms	Conditions
Acute pain	Vertebral compression fracture Disc displacement Osteoporotic sacral fracture Visceral origin (eg, aortic aneurysm)
Positional pain	
Increased with standing and walking and relieved with sitting	Lumbar spinal stenosis
Brought on by bending, lifting, or unguarded movements	Unstable lumbar spine
Persistent pain (gradually increasing, nonpositional)	Tumor Infection

Chapters

quite severe. (Interestingly, only about one-third of older adults with severe hyperkyphosis have vertebral fractures.) The pain from an acute vertebral fracture usually lasts at least 3-4 weeks. The onset of pain is abrupt, and intense pain is felt deep at the site of the fracture. Tenderness is often marked over the involved vertebra. The pain is usually worse on standing and walking, and relieved with lying down. Although the pain commonly radiates to the flank, abdomen, and legs, neurologic sequelae should not occur in patients with spontaneous osteopenic fractures. Symptomatic fractures most often affect the lower thoracic and lumbar vertebrae.

The acute pain resolves slowly. In one study, analgesic use decreased by 16% at day 5 and by 33% at day 14. Patients often have trouble walking for 2 weeks and restrict their activity for approximately 1 month.

The impact of these fractures, and osteoporosis in general, on chronic back pain and the function of older adults is unclear. Patients with these fractures are more apt to have further fractures, are more disabled, and have a higher mortality than those without fractures. An increase in chronic back pain, however, is seen only in patients with extensive fractures.

Osteoporotic Sacral Fractures

Lower back pain in older women may be due to osteoporotic sacral fractures. This pain often occurs spontaneously, usually involving the lower back. Pain can also be felt in the buttock or hip area. Sacral tenderness on physical examination is usually present. The incidence of associated additional osteoporotic fractures is high.

Plain radiographs are usually negative. Technetium bone scans show a characteristic H-shaped uptake over the sacrum. A CT scan shows displacement of the anterior border of the sacrum. Prognosis for recovery is excellent, with no neurologic deficits. The pain usually resolves in 4–6 weeks.

Nonspecific Back Pain

Assessment of back pain in older adults has been limited by a lack of information about the natural history of this condition. In a recent study, 80% of episodes of back pain in adults >70 years old lasted <4 weeks.

This information is very helpful, because certain specific causes of back pain in older adults (tumor, infection, lumbar spinal stenosis, compression fractures, and sacral fractures) are not likely to resolve within 4 weeks. Most episodes of back pain in older adults are self-limited, of short duration, and probably mechanical in origin.

It is likely that this pain is similar to back pain in younger individuals. Back pain in younger individuals is usually due to mechanical causes and has a reassuring natural history. In younger individuals, 50% of patients with mechanical low back pain are better in 1 week, 80% are better in 2 weeks, and 90% are better in 2 months.

Unstable Lumbar Spine

Lumbar degenerative disc disease may produce a *relatively* unstable lumbar spine. Individuals with this condition often have episodes of severe pain in the back or in the distribution of the sciatic nerve. This pain usually comes on suddenly, often after abrupt movements. It usually lasts only minutes to hours but recurs frequently. This pain also arises with significant flexion or extension of the lumbar spine. On physical examination, the patient often has guarded movements of the lumbar spine and pain when moving from the flexed to the extended position. Significant disc space narrowing, vertebral end-plate sclerosis, and osteophytosis at one disc space, out of proportion to the other spaces, is often seen in patients with lumbar spine instability.

ASSESSMENT

See Table 57.3.

History

Pain that is insidious in onset, progressive in its course, nonpositional, associated with night pain and systemic symptoms or signs, and that persists for >1 month should raise concerns about tumor or infection. Nonsystemic

Table 57.4—Physical Examination of Older Adults with Lower Back Pain

Sign	Condition
Paravertebral muscle spasm	Mechanical disease*
Asymmetric range of motion of the lumbar spine	Mechanical disc disease Unstable lumbar spine
Spinal tenderness	Vertebral compression fracture Infection
Weakness of L4–L5 and L5–S1 muscles	Mechanical disc disease Lumbar spinal stenosis
Normal examination of lumbar spine	Osteoporotic sacral fracture Hip disease Tumor Referred visceral pain

*Not caused by tumor, infection, spinal stenosis, or fracture

causes of pain are characterized by intermittent, often positional pain that is worse at onset and that usually improves over time.

Diseases of the hip often result in pain in the back and leg in a distribution that resembles that of back disease. Back disease is more apt to cause pain when an individual goes from the supine to the sitting position. The hip is more apt to be the cause of the pain if the individual has pain in the groin, a limp, or limited range of motion of the hip.

Physical Examination

The physical examination of the back, hips, and legs is essential in the assessment of an older adult with back pain (Table 57.4). The finding of subtle but asymmetric weakness of the hip, ankle, and foot muscles innervated by the lumbar and sacral nerves can help elucidate the cause of back and leg pain.

A thorough back examination begins with the patient in the upright position. The back should be moved through all four planes of movement of the lumbar spine: side flexion to the right, side flexion to the left, forward flexion, and extension. Asymmetric limitation of the range of motion of the lumbar spine, or reproduction of the pain with these maneuvers, often indicates mechanical disease of the lumbar spine. The pain of lumbar spinal stenosis is often produced by spinal extension.

The remainder of the examination is performed with the patient in the supine position. A straight leg raise test can be informative if positive, but a negative test does not exclude any condition. Each patient with a back complaint should have a complete examination of the hips, focusing on the passive range of motion. The examiner should be able to abduct the hip to 40 degrees before the pelvis starts to tilt. The hip should flex beyond 110 degrees, externally rotate 50–60 degrees, and internally rotate 15–20 degrees.

Manual examination of the leg muscles can be helpful. Nerve root irritation from a spinal process should affect all the muscles innervated by these nerve roots. Thus, an individual with lumbar spine disease at the L4–L5 and the L5–S1 level should have weakness of the hip abductor and hip extensor, as well as of the ankle dorsiflexor, great toe dorsiflexor, and ankle evertor. A patient with a peroneal palsy should have weakness of the great toe extensor, ankle dorsiflexor, and ankle evertors, but no involvement of the hip abductors and hip extensors (Table 57.2).

Observation of the patient can be very helpful. Patients with lumbar spinal stenosis often bend forward more and more as they walk, while patients with hip disease are apt to limp.

Laboratory Tests and Imaging

Although not recommended in the evaluation of younger patients in the routine evaluation of low back pain, a plain lumbar spine radiograph can be a helpful test in evaluating back pain in older adults, particularly if there is suspicion of an underlying systemic condition. This single diagnostic tool can demonstrate degenerative disc and joint disease, vertebral compression fractures, deformities such as spondylolisthesis and scoliosis, and systemic disorders such as osteoporosis and Paget disease.

A technetium bone scan is useful in evaluating a suspected infection or neoplasm. CT and MRI have replaced myelography in assessing the neural canal. CT imaging is, in many cases, slightly superior in demonstrating the bony architecture of the spine, whereas the MRI is more sensitive to morphology of soft tissue, including disc, ligamentum flavum, neoplasm, and infection. Either CT or MRI studies are necessary to document spinal stenosis if surgical treatment is contemplated.

The use of diagnostic imaging studies is tempered by the high false-positive rates of these studies in older adults. A diagnostic imaging study simply identifies an anatomic abnormality—it does not demonstrate that this abnormality is the cause of the pain. In one study, 57% of adults ≥60 years old, with no history of lower back pain or sciatica, had abnormal lumbar spine MRIs. Of these individuals, 36% had a herniated nucleus pulposus, and 21% had lumbar spinal stenosis. In another study, only 36% of asymptomatic individuals had normal discs at all levels; the prevalence of disc abnormalities increased in older adults. Other studies have shown similarly high rates of abnormal findings in asymptomatic individuals. These studies reinforce the need to correlate carefully the history and physical examination with the findings on diagnostic imaging studies.

MANAGEMENT

Management of back pain is hampered by the common difficulty of making a definitive diagnosis. Patients can do well, however, with a therapeutic approach that addresses the structural problems most likely to be causing their pain.

Treatment of an unstable lumbar spine is symptomatic. Nonopioid analgesics are often helpful in the early stages. As soon as the acute symptoms subside, a gentle, progressive exercise program should be started that is designed to strengthen and improve the efficiency of the spinal and abdominal musculature. An aquatic program offers the dual benefits of rapid rehabilitation with a low incidence of reinjury. Walking in chest-high water against resistance and performing the flutter kick are two simple aquatic exercises (SOE=D). Design and oversight of an appropriate exercise program can be performed by physical therapy.

Chronic mechanical pain is often caused by excessive vertebral motion that is jarring or repetitive. Management is aimed at eliminating or reducing motion. This can be done internally by strengthening the paraspinous and abdominal muscles, thus providing an internal "brace" for the lumbar spine. It must be stressed that this exercise should be a lifetime commitment. Lumbar sacral corsets and braces provide an external method of immobilizing the lumbar spine. In severe cases in which conservative therapy has not been successful, surgical fusion can be considered (SOE=D).

Analgesia is the most important goal of treatment of vertebral compression fractures, while trying to avoid the complications of the bed rest required because of pain. Braces and corsets are rarely required, because the natural history of the acute pain is relatively brief. Corsets can offer symptomatic relief if the pain is persistent. Spinal extension exercises also may be helpful. Calcitonin[OL] has been demonstrated to decrease the pain associated with acute vertebral fractures. For severe or incapacitating pain unrelieved by other analgesics or calcitonin, low-dose opiates can be helpful, although patients should be warned about potential adverse effects (confusion, drowsiness, constipation).

Vertebroplasty is the percutaneous injection of bone cement into a collapsed vertebra. Two randomized trials demonstrated no difference in pain relief between vertebroplasty and placebo participants who had fracture pain for a median of 9 weeks in one trial and 18 weeks in the other (range 1–52 weeks) (SOE=A). However, in another study, vertebroplasty did significantly reduce pain compared with conservative therapy for these fractures. Although the authors stated that treatment was given for "acute osteoporotic vertebral compression fractures," the average patient who underwent the procedure had pain for 5–6 weeks. Half of patients originally randomized to vertebroplasty did not undergo this procedure, because their pain had resolved spontaneously. The American Association of Orthopedic Surgeons now recommends that vertebroplasty not be used in the treatment of osteoporotic spinal compression fractures (SOE=D). Kyphoplasty resembles vertebroplasty in that bone cement is injected into a vertebra, but with kyphoplasty an attempt is made to restore the height of the collapsed bone. The evidence of benefit of this procedure is uncertain.

Because mechanical encroachment on lumbar nerve roots causes lumbar spinal stenosis, conservative therapy is limited. Epidural corticosteroid injections have been used extensively for the sciatica associated with lumbar spinal stenosis, but a review of controlled trials of this therapy did not demonstrate efficacy of injection over controls.

Lumbar spinal stenosis is the most common indication for spinal surgery in older adults. In a prospective study of surgery for spinal stenosis, the ideal candidates for surgery were found to be those patients with severe narrowing of the spinal canal, minimal associated back pain, no coexisting conditions that affect walking, and symptom duration of <4 years. In two randomized, controlled trials and a high-quality observational study, surgery provided earlier and greater pain relief and improvement in functional status. (SOE=A).

Lumbar interspinous spacers have been used to treat neurogenic claudication in patients with lumbar spinal stenosis. A recent review concluded that these spacers may have a potential beneficial effect in selected patients with degenerative disease of the lumbar spine whose symptoms improve with flexion. Further studies are needed to clearly outline the indication for the use of these devices.

NECK PAIN

Causes

Although neck pain can be due to inflammatory and systemic conditions, it is most often due to mechanical disease of the cervical spine. Inflammatory conditions such as polymyalgia rheumatica and rheumatoid arthritis are characterized by morning stiffness; systemic complaints such as fatigue, fever, and weight loss; and other muscle and joint complaints.

Neck pain has been associated with back pain in a number of studies. The prognosis for resolution of neck pain is worse in older patients and in patients with accompanying back pain. Mechanical disease of the cervical spine can cause neck and occiput pain, scapula and trapezius pain, radicular pain down the arm, as well as spastic paraparesis due to cervical myelopathy.

The referral pain pattern of cervical spine disease has been demonstrated by a number of injection studies. C2–C3 disease is felt in the occiput; C3–C4 and C4–C5 problems are referred into the posterior and lateral aspects of the neck; C5–C6 lesions are referred into the trapezius and upper cervical region; C6–C7 disease is felt in the retroscapular region, often as far down as the mid to lower thoracic region. This referral process produces not only pain in these regions but also local muscle spasm and tenderness, often mistaken for "trigger points."

Irritation of a cervical nerve root produces lancinating pain and numbness in the neck and upper scapular region, radiating into the arm in a dermatomal distribution. Characteristic weakness of the arm muscles (see below) confirms the specific nerve root involved.

Narrowing of the cervical canal can produce the syndrome of cervical myelopathy, which is characterized by clumsiness, weakness, and spasticity of the legs; bladder spasticity; and upper motor neuron signs of the legs (clonus, hyperreflexia, and Babinski signs). Although progressive signs and symptoms call for an aggressive diagnostic and therapeutic approach, the natural history of this problem can be quite variable, and surgical intervention is not always necessary.

Assessment

Mechanical disease of the cervical spine is best diagnosed on physical examination. The cervical spine has four planes of movement: rotation to the right, rotation to the left, flexion, and extension. Asymmetric limitation of the range of motion of the cervical spine in some but not all of these movements, and weakness of the arm muscles innervated by the cervical nerve root, indicate mechanical disease of the cervical spine. The shoulder abductor and elbow flexor muscles are innervated by C5 and C6 nerve roots, the wrist extensor and thumb opponens muscles by C6 and C7, and the elbow extensor and finger abductors muscles by C7 and C8. Weakness of the C7- and C8-innervated muscles is most common with cervical disc disease, because the C7–T1 interspace is the most common site of cervical spine lesions. Individuals with mechanical disease of the cervical spine often awake in the morning with pain in the trapezius and scapular region, do not have full rotation of the cervical spine, and have difficulty with such activities as backing a car out of a driveway.

Diagnostic Imaging

The role of diagnostic imaging tests in the diagnosis and management of neck pain is unclear. A plain radiograph of the cervical spine has limited value, in that 80% of adults ≥55 years old have signs of degenerative cervical disc disease on these films. MRIs of the cervical spine also show degeneration in at least one level in almost 60% of adults ≥40 years old. These anatomic abnormalities call for interventions only if they are consistent with significant historical and physical features of the patient's condition.

Management

There is much controversy about the therapy of mechanical disease of the cervical spine. Two studies from the Netherlands and Finland, done on younger individuals, have had promising results for manual therapy and active neck-muscle training in the treatment of neck pain. In a Cochrane review of the management of neck disorders, the combination of mobilization and/or manipulation along with active exercises was beneficial for persistent mechanical neck disorders. Mobilization and/or manipulation done alone or combined with other treatments such as heat were not effective. These therapies were effective only when combined with an exercise program.

REFERENCES

- Esses SI, McGuire R, Jenkins J, et al. American Associate of Orthopedic Surgeons Clinical Practice Guideline Summary: the treatment of symptomatic osteoporotic spinal compression fractures. *J Am Acad Orthop Surg*. 2011;19(3):176–182.
- Herr K. Pain in the older adult: An imperative across all health care settings. *Pain Manage Nurs*. 2010;11(2 Suppl):S1–S10.
- Klazen CA, Lohle PN, deVries J, et al. Vertebroplasty versus conservative treatment in acute osteoporotic vertebral compression fractures (Vertos II): an open-label randomized trial. *Lancet*. 2010;376(9746):1085–1092.
- Makris UE, Fraenkel L, Han L, et al. Epidemiology of restricting back pain in community-living older persons. *J Am Geriatr Soc*. 2011;59(4):610–614.

CHAPTER 58—DISEASES AND DISORDERS OF THE FOOT

KEY POINTS

- Foot and ankle problems are common in older adults. Early diagnosis and effective treatment are critical to maintaining function and quality of life.
- Long-term effects of common structural foot deformities—including collapsing pes plano valgus, cavus foot, and equinus deformity—cause significant disability in older adults.
- Skin disorders of the foot are common in older adults. Complete assessment of the skin of the foot is necessary to identify skin conditions and potential malignancies.
- Systemic diseases can have long-term effects on the foot and ankle.
- Surgical intervention for treatment of foot deformities can alleviate pain and improve function in older adults who are appropriate surgical candidates. Most surgical interventions in older adults can be performed under local anesthesia.

Foot problems can have a significant effect on the functional capacity of older adults, and negatively impact their quality of life. If left untreated, these problems can lead to inactivity, morbidity, and even death.

Foot problems vary in severity from dry xerotic skin on the plantar surface of the foot to an infected, limb-threatening diabetic foot ulcer in a patient with peripheral arterial disease. In general, most foot problems are musculoskeletal and/or dermatologic in nature, although vascular, neurologic, and systemic diseases can also affect the foot. Complicating the situation is the fact that many patients are not in the habit of inspecting their feet, or may lack the flexibility and mobility to do so effectively. Unless they are experiencing some pain or discomfort, they may not notice or may ignore pathologic changes that are developing.

Therefore, clinicians who are treating older adults should be conscious of the potential for foot problems and make an effort to determine whether any of these conditions, or preconditions, exist. Once identified, specific problems should be treated or the patient referred to the appropriate specialist, depending on the preliminary presentation or diagnosis.

Not all older adults are similarly affected by foot problems. The prevalence of foot problems in older adults varies by level of disability and site of care. Studies of a variety of healthcare settings (including nursing homes, inpatient facilities, and outpatient settings) and examination of age- and morbidity-specific populations have confirmed that the prevalence of foot pathology increases with age. Approximately one-third of the geriatric population has some foot pathology, with a higher incidence in those residing in a medical facility such as a nursing home or hospital.

The most common problems identified by these studies are nail disorders, corns/calluses, hammertoes, plantar fasciitis, hallux valgus, and flat feet. Studies of the geriatric population demonstrate that foot complaints can inhibit daily activities such as getting out of a chair, walking, and climbing stairs. The resulting decrease in mobility can exacerbate other age-related conditions and lead to loss of muscle, a decrease in cardiovascular function, and weight gain. Foot complaints are also associated with increased risk of falling in the aging population.

THE ROLE OF THE PRIMARY CARE CLINICIAN IN FOOT CARE

Because older adults may not always be vigilant when it comes to the health of their lower extremities, primary care physicians should regularly assess their geriatric patients' feet. Practitioners should pay close attention to foot conditions and the complications of systemic diseases, such as arthritic changes, neurologic disorders, diabetes mellitus, peripheral arterial disease, and mental health issues that can manifest as foot symptoms and signs. Primary care clinicians should recognize common foot problems and refer patients for podiatric care and management in a timely and appropriate manner. The health, quality of life, and the functional capacity of older adults can be significantly improved by early detection and comprehensive management of foot problems (SOE=D).

COMMON DEFORMITIES OF THE FOOT

See Table 58.1.

Collapsing Pes Plano Valgus Foot (Pes Planus), Cavus Foot, Equinus Deformity

Most foot deformities derive from the longstanding effects of a pathologic foot. A pathologic foot is one

Table 58.1–Common Disorders of the Foot

Disorder	Definition or Description
Bunion	Prominent and dorsal medial eminence of the first metatarsal; associated with hallux valgus
Calcaneal spur/heel spur	A calcification of the attachment of the plantar fascia, usually at the medial plantar tuberosity of the calcaneus. The spur projects anteriorly and is the consequence of chronic repetitive trauma or stress resulting from biomechanical and pathomechanical change. When ligamentous calcification occurs, inflammation and associated pain at the attachment result. This may be referred to as heel pain syndrome and may be related to plantar fasciitis.
Cystic erosion	Areas of radiolucency usually noted with arthritic changes, such as rheumatoid arthritis, and usually seen in the metatarsal heads with associated joint changes
Digiti flexus	Fixed or flexible flexion at the metatarsal phalangeal joints, ie, hammertoe
Digiti quinti varus	Valgus displacement or splaying of the fifth metatarsal, with a resulting varus or inward deviation of the fifth toe
Dislocation of lesser metatarsal phalangeal joint	Toe joint is out of its socket
Entrapment syndrome	Occurs when a nerve is compressed by ligamentous or other soft-tissue inflammation, resulting in pain and possibly numbness and neuropathic symptoms. The most common sites are the posterior tibial nerve and the intermetatarsal nerves, plantarly.
Equinus	Tight Achilles tendon
Haglund deformity	A hyperostosis of the posterior and superior portion of the calcaneus, enlarging the calcaneus, which can in turn place pressure on the attachment of the Achilles tendon. The presence of the deformity also can produce a pressure area for the heel counter of the shoe. It is easily demonstrated on a lateral radiograph of the foot and can be associated with tendinitis or bursitis, usually resulting from an incompatibility of foot to shoe last.
Hallux abducto valgus	An alternative clinical diagnosis for hallux valgus, or bunion. There is a varus splaying of the first metatarsal with a valgus and rotational deformity of the phalanges of the great toe.
Hallux limitus and rigidus	A degenerative joint change involving the first metatarsal phalangeal joint, resulting from dorsal spurs, with a marked limitation or absence of any range of motion. The difference between hallux limitus and rigidus is based on the radiographic interpretation and difference in function.
Hallux valgus	Deviation of the tip of the great toe, or main axis of the toe, toward the outer or lateral side of the foot, ie, bunion
Hammertoe	Muscle tendon imbalance causing contraction of the proximal or distal interphalangeal joint, or both
Metatarsalgia	Pain in the forefoot near the heads of the metatarsals
Morton neuroma/syndrome	A congenital shortening of the first metatarsal shaft, which creates an abnormal metatarsal arc. Excessive weight is placed on the second metatarsal head during gait and stance. The dynamics and pathomechanics of the foot are modified and can lead to hallux valgus, abducto valgus, or rotational deformity of the hallux.
Periostitis	Inflammation of the periosteum
Pes cavus	Higher than normal arch that is commonly associated with neurologic change. In older adults, excessive pressure is usually placed on the metatarsal heads. With atrophy of the plantar fat pad and displacement, pressure is increased, which can predispose to pain and ulceration.
Pes planus	A flattening of the medial longitudinal arch, in which the calcaneal pitch on a radiograph is usually below 15 degrees (ie, flat feet)
Pes valgo planus	Clinical picture same as that of pes planus, with an addition of pronation, demonstrated by a lateral deviation of the Achilles tendon and an outward and rotational deformity of the foot.
Plantar fasciitis	Inflammation and pain involving repetitive microtrauma to the plantar fascia, particularly at its posterior calcaneal attachment; associated with biomechanical and pathomechanical changes in the function of the foot. It is related to calcaneal spurs, ligamentous calcification, and tissue atrophy.
Subluxation	Deviation of a joint's position
Tailor's bunion	Prominence of the dorsal lateral aspect of the fifth metatarsal head
Tarsal tunnel syndrome	An entrapment neuropathy of the posterior tibial nerve
Tenosynovitis	Inflammation of the synovial sheath of a tendon complex; sometimes associated with a tendon tear
Tibialis posterior dysfunction	Chronic rupture or weakening of the tibialis posterior tendon secondary to long-term pes planus
Valgus position	Frontal plane position in which pressure is inwardly directed in the foot
Varus position	Frontal plane position in which pressure is outwardly directed in the foot

that abnormally distributes weight during walking and other movement, creating stress on the musculoskeletal structure of the foot and often resulting in pain. Over an extended period of time, this physical stress on the foot may result in arthritis, tissue atrophy, and subluxation of foot joints.

This disability is created by two pathologic foot types: collapsing pes plano valgus (low arch morphology) and cavus foot (high arch morphology). Equinus, the effect of a tight heel cord or Achilles tendon, is a deforming force that can be identified in both pes planus and pes cavus foot types.

Collapsing pes plano valgus is generally seen in a foot type with an unstable medial longitudinal arch, which leads to a "flat foot." The instability can occur in the talonavicular joint, the navicular cuneiform joint, and/or the first metatarsal cuneiform joint. This instability causes the forefoot to abduct on the rearfoot, and the rearfoot to go into valgus attitude in respect to the ankle joint. When the patient is standing, the longitudinal arch collapses on the weight-bearing surface, resulting in the subluxation of joints and leading to arthrosis.

Early in life, this deformity is usually quite flexible and can be treated with functional orthoses to help support the arch. However, later in life, the foot becomes more rigid and is better treated with an accommodative orthosis that absorbs the abnormally high pressure on the pes planus foot type. The deformity can be congenital or acquired, but the extent of the deformity depends on activity level, body type, types of shoe worn, etc. Patients with this type of foot often have a number of other associated deformities, including posterior tibial tendon dysfunction, hallux valgus (bunion deformity), lesser metatarsal phalangeal joint dislocations (chronic dislocation of the toe joints), hammertoes, and neuromas.

The cavus foot type is generally rigid and a very poor shock absorber. It also can be congenital. If acquired later in life, it usually has a neurologic origin. Cavus foot often has a component of metatarsus adductus (inward orientation of the metatarsal bones). Older adults with this foot type generally experience loss of the fat pad in both the heel and the submetatarsal head region or ball of the foot. Associated deformities include cocked hallux (hammertoe of the great toe), sagittal dislocation of the metatarsal phalangeal joints, metatarsalgia, midfoot dorsal exostoses (bone spurs), and rigid hammertoe deformities.

An equinus deformity is commonly seen in a pes planus or cavus foot, but it can also be seen in a foot with a normal appearance. Just as a horse bears most of its weight on the front of its hoof, a patient with an equinus deformity bears most of his or her weight on the toes when walking because the deformity prevents weightbearing on the ball or the heel of the foot. Equinus may involve a tightness of either the gastrosoleal complex or the gastrocnemius muscle complex and can cause various symptoms, including Achilles tendinitis, plantar fasciitis, metatarsalgia, and hammertoe deformities.

Common Associated Deformities

Specific associated deformities can develop due to the pathomechanics of the general deformities.

Posterior Tibial Tendon Dysfunction

Posterior tibial tendon dysfunction is a foot deformity that is defined as the gradual tearing and/or rupturing of the tibialis posterior tendon. The tibialis posterior muscle arises from the posterior aspect of the leg, and its tendon runs posteromedially across the ankle joint and inserts primarily into the navicular joint, with small connections to remaining tarsal bones. In a healthy foot, this muscle serves as a powerful inverter and plantar flexor, and the loss of its function creates significant disability, especially in obese patients. This condition causes collapse of the longitudinal arch, which in turn leads to subluxation of the rear-foot tarsal joints, and eventually the ankle joint.

The dysfunction is divided into four stages. Stage I is a tendinitis of the tibialis posterior tendon without foot deformity. Stage II is tearing or rupturing of the tibialis posterior tendon, which creates a flexible and fully reducible deformity. Stage III involves a deformity that has become rigid and arthritic (Figure 58.1). Stage IV occurs when the pronatory forces weaken the deltoid ligament, resulting in a valgus ankle deformity. This can be crippling in older adults.

Conservative treatment ranges from orthoses built to place the foot in a supinatory position to bracing with either an ankle-foot orthosis or a custom brace that provides increased foot control. Surgical treatment may vary, depending on the stage of deformity. Stage

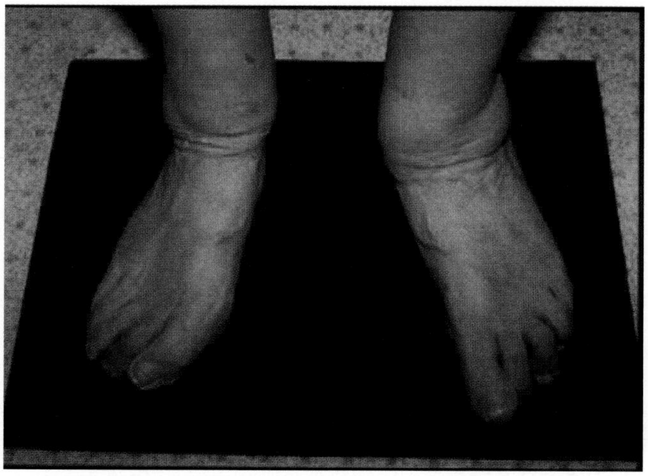

Figure 58.1—Stage 3 tibialis posterior dysfunction

I deformity is treated with synovectomy and repair of the tendon, Stage II requires calcaneal osteotomies and tendon transfers to reconstruct the foot, Stage III involves arthrodesis of the rearfoot, and Stage IV requires a plantar arthrodesis. Stage I and II repairs can improve function and reduce symptoms (SOE=B).

Hallux Valgus

Bunion

One-third of people >65 years old have a hallux valgus deformity, or bunion. The hallux valgus deformity is a subluxation of the first metatarsal phalangeal joint, resulting from the adduction of the first metatarsal and the abduction of the hallux. This deformity progresses throughout a person's lifetime, often leading to hypermobility of the first metatarsal cuneiform joint. The prominence and subluxation can be painful, especially when wearing shoes, because of the pressure applied by the shoes to the bunion deformity.

Chronic hallux valgus deformities are frequently arthritic. These deformities are treated conservatively by adapting the shoe to the deformity, ie, instructing the patient to wear wider shoes with a wider toe box and to use various padding techniques. Surgery may be considered if the deformity is symptomatic and unresponsive to conservative management. The types of procedures undertaken depend on the severity of the deformity and on the patient's health and activity level.

Studies evaluating orthopedic quality-of-life indicators and Short Form-36 after repair of hallux valgus showed that patients experienced a reduction in symptoms and were once again able to wear shoes comfortably. In most instances, this positive outcome was seen regardless of the surgical approach. These findings were consistent over all age ranges (SOE=B).

Hallux Limitus

Hallux limitus is an arthritic condition involving the first metatarsal phalangeal joint. Normal motion of the first metatarsal phalangeal joint generally ranges from 35 to 75 degrees. Hallux limitus occurs when there are clinical findings of arthritis, including crepitus and a decrease in the normal range of motion. Hallux rigidus is present when there is very little motion and the joint is essentially functioning as if it were fused.

The cause of hallux limitus is thought to be sagittal plane instability in the first toe (the first metatarsal has increased dorsi and plantarflexion), resulting in hypermobility. This causes elevation of the first toe and impingement of the joint and, over time, results in an arthritic joint. Traditional treatment consists of orthoses that prevent motion at the first metatarsal phalangeal joint and thereby relieve pain. In a study of >700 patients, more than half were successfully treated with conservative orthotic therapy, indicating that it is a viable approach as an initial treatment (SOE=B).

An alternative approach in patients who still have some motion at the joint is to construct an orthosis with a first ray cut-out. This plantarflexes the first metatarsal and places the joint in a mechanically better position as the patient shifts his or her weight from the heel to the ball of the foot when walking. Surgical treatment of hallux limitus can range from removal of bone spurs (cheilectomy) and joint implants to osteotomies and arthrodesis of the joint. Surgery can successfully reduce symptoms and increase function (SOE=B).

Hammertoe Deformities

Hammertoes are caused by a muscle-tendon imbalance that occurs around the metatarsal phalangeal joint. Hammertoes involve a buckling or contraction at the proximal interphalangeal joint (PIPJ) or the distal interphalangeal joint (DIPJ) of the lesser toes. In a "classic" hammertoe, there is a flexor contracture at the PIPJ. A mallet toe is a hammertoe that contracts at the DIPJ. A claw toe is a hammertoe that contracts at the PIPJ and the DIPJ.

Hammertoes can be flexible and easily reducible, or they can be rigid and nonreducible. Rigid hammertoes are generally more painful and create problems when the patient is wearing shoes. When hammertoes press against the shoe, a callus or corn is created, causing foot pain. Treatment of hammertoes may include padding of the affected area, a wide toe box in shoes or custom shoes, the debridement of calluses, or surgical correction of the deformity (SOE=C).

Chronic Dislocated Metatarsal Phalangeal Joint

The end-stage of a hammertoe deformity is a chronically dislocated joint, a condition that is not uncommon in older adults and is caused by long-term biomechanical pathology in the forefoot. This is also seen sometimes at an earlier age in patients with rheumatoid arthritis. The toe generally dislocates on top of the metatarsal head, which places pressure on the ball of the foot. When this occurs on the second toe, it is usually associated with a hallux valgus deformity and can result in a cross-over deformity (Figure 58.2).

Metatarsal phalangeal joint dislocations are a source of chronic pain and can cause plantar ulcerations, especially in those who suffer from neuropathy. Patients developing metatarsal phalangeal joint dislocations usually require shoes with increased toe box height to reduce dorsal pressure. When shoes can no longer control symptoms and skin breakdown, surgical reconstruction of the joint(s) may be necessary (SOE=A).

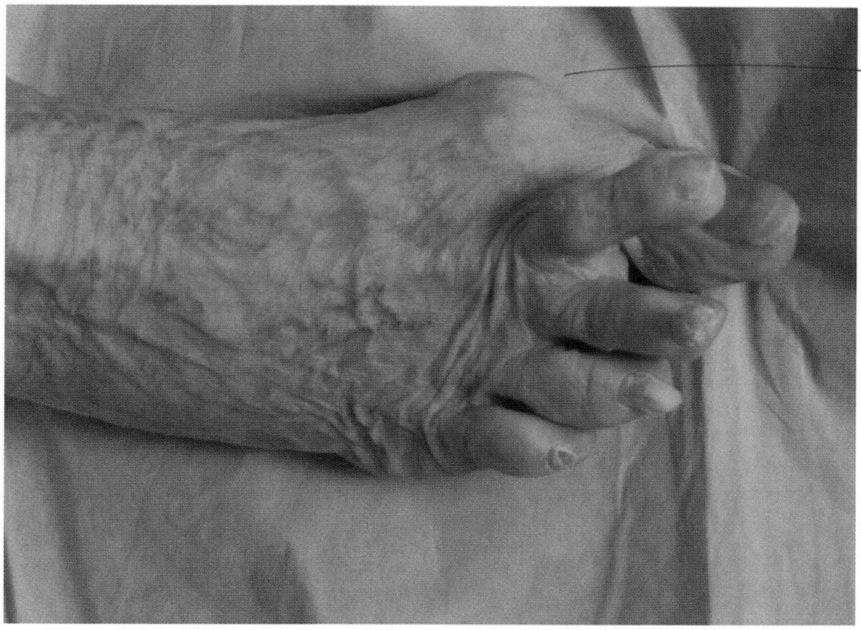

Bunion

Figure 58.2—Hallux abducto valgus with crossover toe deformity

Neuromas

A neuroma is a benign growth of a peripheral nerve, caused by chronic entrapment. Neuromas are often seen in the foot between the third and fourth metatarsal heads, where they are referred to as Morton neuromas. It is theorized that the metatarsal nerve is entrapped by the deep intermetatarsal ligament as it courses underneath the ligament and forms the digital nerve branches.

Conservative treatment of neuromas may involve metatarsal pads, orthoses, corticosteroid injections, cryotherapy, or alcohol injections. Alternatively, the patient may require surgical release of the intermetatarsal ligament or primary excision of the neuroma. A comparative review of surgical intervention consistently demonstrates favorable results, with 80% of patients reporting a high level of satisfaction after surgery (SOE=B).

Plantar Fasciitis and Heel Pain

Heel pain is common in older adults, with studies demonstrating that up to one in seven patients will present with a painful heel. Patients generally have two different symptoms: a painful heel on waking or after rest, or a painful plantar heel while walking.

The first condition, commonly referred to as plantar fasciitis, involves the plantar fascial ligament pulling from the medial tuberosity of the calcaneus as the medial arch collapses. As this process becomes chronic, osseous bleeding causes calcification of the ligament and is seen as a bone spur on radiographic examination. A tight Achilles tendon causes equinus and predisposes patients to this process. Initial treatments include reducing inflammation through the use of oral NSAIDs, steroid injections, and/or physical therapy. Second and more preventive therapies include reducing ligamental strain with inserts, night splints, and stretching exercises.

Heel pain while walking is associated with fat pad atrophy. As the plantar cushion thins, direct bone-to-skin contact occurs due to the lack of the intermediary cushion, causing pain. Direct palpation demonstrates lack of the fat pad, and possible keratotic lesions may be present at pressure points. Symptoms increase during barefoot ambulation and decrease with the use of cushioned shoes or inserts. The only treatment is accommodative shoes and inserts, which act as external shock absorbers.

General Treatment Strategies

Orthoses

Orthoses are external devices that are placed either on the foot or into the shoe to accommodate for a foot deformity or to alter the function of the foot to relieve physical stress on a certain portion of the foot. Orthoses placed on the foot include temporary felt padding or silicone/putty spacers to accommodate for structural deformities (eg, hallux valgus, hammertoes, tailor's bunion).

Orthoses placed in the shoe are either OTC devices or are custom made. OTC devices are generally made of lightweight polyethylene foam, soft plastics, or silicone, and are produced for a certain size of foot. A

Chapters

Table 58.2—Shoe Terms

Term	Definition or Description
Custom-made molded shoes	Made from an impression of the foot either by a plaster cast or foam imprint
Extra depth shoe	Provides additional space in the toe box
Heel counter	Back of the shoe that the heel fits in; shoes with a stiffer and higher heel counter have more stability
Rocker bottom sole	Modification of the sole
Shock-absorbing heel	Hard but absorbent material that provides shock absorption; good for patients with a cavus foot and for obese patients
Thomas heel modification	A distal medial extension of the heel that provides stability of the arch
Toe box	Part of the shoe that contains the toes
Velcro lacing	Hook and loop tape used to secure the shoe closed, rather than conventional laces

custom-made device is constructed from an impression of a person's foot. In the past, impressions were made by plaster casting the foot in a subtalar joint neutral position. Impressions are now being made through computerized assessment or through a foam box. The devices are then made to the impression, taking into account the patient's structural deformities. These devices are generally made from a variety of flexible and rigid plastics.

Shoes

Because of physical changes that occur in the foot as people age, shoes usually do not fit well in older adults and can be a source of foot pain. Studies have indicated that approximately 75% of adults ≥65 years old wear shoes that are too small. It is common for feet to flatten and widen with age, and feet should be measured routinely. Older adults should be advised to purchase a shoe that fits well, and has a sturdy heel counter, a firm beveled sole, and good traction. With recent expansion of the wider shoe size market, shoes that fit well and are structurally sound are available OTC. Athletic and walking sneakers also offer patients accommodative shoes with structural support.

Narrow high heels should be avoided. A wide heel that is <6 cm high can be appropriate for women who have tight heel cords and have been wearing high-heeled shoes all their lives. Older adults wearing heels that are >6 cm high are at a greater risk of falls. Proper shoes and inserts that reduce pressure can decrease pain, protect the foot from injury, and improve function in older adults (SOE=B). See Table 58.2.

Most patients can be fitted with OTC shoes, except when significant structural changes occur or systemic diseases change the foot. Extra-depth shoes can help accommodate foot changes that prevent regular shoe gear usage. In diabetes, intrinsic muscle weakness causes hammering of the digits and bunion formation. Extra-depth shoes have one-and-a-half times the toe box height and soft leather material, which prevents irritation to the dorsal contracted digits. When severe structural changes occur, as seen in patients with end-stage rheumatoid arthritis, a custom molded shoe may be required. These shoes are manufactured from plaster molds of the patient's feet to allow for the severe changes and to prevent skin breakdown.

Surgical Considerations of Foot Deformities

Foot surgery in older adults has increased substantially in the past 30 years, mainly because of the growth of this population segment. Studies have shown that poor surgical outcomes usually reflect the overall health of an individual rather than his or her chronological age. When relief of pain and restoration of function are the goals, surgery may be a better alternative for foot problems that are not alleviated by conservative methods. Most podiatric surgical procedures for older adults can be performed under local anesthesia with monitored sedation, thereby minimizing surgical risk.

SKIN AND NAIL DISORDERS

Skin Neoplasms

Skin neoplasms or lesions on the foot are common in older adults but are rarely malignant. Suspicious lesions require biopsy. Common benign lesions include the following:

- Keratotic lesions: These calluses or corns are often seen over sites of pressure. Common types are heloma durum (hard corn), heloma molle (soft corn), and tyloma (widespread callus).
- Plantar verruca: This is the most common skin disorder of the foot, although these lesions dramatically reduce in incidence with age. This viral infection of the plantar aspect is caused by a strain of the human papilloma virus. Lesions are circular, punctated, flat, and commonly contain thrombosed vessels. It is important to differentiate these lesions from keratotic lesions. Clinically, verrucae demonstrate interrupted skin lines, pinpoint bleeding with debridement, and increased lateral compression pain when compared with keratosis. A cluster of the lesions is referred to

as a mosaic wart. Treatments include application of topical salicylic acid, bleomycin injections, cryotherapy, CO_2 laser treatment, and surgical excision, which must be used with caution in older adults who have reduced circulation and impaired healing. Treatment of verrucoid lesions in older adults may require mixing approaches and treating associated complications, eg, treating hyperkeratosis with keratolytic agents such as urea (SOE=B).

- Epidermal inclusion cysts: These cysts are created by a portion of the epidermis proliferating in the dermis.
- Dermatofibromas: These flat-topped, raised, and firm lesions are generally not treated unless located across a joint or irritated by shoewear. Recurrence rate after excision is high.
- Hemangioma: These common vascular tumors manifest as flat-topped, red lesions that contain abundant capillaries and are typically seen on the plantar aspect of the foot.

Malignant lesions are uncommon in the foot but can easily go undiagnosed and generally have a poor outcome. Pigmented lesions of the foot should be fully evaluated, with biopsies of any suspicious lesions performed. Characteristics of a potentially malignant lesion include a new lesion in a patient ≥60 years old, or a lesion that changes in shape, color, or diameter. Lesions not responding to conservative therapy and slow or nonhealing ulcerations of the foot should be biopsied to exclude a potential underlying neoplasm. Morbidity associated with these lesions increases at age 60 and beyond. Malignant lesions identified in the foot include basal cell carcinoma, Bowen disease, squamous cell carcinoma, and malignant acral lentiginous melanoma.

Xerosis

Excessive dryness, or xerosis, is associated with a lack of hydration and lubrication. The number of sebaceous and sweat glands decrease in older adults and plantar skin lacks sebaceous glands, so it is common for fissures to develop on the heel, resulting in dryness and increased stress in that area.

The goal in managing xerosis is to prevent infection and other complications. Urea cream or solution (10%, 20%, or 40%) or ammonium lactate (12%) may be helpful as a mild and safe keratolytic. A heel sleeve or pad made with mineral oil or a heel cup can help minimize trauma to the heel, thereby reducing the potential for complications. Urea and/or lactic acid–based emollients have been shown to be effective but must be used daily and applied after bathing (SOE=C).

Eczema

Eczema is inflamed skin that is not infected. The most common types in older adults are xerotic eczema, venous stasis eczema, and drug-induced eczema. Treatment is generally a combination of emollients and steroid creams, with or without occlusive dressings.

Nail Disorders

Ingrown Nails and Paronychia

Nail disorders are the most common disorders of the foot.

Onychocryptosis, the incurvation of the edge of the nail plate into the nail groove, is generally seen in the distal portion of the nail groove. This condition can result from long-term improper nail cutting, narrow shoes, and/or genetically incurvated nail matrixes. A chronically ingrown nail is best treated either with a partial nail avulsion or a permanent matricectomy.

Paronychia, a localized infection caused by the nail embedding into the nail groove, requires incision and drainage of the abscess with removal of the nail spicule. All infected granulation tissue is resected. Depending on the presence of cellulitis or comorbidities, antibiotic treatment may be needed. Toes with chronic paronychiae should be radiographed to exclude underlying osteomyelitis, especially in patients with diabetes or peripheral arterial disease.

Onychomycosis

Approximately one-third of the older population has onychomycosis, a fungal infection of the nail plate. An increased incidence is seen in older adults with obesity, immunodeficiency, diabetes, peripheral arterial disease, chronic tinea pedis, and/or psoriasis. By the age of 65, approximately 20% of men and 10% of women are

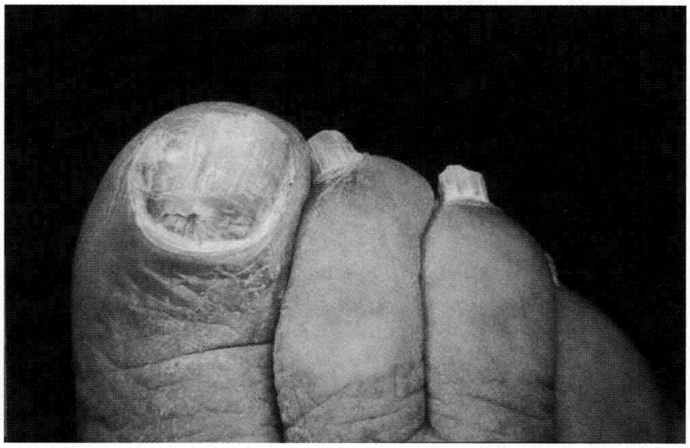

Figure 58.3—Onychomycosis. Nails infected by fungi are often yellow, thickened, and friable, with yellow-brown debris under the nail plate.

Chapters

affected; these values are doubled if the patient has diabetes. Dermatophytes account for 80% of infections, with the remainder caused by saprophytes or yeast.

Onychomycosis results in thickening of the nail plate and can cause pain (Figure 58.3). In patients with neuropathy, onychomycosis can be a source of nail bed ulcerations. Treatment includes topical and oral antifungal medications, as well as permanent excision of the nail plate. A decision to treat is usually made because of one of the following: the cosmetic concern of a yellow friable nail, other comorbidities (particularly diabetes mellitus, in which the break in the epidermal barrier due to the fungal infection can serve as a route for bacterial infections), and occasionally pain.

No topical antifungal agent is effective against onychomycosis (SOE=A). Ciclopirox, a topical nail lacquer applied daily for 1 year, is available to treat onychomycosis. However, in clinical studies, <12% of patients using ciclopirox achieved clear or almost clear toenails. Although newer laser treatments are available, poor therapeutic results are reported in medical literature. Moreover, this procedure is costly and is usually an out-of-pocket expense. Oral antifungals such as terbinafine, fluconazole, and itraconazole are effective for onychomycosis, but their duration of treatment, adverse-event profile, and high rate of relapse after discontinuation warrant careful consideration for use in older adults. These agents are primarily metabolized by the liver and can interact with many medications that are commonly administered to older adults.

Treatment can take 3–4 months, and the rate of relapse is high. Comorbidities such as diabetes, secondary fungal infections, and quality of life should be considered before starting treatment.

SYSTEMIC DISEASES AFFECTING THE FOOT AND ANKLE

Diabetes Mellitus

Diabetes is the number one disease affecting foot health in older adults. Complications of diabetes can cause loss of limbs and significant disability. It has been estimated that 50%–75% of all amputations in patients with diabetes could be prevented by foot health education, periodic clinician assessment, and early intervention. The ocular complications of diabetes can adversely impact the ability of patients to see ingrown toenails, corns, and ulcers. Other complications of diabetes that contribute to poor foot health include neuropathy, vascular insufficiency, dermopathy, atrophy of the muscles and soft tissues, and deformity. Neuropathy, especially sensory impairment, is a precursor to ulcers. Paresthesias, decreased vibratory sense, and loss of sensation are among the most important neuropathic changes that contribute to ulcer formation in older diabetic patients.

Arterial insufficiency causes pallor, a loss or decrease in the posterior tibial and dorsalis pedis pulse, dependent rubor, and decreased capillary filling time in the toes. Severe vascular disease can result in rest pain that typically occurs at night. A loss of the plantar metatarsal fat pad is associated with vascular insufficiency and predisposes to ulcerations at the site of bony prominences or deformities of the foot.

Foot ulcers are a common result of the multiple pathologies found in patients with diabetes. Prevention and early recognition are the most important strategies in managing foot ulcers. Clinicians should ensure that older diabetic patients have their feet examined at least annually. Diabetic patients are often instructed to remove their shoes at all visits so that the clinician can visually inspect the feet and the areas between the toes to ensure there has been no skin breakdown. Patients and caregivers should be instructed in the importance of daily foot inspections. Preventive strategies include optimizing glycemic control, and monitoring and treating peripheral neuropathy, arterial disease, limited joint mobility, bony deformities, hyperkeratosis, and onychodystrophy (SOE=C).

Prevention of foot ulcers in diabetic patients is both cost-effective and limb saving in this high-risk population (SOE=A). Assessing vibratory sensation using the Semmes-Weinstein monofilament and monitoring reflex changes help the clinician determine a patient's risk of development of ulcers. If a diabetic patient's risk is high, the clinician can then take appropriate steps to prevent ulcers, including reducing excessive pressure, shock, and shear by accommodating, stabilizing, and supporting deformities through weight diffusion and dispersion (SOE=C). Early intervention with proper shoes and foot care reduces complications in high-risk feet, as demonstrated by the Lower Extremity Amputation Prevention (LEAP) program and Medicare Loss of Protective Sensation (LOPS) program.

When an ulcer develops despite preventive efforts, the history should focus on duration, inciting event or trauma, prior ulcerations, previous attempts at wound care, and use of pressure off-loading procedures. The examination should include an assessment of the location and depth of the ulcer, the presence of infection, ischemic or neuropathic changes, edema, and the presence of a Charcot joint. Imaging should be performed to exclude osteomyelitis (SOE=B) and may include plain radiography, CT, technetium bone scans, indium scans, and MRIs. Noninvasive vascular studies include Doppler and transcutaneous oxygen tension. Consultation with a vascular specialist may be needed when vascular insufficiency is severe or the wounds are nonhealing.

The general principles of high-risk foot management include debridement, pressure relief, off-loading, avoidance or limitation of weight bearing, proper dressings, treatment of infection with antibiotics, management of ischemia, medical management of comorbidities, and hospitalization and surgical management when necessary. Weight bearing can be modified by the use of crutches and wheelchairs as well as contact casts, walkers, boots, braces, total contact orthotics, modified surgical shoes and boots, and appropriate dressings. Wounds should be reduced by 50% within a 4-week period. If a wound is reducing as planned, then regular follow-up care and prevention are required. Nonreducing wounds require reassessment of the patient's medical condition, and well as his or her vascular, infectious, and nutritional statuses. Adjunctive therapies should be used if there is no response to treatment or correction of medical status.

A wide variety of dressings and topical agents is available; selection is guided by the nature of the ulcer and its complications. Topical agents include saline, antiseptics, topical antibiotics, enzymes, growth factors, and dermal skin substitutes. Vacuum-assisted closure and hyperbaric oxygen chambers can also aid in the closure of difficult-to-heal wounds in diabetic patients (SOE=B). Empiric antibiotic therapy should be started early when infection is suspected. Hospitalization is usually indicated in cases involving osteomyelitis or limb-threatening infection. The choice of antibiotic is based on the clinical symptoms, culture and sensitivity, and the presence of deep infection, bone exposure, or sepsis, as well as whether soft tissue or bone is infected (SOE=B).

Peripheral Arterial Disease

Older adults with peripheral arterial disease demonstrate many of the same signs and symptoms as those with diabetes mellitus. In contrast to neuropathic ulcers, vascular ulcers are extremely painful.

Arthritis

Osteoarthritis is common in older adults. It causes pain, swelling, stiffness, limitation of movement, and deformity in weight-bearing joints. It may be worsened by chronic trauma, strain, or obesity. Gouty arthritis is monoarticular and is most common in the first metatarsal phalangeal joint. In its early stages, it results in intense pain and erythema, followed later by joint damage.

Rheumatoid arthritis affects the hands and feet equally and is usually symmetric in its presentation. It can result in muscle wasting and marked deformity. The metatarsal phalangeal joints become dislocated or subluxed; there is increased protrusion of the metatarsal heads, and walking becomes painful. If conservative treatment with orthotics and special shoes do not relieve the pain, surgery may help to allow less painful ambulation.

References

- Benirschke SK, Meinberg E, Anderson SA, et al. Fractures and dislocations of the midfoot: Lisfranc and Chopart injuries. *J Bone Joint Surg Am*. 2012;94(14):1325–1337.
- Nishide K, Nagase T, Oba M, et al. Ultrasonographic and thermographic screening for latent inflammation in diabetic foot callus. *Diabetes Res Clin Pract*. 2009;85(3):304–309.
- Roddy E, Muller S, Thomas E. Onset and persistence of disabling foot pain in community-dwelling older adults over a 3-year period: a prospective cohort study. *J Gerontol A Biol Sci Med Sci*. 2011;66(4):474–480.
- Vernon W, Borthwick A, Walker J. The management of foot problems in the older person through podiatry services. *Rev Clin Gerontology*. 2011;21(4):331–339.
- Yates B, ed. Merriman's Assessment of the Lower Limb. 3rd ed. Philadelphia, PA: Churchill Livingstone; 2012.

CHAPTER 59—NEUROLOGIC DISEASES AND DISORDERS

KEY POINTS

- Cerebrovascular disease is a leading cause of disability and death among older adults.
- Primary and secondary stroke prevention can significantly decrease the burden of cerebrovascular disease in elderly populations.
- Parkinson disease is diagnosed clinically and can be effectively managed medically.
- Late-life seizures are frequently a symptom of structural damage to the brain or a metabolic imbalance (eg, stroke, tumor, or hyponatremia).

Neurologic diseases and disorders are very common in older adults and become increasingly more common with advancing age. The most prevalent neurologic disorders include Alzheimer disease (AD) and related dementias, gait disorders, cerebrovascular disease, Parkinson disease (PD), and epilepsy. For example, in the United States almost half (40%–50%) of the population >85 years old suffer from dementia, and a similar percentage of hospitalized patients of this age have a gait disorder caused by a neurologic condition. Other U.S. population data include the following: 7.5% of adults 60–79 years old and 15% of those ≥80 years old have had a stroke, 1% of adults >60 years old and 3% of those >80 years old have been diagnosed with PD, and 3% of adults by age 75 and close to 10% of the nursing-home population have been diagnosed with epilepsy.

Neurologic disorders in older adults can be challenging to diagnose, especially considering that multiple neurologic disorders or sequelae in an individual patient are the rule, not the exception. Pharmacologic treatment of neurologic disorders must account for the unique metabolism of older adults and the potential for drug-drug interactions. Furthermore, because neurologic disorders add substantially to the burden of functional dependency, acknowledging the psychosocial aspects of these conditions is also vital in constructing plans to improve functional abilities and quality of life.

CEREBROVASCULAR DISEASES

Stroke is a leading cause of disability and death among older adults. The incidence of stroke increases with advancing age, approximately doubling with each decade. The incidence of stroke for women is 25%–30% lower than that for men in comparable age groups, but it surpasses that of men ≥85 years old. Approximately

Table 59.1—Components of the National Institutes of Health Stroke Scale[a]

Stroke Scale Item	Item Score[b]
Level of consciousness	0–7
Best gaze	0–2
Visual fields	0–3
Facial palsy	0–3
Motor: arms	0–8
Motor: legs	0–8
Limb ataxia	0–2
Sensory	0–2
Best language	0–3
Dysarthria	0–2
Extinction and inattention	0–2
Total	**0–42**

[a] Full details of criteria for scoring each item can be obtained at www.ninds.nih.gov/doctors/NIH_Stroke_Scale.pdf (accessed Oct 2013).

[b] Greater score reflects increased impairment.

80% of strokes are ischemic and 20% hemorrhagic. Besides being the most common acute, serious neurologic disease, stroke is also a leading cause of death. Intracerebral hemorrhage carries a higher rate of morbidity and mortality than ischemic stroke. The fatality rate within 1 month of an acute stroke is 20%–30% across all age groups; mortality is highest among older adults. Survival in part depends on the anatomic location and severity of the stroke. In ischemic stroke, the most important predictor is the severity of neurologic signs, which can be quantified after stroke by use of an instrument such as the NIH Stroke Scale (Table 59.1). This severity scale is widely used to describe the degree of impairment after stroke. In general, a score of <5 in this scale, which ranges from 0 to 42, is associated with a very good prognosis. Individuals with a score >20 have a very poor prognosis and a high likelihood of major complications. Neurologic causes of death include the brain injury itself or resultant brain edema. Common medical causes of death in the setting of stroke are myocardial infarction, arrhythmia, heart failure, aspiration pneumonia, and pulmonary embolism. Age in itself does not influence the gross neurologic aspects of stroke, but older age is associated with lesser recovery in ADLs. Older stroke patients can benefit from formal rehabilitation. See "Rehabilitation," p 139.

Stroke Prevention and Transient Ischemic Attack (TIA)

Throughout the latter half of the 20th century, the incidence of stroke declined in the United States, Canada, and Western Europe. This drop may be attributable to better control of modifiable risk factors, including hypertension, heart disease, diabetes mellitus, cigarette smoking, increased blood lipids, and alcohol use. Hypertension is the most prevalent risk factor for stroke, and its treatment results in a substantially reduced risk of stroke. Treatment of isolated systolic hypertension in older adults reduces the risk of stroke by nearly 40% (SOE=A). See "Hypertension," p 402. Another important risk factor is heart disease, including atherosclerotic coronary heart disease, left ventricular hypertrophy, valvular heart disease and valve replacement, and atrial fibrillation. See "Cardiovascular Diseases and Disorders," p 378. Several studies have confirmed a 2- to 4-fold increased risk of stroke in individuals with diabetes mellitus (SOE=A). Studies suggest that tight control of blood-glucose levels might reduce the risk of stroke in individuals with diabetes mellitus, although the evidence for reduction of other vascular complications (eg, retinopathy, nephropathy) is somewhat more compelling. See "Diabetes Mellitus," p 520. Additionally, aggressive treatment of hypertension and hyperlipidemia in the diabetic population is a crucial component in lowering the risk of stroke. Cigarette smoking independently increases the risk of stroke as much as 3-fold (SOE=A). The incidence of stroke declines significantly even after 2 years of smoking cessation, and after 5 years the level of risk returns to that of nonsmokers.

Special consideration should be given to those suffering a TIA, which is defined as a brief episode of neurologic dysfunction caused by focal ischemia to the brain or spinal cord that does not result in acute infarction. The traditional definition suggested that these deficits could last up to 24 hours, but with newer imaging it is clear that a TIA typically lasts <1–2 hours, and longer episodes are commonly associated with acute infarction. A TIA is a medical emergency. This cohort of individuals represents those at highest risk of going on to develop acute stroke. Among patients with TIA (10%–15%), half have a stroke within the first 48 hours and the other half sometime within the next 3 months. These data emphasize the importance of careful monitoring of those suffering a TIA. Brain imaging, ideally with MRI, is important to determine whether there has been an acute stroke and, if so, the location and type of stroke. Noninvasive imaging of the carotid arteries (Doppler ultrasonography or magnetic resonance angiography), continuous cardiac rhythm monitoring, and an echocardiogram are important tests to complete to better determine the most likely cause of the TIA. Modifiable stroke risk factors should be sought out by testing fasting glucose and lipid levels, monitoring blood pressure, and asking about tobacco use. Treatment for patients with TIA is essentially the same as for patients with acute ischemic stroke, with management plans targeting the conditions found during the evaluation. See treatment of acute ischemic stroke, below.

Small-Vessel Disease

Lacunar disease secondary to occlusion of small penetrating vessels is presumably the consequence of lipohyalinosis (lipid deposition and hyalinization) or local arteriolosclerosis. Small vessels supply deep white and gray matter structures such as the internal capsule, basal ganglia, and thalamus and pons; occlusion of these small vessels can result in several well-defined clinical syndromes, including pure motor hemiplegia, pure hemisensory stroke, ataxic hemiparesis, and dysarthria–clumsy hand syndrome. Lacunar ischemic strokes are typically <1 cm in size. Risk factors include hypertension and diabetes mellitus. The most effective means of managing lacunar disease is aggressive treatment of these risk factors (SOE=B). Although antiplatelet agents (eg, aspirin) are prescribed for stroke prevention in patients who have suffered lacunar strokes, they have not been shown to prevent lacunar strokes specifically. Lacunar strokes can occur independently or concurrently with large-vessel cerebrovascular disease.

Large-Vessel Disease

A lesion at the origin of the internal carotid artery, most commonly secondary to atherosclerosis, can lead to transient monocular blindness (ie, amaurosis fugax) or a cerebral hemispheric deficit (eg, hemiparesis, hemisensory loss, aphasia, apraxia, homonomous hemianopia), because both the retina and cerebral hemispheres derive their blood supply from the internal carotid artery. Large-vessel disease can be identified by noninvasive imaging of the carotid arteries (B-mode ultrasonography and Doppler ultrasonography or magnetic resonance angiography) or conventional angiography. For patients with ≥70% symptomatic stenosis, carotid endarterectomy significantly reduces subsequent stroke risk (number needed to treat [NNT] =15 over 2–6 years of follow-up), provided that the patient has few comorbidities and that endarterectomy is performed at an institution and by a surgeon with extensive experience with the procedure (SOE=A). The optimal treatment for symptomatic carotid stenosis of <70% or of asymptomatic carotid stenosis remains unclear; treatment options include carotid endarterectomy, endovascular treatment, or medical management. Medical management should target modifiable risk factors and should include daily use of an antiplatelet agent.

Large-vessel disease can affect the vertebral and basilar arteries. Syndromes associated with vascular lesions in the posterior circulation (ie, vertebral and basilar arteries) can result in dysfunction of the cranial nerves, descending motor or ascending sensory tracts within the brain stem, cerebellar and vestibular pathways, and visual cortex. Signs and symptoms can include crossed cranial nerve and long-tract findings (eg, complete facial palsy ipsilateral to the lesion and hemiparesis involving the contralateral arm and leg), vertigo, double vision, ataxia, dysarthria, hemianopia or cortical blindness, Horner syndrome (ipsilateral miosis, anhidrosis, and mild ptosis), stupor, or coma. Treatment of posterior circulation large-vessel disease is typically medical, but as new technology emerges, endovascular therapies may be a potential option in the future (SOE=D).

Aspirin is the mainstay of antiplatelet therapy for secondary atherosclerotic stroke prevention (SOE=A; relative risk reduction 15%–20%; NNT approximately 60 for prevention of one stroke over 1 year of therapy). Studies on the use of aspirin in stroke prevention suggest that dosages >325 mg/d do not add therapeutic benefit, but the minimal necessary dosage has not been definitively determined. Many clinicians routinely prescribe 81–325 mg/d, although even the lower dosage can cause GI irritation and blood loss. Other antiplatelet medications are available but have not shown consistent superiority to aspirin. These agents include sustained-release dipyridamole combined with aspirin and clopidogrel. Clopidogrel 75 mg/d is an alternative for patients who cannot tolerate aspirin. Combining clopidogrel and aspirin does not provide additional benefit in the secondary prevention of stroke (SOE=B). In two large trials, no benefit was found for the use of warfarin over aspirin for secondary stroke prevention (SOE=A) in the setting of large-vessel disease.

Cardioembolic Stroke

Atrial fibrillation is associated with a 4- to5-fold increased risk of ischemic stroke due to thrombus formation in the left atrial appendage and cardioembolism to cerebral vessels. Cardioembolic stroke due to atrial fibrillation accounts for 10% of all ischemic strokes. Persistent and paroxysmal atrial fibrillation are associated with similar risks of ischemic stroke. A meta-analysis of stroke prevention trials in the setting of non-valvular atrial fibrillation has shown an average relative risk reduction of 64% for warfarin and 19% for aspirin when compared with placebo. (See atrial fibrillation and its management in "Cardiovascular Diseases and Disorders," p 378.)

Treatment of Acute Ischemic Stroke

The current protocol for care of the older stroke patient includes optimizing hydration status; controlling blood pressure while avoiding hypotension; preventing deep-vein thrombosis; detecting and treating coronary ischemia, heart failure, and cardiac arrhythmias; and starting long-term treatment with antiplatelet agents or oral anticoagulation (depending on the presumed cause) to prevent recurrent stroke. Body temperature and blood glucose should be normalized in the acute setting. Dehydration on presentation is common, but rehydration should be gradual to reduce the risk of cerebral edema. Immediately after an ischemic cerebral infarction, treatment of hypertension should be delayed (unless blood pressure is very high, eg, >220/120 mmHg) until the situation stabilizes. Even when treatment has been delayed temporarily, the eventual goal is to reduce blood pressure gradually (eg, a goal of 15% reduction over the first 24 hours) while avoiding orthostatic hypotension. The target systolic blood pressure should be 10–20 mmHg higher than the baseline pressure; if the baseline is unknown, systolic pressure should not be lowered below 160 mmHg. Patients with acute ischemic stroke who are treated with thrombolytic agents require careful blood-pressure monitoring, especially during the first 24 hours of treatment. Patients with a history of ischemic heart disease or arrhythmia, and patients with embolic strokes should be monitored with telemetry for at least 48 hours. For large, cardioembolic strokes (eg, involving most of the middle cerebral artery territory or involving both middle and anterior cerebral artery territories), anticoagulation therapy is usually not initiated until at least 48 hours after onset because of a high risk of hemorrhagic transformation. Earlier anticoagulation does not improve outcome in these patients.

The only medication approved by the FDA for the treatment of acute, ischemic stroke is recombinant tissue-plasminogen activator (rt-PA [alteplase]). Infusion of this medication within 3 hours of stroke onset approximately doubles the chances of a favorable outcome at 3 months (SOE=A; very limited data in older adults). However, the benefits of rt-PA must be weighed against the increased risk of intracranial hemorrhage, which can be fatal or result in worsened neurologic status. Overall, the literature suggests that 32% have a better outcome, as measured by >1-point improvement in the modified Rankin scale (ie, a clinically meaningful improvement), when compared with placebo. Intracerebral hemorrhage occurs in 6% of patients and is fatal in approximately half of these individuals. Most hemorrhagic events occur among patients with severe strokes (NIHSS score >25). Use of rt-PA requires careful assessment by a clinician experienced in the treatment of stroke. rt-PA should be considered in all patients who present within 3 hours of onset of neurologic deficit and in whom CT confirms the absence of intracranial hemorrhage. Major contraindications include major surgery within the previous 2 weeks, previous intracranial hemorrhage, sustained systolic blood pressure >185 mmHg or diastolic >110 mmHg despite treatment, symptoms of subarachnoid hemorrhage, recent urinary or GI tract bleeding, coagulopathy, thrombocytopenia, or INR >1.7. The NIH Stroke Scale is helpful for stratifying ischemic stroke patients according to risk and benefit for rt-PA. Patients with scores <5 generally have a favorable outcome regardless of treatment; patients with scores >25 have a substantially increased rate of hemorrhagic complications. Although older adults experience higher rates of bleeding complications than those <65 years old (SOE=A), the increased risk does not automatically preclude treatment. Recently, the window for use of rt-PA in acute stroke was increased to include selected patients able to receive treatment 3–4.5 hours after the onset of symptoms. This American Heart Association recommendation was based on results from the European Cooperative Acute Stroke Study 3 (ECASS 3), which identified continued benefit in this time window. Exclusionary criteria included age >80 years, NIHSS >25, and history of both stroke and diabetes.

Intracerebral Hemorrhage

Intracerebral hemorrhage accounts for 15%–20% of all strokes. Approximately 80% occur between the ages of 40 and 70 years. Studies of racial distribution suggest that black Americans and Asian Americans may be at slightly higher risk than white Americans.

The most common risk factor for intracerebral hemorrhage is hypertension, which is present in 75%–80% of cases. Excessive use of alcohol is also associated with a higher incidence. Common locations for hypertensive bleeds are the putamen, thalamus, cerebellar hemisphere, pons, and cerebrum. In older adults, a common cause of cerebral lobar hemorrhage is cerebral amyloid angiopathy, which usually occurs without systemic amyloidosis. In these cases, intracranial bleeds tend to be recurrent. Hemorrhage can be complicated by the use of antiplatelet agents and anticoagulants. Other secondary causes of intracerebral hemorrhage should not be overlooked; these include trauma, arteriovenous malformations, and aneurysms. Acute treatment is supportive, with interim control of severe hypertension and discontinuation of anticoagulant medications. Large lobar or intraventricular hemorrhages can be considered for neurosurgical drainage.

The decision to restart anticoagulation or antiplatelet medications after intracerebral hemorrhage can be difficult. It depends on many factors, including but not limited to, the reason the medications were started, the cause of the hemorrhage, the risk of future ischemic events, and the neurologic state of the patient. In those at high risk of future ischemic cerebrovascular events, such as those with mechanical heart valves or atrial fibrillation and prior stroke, restarting anticoagulation 7–10 days after hemorrhage appears to be safe (SOE=B).

Subdural Hematoma

A subdural hematoma is a collection of blood between the dura and the arachnoid. It is usually due to head trauma, although the trauma may be mild, particularly in older adults. In approximately 15% of cases, the hematomas are bilateral. Some older adults suffer from chronic subdural hematoma that may be symptomatic. The incidence of chronic subdural hematoma increases with age, from 0.13 per 100,000 person-years for those in their 20s to 7.4 per 100,000 person-years for those in their 70s. In 50% of chronic subdural hematomas, there is no history of head injury, although other risk factors include clotting disorders, shunting procedures (eg, ventriculoperitoneal shunting for normal-pressure hydrocephalus separating the blood vessels from the dura, resulting in tears), and seizures. The symptoms of chronic subdural hematoma are headache, slight to moderate cognitive impairment, and focal neurologic signs (eg, hemiparesis, hemisensory loss). Some individuals may have seizures. Neuroimaging studies reveal an extra-axial collection of blood or fluid (eg, subdural hygroma). Treatment varies depending on whether the hematoma is symptomatic or an incidental finding on a neuroimaging study. If symptomatic and the patient's condition is worsening, then removal of the clot may be attempted.

HEADACHES

The prevalence of headaches appears to diminish with age. One study demonstrated that although 74% of men and 92% of women 21–34 years old have headaches, these proportions drop to 22% and 55% after the age of 75 years. Headache is one of the most common medical complaints in young persons, and yet one study suggests that it is the tenth most common symptom in older women and the fourteenth most common symptom in older men. The incidence of migraine, the most common cause of headaches in younger adults, also declines with age, with only 2% of people developing their first migraine after age 50.

New onset or persistent headaches are more likely to represent systemic or intracranial lesions (ie, nonbenign conditions) in older than in younger adults. In one study, 10% of headaches among younger patients represented systemic or intracranial lesions; in older adults, this proportion was 34%. These nonbenign conditions include intracranial masses (eg, primary or secondary tumors, subdural hematomas), cervical spondylosis, COPD, carbon monoxide poisoning, and giant cell arteritis. In addition, many commonly used medications can cause headaches that are dull, diffuse, and nondescript, including vasodilators (eg, nitrates), antihypertensives, antidepressant medications, and stimulants.

An important secondary cause of headache specific to older adults is giant cell (temporal) arteritis. This disease does not appear to develop in those <50 years old and peaks in incidence between the ages of 70 and 80. Women are affected twice as often as men. Pain may be centered at the temporal or occipital arteries. Palpation of the scalp arteries may reveal focal tenderness and nodularity. Complaints of visual changes, low-grade fever, polymyalgia, and constitutional symptoms further suggest the diagnosis. For diagnosis and treatment, see giant cell arteritis and temporal arteritis in "Musculoskeletal Diseases and Disorders," p 453.

The common primary headache disorders can be classified into migraines (with or without aura) and tension-type headaches. Migraines are headaches of moderate to severe intensity associated with nausea, vomiting, or photophobia. Half of the time they are unilateral and throbbing, but commonly the pain is bilateral. Auras, when they occur, usually precede the headache and are manifested by transient neurologic symptoms that can be localized to the cerebral cortex or brain stem. Visual phenomena are among the most common types of auras. Migraine headaches in older adults typically present as they do in younger people, but atypical presentations have been described. These include migraine auras without headache (acephalic migraine). The occurrence of an isolated visual or sensory aura in the absence of a headache can be diagnostically challenging, because it can mimic signs of a transient ischemic attack. In contrast to migraines, tension-type headaches are often more diffuse, less severe in intensity, have a pressing or a tight quality, and are much less often associated with nausea or vomiting.

The treatment of migraine headaches can be categorized as either abortive (treating an attack that has already begun) or preventive. Apart from various OTC preparations that include NSAIDs, migraine-specific abortive therapies include ergotamines or triptans (eg, sumatriptan), which act by central serotonergic mechanisms. These medications are mild vasoconstrictors and contraindicated in patients with uncontrolled hypertension, stroke, or coronary artery disease. Generally, safety data in geriatric populations are lacking. Preventive therapies for migraine include nonselective β-blockers (eg, propranolol[OL]), valproic acid, topiramate, tricyclic antidepressants[OL], and calcium channel blockers (eg, verapamil[OL]). The choice of agent should be guided by an effort to avoid adverse events and drug interactions. Treatment of muscle tension headaches includes NSAIDs[OL] as abortive agents and low doses of tricyclic antidepressants[OL] as preventive medication in chronic muscle tension headaches. Each of the medications above may be contraindicated by comorbidities or existing medication regimens.

Movement Disorders

A movement disorder can be defined simply as abnormal involuntary movements. These movements result not from weakness or sensory deficits but from dysfunction of the basal ganglia or the extrapyramidal motor system. Movement disorders can be classified as hypokinetic (paucity of movement) or hyperkinetic (excessive movement). The hypokinetic movement disorders include Parkinson disease (PD) and the related Parkinson plus disorders (eg, multiple systems atrophy, progressive supranuclear palsy). Hyperkinetic movement disorders include conditions that produce chorea (eg, Huntington disease), dyskinesias (eg, tardive dyskinesias), dystonia, and tremor (eg, essential tremor). Movement disorders are especially common among older adults.

Parkinson Disease (PD)

PD is a progressive neurodegenerative disease first causing cell death in brain-stem nuclei, especially the substantia nigra, resulting in reduced basal ganglia dopamine levels. These changes cause a constellation of clinical signs, including tremor at rest, bradykinesia, rigidity, and postural instability. The pathologic hallmark of the disease is the Lewy body, an intracellular inclusion body found in the substantia nigra. As the disease progresses, neurodegeneration and Lewy body pathology extends into the cortex (limbic and neocortex), with associated cortical Lewy bodies causing neuropsychiatric and cognitive symptoms (ie, PD with dementia).

The incidence and prevalence of PD increase with age. Prevalence rates in the United States rise from 1% of the population at age 60 to 3% of the population at age 80. Aging, environmental factors, and genetics are thought to be involved in the pathogenesis of PD. Risk factors associated with an increased risk of PD include exposure to pesticides, welding as a profession, exposure to manganese, age, and family history. Smoking and caffeine consumption have been associated with a decreased risk. In a small proportion of cases (5%–10%), the disease clusters within families and has a genetic basis. Approximately 10 genes have been associated with PD, either as causative mutations or susceptibility genes in these families. The disease most commonly appears between the ages of 50 and 79 years. Dementia in PD occurs in 30%–40% of PD patients and is more common with longer duration of disease, more severe motor symptoms, an akinetic-rigid presentation, and older age of onset of motor symptoms.

The disease begins insidiously and asymmetrically. The clinical manifestations include tremor, usually in one hand or sometimes in both, classically involving the fingers in a pill-rolling motion. The tremor (slow frequency, usually 3–5 Hz) is present at rest and typically resolves or decreases with active, purposeful movement. Muscular rigidity is usually readily evident on passive movement of a limb. Passive movement may demonstrate a smooth resistance or superimposed ratchet-like jerks (ie, cogwheel phenomenon). The term *bradykinesia* is often used to describe either a slowness in initiating movement (ie, a paucity of spontaneous movements) or movements themselves that are slow, and the term *freezing* is used to describe sudden interruption of movement. Other clinical features of PD may include micrographia (small handwriting), festinating gait (inadvertently taking progressively smaller steps and falling forward), hypophonic speech (low volume to voice), masked facies (decreased facial expression and diminished eye blinking), and drooling due to decreased swallowing ability. An erect posture is not readily assumed or maintained, and impaired postural reflexes can be elicited with a pull test (pulling the patient backward and asking them to catch their balance). Impaired postural balance is a feature present later in the course of idiopathic PD, and the presence of early postural imbalance and frequent falls often signals a Parkinson plus syndrome. Mood abnormalities, usually depression or anxiety, are common, as are cognitive impairment and dementia, involving speed of thinking, memory retrieval, attention, and visual-spatial abilities. It is common for patients with PD to report constipation, seborrhea, myalgia, urinary incontinence, and impotence.

Patients with parkinsonism can present for a multitude of reasons, but the most common are tremor and changes in gait. Distinguishing between the parkinsonian resting tremor and other types of tremor such as essential tremor can be at the crux of making the diagnosis. Another early diagnostic challenge may be distinguishing mild early parkinsonism from the changes that can accompany aging (eg, general slowing, loss of balance, stiffness, difficulty walking, stooped posture). However, the bradykinesia and rigidity of PD are usually asymmetric at onset, typically presenting in one upper extremity. In addition, tremor at rest is not a feature of normal aging, and although older adults may complain of stiffness, true extrapyramidal rigidity is otherwise uncommon. The diagnosis of PD is made clinically by demonstrating the classic features described above and excluding other possible causes. A positive response to dopaminergic medications such as levodopa supports a diagnosis of idiopathic PD. Neuroimaging should be considered in atypical presentations such as the abrupt onset of tremor, focal weakness, sensory disturbances, or reflex abnormalities. Falls early in the course of the disease may alert the clinician to one of the Parkinson plus syndromes (see progressive supranuclear palsy, below), as opposed to idiopathic PD.

Once the diagnosis is made, treatment programs are multifactorial and must be individualized. Nonpharmacologic therapy includes a regular exercise program. Many older adults benefit from a course of physical therapy aimed at restoring their confidence in walking and maintaining balance, as well as instruction in how to manage unpredictable and disabling freezing episodes. Physical therapists can also help, when needed, with selection of appropriate canes or walkers. A home visit by an occupational therapist can help to plan the appropriate placement of wall rails, grab bars, and other such assistive devices that reduce the possibility of falling. If patients are functionally disabled by their tremors, bradykinesia, or rigidity, then pharmacologic treatment should be initiated.

The most effective pharmacologic treatment of patients with PD is levodopa combined with carbidopa (SOE=A). Levodopa is converted to dopamine in both the CNS and the periphery via dopa decarboxylase. Peripheral conversion is reduced by combining levodopa with carbidopa (a dopa decarboxylase inhibitor), which does not cross the blood-brain barrier. This formulation decreases adverse events associated with peripheral conversion. Treatment usually begins with a half tablet of the 25/100 combination (ie, 25 mg carbidopa to 100 mg levodopa) q8–12h. Every 1–2 weeks, the dose can be increased by one-half tablet, to reach a dosage of one full tablet three times a day (commonly 30 minutes before meals). The duration of action of this formulation is typically 4 hours. If disabling bradykinesia, rigidity, postural instability, or tremor is still present, the dosage can be gradually increased further, with cautious observation for adverse events. Older adults, particularly if cognitively impaired, rarely tolerate levodopa doses of >1,000 mg/d. The controlled-release form (25/100 and 50/200) generally requires a slightly higher total daily dose. Common adverse events of levodopa-carbidopa include nausea, abdominal cramping, orthostatic hypotension, and visual hallucinations.

After 5 years of treatment for PD, up to 50% of patients develop motor fluctuations (fluctuations in motor symptoms and medication effects) or dyskinesias (involuntary choreiform movements). These complications are more common in younger PD patients (ie, <75 years old). Patients are described as "on" (symptoms well controlled), "on with dyskinesias" (symptoms controlled but complicated by dyskinesias), or "off" (parkinsonism not well controlled). End-of-dose "off" symptoms are most common and can be treated by increasing the dosing frequency of levodopa to every 3–4 hours or by adding an enzyme inhibitor such as rasagiline or entacapone (both described below) to increase the duration of action of levodopa. Peak dose dyskinesias are common and are treated by increasing the interval between levodopa doses and lowering the total daily dose of dopaminergic medications. The incidence and severity of dyskinesias can be reduced by introducing a dopamine agonist (described below) early in the treatment of PD, either as monotherapy or in combination with levodopa when daily dosages exceed 400 mg/d. This is an important consideration in younger patients (<75 years old) expected to have a long duration of disease and treatment.

Enzyme inhibitors include the catechol-O-methyl-transferase (COMT) inhibitor entacapone. COMT inhibitors block breakdown of levodopa, thereby increasing bioavailability at the synapse. Entacapone increases the duration of action of levodopa, resulting in greater "on" time for a given dose of levodopa, but it can also exacerbate dyskinesias (SOE=A). Adverse events of COMT inhibitors are similar to those of levodopa. A second class of enzyme inhibitors are the monoamine oxidase B (MAO-B) inhibitors, which also block one of the enzymes responsible for dopamine breakdown. Rasagiline is a newer selective MAO-B inhibitor that has been approved by the FDA as early monotherapy or as adjunct therapy (SOE=A). Selegiline is an older MAO-B inhibitor that delayed the need for additional antiparkinsonian agents in controlled trials (SOE=B). A neuroprotective role of MAO-B inhibitors in PD has been investigated but has not been established. Although chemically related to nonselective monoamine oxidase inhibitors, the selective MAO-B inhibitors, rasagiline and selegiline, do not require dietary restrictions. MAO-B inhibitors are generally well tolerated, although some patients can experience adverse events, including nausea, insomnia, confusion, anxiety, and feeling "revved up." Other medications used to treat motor symptoms of PD include amantadine and anticholinergic medications such as trihexyphenidyl. Amantadine has multiple pharmacologic properties but can provide mild improvement in PD motor symptoms and can decrease dyskinesias (SOE=B). Older adults, especially with impaired renal clearance, can develop confusion and hallucinations with amantadine. Anticholinergic medications improve PD tremor, but adverse events such as dry mouth, urinary retention, and confusion outweigh benefits in most older adults.

For younger PD patients with milder disease and no signs of dementia, dopamine agonists may be used initially as monotherapy or added when the levodopa dosage exceeds 400 mg/d (SOE=A). A cautious induction period and slow titration are required with dopamine agonists, because nausea, orthostatic hypotension, and hallucinations are common adverse events. When compared with levodopa, dopamine agonists are less effective in controlling motor symptoms and are associated with more adverse events. Currently used dopamine agonists include ropinirole (given in starting dosages of 0.25 mg/d and increased as needed to dosages of 6–8 mg/d) and pramipexole (given in starting dosages of 0.125 mg/d and increased as needed to dosages of 4.5 mg/d). A three-times-a-day dosage schedule is used for the immediate-release form of both medications, and a controlled-release, once-a-day formulation is now available for both. Rotigotine transdermal patch is also available; the starting dosage is 2 mg/24 hours, increasing to a maximum of 8 mg/24 hours. All dopamine agonists, and to a lesser extent levodopa, have been associated with sudden sleep attacks in which patients may fall asleep abruptly while driving. Additionally, all these medications have been associated with compulsive behaviors such as pathologic gambling. Patients should be warned of these rare but potentially serious adverse events, and clinicians should ask about these behaviors during routine follow-up visits.

A major factor influencing the treatment of PD is the propensity of older adults to develop confusion and psychosis on antiparkinsonian medications. In general, the therapeutic regimen should be kept simple. Rather than small dosages of multiple medications, higher dosages of one or two medications is less likely to result in toxic adverse events. Levodopa provides the most improvement in the motor manifestations of PD relative to its toxic effects on the CNS, whereas medications with anticholinergic properties (eg, trihexyphenidyl, amantadine) provide the least benefit. The dopamine agonists (ropinirole, pramipexole) fall in between. Although psychosis can be treated effectively with clozapine or quetiapine, which have fewer extrapyramidal adverse events than other antipsychotic agents, confusion and disorientation can be treated more simply by lowering the dosages of antiparkinsonian medications. In this setting, anticholinergic medications should be the first to be discontinued, followed by enzyme inhibitors, dopamine agonists, and finally levodopa.

Other nonmotor symptoms are common in patients with PD, including sleep disorders (eg, restless legs syndrome, rapid-eye movement sleep behavior disorder), autonomic dysfunction (orthostatic hypotension, incontinence, constipation), and cognitive impairment. Many of these symptoms can be managed with medications, including the cholinesterase inhibitor rivastigmine, which has been FDA approved for the treatment of the dementia associated with PD (SOE=A). In 2010, the American

Table 59.2—Early Features that Distinguish Parkinsonian Syndromes

Condition	Asymmetric onset	Rest tremor	Levodopa response	Falls in first year	Early dementia	Postural hypotension	Cerebellar/ UMN signs
Parkinson disease	+	+	+	-	-	-	-
Medication-induced parkinsonism	-	+/-	+/-	-	-	-	-
Vascular parkinsonism	+/-	-	-	+/-	+/-	-	+/-
Dementia with Lewy bodies	+/-	+/-	+/-	+/-	+	+/-	-
Progressive supranuclear palsy	-	-	-	+	+/-	-	+
Multiple system atrophy	+/-	-	+/-	+/-	-	+	+

Note: + = usually or always present, +/- = sometimes present, - = absent
UMN = upper motor neuron

SOURCE: Adapted with permission from Reuben DB, Herr K, Pacala JT, et al. *Geriatrics At Your Fingertips*, 15th ed. New York: American Geriatrics Society; 2013:199 and from Christine CW, Aminoff MJ. Clinical differentiation of parkinsonian syndromes: prognosis and therapeutic relevance. *Am J Med.* 2004;117:412–419.

Academy of Neurology developed and published quality measures for the care of patients with PD to guide and improve patient care. Many of these quality measures focus on the recognition and management of nonmotor symptoms of PD.

Surgical options can be considered for PD patients who have symptoms that cannot be controlled by medical therapies. Deep brain stimulation (DBS) of the globus pallidus or subthalamic nucleus is most effective for patients who have motor fluctuations and dyskinesias despite medical therapy, and who have few comorbidities and no dementia. DBS significantly increases "on" time and decreases troubling dyskinesias (SOE=B).

Parkinsonian Syndromes

The parkinsonian syndromes (also termed Parkinson plus syndromes) are a group of disorders with some motor features of PD (ie, resting tremor, bradykinesia, rigidity, postural imbalance) but that also have additional distinct and distinguishing features. As a group, these disorders are much less responsive to pharmacologic treatment with dopaminergic medications than idiopathic PD. The parkinsonian syndromes described in this chapter include multiple system atrophy (MSA), and progressive supranuclear palsy (PSP). Dementia with Lewy bodies is another Parkinson plus syndrome described elsewhere (see atypical dementias in "Dementia," p 256). Other parkinsonian syndromes include vascular parkinsonism, in which small-vessel ischemic strokes in the basal ganglia produce parkinsonism, and medication-induced parkinsonism, in which dopamine-receptor blocking medications (eg antipsychotic or antiemetic drugs) produce parkinsonism. For a comparison of characteristic features of PD and these parkinsonian syndromes, see Table 59.2.

A histopathologic understanding of three parkinsonian syndromes, olivopontocerebellar atrophy, Shy-Drager syndrome, and striatonigral degeneration, has permitted these overlapping syndromes to be included within the rubric of one disease named multiple system atrophy (MSA). MSA produces degeneration in three areas, specifically the basal ganglia, cerebellum, and autonomic nervous system. MSA is characterized by parkinsonism, autonomic failure (eg, severe orthostatic hypotension, constipation, incontinence, impotence, impaired sweating or temperature control), and cerebellar dysfunction (eg, ataxia, dysmetria). Other features that can accompany MSA are upper motor neuron signs, severe dysarthria, stridor, dystonia, and restless legs syndrome. The diagnosis is clinical, and MSA can initially be indistinguishable from idiopathic PD, but the degree of autonomic dysfunction, disappointing response to levodopa, and cerebellar signs all support a diagnosis of MSA. The mean age of onset for MSA is 55 years; it is slightly more common in men, and it progresses to death in approximately 7 years on average. MSA accounts for approximately 3% of cases of parkinsonism.

Orthostatic hypotension is often the most disabling symptom of MSA. Nonpharmacologic treatment of the autonomic dysfunction includes eating small meals, getting up slowly, and avoiding excessive straining during bowel movements. Compressive clothing and elastic stockings, increased salt and fluid intake, and sleeping in a reverse Trendelenburg position can ameliorate some of the orthostatic symptoms. Medications that are sometimes useful in treating the orthostatic hypotension include midodrine and fludrocortisone[OL]. Use of these medications occasionally results in supine hypertension, which requires close blood-pressure monitoring. Levodopa can initially help symptoms of rigidity and bradykinesia, but dopamine replacement may worsen the orthostatic hypotension.

Progressive supranuclear palsy (PSP) accounts for approximately 4% of cases of parkinsonism. PSP is marked by an akinetic-rigid form of parkinsonism (ie, bradykinesia and rigidity) with early loss of postural balance causing frequent falls (typically falling backward). As the disease progresses, supranuclear gaze palsy becomes apparent, and patients eventually develop spasticity, dystonia, dysarthria, dysphagia, and a subcortical-frontal dementia. Onset is usually during the late 50s or early 60s. The pathogenesis is unknown. The disease usually progresses rapidly, with marked incapacity occurring within 3–5 years and death within 6–8 years, generally as a result of aspiration, infection, or complications of immobility. Progressive supranuclear palsy derives its name from progressive impairments of voluntary, vertical gaze. Most patients develop eye movement restrictions approximately 3–4 years into the disease course. Patients are unable to voluntarily look downward or upward (upward gaze is less severely involved). Limitation of voluntary gaze is termed supranuclear, because the vestibular nuclei are still able to direct eye movements reflexively: when the examiner abruptly tips the head, the eyes can be driven to look downward or upward.

As the disease progresses, its appearance differentiates it from that of idiopathic PD. Resting tremor is typically absent or very subtle, and the rigidity is more pronounced in the neck and trunk (axial rigidity). Patients with PSP often have a fixed facial expression due to facial dystonia that causes them to keep their eyebrows elevated in a "surprised look." The dysarthria of PSP is distinct from that of PD, with mixed spastic (strangled) and hypophonic features. Gait is disturbed early in the course, and falls are frequent in most patients. Cognition is often affected, with personality changes and impaired judgment and executive cognitive function. For example, patients may laugh or cry at inappropriate times. Unlike in MSA, other than urinary incontinence, autonomic dysfunction is atypical. No effective pharmacologic treatment is available. Treatment with levodopa may partially reduce the rigidity, although the dramatic response to levodopa that is experienced by patients with PD is lacking.

Hyperkinetic Movement Disorders

Chorea is a flowing, continuous, random movement that migrates from one part of the body to another. A variety of conditions are associated with chorea in older adults. The pathologic basis for chorea is dysfunction of the striatum. Huntington disease is the most common cause of chorea in adults. Typically a patient's family history will suggest an autosomal dominant mode of inheritance, and other family members may have a genetically confirmed diagnosis. However, sometimes family history is lacking, or the patient may have a late onset of the disease with mild features. The diagnosis of Huntington disease can be made by confirming an increased number of CAG repeats in the huntingtin gene. Drug-induced chorea (from levodopa, anticonvulsants, antipsychotics, estrogen) is common and first treated by reducing or removing the offending agent. Chorea can arise from ischemic injury to the basal ganglia (ie, vascular chorea). Idiopathic choreiform movements can occur as an isolated symptom in adults ≥60 years old and are termed senile chorea, if other causes of chorea have been excluded.

Chorea can be treated with dopamine-receptor blocking medications (eg, haloperidol[OL]), but a potential adverse effect is the development of tardive dyskinesia. Tetrabenazine blocks the storage and transport of dopamine presynaptically; it is currently FDA approved for the treatment of chorea in Huntington disease (SOE=A) and can be used to treat other causes of chorea. It is not associated with an increased risk of tardive dyskinesia. Patients taking tetrabenazine need to be monitored closely for signs of depression and parkinsonism.

Dystonia is a hyperkinetic movement disorder that results in sustained muscle contractions causing twisting movements or abnormal postures. Dystonia can occur as an isolated disorder, on a genetic basis, or as part of another movement disorder (eg, PD, corticobasal degeneration). Common focal dystonias seen in older adults include cervical dystonia (spasmodic torticollis), blepharospasm, spasmodic dysphonia, or focal hand dystonia (writer's cramp). Medications such as anticholinergics (eg, trihexyphenidyl) or muscle relaxants (eg, baclofen) can be tried, but improvement in symptoms is typically limited. Botulinum toxin injections of contracted muscle can provide effective, but temporary, relief of dystonia.

Drug-Induced Movement Disorders

Several different types of involuntary movements can arise as a result of the use of medications. It is important to distinguish among effects of medications that are acute, chronic but reversible, and chronic and irreversible. One acute effect that can occur with antipsychotic medications is an acute dystonic reaction resulting in oral, lingual, or nuchal dystonia. If the dystonia is severe enough, treatment with intravenous diphenhydramine or lorazepam may be required, although this approach in older adults should be exercised with caution, given the propensity of these agents to produce somnolence or confusion. Fortunately, acute dystonia occurs less frequently in older than in younger adults. Chronic reversible drug effects (effects that resolve when the causative medication is discontinued) include action tremor (eg, lithium, theophylline, valproic acid), parkinsonism (eg, antipsychotic, antiemetic medications), chorea (eg, anticonvulsant medications, estrogen, levodopa), or dystonia (dopamine replacement therapy in PD). Chronic irreversible drug effects or tardive phenomena often begin after the medication (usually an antipsychotic medication) has been used for weeks to months. Movements can include orobuccal dyskinesias, dystonia, akathisia (sensation of needing to move), myoclonus, and tics. Advanced age and duration of treatment with antipsychotic medications are the only well-established risk factors for developing tardive movement disorders. Once the diagnosis of a tardive phenomenon is established, the dosage of medication should be reduced or the medication should be discontinued. Treatment for tardive dyskinesia or tardive dystonia includes anticholinergic agents (eg, trihexyphenidyl[OL]), baclofen[OL], and tetrabenazine[OL], each of which must be used with caution in older adults. In cases of severe tardive dystonia in which there is neck jerking or sustained eye closure, intramuscular injections of botulinum toxin[OL] can reduce the frequency and severity of movements.

Essential Tremor

Essential tremor (ET) is the most common form of abnormal tremor. The tremor of ET is an action tremor, which is present when the limbs are in active use (eg, while writing or holding a cup). The tremor most commonly involves the arms, although the head and voice can be affected also. Other areas of the body that can be affected include the chin, tongue, and legs. The tremor is often slightly worse in one arm than in the other. One of the striking features of the tremor is that it has varying amplitude so that during some moments, the tremor is mild or even absent and during others it is severe. The tremor disappears when the arms are relaxed, ie, when the person is sitting with hands in the lap or when standing or walking with arms held at the sides. Functionally, the tremor can interfere with many daily activities, such as eating, writing, or fastening buttons. Stress or anxiety can exacerbate the tremor. The frequency of the tremor is in the 4–12 Hz range, which is faster than the resting tremor in PD.

The prevalence of the disorder increases with advancing age, with as many as 5% of adults >60 years old affected. The age of onset seems to have a bimodal distribution, with peaks in the teens and 20s and in the 50s through the 70s. Prevalence rates among men and women are similar, although head tremor may be more common in women. Affected individuals commonly report that they have an affected relative, suggesting a familial or genetic cause in some patients. Familial forms of the tremor have been linked to regions on chromosomes 2p and 3q. Familial and sporadic forms of essential tremor have no apparent clinical differences. The cause of the sporadic form of the illness is not known. Alcohol may decrease the severity of ET.

The main indication for treatment of ET is functional disability due to the tremor (eg, difficulty writing, drinking from a cup or spoon, trouble holding objects). It is important to educate the patient on exacerbating factors such as caffeine, stress, and fatigue. The first-line options for pharmacologic treatment of ET are nonselective β-blockers (propranolol[OL], nadolol[OL]) or primidone[OL] (SOE=B). Each provides an approximately 30%–50% improvement in the severity of tremor in most patients. Other medications have been described as effective in some patients, including baclofen[OL], gabapentin[OL], mirtazapine[OL], and topiramate[OL], but results have not been consistent (SOE=C or D). Some patients with severe, medically refractory tremor may undergo DBS. DBS stimulation in the ventral intermediate nucleus of the thalamus provides significant improvement in tremor control in most patients (SOE=B). Potential adverse events are similar to those of DBS in PD that has been described previously.

EPILEPSY

A seizure is a paroxysmal, excessive, and synchronous discharge of cortical neurons that results in a transient change in motor function, sensation, or mental state. Recurrent seizures are the defining feature of epilepsy. Depending on whether the seizure discharges involve only a portion of the cortex or the entire cortex, seizures are broadly classified as partial or generalized. Partial seizures are subdivided on the basis of whether or not the seizure is associated with impaired consciousness. Simple partial seizures do not impair consciousness, and most often are associated with focal rhythmic motor twitching. Complex partial seizures are associated with altered consciousness and commonly amnesia for the event. Automatisms and other motor manifestations can occur with complex partial seizures. Generalized seizures in older adults are almost invariably convulsive (ie, generalized tonic-clonic seizures or "grand mal" seizures).

New-onset seizures are seen in a bimodal pattern with respect to age, with an initial peak in incidence within the first year of life and a second peak after the age of 60 years. Disease-specific causes of seizures are more common in older adults, and one-half or more of older adult patients with new-onset seizures have an underlying discernible cause. Common causes include cerebrovascular disease, space-occupying lesions, brain trauma, alcohol withdrawal, and neurodegenerative diseases. The incidence of partial seizures (which frequently have an underlying cause) increases in older adults, whereas the incidence of generalized tonic-clonic seizures (which are more often idiopathic) remains constant with respect to age.

Because of this propensity for new-onset cases of seizures to be harbingers of focal lesions, it is important that older adults undergo diagnostic evaluation to exclude an underlying treatable cause. The neurologic history and examination should aim to clinically characterize the seizure and localize its source, as well as to elicit other signs of a focal lesion or a metabolic disturbance (eg, uremia, hepatic failure). Blood studies (comprehensive metabolic panel, magnesium, calcium), brain imaging (MRI is preferable to CT), and electroencephalography play important roles. Brain imaging should be performed with and without contrast.

Once the appropriate evaluation is done, the decision to begin an anticonvulsant should not be taken lightly. On average, 30% of patients with a single unprovoked seizure have another seizure, but 70% do not. The presence of a focal brain abnormality on brain imaging or epileptic changes on an electroencephalogram (EEG) raises the likelihood of recurrence and should prompt consideration of pharmacologic therapy. If a patient has a second unprovoked seizure, then the probability of further seizures increases to 70%, and pharmacologic therapy should be initiated if possible.

The treatment of epilepsy in older adults is particularly challenging. The prevalence of adverse drug-disease and drug-drug interactions increases with age. One example of a drug-disease interaction is that between anticonvulsants such as divalproex sodium or carbamazepine and hepatic disease, given the tendency of these agents to exacerbate preexisting liver dysfunction, particularly in older adults. Caution should also be taken with the newer anticonvulsants levetiracetam and gabapentin in patients with renal failure, because they are cleared renally.

In terms of drug-drug interactions, many of the anticonvulsant medications are metabolized via the cytochrome P450 system, especially the older agents (eg, phenytoin and carbamazepine). Before starting any new medication in patients taking anticonvulsant agents, the possibility of an interaction should be investigated. Further, age-related changes in renal and hepatic function can alter drug metabolism significantly, so that older adults often need lower dosages of anticonvulsant medications. A sizable fraction of many anticonvulsant medications is bound to plasma proteins. Because aging decreases albumin synthesis, free (unbound) levels of anticonvulsant medications (eg, phenytoin) may need to be monitored. Older adults can be particularly sensitive to adverse events of medications. For example, anticonvulsant medications can intensify an underlying dementia, exacerbate mild cognitive decline, or worsen a gait disorder. A clinical pharmacist can help resolve complex issues of drug interactions, dosages, and adverse events. Finally, older adults may have difficulty with adherence for a variety of reasons. It is particularly important when treating older adults to involve caregivers so that the goals of the treatment, adverse events, and monitoring of response are understood.

Most anticonvulsant medications are started slowly and the dosages increased gradually (Table 59.3). There is recent evidence that several newer anticonvulsants (ie, lamotrigine, levetiracetam, gabapentin) may be better tolerated and have fewer drug-drug interactions, yet provide good seizure control in older adults (SOE=C or D). Medication dosing should be determined more by seizure control and adverse events than by serum concentrations. If monotherapy has not adequately controlled the seizures and the dosage has been maximized, then monotherapy with another agent should be tried before resorting to combination therapy. The common causes of breakthrough seizures in individuals known to be epileptic are infections, metabolic disturbances, sleep deprivation, and medication noncompliance.

Rarely, partial seizures can present in patients as nonconvulsive status epilepticus (NCSE). This is defined as continuous electrical seizure activity without outward convulsion. After a seizure, it is important to distinguish between NCSE and a postictal state. If a patient is not improving gradually or is demonstrating focal neurologic signs such as eye deviation or nystagmus, evaluation with an EEG to exclude NCSE is warranted. An EEG is also warranted in the routine evaluation of a delirious patient with no apparent cause or who does not improve after the proposed underlying cause has been treated.

Surgery for epilepsy has become an increasingly common choice of patients whose seizures have proved refractory to pharmacologic management. The utility of surgery in older adults is not known.

Discontinuing anticonvulsant medications should be considered if the patient has not had a seizure for several years, particularly if the original seizure activity was a single or poorly characterized event and if a recent EEG does not show epileptic activity.

MOTOR NEURON DISEASE

Amyotrophic lateral sclerosis (ALS) is a neurodegenerative condition involving the cell bodies of both upper and lower motor neurons. It is characterized clinically by a progressive weakness and wasting of skeletal muscles, often in combination with dysarthria, dysphagia, and respiratory failure. The incidence increases with age but reaches a plateau in the 60s. To date, age remains the single most clearly identifiable risk factor for this progressive and fatal disorder.

Table 59.3—Anticonvulsant Therapy in Older Adults

Medication	Dosage (mg)	Target Blood Level (mcg/mL)	Comments (Metabolism, Excretion)
Carbamazepine[a]	200–600 q12h	4–12	Many drug interactions, also a mood stabilizer, may cause SIADH, thrombocytopenia, leukopenia (L, K)
Gabapentin	300–600 q8h	NA	Used as adjunct to other agents, adjust dosage on basis of CrCl (K)
Lamotrigine[a]	100–300 q12h	NE	Prolongs PR interval; risk of severe, potentially fatal rash that depends on speed of titration (risk virtually disappears with slow titration); when used with valproic acid, begin at 25 mg q48h, titrate to 25–100 mg q12h (L, K)
Levetiracetam	500–1,500 q12h	NE	Reduce dosage in renal impairment: CrCl 30–50 mL/min: 250–750 q12h CrCl 10–29 mL/min: 250–500 q12h CrCl <10 mL/min: 500–1,000 q24h
Oxcarbazepine	300–1,200 q12h	NE	Can cause hyponatremia, leukopenia (L)
Phenobarbital	30–60 q8–12h	20–40	Many drug interactions; not recommended for use in older adults (L)
Phenytoin	200–300 q24h	10–20[b]	Many drug interactions; exhibits nonlinear pharmacokinetics (L)
Pregabalin	50–200 q8–12h	NA	Indicated as adjunct therapy for partial-onset seizures only; not well studied in older adults (K)
Tiagabine	2–12 q8–12h	NA	Adverse-event profile in older adults less well described (L)
Topiramate	25–100 q12–24h	NE	Can affect cognitive functioning at high dosages (L, K)
Valproic acid	250–750 q8–12h	50–100	Can cause weight gain, tremor, hair loss; several drug interactions; mood stabilizer; monitor liver function tests and platelet counts (L)
Zonisamide	100–400 q24h	NA	Anorexia; contraindicated in patients with sulfonamide allergy (K)

NOTE: SIADH = syndrome of inappropriate secretion of antidiuretic hormone; L = metabolized via liver; K = metabolized via kidneys; NA = not available; CrCl = creatinine clearance; NE = therapeutic range has not been established

[a] 2009 FDA warning regarding increase in suicidal thoughts and behaviors among all populations treated with anticonvulsant agents, including those used as mood stabilizers

[b] Phenytoin is extensively bound to plasma albumin. In cases of hypoalbuminemia or marked renal insufficiency, calculate adjusted phenytoin concentration (C):

$$C_{adjusted} = \frac{C_{observed}\ (\text{mcg/mL})}{0.2 \times \text{albumin (g/dL)} + 0.1}$$

If creatinine clearance <10 mL/min, use:

$$C_{adjusted} = \frac{C_{observed}\ (\text{mcg/mL})}{0.1 \times \text{albumin (g/dL)} + 0.1}$$

Obtaining a free phenytoin level is an alternative method of monitoring phenytoin in cases of hypoalbuminemia or marked renal insufficiency.

SOURCE: Adapted with permission from Reuben DB, Herr K, Pacala JT, et al. *Geriatrics At Your Fingertips*, 15th ed. New York: American Geriatrics Society; 2012:202–203.

Patients commonly present with gait disturbance, falls, foot drop, weakness in grip, dysphagia, or dysarthria. On neurologic examination, patients may have a combination of upper motor neuron signs (eg, hyperreflexia, clonus, extensor plantar responses) and lower motor neuron signs (eg, weakness, atrophy, fasciculations). Weakness of the face, tongue, and palate are common (bulbar weakness), but the extraocular muscles are usually spared. The electromyogram demonstrates findings consistent with diffuse denervation and poor recruitment of motor units. The differential diagnosis includes lesions at the level of the foramen magnum, a combination of cervical myelopathy associated with cervical and lumbar polyradiculopathies, or a motor predominant peripheral polyneuropathy in a patient with CNS lesions. The prognosis is poor with survival time averaging 2–3 years. The presence of bulbar signs carries a poorer prognosis.

Although most new cases of ALS are in older adults, it is less common than several other neurologic disorders in this population. Therefore, gait disturbance and focal motor weakness may frequently be incorrectly attributed to the more common conditions. Older adults are also more likely to have coexisting neurologic disorders that might explain symptoms of weakness, adding to the challenge of and delay in diagnosing ALS. In one study, those >65 years old were diagnosed after 19 months, while those <65 years old were diagnosed after 3 months.

Treatment is predominantly supportive. Riluzole, which has demonstrated modest effects on survival or time to tracheostomy (SOE=A), is in widespread use. Riluzole is thought to protect against glutamate toxicity, which may be involved in the pathogenesis of ALS. Follow-up in a dedicated multidisciplinary ALS or muscular dystrophy clinic has also been shown to improve quality of life of ALS patients. In these settings, patients can receive multidisciplinary care from a team, including a neuromuscular subspecialist; physical, occupational, and speech therapists; and a social worker.

Myelopathy

In older adults, myelopathy or spinal cord dysfunction can be the result of compression of the spinal cord or intrinsic spinal cord lesions. The cervical region is affected most commonly. Intrinsic spinal cord lesions can be caused by spinal cord tumors, vascular events (eg, infarcts or hemorrhages), or trauma (eg, central cord syndrome). Extrinsic compressive lesions are more prevalent; common causes among older adults are cervical spondylosis (with resultant osteophyte formation and degenerative disc disease), disc prolapse or herniation, rheumatoid arthritis resulting in vertebral body subluxation, meningioma, or spinal metastases. Nearly 80% of adults ≥70 years old have radiographic evidence of osteophyte formation with some narrowing of the spinal canal, but most are asymptomatic. Cervical spinal stenosis most often arises from spondylosis but may be worsened by disc protrusion or a congenitally narrow canal. Narrowing of the cervical canal can lead to neck stiffness and pain; radicular pain, sensory loss, or weakness in the arms; and weakness and upper motor neuron signs (eg, hyperreflexia, spasticity, Babinski sign) in the legs. Narrowing of the lumbar canal can lead to lower back pain; radicular pain, sensory loss, or weakness in the legs; and typically lower motor neuron signs in the legs. Lumbar spinal stenosis causes neurogenic claudication, which manifests as increasing pain and weakness and numbness with walking, with relief by flexion at the waist or sitting. See also "Back and Neck Pain," p 465.

MRI can be helpful for diagnosis, but results must be viewed with caution because abnormal MRI findings are common in asymptomatic older adults. If the patient cannot tolerate MRI because of the presence of implanted metallic objects, a pacemaker, or severe claustrophobia, then spinal CT with intrathecal contrast can be performed.

Conservative management, particularly if neck pain is present, includes activity modification, neck immobilization with a cervical collar, massage, heat treatment, physical therapy, and medications (eg, muscle relaxants and pain medications, including NSAIDs). Decompressive surgery is recommended for persistent pain or a progressive neurologic deficit. Older adults are more prone to have multiple levels of involvement, and some studies have suggested the prognosis after surgery of older adults is poorer than that of younger patients. See also "Back and Neck Pain," p 465.

Radiculopathy

Radiculopathy results from compression of a spinal root as it exits the spinal canal. Among older adults, this can be the result of herniated discs or osteophyte formation. Symptomatic nerve root compression may result in complaints of pain radiating down the neck, back, arm, or leg, and on neurologic examination, this can be accompanied by motor and sensory deficits as well as by diminution of reflexes in the distribution of a particular spinal root or roots. See also "Back and Neck Pain," p 465.

Peripheral Neuropathy

The prevalence of peripheral neuropathy in older adults has been estimated to be as high as 20%, and some degree of subclinical decrease in peripheral nerve function on electromyography is probably universal in healthy older adults. Peripheral neuropathy can be particularly devastating in older adults because of gait impairment due to sensory and motor deficits with a resulting propensity to fall. In developed countries, diabetic neuropathy is the most common form of neuropathy; up to 60% of individuals who have diabetes mellitus and who are ≥60 years old have a peripheral neuropathy. Several types of neuropathy are associated with diabetes mellitus, including a distal symmetric neuropathy; asymmetric neuropathies that may involve cranial nerves, roots, or plexi; and mononeuropathy multiplex. Other common causes of peripheral neuropathy in older adults are medications (eg, amiodarone, colchicine, phenytoin, lithium, vincristine, isoniazid), alcohol abuse, nutritional deficiencies (eg, deficiencies of vitamins B_6 and B_{12}, thiamine, folate, and niacin), renal disease (ie, uremia), monoclonal gammopathy (eg, multiple myeloma or monoclonal gammopathy of undetermined significance), and neoplasia (eg, infiltration of peripheral nerves by malignant cells or paraneoplastic syndromes).

The history and physical examination are the most important tools in diagnosis of a peripheral neuropathy. Questions should be geared toward identifying possible causes and risk factors of the individual patient. If the patient is not known to be diabetic, risk factors for diabetes and possible insulin resistance should be assessed. The past history and review of systems can give clues to a systemic disease that could contribute to a peripheral nerve disorder. A history of gastric bypass, eating disorder, or hemodialysis could indicate a possible nutritional deficiency. A thorough medication history should be taken to look for possible causes. A social history can provide evidence of a possible toxic exposure, such as alcohol or an occupational exposure.

Electrodiagnostic studies are considered an extension of the neurologic examination. They can yield valuable information in classifying the neuropathy to help narrow a complicated differential diagnosis. First, they can differentiate between a single or multiple mononeuropathy or a polyneuropathy. Next, they can help classify a polyneuropathy as axonal, demyelinating, or mixed. This is important because certain neuropathies affect nerves in characteristic ways. For instance, a diabetic neuropathy is predominantly an axonal neuropathy, as are many of the toxic neuropathies such as alcohol and heavy metal exposure. In contrast, the hereditary and immune-mediated neuropathies more commonly cause peripheral demyelination.

Treatment of the neuropathy depends on the underlying cause and ranges from withdrawal of the causative agent (eg, alcohol, medications) to nutritional supplementation (eg, in nutritional deficiency), to treatment of a primary cancer (in the case of paraneoplastic neuropathy). There is evidence that optimizing glucose control can lessen the severity of diabetic neuropathy.

Treatment of neuropathic pain includes the use of tricyclic antidepressants[OL] or anticonvulsant medications such as gabapentin, and pregabalin. Gabapentin and pregabalin are approved for use in treatment of post-herpetic neuralgia, and pregabalin is also approved for use in diabetic neuropathy and fibromyalgia (SOE=A). Topical agents include capsaicin cream and local anesthetic medications (eg, lidocaine patch). Another option approved for use in diabetic neuropathy is the serotonin-norepinephrine reuptake inhibitor antidepressant duloxetine. See "Persistent Pain," p 119.

MYOPATHY

Myopathies are characterized by proximal muscle weakness, wasting, and diminished or absent reflexes. They can be accompanied by increases in serum concentrations of muscle enzymes (eg, creatine kinase) and a myopathic pattern on electromyogram and on muscle biopsy. Older adults may attribute mild to moderate muscle weakness to aging and therefore may not immediately consult a clinician. Proximal muscle weakness, which results in difficulty rising from a chair, climbing stairs, or washing one's hair, is particularly likely to be falsely attributed to aging or arthritis.

The most common myopathies in older adults are polymyositis, endocrine myopathies, and toxic myopathies. Polymyositis, a disorder of skeletal muscle with diverse causes, is characterized by lymphocytic infiltration of the muscles. Muscle biopsy usually shows signs of degeneration, regeneration, and infiltration by lymphocytes. Prednisone treatment should be used with caution in older adults because of its propensity to produce psychosis. In thyrotoxic myopathy, weakness and wasting are greatest in the pelvic girdle muscles and to some extent in the muscles of the shoulder region. Reflexes can be normal, and the diagnosis is based on the distribution of muscle weakness in an individual with thyrotoxicosis. The myopathy improves after the underlying endocrine disorder is treated. Hypothyroidism can also cause a myopathy that improves with thyroid replacement therapy. Creatine kinase levels are significantly increased in the myopathy associated with hypothyroidism. Finally, several medications are known to cause myopathy, including corticosteroids, lipid-lowering agents, colchicine, and procainamide.

RESTLESS LEGS SYNDROME

See "Sleep Problems," p 285.

REFERENCES

- Bril V, England J, Franklin GM, et al. Evidence-based guideline: treatment of painful diabetic neuropathy. Report of the American Academy of Neurology, the American Association of Neuromuscular and Electrodiagnostic Medicine, and the American Academy of Physical Medicine and Rehabilitation. *Neurology*. 2011;76(20):1758–1765.
- Brott TG, Halperin JL, Abbara S, et al. 2011 ASA/ACCF/AHA/AANN/AANS/ACR/ASNR/CNS/SAIP/SCAI/SIR/SNIS/SVM/SVS guideline on the management of patients with extracranial carotid and vertebral artery disease: executive summary. *Vasc Med.* 2011;16(1):35–77.
- Goldstein LB, Bushnell CD, Adams RJ, et al. Guidelines for the primary prevention of stroke: a guideline for healthcare professionals from the American Heart Association/American Stroke Association. *Stroke*. 2011;42(2):517–584.
- Saccomano SJ. Ischemic stroke: the first 24 hours. *Nurse Pract.* 2012;37(10):12–18.
- Vernon GM. Parkinson's disease and the nurse practitioner: diagnostic and management challenges. *J Nurse Pract.* 2009;5(3):195–206.

CHAPTER 60—INFECTIOUS DISEASES

KEY POINTS

- Immune function wanes with age, and resistance is compromised in older adults not only as a consequence of age-related declines in immunity (ie, immune senescence) but also more importantly because of comorbid disease.
- Accepted thresholds for "fever" generally do not apply in infected older adults because of their altered febrile response to infection. Fever can be redefined in frail older patients (temperature >2°F over baseline or oral temperature >99°F) to enhance its diagnostic utility.
- Applying minimal criteria for starting antibiotic therapy in residents of long-term care facilities is likely to reduce inappropriate antibiotic use without jeopardizing patient safety.
- First-line therapy should be selected carefully in older patients with pneumonia because of the associated high mortality rates and because the causes of pneumonia differ in older versus younger patients.
- The response to aggressive, highly active antiretroviral therapy is similar in younger and older adults with HIV infection, but diseases associated with advancing age develop earlier in HIV-infected adults, even those with prolonged suppression of HIV replication.

Infection is the major cause of mortality in 40% of those ≥65 years old, and it contributes to death in many others. Infection is also a significant cause of morbidity in older adults, often exacerbating underlying illness or leading to hospitalization. Pneumonia and other respiratory tract infections, urinary tract infection, and sepsis are all in the top 20 diagnosis-related groups paid by Medicare. Further, older adults are often a "sentinel" population in which new infections (eg, West Nile virus), newly more virulent strains (*Clostridium difficile* colitis), or the return of annual epidemics (eg, influenza) are first noted. Associations of infection and inflammation with age-related chronic diseases suggest that infectious diseases may play an even larger role in the morbidity and mortality of the older adult population than previously realized. This chapter explores the biological, cultural, and societal factors that influence susceptibility to infection, the presentation of disease, and management suggestions for several common infectious disease syndromes in older adults.

PREDISPOSITION TO INFECTION

The immune system undergoes an age-related decline, often termed immunosenescence, putting older adults at higher risk of development of infectious diseases, which are also more severe in course. Vaccine efficacy is also lower in older adults because of this phenomenon. Changes in adaptive immunity because of thymic involution involve depressed T-cell functions. B cells in older adults can produce antibodies with lower affinity, leading to weakened immunogenicity of vaccines. Deficits of innate immunity include decreased macrophage activity, causing infections to have a longer duration. Macrophages also regulate adaptive immune response, which can be dysfunctional in older adults (Table 60.1).

Although age itself influences immune function, nonspecific host-resistance factors that change with age also increase the risk of infection in older adults. For example, poor skin integrity predisposes to skin and soft-tissue infection, impaired cough or gag reflexes increase the risk of pneumonia, and increased gastric pH and decreased GI motility predispose to diarrheal illnesses. However, all of these changes associated with aging have far less influence on risk of infection than comorbid diseases. Diabetes mellitus, chronic renal insufficiency, heart failure, chronic edema due to venous insufficiency, COPD, and stroke are but a few examples of age-related comorbid illnesses that increase risk of infection. Comorbidity further influences the outcomes of and management strategies for infection in older adults. For example, community-acquired pneumonia in otherwise healthy adults <50 years old is typically treated on an outpatient basis and rarely causes mortality; however, in older adults with community-acquired pneumonia and multiple comorbid conditions, the greatly increased risk of morbidity and mortality often necessitates hospitalization. In addition, cognitive impairment and other barriers to adherence may increase the difficulty of treating older patients, increasing complications and costs.

A major influence on immune function in older adults is nutritional status. Protein and calorie undernutrition is present in 30%–60% of adults ≥65 years old on admission to the hospital. Among outpatients, 11% of older adults are malnourished, 90% of which is due to reversible underlying conditions such as depression, poorly controlled diabetes mellitus, and adverse events of medication (SOE=B). Delayed wound healing, increased risk of nosocomial infection, extended lengths of hospital stay, and increased

Table 60.1—Changes in Immune Function Associated with Aging

Type of Immunity	Change With Age	Comment
Innate immunity		
Skin, mucous membranes	↓↓↓	Skin thins and dries with aging
Polymorphonuclear neutrophils		
Adherence, chemotaxis	—	
Ingestion	—	
Intracellular killing	↓	Most changes are due to comorbidity
Adaptive immunity		
Thymic hormones	↓↓↓	
Lymphocyte subsets		
T cells	↓↓↓	Shift from naive to memory subtypes
Natural killer cells	↓↓	Number increases but function declines
Lymphocyte functions		
Proliferative responses	↓↓	
Senescent phenotype	↑↑↑	Refers to oligoclonal expansion of CD8 cells that have replicative senescence, are CD28 negative, and secrete high quantities of proinflammatory cytokines
Cytokine production, secretion		
IL-2, IL-2 receptor	↓↓↓	After stimulation
Interferon-γ	↑	Primarily basal secretion
Prostaglandin E_2	↑↑	Basal and stimulated
Delayed-type hypersensitivity	↓↓	
Autoimmunity	↑↑	Autoantibodies common but of unclear significance

NOTE: — = no age-related changes; ↑ = mild increase; ↑↑ = moderate increase; ↑↑↑= marked increase; ↓= mild decrease; ↓↓ = moderate decrease; ↓↓↓= marked decrease; IL=interleukin

mortality are all associated with malnutrition. Even mildly undernourished older adults (ie, those with a serum albumin of 3–3.5 g/dL) have evidence of immune compromise, poor vaccine responses, and diminished cytokine responses to specific challenges. Nutritional interventions may boost immune function in some older adults, but this remains controversial. Some studies suggest a clinical benefit, particularly in older adults with subclinical nutritional deficiencies, whereas others do not. Differences in study design, population enrolled, duration of follow-up, and definitions of infection (self-reported versus clinician diagnosed) may account for many of these differences. See also "Malnutrition," p 209.

Residing in long-term care or nursing facilities also places older adults at increased risk of epidemic diseases such as influenza. Widespread antibiotic use in these settings increases the likelihood of acquiring diseases caused by antibiotic-resistant organisms; methicillin-resistant *Staphylococcus aureus*, vancomycin-resistant enterococci, and multiply resistant gram-negative rods are more common causes of infection in institutionalized than in community-dwelling older adults. Resistance issues are augmented in the nursing home by debilitated hosts, close proximity of residents, poor staff compliance with prevention strategies (eg, influenza immunization), and difficulties in implementing infection-control measures in long-term care.

Because of the many risk factors predisposing older adults to infections, maintaining up-to-date immunizations is very important. Adults >65 years old should receive yearly influenza vaccination as well as one-time pneumococcal and zoster vaccinations. Other immunizations need updating based on previous vaccination status and current evidence of sustained immune response from previous infection (Table 60.2).

DIAGNOSIS AND MANAGEMENT OF INFECTIONS

Presentation

Older adults often present without typical signs and symptoms, even in severe infection. Fever, the most readily recognized feature of infection, may be absent in 30%–50% of frail older adults with serious infections, even pneumonia or endocarditis. The cause of impaired febrile responses in older adults is incompletely understood, but diverse mechanisms of thermoregulation are involved, including a reduced basal body temperature in many older adults and blunted thermogenesis by brown adipose tissue.

Given the sensitivity, specificity, and positive and negative predictive values, fever in older nursing-home residents can be redefined appropriately as a temperature >2°F (1.1°C) over baseline (if a baseline

Table 60.2—Immunization Schedule for Adults ≥65 Years Old

Vaccine	Dose Recommendation
Influenza	1 dose annually of standard or high-dose trivalent inactivated vaccine
Tetanus, diphtheria, pertussis (Td/Tdap)[a]	Substitute 1-time dose of Tdap for Td booster, then boost with Td every 10 years
Varicella	2 doses unless immune or previous receipt of 2 vaccine series
Zoster	1 dose
Pneumococcal (polysaccharide)	1 dose
Meningococcal	1 or more doses based on risk factors
Hepatitis A	2 doses based on risk factors
Hepatitis B	3 doses based on risk factors

[a] There is no commercially available Tdap preparation that has been FDA approved for patients ≥65 years old, but in light of recent pertussis outbreaks, the CDC recommends vaccination with Tdap in those ≥65 years old who have or anticipate having close contact with an infant <12 months old. The CDC also state that other adults ≥65 years old may be given a single dose of Tdap.

SOURCE: Updated Recommendations for Use of Tetanus Toxoid, Reduced Diphtheria Toxoid and Acellular Pertussis (Tdap) Vaccine from the Advisory Committee on Immunization Practices, 2010. *MMWR.* 2011;60(1):13–15. Recommended Adult Immunization Schedule, United States, 2011. Available at: http://www.cdc.gov/vaccines/schedules/index.html (accessed Oct 2013).

Table 60.3—Defining Fever in Frail, Older Residents of Long-Term Care Facilities

Definition	Sensitivity	Specificity	(+) Likelihood Ratio	(–) Likelihood Ratio
T >101°F (38.3°C)	40.0%	99.7%	133	0.6
T >100°F (37.7°C)	70.0%	98.3%	41	0.3
T >99°F (37.2°C)	82.5%	89.9%	8	0.2

NOTE: (+) Likelihood ratio = sensitivity / (1– specificity); (–) Likelihood ratio = (1– sensitivity) / specificity; T = temperature

SOURCE: Data from Castle SC, Yeh M, Toledo S, et al. Lowering the temperature criterion improves detection of infections in nursing home residents. *Aging Immunol Infect Dis.* 1993;4(2):67–76.

is available) or, perhaps more practically, an oral temperature >99°F (37.2°C) or a rectal temperature >99.5°F (37.5°C) on repeated measures (SOE=B). This definition of fever has a sensitivity of 82.5% in nursing-home residents, and the specificity remains high at 89.9% (Table 60.3). These data were generated in a cohort of frail, older, male veterans in a nursing home. It would seem reasonable to apply the same definitions to frail, older adults of either sex in the community, although the performance characteristics of this definition of fever in otherwise healthy older adults have not been validated.

The absence of fever is only one way that infectious diseases can present atypically in older adults. For example, pneumonia can be signaled by a nonspecific decline in baseline functional status, such as confusion or falling, without cough, sputum production, or shortness of breath. Anorexia and decreased oral intake may be the primary manifestation of infection, or exacerbation of an underlying illness (eg, atrial fibrillation) may become the predominant feature. Cognitive impairment, when present, further contributes to the often confusing presentation of infections in older adults. Many cognitively impaired older adults are unable to communicate symptoms accurately, and clinicians must be ready to pursue objective assessments such as laboratory and radiologic evaluations at a lower threshold, unless advance directives indicate otherwise.

Antimicrobial Management

Drug distribution, metabolism, excretion, and interactions can be altered with age. Aging in the absence of any comorbid disease is associated with decreased renal function, and antibiotic dosages may need to be reduced in older adults. See "Pharmacotherapy," p 81. Furthermore, antibiotics interact with many other medications commonly prescribed for older adults. Digoxin, warfarin, oral hypoglycemic agents, theophylline, antacids, lipid-lowering agents, antihypertensive medications, and H_2-receptor antagonists all have significant interactions with commonly prescribed antimicrobials. Drug concentrations can increase (eg, enhanced digoxin toxicity associated with macrolides, tetracyclines, and trimethoprim) or decrease (eg, reduced absorption of some fluoroquinolones with antacids) with concomitant medication administration. Atrophic gastritis, a common problem in older adults, and H_2 blockers or proton-pump inhibitors can reduce the absorption of some antimicrobials, such as ketoconazole or itraconazole. Finally, adherence to prescribed regimens may be limited as a consequence of poor cognitive function, impaired hearing or vision, multiple medications, and financial constraints.

The choice and timing of antibiotics may also be important. In sepsis, pneumonia, and other severe infections, an increasing body of evidence suggests that broad coverage is warranted initially because

Table 60.4—Suggested Minimal Criteria for Initiation of Antibiotic Therapy in the Long-Term Care Setting

Condition	Minimal Criteria
Urinary tract infection, without catheter	Fever *and* one of the following: new or worsening urgency, frequency, suprapubic pain, gross hematuria, costovertebral angle tenderness, incontinence
Urinary tract infection, with catheter	Fever or one of the following: new costovertebral angle tenderness, rigors, or new-onset delirium
Skin and soft-tissue infection	Fever or one of the following: redness, tenderness, warmth, new or increasing swelling of affected site
Respiratory infection	■ Fever ≥102°F (38.9°C) *and* one of the following: RR >25, productive cough ■ Fever >100°F (37.8°C) and <102°F (38.9°C) *and* one of the following: RR >25, pulse >100, rigors, new-onset delirium ■ Afebrile with COPD *and* new or increased cough with purulent sputum ■ Afebrile without COPD *and* new or increased cough *and* either RR >25 or new-onset delirium
Fever without source of infection	■ At least one of the following: new-onset delirium, rigors ■ If these are not present, evaluate without initiating antibiotics. ■ Antibiotics probably should not be instituted as a diagnostic test, but if initiated as such, discontinue in 3–5 days if no improvement and evaluation negative.

NOTE: RR = respiratory rate (per minute)

SOURCE: Data from Loeb M, Bentley DW, Bradley S, et al. Development of minimum criteria for the initiation of antibiotics in residents of long-term-care facilities: results of a consensus conference. *Infect Control Hosp Epidemiol.* 2001;22:120–124.

outcomes (ie, mortality, length of stay in intensive care) are improved when the offending organism is covered by the *initial* antibiotic regimen. In older adults with pneumonia, data suggest that delaying the start of therapy for ≥4 hours after admission to the hospital is associated with an increased risk of mortality (SOE=B). "De-escalation," a narrowing of antibiotic choice to specific therapy if the offending organism is identified by culture or other diagnostic studies, is essential for antibiotic stewardship and should be done whenever possible. Unfortunately, diagnostic studies (eg, obtaining sputum) are often difficult in older adults or are unavailable in long-term care settings. These factors and the atypical presentation of infection noted above often lead to early initiation of antimicrobials in older adults, particularly in long-term care. However, this practice results in inappropriate use of antibiotics in up to 75% of cases in long-term care. The use of strict, minimal criteria for initiation of antimicrobials in long-term care is most likely to reduce inappropriate antibiotic use without jeopardizing patient safety (Table 60.4) (SOE=C).

PREVENTION OF INFECTIONS

This is an exciting time for the prevention of infection in older adults. Immunizations, which historically been centered on children, have become an area of increasing research in older adults. In 2010, the FDA licensed the first high-dose influenza vaccine for adults ≥65 years old. Clinical trials are underway to determine if the increased immunogenicity in the phase III studies will correlate with increased clinical protection. The FDA has also licensed a conjugate pneumococcal vaccine (PCV-13) for use in adults ≥50 years old. The Advisory Committee on Immunization Practices has not yet recommended this vaccine for adults ≥50 years old, because effectiveness studies are currently underway. One other major change in the U.S. immunization recommendations includes the use of tetanus, diphtheria, acellular pertussis (Tdap) vaccine in older adults to protect children from pertussis infection.

INFECTIOUS SYNDROMES

Bacteremia and Sepsis

Bacteremia is a common cause of hospitalization in older adults. Older adults with bacteremia are less likely than their younger counterparts to have chills or sweating, and fever is often absent. Gastrointestinal and genitourinary sources of bacteremia are more common; thus, the causative bacteria are more likely to be gram-negative rods or enterococci in older adults versus younger patients.

Bacteremia carries a poor prognosis in older adults. For example, nosocomial gram-negative bacteremia carries a mortality rate of 5%–35% in young adults, but 37%–50% in older adults. Major contributing factors include coexisting diseases that reduce physiologic reserve and the more common use of invasive devices (eg, intravenous or urinary catheters) that make eradication of organisms difficult.

The management of bacteremia and sepsis in older and younger patients is similar. Rapid administration of appropriate antibiotics aimed at the most likely sources is essential, and early "goal-directed" therapy for volume resuscitation has proven benefit in populations of all ages with sepsis (SOE=B).

Pneumonia

Patients aged ≥65 years old account for >50% of all pneumonia cases, and annual hospitalization rates for pneumonia range from 12 per 1,000 among community-dwelling adults ≥75 years old to 32 per 1,000 among nursing-home residents. In fact, the cumulative 2-year risk of pneumonia for long-term care residents is approximately 30%. Mortality caused by pneumonia in older adults is three to five times that in young adults, but the rate is profoundly influenced by comorbidity. Comorbidity, defined in one study as cancer, collagen vascular disease, or advanced liver disease, was the strongest independent predictor of mortality in community-acquired pneumonia in older adults, with a relative risk (RR) of 4.1. Other independent risk factors for pneumonia-related mortality include age ≥85 years old; debility (decreased motor function); serum creatinine >1.5 mg/dL; and the presence of hypothermia (<36.1°F), hypotension (<90 mmHg systolic), or tachycardia (>110 beats per minute) on admission (SOE=A). Long-term follow-up data also suggest that community-acquired pneumonia in older adults indicates a higher risk of subsequent all-cause mortality over the next 12 years, as a consequence of both recurrent pneumonia (RR 2.1 [1.3–3.4]) and cardiovascular disease (RR 1.4 [1.0–1.9]) (SOE=A).

The causes of pneumonia in younger and older adults differ. In older patients, *Streptococcus pneumoniae* is still the predominant organism, but gram-negative bacilli (eg, *Haemophilus influenzae, Moraxella catarrhalis, Klebsiella* spp) are much more common than in younger adults, particularly in patients with COPD or who reside in long-term care facilities. *Staph aureus* and respiratory viruses are also common causes of community-acquired pneumonia in nursing-home residents. Obtaining a microbiologic diagnosis is often difficult in older adults who rarely produce sputum. Blood cultures should be obtained before antimicrobial therapy but are positive in only 10%–15% of patients. An often overlooked diagnostic test for pneumonia is that of urinary antigen testing for *Strep pneumoniae* (sensitivity 70%–80%; specificity 77%–97%) or *Legionella pneumophila* (sensitivity 70%–80%; specificity 77%–97%). Importantly, the sensitivity of these tests is not affected for some time (up to 24 hours) after the initiation of antimicrobial therapy. The test for legionellosis detects only serogroup 1, which causes 80% of all *Legionella* infection.

Guidelines for pneumonia therapy have evolved to account for the emergence of resistant bacteria, particularly drug-resistant *Strep pneumoniae*, and the recognition of comorbidities, healthcare setting versus community-acquired illness, and specific pathogens of interest in certain settings (eg, *Staph aureus* after viral influenza infection). Because of their ease of administration and broad activity versus respiratory pathogens, respiratory fluoroquinolones are used often in older adults, and they are one of the first-line therapies suggested by more recent guidelines. Guidelines of the Infectious Diseases Society of America for treatment of community-acquired pneumonia suggest the following as first-line therapy in adults ≥60 years old with or without comorbidity: a β-lactam/β-lactamase combination or advanced-generation cephalosporin (eg, ceftriaxone or cefotaxime) with or without a macrolide. Alternatively, one of the newer fluoroquinolones with enhanced activity against *Strep pneumoniae* (eg, levofloxacin, moxifloxacin, gemifloxacin) may be used. However, several notes of caution are needed regarding fluoroquinolone use in older adults: first, fluoroquinolones kill bacteria better at higher concentrations, and outcomes are better in older adults when high drug concentrations are present (SOE=B). Thus, full-dosage therapy should be provided (ie, the adage of "start low, go slow" often invoked for drug therapy in older adults is *not* appropriate for this class of drugs). Second, if tuberculosis (TB) is a realistic possibility, fluoroquinolone use should be reserved. Use of fluoroquinolones to treat community-acquired pneumonia can lead to delayed diagnosis of TB (by an average of >40 days) and to fluoroquinolone resistance in the organism. Finally, significant adverse events, including dizziness and cardiac conduction abnormalities (QT prolongation), may limit the use of fluoroquinolones in certain older adults; however, the overall safety of fluoroquinolones in older adults without underlying conduction abnormalities or specific contraindications is quite good (SOE=B).

Nursing-home–acquired pneumonia or hospital-acquired pneumonia in older adults requires broader initial therapy than does community-acquired pneumonia because of the broader spectrum of organisms causing infection. In the nursing-home setting, polymicrobial infection, often due to aspiration, and *Staph aureus* are much more common than in the community setting. In the hospital setting, gram-negative bacilli predominate, but *Staph aureus* is more common as well and is more likely to affect specific antibiotic choices because of resistance. Outcomes data suggest that response to therapy is greater when the initial antibiotic regimen covers the offending agent. Thus, initial regimens should be broadly inclusive, followed by step-down therapy to more narrow coverage if the causative agent is identified. Importantly, if patients are known to be colonized with methicillin-resistant *Staph aureus* (MRSA), initial regimens should include vancomycin or linezolid until MRSA is excluded as the causative agent. Further, data suggest that patients with clinically improving hospital-acquired pneumonia not caused by nonfermenting gram-negative bacilli (eg, *Pseudomonas, Stenotrophomonas*) can be treated with shorter courses of antibiotics (7 or 8 days, rather than the 2 weeks commonly used in the past). Shorter courses (8 days versus 15 days) of antibiotics are associated with equivalent efficacy and less antibiotic resistance (SOE=A).

The prevention of pneumonia in older adults is a complex issue, and a multipronged approach is most likely to be effective. Immunization of at-risk individuals is by far the most well-studied measure. Annual influenza vaccine and pneumococcal vaccine should be administered to all older adults (see "Prevention," p 70). In addition to vaccines, smoking cessation and aggressive treatment of comorbidities (eg, minimizing aspiration risk in patients after stroke, limiting use of sedative hypnotics) can reduce the risk of infection. Finally, system changes with attention to infection control (isolation, cohorting, skin testing for TB with purified protein derivative, and immunization policies for staff/visitors) can be particularly effective in the nursing home.

Influenza

Influenza results in approximately 40,000 deaths annually in the United States, nearly all of which are in the older adult population. The clinical syndrome of influenza is easily recognized by most clinicians, particularly in the setting of local activity or outbreak settings frequently seen in the nursing home. Although some controversy exists with regard to the effectiveness of influenza vaccine in frail older adults, the bulk of the data suggests the vaccine is 60%–80% efficacious in older adults for preventing severe disease, hospitalization, and death. Therefore, annual immunization is recommended for all adults (SOE=A). The FDA has approved a high-dose influenza vaccine for adults ≥65 years old. This vaccine produces higher antibody responses, but it is unknown if this provides better clinical protection. Hence, the CDC recommends either standard or high-dose vaccine for adults ≥65 years old.

Several medications are available for treatment and prophylaxis of influenza. M2 inhibitors (amantadine and rimantadine) block the M2 ion channel of influenza and are effective only against influenza A; their use is limited by widespread resistance (>90% of the most virulent strains). Further, amantadine is particularly difficult to use in older adults because of the extensive dosage adjustments required for small changes in kidney function and marked adverse events, particularly CNS symptoms. In contrast, neuraminidase inhibitors (zanamivir and oseltamivir) are effective against both influenza A and B; they inhibit the virus by interfering with an essential enzyme, neuraminidase, that cleaves sialic acid to expose host cell receptors for the virus. Oseltamivir, a capsule, is preferred over zanamivir in older adults because zanamivir must be inhaled, and it is difficult for many older adults to properly use the product. Treatment of influenza is effective if started in the first 48 hours, but it is most effective if started within 24 hours of symptom onset (SOE=A). Oseltamivir and zanamivir can also be used for prevention in outbreak situations (eg, in long-term care) when combined with appropriate vaccination strategies (SOE=A).

Urinary Tract Infection

Urinary tract infection (UTI) is among the most common of clinical illnesses in older adults, with an incidence of 10.9 per 100-person years in men and 14 per 100 person-years in women ≥65 years old. Gram-negative bacilli (eg, *Escherichia coli, Enterobacter* spp, *Klebsiella* spp, *Proteus* spp) are most common, but there is an increase in more resistant isolates, such as *Pseudomonas aeruginosa*, and in gram-positive organisms, including enterococci, coagulase-negative staphylococci, and *Streptococcus agalactiae* (group B strep). In patients with indwelling catheters, the microbes listed still predominate, but it is also common to encounter additional organisms, including enterococci, *Staph aureus*, and fungi, particularly *Candida* spp. The organisms colonizing urinary catheters commonly develop biofilms, and infections are difficult to resolve with the same urinary catheter in place.

Asymptomatic Bacteruria Versus Urinary Tract Infection

Up to 15% of women in the community and 40% of women in nursing homes have asymptomatic bacteruria; the incidence in men is approximately half that in women. Rates are even higher with the use of condom catheters (87%) or Foley catheters (nearly 100%). Numerous studies have suggested that there is no clinical benefit from the treatment of asymptomatic bacteruria, and that treatment is associated with significant adverse events, expense, and the potential for selection of resistant organisms. Thus, no treatment is recommended (SOE=A). The clinical difficulty is deciding what is symptomatic and, thus, when a urine culture should be ordered, particularly in the nursing-home setting. The presentation of infection can be quite subtle in older adults, and a change in functional status often prompts the collection of a urine specimen even in the absence of fever, dysuria, or other typical clinical features. Similarly, empiric antimicrobial therapy should be started only when infection is documented or highly suspected.

Urinary Tract Infection in Women

In contrast to asymptomatic bacteruria, symptomatic UTI requires therapy. Therapy is based on the location of infection (upper versus lower tract disease) and the likely causative agent. Lower-tract UTI (ie, cystitis), characterized by dysuria, frequency, and urgency (not fever, which generally indicates upper-tract disease), is often treated in young women for 1–3 days, and 3–7 days of therapy is probably sufficient for uncomplicated cystitis in older women (SOE=B). Randomized trials in older women indicate that fluoroquinolones are more efficacious than trimethoprim-sulfamethoxazole (TMP-SMX), likely because resistance rates of *E coli* to TMP-SMX are 10%–20% in most areas of the United States; however, with wider use of fluoroquinolones, resistance to these agents is also increasing. Other reasonable choices in some settings include amoxicillin (particularly for enterococcal infection) and first-generation cephalosporins in patients with multiple antibiotic intolerances. Culture is not required unless first-line therapy is not effective (SOE=A).

Upper UTI (ie, pyelonephritis), characterized by fever, chills, nausea, and flank pain, is commonly accompanied by lower-tract symptoms and requires a longer period of therapy (7–21 days). Because of the excellent bioavailability of many antibiotics, particularly the fluoroquinolones, intravenous therapy is not essential if the patient can tolerate oral medications. In a study comparing fluoroquinolones with TMP-SMX for upper-tract UTI in younger women (18–58 years old), fluoroquinolones were more effective (microbiologic cure rate 99% versus 89% for TMP-SMX; clinical cure rate 96% versus 83% for TMP-SMX) because of the presence of organisms resistant to TMP-SMX. This is likely to be true in older adults as well. Intravenous administration of antibiotics remains the standard of care for patients with suspected urosepsis, those with upper-tract disease due to relatively resistant bacteria such as enterococci, or those unable to tolerate oral medications. Culture and sensitivity data are more useful in guiding antimicrobial therapy in upper-tract UTIs than in lower-tract disease and should be obtained in most cases (SOE=A).

Prophylactic antibiotics intended to prevent frequently recurrent UTIs in older women are not recommended because of the high incidence of the development of resistant organisms. Several measures may decrease the frequency of recurrence, including intravaginal or systemic estrogen replacement that changes the vaginal flora, thus reducing the risk of UTI, or perhaps ingestion of cranberry juice (≥300 mL/d).

Urinary Tract Infection in Men

Prostatic disease (primarily hyperplasia) or functional disability, such as autonomic neuropathy from diabetes mellitus with incomplete bladder emptying, account for most lower and upper UTIs in older men. Thus, short-course therapy for UTIs in older men is inappropriate. Therapy should last at least 14 days, and if prostatic involvement is suspected (ie, acute or chronic prostatitis), at least 6 weeks (SOE=B). The causative organisms and treatment choices are similar to those outlined above for older women. Fluoroquinolones and TMP-SMX are most widely used when prostatic involvement is suspected and culture data confirm the organism's susceptibility because, of the available agents, these two penetrate the prostate best. Because treatment for all UTIs in men is generally longer than in women and the prostate is a common reservoir for recurrent UTIs, culture and sensitivity data should guide therapy for virtually all UTIs in men (SOE=C).

Tuberculosis

Worldwide, approximately 1.7 billion people are infected with *Mycobacterium tuberculosis*, 16 million in the United States. Adults ≥65 years old account for one-fourth of all active TB cases in the United States. The vast majority of active TB in older adults is in community-dwelling adults, but the rate of infection in long-term care residents is much higher: skin-test studies show prevalence rates of skin-test reactivity in the range of 30%–50%. This high prevalence is due to exposure to *M tuberculosis* in the early 1900s, when it was estimated that 80% of all individuals were infected by age 30. Most active cases of TB in older adults are, therefore, due to reactivated disease, but primary infection may account for 10%–20% of cases and is of particular concern in nursing-home outbreaks.

As with most other infections, TB may not present in classical fashion (ie, cough, sputum, fever, night sweats, weight loss) in older adults. Often fatigue, anorexia, decreased functional status, or low-grade fever are presenting manifestations. Most tuberculous disease in older adults occurs with lung involvement (75%), and pneumonic processes in older adults, particularly those that occur in a postacute manner, should raise a high index of suspicion for *M tuberculosis* infection. Older adults are more likely than their younger counterparts to have extrapulmonary disease. Other sites include miliary (disseminated) disease, tuberculous meningitis or osteomyelitis, and urogenital disease, but virtually any body structure or organ system can be involved and can account for the major presenting symptom.

A diagnosis of active disease usually requires isolation of the organism from sputum, urine, or other clinical specimen. Current techniques have improved the speed of diagnosis, particularly for identifying the species of *Mycobacterium* after isolation. This is now typically accomplished within 24 hours of obtaining a positive culture by use of DNA probes. Direct polymerase chain reaction of clinical specimens or other rapid diagnostic techniques are not available or reliable in most local laboratories, but such tests can be available in research settings. They are most likely to be helpful for establishing a diagnosis from cerebrospinal or pleural fluid, which yields positive cultures in only 10%–15% of cases.

The most confusing area of TB diagnostics is typically interpretation of the results of purified-protein derivative (PPD) skin tests. In all populations, induration of ≥15 mm 48–72 hours after placement of a 5-tuberculin-unit PPD indicates a positive test. Induration ≥10 mm is considered a positive test in nursing-home residents, recent converters (previous PPD <5 mm), immigrants from countries with high endemicity of *M tuberculosis* infection, underserved populations in the United States (homeless people, black Americans, Hispanic Americans, and Native Americans), and those with specific risk factors (eg, gastrectomy, >10% below ideal body weight, chronic kidney failure, diabetes mellitus, or immunosuppression, including that caused by corticosteroids or malignancy). In individuals infected with HIV, those with a history of close contact with people with active *M tuberculosis*, and those with chest radiographs consistent with *M tuberculosis* infection, ≥5 mm induration is considered a positive PPD test. Anergy panel testing in conjunction with PPD testing is of little value and is not recommended (SOE=C).

Long-term care facilities should use a two-step procedure for PPD testing during the initial evaluation of residents (SOE=C). Two-step testing requires retesting of patients with <10 mm induration within 2 weeks. If the second skin test results in ≥10 mm of induration or the increase in the size of the induration from the first to the second skin test is ≥6 mm, the patient is considered PPD positive. See "Nursing Home Care," p 153.

The treatment of active TB in older adults is similar to that in young adults. Four-drug therapy (usually isoniazid [INH], rifampin, pyrazinamide, and ethambutol or streptomycin) is recommended as initial therapy, with tapering to one of several two- or three-drug regimens once susceptibility testing is available. The most common regimen is INH, rifampin, and pyrazinamide for 2 months, followed by INH and rifampin for an additional 4 months. Adjustments in routine drug treatment protocols are often needed, however, because of comorbidities and drug tolerance in older adults.

Prophylaxis with 9 months of INH for asymptomatic individuals with a positive PPD should be provided *regardless of age* in adults who are recent converters (defined in adults >35 years old with a PPD that has gone from <10 mm to ≥15 mm within 2 years), or regardless of duration of PPD positivity if an individual has any of the specific risk factors highlighted above. Patients with a positive PPD of unknown duration should receive INH prophylaxis, even those >35 years old (as opposed to recommendations in the 1990s). Older adults should be monitored closely for symptoms and signs of peripheral neuropathy (due to INH and preventable by coadministration of pyridoxine) and hepatitis (due to treatment with INH, rifampin, or pyrazinamide). Shorter-course therapy with 2 months of rifampin and pyrazinamide is effective but has a much higher incidence of hepatotoxicity than INH treatment and thus should be used only in very specific circumstances (SOE=B).

Infective Endocarditis

Since the early part of the 20th century, infective endocarditis has undergone a transformation from a disease of young adults primarily due to rheumatic or congenital valve anomalies to one of older adults associated with degenerative valvular disorders and prosthetic valves. Native-valve endocarditis is typically caused by viridans streptococci and *Staph aureus*, and occasional infections are due to HACEK organisms (a group of typically nonfermenting gram-negative rods that primarily inhabit the oral cavity and include the genera *Haemophilus, Actinobacillus, Cardiobacterium, Eikenella,* and *Kingella*). Gastrointestinal and genitourinary organisms, such as enterococci and gram-negative rods, are more common in native-valve infective endocarditis in older adults, and coagulase-negative staphylococci are a common cause of prosthetic-valve endocarditis, particularly in the first 60 days after placement of a prosthetic valve.

The diagnosis of endocarditis is often difficult in older adults. Fever is less common in older adults than in younger ones, occurring in 55% versus 80%, respectively, as is leukocytosis, occurring in 25% versus 60%. Rates of positive blood cultures do not vary by age; however, degenerative, calcific valvular lesions and prosthetic valves lower the sensitivity of transthoracic echocardiography to 45% in older patients (versus 75% in younger patients). Transesophageal echocardiography (TEE) improves the diagnostic yield for infective endocarditis, but the lack of positive findings on TEE never excludes it. TEE is of particular value in resolving *Staph aureus* bacteremia. Positive findings on TEE support prolonged antibiotic administration (4–6 weeks) versus short-course (2 weeks) therapy. However, TEE is invasive and expensive. Interestingly, age does not appear to play a major role in mortality risk, with a 2-year survival of 75% for infective endocarditis in all age groups unless major comorbidities are also present.

Antibiotic treatment of infective endocarditis is directed at the identified pathogen or at the most likely causes if blood cultures are negative. Therapy is administered intravenously for 2–6 weeks. Surgical therapy should be considered in cases of severe valvular dysfunction, recurrent emboli, marked heart failure, myocardial abscess formation, fungal endocarditis, or when appropriate antibiotic treatment does not yield negative blood cultures.

Recommendations for endocarditis prophylaxis for dental procedures were revised in 2007, focusing on providing prophylaxis only in the highest-risk patients and eliminating recommendations for prophylaxis for those undergoing gastrointestinal or genitourinary procedures.

Prosthetic Device Infections

Permanent implantable prosthetic devices are common in older adults. Prosthetic joints, cardiac pacemakers, artificial heart valves, intraocular lens implants, vascular grafts, penile prostheses, and a variety of other devices are placed more often in older than in younger adults. A discussion of all prosthetic device infections (PDIs) is beyond the scope of this chapter, but several general concepts can be summarized.

PDIs are usually separated into early versus late infections because the causative agents differ significantly. Early PDIs, most commonly defined as occurring <60 days after device implantation, are primarily due to contamination at the time of implantation or to events associated with the acute hospitalization (ie, occult bacteremias caused by intravenous catheters). Thus, coagulase-negative staphylococci predominate, and *Staph aureus* and diphtheroids are common as well; gram-negative bacilli and fungi are relatively rare causes of early PDI. Late PDIs are usually caused by organisms that commonly cause transient bacteremia (in older adults this is most often skin, respiratory, gastrointestinal, or genitourinary organisms). Staphylococci, including coagulase-negative staphylococci, play a major role in both early and late PDIs, although their relative importance is greater in early PDIs. Thus, empiric staphylococcal therapy should be provided in either early or late PDIs if a specific causative agent is not identified.

In general, hardware removal is required to clear PDIs. However, early antibiotic treatment, in some instances combined with aggressive surgical drainage, can be successful. Small studies in prosthetic joint infection suggest that initial debridement and culture and a brief course (2 weeks) of intravenous antibiotics followed by combination oral two-drug therapy that includes rifampin may obviate the need for device removal. Until more definitive data are available, it is prudent to restrict this approach to patients with a short duration of symptoms (<3 weeks), those who are likely to have difficulty tolerating another surgical procedure, or those in whom return to full functional status is not a realistic goal because of comorbidities. In those older adults in whom full function is the goal, the best chance for cure is a two-stage procedure in which the device is removed and antibiotics are given for an extended period (6–8 weeks), followed by delayed reimplantation. Of course, for life-saving devices, such as mechanical valves or implantable defibrillators, this is not an option. Infected prosthetic devices are usually surrounded by microbial biofilms, such as microbe-derived glycocalyx. Biofilms reduce antibiotic penetration and thus greatly increase the concentrations of antibiotic needed for bactericidal activity. Furthermore, many conditions associated with infected prostheses are also accompanied by poor blood flow to the area. Therefore, it is preferable to use bactericidal antibiotics, often in combination with a second agent that penetrates biofilms and poorly perfused areas (eg, rifampin for staphylococci).

Bone and Joint Infections

Native bone and joint infections in the absence of prostheses occur in older adults. Septic arthritis is more likely to occur in joints with underlying pathology (eg, rheumatoid changes, gout, osteoarthritis), and early arthrocentesis is indicated in any mono- or oligo-articular syndrome to exclude infection. *Staphylococcus aureus* is the most likely pathogen; infections are only rarely due to gram-negative bacilli and streptococci. Aggressive antibiotic therapy combined with serial arthrocentesis may be as effective as open surgical drainage in uncomplicated septic arthritis, while also preserving better joint function. Surgical drainage is required if this more conservative strategy is not successful.

Osteomyelitis in older adults can be due to hematogenous seeding from a bacteremia or contiguous spread from an adjacent focus. *Staphylococcus aureus* is the predominant organism, but gastrointestinal and genitourinary flora are again more common in older adults, emphasizing the advantage of a specific microbiologic diagnosis to guide therapy. Pressure ulcer infections and diabetic foot infections are very common, particularly in institutionalized older adults, and they commonly require surgical consultation combined with aggressive antimicrobial therapy aimed at mixed aerobic and anaerobic bacteria. Osteomyelitis requires definitive treatment with aggressive debridement/amputation of the infected bone with up to 8 weeks of appropriate (and often intravenous) antimicrobial therapy in consultation with an infectious diseases specialist.

HIV Infection and AIDS

HIV infection in older adults was initially limited to those who had received blood transfusions for surgical procedures. However, increasing numbers of older Americans with HIV have acquired their infection via sexual activity. In addition, improvements in treatment have resulted in a large population of adults aging with HIV infection. By 2015, >50% of U.S. adults infected with HIV will be ≥50 years old. Older adults constitute approximately 10% of all new diagnoses of AIDS in the United States, but this group and their clinicians often suffer from a lack of HIV awareness. Nonspecific symptoms such as forgetfulness, anorexia, weight loss, and recurrent pneumonia are often dismissed as age related, delaying HIV testing. Untreated HIV infection in older adults tends to pursue a more rapid downhill course, perhaps because of impaired T-cell replacement mechanisms with advanced age and the impact of additional comorbidities. However, if older adults are treated with aggressive highly active antiretroviral therapy (HAART), the antiviral response is similar to that seen in young adults. In fact, older adults often are more adherent with complicated HAART regimens than young adults. However, despite this response, increasing data suggest immune reconstitution is less robust in older adults with HIV infection. Recommendations are becoming more aggressive with regard to threshold for initiation of HAART; however, these recommendations have been in a state of flux for the past several years, and it is suggested that all patients with HIV be under the care of an infectious diseases specialist to decide when to begin therapy and what agents are most appropriate.

Treatment regimens and prophylaxis of opportunistic infections with HAART are similar to those used in younger patients. Indications that HIV therapies can accelerate atherosclerosis and glucose intolerance suggest that an aggressive approach to prevention of cardiovascular disease in older HIV-infected adults is warranted and may lead to specific recommendations in older adults if associations of metabolic changes with specific HIV therapies become clearer. Other age-related comorbidities are also more common in HIV-infected individuals, even those with well-controlled viral replication (ie, a peripheral blood viral load <50 copies/mL). Many types of cancer, osteoporosis, and cirrhosis are all more prevalent in this population and appear to develop about a decade earlier in HIV-infected individuals versus appropriately matched, uninfected controls. Older adults appear to be more susceptible to specific complications associated with HIV infection, such as encephalopathy. Finally, older HIV-infected adults are more likely than uninfected, age-matched adults to have multiple comorbidities, which increases the complexity of their care and the potential for medication interactions.

HIV prevention is rarely discussed in the geriatric community but is important if the trend of increasing sexual acquisition of HIV in older adults is to be reversed. Most older women do not believe that they are at risk of HIV infection, yet heterosexual activity is the primary mode of infection in this group. The concept of HIV-risky behavior is not well known among older adults, because HIV was not a problem during their adolescence or young adulthood. Older adults must be included in educational programs aimed at ensuring safe sexual practices and increasing awareness of the benefits of testing and effective HIV therapy.

Miscellaneous Infectious Syndromes

Bacterial meningitis is most common at the age extremes of life, and most meningitis-associated fatalities are in older adults. *Streptococcus pneumoniae* remains the most common cause in older adults, but gram-negative bacilli (20%–25%), *Listeria* spp (up to 10%), and TB are more common than in young adults. Because many *Strep pneumoniae* are now resistant to β-lactam antibiotics (up to 30% penicillin resistance and 10% ceftriaxone resistance nationwide), ceftriaxone or cefotaxime *plus* vancomycin are recommended as empiric therapy for bacterial meningitis in older adults until a specific isolate can be tested for antimicrobial susceptibility. Ampicillin is the drug of choice for *Listeria* spp, and more resistant gram-negative rods (eg, *Pseudomonas* spp) require ceftazidime or an extended-spectrum penicillin with or without intrathecal aminoglycoside therapy.

Neurosyphilis remains one of the most perplexing diagnoses in medicine. It is often raised as a possible underlying process in stroke or dementia in older adults. Syphilis should also be considered in unilateral deafness, gait disturbances, uveitis, and optic neuritis. In reality, there is no gold-standard test to exclude neurosyphilis. Neurosyphilis can only be "ruled in" by such tests. However, suspicion is often first raised when a serum rapid plasma reagent or Venereal Disease Research Laboratory test (VDRL) is positive. A reasonable diagnostic evaluation after discovery of such a positive test includes confirmation of nonspecific tests (rapid plasma reagent and VDRL) with a specific test (microhemagglutination-*Treponema pallidum*, or fluorescent treponemal antibody absorption); if tests are confirmed, lumbar puncture should be performed for cell counts, glucose, protein, and cerebrospinal fluid (CSF) VDRL. A positive VDRL on CSF is diagnostic of neurosyphilis, but the sensitivity of this test is approximately 75% in most series. Other diagnostic tests are controversial. The ratio of intrathecal to serum-specific treponemal antibody (standardized to the total IgG in CSF and serum) may also be helpful, with ratios of ≥3 indicating likely infection. In the absence of these tests, it must be the judgment of the clinician as to whether minor abnormalities in CSF (eg,

Table 60.5—Evaluation of Fever of Unknown Origin in Older Adults

1	Confirm fever; conduct thorough history (include travel, *Mycobacterium tuberculosis* exposure, medications, constitutional symptoms, symptoms of giant cell arteritis) and physical examination. Discontinue nonessential medications.
2	Initial laboratory evaluation: CBC with differential, liver enzymes, erythrocyte sedimentation rate, blood cultures × 3, PPD skin testing, thyrotropin, antinuclear antibody, consider antineutrophilic cytoplasmic antibody or HIV-antibody testing in specific cases.
3	a) Chest or abdomen or pelvic CT scan—if no obvious source *or* b) Temporal artery biopsy—if symptoms or signs consistent with giant cell arteritis or polymyalgia rheumatica and increased erythrocyte sedimentation rate *or* c) Site-directed evaluation on basis of symptoms or laboratory abnormalities, or both.
4	If 3a is performed and no source is found, then 3b, and vice versa.
5	Bone marrow biopsy—yield best if hemogram abnormal—send for hematoxylin and eosin stain, special stains, cultures, *or* liver biopsy—very poor yield unless abnormal liver enzymes or hepatomegaly
6	Indium-111 labeled WBC or gallium-67 scan—nuclear scans can effectively exclude infectious cause of fever of unknown origin if negative.
7	Laparoscopy or exploratory laparotomy
8	Empiric antibiotic trial—typically reserved for antituberculosis therapy in rapidly declining host or high suspicion of tuberculosis (ie, prior positive PPD)

NOTE: PPD = (tuberculin) purified protein derivative

low-level pleocytosis) and the clinical picture support the diagnosis and warrant therapy for neurosyphilis. Optimal treatment of neurosyphilis remains penicillin G, but a study in HIV-infected patients suggests that ceftriaxone may be an acceptable alternative.

Advancing age is the major risk factor for reactivated varicella-zoster virus herpes zoster (or "shingles"); the most disabling complication, post-herpetic neuralgia, is common in older adults. See "Dermatologic Diseases and Disorders," p 350, for diagnosis and treatment. Zoster vaccine is recommended for all immunocompetent adults ≥60 years old, and it reduces the risk of zoster and post-herpetic neuralgia by >50% (SOE=A).

Facial nerve palsy (Bell's palsy) is common in older adults and associated with at least three infectious causes: herpes simplex virus, varicella zoster virus, and *Borrelia burgdorferi* (which causes Lyme disease). There are no strong data at present to suggest benefit of antiviral therapy for facial nerve palsies due to herpes simplex virus, but trials are underway. If facial nerve palsy is seen as part of an episode of varicella zoster virus, treatment is indicated. If Lyme disease is suspected clinically, the patient should receive oral amoxicillin 500 mg q6h for 14 days, oral doxycycline 100 mg q12h for 14 days, or intravenous ceftriaxone 2 g/d for 14 days.

Gastrointestinal infections are common among older adults. Diverticulitis, appendicitis, cholecystitis, intra-abdominal abscess, and ischemic bowel can present diagnostic dilemmas in the absence of fever or increased WBC counts. A high index of suspicion is necessary in older adults. CT or labeled WBC studies are most likely to be of value in establishing the diagnosis of intra-abdominal infection, and ultrasonography is an easy, readily available tool to assist in diagnosing cholecystitis, appendicitis, or abscess. Ischemic bowel often requires angiography.

Infectious diarrhea is also common in older adults. Older patients with achlorhydria are at particular risk because a lower bacterial inoculum is necessary to cause disease. Decreased intestinal motility associated with specific medications and advanced age may further increase susceptibility to infection. Epidemics occurring in the long-term care setting are commonly due to *E coli*, viruses, salmonellae, or *Shigella* spp. Frequent use of antimicrobials in older adults also increases the risk of *C difficile* colitis, and the risk of severe disease is greatest in this age group. Recently, *C difficile* infection has increased in incidence and severity, most prominently affecting older adults. The reasons for this are uncertain but likely relate to spread of more virulent strains, widespread use of fluoroquinolone antibiotics, and perhaps proton-pump inhibitors (SOE=B). Data suggest vancomycin is more effective than metronidazole for *C difficile* disease and should be used as first-line therapy when severe disease is present. Metronidazole is still suggested as first-line therapy for mild to moderate disease. Relapse is more common in older adults and may require tapering of vancomycin (to be done over several months). A new treatment option, fidaxomicin, a macrocyclic antibiotic, was approved in May 2011 for the treatment of ***C difficile***–associated diarrhea at a dosage of one 200-mg tablet PO q12hr. Ongoing research is needed to establish efficacy and safety. Alternatively, intestinal microbiota transplantation, also known as fecal bacteriotherapy or fecal transplant, has recently regained interest. The concept of intestinal microbiota transplantation is based on the rationale of restoring the balance of colonic flora that has been disturbed by outside influences (eg, antimicrobial therapy, acid-suppressive therapy, GI surgery). Implantation is done by enema or nasogastric tube and has been shown to have low recurrence rates. Prevention of *C difficile* disease is mainly accomplished by reducing the unneeded antibiotics and the duration of needed antibiotic use. This is highlighted by data showing that one of every three courses of antibiotics in nursing-home residents results in *C difficile* disease. See "Gastrointestinal Diseases and Disorders," p 408.

Fever of Unknown Origin

Fever of unknown origin (FUO) is defined as temperature >38.3°C (101°F) that lasts for at least 3 weeks and is undiagnosed after 1 week of medical evaluation. Several studies have examined this syndrome in older patients and demonstrated differences between older and younger adults. The cause of FUO can be determined in >90% of cases in older adults, and one-third have treatable infections, such as intra-abdominal abscess, bacterial endocarditis, TB, perinephric abscess, or occult osteomyelitis, with an incidence of infection similar to that in younger patients. In contrast, collagen vascular diseases are more common causes of FUO in older than in younger patients. These are primarily due to giant cell arteritis, polymyalgia rheumatica, and polyarteritis nodosa but rarely to Wegener granulomatosis. In several published series, 28% of all FUOs in older adults were due to collagen vascular diseases. Neoplastic disease accounts for another 20%, but with rare exceptions, fever due to cancer is primarily caused by hematologic malignancies (eg, lymphoma and leukemia) and not solid tumors. Medications are another cause of FUO in older adults. Rare causes in this age group include deep-vein thrombosis with or without recurrent pulmonary emboli and hyperthyroidism.

For a diagnostic approach to FUO in older adults, see Table 60.5.

References

- High K, Bradley S, Mehr D, et al. Clinical practice guideline for evaluation of fever and infection in long-term care facilities: 2008 update by the Infectious Diseases Society of America. *Clin Infect Dis.* 2009;48(2):149–171.
- Hooten TM, Bradley SF, Cardenas DD, et al. Diagnosis, prevention, and treatment of catheter-associated urinary tract infection in adults: 2009 International Clinical Practice Guidelines from the Infectious Diseases Society of America. *Clin Infect Dis.* 2010; 50(5):625–663.
- Mokabberi R, Haftbaradaran A, Ravakhah K. Doxycycline vs. levofloxacin in the treatment of community-acquired pneumonia. *J Clin Pharm Ther.* 2010;35(2):195–200.
- Muzzi-Bjornson L, Macera L. Preventing infection in elders with long-term indwelling urinary catheters. *J Am Acad Nurse Pract.* 2011;23(3):127–134.

CHAPTER 61—ENDOCRINE AND METABOLIC DISORDERS

KEY POINTS

- Thyrotropin (thyroid-stimulating hormone) is an adequate screening test for thyroid function in a healthy older adult outpatient population, but both free T_4 and thyrotropin should be used to evaluate thyroid status in sick older adults.
- Chronic adrenal insufficiency presents with nonspecific symptoms such as anorexia, nausea, weight loss, abdominal pain, weakness, hypotension, and impaired function. It should be considered as a cause of unexplained cachexia, mobility disability, and hypotension, even in the absence of hyponatremia and hyperkalemia.
- Vitamin D deficiency is common and not only contributes to bone loss due to osteoporosis and osteomalacia but also has been associated with muscle weakness and falls.
- The most common causes of hypercalcemia are primary hyperparathyroidism in outpatients, and malignant hypercalcemia (eg, caused by squamous cell cancers, breast cancer, myeloma, and lymphoma) in the inpatient setting.
- There is little evidence of long-term clinical benefit from supplementation with dehydroepiandrosterone (DHEA), testosterone, and growth hormone in older adults.

Impaired homeostatic regulation, a hallmark of aging, occurs in many endocrine systems but may become manifest only during stress. For example, fasting blood glucose concentrations change little with normal aging, increasing 1–2 mg/dL per decade of life. In contrast, glucose concentrations after glucose challenge (eg, postprandially) increase much more in healthy older adults than in young adults. In some cases, a loss of function in one aspect of endocrine function can result in a compensatory change in endocrine regulation and be associated with changes in catabolism that maintain homeostasis. For example, decreased testosterone production by the testes, which is seen in many older men, may be partially compensated for by an increase in secretion of pituitary luteinizing hormone and offset by a decrease in metabolism of testosterone. In other instances, compensatory changes or changes in hormone catabolism do not fully offset age-related impairment in endocrine functions, as illustrated by the age-related decline in basal serum aldosterone concentrations. In this case, a decline in aldosterone clearance fails to offset the decrease in aldosterone secretion.

As with diseases in other organ systems, endocrine disorders in older adults often have nonspecific, muted, or atypical symptoms and signs. Some of these presentations are well-defined syndromes that are seen almost exclusively in older adults, such as apathetic thyrotoxicosis or hyperosmolar nonketotic state in patients with type 2 diabetes mellitus. However, more commonly, endocrine disorders present with subtle, nonspecific symptoms, such as cognitive impairment or reduced functional status, or an absence of any complaints. Indeed, the diagnosis of endocrinopathies such as primary hyperparathyroidism, type 2 diabetes mellitus, hypothyroidism, and hyperthyroidism in older adults is commonly established as a result of abnormalities found on routine laboratory screening.

Laboratory evaluation of older adults for endocrine disorders can be complicated by coexisting medical illnesses and medications. For example, the presence of serious acute or chronic nonthyroidal illness can lead to the mistaken impression of a thyroid disorder because of the increase or decrease in T_4 concentrations and sometimes increased or decreased thyrotropin concentrations in sick but euthyroid older adults. As a result of biological and assay variability, hormone concentrations may vary considerably in the short term. Therefore, abnormal hormone measurements should always be repeated to confirm endocrine dysfunction, and a stimulatory or suppression test may be required to firmly establish a diagnosis of endocrine hypofunction or hyperfunction, respectively. Furthermore, ranges of normal laboratory values for endocrine testing are commonly established in younger adults, and even age-adjusted norms for laboratory tests may be confounded by the inclusion of older adults who are ill. Consequently, normal ranges for healthy older adults are not available for most laboratory tests.

THYROID DISORDERS

With aging, a decrease in T_4 secretion is balanced by a decrease in T_4 clearance, resulting in unchanged circulating T_4 concentrations. T_3 concentrations are unchanged until extreme old age, when they decrease slightly. However, T_3 concentrations are commonly decreased in nonthyroidal illness because of decreased peripheral conversion of T_4 to T_3. The distribution of thyrotropin concentrations shifts toward a higher level with increasing age, with the 97.5th percentile of thyrotropin distribution of 7.5 mIU/L in adults ≥80 years old, contributing to the higher prevalence of biochemical hypothyroidism. Furthermore, this shift toward higher thyrotropin concentrations with age appears also to apply to extremely long-lived individuals. Nonspecific, atypical, or asymptomatic presentations of thyroid disease are common in older adults. Laboratory testing in the stable outpatient using thyrotropin measurements is the most reliable way to identify hypothyroidism or hyperthyroidism in older adults who are not acutely ill. Screening for thyroid disease by measurement of thyrotropin every 2 years is recommended for older adults (SOE=C). In addition, the prevalence of hypothyroidism or hyperthyroidism is sufficiently high to warrant thyrotropin testing in all older adults with a recent decline in clinical, cognitive, or functional status, or on admission to a nursing home. However, the results of thyroid function testing can be confusing in euthyroid patients with significant concurrent illnesses, as discussed below.

Hypothyroidism

Most prevalence estimates of hypothyroidism in older adults range from 0.5% to 5% for overt disease, depending on the population studied. As in younger people, most cases of hypothyroidism in older people are due to chronic autoimmune thyroiditis (Hashimoto disease). Symptoms of hypothyroidism are often atypical in older adults. Some clinical features of hypothyroidism (eg, dry skin, decreased skin turgor, slowed mentation, weakness, constipation, anemia, hyponatremia, arthritis, paresthesias, peripheral neuropathy, gait disturbances, edema, and increased myocardial fraction of creatine kinase) can misleadingly suggest other diseases. Furthermore, these symptoms usually have an insidious onset and a slow rate of progression. As a result, the diagnosis of hypothyroidism is recognized on clinical examination in only 10%–20% of cases in older adults, and laboratory screening is necessary to detect most cases of hypothyroidism in this population. In addition, older adults with mild hypothyroidism who develop serious nonthyroidal illness may rapidly become severely hypothyroid, a situation that increases susceptibility to myxedema coma. Demented older adults with hypothyroidism rarely recover normal cognitive function with thyroid replacement, but cognition, functional status, and mood may improve with treatment of the hypothyroidism.

Subclinical hypothyroidism, characterized by increased serum thyrotropin and normal free T_4 concentrations, has been reported in up to 15% of people ≥65 years old, and is more common in women. However, up to 70% of these individuals actually have values within their age-specific 97.5th percentile, and people with exceptional longevity have higher thyrotropin levels than those aged 70 years.

In younger adults, some data have linked subclinical hypothyroidism to increased of cardiovascular disease and to cognitive and neuromuscular dysfunction. The relative risk of coronary heart disease and cardiovascular and all-cause mortality is increased among adults with subclinical hypothyroidism who are <65 years old but not in those ≥65 years old. In older adults, a mildly low activity of thyroid hormone may be beneficial, with increased thyrotropin levels and low levels of free T_4 associated with improved survival risk. Randomized trials of T_4 supplementation in older adults with subclinical hypothyroidism have not shown a consistent improvement in symptoms, although people with thyrotropin concentrations >10 mIU/L may derive symptomatic benefit. Based on the foregoing, T_4 supplementation in older adults with mildly increased thyrotropin levels may be of limited clinical benefit or even harmful. However, adults with thyrotropin levels ≥10 mIU/L are at increased risk of coronary heart disease events and mortality regardless of age. It is unknown whether these risks can be ameliorated with thyroxine replacement.

By itself, an increased thyrotropin concentration is usually due to primary hypothyroidism, but thyrotropin concentrations may be transiently increased during recovery from acute illnesses. Therefore, the diagnosis of hypothyroidism should be confirmed by the combination of an increased thyrotropin concentration and a decreased free T_4 or free T_4 index (total T_4 × thyroid uptake [an estimate of thyroid hormone binding]), or by demonstration of a persistently increased thyrotropin concentration, or both. Potentially confusing scenarios in the diagnosis of hypothyroidism may occur in the *nonthyroidal illness syndromes*, which may present with low serum total T_4 levels ("low T_4 syndrome") without increased thyrotropin concentrations in euthyroid patients with severe nonthyroidal illnesses. Free T_4 concentrations are usually normal in the low T_4 syndrome, with increased concentrations of reverse T_3. Serum thyrotropin levels may also be low in the nonthyroidal illness syndrome. However, the most common alteration in thyroid hormone levels in nonthyroidal illness is a decrease in serum T_3 levels (*low T_3 syndrome*), occurring even in mild nonthyroidal illnesses. In the past, patients with the nonthyroidal illness syndrome were thought to be euthyroid, but some may actually have developed *transient* secondary hypothyroidism. Thyroid hormone supplementation has not been shown to be beneficial in these patients, and it may be harmful. An inappropriately normal or low thyrotropin concentration found in conjunction with a low free T_4 concentration suggests *secondary hypothyroidism*, which may be differentiated from the low T_4 syndrome by the presence of hypopituitarism (deficiencies in other pituitary hormones) and decreased reverse T_3 concentrations (versus increased reverse T_3 in nonthyroidal illness). Rarely, older adults with primary hypothyroidism can also have inappropriately normal thyrotropin concentrations resulting from suppression of thyrotropin by fasting, acute illnesses, and medications such as dopamine, phenytoin, or glucocorticoids. To minimize confusion between thyroid disease and the nonthyroidal illness syndrome, thyroid function testing in seriously ill patients should be performed only if thyroid dysfunction is strongly suspected.

T_4 replacement is usually started at a low dosage (eg, 25 mcg/d) in older adults, increasing the dosage every 4–6 weeks until thyrotropin concentrations reach the normal range. However, in patients with severe cardiac disease, it is sometimes prudent to begin replacement therapy at even lower dosages (eg, 12.5 mcg/d) if patients are asymptomatic or have minimal symptoms of hypothyroidism (SOE=D). In these patients, thyroid replacement should not be withheld for fear of exacerbating cardiac disease; instead, the goal is to reduce or eliminate symptoms of hypothyroidism while minimizing the potential for exacerbating cardiac symptoms, such as angina. Older adults who are severely hypothyroid at presentation should receive larger initial T_4 replacement doses of 50–100 mcg, or as high as 400 mcg IV for those with myxedema stupor or coma, even if there is preexisting heart disease (SOE=D). Older adults with severe hypothyroidism or myxedema stupor or coma should also be tested to exclude concomitant adrenal insufficiency as well as given stress doses of glucocorticoids before receiving T_4 to avoid precipitating an adrenal crisis with T_4 replacement.

Thyroid hormone requirements decrease with aging because of a decreased clearance rate, and T_4 replacement dosages are as much as a third lower in older than in younger adults. The average T_4 replacement dosage in older adults is approximately 110 mcg/d. Thyroid hormone is best taken fasting to avoid reduced absorption related to food and other medications (eg, calcium, iron, or soy). Over-replacement of thyroid hormone should be avoided, because osteopenia related to increased bone turnover and exacerbation of heart disease may occur. With correction of the hypothyroid state, the clearance rate of medications such as anticonvulsants, digoxin, and opioid analgesic agents may be affected, necessitating dosage adjustments.

Hyperthyroidism

Hyperthyroidism develops in 0.5%–2.3% of older adults, and 15%–25% of all cases of thyrotoxicosis are in adults ≥60 years old. In the United States, most cases in older adults are due to Graves disease, but toxic multinodular goiter and autonomously functioning adenomas are more common in older than in young adults, especially in populations with low iodine intake.

Hyperthyroidism often presents with vague, atypical, or nonspecific symptoms in frail older adults. Many findings that are common in younger adults (eg, tremor, hyperkinesis, heat intolerance, tachycardia, frequent bowel movements, ophthalmopathy, increased perspiration, goiter, brisk reflexes) are less common or absent in older adults, whereas other manifestations, such as atrial fibrillation, heart failure, muscle atrophy, and weakness, are more common in older adults. Older adults can present with *apathetic thyrotoxicosis*, a well-known clinical presentation of hyperthyroidism that is rarely seen in younger adults, in which the usual hyperkinetic presentation is replaced by depression, inactivity, lethargy, or withdrawn behavior, often in association with symptoms such as anorexia, weight loss, constipation, muscle weakness, or cardiac symptoms. A low thyrotropin concentration is associated with a 3-fold higher risk of developing atrial fibrillation within 10 years, and hyperthyroidism is present in 13%–30% of older adults with atrial fibrillation. Hyperthyroidism is a cause of secondary osteoporosis and should be considered in the evaluation of patients with decreased bone mass.

A highly sensitive thyrotropin test is adequate as an initial test for hyperthyroidism in relatively healthy older adults, but the diagnosis should be confirmed with a free T4 test. Most asymptomatic older adults with low serum thyrotropin concentrations are clinically euthyroid and have normal T_4 and T_3 concentrations, with normal thyrotropin on repeat testing 4–6 weeks later. *T_3 thyrotoxicosis*, with increased T_3 but normal T_4 concentrations, is seen in a minority of hyperthyroid patients, but it is more common with aging, especially in older adults with toxic adenomas or toxic multinodular goiter. However, in contrast to young adults, many older adults with hyperthyroidism do not have increased T_4 or T_3 concentrations, probably because of decreased conversion of T_4 to T_3 associated with aging and concomitant nonthyroidal illness. The reduction in T_4 and T_3 conversion in nonthyroidal illness is mediated by a decrease in T_4-5′-deiodinase activity, although the specific factors mediating changes in enzymatic activity are unknown. Diagnostic confusion can occasionally occur in euthyroid patients with nonthyroidal illness or medications causing increased T_4 concentrations (*high T_4 syndrome*). The high T_4 syndrome can develop with medications or illnesses that decrease the conversion of T_4 to T_3 (high-dose glucocorticoids or β-blocking agents, acute fasting) or that increase circulating concentrations of thyroid-binding globulin (estrogens, clofibrate, hepatitis).

Subclinical hyperthyroidism is present in approximately 2% of older adults without known thyroid disease. In patients with a thyrotropin <0.1 mIU/L, 1%–2% per year develop overt hyperthyroidism, whereas overt disease develops uncommonly in those with thyrotropin concentrations between 0.1 and 0.45 mIU/L. Thyrotropin concentrations normalize over time in many of these patients, although persistence of subclinical hyperthyroidism is the most common outcome.

There is good evidence for an association between subclinical hyperthyroidism and atrial fibrillation for thyrotropin concentrations <0.45 mIU/L (SOE=A), as well as for people with thyroid function in the high-normal range. Subclinical hyperthyroidism can increase left ventricular mass and cardiac contractility and can cause delayed diastolic relaxation, but these effects are of uncertain clinical importance. Subclinical hyperthyroidism is associated with modestly increased cardiovascular and all-cause mortality in some, although not all, studies. Subclinical hyperthyroidism can accelerate bone mineral density loss, especially in people with a thyrotropin concentration <0.1 mIU/L, but even thyroid function within the high-normal range is associated with reduced bone mineral density and increased risk of nonvertebral fractures. In postmenopausal women, ongoing bone losses associated with thyrotropin concentrations <0.1–0.2 mIU/L are stabilized by treating the hyperthyroidism. In some, but not all, population-based studies, neuropsychiatric symptoms and cognitive impairment have increased in older adults with subclinical hyperthyroidism. Treatment of hyperthyroidism should be considered in older adults with thyrotropin concentrations <0.1 mIU/L due to Graves or nodular thyroid disease (SOE=C). Evidence is insufficient to recommend treating older adults with thyrotropin concentrations between 0.1 and 0.45 mIU/L, although treatment consideration has been advocated based on increased risk of atrial fibrillation in this group.

Thyroid scanning and measurement of radioactive iodine uptake may be useful in confirming hyperthyroidism and defining the cause. It is important to identify hyperthyroid patients with low radioactive iodine uptake, because these patients do not respond to radioactive iodine therapy or antithyroid medications and are treated symptomatically. Radioactive iodine therapy is the treatment of choice for most older adults with hyperthyroidism due to Graves disease or toxic nodular thyroid disease. Radioactive iodine treatment is usually curative in patients with toxic adenoma, but higher or repeated doses are often necessary for patients with toxic multinodular goiter. Antithyroid drugs such as methimazole are given before radioactive iodine, to control symptoms and to avoid a worsening of thyrotoxicosis due to transient release of thyroid hormone after radioactive iodine. β-Blocking agents are helpful to manage symptoms such as tachycardia, tremor, and anxiety[OL], but patients should be monitored for changes in cardiopulmonary function. After radioactive iodine therapy, patients should be monitored by serial measurements of thyrotropin concentration for the eventual development of hypothyroidism and for persistent or recurrent hyperthyroidism. With resolution of hyperthyroidism, the clearance rate of other medications may decrease, necessitating dosage adjustments to avoid excessive drug concentrations.

Nodular Thyroid Disease and Thyroid Cancer

The incidence of multinodular goiter increases with age. Multinodular goiters often have autonomously functioning areas, so that administration of exogenous thyroid hormone to suppress these goiters can cause iatrogenic hyperthyroidism. Older adults with multinodular goiter can develop iodine-induced thyrotoxicosis after receiving radiocontrast or amiodarone.

Approximately 90% of women ≥70 years old and 60% of men ≥80 years old have thyroid nodules. Most of these nodules are nonpalpable but are detected incidentally on highly sensitive ultrasound or imaging studies done for other reasons (eg, carotid duplex ultrasound to assess carotid artery atherosclerosis). Thyroid nodules are more likely to be malignant in adults ≥60 years old, especially men. Thyroid cancer is present in 4%–6.5% of thyroid nodules, and incidentally discovered nonpalpable nodules are as likely to be malignant as palpable nodules. The incidence of differentiated thyroid cancers is similar in older and younger adults, whereas thyroid lymphomas are more common and anaplastic thyroid carcinomas are found almost exclusively in older adults. However, even well-differentiated papillary and follicular carcinomas are more aggressive and are associated with increased mortality in older adults.

Ultrasound is the most sensitive test to detect thyroid nodules. Screening ultrasonography of the thyroid is not indicated in the general population. The procedure should be performed when there is unexplained cervical lymphadenopathy or when risk factors for thyroid cancer are present (Table 61.1). Additionally, ultrasound is warranted in patients with normal or high thyrotropin concentrations and one or more palpable thyroid nodules (SOE=A). However, autonomously functioning thyroid nodules are rarely malignant, so no further evaluation for cancer is required in patients with low thyrotropin concentrations and a "hot" nodule on radionuclide thyroid scanning that corresponds to a palpable nodule.

Table 61.1—Indications for Thyroid Ultrasonography

Screening

- History of head and neck irradiation
- Multiple endocrine neoplasia type 2
- Family history of thyroid cancer

Diagnosis

- Unexplained cervical lymphadenopathy
- Guidance for fine-needle aspiration of single or multiple thyroid nodules
- Identification of nodular characteristics suspicious of cancer
- Thyroid nodule discovered incidentally on CT, MRI, or 2-deoxy-2[18F]fluoro-d-glucose positron emission tomography (18FDG-PET scanning)

Referral to endocrinology is appropriate for older adults interested in pursuing treatment.

Disorders of Parathyroid and Calcium Metabolism

Important changes occur with aging in several systems that regulate calcium homeostasis, ultimately leading to decreased bone mass and in some cases osteoporosis in older adults (Table 61.2). The net effect of these changes is to increase circulating concentrations of parathyroid hormone (PTH), which increases 30% between 30 and 80 years of age. Serum calcium concentrations remain normal as a result of the increase in PTH, but the balance between bone resorption and bone formation is changed in favor of resorption, resulting in decreased bone mass and increased risk of osteoporosis with aging.

Table 61.2—Causes of Age-Related Changes in Calcium Homeostasis

Decreased concentrations of 1,25(OH)D
- Decreased renal 1α-hydroxylase activity, leading to decreased renal parathyroid hormone responsiveness
- Decreased vitamin D synthesis by the skin
- Decreased sunlight exposure (housebound and institutionalized older adults)

Decreased intestinal absorption of dietary calcium
- Inadequate dietary calcium and vitamin D intake
- Decreased intestinal responsiveness to 1,25(OH)D
- Decreased gastric acid secretion
- Lactase deficiency (avoidance of dairy products)

Increase in serum parathyroid hormone concentrations
- Slight decrease in serum calcium concentrations
- Decreased renal clearance of parathyroid hormone
- Decreased concentrations of 1,25(OH)D

Vitamin D Deficiency

Vitamin D deficiency, defined as a circulating 25(OH)D level <20 ng/mL, is extremely common, affecting 20%–100% of older community-dwelling adults. Exposure to natural sunlight is the major source of vitamin D, but many older people do not receive adequate sunlight to maintain vitamin D sufficiency and even with adequate exposure to sunlight, the synthesis of vitamin D in skin declines progressively with aging. In addition, dietary calcium intake is inadequate in most older adults. However, as a consequence of factors mentioned in Table 61.2, older adults are less able than younger adults to compensate by increasing their intestinal absorption of ingested calcium. Increased bone turnover and bone loss, especially of cortical bone, is a major consequence of secondary hyperparathyroidism in vitamin D–deficient older adults. Furthermore, vitamin D deficiency is associated with muscle weakness and can contribute to fall risk in some individuals.

Although population screening for vitamin D deficiency is not recommended in current guidelines, 25(OH)D levels should be obtained in older adults at high risk of vitamin D deficiency, including those with obesity, a history of falls, nontraumatic fractures, osteoporosis, or intake of medicines such as anticonvulsant drugs. The main form of vitamin D in circulation, 25(OH)D is measured in serum to evaluate vitamin D status. Measurements of $1,25(OH)_2D_3$, the active metabolite of vitamin D, are not useful to assess vitamin D status in most individuals, because levels are normal or increased in vitamin D–deficient individuals with secondary hyperparathyroidism. Levels of $1,25(OH)_2D_3$ are mostly used clinically in patients with late-stage chronic kidney disease.

The Institute of Medicine (IOM) report published in 2010 provides recommended dietary reference intakes for calcium and vitamin D intended to optimize the health of the general population, not to treat diagnosed vitamin D deficiency states. The IOM recommended maintaining 25(OH)D concentrations >20 ng/mL, with the goal of assuring vitamin D levels adequate for bone health in at least 97.5% of the population. Other experts advocate a minimum level of 30–32 ng/mL in older adults to minimize falls and fracture risk. Many older people have 25(OH)D concentrations below 30 ng/mL, including most postmenopausal women taking medication for osteoporosis. Despite the lack of consensus on the 25(OH)D concentration required for optimal bone health, there is general agreement that levels <20 ng/mL are suboptimal for bone health, and that the optimal serum 25(OH)D concentrations for outcomes other than bone health have not been established.

Evidence for the 25(OH)D concentration required for vitamin D sufficiency comes from studies showing an inverse relationship between circulating PTH and 25(OH)D concentrations that begins to plateau at 25(OH)D levels between 30 and 40 ng/mL, suggesting secondary hyperparathyroidism associated with vitamin D deficiency at 25(OH)D levels below these values. However, other experts, including the authors of the IOM report, cite studies showing suppression of PTH across a wide range of 25(OH)D levels from 15 to 50 ng/mL. Treating postmenopausal women with vitamin D sufficient to boost 25(OH)D concentrations from 20 to 32 ng/mL increased intestinal calcium transport in one study, although others found no increase in intestinal calcium absorption across a range of circulating 25(OH) D levels.

Severe vitamin D deficiency is associated with proximal muscle weakness, myalgias, and gait impairment. A recent meta-analysis of double-blind randomized controlled trials (RCTs) in adults > 65 years old (n=8 for falls, n=12 for nonvertebral fractures) found a significant dose-response relationship between reduction in falls and both the level of vitamin D supplementation (<700 IU/d versus 700–1000 IU/d), and the 25(OH)D levels in study participants (<24 ng/mL versus ≥24 ng/mL), whereas other experts evaluating the same data found no significant dose-response relationship.

With regard to fracture risk, some studies found that supplementation of vitamin D at doses sufficient to achieve 25(OH)D levels of 28–40 ng/mL was necessary to minimize fracture risk (levels reached only in trials in which 700–800 IU/d of vitamin D_3 was given). A recent meta-analysis of 12 double-blind RCTs for nonvertebral fractures and 8 RCTs for hip fractures comparing vitamin D with or without calcium supplementation versus calcium or placebo found a pooled RR of 0.86 (95% CI, 0.77–0.96) for prevention of nonvertebral fractures and 0.91 (95% CI, 0.78–1.05) for hip fracture prevention. The effect on fracture reduction was seen only at dosages >400 IU/d of vitamin D, which reduced nonvertebral fractures by 29% in community-dwelling older adults and 15% in institutionalized older adults. Furthermore, reduction of nonvertebral fractures was found only when vitamin D supplementation was sufficient to achieve 25(OH)D levels of ≥30 ng/mL.

How much vitamin D should be prescribed for older adults? The IOM report recommended dietary intakes of 800 IU/d of cholecalciferol (vitamin D_3) for men and women >70 years old; other experts recommend intakes of at least 800 IU/d. However, at least 1,500–2,000 IU/d may be required to increase the circulating level of 25(OH)D above 30 ng/mL (SOE=A). Maintaining adequate calcium intake (1,000–1,500 mg/d from the diet and supplements) is also important for bone health and prevention of secondary hyperparathyroidism, although recent meta-analyses suggest that calcium supplementation with or without vitamin D may increase the risk of cardiovascular events. In this regard, it is important to consider daily dietary intake of calcium (primarily in dairy products), which in some individuals may be considerable, obviating the need to use calcium supplements. High-dose supplementation may cause vitamin D intoxication with hypercalcemia, hypercalciuria, impairment of kidney function, and bone loss, but dosages of 10,000 IU/d do not cause toxicity when taken for up to 5 months. The maximum tolerable intake for maintenance therapy in the general population is 4,000 IU/d. However, a higher intake of 10,000 IU/d may be needed to correct vitamin D deficiency in some individuals, eg, those with celiac disease (SOE=A). Vitamin D–deficient older adults should be treated with 50,000 IU/week of vitamin D_2 or vitamin D_3 for 8–12 weeks or an equivalent daily dose of 6,000 IU of vitamin D_2 or vitamin D_3 with the goal of achieving a blood level of 25(OH)D >30 ng/mL, followed by 1,000–1,500 IU/d (occasionally higher dosages) for maintenance therapy (SOE=A). Obese individuals and those with malabsorption syndromes who are vitamin D–deficient may require vitamin D dosages 2- to 3-fold higher, ie, at least 6,000–10,000 IU/d of vitamin D to achieve a 25(OH)D level >30 ng/mL, followed by maintenance therapy of 3,000–6,000 IU/d (SOE=A). A few patients who are unable to take daily oral supplements may benefit from oral vitamin D at 100,000 IU every 6 months with minimal risk of hypercalcemia. See also prevention and treatment of osteoporosis in "Osteoporosis," p 243.

Hypercalcemia

Primary hyperparathyroidism and malignancy are the most common causes of hypercalcemia in older adults. The annual incidence of primary hyperparathyroidism is approximately 1 per 1,000, and the disease is 3-fold more prevalent in women than in men. Most patients with primary hyperparathyroidism are asymptomatic, and the diagnosis is made after an incidental finding of hypercalcemia. When the disease is symptomatic, older adults are more likely than younger adults to present with neuropsychiatric symptoms such as depression and cognitive impairment, neuromuscular symptoms such as proximal muscle weakness, or osteoporosis. For typical laboratory findings in primary hyperparathyroidism and other common causes of hypercalcemia, see Table 61.3. The diagnosis of primary hyperparathyroidism is confirmed with an increased or high normal PTH concentration, by the use of an assay for intact PTH, in the presence of hypercalcemia. Parathyroid surgery is the treatment of choice for symptomatic primary hyperparathyroidism and for asymptomatic patients with total serum calcium concentrations >1 mg/dL above the normal range, creatinine clearance reduced

Table 61.3—Typical Laboratory Results in the Differential Diagnosis of Hypercalcemia

Laboratory Test	Primary Hyperparathyroidism	Humoral Hypercalcemia of Malignancy	Local Osteolytic Hypercalcemia
Serum calcium	↑	↑ or ↑↑	↑ or ↑↑
Serum phosphate	↓or low-normal	↓	↑
Urine calcium	↑	↑	↑
Parathyroid hormone	↑	↓↓	↓↓
Parathyroid hormone-related peptide	0	↑	0

NOTE: The diagnosis of malignancy-related hypercalcemia is normally straightforward, and extensive diagnostic testing is rarely required. ↑ = increased; ↑↑ = markedly increased; ↓ = decreased; ↓↓ = markedly decreased; 0 = undetectable

to <60 mL/min, or markedly decreased bone density (T score below −2.5 at any site on bone densitometry) (SOE=C). Referral to endocrinology should be made for treatment decisions.

Patients with serum calcium concentrations <1 mg/dL above the normal range who are asymptomatic and managed conservatively should avoid lithium carbonate, thiazide diuretics, volume depletion, and immobilization. Baseline assessment in these patients should include blood pressure; serum calcium, phosphate, and creatinine; creatinine clearance; and bone densitometry. Follow-up assessments should include serum calcium and creatinine every 12 months, and bone densitometry (at 3 sites) every 12–24 months (SOE=C). In addition, these patients should be followed clinically for the development of nephrolithiasis, fractures caused by minimal trauma, and neuropsychiatric or neuromuscular symptoms. At present, no medications are approved specifically for the treatment of primary hyperparathyroidism. Medical management options for primary hyperparathyroidism include the bisphosphonate alendronate, which improves bone mineral density in patients with primary hyperparathyroidism without consistently affecting calcium or PTH concentrations[OL] (SOE=A). However, it is unknown whether alendronate or other bisphosphonates reduce fracture risk in these patients. The selective estrogen receptor modulator raloxifene reduces bone turnover in patients with primary hyperparathyroidism[OL], but data on the skeletal effects of raloxifene are very limited. Cinacalcet, a calcimimetic agent that inhibits parathyroid cell function, reduces or normalizes serum calcium concentrations and reduces PTH concentrations during long-term treatment of primary hyperparathyroidism[OL], but bone mineral density is not increased. Accordingly, the role of cinacalcet is limited to the management of symptomatic hypercalcemia in patients who are not candidates for parathyroid surgery. Estrogen–progestin therapy increases bone mineral density in postmenopausal women with primary hyperparathyroidism, but it should not be used as first-line medical therapy because of its associations with increased risk of coronary heart disease, breast cancer, and stroke (see section on estrogen replacement therapy, below).

In hospitalized patients, the most common cause of hypercalcemia is a malignancy that produces PTH-related peptide (PTHrp), with hypercalcemia resulting primarily from increased net bone resorption. The presence of an underlying cancer is usually evident on examination and routine diagnostic testing. Squamous cell cancers of the lung or head and neck are common causes of hypercalcemia due to PTHrp production. Other common malignancies associated with hypercalcemia include breast cancer, lymphoma, and myeloma, although the mechanisms of the hypercalcemia associated with these malignancies are usually not PTHrp-mediated and may be responsive to glucocorticoid treatment. Acute treatment for hypercalcemia of malignancy includes volume replacement with intravenous saline. A parenteral bisphosphonate such as pamidronate or zoledronic acid should be given, along with treatment for the underlying malignancy, if possible. In addition to their usefulness in the treatment of hypercalcemia, high-potency bisphosphonates such as zoledronic acid may decrease bone pain and the risk of pathologic fractures in patients with osteolytic bone metastases from a variety of cancers (SOE=A). Nephrotoxicity associated with these agents may be minimized by adhering to recommended dosages and infusion times. However, these agents should be used cautiously if at all in people with a creatinine clearance of ≤30 mL/min. Cancer patients receiving repetitive dosing of parenteral bisphosphonates who have had recent dental extractions, dental implants, poorly fitting dentures, or preexisting disease, or receiving high-dosage glucocorticoid treatment are at risk of osteonecrosis of the jaw.

Paget Disease of Bone

Paget disease is characterized by localized areas of increased bone remodeling, resulting in a change in bone architecture and an increased tendency to deformity and fracture. Its prevalence increases with aging, affecting 2%–5% of people ≥50 years old.

Paget disease is usually asymptomatic and is often diagnosed as an incidental finding on radiographs or during evaluation for an unexplained increase in serum alkaline phosphatase. The most commonly affected sites are the pelvis, spine, femur, tibia, and skull. When Paget disease is symptomatic, pain is the most common presenting symptom, either localized to the affected bones or resulting from secondary osteoarthritic changes, often in the hips, knees, and vertebrae. When bone deformities occur, the long bones of the legs are usually affected, often with bowing. Skull involvement may result in compression of the eighth cranial nerve and sensorineural hearing loss. The most devastating complication of Paget disease is malignant transformation of the affected bone, especially the development of osteosarcoma. The primary indication for treatment in asymptomatic patients is active disease in areas where complications may occur, including the skull, weight-bearing bones, and bone adjacent to major joints, which may increase the risk of secondary osteoarthritis (SOE=C). In asymptomatic patients with a normal serum alkaline phosphatase (SAP), a bone scan may be useful to identify active sites of disease. Bisphosphonates suppress the accelerated bone turnover and bone remodeling that is characteristic of Paget disease, and newer-generation aminobisphosphonates (eg, zoledronic acid, pamidronate, alendronate, or risedronate) are the treatment of choice (SOE=C). These agents are effective in treating bone pain associated with Paget disease (SOE=A), and sustained biochemical remissions are achieved with high-potency bisphosphonates in many patients.

An unblinded RCT, the Paget's disease Randomized trial of Intensive versus Symptomatic Management (PRISM) study, compared the effects over a 3-year period of intensive bisphosphonate therapy to normalize SAP levels versus bisphosphonate treatment only for symptoms of Paget disease. Although intensive therapy was more effective than symptomatic therapy in lowering SAP levels, except for a higher NSAID requirement in the symptomatic treatment group, no significant differences were found for any other end point, including fracture occurrence, bone pain, bodily pain, quality of life, hearing threshold, or orthopedic surgery. However, the study was insufficiently powered to detect a reduction in fracture rate of <50% in the intensive versus the symptomatic treatment group. At present, there is little evidence that bisphosphonate treatment reduces complications such as the development and progression of osteoarthritis related to Paget disease, and the effects of treatment on other long-term clinical outcomes remain uncertain.

Calcium and vitamin D should be administered concomitantly with bisphosphonates to prevent hypocalcemia[OL]. NSAIDs may be useful in treating secondary osteoarthritis. During treatment, patients should be monitored clinically for changes in bone pain, joint function, and neurologic status. SAP levels should be monitored to assess the initial and ongoing response to bisphosphonate therapy. It is not usually necessary to measure other markers of bone turnover such as serum osteocalcin or urinary N-telopeptide.

HORMONAL REGULATION OF WATER AND ELECTROLYTE BALANCE

Unlike young adults, older adults are predisposed to both volume depletion and free water excess. This impairment in regulation of volume status and osmolality is multifactorial, reflecting decreased total body water content as well as changes in antidiuretic hormone (ADH) secretion, osmoreceptor and baroreceptor systems, urine-concentrating capability, renal hormone responsiveness, and thirst sensation. ADH secretion tends to be excessive in older adults, with normal to increased basal ADH concentrations, increased ADH responses to osmoreceptor stimuli such as hypertonic saline infusion, and decreased ethanol-induced inhibition of ADH secretion. This state of relative ADH excess seen with aging, when combined with renal insufficiency, heart failure, hypothyroidism, or diuretic use, predisposes older adults to hyponatremia by impairing free water clearance. Even when mild and apparently asymptomatic, hyponatremia is associated with deficits in gait and attention, falls, and increased fracture risk in older adults (SOE=A). The syndrome of inappropriate antidiuretic hormone (SIADH) is the most common cause of hyponatremia in older adults. Most cases of SIADH are mild and relatively asymptomatic, but even mild chronic hyponatremia (serum sodium of 120–132 mEq/L) may increase the risk of falls, gait impairment, and difficulty sustaining attention in older adults. Medications causing SIADH include the SSRIs, sulfonylureas, carbamazepine, oxcarbazepine, and tricyclic antidepressants.

Treatment of mild hyponatremia should focus initially on identifying and treating the underlying cause(s) of hyponatremia (eg, treatment of hypothyroidism or adrenal insufficiency). Hypovolemic hyponatremia is usually managed with isotonic saline administration for intravascular volume expansion, whereas fluid restriction is often tried first for patients with euvolemic or hypervolemic hyponatremia. However, fluid restriction may be poorly tolerated or unacceptable to patients. Vasopressin receptor antagonists such as tolvaptan or conivaptan may be used as an alternative to fluid restriction or in addition to it. These agents cause a free water diuresis without increasing sodium excretion. Although correcting hyponatremia with tolvaptan improved performance on the mental component of the Medical Outcomes Study SF12 at 1 month, clinically significant long-term benefits of vaptan treatment have not been established. Vasopressin receptor antagonists should not be used in hypovolemic patients.

Older adults are at increased risk of volume depletion. With aging, basal aldosterone secretion declines disproportionately to the decrease in clearance, with a net reduction in circulating aldosterone concentrations of about 30% by the age of 80 years. At the same time, atrial natriuretic hormone secretion (and renal responsiveness to this hormone) increases with aging. Atrial natriuretic hormone inhibits aldosterone production and causes natriuresis and diuresis through its effects on the kidneys. Taken together, these changes predispose older adults to volume depletion by decreasing the ability of the kidneys to conserve sodium under conditions of fluid deprivation. Baroreceptor ADH responses to hypotension and hypovolemia are decreased in older adults, placing them at additional risk of dehydration. Moreover, renal responsiveness to ADH is decreased with aging, resulting in a decreased ability of the kidneys to maximally concentrate urine. Finally, even healthy older adults have decreased thirst sensation and may not be aware that they are becoming dehydrated. Demented and immobile older adults are at the highest risk of severe dehydration and hypernatremia.

In addition to predisposing to volume depletion, age-related hyporeninemic hypoaldosteronism also increases the risk of hyperkalemia, especially in older adults with diabetes mellitus or renal insufficiency. The addition of ACE inhibitors, NSAIDs, β-blocking agents, and diuretics with aldosterone-antagonist properties may lead to potentially lethal hyperkalemia in some of these patients. See "Kidney Diseases and Disorders," p 420.

Disorders of the Adrenal Cortex

Basal serum cortisol concentrations do not change with aging, because decreased cortisol secretion is balanced by a decrease in clearance. Stimulation of cortisol production by adrenocorticotropic hormone (ACTH) is unchanged, and cortisol and ACTH responses to stress and secretagogues are unimpaired with aging. Clinically, acute cortisol responses to stress may be higher and more prolonged in older than in younger adults. Accordingly, in nonemergent situations, adrenal function testing should be deferred at least 48 hours after major stressors, such as surgery or trauma. In older adults with a normal ACTH stimulation test in whom adrenal insufficiency is suspected, endocrinology consultation is recommended to assist with further testing.

Hypoadrenocorticoidism

Chronic glucocorticoid therapy is the most common cause of adrenal failure in older adults because of chronic suppression of adrenal function. Recovery of adrenal axis function is variable and may take several months to a year. Autoimmune-mediated adrenal failure is less common in older than in younger adults, but tuberculosis, adrenal metastases, and adrenal hemorrhage in anticoagulated patients are more common causes of adrenal insufficiency in older adults. Additionally, prolonged use of megestrol acetate (eg, as an appetite stimulant) may cause hypoadrenocorticoidism. Older adults with chronic adrenal insufficiency may present with nonspecific symptoms such as anorexia, nausea, weight loss, abdominal pain, weakness, hypotension, or impaired functional status, and hyponatremia and hyperkalemia may not always be present. Accordingly, a high index of suspicion is required to make the diagnosis. Chronic adrenal insufficiency should be considered in patients with unexplained cachexia, mobility impairment, and hypotension. When adrenocortical insufficiency is suspected, the ACTH stimulation test should be performed (SOE=A) and therapy initiated (SOE=D). A normal serum cortisol response 30 or 60 minutes after administration of 250 mcg of ACTH (cosyntropin) is 18–20 mcg/dL. A serum ACTH concentration should be obtained before administration of cosyntropin to distinguish secondary adrenal insufficiency (decreased pituitary ACTH secretion), which is characterized by a low or normal ACTH concentration, from primary adrenal insufficiency, which is associated with a high ACTH concentration. Patients with recent onset ACTH deficiency (eg, within 4 weeks of pituitary surgery) may still be capable of mounting a response to ACTH stimulation. In older adults who are stopping chronic glucocorticoid therapy, the replacement regimen should be tapered gradually (SOE=D), and stress dose coverage should be given for major surgery and other acute physiologic stresses until adrenocortical function has returned to normal (SOE=D). Recovery of the hypothalamic-pituitary-adrenal axis may take >9 months.

Hyperadrenocorticoidism

Exogenous glucocorticoids are the most common cause of hyperadrenocorticism in older adults, often causing adverse events, including psychiatric and cognitive symptoms, osteoporosis, myopathy, and

Table 61.4—Screening Tests for Hormone Hypersecretion in Patients with Adrenal Incidentalomas

Indications	Test	Diagnosis
Cushing syndrome manifestations	24-hour urine free cortisol	Functional adrenocortical adenoma
Before major surgery	1-mg overnight dexamethasone suppression test	
All patients with incidentaloma	24-hour urine metanephrines and catecholamines	Pheochromocytoma
Before major surgery	Plasma metanephrines	
Hypertension	Serum potassium	Primary aldosteronism
Hypokalemia	Ratio of plasma aldosterone concentration to plasma renin activity	

glucose intolerance. For patients beginning long-term glucocorticoid therapy, baseline and follow-up bone densitometry measurements are indicated, and calcium, vitamin D, and antiresorptive treatments such as alendronate, risedronate, or zoledronic acid should be started as appropriate for prevention or treatment of glucocorticoid-induced osteoporosis. Management of subclinical glucocorticoid hypersecretion should be coordinated with an endocrinologist.

Adrenal Neoplasms

In autopsy studies, the prevalence of clinically inapparent adrenal masses (*adrenal incidentalomas*) ranges from <1% in people <30 years old to ≥10% in older adults. Most adrenal incidentalomas are benign adrenocortical adenomas, although pheochromocytomas and adrenocortical carcinomas are also found. It is important to exclude pheochromocytoma, because it is not uncommon and potentially life-threatening.

The goals of assessment are to determine whether the tumor is functional (hormone-secreting) (Table 61.4) and whether it is benign or malignant. Screening for *subclinical glucocorticoid hypersecretion* is controversial. Many adrenocortical adenomas have a degree of functional autonomy, and some patients may be at increased risk of new vertebral fractures and develop hypertension, insulin resistance, and other metabolic derangements. However, it is unclear whether subclinical glucocorticoid hypersecretion is associated with long-term morbidity, or whether adrenalectomy or medical management of metabolic derangements improves outcomes. Moreover, screening all older adults with adrenal incidentalomas for glucocorticoid hypersecretion would yield a high proportion of false-positive results. Accordingly, it may be prudent to limit testing to patients with a symptom complex suggesting hyperadrenocorticism and to patients scheduled for major surgery who are at risk of postoperative adrenal crisis (SOE=D).

The assessment of malignancy risk in patients with adrenal incidentaloma is based on lesion size, its imaging characteristics, and its rate of growth. The prevalence of adrenal cortical carcinoma in these patients increases from 2% of lesions <4 cm to 25% of lesions >6 cm. Some experts suggest removal of masses >4 cm; however, the size threshold clearly indicating malignancy is unknown. Surgical excision is generally recommended for adrenal masses with other imaging characteristics suggesting malignancy, including high density, irregular shape, unilaterality, tumor calcification, and rapid growth rate, suggesting that the mass is not an adenoma (SOE=B). However, the patient's treatment preferences and clinical condition must be considered before recommending treatment. In patients followed expectantly for masses >2 cm without clearly benign features, imaging should be repeated in 3–6 months to identify rapidly growing tumors that are more likely to be malignant (SOE=B).

Adrenal Androgens

In contrast to the changes seen in cortisol concentrations with aging, circulating concentrations of the principal adrenal androgen, dehydroepiandrosterone (DHEA), decline progressively with aging, and in octogenarians are only 10%–20% of concentrations in young adults. Low DHEA concentrations are associated with poor health, whereas DHEA concentrations are positively correlated with some measures of longevity and functional status. Given these associations, there has been interest in the potential therapeutic effects of DHEA administration in older adults.

Most studies involving physiologic to mildly supraphysiologic DHEA supplementation in middle-aged and older adults have not found clinically meaningful beneficial effects on body composition. Although DHEA may increase bone mineral density in postmenopausal women (and not in older men), these effects are minimal in comparison with established treatments for osteoporosis. In RCTs of DHEA supplementation alone for up to 2 years in older adults with low DHEA concentrations, improvements were not detected in measures of physical performance, well-being, mood, quality of life, and cognition. In one RCT in frail older women, exercise together with DHEA supplementation improved some measures of lower extremity strength and function, but the clinical significance of this finding is unknown.

Potential risks of DHEA treatment include decreased circulating high-density lipoprotein cholesterol levels in older women, raising the possibility of potential long-term atherogenic effects. Furthermore, DHEA is metabolized to estrogens and to androgens such as testosterone and dihydrotestosterone, and its effects on the risk of breast cancer in women and prostate cancer in men are unknown. Finally, higher dosages of DHEA can cause androgenization in some women and gynecomastia in men. Thus, the safety and efficacy of DHEA supplementation in older adults have not been established, and its use is inappropriate other than in clinical studies.

Women with adrenal insufficiency or who are surgically menopausal develop severe androgen deficiency and may present with symptoms of decreased libido, energy, and well-being despite optimal glucocorticoid and (in primary adrenal insufficiency) mineralocorticoid replacement. In middle-aged women with adrenal insufficiency, DHEA supplementation appears to have small beneficial effects on health-related quality of life and depression, but no significant effects on anxiety and sexual well-being. Androgen replacement therapy (eg, with DHEA or testosterone) may be justifiable in these women to treat severe androgen deficiency with symptoms of impaired mood and well-being. However, widespread use of androgen supplementation in women, including testosterone treatment for hypoactive sexual desire in nonsurgical postmenopausal women, is not recommended. Although testosterone appears to improve measures of sexual desire and function in estrogen-replete postmenopausal women, concerns remain regarding concomitant long-term estrogen therapy as well as the lack of a clearly defined clinical syndrome, data regarding the long-term safety of testosterone therapy, and age-based normative data for serum testosterone concentrations. However, a trial of testosterone treatment may be warranted in selected postmenopausal women with hypoactive sexual desire in whom nonpharmacologic management is unsuccessful and who have no contraindications to testosterone[OL] (SOE=B). See "Disorders of Sexual Function," p 446.

TESTOSTERONE

Total and free testosterone levels and testosterone secretion are lower in healthy older men than in younger men. Many healthy older men exhibit moderate primary testicular failure, with decreased sperm production, testosterone levels, and testosterone secretory responses to gonadotropin administration. In addition, many of these men also have inappropriately normal (ie, not increased) gonadotropin levels in the presence of low testosterone levels, suggesting secondary (hypothalamic or pituitary) testicular failure. Overt testicular failure is common in chronically ill and debilitated older men or in men receiving chronic glucocorticoids or opioids, manifested by testosterone levels well below the normal range and symptoms suggesting androgen deficiency, including decreased libido and impotence, gynecomastia, and hot flushes. Testosterone replacement therapy may generally be warranted in these severely clinically and biochemically androgen-deficient patients, as it would be in hypogonadal young men. However, it is more common to encounter older men with low-normal or mildly decreased serum testosterone levels and nonspecific manifestations, such as decreased libido and potency, reduced energy, depressed mood, weakness, decreased muscle mass, osteopenia, metabolic syndrome, and memory loss. In most cases, these manifestations have multiple causes, but it has been hypothesized that declining testosterone levels with aging contribute to their development, and that testosterone supplementation can help to prevent or treat these disorders.

Symptoms such as poor morning erections, diminished sexual desire, and erectile dysfunction correlate with low testosterone levels in middle-aged and older men. Male hypogonadism should be diagnosed only in men with signs and symptoms suggesting androgen deficiency, as well as unequivocally low serum testosterone levels. Men with suspected hypogonadism should be evaluated initially with a morning serum total testosterone level using a reliable assay. The diagnosis should be confirmed by repeating measurement of morning total testosterone, or preferably, if available, a morning serum free or bioavailable (non–sex hormone–binding globulin-bound) testosterone level either measured by equilibrium dialysis or calculated from measurements of total testosterone and sex hormone–binding globulin (SHBG) (SOE=C).

The potential short-term benefits and risks of testosterone supplementation in older men with low-normal or mildly decreased serum testosterone levels in randomized, placebo-controlled studies of up to 3 years' duration are summarized in Table 61.5. However, it is unknown whether these potential benefits and risks are clinically important or whether longer-term potential benefits outweigh risks. In one RCT in older, functionally impaired men with low total testosterone levels and a high prevalence of hypertension, diabetes, hyperlipidemia, and obesity, testosterone-treated men experienced significantly more cardiovascular events than men receiving placebo. However, the small study size and high-risk population limit the generalizability of these findings; cardiovascular events were not increased in another

Table 61.5—Potential Short-Term Benefits and Risks of Testosterone Supplementation in Older Men with Low-Normal or Mildly Decreased Testosterone Concentrations

Study End Point	Effect of Testosterone
Lean body mass	Increased
Fat mass	Decreased
Bone mineral density	Variable; increased at lumbar spine and hip in some studies
Strength	Improved grip strength in some studies Inconsistent effect on leg muscle strength
Physical function	Inconsistent effects; improved performance of functional tasks in some studies; improvement more likely in older, more frail men in one study
Sexual function	Variable; most consistent findings are activation in sexual behavior and increased libido
Mood	Variable; mood and subjective well-being improved in some studies; inconsistent effects on depression
Cognitive	Inconsistent effects; in some studies, some cognitive domains improved (eg, verbal memory, visual memory, spatial ability, executive function); worsened effect of practice on verbal fluency
Quality of life	Inconsistent effects; some studies show significant improvement of physical function domain and improvement in subjects with more somatic symptoms at baseline
Lipid profile	Variable; total, low-density lipoprotein cholesterol and high-density lipoprotein cholesterol unchanged or decreased
Coronary heart disease	In men with established disease, improved ECG evidence of exercise-induced coronary ischemia (in most studies); variable effect on angina pectoris May increase risk of cardiovascular events in older men with extensive history of cardiovascular disease and immobility
Prostate	Prostate-specific antigen (PSA) increased slightly in many patients; significantly higher incidence of prostate-related event (increased PSA, prostate cancer, prostate biopsy) in testosterone-treated men than in placebo-treated men
Hematocrit	Increased 2.5%–5% versus baseline
Long-term clinical outcomes	Unknown

NOTE: This table summarizes results of placebo-controlled studies.

RCT of testosterone treatment in frail to intermediately frail older men. Thus, caution is suggested when using testosterone treatment in frail older men with established cardiovascular disease or cardiovascular risk factors.

After an explicit discussion of the uncertain risks and benefits of testosterone therapy, a trial of testosterone supplementation may be appropriate in older men with unequivocally low serum total testosterone levels (eg, <2.8 ng/mL) or decreased free or bioavailable testosterone levels, and clinical features suggesting hypogonadism (eg, osteoporosis, muscle wasting or weakness, mild anemia of unclear cause, loss of libido)[OL] (SOE=C). Clinicians should aim to achieve total testosterone levels in the lower part of the normal range for young men (eg, 400–500 ng/dL). Androgen replacement therapy is inappropriate in asymptomatic older men with low-normal total or free testosterone levels who do not have clinical manifestations consistent with androgen deficiency. Notably, bisphosphonates are clearly efficacious in treating older men with low testosterone and osteoporosis, so testosterone therapy is not appropriate in older men who have no manifestations of hypogonadism other than osteoporosis. Furthermore, testosterone administration is contraindicated in patients with prostate cancer and breast cancer, and should be avoided in men with an undiagnosed prostate nodule or induration on digital rectal examination, consistently increased prostate-specific antigen (PSA), erythrocytosis, severe lower urinary tract symptoms due to benign prostatic hyperplasia, or uncontrolled severe heart failure (SOE=C). For available preparations of testosterone, see Table 61.6.

Table 61.6—Testosterone Preparations Available in the United States for Hypogonadal Older Men

Preparation	Initial Treatment Dosage
Testosterone enanthate or cypionate	75 mg IM every week, or 150 mg IM every 2 weeks
Nonscrotal transdermal patch	2 or 4 mg transdermal every night
Gel	1% gel: 5–10 g transdermal every day 1.62% gel: 20.25–81 mg every day 2% gel: 10–70 mg every day
Buccal tablet	30 mg applied to buccal mucosa q12h
Testosterone pellets	150–450 mg SC every 3–6 months
Solution	30–120 mg applied to axilla once daily

Men should be monitored closely for efficacy as well as for adverse events of testosterone treatment, including new or worsening snoring, observed apnea during sleep, or excessive daytime sleepiness that may suggest obstructive sleep apnea syndrome. Routine monitoring for potential adverse effects of testosterone should be performed before initiation of therapy, 3–6 months after initiation, and then annually thereafter (SOE=C); monitoring should include measurement of serum hematocrit (to check for erythrocytosis), serum PSA and digital rectal examination (to assess for prostatic disease), and inquiry about lower urinary tract symptoms. Serum testosterone levels should also be monitored to assess the adequacy of delivery, especially in men receiving transdermal testosterone formulations (patch or gel). An increase in the PSA concentration to >4 ng/mL or an increase of >1.4 ng/mL over baseline within any 12-month period after starting testosterone therapy can indicate the presence of previously undetected prostate cancer, and testosterone should be discontinued until the prostate has been fully evaluated (SOE=C). However, there is no direct evidence that testosterone therapy increases risk of prostate cancer or symptomatic benign prostatic hyperplasia. See also "Disorders of Sexual Function," p 446.

ESTROGEN THERAPY

Many of the symptoms and signs of hormone deficiency mimic physiologic changes associated with aging. The fact that many hormones also decline with aging has led to an enthusiasm for attempting to reverse unwanted changes associated with aging by the use of hormonal replacement. Based on very compelling epidemiologic data, replacement of estrogen, with or without progesterone, was once the standard of care for postmenopausal women, but is no longer because of more recent data from randomized clinical trials demonstrating significant adverse events from such therapy. Estrogen therapy is now largely limited to treatment of menopausal symptoms (see treatment of menopausal symptoms in "Gynecologic Diseases and Disorders," p 431).

Three meta-analyses of observational studies have demonstrated an association of estrogen therapy in women with a reduction in heart disease by half. However, a few long-term prospective studies of secondary prevention demonstrated increased mortality in the first year on therapy, with improved survival in years 2 through 5, leading to no net benefit. In another trial of women with coronary artery disease, no benefit from estrogen was found for angiographic changes of atherosclerosis. The Women's Health Initiative (WHI) is a set of clinical trials to test primary prevention of coronary artery disease with estrogen and estrogen–progesterone combinations. The estrogen–progesterone arm was discontinued early because of the increased risk of coronary disease, breast cancer, stroke, and deep-vein thrombosis (SOE=A); the estrogen-alone arm of the study was discontinued because of increased risk of stroke (SOE=A). Post-hoc analysis of the WHI data suggest that risk of cardiovascular events was increased in older women and with increased years since menopause.

Although observational studies also suggested that estrogen may have a role in preventing dementia, a placebo-controlled trial of estrogen replacement given for 1 year to 120 women with early to moderate Alzheimer dementia found no improvement in affective or cognitive outcomes. In the WHI, in a study to assess primary prevention, women in the estrogen arm had clinically important declines in their Mini–Mental State Examination scores or transition to mild cognitive impairment or dementia.

The risks of breast cancer, endometrial cancer, and deep-vein thrombosis/pulmonary emboli associated with the use of estrogen have been well established; these results were confirmed in the WHI trial. A recent study to assess change in risk approximately 3 years after the WHI trials were discontinued demonstrated continued increased risk with previous estrogen use due to fatal and nonfatal malignancies. The risk of breast cancer was similar to that in the nontreatment arm at the 3-year follow-up and the previously demonstrated beneficial effects on colon cancer had dissipated, but risk of lung cancer was higher than in the nontreatment arm. Overall mortality was similar in the estrogen and placebo groups. See also estrogen therapy for osteoporosis prevention in "Osteoporosis," p 243.

GROWTH HORMONE

Growth hormone secretion declines with aging, and by 70–80 years of age, about half of adults have no significant growth hormone secretion over 24 hours. A corresponding decline occurs in concentrations of insulin-like growth factor 1, which mediates most of the effects of growth hormone; in 40% of adults 70–80 years old, it falls to concentrations comparable to those in growth hormone–deficient children.

Adults with growth hormone deficiency due to hypothalamic-pituitary disease exhibit decreased muscle strength, lean body mass, and bone density; increased abdominal obesity; unfavorable lipid profiles; and an increased risk of cardiovascular disease. Many of these clinical consequences of growth hormone deficiency improve with growth hormone replacement, but not all studies have demonstrated improvements in muscle strength, and the effects on cardiovascular risk are unknown. Older adults without hypothalamic-pituitary disease have many of the same conditions, which leads to the hypothesis that growth hormone supplementation may have a beneficial effect on these clinically important age-related disorders. Randomized controlled trials of short-term growth hormone supplementation in older adults have reported increased lean body mass (change in lean body mass, 2.1 kg [CI, 1.3 to 2.9]) and decreased fat mass (change in fat mass, –2.1 kg [CI 95%, –2.8 to –1.35]). However, growth hormone was not found to augment improvements in muscle strength achieved with exercise alone, no improvements in functional status were demonstrated, and there were no significant improvements in bone density or lipid levels after adjustment for body composition changes (SOE=A). Furthermore, significant adverse events were common, including carpal tunnel syndrome, arthralgias, edema, and gynecomastia. The long-term efficacy and safety of growth hormone administration in older adults are unknown. Short-term growth hormone supplementation may improve nitrogen balance in older adults with severe illness and catabolic states. However, growth hormone is very expensive, and at present it is not recommended for clinical use in older adults who do not have established hypothalamic-pituitary disease.

MELATONIN

Melatonin, a hormone secreted by the pineal gland, is thought to be involved in the regulation of circadian and seasonal biorhythms. Melatonin secretion is inhibited by exposure to light, resulting in a marked circadian variation in circulating melatonin concentrations. Its sedative effects suggest a role in sleep induction. Most studies show that plasma melatonin concentrations decline throughout life after early childhood, but the physiologic significance of this decline in melatonin secretion is unclear. Numerous claims have been made in the lay press regarding the "antiaging" benefits of melatonin supplementation for various conditions, including insomnia, immune deficiency, cancer, and the aging process itself. In placebo-controlled trials up to 6 months, sustained-release melatonin reduced the time to sleep onset in older adults with insomnia, and 2 days of treatment with sustained-release melatonin did not impair psychomotor function, memory recall, and driving skills in older adults. In patients with dementia, a Cochrane review did not find evidence that melatonin is effective for cognitive impairment, although it may be effective for the treatment of dementia-related mood and behavior disturbances. The longer-term risks and benefits of melatonin supplementation have not been established for insomnia or any other indication.

REFERENCES

- Donangelo I, Braunstein GD. Update on subclinical hyperthyroidism. *Am Fam Physician.* 2011;83(8):933–938.
- Gordon CM, Hanley DA, Heaney RP, et al. Evaluation, treatment, and prevention of vitamin D deficiency: an Endocrine Society Clinical Practice Guideline. *J Clin Endocrinol Metab.* 2011;96(7):1911–1930.
- Song JH, Mayo-Smith WW. Incidentally discovered adrenal mass. *Radiol Clin North Am.* 2011;49(2):361–368.
- Wu B, Haigh PI, Hwang R, et al. Underutilization of parathyroidectomy in elderly patients with primary hyperparathyroidism. *J Clin Endocrinol Metab.* 2010;95(9):4324–4330.

CHAPTER 62—DIABETES MELLITUS

KEY POINTS

- Diabetes mellitus, one of the most common chronic conditions in older adults, results in decreased life expectancy, numerous complications and comorbidities, a higher risk of other common geriatric conditions (eg, polypharmacy, urinary incontinence, falls, cognitive impairment, depression, and chronic pain), functional impairment, and disability.
- Both diabetes and impaired glucose tolerance are important to identify and address by changes in lifestyle.
- Because of the great heterogeneity in the older population, treatment goals for older diabetic patients must be carefully individualized.
- Although the target blood pressure is debated, attempts to lower blood pressure are important for older hypertensive diabetic patients.
- Diabetes self-management is an important part of diabetes care, and annual self-management training is a covered benefit under Medicare Part B.

Diabetes mellitus is a group of metabolic disorders characterized by hyperglycemia due to abnormalities in insulin secretion, insulin action, or both. It is one of the most common chronic diseases affecting older adults. The CDC estimates that among people ≥65 years old, 10.9 million, or 26.9%, have diagnosed or undiagnosed diabetes. Because the general population is aging and rates of obesity are increasing among middle-aged adults, people ≥65 years old will constitute the majority of diabetic adults in the United States and in other developed countries in the coming decades. In the United States, people ≥65 years old now account for more than 40% of all people with diabetes. In the coming years, the largest percent increase in diabetes prevalence in any age group will be among those >75 years old.

The age-adjusted prevalence of diabetes mellitus is higher among black Americans and Hispanic Americans than white Americans. Further, black Americans suffer from complications of diabetes at disproportionately higher rates than white Americans. Research is only starting to decipher the effects of race on diabetes development and outcomes.

Because diabetes may be asymptomatic for many years, some people with diabetes mellitus are unaware of their condition. Despite the early asymptomatic period, diabetes mellitus is a serious condition associated with significant morbidity and a shortened survival. Older adults with diabetes can expect a 10-year reduction in life expectancy and a mortality rate nearly twice that of people without this disease. In addition, older adults disproportionately experience the clinical complications and comorbidities associated with diabetes. These complications include atherosclerosis, neuropathies, loss of vision, and renal insufficiency. The rates of myocardial infarction, stroke, and kidney failure are increased approximately 2-fold, and the risk of blindness is increased approximately 40% in older adults with diabetes. Most patients ≥65 years old who require dialysis have diabetes.

Research is accumulating about important clinical consequences of diabetes that are common in older adults and have serious consequences to health status and quality of life. When diabetes is poorly controlled in older adults, hyperglycemia alone can be the cause of insidious decline characterized by fatigue, weight loss, muscle weakness, and reduced function. Older adults with diabetes are at higher risk than those without diabetes for geriatric syndromes, including incontinence, falls, frailty, cognitive impairment, and depressive symptoms; they also have a higher prevalence of functional impairment and disability. Mobility problems are about 2 to 3 times more likely, and disability in ADLs is about 1.5 times more likely in older adults with diabetes than in those without.

PATHOPHYSIOLOGY OF DIABETES IN OLDER ADULTS

The American Diabetes Association (ADA) classifies diabetes mellitus affecting older adults into three types. Type 1 is the result of an absolute deficiency in insulin secretion due to autoimmune destruction of the β cells of the pancreas. Type 2 is most commonly due to tissue resistance to insulin action and relative insulin deficiency. A third category is reserved for other specific types of diabetes: injuries to the exocrine pancreas; endocrinopathies characterized by excesses of hormones, such as growth hormone, cortisol, glucagon, and epinephrine, which antagonize insulin action; drug- or chemical-induced diabetes; and infections leading to the destruction of the β cells of the pancreas.

In about 90% of cases, older adults with diabetes have the type 2 form of the disease. Most older adults with type 2 diabetes have had years of abnormal glucose metabolism, with decreased glucose intolerance and/or impaired fasting glucose, and insulin resistance. This "prediabetes" syndrome is also associated with increased risk of atherosclerotic disease, as well as development of type 2 diabetes. Prediabetes is important to recognize and evaluate in order to manage associated atherosclerosis risk factors such as hypertension and dyslipidemia that commonly occur with prediabetes.

The prevalence of both type 2 diabetes and glucose intolerance increases with age. The reasons for this are not fully known; there appears to be an interaction among several factors, including genetics, lifestyle, and aging influences. Obesity and decreased physical activity, common among older adults, contribute to impairments in insulin action. Glucose intolerance has also been shown to be related to age-associated decline in pancreatic β-cell function and in the insulin-signaling mechanisms that limit the mobilization of glucose transporters needed for insulin-mediated glucose uptake and metabolism in muscle and fat. Changes in body composition that occur with aging, such as increased visceral fat leading to insulin resistance, can also contribute to changes in carbohydrate metabolism. Decreased levels of physical activity in some older adults can exacerbate age-related changes in body composition and increased carbohydrate intolerance. An altered inflammatory environment with aging can also contribute to the higher rates of diabetes in older adults.

In addition to intrinsic physiologic mechanisms, external factors can contribute to glucose intolerance and type 2 diabetes. Some medications commonly taken by older adults—diuretics, sympathomimetics, glucocorticoids, niacin, and olanzapine—change carbohydrate metabolism and increase glucose concentration. Concurrent illnesses, such as infections, myocardial infarction, and stroke, as well as other physiologic stresses can lead to worsened hyperglycemia. The heterogeneity in the severity of hyperglycemia among older adults with type 2 diabetes is related to the varying contributions of these factors in each individual.

The pathophysiology of the complications of diabetes is similar in younger and older adults. Prolonged hyperglycemia leads to glycosylation of proteins; the accumulation of these abnormal proteins can cause tissue damage. Also, metabolic products of the aldose-reductase system, such as sorbitol, accumulate in the presence of hyperglycemia. These products can impair cellular energy metabolism and contribute to cell injury and death.

Physiologic changes that develop with diabetes and its complications can interact with physiologic changes associated with aging to further decrease physiologic reserve. Type 2 diabetes and obesity are associated with inflammatory dysregulation, which can also be associated with aging and lead to clinical sequelae such as sarcopenia. Aging is associated with decreased physiologic reserve in multiple organ systems (eg, renal, cardiovascular, CNS), which may interact with end-organ damage due to diabetes, resulting in increased vulnerability to physiologic stressors.

DIAGNOSIS AND EVALUATION

In 2009, an international group of diabetes experts recommended using a hemoglobin A_{1c} (HbA_{1c}) level of ≥6.5% to diagnose diabetes; the ADA participated in that decision and formally adopted this recommendation in 2010. This decision was based on the ease of performing the HbA_{1c} test, which can facilitate diagnosis of more people with diabetes. Only an HbA_{1c} test that meets standards of the National Glycohemoglobin Standardization Program (NGSP) can be used for diagnosis (pinprick tests are not acceptable). Although epidemiologic studies demonstrate that the tests identify somewhat different groups of people, the groups are similar. None of the diagnostic criteria include any adjustments for age. The four ways to establish the diagnosis of diabetes mellitus are summarized below; each must be confirmed, on a subsequent day, preferably by the same method:

- HbA_{1c} ≥6.5% using an assay standardized to the NGSP
- Symptoms of polyuria, polydipsia, and unexplained weight loss plus a random plasma glucose concentration of ≥200 mg/dL (11.1 mmol/L)
- A plasma glucose concentration after an 8-hour fast of ≥126 mg/dL (7 mmol/L)
- A plasma glucose concentration of ≥200 mg/dL (11.1 mmol/L) measured 2 hours after ingestion of 75 g of glucose in 300 mL of water administered after an overnight fast

Older adults with a fasting blood glucose of 100–125 mg/dL (5.6–6.9 mmol/L), a 2-h plasma glucose of 140–199 mg/dL (7.8–11.0 mmol/L) after a 75-g oral glucose tolerance test, or an HbA_{1c} of 5.7%–6.4% are considered to have prediabetes. Some older adults have isolated postchallenge hyperglycemia but do not have high fasting blood glucose concentrations; many of these people would be diagnosed as having type 2 diabetes by oral glucose tolerance testing criteria. Isolated postchallenge hyperglycemia does appear to confer increased risk of atherosclerotic complications but not as much as diagnosed type 2 diabetes.

Several diabetes prevention trials demonstrated that in people with prediabetes, progression to type 2 diabetes can be prevented by medications and lifestyle changes (SOE=A). Lifestyle changes were found to be slightly more efficacious in older than in younger adults and superior to medications in the older group. These results demonstrate the importance of preventive measures and lifestyle changes in older adults who are at risk of developing type 2 diabetes.

MANAGEMENT

General Principles

Older adults with diabetes require a comprehensive evaluation, which in the primary care setting may be done over several patient visits. For patients with significant functional impairments and comorbidities, including those with psychosocial problems and caregiver requirements, a formal, comprehensive geriatric assessment may be needed. Regardless of how the comprehensive evaluation of an older adult with diabetes mellitus is handled, four issues deserve special attention.

First, the history and physical examination must include evaluation of risk factors for atherosclerotic disease and the presence of all comorbid diseases. Diabetes is a well-established risk factor for atherosclerotic cardiovascular disease, so other risk factors such as smoking, family history, hypertension, and hyperlipidemia should also be explored. Diabetes is also associated with multiple vascular complications that may be subclinical or clinical. The presence of coronary artery disease, peripheral vascular disease, neuropathy, foot problems, and medical eye disease must be determined. In many cases, subspecialty consultation (as for retinopathy) and laboratory or diagnostic testing is indicated. In addition, older adults with diabetes are also likely to have prevalent chronic diseases that are not necessarily associated with their diabetes, such as osteoarthritis.

Second, a thorough medication history is important. As previously stated, certain medications can contribute to hyperglycemia. More often, older adults may be on multiple medications for multiple comorbidities and may experience adverse drug events or trouble with medication management or finances, which will affect formulating the treatment plan.

Third, an assessment of functional status is important to help determine whether the patient is able to independently manage his or her diabetes, or whether caregiver input is also needed. Functional assessment will also assist the clinician and patient in setting diabetes management targets and assessing the patient's ability to increase physical activity.

Fourth, older adults should be screened for the use of multiple medications, depression, cognitive impairment, urinary incontinence, injurious falls, and pain. Multiple observational studies have shown that these geriatric conditions are more common in older adults with diabetes than without (SOE=B). Finally, each patient's needs for diabetes education and self-management support, including whether to involve a caregiver, should be assessed.

The clinician develops goals for diabetes management and individualized clinical targets with each older adult with diabetes, involving the caregiver when appropriate. The goals of diabetes management in older adults include the following:

- control of hyperglycemia and its symptoms
- evaluation and treatment of associated risks for atherosclerotic and microvascular disease
- evaluation and treatment of diabetes complications
- support for diabetes self-management and education
- maintenance or improvement of general health status

Although these goals are similar for older and younger people with diabetes, the management of older patients is complicated by the medical and functional heterogeneity of this group. In fact, this heterogeneity is a key consideration in developing individualized diabetes management interventions and clinical targets for older patients with diabetes. Some may have developed diabetes in middle age and have developed multiple related comorbidities. Some may be recently diagnosed but have had undiagnosed diabetes for years and have complications at diagnosis. Others may have just converted from impaired glucose tolerance to diabetes and may have few complications or comorbidities. In addition to medical heterogeneity, older adults with diabetes are heterogeneous in their functional status. Many are active with excellent function. Others may be disabled and frail, with advanced cognitive impairment, multiple comorbidities and complications, and significant functional limitations. Many others are in between, with mild or early functional limitations, several related comorbidities, and multiple risks for worsening morbidity. Several researchers have pointed out the burden that some patients with diabetes complications and other comorbidities experience trying to cope with self-management of multiple chronic diseases.

Another consideration in treating older adults with diabetes is life expectancy and the time needed for clinical benefit from a specific intervention. Clinical trials have demonstrated that approximately 8 years are needed before the benefits of glycemic control are reflected in reduced microvascular complications such as diabetic retinopathy or kidney disease, but that only 2–3 years are required to see benefits from better control of blood pressure and lipids (SOE=A). It is important to remember that the median remaining life expectancy for a 70-year-old woman is 14 years, which is plenty of time for the development of diabetes complications.

Therefore, for a person in his or her early 70s who is newly diagnosed or highly functional, diabetes management is no different from that of younger people. However, management must be designed to fit the clinical status of older adults who are significantly functionally impaired or who have multiple comorbidities that limit life expectancy or that significantly increase the risks of hypoglycemia. In all cases, patient preferences and quality of life must be considered.

Solid evidence supports the effectiveness of several components of diabetes care, including control of lipids and blood pressure, control of hyperglycemia, aspirin use, smoking cessation, appropriate eye and foot care, prevention of nephropathy, diabetes education and self-management support for medication adherence, appropriate nutrition, weight loss if indicated, and increased physical activity (SOE=A). Home monitoring of blood glucose has not been found to be cost-effective (SOE=A). Very few of the data supporting these interventions were obtained from research studies of older people. In addition, debates continue about the targets for glycemic and blood pressure control; there is less debate about low-density lipoprotein (LDL) cholesterol targets (targets are further discussed in a following section). It is likely that many management guidelines can be generalized to many older adults with diabetes, particularly those who are healthy and functional. For some older patients, particularly those with severe comorbidities and disabilities, aggressive management is not likely to provide benefit and may even result in harm, such as hypoglycemia with aggressive glycemic control or hypotension with aggressive blood-pressure control.

Patient preferences regarding management interventions are also important to elicit and consider, because the patient is the one who will ultimately manage his or her diabetes and comorbid conditions. Some patients do not want to follow some management recommendations. Some fear dependency and the need for assistance more than death. Some find certain medications or monitoring activities burdensome.

Therefore, it is important to establish individual goals for diabetes management and clinical targets with patients; to reevaluate the clinical, functional, and social status of the patient if these goals and targets are not being met; and to determine if caregiver support or specialty input is needed. A practical clinical method of individualizing and prioritizing diabetes care is to assess goals and preferences, assess patient longevity and functional status, consider the time needed for treatment impact, screen for geriatric syndromes, and assist patients with decision making and prioritization of treatment strategies.

In 2003, the California Healthcare Foundation (CHF) and the American Geriatrics Society (AGS) collaborated to develop one of the first set of guidelines for improving the care of older adults with diabetes mellitus. Since this guideline was developed, ideas such as individualizing glycemic targets and evaluating geriatric conditions and common comorbidities such as falls and gait disorders, depression, cognition and functioning in older adults with diabetes are now widely accepted. Since then, several landmark studies, most importantly the Action to Control Cardiovascular Risk in Diabetes (ACCORD), the VA Diabetes Trial (VADT), and the Action in Diabetes and Vascular Disease: Preterax and Diamicron Modified-Release Controlled Evaluation (ADVANCE) trials) have included older adults with prevalent diabetes and comorbidities and have added to the evidence base about management of the types of patients that are commonly seen in an office practice. The references (at end of chapter) include the 2003 CHF/AGS Guidelines, the ADVANCE and ACCORD findings about treatment of hypertension in patients with diabetes, and an excellent review of the evidence base for diabetes management and its gaps regarding treatment of older adults.

Atherosclerotic Complications

Older adults with diabetes are at high risk of atherosclerosis and its complications. In fact, virtually all older adults with diabetes have either clinical or preclinical atherosclerotic disease. Therefore, interventions that reduce the risk of atherosclerotic diseases are extremely important. Smoking cessation counseling and pharmacologic intervention should be offered to any older adult with diabetes who smokes. Daily aspirin therapy should be offered to older adults with diabetes if there is not a contraindication to aspirin. Available evidence suggests that dosages from 81 to 325 mg/d are appropriate.

A number of randomized controlled trials (RCTs) provide strong evidence that the management of hypertension in older adults reduces cardiovascular events and mortality; some of these studies included substantial numbers of older adults with diabetes (SOE=A). The best target blood pressure for older diabetic patients is not clear, but experts suggest that in most patients the target blood pressure should be <140/80 mmHg. In 5 major RCTs of blood-pressure control that included people with diabetes, levels <140/80 mmHg were achieved in only one. However, in the ADVANCE trial, with 11,140 people in multiple sites around the world with a mean age of 66 years, a mean blood pressure of 136/73 mmHg was achieved in the intensive treatment group. The relative risk of cardiovascular death decreased 18% in the intensive group; the relative risk of all-cause death decreased 14% (ARR=1.3%, NNT=79 for all-cause mortality over

5 years) (SOE=A). However, there was no difference in new cardiovascular events. In the ACCORD study, a blood pressure of <119/70 mmHg was achieved in the intensive treatment arm versus 140/70 mmHg in the standard treatment arm. No significant benefit of intensive blood pressure on cardiovascular outcomes was observed (SOE=A). Current targets for hypertension management in diabetes continue to be debated, but <140/70 mmHg appears to be appropriate based on current evidence. Although observational studies suggest that lowering blood pressure to <130/70 mmHg may provide increased benefit, these two studies taken together cannot support blood pressure targets more specific than <140/80 mmHg. Because some older adults may not be able to tolerate aggressive blood-pressure lowering, hypertension should be treated gradually to avoid complications. Patient preference and adverse events of medication should be considered. There is concern that overtreatment of hypertension in older adults with diabetes could increase risk of cardiac events or falls. The evidence for these adverse events is mixed, but management to <140/80 mmHg is now most consistent with available evidence. Evidence for medication choice in older adults with diabetes suggests that most classes chosen (diuretics, ACE inhibitors, β-blockers, and calcium channel blockers) have comparable effectiveness in reducing cardiovascular disease and mortality. Evidence suggests that ACE inhibitors (SOE=A) and angiotensin II receptor blockers (SOE=B) have additional cardiovascular and renal benefit for people with diabetes.

Evidence supports the use of lipid-lowering therapy; RCTs and a meta-analysis have confirmed the benefit of the statin drugs, particularly for secondary prevention of cardiovascular events (SOE=A). In general, most studies with statin management suggest that patients with diabetes benefit more from cholesterol lowering than those without diabetes, and secondary prevention is particularly beneficial. Analyses have calculated NNTs of 14 to 46 for prevention of one major cardiovascular event over 5 years of lipid-lowering treatment in diabetic patients. However, some controversy still exists regarding the treatment of cholesterol in older adults with diabetes for primary prevention. The one major study (Prospective Study of Pravastatin in the Elderly at Risk, or PROSPER) of statin treatment in older adults, which included some people with diabetes, did not find benefit for primary prevention.

Even with statin therapy, rates of cardiovascular events remain high, and observational and pilot research suggests broader targeting of dyslipidemia. However, ACCORD tested the use of fenfibrate in addition to a statin and found no benefit (SOE=A).

Lipid abnormalities should be corrected in older adults with diabetes when appropriate after considering the individual's overall health status. Evidence suggests that the target LDL level is <100 mg/dL (SOE=B). Dietary modification can be tried for 6 months if the LDL level is <100–129 mg/dL. If the LDL level is ≥130 mg/dL, pharmacologic therapy is indicated in addition to lifestyle modifications in diet and activity level. Older adults are always at risk of adverse drug events, so when an older adult with diabetes is prescribed a statin or niacin, or when the dosage is increased, an alanine aminotransferase concentration should be measured within 12 weeks of starting the medication or changing the dosage. Also, some people may develop muscle inflammation with the statins, so symptoms of muscle pain and weakness in the presence of statin therapy must be evaluated. Recent evidence has suggested several problems with high-dose statin use, including increased muscle toxicity (with high-dose simvastatin) and increased risk of new-onset diabetes (SOE=A). This is of some concern because target LDL levels are not achieved in some people with regular doses of a statin. If a fibrate has been started or increased, liver enzymes should be evaluated annually.

Microvascular Complications

Microvascular complications of diabetes are major problems among older adults with diabetes and can be important contributors to disability. Diabetic retinopathy can result in decreased vision. Other eye conditions, such as glaucoma and cataracts, are also extremely common in older adults with diabetes. Any older adult with new-onset diabetes should have a screening dilated-eye examination by an eye-care specialist. If there is presence of retinopathy, other eye disease, ocular symptoms, poorly controlled hyperglycemia, or poorly controlled hypertension, a dilated-eye examination should be done every year. If there is no ocular disease or high risk, eye examinations can be performed every other year (SOE=D).

Serious foot problems and amputations are more common among older adults with diabetes than those without diabetes. These patients should have a careful foot examination at least annually or more frequently if there is evidence of any problems. To screen for kidney disease, a test for the presence of microalbuminuria should be performed at diagnosis and annually if no abnormalities are detected. Finally, given a higher mortality rate among diabetic patients who develop pneumonia, pneumococcal vaccination is strongly recommended.

Hyperglycemia

Control of hyperglycemia in diabetes is important to prevent the symptoms of uncontrolled hyperglycemia, such as weight loss, fatigue, sometimes the classic polyuria and polydipsia, and possibly increased infections. Treatment of hyperglycemia in type 2 diabetes to prevent vascular complication is more controversial. There is evidence that control of hyperglycemia to near-normal levels may prevent retinal and renal complications, but the effects may be modest, and RCTs have failed to support the hypothesis that intensive glycemic control prevents cardiovascular disease (SOE=A). The risks and benefits of intensive glycemic control are actively debated, and the most appropriate HbA_{1c} target for people of all ages with type 2 diabetes is unclear. One RCT was stopped early because of an increased mortality rate in the intensively treated group (SOE=A). RCTs of treatment of hyperglycemia near normal levels in older adults with diabetes did not demonstrate that this would prevent cardiovascular disease. They did, however, find that control of hyperglycemia to a target HbA_{1c} <7% in those with longstanding diabetes reduced microalbumin and lower rates of microvascular complications (SOE=A).

The VADT and ADVANCE trials did find that control of hyperglycemia to a target HbA_{1c} <7% in patients with long-standing diabetes reduced microalbuminuria, and analyses of ACCORD also show lower rates of microvascular complications (SOE=A). Given these findings, glycemic targets for all patients with diabetes are unclear and continue to be debated. The ADA has a position paper that has reviewed these studies and their implications in detail. Management of hyperglycemia to an HbA_{1c} level between 7.0% and 8.5%, depending on the individual patient's management plan and the duration of his or her diabetes, is reasonable (SOE=C).

There are many options for drug therapy in older adults with type 2 diabetes, with no clearly preferred algorithm. Few comparisons of the medications are available, and most studies have focused on decreasing hyperglycemia, an intermediate outcome. Little information is available about adverse drug events other than hypoglycemia.

Hyperglycemia-lowering regimens can consist of any of several classes of drugs (Table 62.1 and Table 62.2), used alone or in combination. The regimen should be adjusted over the course of the illness as goals change, the disease progresses, or complications develop. Sulfonylurea preparations have a long record of safety and effectiveness. Hypoglycemia is a serious adverse event, and these medications must be used cautiously in older adults with significant hepatic and renal insufficiency, because the liver is the primary site of metabolism and excretion is via the kidneys. α-Glucosidase inhibitors impair the breakdown of carbohydrates in the gut and limit absorption; the residual carbohydrates in the intestinal lumen are responsible for diarrhea observed in about 25% of older adults who use these medications. The biguanide preparations also have GI adverse events and can theoretically cause lactic acidosis in older adults with renal insufficiency. However, a Cochrane review of metformin found no significantly increased risk of lactic acidosis. If an older adult is taking metformin, serum creatinine concentration should be measured at least annually and with any increase in dosage. For those ≥80 years old or those suspected to have reduced muscle mass, renal function should be assessed thoroughly, either through a timed urine collection or application of a formula that corrects serum creatinine for age.

Another class of drugs, the thiazolidinediones, although apparently well tolerated by most patients, carries black box warnings because of a risk of worsening of heart failure and other cardiovascular complications. In a recent meta-analysis of 42 clinical studies, data indicated that one of these drugs (rosiglitazone) is associated with an increased risk of myocardial ischemic events, such as heart attack and stroke. As of September 2010, the FDA has restricted the use of rosiglitazone to patients with type 2 diabetes whose diabetes is not controlled on other medications. Restricted access to rosiglitazone will be accomplished through the use of a risk evaluation and mitigation strategy. Complete details of the FDA safety alert are available at: www.fda.gov/Safety/MedWatch/SafetyInformation/SafetyAlertsforHumanMedicalProducts/ucm226994.htm (accessed Oct 2013).

The DPP-4 enzyme inhibitors, and newer injectable agents such as exenetide, are effective in lowering glucose but have a limited role in routine care of older adults with diabetes. These drugs are contraindicated in significant chronic kidney disease, and exenetide is associated with hypoglycemia. Both are expensive and confer no benefit over the usual oral hypoglycemics.

Finally, insulin can be used effectively in older adults with type 2 diabetes. Good glycemic control can often be achieved with one or two injections a day of an intermediate-acting insulin preparation. The greatest risk of insulin therapy is hypoglycemia, and evidence suggests that frail older adults are at higher risk of serious hypoglycemia than are healthier, more functional older adults. The management plan for an older adult with diabetes who experiences severe or frequent hypoglycemia should be evaluated, and an appropriate higher glycemic target set. Hypoglycemia is increasingly being recognized as a relatively uncommon but important problem among older adults with diabetes. It is thought to have played a role in the excess mortality in the ACCORD trial. Long-acting sulfonylureas can cause hypoglycemia. In patients with a history of hypoglycemia, or those with multiple comorbidities and poor functional status who are at risk of hypoglycemia, short-acting sulfonylureas or oral hypoglycemics that do not cause hypoglycemia should

Table 62.1—Non-Insulin Agents for Treating Diabetes Mellitus

Medication	Dosage	Formulations	Comments (Metabolism)
Oral Agents			
Biguanide			Decrease hepatic glucose production; lower HbA_{1c} by 1%–2%; do not cause hypoglycemia
Metformin (generic or Glucophage)	500–2,550 mg divided	T: 500, 850, 1,000	Avoid in patients with eGFR <30 mL/1.73 m^2, heart failure, COPD, increased liver enzymes; hold before contrast radiologic studies; may cause weight loss (K)
(Riomet [oral solution])		100 mg/mL	
(generic or Glucophage XR, Fortamet, Glumetza)	1,500–2,000 mg/d	T: ER 500, 750, 1000	Same as above
2nd-Generation Sulfonylureas			Increase insulin secretion; lower HbA_{1c} by 1%–2%; can cause hypoglycemia and weight gain
Glimepiride (generic or Amaryl)	4–8 mg once (begin 1–2 mg)	T: 1, 2, 4	Numerous drug interactions, long-acting (L, K)
Glipizide (generic or Glucotrol)	2.5–40 mg once or divided	T: 5, 10	Short-acting (L, K)
(generic or Glucotrol XL)	5–20 mg once	T: ER 2.5, 5, 10	Long-acting (L, K)
Glyburide (generic or Diaβeta, Micronase)	1.25–20 mg once or divided	T: 1.25, 2.5, 5	Long-acting, increased risk of hypoglycemia; not recommended for use in older adults (L, K)
Micronized glyburide (Glynase)	1.5–12 mg once	T: 1.5, 3, 4.5, 6	Long-acting, increased risk of hypoglycemia; not recommended for use in older adults (L, K)
α-Glucosidase Inhibitors			Delay glucose absorption; lower HbA_{1c} by 0.5%–1%; can cause hypoglycemia and weight gain
Acarbose (generic or Precose)	50–100 mg 3 times/d with first bite of meal; start with 25 mg/d	T: 25, 50, 100	GI adverse events common, avoid if Cr >2 mg/dL, monitor liver enzymes (gut, K)
Miglitol (Glyset)	25–100 mg 3 times/d with first bite of meal; start with 25 mg/d	T: 25, 50, 100	Same as acarbose but no need to monitor liver enzymes (L, K)
DPP-4 Enzyme Inhibitors			Protect and enhance endogenous incretin hormones; lowers HbA_{1c} by 0.5%–1%; do not cause hypoglycemia, weight neutral
Linagliptin (Tradjenta)	5 mg	T: 5	(L)
Saxagliptin (Onglyza)	5 mg; 2.5 mg if CrCl <50 mL/min	T: 2.5, 5	(K)
Sitagliptin (Januvia)	100 mg once daily as monotherapy or in combination with metformin or a thiazolidinedione; 50 mg/d if CrCl 31–50 mL/min; 25 mg/d if CrCl <30 mL/min	T: 25, 50, 100	
Meglitinides			Increase insulin secretion; lower HbA_{1c} by 1%–2%; can cause hypoglycemia and weight gain
Nateglinide (Starlix)	60–120 mg 3 times/d before meals	T: 60, 120	Give 30 minutes before meals
Repaglinide (Prandin)	0.5 mg 3 times/d before meals if HbA_{1c} <8% or previously untreated; 1–2 mg 3 times/d before meals if HbA_{1c} ≥8% or previously treated	T: 0.5, 1, 2	Give 30 minutes before meals, adjust dosage at weekly intervals, potential for drug interactions, caution in hepatic or renal insufficiency (L)
Thiazolidinediones			Insulin resistance reducers; lower HbA_{1c} by 0.5%–1.5%; increased risk of heart failure; avoid if NYHA Class III or IV cardiac status; discontinue if any decline in cardiac status; weight gain; check liver enzymes at start, every 2 months during first year, then periodically; avoid if clinical evidence of liver disease or if serum ALT levels >2.5 times upper limit of normal; may increase risk of fractures in women (L, K)

Table 62.1—Non-Insulin Agents for Treating Diabetes Mellitus (continued)

Medication	Dosage	Formulations	Comments (Metabolism)
Pioglitazone (generic or Actos)	15 or 30 mg/d; max 45 mg/d as monotherapy, 30 mg/d in combination therapy	T: 15, 30, 45	
Rosiglitazone (Avandia)	4 mg q12–24h	T: 2, 4, 8	*Restricted access:* Because of data suggesting higher cardiovascular risk, people with type 2 diabetes who are not currently taking rosiglitazone can be prescribed the medication only if glycemic control cannot be achieved with an alternative medication. Rosiglitazone will continue to be available to those who are currently taking it only if they appear to be benefiting and understand the risks.
Combinations			
Glipizide and metformin (generic or METAGLIP)	2.5/250 mg once; 20/2,000 in 2 divided doses	T: 2.5/250, 2.5/500, 5/500	Avoid in patients >80 years old, Cr >1.5 mg/dL in men, Cr >1.4 mg/dL in women; see individual drugs (L, K)
Glyburide and metformin (generic or Glucovance)	1.25/250 mg initially if previously untreated; 2.5/500 mg or 5/500 mg q12h with meals; maximum 20/2,000/d	T: 1.25/250, 2.5/500, 5/500	Starting dose should not exceed total daily dose of either drug; see individual drugs (L, K)
Linagliptin and metformin (Jentadueto)	2.5/500 to 2.5/1,000 2 times/d	T: 2.5/500, 2.5/850, 2.5/1,000	
Pioglitazone and glimepiride (Duetect)	30/2 mg initially; max 45/8 mg	T: 30/2, 30/4	See individual drugs.
Pioglitazone and metformin (ACTO plus met)	15/850 mg q12–24h	T: 15/850	See individual drugs.
Repaglinide and metformin (PrandiMet)	1/500 mg to 4/1,000 mg twice q12h or q8h before meals; maximum 10/2,500 mg/d	T: 1/500, 2/500	See individual drugs.
Rosiglitazone and glimepiride (Avandaryl)	1 or 2 tab/d; max 8 mg/4 mg	T: 4/1, 4/2, 4/4, 8/2, 8/4	See individual drugs.
Rosiglitazone and metformin (Avandamet)	4/1,000–8/2,000 in 2 divided doses	T: 1/500, 2/500, 4/500, 2/1,000, 4/1,000	Avoid in patients >80 years old, Cr >1.5 mg/dL in men, Cr >1.4 mg/dL in women; see individual drugs (L, K)
Saxagliptin and metformin (Kombiglyze XR)	5/1,000–2,000 once	T: ER 5/500, 5/1,000, 2.5/1,000	See individual drugs.
Sitagliptin and metformin (Janumet)	Begin with current doses; maximum 100/2,000 mg in 2 divided doses	T: 50/500, 50/1,000	See individual drugs.
Injectable Agents			Hypoglycemia common if combined with sulfonyl urea or insulin
Exenatide *(*Byetta*)*	5–10 mcg SC twice daily with meals	1.2-, 2.4-mL prefilled pen	Incretin mimetic; lowers HbA_{1c} by 0.4%–0.9%; nausea and hypoglycemia common; less weight gain than insulin; avoid if CrCl <30 mL/min (K)
Long-acting exenatide (Bydureon)	2 mg once weekly		
Liraglutide (Victoza)	0.6–1.8 mg SC once daily	0.6, 1.2, 1.8 (6 mg/mL) in prefilled, multidose "pen"	Glucagon-like peptide-1 (GLP-1) receptor agonist; lowers HbA_{1c} by 1%; risks include acute pancreatitis and possibly medullary thyroid cancer
Pramlintide (Symlin)	60 mcg SC immediately before meals	0.6 mg/mL in 5-mL vial	Amylin analog; lowers HbA_{1c} by 0.4%–0.7%; nausea common; reduce pre-meal dose of short-acting insulin by 50% (K)

NOTE: eGFR = estimated glomerular filtration rate; ALT = alanine aminotransferase; Cr = creatinine; CrCl = creatinine clearance; ER = extended release; K = renal elimination; L = hepatic elimination; SC = subcutaneously; T = tablet

SOURCE: Reuben DB, Herr KA, Pacala JT, et al. *Geriatrics At Your Fingertips*, 15th ed. New York: American Geriatrics Society; 2013:101–104. Reprinted with permission.

Table 62.2—Insulin Preparations

Preparations	Onset	Peak (hours)	Duration (hours)	Number of Injections or Inhalations/day
Rapid-acting				
Insulin glulisine (Apidra)	20 min	0.5–1.5	3–4	3
Insulin lispro (HumaLog)	15 min	0.5–1.5	3–4	3
Insulin aspart (NovoLog)	10–20 min	1–3	3–5	3
Insulin aspart protamine and insulin aspart (NovoLog Mix 70/30)	10–20 min	1–4	18–24	2
Insulin lispro protamine and insulin lispro (HumaLog mix 75/25)	15–30 min	1.6–5	14–24	2
Regular (eg, Humulin, Novolin)[a]	0.5–1 h	2–3	5–8	1–3
Intermediate or long-acting				
NPH (eg, Humulin, Novolin)[a]	1–1.5 h	4–12	24	1–2
Insulin detemir (Levemir)	3–4 h	6–8	6–24 depending on dose	1–2
Insulin glargine (Lantus)[b]	1–2 h	—	24	1
Isophane insulin and regular insulin injectable (Novolin 70/30)	30 min	2–12	24	1–2

NOTE: NPH = neutral protamine Hagedorn (insulin)

[a] Also available (not in United States) as mixtures of NPH and regular in 50:50 proportions.

[b] To convert from NPH dosing, give same number of units once a day. For patients taking NPH q12h, decrease the total daily units by 20% and titrate on basis of response. Starting dosage in insulin-naive patients is 10 U once daily at bedtime.

SOURCE: Reuben DB, Herr KA, Pacala JT, et al. *Geriatrics At Your Fingertips*, 15th ed. New York: American Geriatrics Society; 2013:105. Reprinted with permission.

be used. In addition, referral to subspecialty diabetes care or more frequent contact with the healthcare team may be needed. Psychosocial reasons for hypoglycemia must be investigated and treated, such as an inability to understand self-management because of cognitive problems, inadequate diabetes knowledge, difficulty in implementing therapy because of disability, or lack of caregiver support.

Education and Self-Management Support

Because diabetes is a disease for which the patient and/or family caregivers bear the primary responsibility for management and ultimate control, it is imperative that the patient understands the mechanisms and management of the metabolic derangements and becomes fully involved in diabetes self-management, ie, monitoring and treating the disease and its complications. Therefore, education about diabetes, and particularly diabetes self-management, are key components of effective care. Often, basic education can be accomplished in the primary care setting. Patients with diabetes and other comorbidities may need referral to a diabetes educator for one-on-one counseling or group classes, enrollment in a comprehensive diabetes disease management program, or specialty physician care. Annual diabetes self-management training is a covered benefit under Medicare Part B. Diabetes mellitus education programs may be particularly important in older adults with diabetes who are members of minority groups, particularly black Americans or Hispanic Americans. It is extremely important to recognize when caregiver involvement in diabetes self-management activities is required. The caregiver must be highly involved and educated about diabetes and its self-management when the patient is cognitively impaired, is significantly disabled or frail, or when communication issues exist, eg, the patient has limited proficiency in English.

Diabetes self-management and support must cover several important areas. The older patient, and caregiver if appropriate, must be educated about hypo- and hyperglycemia, including precipitating factors, prevention, symptoms, monitoring, treatment, and indications for notifying the clinician. Although hypoglycemia is unusual in older adults when they are treated with sulfonylurea or insulin, they are still at higher risk than middle-aged adults with diabetes. When appropriate, the patient and caregiver should be taught blood-glucose self-monitoring, and their technique should be reassessed and reinforced periodically.

Diet and physical activity remain important components of the initial and ongoing management of patients with diabetes. Specific dietary recommendations must be tailored for each individual and focus on strategies that improve glycemic control as well as lipids and blood pressure. An individual meal plan of regular, well-balanced meals consisting of healthy food in the correct amounts with the goal of keeping weight under control is key to diabetes management. Physical activity programs should also be individualized. The patient should be assessed regularly for level of physical activity and informed about the benefits of exercise and available resources for becoming more active.

An older adult with diabetes who is prescribed a new medication and any caregiver should be educated on the purpose of the medication, how to take it, and the adverse events that are common or important, with reassessment and reinforcement periodically as needed. Finally, every older adult with diabetes and any caregiver should be educated about risk factors for foot ulcers and amputation. Physical ability to provide foot care should be evaluated, with periodic reassessment and reinforcement.

For patient education to be an effective tool in diabetes management, it must take into account the level of adjustment to the disease. In addition, it is critical that the patient and/or family and caregivers understand not only "what" needs to be done but "why" it needs to be done. Self-efficacy strengthening and coping skills training should also be addressed. Support groups, such as those available through the ADA, can be extremely helpful for the older patient and/or family and caregivers.

References

- The American Diabetes Association. Clinical Practice Recommendations 2011. *Diabetes Care.* 2011;34(Suppl 1).
- Beckwith S. Structured assessment of diabetic residents. *Nurs & Residential Care.* 2011;13(1):19–20-25.
- Cigolle CT, Blaum CS, Halter JB. Diabetes and cardiovascular disease prevention in older adults. *Clin Geriatr Med.* 2009;25(4):607–641.
- Skyler J, Bergenstal R, Bonow R, et al. Intensive glycemic control and the prevention of cardiovascular events: implications of the ACCORD, ADVANCE, and VA Diabetes Trials. A Position Statement of the American Diabetes Association and a Scientific Statement of the American College of Cardiology Foundation and the American Heart Association. *J Am Coll Cardiol.* 2009;53(3):298–304.
- Whitehouse C. Sexuality in the older female with diabetes mellitus: A review of the literature. *Urol Nurs.* 2009;29(1):11–19.

CHAPTER 63—HEMATOLOGIC DISEASES AND DISORDERS

KEY POINTS

- The reserve capacity of hematopoiesis diminishes with advancing age.
- The possibility of a multifactorial cause should be considered when a patient with anemia of chronic disease has a hemoglobin (Hb) of <10 g/dL.
- Data from the National Health and Nutrition Examination Survey III (NHANES III) indicate that about 35% of all anemia among older adults in the United States results from nutrient deficiencies (iron, vitamin B12, and/or folate), 45% of all anemia is attributable to chronic disease(s), and 20% is unexplained despite an exhaustive evaluation.
- Coagulation enzyme activity increases with increasing age. This biochemical hypercoagulability can lead to increased thrombotic events in older adults.
- The incidence of myelodysplasia and acute myeloid leukemia increases with age. Age-related defects in lymphopoiesis are thought to be the basis of the myeloid dominance of adult leukemia.
- Polycythemia vera, essential thrombocythemia, and idiopathic myelofibrosis occur primarily in older adults and have a slow rate of spontaneous transformation to leukemia.

HEMATOPOIESIS

Hematopoietic Stem Cells and Aging

The hematopoietic system derives from a small pool of hematopoietic stem cells (HSCs) that can either self-renew or differentiate along one of several lineages to form mature RBCs, WBCs, or platelets. HSCs differentiate into mature cells through an intermediate set of committed progenitors and precursors, each with decreasing self-renewal potential and increasing lineage commitment. Hematopoiesis is tightly regulated by a complex series of interactions between HSCs, their stromal microenvironment, and diffusible regulatory molecules, the hematopoietic growth factors (HGFs) that effect cellular proliferation. The orderly development of the hematopoietic system in vivo and the maintenance of homeostasis require that a strict balance be maintained between self-renewal, differentiation, maturation, and cell loss. Accumulated DNA damage has been proposed as the principal and unifying mechanism underlying age-dependent HSC decline.

Hematopoietic Response with Aging

Human aging is associated with reduced reserve capacity for hematopoiesis. This hematopoietic property appears to be caused by a series of factors that coincide with alterations across all HSC lineages. Age-related deficient lymphopoiesis is characterized by decreased competence in both the innate immune system (decreased natural-killer activity, decreased phagocytic ability of neutrophils and macrophages, and a proinflammatory state) and the adaptive immune system (decreased numbers of memory B and T cells), the expansion of myeloid elements, and the occurrence of a mild to moderate normocytic anemia. Numerous animal studies have shown a reduced ability of the aged hematopoietic system to respond to stimulation. Studies in people have not been as conclusive. (See also "Biology," p 8.) Some of these abnormalities, not evidenced in the basal state, become apparent in the stimulus-driven state. In addition to being of a lower magnitude, the aged response is also more variable. Given a comparable stress, hematologic abnormalities are likely to occur earlier and to be of greater severity in older than in younger adults. Thus, the rate of return of the hemoglobin to normal after phlebotomy is blunted, and the ability to mount a granulocyte response to infection is reduced. The relative contributions of age per se and age-related comorbidities to this suboptimal response are unclear. Retrospective analysis of bone marrow transplantations has established donor age to be the only donor parameter significantly associated with survival of the human recipients, which is consistent with the presence of an age-related defect in the donor HSCs. This finding is also consistent with the decrease in the number of functionally competent HSCs seen in aging mice.

Although there is no significant change in basal blood cell counts with aging, the prevalence of anemia tends to increase modestly. This is more evident in men ≥75 years old, who in cross-sectional studies have lower hemoglobin values than their younger counterparts (≤65 years old). The mechanism for the difference is unclear but is thought to reflect the presence of comorbid illness or reduced erythropoietin (EPO) drive, or both, as a result of declines in androgen. Older adults do not appear to have an impaired ability to increase hematocrit in response to exogenous EPO or to increase granulocyte count after administration of granulocyte colony-stimulating factor. The severity of neutropenia after chemotherapy in older cancer patients is greater in those who are underweight and malnourished than in those who are not. Although aging reduces hematopoietic reserve, it is of clinical relevance only in the presence of comorbidities.

Aging does not appear to affect the circulating concentrations of EPO and other HGFs; the increase in response to anemia or infection in older adults is equivalent to that in their younger counterparts. However, in response to stress, the blunted hematopoietic response seen with age has been attributed to an impaired ability to release HGFs. This might explain the age-related reduced neutrophil response to infection seen in animal studies and may contribute to increased infection-induced morbidity with aging. The production of certain growth factors, particularly interleukin-6 (IL-6), appears to increase with aging, leading to the notion that aging is accompanied by dysregulation of growth factor production, with overproduction of some cytokines and underproduction of others.

ANEMIA

Anemia, clearly the most common age-related hematologic abnormality, is seen in both older men and women. According to World Health Organization criteria, anemia is diagnosed if the hemoglobin concentration is <13 g/dL in men and <12 g/dL in women. Studies have shown a high prevalence of anemia in older adults who are hospitalized, seen in geriatric clinics, or institutionalized. However, if stringent criteria are used to select apparently healthy participants, the prevalence drops. Results from NHANES III in the United States indicated that the prevalence of anemia in community-dwelling adults >65 years old was 11% in men and 10.2% in women. In several studies, the prevalence of anemia in the population >80 years old is reported as being 18%–22% in men and 12%–16% in women.

In the general population, the annual incidence of anemia is estimated to be 1%–2%. In contrast, the incidence of anemia in a well-defined population of white people >65 years old attending the Mayo Clinic was reported to be 4- to 6-fold higher. In this study, in every age group >65 years old, the incidence of anemia in men was higher than that in women.

Most anemia among NHANES III participants was mild; only 2.8% of women and 1.6% of men had a hemoblobin of <11 g/dL. NHANES III also found that of all anemia cases among older adults in the United States, 35% resulted from nutrient deficiencies (iron, vitamin B_{12}, and/or folate), 45% was attributable to chronic disease(s), and 20% was unexplained despite an exhaustive evaluation. Several theories have been put forward to explain possible etiologies for these cases of unknown cause, including reduced pluripotent HSC reserve, decreased production of HGFs, reduced sensitivity of HSCs to HGFs, marrow microenvironment abnormalities, unrecognized anemia of chronic disease, occult renal failure, and undiagnosed myelodysplasia. It is also possible that age-associated increases in levels of proinflammatory cytokines, such as IL-6, may reduce the responses of stem cells to growth factors, including EPO. Results from the InChianti study examined levels of hemoglobin, EPO, and inflammatory molecules (C-reactive protein, IL-6, IL-1, IL-1b, and tumor necrosis factor alpha [TNF-α]) in 1,453 older adults. In this population, the proinflammatory markers increased with age, with a commensurate increase in the EPO level in individuals with a normal hemoglobin and an inappropriately low EPO level in those with anemia. Patients whose anemia was categorized as "unexplained" characteristically had lower than expected proinflammatory markers and low EPO levels.

The importance of anemia in older adults has implications not only relative to the underlying cause but also that may be a direct consequence of its presence. Studies have shown a reverse J-shaped relationship between anemia and morbidity and mortality (ie, outcomes are worse with hemoglobin concentrations both <12 g/dL and >15 g/dL), although direct causality between anemia and mortality and morbidity has not been rigorously established. It is postulated that even mild anemia in older adults leads to increases in cardiac output, local tissue hypoxia, aggravation of already extant comorbidities, and functional decline. Along these lines, anemia in older adults is associated with impaired performance-based mobility function, impaired cognitive performance, the occurrence of depressive symptoms, and a decrease in quality of life metrics. Of great physical consequence is that anemia is associated with increases in muscle weakness, severity of frailty, risks of falls, and mortality. Women >65 years old with hemoglobin concentrations <11 g/dL have an increasingly higher risk of all-cause mortality than those whose hemoglobin concentrations were ≥12 g/dL. This increased risk of mortality among the older anemic patient is independent of the presence of other identified comorbidities such as malignancy, peptic ulcer disease, and infection.

Evaluation of Anemia

The presence of multiple pathologies in older adults often makes the evaluation of anemia challenging. Attempting to define the cause of anemia when the hemoglobin concentration is between 12 and 14 g/dL rarely yields a definitive cause. Even when the hemoglobin concentration is 12 g/dL, a decision as

Table 63.1—Physiologic Classification of Anemia

Hypoproliferative	Ineffective	Hemolytic
■ Iron-deficient erythropoiesis Iron deficiency Chronic disease	■ Macrocytic Vitamin B_{12} Folate Myelodysplastic syndrome (refractory anemia)	■ Immunologic Idiopathic Secondary
■ Erythropoietin lack Renal Endocrine	■ Microcytic Thalassemia Sideroblastic	■ Intrinsic Abnormal hemoglobin Metabolic
■ Stem-cell dysfunction	■ Normocytic Myelodysplastic syndrome	■ Extrinsic Mechanical
■ Aplastic anemia		

SOURCE: Data from Chatta GS, Lipschitz DA. Aging and hematopoiesis. In: Hazzard WR, Blass JP, Ettinger WH Jr., et al., eds. *Principles of Geriatric Medicine and Gerontology*. 5th ed. New York: McGraw-Hill Health Professions Division; 2003:763–770.

to how aggressively to evaluate a patient must depend on clinical judgment. Once a decision has been made to investigate a low hemoglobin concentration in an older adult, the principles involved in assessment and evaluation are similar to those used in patients of any age.

For a summary of the causes of the various anemias seen in older adults, see Table 63.1. The approach to the patient with anemia should evaluate renal, hepatic, endocrine, and marrow function. The initial evaluation should include physical examination of these organ systems, medication history, a CBC, a reticulocyte production index, and fecal blood testing. Microcytosis (mean corpuscular volume [MCV] <84) indicates an impairment of hemoglobin synthesis, and macrocytosis (MCV >100) can be caused by reticulocytosis or more commonly by an abnormality in nuclear maturation. Iron deficiency and vitamin B_{12} deficiency can coexist, resulting in confusing RBC indices. RBC production is estimated from the reticulocyte production index (a mathematical manipulation of the uncorrected reticulocyte count that adjusts for the abnormal hemoglobin concentration or hematocrit and the circulating reticulocyte life span) or the absolute reticulocyte count as determined on an automated cell counter. Hemolytic anemia usually has a reticulocyte production index >3, whereas a lack of production is indicated by a reticulocyte production index of <2. Decreased production is caused by the hypoproliferative anemias or by ineffective erythropoiesis. An increased lactate dehydrogenase (LDH) concentration and indirect hyperbilirubinemia result from the increased destruction of RBC precursors in the marrow and can be used to distinguish ineffective erythropoiesis from hypoproliferative anemia. For an approach to the laboratory evaluation of anemia, see Figure 63.1 and Figure 63.2. A significantly increased reticulocyte count, indirect hyperbilirubinemia, and an increased LDH level are diagnostic of hemolytic anemia. A low reticulocyte count, increased indirect bilirubin, and an increased LDH concentration suggest ineffective erythropoiesis. In older adults with ineffective erythropoiesis, macrocytosis strongly suggests vitamin B_{12} or less commonly, folate deficiency, and microcytosis should suggest sideroblastic anemia.

The Hypoproliferative Anemias

Iron is the only nutrient that limits the rate of erythropoiesis. Thus, an inadequate iron supply for erythropoiesis is the most common cause of anemia in older adults, resulting in a hypoproliferative anemia. This is diagnosed by the presence of a decreased serum iron and a decreased transferrin saturation (serum iron divided by the total iron binding capacity, expressed as a percentage), and a normal or increased serum ferritin concentration. Serum iron levels and transferrin saturation is regulated by the release of iron from its storage sites. Absolute iron deficiency (another kind of iron-restricted anemia usually caused by blood loss, malabsorption, or nutritional deficiency) is the most common cause of iron-deficient erythropoiesis in younger people. Blood-loss anemia, the anemia of inflammation or chronic disease, and the anemia associated with protein-energy malnutrition are the most prevalent anemias in older populations. Nutritional iron deficiency is very rare in the older age group, despite the prominence of other nutritional problems.

When unexplained iron deficiency does occur, it is almost exclusively due to blood loss from the GI tract. Typical findings in blood-loss anemia are low iron, low serum ferritin, and high total iron binding capacity, reflecting absent iron stores. Medication-related gastritis, angiodysplasia, and benign tumors are common causes but should be considered only after a malignancy has been excluded. Rarely, iron deficiency can result from malabsorption or urinary losses of iron, which occurs in the face of intravascular hemolysis. Iron deficiency can be treated with either parenteral iron preparations or with oral iron preparations. Some

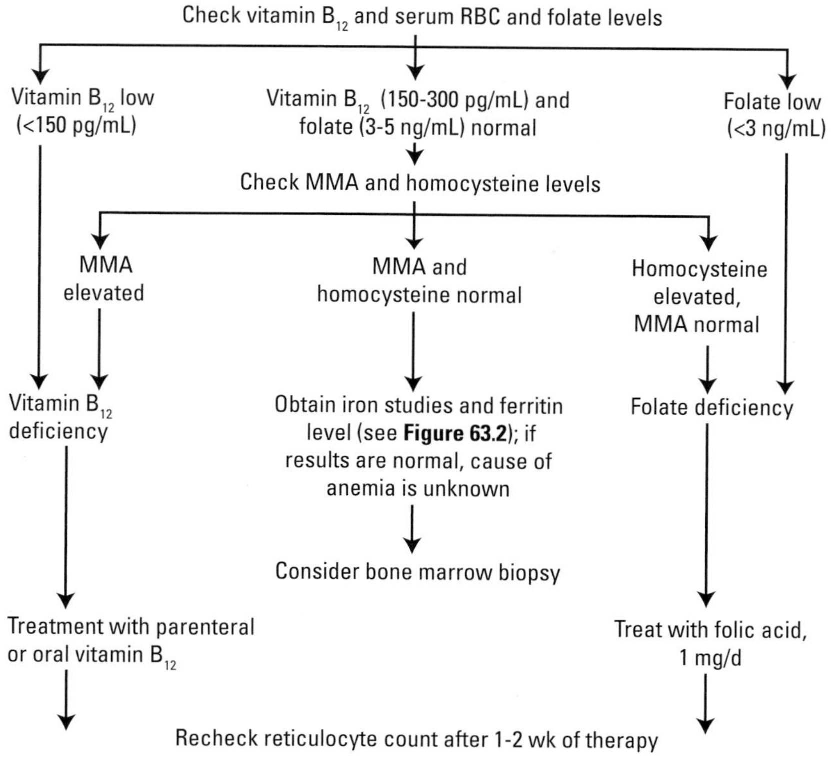

Figure 63.1—Evaluation of Hypoproliferative Anemia Due to Possible Iron Deficiency

SOURCE: Adapted from Reuben DB, Herr K, Pacala JT, et al. Geriatrics At Your Fingertips, 15th ed. New York: American Geriatrics Society; 2013:143. Reprinted with permission.

of the parenteral preparations can be administered intramuscularly; however, this mode of administration is often painful, may leave unsightly blue-black discoloration at the injection site, and requires a significant muscle mass as the target site for injection. Intravenous parenteral administration is indicated only if the patient is also receiving an erythrocyte-stimulating agent during dialysis, or if the use of oral iron preparations is untenable. There is no significant difference among the oral iron preparations in regards to either efficacy or adverse-event profile, although one type of preparation may be better tolerated than another by an individual patient. Oral iron absorption requires that the upper portion of the small bowel be intact and appropriately acidified by gastric secretions. In the presence of achlorhydria from gastric resection or atrophic gastritis, or medications that suppress gastric acid secretion, medicinal iron absorption may be significantly impaired. Although unusual, the incidence of celiac disease, a disease that is characteristically associated with iron malabsorption, is increased in the older population. Common dose-related adverse events of oral iron preparations include mild nausea and constipation. For this reason, the frequency and dosage of administration may require adjustment to ensure compliance. Tablets containing a lower elemental dose of iron (15–20 mg) may be better tolerated than higher dose preparations. Iron elixir and liquid iron drops may be better absorbed, because the availability of elemental iron for absorption does not require tablet dissolution in the GI tract; however, the adverse-event profile is similar to that for tablet preparations.

The terms *anemia of inflammation* or *anemia of chronic disease* are often used to explain an anemia associated with some other major disease process. Examples include cancer, collagen vascular disorders, rheumatoid arthritis, and inflammatory bowel disease. Occasionally, the anemia may be the initial manifestation of an occult disease. It is critical that this condition be distinguished from iron-deficiency (blood-loss) anemia to avoid unnecessary GI tests and to prevent the inappropriate prescribing of oral iron therapy.

The pathophysiology of the anemia of inflammation or chronic disease is complex and is due to an inability of macrophages to release iron from the breakdown of senescent RBCs. As a consequence, the serum iron decreases and, as with blood-loss anemia, the iron supply is inadequate for erythropoiesis. In contrast to blood-loss anemia with absent iron stores, iron stores are normal or increased in the anemia of inflammation or chronic disease. Laboratory features include a mild anemia, a low serum iron, low transferrin saturation, and normal

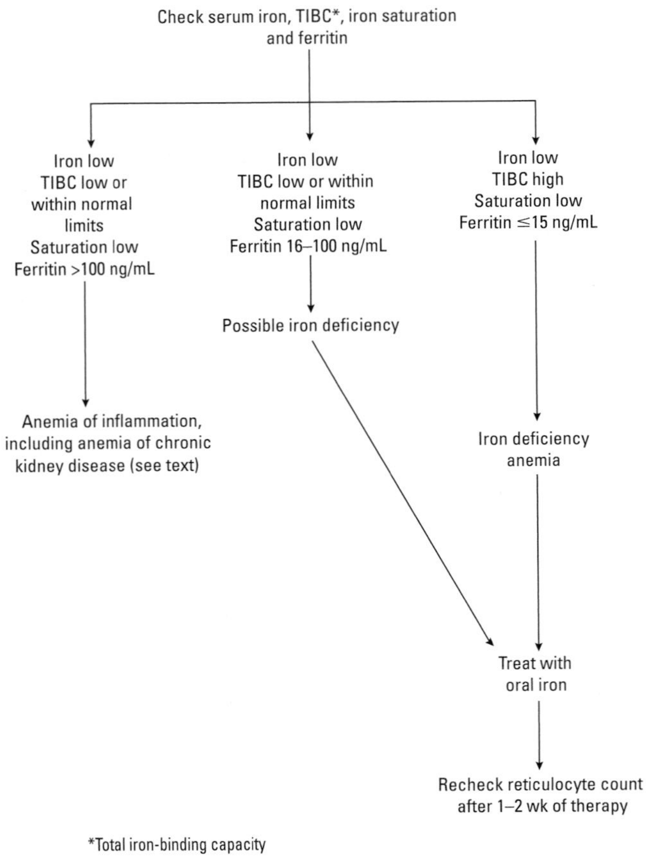

Figure 63.2—Evaluation of Hypoproliferative Anemia Due to Possible Vitamin B_{12} or Folate Deficiency

SOURCE: Balducci L. Epidemiology of anemia in the elderly: Information on diagnostic evaluation. J Am Geriatr Soc. 2003;51(3 Suppl):S2-9. Reprinted with permission.

to increased iron stores (ferritin >100 ng/mL). However, laboratory parameters often can be equivocal, and it may be difficult to distinguish between iron deficiency and defective iron utilization. In this setting, measuring an erythrocyte sedimentation rate or C-reactive protein level may be helpful, because these will often be increased in the presence of an occult inflammatory condition. Hepcidin, a 25 amino acid peptide produced in the liver, has been implicated in the pathogenesis of anemia of chronic disease. Hepcidin functions as a direct mediator of iron homeostasis, regulating both intestinal iron absorption as well as release of macrophage iron to erythroid progenitors. Although hepcidin levels have been reported to be increased nearly 100-fold in association with anemia of chronic disease, studies on the clinical utility of hepcidin are limited by the availability of a suitable clinical assay. The possibility of a multifactorial causation, including blood loss, malnutrition, or hemolysis, should always be considered when the anemia of inflammation or chronic disease is associated with a hemoglobin concentration of <10 g/dL. In this circumstance, laboratory investigations commonly have equivocal results; hence, a bone marrow examination may be required. Clinical judgment is critically important in deciding how aggressive the evaluation for anemia ought to be.

Decreased EPO production accounts for the anemia of end-stage renal disease and is implicated in some anemias of cancer and chronic diseases. Many cancer patients have anemia independently of any myelosuppressive therapy. The anemia is characterized by an inability to use iron stores and an inadequate EPO response, indicated by inappropriately low EPO levels. In addition, a component of the erythroid suppression is mediated by cytokines such as IL-1, TNF-α, and transforming growth factor beta. Although the precise incidence of cancer-related anemia is not known, a number of studies have documented a decrease in transfusion frequency after treatment with EPO. Depending on symptoms, erythroid support is recommended for patients with hemoglobin concentrations <10 g/dL. The currently available alternative to packed red cell transfusions is the use of erythropoiesis-stimulating agents, including epoetin alfa, epoetin beta, and darbopoetin. All of these products are types of recombinant human EPO that bind to EPO receptors on red cell precursors, which results in the increased proliferation and production of mature RBCs. EPO treatment can be started after excluding hemolysis and iron deficiency and bleeding especially in symptomatic older adults. Oral iron replacement should be added to the regimen if ferritin levels fall to <100 ng/mL or transferrin saturation to <20%. Although it is generally accepted that there is no advantage to administering parenteral iron replacement in patients not receiving hemodialysis, an exception to this may be in the older patient in whom iron absorption is impaired. (A temporary cessation of therapy followed by a 25% dosage reduction is indicated if the hemoglobin concentration approaches 12 g/dL or the rate of rise is >1 g/dL every 2 weeks. If the hemoglobin concentration remains <10 g/dL and does not increase by 1 g/dL after 4 weeks, or the hemoglobin concentration falls to <10 g/dL, a 25% increase in dosage is in order.) If the target range of hemoglobin >10 g/dL is not achieved after appropriate dosage adjustments over 12 weeks, the patient should be reevaluated for infection, iron restriction, or the presence of a non-epoetin-alfa–responsive anemia. If after reassessment and iron replacement, the patient remains refractory to treatment, epoetin alfa therapy should be discontinued. Although it is difficult to prospectively identify responders, it has been reported that patients with endogenous EPO levels <500 mU/mL are most likely to respond. Marrow failure due to interference with the proliferation of hematopoietic cells is seen in older adults. The disorder is generally associated with suppression of all marrow elements and is suggested by the presence of peripheral pancytopenia. Common causes include medications, immune damage to the stem-cell population, intrinsic marrow lesions, and marrow replacement by malignant cells or fibrous tissue. The latter is usually associated with a myelophthisic blood picture (nucleated RBCs, giant platelets, and metamyelocytes) as a reflection of the disruption of marrow stromal architecture. The presence of pancytopenia and the absence of iron-deficient erythropoiesis is an indication for bone marrow aspiration and biopsy. Occasionally, isolated suppression of erythropoiesis occurs, which is referred to as *pure red cell aplasia*. This disorder can be related to medication or caused by benign or malignant abnormalities of lymphocytes, including thymoma, or by presence of a viral infection (eg, parvovirus B19). These patients have isolated anemia, an increased serum iron, and an absence of erythroid precursors on bone marrow examination. Patients with parvovirus infection typically have reduced red cell precursors, and if present these precursors may have peculiar intranuclear inclusion bodies.

Ineffective Erythropoiesis

Macrocytic anemias in older adults result from vitamin B_{12} and folate deficiency. The prevalence of pernicious anemia increases with advancing age. Pernicious anemia results from malabsorption of vitamin B_{12} as a consequence of the action of antibodies against gastric parietal cells and intrinsic factor. Atrophic gastritis and decreased secretion of intrinsic factor occur, resulting in failure of vitamin B_{12} absorption. Pernicious anemia is most common in adults >60 years old and is more common in women. Although cobalamin deficiency is common with aging, anemia secondary to this is rare (see the section on vitamin B_{12}, folate, and homocysteine, below). The presence of macrocytosis, hypersegmented neutrophils in the peripheral smear, a decreased reticulocyte index, an increased LDH level, and indirect hyperbilirubinemia suggest a diagnosis of megaloblastic anemia. The bone marrow classically shows giant metamyelocytes, hypersegmented neutrophils, and enlarged erythroid precursors with more hemoglobin than would be expected from the immaturity of their nuclei (nuclear-cytoplasmic dissociation). Chronic pancreatitis and diseases of the distal ileum (blind-loop syndrome) can cause vitamin B_{12} deficiency. An increased prevalence of B_{12} deficiency also has been reported in patients with diabetes taking metformin and in those on chronic proton-pump inhibitors. The Schilling test can distinguish a deficiency of intrinsic factor from an abnormality in the ability of the ileum to absorb the vitamin B_{12}–intrinsic factor complex; however, it is no longer commonly done because of expense and inconvenience (versus simply replacing B_{12}). Folate deficiency of sufficient severity to cause anemia in older adults is rare. Alcohol and various drugs also interfere with folate absorption and metabolism. Vulnerability to deficiency is significantly greater when folate requirements are increased as a result of inflammation, neoplastic disease, or hemolytic anemia.

The major causes of ineffective erythropoiesis and microcytosis are thalassemia and the sideroblastic anemias. Although thalassemia is generally diagnosed at an earlier age, there are reports of its initial detection in older adults. Mild anemia, a disproportionately low MCV, and the absence of iron deficiency usually point to a diagnosis of thalassemia trait, a condition of little or no clinical consequence. Iron supplements have no role in the treatment of thalassemia trait; on the contrary, they can be detrimental. Acquired sideroblastic anemia, which is primarily a disease of older adults, is a heterogenous group of disorders characterized by the presence of iron deposits in the mitochondria of normoblasts. Referral to a hematologist for bone marrow evaluation should be recommended.

Myelodysplastic Syndromes

The *myelodysplastic syndromes* (MDS) are a group of stem-cell disorders characterized by disordered hematopoiesis that occur primarily in the older age group. This group of disorders are classified as refractory anemia with ringed sideroblasts, MDS with isolated del (5q), refractory cytopenia with multilineage dysplasia, refractory anemia with excess blasts-1 or -2, and myelodysplastic syndrome, unclassified. Refractory anemia and refractory anemia with ringed sideroblasts account for 25%–30% of MDS. Refractory anemia commonly presents as a macrocytic anemia with marrow erythroid hyperplasia and relatively normal myeloid and megakaryocytic lineages. Cytogenetic abnormalities are relatively common in MDS, and one of particular interest in older adults is deletion of the long arm of chromosome 5 (5q−). The median age at presentation is 66 years, and the 5q− syndrome is characterized by macrocytic anemia, modest leukopenia, normal or increased platelet counts, and marrow erythroid hypoplasia or hyperplasia; it is also more common in women. Sometimes older patients develop a stem-cell disorder that is characterized by anemia and megaloblastic erythroid precursors, dysplastic myeloid cells, and hyperplasia in the marrow. This may evolve into an "erythroleukemia" (also referred to as M6 leukemia), with an associated pancytopenia and the presence of nucleated RBCs and immature myeloid and megakaryocytic precursors in the circulation. Referral to a hematologist should be recommended to consider further evaluation and treatment options.

Hemolytic Anemias

The causes of hemolytic anemia in older adults are different than those in younger people. Although most patients with congenital disorders will have been previously identified, an occasional older adult with congenital hemolytic anemia can present for the first time with symptoms related to cholelithiasis. Autoimmune hemolytic anemia is the most common cause in the older age group. The diagnosis is made by finding spherocytes or red cell clumping on a peripheral blood smear, a high serum LDH and low plasma haptoglobin, and a positive direct antiglobulin test. In younger patients, a cause of the autoimmune hemolysis is only rarely identified. In contrast, in older adults, the anemia is more likely to be associated with a lymphoproliferative disorder (non-Hodgkin lymphoma or chronic lymphocytic leukemia), collagen vascular disease, or drug ingestion. Corticosteroids and splenectomy are usually effective in patients with red cell antibodies of the IgG type that most frequently cause a warm autoimmune hemolysis. Patients with red cell antibodies of the IgM variety usually have cold reactive antibodies and are typically refractory to splenectomy and corticosteroids. These patients can usually be treated by simply keeping them warm and administering warmed blood products. In the case of cold reactive antibody disease that is difficult to manage, physical removal of the IgM antibodies by plasmapheresis may be indicated. Long-term responses have been seen with the administration of rituximab. Microangiopathic hemolytic anemia occurs secondary to either disseminated intravascular coagulation (DIC) or as a manifestation of the syndrome of thrombotic thrombocytopenic purpura (TTP). DIC is usually associated with severe infections or disseminated cancer and presents with not only hemolysis but also a consumptive coagulopathy. The presence of red cell fragmentation, thrombocytopenia, a prolonged prothrombin time, a prolonged partial thromboplastin time, and hemosiderinuria suggests this diagnosis. Treatment of DIC entails treating the underlying disorder as well as providing blood product support, including fresh frozen plasma and cryoprecipitate as needed. TTP is characterized by the pentad of fever, intravascular hemolysis, thrombocytopenia, neurologic symptoms, and renal dysfunction. In contrast to DIC, in TTP both the prothrombin time and partial thromboplastin time are normal. Early diagnosis is imperative, because TTP responds very well to treatment with plasmapheresis.

Hemolysis is frequently associated with implantation of prosthetic heart valves. The incidence of hemolysis varied from 5% to 35%, and is affected by a variety of factors, mostly related to the type of valve implanted and to the hemodynamic conditions after implantation. In a report of 278 patients, mild subclinical hemolysis was identified at 12 months in 26% of patients with a mechanical prosthesis and in 5% with a bioprosthesis. On multivariate analysis, independent predictors of the presence of subclinical hemolysis were mitral valve replacement, use of a mechanical prosthesis, and double valve replacement. Among mechanical valve recipients, double versus single valve replacement and mitral versus aortic valve replacement were correlated with the presence of hemolysis; double valve recipients also showed a more severe degree of hemolysis (SOE=B). Valve-associated anemia is seldom severe. The amount of hemolysis is assessed based on serum levels of LDH and haptoglobin, and on the presence and amount of reticulocytes and schistocytes in the peripheral blood. Treatment of hemolysis includes the supplementation of iron and folate when their deficiency is evident. The use of β-blockers appears to decrease the severity of hemolysis, likely through induction of bradycardia and negative inotropic effects.

VITAMIN B_{12}, FOLATE, AND HOMOCYSTEINE

Older adults are more likely than younger ones to have lower concentrations of vitamin B_{12} and folate. In epidemiologic studies, approximately 10% of apparently healthy adults ≥70 years old were found to have low vitamin B_{12} levels, and 5%–10% were found to have low folate levels (SOE=A). Low vitamin B_{12} and folate levels are not necessarily accompanied by macrocytosis or evidence of megaloblastic anemia. Atrophic gastritis leading to vitamin B_{12} malabsorption is the likely cause in most cases of vitamin B_{12} deficiency. Although gastritis can also contribute to low folate levels in older adults, alcohol abuse, drug interactions with folate absorption, and inadequate dietary intake are the most common causes of low folate levels. Some evidence suggests that low vitamin B_{12} levels may contribute to cognitive decline in older adults (SOE=C). There is no question that severe vitamin B_{12} deficiency can result in cognitive loss and significant neurologic deficits. However, in most demented patients, B_{12} deficiency is not the cause of their dementia. Nevertheless, aggressive replacement should always be undertaken when a patient with dementia presents with low levels of vitamin B_{12} or folate.

Even in patients with atrophic gastritis, oral vitamin B_{12} is generally adequate; 10% will be absorbed by mass action alone and not require the presence of intrinsic factor. Thus, a daily dose of 1 mg (1,000 mcg) of vitamin B_{12} will replete a person with concentrations in the low-to-normal range. Parenteral replacement should be used in severe vitamin B_{12} deficiencies, ie, concentrations <100 pg/mL or in those with neurologic symptoms. It has been suggested that in older adults with low normal B_{12} concentrations (<350 pg/mL), methylmalonic acid (MMA) concentrations be checked to exclude metabolically active B_{12} deficiency. Kidney failure can artificially increase the serum MMA concentration. In those patients with low-normal B_{12} concentrations and macrocytosis (with or without anemia) or neurologic changes, vitamin replacement should be considered, particularly if the MMA concentration is increased. Folic acid can be replaced in dosages ranging from 400 to 500 mg/d. At these dosages, homocysteine concentrations decrease (analogous to the decrease in MMA when B_{12} is replaced).

Low concentrations of vitamin B_{12} or folate are accompanied by increased concentrations of homocysteine. Epidemiologic studies initially found that B_{12} and folate deficiencies with high levels of homocysteine are associated with cardiovascular disease; however, subsequent trials of homocysteine lowering through vitamin therapy did not reduce end points such as stroke and myocardial infarction (SOE=A), and may increase cancer risk. Increased homocysteine levels are common in patients with renal impairment, and for this reason, should be interpreted with caution.

PLATELETS AND COAGULATION

Bleeding diatheses are not uncommon in older adults. Unexplained bruises, recurrent nosebleeds, GI losses, or excessive blood loss during surgery or after dental extraction are common presentations. In these patients, screening platelet counts and coagulation studies should be obtained. Tests of platelet aggregation are useful in detecting disorders of platelet function.

Thrombocytopenia is a common cause of bleeding problems in older adults. A platelet count <150,000/µL is considered significant, but bleeding usually occurs at much lower levels. Common causes include decreased production of platelets in the bone marrow, sequestration in enlarged spleens, and increased peripheral destruction. Decreased production of platelets occurs in the leukemias, marrow aplasia, or most commonly in older adults in association with medications that suppress platelet production. The major cause of increased peripheral destruction is immune thrombocytopenia. A lymphoma, collagen vascular disease, or a drug-induced cause is common in older adults with autoimmune thrombocytopenia. Treatment of thrombocytopenia depends on the cause. For decreased production, platelet transfusion should be considered if there is significant blood loss, irrespective of the platelet count. Generally, bleeding occurs when the count drops to ≤20,000/µL. Because immune thrombocytopenia is usually secondary in older adults, the initial approach is to identify and treat the primary cause. If no cause is found, a trial of corticosteroids is warranted. Isolated thrombocytopenia in older adults should prompt an evaluation to exclude MDS, particularly when the low platelet count is thought to be secondary to inadequate production. DIC and TTP are also important causes of thrombocytopenia in the older age group, and they should be recognized and treated appropriately.

Platelet function disorders (thrombopathy), although uncommon, can cause significant bleeding in older adults on aspirin therapy and in patients receiving non-aspirin NSAIDs. It is important to point out, however, that platelet dysfunction may be severe enough to cause bleeding without drug exposure. Also, platelet-inhibiting drugs may cause bleeding in the absence of a primary platelet disorder. Platelets exposed to aspirin (an irreversible inhibitor of cyclo-oxygenase) are impaired for their lifetime. In contrast, platelets exposed to NSAIDs (reversible cyclo-oxygenase inhibitors) are only transiently affected. For this reason, bleeding risk may be higher in patients receiving aspirin than in those receiving NSAIDs. In addition to these analgesic medicines, platelet function can be impaired by the administration of drugs used to prevent or treat acute cardiovascular events. Dipyridimole (an adenosine deaminase inhibitor) is commonly used in combination with aspirin and may increase bleeding risk beyond that seen in patients treated with aspirin alone. Clopidogrel and prasugrel are irreversible P2Y12 inhibitors that are used either alone or with aspirin, impair platelet function, are associated with occurrence of TTP, and may predispose to either bleeding or thrombosis. Ticagrelor is a reversible inhibitor of P2Y12 and has an adverse-event profile similar to that of prasugrel. It is unknown whether this drug is associated with TTP. Platelet glycoprotein IIb/IIIa inhibitors (abciximab, eptifibatide, tirofiban) are used in patients with acute coronary syndromes and can be associated with the immediate onset of profound and transient thrombocytopenia and may be associated with life-threatening bleeding.

Bleeding can also occur because of clotting factor deficiencies, which in older adults are usually acquired and caused by the presence of circulating clotting factor inhibitors. Rarely, older male patients may present for the first time with mild hemophilia and, even more rarely, older female patients may present as hemophilia carriers with minimal decreases in coagulation factor VIII or factor IX levels. The most common acquired factor deficiency is caused by an inhibitor to factor VIII. The onset is often sudden. Titers of antifactor VIII antibodies can be very high, and presentation is with bleeding into joints and muscle, similar to that in hemophilia A. Treatment involves factor replacement; depending on the severity, prednisone or cyclophosphamide may also be needed. Deficiency of the vitamin K–dependent clotting factors tends to occur in older adults with major illnesses. Disorders of the hepatobiliary tree, antibiotics that neutralize bowel bacteria (a major source of vitamin K), malabsorption, and severe malnutrition are the common causes. The deficits are readily treated with vitamin K.

Liver disease must always be considered in patients who present with excessive bleeding. The prothrombin time is prolonged even in mild to moderate liver disease. The partial thromboplastin time remains normal until liver disease becomes severe. Except for factor VIII (which is produced by endothelial cells), all clotting factors are reduced in liver disease. Liver disease is also associated with DIC; fibrin degradation products are not cleared as well, and platelet function can be affected. The treatment of a bleeding diathesis in liver disease is fresh frozen plasma.

Chronic Myeloproliferative Disorders

The Philadelphia chromosome–negative chronic myeloproliferative disorders—polycythemia vera (PV), essential thrombocythemia (ET), and idiopathic myelofibrosis (IMF)—have overlapping clinical features but exhibit different natural histories and different therapeutic requirements. All three disorders are seen primarily in the older age group and are characterized by the involvement of a multipotent hematopoietic progenitor cell, marrow hypercellularity, overproduction of one or more marrow lineages, thrombotic and hemorrhagic diatheses, exuberant extramedullary hematopoiesis, and a slow rate of spontaneous transformation to acute leukemia. Thus, PV, ET, and IMF have a long natural history, distinguishing them from chronic myeloid leukemia, the Philadelphia chromosome–positive myeloproliferative disorder, which progresses and transforms much more rapidly. The main cause of morbidity and mortality in PV and ET is thrombosis, which occurs more commonly in older adults or in those with previous vascular complications. Severe bleeding is rare and limited to patients with a very high platelet count or to those taking antiplatelet drugs. Cytotoxic therapy is effective in preventing thrombosis but increases the risk of leukemic transformation (SOE=A). Because there is no curative therapy for PV and ET, the goals of therapy are to minimize thrombotic risk and to prevent progression to marrow fibrosis or acute leukemia, or both.

Several different treatment strategies for PV have been tested in randomized clinical trials. In the PV Study Group (PVSG-01) trial, 431 patients were randomized to one of the following: phlebotomy alone, 32P (a myelosuppressive agent) plus phlebotomy, or chlorambucil plus phlebotomy. The median survival time in the three arms was 13.9 years, 11.8 years, and 8.9 years, respectively. In the phlebotomy-only arm, thrombotic deaths were higher, particularly in the first 2–3 years. In the other two arms, the incidence of leukemic transformation was higher. The risk of thrombotic events is highest in those ≥60 years old and in those with a prior history of thrombosis. Given these findings, current treatment recommendations include:

- Phlebotomy in all patients to maintain hematocrit <0.45
- Myelosuppressive agents like hydroxyurea in patients at high risk of thrombosis (>60 years old) and in those with excessive phlebotomy requirements
- Hydroxyurea and an antiplatelet agent for symptomatic thrombocytosis

32P, busulfan, interferon, and anagrelide remain as viable options in these patients; however, they are usually reserved for patients with disease that is difficult to control. Both 32P and busulfan have been associated with an increased risk of treatment-related leukemia. Patients receiving anagrelide have been reported to have an increased risk of developing myelofibrosis. Pegylated interferon is effective but may not be well tolerated.

Additionally, given the results of the European Collaboration on Low-dose Aspirin in Polycythemia Vera trial, low-dose aspirin is recommended for all patients with PV. In this trial, 531 patients with PV were randomized to receive either no aspirin or low-dose aspirin. In those treated with aspirin, cardiovascular mortality was reduced by 59%, with a nonsignificant risk of increased bleeding.

The incidence of thrombotic and hemorrhagic complications in ET was analyzed in 1,850 patients from 21 retrospective cohort studies. Rates of thrombosis ranged from 7% to 17%, and rates of hemorrhage from 8% to 14%. Age >60 years, a prior thrombotic event, and a long duration of thrombocytosis are the major risk factors for thrombotic events. Consensus-based practice guidelines for ET include observation in asymptomatic low-risk patients with platelet counts $<1{,}500 \times 10^9$/L, and hydroxyurea plus aspirin in high-risk patients with platelet counts $\geq 1{,}500 \times 10^9$/L (SOE=A). Anagrelide is also very effective at reducing high platelet counts. However, a randomized trial comparing hydroxyurea plus aspirin to anagrelide plus aspirin demonstrated that hydroxyurea was more effective and associated with less adverse events. Hydroxyurea appears to be associated with a better overall survival, less serious hemorrhagic events, and fewer fibrotic transformations than anagrelide. ET, like PV, has a long natural history with a low incidence of leukemic transformation. In contrast, IMF progresses much more rapidly, with median survival of 3.5–5.5 years.

Hematologic Malignancies, Lymphomas, and Multiple Myeloma

See "Oncology," p 540.

References

- den Elzen WP, Willems JM, Westendorp RG, et al. Effect of anemia and comorbidity on functional status and mortality in old age: results from the Leiden 85-plus Study, *CMAJ*. 2009;181(3–4):151–157.
- Estey E. Acute myeloid leukemia and myelodysplastic syndromes in older patients. *J Clin Oncol.* 2007;25(14): 1908–1915.
- Herishanu Y, Katz BZ, Lipsky A, et al. Biology of chronic lymphocytic leukemia in different microenvironments: clinical and therapeutic implications. *Hematol Oncol Clin North Am.* 2013;27(2):173–206.
- Killen JP, Brenninger VL. Vitamin B_{12} deficiency. *N Engl J Med.* 2013;368(21):2040–2041.

CHAPTER 64—ONCOLOGY

Key Points

- Older adults and black Americans of all ages are more likely to develop cancer and present with more advanced disease.
- Older age has a variable association with the aggressiveness and growth rate of malignant tumors.
- There has been no demonstrated age-associated resistance to chemotherapy.
- Although some acute toxicities (eg, nausea, vomiting, and hair loss) are less prominent in older adults, other toxicities such as diarrhea and neuropathy are more common.
- Surgery, radiation, chemotherapy, and biologic therapies are safe and effective treatment interventions for older cancer patients when appropriate precautions are taken based on the patient's comorbidities, vital organ functions, and medications.
- Geriatric assessment can help determine which older patients are more likely to benefit from aggressive cancer treatment and which are most likely to experience toxicity from cancer treatment.

Cancer is a disease associated with aging—most cancer diagnoses and deaths are in people >65 years old. Currently, the median age of patients with a new cancer diagnosis is 70 years. On the basis of the aging of the U.S. population and the known association between cancer and aging, a dramatic increase in the number of new cancer diagnoses is projected for the next 20 years. It is anticipated that patients ≥65 years old will account for 70% of all cancer diagnoses by the year 2030.

According to the National Cancer Institute's Surveillance, Epidemiology and End Results data, over 70% of cancer deaths were in people >65 years old. One in four deaths in the United States is caused by cancer. Overall cancer incidence rates decreased in the most recent time period in both men (1.3% per year from 2000 to 2006) and women (0.5% per year from 1998 to 2006), largely due to decreases in the three major cancer sites in men (lung, prostate, and colorectum) and two major cancer sites in women (breast and colorectum). Among men, death rates for all races combined decreased by 21.0% between 1990 and 2006, with decreases in lung, prostate, and colorectal cancer rates accounting for nearly 80% of the total decrease. Among women, overall cancer death rates between 1991 and 2006 decreased by 12.3%, with decreases in breast and colorectal cancer rates accounting for 60% of the total decrease. Although progress has been made in reducing incidence and mortality rates and improving survival, cancer still accounts for more deaths than heart disease in people <85 years old. After age 85, heart disease becomes the number one killer, and the risk of cancer declines for reasons that are not defined. Because of the paucity of older adults in clinical trials, it is not clear how much of the improvement in treatment has translated to the benefit of older patients. However, when such data have been evaluated (eg, for colon cancer, breast cancer) within clinical trials, it appears that treatment that is effective in younger patients is also effective in older patients (SOE=A). The older patients in clinical trials, however, tend to be healthy (ie, other than having cancer) and are therefore without significant comorbidities or functional impairment.

Although cancer has long been recognized as a disease of older people, emphasis on the interactions of cancer and aging is a recent development. Experimental data and clinical experience have indicated that tumors are not resistant to treatment by virtue of age alone. However, age is associated with reductions in certain organ functions, and these deficiencies in physiologic reserve might be magnified by comorbid conditions. Cancer treatments can therefore be associated with an increase in adverse events, and treatment should be tailored to the individual, taking into consideration potential increased toxicities and balancing this with expectations of survival in the context of comorbidities. Although we have much to learn about providing optimal management of cancer in older adults, especially those who are vulnerable or frail, some research has shown that geriatric assessment can help identify older patients who would most benefit from aggressive treatment and those who are at most risk of toxicities from cancer treatment.

Four questions form the basis of this new emphasis:

- Why are tumors more common in older adults?
- Is there a difference in tumor aggressiveness with advancing age?
- Should treatment be different for older patients?
- How can cancer treatment be best individualized for older patients?

Cancer Biology and Aging

Numerous explanations have been offered as to the biologic connection between cancer and aging, including extended exposure to carcinogens, increased DNA instability resulting in a higher mutation potential, telomere shortening, immune dysregulation, and increased susceptibility to oxidative stress. While these explanations for the link between cancer and aging are plausible, they do not pinpoint the reason why one older adult is more susceptible to cancer than another. Furthermore, the association between cancer and aging is complex. Population-based studies demonstrate a steady rise in the probability of developing cancer across the strata of age, but few studies have examined cancer prevalence and mortality in the highest age groups.

Explaining the Increased Prevalence of Cancer with Age

The prevalence of cancer increases with age for at least three reasons. First, cancers, particularly those that occur in people >65 years old, are thought to develop over a long period, perhaps decades. This is best exemplified by the current understanding of colon cancer, which has been shown to develop because of an accumulation of several damaging genetic events occurring in a stochastic manner over time. Colon cancer, which occurs via an intermediate precursor (the adenomatous polyp), is an example of the multi-step genetic changes required over time for cancer development. In colon cancer, mutations in tumor suppressor genes such as inactivation of the *APC* and *DCC* genes and subsequent additional genetic defects in the oncogenes such as *K-Ras* promote the accumulation of mutations that lead to carcinogenesis. If mutations are acquired at a constant rate, older people are more likely to have lived long enough to develop the 8 to 10 genetic lesions it takes to develop a malignancy. In contrast, lymphomas are just as likely to occur in young as in old people. Lymphocytes normally undergo gene rearrangements and mutations to generate antigen receptors, and these processes appear to be particularly vulnerable to errors that can lead to lymphoma at any age.

A second reason for the greater prevalence of cancer with advancing age is that DNA repair mechanisms are thought to decline with age. As a consequence, cells can accumulate damage. Normally, a dividing cell pauses in G1 (the gap after mitosis [M] and before DNA replication [S]) and in G2 (the gap after S and before M) to take inventory and repair any damage before proceeding to the next phase. These are the G1 and G2 checkpoints. Older cells may fail to detect or repair damage and fail to accurately control DNA replication. This leads to aneuploidy and uncontrolled proliferation. In younger people, these aberrations can trigger the death of the cell; in older people, the errors may be tolerated and fail to signal cell death. Cells without functioning checkpoints are vulnerable to loss of growth control. Telomere dysfunction and increased epigenetic gene silencing have also been implicated in the pathogenesis of cancers. Telomeres are essential for chromosomal stability; with aging, their length progressively shortens, which interferes with cell division. This instability at the cellular level increases the rate of somatic mutations that predispose to cancer and other disorders like aplastic anemia. Paradoxically, human cancers have developed mechanisms to maintain telomere length for survival. Autophagy is interrupted with aging, which leads to the accumulation of damaged proteins and mitochondria, which in turn are a source of reactive oxygen species and contribute to cancer.

A third contribution to increased cancer incidence in older people may be a decline in the function of the immune system, particularly in cellular immunity. A number of findings suggest that the immune system can recognize and control certain cancers. A decline in immune function may lead to the emergence of a cancer in an older adult that was controlled when that person was younger.

The Different Characteristics of Cancer with Age

A long-held but incompletely documented clinical dogma that cancers in older people are less aggressive or slower growing has not been consistently supported by epidemiologic data from tumor registries or large clinical trials. Such data can be confounded by geriatric problems that shorten survival independently of the cancer (eg, comorbidity, multiple medications, clinician or family bias regarding diagnosis and treatment in older adults, and age-associated life stresses). These factors may counter any primary influence that aging might have on tumor aggressiveness. Despite these uncertainties, however, there is experimental support for the contention that tumor aggressiveness declines with age. Data obtained from laboratory animals with a wide range of tumors under highly controlled circumstances demonstrate slower tumor growth, fewer experimental metastases, and longer survival in old mice. Tumor growth involves several levels of interaction between the tumor and the host. It may be that tumor angiogenesis is impaired in older people, thereby controlling the rate of tumor growth. The clinical importance of this work is limited, inasmuch as it is difficult to know in any given individual whether the course of the disease will be characterized by an indolent or aggressive pattern of growth.

Breast cancer is the most notable clinical example of an age-associated decline in tumor aggressiveness. Older patients are more likely to have more favorable histologic types, higher levels of estrogen- and progesterone-receptor expression, lower growth fraction, and less frequent metastases. In a published series on breast cancer patients with primary tumors of ≤1 cm in diameter, the single most important predictor of metastasis to axillary nodes has consistently been found to be patient age: patients <50 years old have the highest likelihood of spread, whereas those >70 years old have the lowest likelihood of spread. Stage for stage in breast cancer, older patients seem to have longer survival times than younger patients (SOE=A).

By contrast, Hodgkin disease seems to be a more aggressive disease in older patients. The most likely reason for the age-associated differences in prognosis is that Hodgkin disease is a different disease in patients ≥45 years old than in younger patients. Incidence data demonstrate two distinct peak incidence rates, one at age 32 years and one at age 84 years. The frequency of particular histologic subtypes of Hodgkin disease is different in younger and older patients: nodular sclerosis is the most common subtype in younger patients, while mixed cellularity is the most common in older patients. In all reported treatment series, older age is an independent prognostic factor. Additional study is necessary to document age-associated differences in tumor cell biology.

Acute leukemia, like Hodgkin disease, appears to be a different disease in older people; the MDR1 drug resistance pump (which eliminates toxins, including certain cancer chemotherapy agents, from the cell) is more commonly expressed, response to treatment is less, and survival time is shorter than in younger patients.

However, for most cancer types, the molecular biology and clinical behavior of the tumor is similar across the age span.

Ethnic Differences in Cancer Incidence and Mortality

As the demographics of the U.S. population changes, additional information is needed on incidence and on natural history differences in cancers that develop in different ethnic and racial groups. There is a lack of basic data about aging minority populations. This is largely due to small sample sizes of these populations and to language barriers that prevent certain racial and ethnic groups from participating in survey research. The U.S. Census Bureau estimates that by 2050, Hispanic Americans will account for nearly 25% of the population, and black Americans, Asian Americans, and Native Americans combined will total another 25%. By the year 2050, under current projections, our numbers in minority populations are expected to outpace that number of white Americans. While the number of older white Americans is anticipated to double to 62 million, the number of older black Americans will nearly quadruple to over 9 million. Older Hispanics will total about 12 million, 11 times as many as in 1990. The number of American Indian and Alaska Natives will grow to 562,000, while the number of older Asian and Pacific Islanders will approach 7 million.

Cancer incidence and death rates are lower in other racial and ethnic groups than in white and black Americans for all cancer sites combined and for the four most common cancer sites. Overall, black Americans have the highest cancer incidence and mortality rates. Cancer incidence among black Americans is 10% higher than among white Americans, 50%–60% higher than among Hispanic Americans and Asian Americans, and more than twice as high as among Native Americans. Black Americans with cancer have shorter survival times than white Americans at all stages of diagnosis. Relative 5-year survival rates are higher among people diagnosed at younger ages (52% among black Americans diagnosed before age 45) than in those diagnosed at older ages (43% among those diagnosed after age 75). The cancer death rate for black Americans is about 30% higher than for white Americans and more than twice as high as for Hispanic Americans, Asian Americans, and Native Americans.

The factors contributing to the ethnic differences are not defined. However, certain data suggest that when the quality of the health care delivered to white and black Americans is similar, disease outcomes in the two groups are comparable (SOE=B).

Principles of Cancer Management

Randomized clinical trials are the most reliable method of studying medical intervention, and treatment decisions are best founded on their results. However, despite efforts from the cooperative oncology groups, patients entered into trials are by and large younger and presumably healthier than the typical older patient with the same disorder. Only 3% of older patients are treated in clinical trials. There is little evidence of efficacy and tolerability of cancer treatment in older patients, especially those who are >75 years old and/or vulnerable because of comorbidities. Furthermore, common end points of these trials are length of survival (for therapeutic interventions) or disease-specific deaths (for prevention studies), which are not always the most appropriate outcomes for older patients (because of their inherently limited life expectancies on the basis of age alone). More and more, clinical researchers are addressing issues of geriatric oncology. New, geriatrics-oriented trials are focusing more on symptom reduction and quality-of-life outcomes than on life expectancy. Surveys have indicated that many older adults, when fully informed, most often choose life-extending treatments, even at the risk of toxicity. Because of physiologic changes in older adults, there is potential for an increase in adverse events associated with standard chemotherapy and other cancer management options. However, for the most part, tumors are not more resistant to treatment in older adults (SOE=B), and acute toxicities (eg, nausea, vomiting, hair loss) may be less prominent in this population (SOE=B). Thus, although quality of life remains a primary treatment consideration, efforts at extending life should not be denied older adults on the basis of age alone.

Oncologists are often faced with the challenge of making management decisions in older adults in the absence of evidence-based guidelines. Aging is associated with a multitude of physiologic changes, which in turn are magnified by medical comorbidities and other geriatric problems. Appropriate treatment for cancer can be safe and effective in older adults if an adequate assessment is done and appropriate precautions are undertaken. Unfortunately, the fear of treatment-related adverse events and lack of evidence-based data leads to the undertreatment of cancer and decreased survival in this population. Life expectancy based on chronologic age is heterogeneous with comorbidities, disability, and geriatric syndromes having a substantial impact. After estimating the life expectancy, it should be determined whether the benefit of the suggested treatment will likely occur in the remaining life span. This consideration is especially important when making treatment decisions about adjuvant therapy.

Assessment of the Older Cancer Patient

Data regarding the application of the geriatric assessment to patients with cancer and the use of it to determine the capacity of patients to tolerate treatment are growing. Several abbreviated versions of geriatric assessment are being evaluated for their ability to predict treatment tolerability. Even these sophisticated tools need to be applied and interpreted with good clinical judgment. An 85-year-old man who was mowing his lawn last month but now presents with a tumor-related decline in function is much more likely to tolerate therapy than a person whose baseline level of activity was poor.

Although data are growing, few oncology trials that have provided evidence for cancer treatment in older adults have included geriatric assessment. Geriatric assessment provides an assessment of the global health of the patient, including an evaluation of the functional status, comorbid medical conditions, cognition, nutrition, polypharmacy, psychological status, social support, and geriatric syndromes. Each domain is an independent predictor of morbidity and mortality in older patients. Geriatric assessment can detect issues pertinent to cancer management that would go unrecognized otherwise. Geriatric assessment requires a multidisciplinary approach and analysis of the data to create a personalized plan. Incorporation of a geriatric assessment into care of older patients improves outcomes by preventing disability and reducing hospitalizations and may prove to be beneficial for older cancer patients. Recent studies have shown that geriatric assessment is feasible in oncology clinical assessment and cooperative group clinical trials, and that factors within geriatric assessment can predict toxicity from chemotherapy. Geriatric assessment can help stratify patients into "fit," "vulnerable," and "frail" subgroups. This stratification scheme can help to identify patients who would most benefit from standard treatments and those who would be at the highest risk of toxicity.

See also "Assessment," p 48.

Treatment Options for Older Patients with Cancer

Current forms of cancer treatment include surgery, radiation, chemotherapy, hormone manipulation, and biologic therapy. Age alone does not preclude any of these approaches, but because of normal changes with age in certain organs and also age-associated conditions (comorbidities), special considerations are warranted.

Cancer Screening

Studies that have contributed to the evidence on which the recommendations are based have included younger individuals, which make it difficult to generalize the findings to the oldest old. Thus, there are no clear guidelines for how to proceed with cancer screening in those >85 years old. Older adults, particularly those ≥85 years old, are underrepresented in most studies that contribute to the body of evidence used to establish cancer screening guidelines. There is no consensus about the value of cancer screening tests in the oldest old, especially because the increased prevalence of comorbid disease in old age may reduce the chance that the benefits of screening will exceed the harms of screening. Thus a paradox exists. The USPSTF evidence-based guidelines (http://www.ahrq.gov/clinic/uspstfix.htm) are based on the premise that screening will improve patient outcomes. However, screening in those ≥85 years old seems contradictory, because there is very little data that provide evidence that cancer screening tests are of any benefit for this age group. Many national organizations that publish screening guidelines do not address old age at all and do not have any upper age limits for prostate-specific antigen, mammography, Pap smear, and most recently, colorectal cancer screening.

For a complete discussion of issues in cancer screening, along with recommendations for older adult populations, see "Prevention," p 70.

Chemotherapy

Aging can be associated with changes in key pharmacologic parameters of antineoplastic agents and in the susceptibility to end-organ toxicity (Table 64.1).

Table 64.1—Chemotherapy Issues in Geriatric Oncology

Issue	Comments
General	■ Comorbidities and multiple medications add complexity.
Pharmacokinetic changes	■ A progressive delay with age in the elimination of renally excreted medications, due to a reduction in glomerular filtration rate, can account in part for more severe toxicity.
Pharmacodynamic changes	■ Possible enhanced resistance with age to antitumor agents.
	■ Increased expression of the multidrug resistance gene has been reported in some older adults.
	■ Other proteins that result in drug efflux have been shown to have prognostic importance, but age-associated changes have not been described.
	■ Increased tumor hypoxia with age has been observed in a murine model.
Toxicity	■ Mucositis, cardiotoxicity, and peripheral and central neurotoxicity become more common and more severe with aging (SOE=B).
	■ Cardiotoxicity is a complication of anthracyclines and anthraquinones, mitomycin C, and high-dose cyclophosphamide; incidence of cardiotoxicity increases with age.
	■ Peripheral neurotoxicity with vincristine is more common and more severe in older adults.
	■ The incidence of cerebellar toxicity from high-dose cytosine arabinoside increases with age.
Myelotoxicity	■ Chemotherapy-related myelotoxicity can become more severe and more prolonged with aging, but moderately toxic treatment regimens, such as CMF (cyclophosphamide, methotrexate, fluorouracil), cisplatin and fluorouracil, and cisplatin and etoposide are tolerated by many patients ≥70 years old without life-threatening neutropenia or thrombocytopenia (SOE=A).
	■ However, infections are markedly increased among older acute leukemia patients undergoing intensive induction treatment; in these cases, it is possible that the disease itself, rather than an age-associated change in "marrow reserve," is responsible for the depletion of hematopoietic stem cells.
Recent advances	■ Granulocyte colony-stimulating factor and granulocyte-macrophage colony-stimulating factor have reduced the incidence of neutropenic infections in patients receiving intensive treatment, and their effectiveness does not appear to be diminished with advancing patient age.
	■ Certain new medications or new formulations may be particularly suitable for older patients, eg, oral etoposide and fludarabine, gemcitabine, vinorelbine, capecitabine, paclitaxel protein-bound particles, and liposomal doxorubicin.

The most consistent pharmacokinetic change of aging is a progressive delay in the elimination of renally excretable medications because of a reduced glomerular filtration rate. The prolonged half-life of these agents can account in part for more severe toxicity. In a study of 65-year-old women with metastatic breast cancer, dosages of methotrexate and cyclophosphamide were modified according to creatinine clearance. As a consequence, myelotoxicity was markedly reduced without compromise of therapeutic effect.

Owing to differences in their pharmacokinetics and pharmacodynamics, certain medications can be particularly suitable for treating older patients. Oral etoposide provides valuable palliation for small-cell cancer of the lung and large-cell lymphoma, with minimal risk of complications. Fludarabine, which is very active in lymphoproliferative neoplasms, induces apoptosis of cancer cells, a process that can be altered in malignancies occurring in older adults. Vinorelbine and gemcitabine active against lung and breast cancer and are well tolerated and effective in older adults.

Hormonal Therapy

Hormonal treatment is effective in cancers of the breast, prostate, and endometrium. Most of these are well tolerated by older adults and commonly are the treatment of choice in this age group. However, adverse events of hormonal therapies should be considered in older patients. Tamoxifen, a selective estrogen-receptor modulator, has antagonistic and partial agonistic effects. It is a useful therapy in adjuvant treatment of breast cancer and also has estrogen-like positive effects on cardiovascular risk factors and bone disease. Aromatase inhibitors are oral medications that have been proved to be more efficacious than tamoxifen in the adjuvant and metastatic treatment for breast cancer. Although well-tolerated, osteoporosis and fractures are more common in patients on aromatase inhibitors. Hormonal therapies are the first-line of treatment for patients with systemic prostate cancer. The most commonly used hormonal therapies significantly decrease testosterone levels. Because prostate cancer can be an indolent and chronic disease, older men can be subjected to adverse events of hormonal therapies for many years. Growing evidence shows that hormonal therapy is associated with metabolic syndrome, cardiovascular disease, osteoporosis/fractures, and physical performance issues in older men. The decision to start hormonal treatment should not be taken lightly and should include an assessment of life expectancy, prostate cancer severity, and overall health status.

Biologic and Targeted Therapies

Over the last decade, the options for biologic and targeted therapies for cancer have grown significantly. These options have significantly changed the field of oncology. Immunotherapy, or modulation of immune response, is a particularly attractive option in treating older adults, whose natural defenses against cancer can be impaired by immune senescence. Only a limited number of options are clinically available, and these are still clearly inadequate to restore a normal immune response in older adults. Targeted therapies involve options that influence the activity of a specific receptor that is involved in cancer signaling. These options, including monoclonal antibodies or small molecule inhibitors, are used with chemotherapy or as a single agent, depending on the stage and type of cancer. Adverse-event profiles tend to be different for these agents. For example, many agents (such as the monoclonal antibody bevacizumab and the oral agents sunitinib and sorafenib) target the vascular endothelial growth factor (VEGF) receptor, thereby limiting tumor-related angiogenesis. These agents are associated with hypertension and thromboembolism, which can be a significant issue in patients who already have a history of these conditions. Hypertension can be particularly hard to control, and close interdisciplinary care and communication are necessary to prevent complications.

Several immunotherapy options are available for selected cancers. Recombinant α-interferon at moderate dosages (eg, 3 million units, three times weekly) is reasonably well tolerated by patients of all ages. At higher dosages, α-interferon causes myelodepression, severe fatigue, flu-like illness, malaise, fever, neuropathy, and abnormalities of liver enzymes. Delirium, depression, and dementia after α-interferon use have been reported in patients ≥65 years old. More information on the safety of α-interferon in older patients would be desirable. This is particularly important because interferon has been shown to be effective therapy for chronic myeloid leukemia, hairy cell leukemia, and multiple myeloma, hematologic malignancies that are more common among older adults (SOE=A). It may also prolong survival after chemotherapy for follicular lymphoma and has been used in renal cell carcinoma. It is being tested at higher, more toxic dosages in patients with stage II melanoma after surgical resection of the primary lesion. About 15% of patients with metastatic melanoma can experience a partial response from α-interferon. However, because of adverse events, interferon is often not chosen as a first-line treatment.

Interleukin-2 is used to treat metastatic melanoma and renal cancer. When administered daily at 3 million units/m^2, it may produce partial responses in about 15% of patients and complete remissions, many of which are long lasting, in about 5% of patients. Interleukin-2 can produce severe dose-related toxicity, including capillary leak syndrome, hypotension, adult respiratory distress syndrome, cardiac arrhythmias, peripheral edema, renal failure (prerenal), cholestatic liver dysfunction, skin rashes, and thrombocytopenia. These complications can be life-threatening in any patient, and initiation (especially when other options are available) should be undertaken cautiously.

Monoclonal antibodies directed against CD20 (rituximab) expressed on B-cell lymphomas and against HER-2/*neu* (trastuzumab) expressed on breast cancer and other epithelial malignancies are effective treatments. These humanized antibodies generally have mild toxicities. Patients can develop hypotension or shortness of breath with the first infusion because of complement fixation. Symptoms abate when the infusion rate is slowed down, and such symptoms rarely recur. Although monoclonal antibodies and targeted therapies are thought to be safer than chemotherapy because of decreased risk of myelosuppression, toxicities do occur and supportive mechanisms for older patients should be considered. Of note, many of the newer agents are administered as oral agents. Nonadherence is linked to adverse cancer outcomes, and therefore close monitoring is important.

Radiation Therapy

Radiation therapy provides palliation for virtually all cancers, and it may be part of a treatment plan for lymphomas and cancers of the prostate, bladder, cervix, esophagus, breast, and head and neck area. In combination with cytotoxic chemotherapy, radiation therapy has allowed organ preservation in cancers of the anus, bladder, and larynx, and in extremity sarcomas. A central issue for radiation therapy in older adults is safety. There has been a trend for almost five decades to use radiation therapy as an alternative to surgery in poor surgical candidates, mainly patients ≥65 years old, with the implied expectation that such an approach is less toxic. In fact, published reports have indicated that radiation therapy is both safe and effective in older patients (SOE=A). However, concern remains when treatment involves irradiation of the whole brain (fear of neurologic sequelae, including dementia) or pelvis (fear of marrow aplasia, myelodysplasia, or radiation enteritis), but no systematic investigation has categorically substantiated these concerns.

Advances in radiation therapy include techniques that allow a more restricted radiation field (such as stereotactic techniques for brain and lung), new applications of brachytherapy (insertion of radiation sources into the tumor bed), the development of radiosurgery (gamma ray knife, a precisely focused external beam of radiation) that allows destruction of small lesions (diameter ≤4 cm) of the CNS without craniotomy, and the development of new radiosensitizers.

Surgery

Concerns related to cancer surgery in older adults are safety and rehabilitative potential. Several reports indicate that age itself is not a risk factor for elective cancer surgery, but the length of hospital stay and the time to full recovery become longer with advancing age. Similar results have been reported both from referral centers and community hospitals.

Advances in anesthesia and surgery have benefited older patients. Included among these are endoscopic procedures that provide valuable palliation for the many tumors of the GI tract, and the more widespread use of spinal anesthesia for major abdominal interventions, with a substantial decline in perioperative complications and mortality. More widespread use of laparoscopic surgical techniques and application of laser and photodynamic therapy is also broadening the surgical armamentarium and providing more older patients with potential palliation and cure.

The trend to manage cancer without deforming surgery can preclude the need for complex rehabilitation and can be of special value for older adults. Organ preservation without compromise of treatment outcome is obtainable for cancer of the anus and larynx, and is being studied for cancers of the oropharynx, esophagus, bladder, and vulva. Also, the use of initial (neoadjuvant) chemotherapy before primary surgery has been effective in patients with large primary breast and lung cancers. Such an approach results in less extensive and potentially more curative surgical procedures.

See also "Perioperative Care," p 102.

Quality-of-Life Issues

Several studies have determined that the perception of quality of life is highly subjective and poorly reproduced by external observers, even by those who have close relationships with the patient or by healthcare providers who are very familiar with the patient's physical condition. Furthermore, there is considerable discrepancy between the clinician's determination of the patient's quality of life and the patient's own assessment, with clinicians tending to underestimate the patient's quality of life (SOE=B).

Early assessments of quality of life focused on functional status and freedom from pain, but these factors, although important, are inadequate for evaluating far-reaching consequences of serious diseases on all domains of life. In the past decade, several instruments for measuring quality of life have been validated and used successfully to study specific problems, such as the effects on quality of life of intensive care, the consequences of limb amputation or of partial and total mastectomy, and iatrogenic impotence. These instruments are questionnaires querying an individual to rate his or her own well-being in several dimensions with a categorical or a visual analog scale. Unfortunately, these instruments have not been adjusted to the special needs of older adults. While it is reasonable to assume that the importance of some factors, such as professional or job satisfaction, may decline with age, the importance of others, including social support and the perception of family burden, can become more prominent.

Other problems related to assessing quality of life include the complexity of some questionnaires, which can overwhelm some older adults. In addition, little progress has been made in the assessment of quality of life in cognitively impaired individuals. Studies of pain in demented individuals have demonstrated the reliability of repetitive behavioral testing in assessing discomfort, even in patients with cognitive impairment. Perhaps the same principles can be applied to assessing quality of life in demented patients.

At present, the main application of quality-of-life assessment in clinical decision making concerns the choice between interventions yielding comparable survival. An area of potential use is in medical decisions involving limited survival benefits at the price of a decline in quality of life. At present, the value of this trade-off is evaluated with measures known as "quality of life adjusted survival" or "quality-adjusted time without symptoms or toxicity," both of which may be important to consider for adults ≥70 years old. Research is needed in the melding of geriatric assessment and quality of life instruments.

SPECIFIC CANCERS

The three most commonly diagnosed types of cancer among women are cancers of the breast, lung and bronchus, and colorectal area, accounting for 52% of estimated cancer cases in women. Breast cancer alone is expected to account for 28% of all new cancer cases among women. Among men, cancers of the prostate, lung and bronchus, and colorectum account for 52% of all newly diagnosed cancers. Prostate cancer alone accounts for 28% of incident cases in men. Based on cases diagnosed between 1999 and 2005, an estimated 92% of these new cases of prostate cancer are expected to be diagnosed at local or regional stages, for which the 5-year relative survival approaches 100%.

Breast Cancer

Worldwide, nearly a third of breast cancer cases are seen in patients >65 years old, and in more developed countries this proportion rises to more than 40%. Advanced age at diagnosis of breast cancer is associated with more favorable tumor biology as indicated by increased hormone sensitivity and lower grades and proliferative indices. However, older patients are more likely to present with larger and more advanced tumors. Furthermore, there seem to be no major differences in outcomes in stage-matched patients as age increases. Nevertheless, older patients are less likely to be treated according to accepted treatment guidelines, and undertreatment can have an adverse impact on overall outcome. The explanation for these age-related differences in approach to treatment is complex and includes physician and patient bias, psychosocial issues, cost, and proximity to treatment centers. Underlying complexities due to health status also influence decision-making for treatment. Despite the fact that breast cancer occurs mainly in older patients, this population is under-represented in clinical trials. Less than 5% of participants included in clinical trials that evaluate adjuvant chemotherapy are ≥75 years old. Age is a significant predictor of whether older patients with breast cancer are offered entry into clinical trials, when in fact older patients are just as likely as younger patients to participate if given the opportunity. Because comorbidities and functional status significantly affect prognosis and treatment choice, thorough consideration must be given to the overall health of older patients.

For patients with localized cancer, the evidence supports surgical treatment when compared with primary hormonal treatment. Breast conservation treatment, consisting of breast-conserving surgery (lumpectomy or partial mastectomy) and postoperative radiotherapy, is now recommended as the standard of care for patients of all ages with early disease. As in younger patients, total mastectomy remains a surgical option for patients who prefer it over breast conservation treatment, and for those who decline or are not candidates for postoperative breast radiotherapy. Mastectomy is also indicated in patients with large primary lesions. Axillary lymph node dissection should be done in patients with clinical evidence of axillary lymph node involvement. However, for those without clinical lymph node involvement, the indication for upfront axillary lymph node dissection has been less clear for the older population. Sentinel lymph node dissection has been introduced as an alternative to axillary lymph node dissection. Sentinel lymph node biopsy has been shown to be a safe and accurate method of predicting axillary status in patients with breast cancer, including those ≥70 years old. Sentinel lymph node biopsy is now widely considered an acceptable treatment option in patients of all ages with tumor size <2–3 cm and no clinical evidence of axillary involvement. Findings from such biopsies in older patients with breast cancer could significantly affect subsequent treatment decisions, including adjuvant systemic treatment. Controversy exists regarding the need for complementary axillary lymph node dissection after a positive sentinel lymph node is found. Data suggest that sentinel node sampling is just as accurate as axillary dissection but considerably less toxic (SOE=A).

Controversy surrounds several critical issues in the management of this most common malignancy in older women. These issues include postoperative irradiation after lumpectomy, adjunct hormonal treatment, and initial management of metastatic breast cancer.

Postoperative Irradiation after Lumpectomy: Although irradiation after lumpectomy is safe in women ≥65 years old, it may be a source of significant inconvenience and cost. The value of postoperative irradiation has been questioned because the local recurrence rate of breast cancer may decrease with age, and the inconvenience of daily radiation treatment protocols may outweigh the limited benefits for some.

Adjunct Hormonal Treatment: Adjunct treatment with tamoxifen for at least 2 years prolongs both the disease-free survival and the overall survival of postmenopausal women (SOE=A). The benefits and risks of more prolonged treatment, especially for women >70 years old, remain controversial. Aromatase inhibitors are currently licensed as second-line hormonal treatment for those on tamoxifen whose cancer has progressed. Aromatase inhibitors are used as first-line treatment in women with estrogen receptor–positive tumors, and the medication is given for at least 5 years. Aromatase inhibitors are both more effective and less toxic than tamoxifen (SOE=A). In women currently on tamoxifen, it is recommended that tamoxifen treatment be continued for a 5-year duration, followed by 5 years of an aromatase inhibitor.

Initial Management of Metastatic Breast Cancer: Women ≥65 years old with metastatic, hormone receptor–positive breast cancer are likely to have effective palliation with hormonal therapy, such as tamoxifen. Hormonal treatment has been shown to benefit older women with hormone receptor–poor tumors, but chemotherapy has also been shown to be safe and effective in this group of patients. Generally, single agents are used and treatment is begun at full dosage with modifications based on any toxicities that develop. In frail older adults, treatment can usually begin safely at 75% of the recommended dosage.

Lung Cancer

Lung cancer is the leading cause of cancer-related death in Western countries for both men and women. More than 40% of patients diagnosed with lung cancer are ≥70 years old. Management options for lung cancer are based on the cell type. Non–small-cell cancer constitutes around 80% of all lung cancers, while small-cell cancer makes up the remaining. Most patients with lung cancer present with stage 4 disease, in which the goal of therapy is palliative. Lung cancer is becoming increasingly common in older women for reasons that are not completely understood. The increase may possibly be due to higher smoking rates among women. In addition, some data suggest that women are at greater risk (than men) of developing lung cancer per unit of tobacco exposure. Early recognition and surgical resection remain the best chance for cure. For patients with lesions in a location that precludes surgery, localized radiation can result in long-term survival. Over the past decade, chemotherapy has produced clinical responses and provided effective palliation for a portion of patients with metastatic disease. A meta-analysis of over 50 trials comparing chemotherapy to best supportive care indicated that chemotherapy is not associated with a worse outcome in older adults and thus paved the way for exploration of better suited regimens. Combination chemotherapy with a platinum doublet continues to remain the standard of care for patients in the "young-old" age category who are candidates. Retrospective analysis of large randomized, controlled trials that have investigated the role of a platinum-based chemotherapy for older patients noted a similar survival benefit as in the young, with a predictable increase in toxicity. Survival was prolonged, with the added increment measured in weeks to months. However, results from these trials cannot be extrapolated to the general older adult population, because the trials are potentially biased by selection criteria that govern enrollment. New chemotherapeutic agents, such as vinorelbine and gemcitabine, and more established agents such as paclitaxel or docetaxel used in lower-dose weekly schedules, have proved to produce responses, improve quality of life, and prolong overall survival by a few months for older patients with lung cancer (SOE=A).

Colon Cancer

Two-thirds of colon cancer cases are seen in adults ≥65 years old. With advancing age, there is a greater likelihood of right-sided lesions and presentations with anemia rather than pain. Colonoscopy has become the mainstay of diagnosis, primarily because it enables direct visualization of the entire colon and biopsy. Surgical excision may be adequate for lesions confined to the colon, but if regional nodes are involved, postoperative adjuvant chemotherapy (usually 5-fluorouracil plus leucovorin) has reduced recurrence by 40%–50% (SOE=A). The addition of oxaliplatin to 5-fluorouracil for adjuvant chemotherapy has improved outcomes for younger patients with regional nodes after resection (ie, stage III disease). Trials that have evaluated this regimen for patients included very few older patients, so more data are necessary.

The standard of care in patients with stage 4 disease is systemic chemotherapy with or without targeted therapy and surgical intervention when appropriate for curative intent or symptom management. Survival of patients with metastatic disease in the liver or other organs has improved significantly because of new medications, such as irinotecan and oxaliplatin, that have induced partial remissions in a subset of patients. Survival has increased from 6 months on average to >2 years for patients who can tolerate treatment. Active debate continues on the use of combination therapy versus monotherapy in the management of older patients with metastatic colon cancer because of a similar overall survival benefit noted in several trials. Capecitabine, an oral 5-fluorouracil pro-drug, is an option for older patients, especially those who are wary of infusional regimens. New medications that target a tyrosine kinase (an integral enzyme for cellular proliferation) within tumor cells and neutralize vascular endothelial growth factor (VEGF) (thought to promote angiogenesis) have improved outcomes. Bevacuzimab, a VEGF antibody, has been shown to improve overall survival of older adults when used in combination with standard chemotherapy (SOE=A). The incidence of arterial thromboembolic events increased with age, and caution must be used when prescribing this in older adults.

Age per se should not be considered a contraindication for surgery. In patients with hepatic metastasis only, hepatic resection can offer a chance of long-term survival. In selected older patients, this procedure is safe and feasible with a similar survival benefit (SOE=B). Unfortunately, older patients who undergo this procedure are less likely to receive perioperative chemotherapy. Surgical excision of solitary hepatic lesions offers a survival advantage for selected patients, primarily those with smaller lesions, five or fewer lesions confined to a single hepatic lobe, and a longer interval from original tumor resection until the diagnosis of hepatic metastasis. See also Colonic Polyps and Colon Cancer in "Gastrointestinal Diseases and Disorders," p 408.

Prostate Cancer

Prostate cancer affects older men disproportionately. The estimated prevalence of prostate cancer in men ≥75 years old is over 1 million, with more than 60% of all new cases diagnosed in men >65 years old. Because of the long natural history of the disease, the case fatality rate is low in the young. It is notable, however, that 70% of men who die of prostate cancer are ≥75 years old. Advanced prostate cancer cannot be cured and affects patients whose disease has spread beyond the prostate and/or are symptomatic, as well as patients with biochemical recurrence only (a rise in prostate-specific antigen with no evidence of disease). Androgen-deprivation therapy (ADT) is used in the initial management of these patients and is associated with a multitude of adverse events, including hot flashes, sexual dysfunction, osteoporosis, and metabolic syndrome. ADT consists of gonadotropin releasing–hormone agonist or antagonist as well as an antiandrogen (pills that block the androgen receptor), and their effects lie in their ability to lower the testosterone levels available to the cancer cells. Given the significant consequence of ADT in older men, serious consideration must be undertaken with the patient regarding risks versus benefits before beginning therapy. For older patients with indolent cancer characteristics and no clinical symptoms, active surveillance should be considered.

In older men, when the disease has progressed on ADT (castrate-resistant prostate cancer), standard-dose chemotherapy is docetaxel at 75 mg/m^2 every 3 weeks. Subset analysis of the index trials has established that older men >75 years old had an equivalent response to that of the younger population with a predictable increase in toxicity. A lower dosage of docetaxel (ie, 30 mg/m^2 on a weekly basis) has been studied in an attempt to address the issue of myelosuppression and other adverse events seen with standard-dose chemotherapy. Results from these studies indicate that this schedule has a modest effect on the progression-free survival but does not impact overall survival. Several new regimens have been approved for treatment of castrate-resistant prostate cancer. Abiraterone, which selectively blocks the cytochrome P450 C17 and thereby inhibits androgen biosynthesis, has been shown to improve overall survival in this setting. The trial that led to its approval included patients >75 years old (28% of the study population) who had similar benefit. Overall survival was also improved with sipuleucel-T, an autologous active cellular-based immunotherapy, when compared with placebo in a trial in which the median age was 72 years old (SOE=A).

See also "Prostate Disease," p 437.

Hematologic Malignancies, Lymphomas, and Multiple Myeloma

Leukemias

Acute myeloid leukemia (AML) after myelodysplastic syndromes, as is seen more commonly among older adults, is more likely to be refractory to treatment and to have a smoldering course, for which only supportive care is administered. What is not clear is whether the prevalence of unfavorable cytogenetic abnormalities and of multilineage neoplastic involvement increases with age in de novo AML. The subset of patients with myelodysplasia who do not have excess blasts or overt leukemia but are neutropenic and have recurrent infections may benefit from intermittent treatment with granulocyte colony-stimulating factor.

In a trial with older patients with AML, delayed treatment was much less effective than immediate treatment. Although this study established the value of timely chemotherapy, the choice of treatment (whether full-dose induction or low-dose cytarabine) remains controversial. In one study, the survival of older patients with leukemia treated with low-dose cytarabine was superior to the survival of those receiving standard induction, because of lower treatment-related mortality. However, others have obtained different results and claimed the superiority of standard treatment.

Chronic lymphocytic leukemia is the most common form of leukemia in the Western world; about 12,500 cases are diagnosed each year in the United States. The incidence is declining for unknown reasons. The median age at diagnosis is 61 years. The diagnosis is most often made incidentally when a peripheral WBC count reveals leukocytosis with a small-lymphocyte count >4,000/μL. Treatment is generally instituted only to control a life-threatening or symptomatic complication. The major complications are infection and marrow failure. Because about 25% of patients develop autoimmune anemia or thrombocytopenia sometime in the course of the disease, it is important to investigate the mechanism of any decline in peripheral blood cell counts. Autoimmune mechanisms can be treated with glucocorticoids or splenectomy, whereas marrow infiltration by tumor cells requires antitumor therapy. Chlorambucil and fludarabine are the two most active agents. Median survival varies with the stage of disease. Once anemia or thrombocytopenia develops as a consequence of marrow failure, median survival is about 18 months.

Non-Hodgkin Lymphoma

Although there are about 38 named varieties of lymphoma, the two most common forms (diffuse large B-cell lymphoma and follicular lymphoma) account for about 75% of cases. The prognosis of non-Hodgkin lymphoma worsens with age, but the explanation remains unclear. It is likely that older adults are more susceptible to the complications of intensive treatment.

The treatment of older adults with diffuse large B-cell lymphoma has improved in recent years. In this group, 60%–70% of patients obtain a durable complete remission with combination chemotherapy (eg, cyclophosphamide, doxorubicin, vincristine, prednisone [CHOP]) plus rituximab (a monoclonal antibody against CD20 on B cells). Administration of lower-than-normal dosages results in a poorer

Chapters

outcome. Hematopoietic growth factors can lessen the hematopoietic toxicity of treatment.

The treatment of follicular lymphoma is more controversial. Localized forms of the disease (seen in 15% of patients) are curable with radiation therapy. In the 85% of patients with more advanced disease, single agent and combination chemotherapy can sometimes induce long, complete remissions (median duration 6–7 years). However, in patients with other serious morbidities and a remaining life expectancy of 5 years, treatment may not be needed because of the indolent nature of the disease progression.

Hodgkin Disease

Hodgkin disease exhibits a curious bimodal age-incidence curve, with a second peak late in life. Compared with younger patients, older patients with advanced disease may respond less well to therapy and have poorer survival rates (SOE=C). Several factors can contribute to this poorer prognosis: more extensive disease at presentation, biologic variations from true Hodgkin disease, greater toxicity with standard treatment regimens, and less aggressive treatment. Older adults can usually tolerate full doses of doxorubicin, bleomycin, vinblastine, and dacarbazine (ABVD) without life-threatening bone-marrow toxicity.

Multiple Myeloma and Monoclonal Gammopathy of Uncertain Significance (MGUS)

Multiple myeloma is diagnosed in about 19,900 people each year in the United States. The median age at diagnosis is 68 years; it is rare in people <40 years old. The incidence in black Americans is twice that in white Americans. The classic triad of myeloma is marrow plasmacytosis (>10%), lytic bone lesions, and a serum or urine (or both) monoclonal gammopathy. Monoclonal gammopathy is common in older adults, estimated at 6% of those ≥70 years old. When an abnormal paraprotein is discovered on serum immunoelectrophoresis, the best diagnostic test to distinguish myeloma from MGUS is a skeletal survey. If the skeletal survey is normal, a bone marrow biopsy is still indicated to determine the presence of marrow plasmacytosis. Patients with MGUS have marrow plasma cells constituting <10% of the total cell number; do not have lytic bone lesions; and usually do not have other features of myeloma, including hypercalcemia, renal failure, anemia, or susceptibility to infection. MGUS progresses to multiple myeloma or a related malignancy at a rate of 1% per year (SOE=B).

Patients with myeloma require treatment when the lytic bone lesions become symptomatic or progressive, infections are recurrent, or the serum paraprotein increases. Standard treatment consists of lenalidomide plus dexamethasone for those who will go on to receive high-dose therapy plus an autologous stem-cell transplant. For those who are not transplant candidates, intermittent pulses of an oral alkylating agent (eg, melphalan), prednisone, and lenalidomide are given for 4–7 days every 4–6 weeks. Supportive care includes bisphosphonates to decrease bone turnover, erythropoietin and other hematinics for the anemia, intravenous immunoglobulin for recurrent infections, radiation for specific symptomatic bone lesions, maintenance of hydration to preserve renal function, and adequate analgesia.

PRINCIPLES OF MANAGEMENT

Both the incidence and prevalence of cancer increase with age, and older adults more often present with advanced-stage disease. Screening older populations for colon and breast cancer can lead to early detection of more curable lesions. Older patients can have less physiologic reserve than younger patients, but unless a specific comorbid illness is influencing baseline organ function, cancer treatments with curative or palliative potential should be offered to most patients in most settings, regardless of age. Curative surgical procedures may require more prolonged convalescence, but recovery from most procedures is expected. Radiation therapy is safe and effective in the same settings in which it is used in younger patients. Chemotherapy may need to be adjusted to the individual patient's level of tolerance of the adverse events, but usually the changes should be made in the face of toxicities that actually develop rather than on toxicities anticipated to develop. Biologic therapies also are generally safe.

See also "Dermatologic Diseases and Disorders," p 350, for the diagnosis and treatment of skin cancers, and "Persistent Pain," p 119, and "Palliative Care," p 111, for the management of pain and end-of-life care.

REFERENCES

- Austin S, Martin MY, Kim Y, et al. Disparities in use of gynecologic oncologists for women with ovarian cancer in the United States. *Health Serv Res.* 2013;48(3):1135–1153.
- Hemmerich JA, Ahmad FS, Meltzer DO, et al. African American men significantly underestimate their risk of having prostate cancer at the time of biopsy. *Psychooncology.* 2013;22(2):338–345.
- Hurria A, Togawa K, Mohile SG, et al. Predicting chemotherapy toxicity in older adults with cancer: a prospective multicenter study. *J Clin Oncol.* 2011;29(25):3457–3465.
- Pal SK, Katheria V, Hurria A. Evaluating the older patient with cancer: understanding frailty and the geriatric assessment. *CA Cancer J Clin.* 2010;60(2):120–132.

Normal Laboratory Values*

Referenced in the Questions and Critiques

BLOOD, PLASMA, SERUM CHEMISTRIES

Alanine aminotransferase (ALT) 0–35 U/L

Aspartate aminotransferase (AST) 0–35 U/L

Bicarbonate (CO_2) 21–30 mEq/L

Blood gas studies:

- PO_2 83–108 mmHg
- PCO_2 Women: 32–45 mmHg; Men: 35–48 mmHg
- pH 7.35–7.45
- Oxygen saturation 95%–98%

Blood urea nitrogen (BUN) 8–20 mg/dL

Calcium 8.8–10.3 mg/dL

Calcium, ionized 4.5–5.6 mEq/L

Carcinoembryonic antigen <2.5 ng/mL

Chloride 98–106 mEq/L

Cholesterol:

- Total Desirable: <200 mg/dL
- High-density lipoprotein (HDL) Desirable: >39 mg/dL
- Low-density lipoprotein (LDL) Recommended: <130 mg/dL, lower for those with CHD risk factors or vascular disease; evidence limited for adults ≥85 yr old
  - Moderate risk: 130–159 mg/dL
  - High risk: ≥160 mg/dL

Creatinine 0.7–1.5 mg/dL

Creatine kinase Women: 26–140 U/L; Men: 38–174 U/L

Digoxin (therapeutic level) 0.8–2.0 ng/mL for rate control; 0.6–0.8 for heart failure

Ferritin 20–250 ng/mL

Folate 2.2–17.3 ng/mL

Glucose Fasting: 70–105 mg/dL
2-hour postprandial: <140 mg/dL

Hemoglobin A_{1c} 5.3%–7.5%

Homocysteine 5–15 μmol/L

Iron 50–150 mcg/dL; iron saturation ([iron/iron-binding capacity] × 100) ≤10% abnormal

Iron-binding capacity, total 250–450 mcg/dL

Lactate dehydrogenase 60–100 U/L

Methylmalonic acid (MMA) 0.08–0.56 μmol/L

Magnesium 1.8–3.0 mg/dL

Parathyroid hormone 10–65 pg/mL

Phosphatase, acid 0.5–5.5 U/L

Phosphatase, alkaline 20–135 U/L

Phosphorus (≥60 yr old) Women: 2.8–4.1 mg/dL
Men: 2.3–3.7 mg/dL

Potassium 3.5–5 mEq/L

Prostate-specific antigen (PSA) <4 ng/mL

Protein, total 6.4–8.3 g/dL

- Albumin 3.5–5.5 g/dL
- Globulin 2.0–3.5 g/dL

Rheumatoid factor, latest test >1:80 is abnormal

Sodium 136–145 mEq/L

Testosterone:

- Women <3.5 nmol/L (<100 ng.dL)
- Men 10–35 nmol/L (300–1,000 ng/dL)

Thyrotropin (TSH) 0.5–5.0 μU/mL

Thyroxine (T_4) Total: 5–12 mcg/dL; Free: 0.9–2.4 ng/dL

Triglycerides Recommended: <150 mg/dL

Uric acid 2.5–8.0 mg/dL

Vitamin B_{12} 200–950 pg/mL

25(OH) vitamin D (total) 30–75 mcg/L

HEMATOLOGY

RBC count Women: 4.2–5.4 × 10^6/μL; Men: 4.7–6.1 × 10^6/μL

Erythrocyte sedimentation rate (Westergren) 0–35 mm/h

Hematocrit Women: 33%–43%; Men: 39%–49%

Hemoglobin Women: 11.5–15.5 g/dL; Men: 14–18 g/dL

WBC count and differential 4,800–10,800/μL

- Segmented neutrophils 54%–62%
- Band forms 3%–5%
- Lymphocytes 23%–33%
- Monocytes 3%–7%
- Eosinophils 1%–3%
- Basophils <1%

Mean corpuscular hemoglobin 28–32 pg

Mean corpuscular volume 86–98 fL (86–98 mm^3)

Platelet count 150,000–450,000/μL

URINE

Creatinine clearance 90–140 mL/min

Creatinine, urine Women: 11–20 mg/kg/24 h
Men: 14–26 mg/kg/24 h

Urine, postvoid residual volume <50 mL, normal; >200 mL, abnormal; 50–200 mL, equivocal

---

* Note: Because normal ranges vary among laboratories, data in this table may not conform with that of all laboratories.

go thru these

INDEX OF QUESTION NUMBERS BY PRIMARY TOPIC

Addictions 8, 15
Anxiety Disorders 88, 92
Assessment 51, 94

Back and Neck Pain 103, 122
Behavior Problems in Dementia 17, 29, 79
Biology 16, 113

Cardiovascular Diseases and Disorders 26, 49
Community-Based Care 63, 100
Complementary and Alternative Medicine 40, 89
Cultural Aspects of Care 42, 118

Delirium 1, 22
Dementia 3, 7, 59, 74
Demography 81, 104
Depression and Other Mood Disorders 14, 56
Dermatologic Diseases and Disorders 33, 71
Diabetes Mellitus 25, 101
Diseases and Disorders of the Foot 43, 72
Dizziness 53, 75

Eating and Feeding Problems 31, 65
Endocrine and Metabolic Disorders 20, 123

Falls 9, 23
Finance 12, 80
Frailty 9, 52

Gait Impairment 62, 73
Gastrointestinal Diseases and Disorders 54, 108
Gynecologic Diseases and Disorders 19, 21, 57

Hearing Impairment 10, 55
Heart Failure 58, 110
Hematologic Diseases and Disorders 45, 95
Hospital Care 27, 106
Hypertension 66, 117

Infectious Diseases 30, 48
Intellectual and Developmental Disabilities 39, 120

Kidney Diseases and Disorders 18, 76

Legal and Ethical Issues 93, 116

Malnutrition 2, 16, 107
Mistreatment of Older Adults 4, 119
Multimorbidity 37
Musculoskeletal Diseases and Disorders 11, 114

Neurologic Diseases and Disorders 77, 86
Nursing-Home Care 28, 99

Oncology 90, 91
Oral Diseases and Disorders 97, 124
Osteoporosis 111, 115, 125
Outpatient Care Systems 64, 105

Palliative Care 41, 98
Perioperative Care 1, 121
Persistent Pain 34, 112
Personality and Somatic Symptom Disorders 35, 85
Pharmacotherapy 36, 68
Physical Activity 13, 96
Pressure Ulcers and Wound Care 47, 70
Prevention 50, 84
Prostate Disease 69, 90
Psychotic Disorders 44, 59

Rehabilitation 31, 87
Respiratory Diseases and Disorders 5, 102

Sexual Function Disorders 24, 38
Sleep Problems 60, 83
Syncope 46, 61

Transitional Care 6, 32

Urinary Incontinence 82, 109

Visual Impairment 67, 78

QUESTIONS

Directions: Each of the questions or incomplete statements below is followed by four or five suggested answers or completions. For self-assessment question answer sheet to print for use with the *GNRS4* Book version, please visit *GNRS4* on www.geriatricscareonline.org. The repeated questions with answers and supporting critiques are located on p 587 The table of Normal Laboratory Values on the previous page may be consulted for any of the questions in this book.

1. A 72-year-old man with an 80 pack-year smoking history is admitted to the surgical intensive care unit (SICU) for exacerbation of COPD after elective cholecystectomy. He has no history of dementia, depression, or other cognitive disorder; score on the Mini–Mental State Examination 1 month ago was 30 of 30. He is started on inhaled albuterol prn, fluticasone/salmeterol, intravenous dexamethasone, intravenous ceftriaxone, and supplemental oxygen. He becomes increasingly anxious. Oxygen saturation decreases, and he is started on lorazepam 0.5 mg IV. Oxygen saturation reaches 93% with 35% venturi mask. He improves overnight and into the next day.

At the beginning of day 3 in the SICU, staff notes that he is inattentive and more confused. He becomes fatigued during the day and increasingly confused and hypervigilant toward evening and overnight. He refuses breathing treatments and pulls out intravenous lines; he undergoes intubation for airway protection. On day 12 in the SICU, he undergoes tracheotomy. He is discharged from the SICU on day 15, with symptoms and signs of delirium.

Which of the following may have prevented the prolonged stay in the SICU?

(A) Substituting methylprednisolone for dexamethasone
(B) Substituting haloperidol for lorazepam
(C) Substituting an intravenous opioid for lorazepam
(D) Substituting nonpharmacologic approaches to anxiety for lorazepam
(E) Starting anxiolytics before arrival in the SICU

2. The daughter of an 86-year-old woman wants to discuss her mother's weight loss. The mother had always been moderately obese, but she has steadily lost >10% of her weight over the last 6 months. The patient lives in a dementia-care unit and has slowly progressive, mild to moderate stage dementia.

Which of the following is the best response regarding weight loss in an older adult living in an institutional setting?

(A) Unintended weight loss in an obese adult often improves outcomes.
(B) Unintended weight loss requires evaluation.
(C) The patient should be given protein supplements.
(D) Weight loss in older adults is normal.

3. Which of the following is true of the 2011 National Institute of Aging and the Alzheimer's Association (NIA–AA) criteria for diagnosis of Alzheimer disease?

(A) Diagnosis of definite Alzheimer disease can be based on neuroimaging findings and markers in cerebrospinal fluid.
(B) Diagnosis of possible Alzheimer disease is reserved for individuals with no memory impairment but with impairment in other cognitive domains.
(C) The criteria now include a formal diagnostic framework for the symptomatic, predementia phase of Alzheimer disease.
(D) Functional decline is not a criterion for Alzheimer disease.

4. An 80-year-old man is brought to the emergency department by police after he was found wandering several blocks from his apartment in the middle of the night. He tells the admitting clinician, "I'm fine. I was taking a walk and got lost." Review of systems is positive only for urinary frequency. When asked about his home medications, he says "it's all there in the chart." His last visit to the primary care clinic was >1 year ago, at which time his medications were listed as glipizide, atenolol, and warfarin. He reports independence in all basic and instrumental activities of daily living (ADLs and IADLs). The patient was evaluated in the emergency department 3 times in the last 3 months for dizziness, back pain, and an INR of 5. He says he has no close family or friends and has no emergency contacts listed in the electronic medical record. Several referrals have been made to home-health agencies, but they report that the patient refuses all nursing and physical therapy visits.

On examination, temperature is 37.7°C (98.0°F), BMI is 16 kg/m^2, blood pressure is 160/90 mmHg, heart rate is 90 beats per minute, and O_2 saturation is 99% on room air. He appears thin and is dressed in a worn bathrobe that smells of urine. Examination of heart, lungs, and abdomen is unremarkable. He becomes irritable and refuses to answer any questions from the Mini–Mental State Examination.

Laboratory findings:

WBC	13,000/µL
Serum glucose	300 mg/dL
Hemoglobin A_{1c}	11%
INR	0.9
Urinalysis	>50 WBC, + nitrites
Urine culture	>100,000 CFU gram-negative rods

The patient is admitted to the hospital, and therapy with antibiotics is initiated for presumed urinary tract infection. His WBC count normalizes, and repeat urinalysis and urine culture are negative. With daily insulin injections and resumption of warfarin, the hyperglycemia resolves and the INR is in the therapeutic range. The patient is medically stable and insists on returning home, but the floor nurse reports that he is unable to self-administer insulin.

Which of the following is the most appropriate next step for determining a safe discharge plan for this patient?

(A) Referral to a home-health agency for evaluation of home safety
(B) Formal evaluation of decision-making capacity
(C) Referral to Adult Protective Services
(D) Evaluation for depression
(E) Evaluation for dementia

5. An 84-year-old woman is admitted to the hospital because of an exacerbation of COPD. Initial therapy included albuterol/ipratropium nebulizer, intravenous corticosteroids, antibiotic therapy, and supplemental oxygen at 2 L/min, but she has become progressively more dyspneic overnight. History includes COPD and hypertension.

On physical examination, respiratory rate is 26 breaths per minute and O_2 saturation is 91%; vital signs are otherwise stable. There is a faint expiratory wheeze and distant breath sounds. She is speaking in partial sentences. Arterial blood gas shows pH of 7.32, pCO_2 of 51 mmHg, and pO_2 of 70 mmHg. Her code status is "Do Not Intubate," but she is willing to go to the intensive care unit.

Which of the following is the most appropriate next step in caring for this patient?

(A) Inhaled corticosteroids via nebulizer
(B) ECG
(C) Noninvasive positive-pressure ventilation
(D) Pulmonary function tests
(E) Repeat measurement of arterial blood gas

6. A 78-year-old man is being discharged to his home from the hospital after treatment for angina. He was hospitalized 3 months ago for a similar illness. History includes hypertension, hyperlipidemia, and mild cognitive impairment.

Which of the following has *not* been shown to reduce risk of readmission?

(A) Comprehensive discharge planning and home follow-up program
(B) Transitions in care/patient coaching intervention
(C) Reengineered discharge intervention
(D) Telehealth discharge intervention

7. A 73-year-old woman is admitted to the hospital with shortness of breath and syncope. History is significant for Alzheimer disease, stroke, and seizure disorder. Medications include carbamazepine 300 mg q12h, lisinopril 10 mg/d, aspirin 325 mg/d, citalopram 20 mg/d, and donepezil 23 mg/d.

On examination, blood pressure is 120/75 mmHg and heart rate is 57 beats per minute.

Which of the following is the most likely cause of her symptoms?

(A) Drug interaction between carbamazepine and donepezil
(B) Drug interaction between carbamazepine and citalopram
(C) Adverse effect from donepezil
(D) Adverse effect from lisinopril

8. An 82-year-old woman comes to the office to establish care. She is accompanied by her daughter, who is concerned that her mother's use of diazepam is related to recent falls and problems with balance. History includes osteoporosis and knee osteoarthritis. Medications include alendronate, calcium, acetaminophen, and diazepam. The patient has been taking diazepam for many years, usually 10 mg q8h. She acknowledges having felt stressed during much of her life but says that she is not anxious or depressed now.

On examination, vital signs are stable, and there are no orthostatic changes in blood pressure. There is some bruising on her elbows and hips, and osteoarthritic changes are noted in both knees. There is no evidence of delirium or cognitive impairment. Her gait is somewhat slow, and she needs to take a couple of steps to make a 180-degree turn. She describes some bilateral knee pain when she rises. She can remain in semi-tandem stance for <10 sec and cannot perform a tandem stance.

Which of the following is the most appropriate first step in addressing the patient's benzodiazepine use?

(A) Refer patient to residential treatment program.
(B) Refer patient for psychiatry consultation.
(C) Recommend gradual taper of the benzodiazepine dosage.
(D) Recommend switch to a shorter-acting benzodiazepine.

9. A 75-year-old woman is brought to the office by her daughter. The mother has been falling, most often when rising from the toilet or attempting to climb stairs. History includes sarcopenia and frailty. She has no neurologic or metabolic abnormalities. Exercise was recommended in a previous office visit. Despite the daughter's efforts, the patient is reluctant to spend time and energy on the exercise program. The daughter asks for help prioritizing the exercises; in particular, she wants to know which exercises are most important in preventing falls.

Which of the following is most effective for preventing falls?

(A) Strengthening exercise
(B) Aerobic exercise
(C) Balance exercise
(D) Multicomponent exercise

10. A 74-year-old woman comes to the office for a routine examination. When asked about her hearing, she indicates that she cannot always understand what people are saying because they mumble. This is a problem, especially at work. She appears to struggle to hear the questions, and she seems more withdrawn and confused than in the past.

Which of the following is the most appropriate next step?

(A) Explain that hearing loss is inevitable as people age and there is no effective treatment.
(B) Screen for hearing impairment and hearing handicap.
(C) Screen for dementia.
(D) Refer the patient to an otolaryngologist.

11. A 78-year-old man comes to the office to establish care. History includes tophaceous gout, type 2 diabetes mellitus, hypertension, and benign prostatic hyperplasia. He adheres to a low-purine diet and has taken allopurinol for >10 years; his current dosage is 300 mg/d, which he takes exactly as prescribed. Each year he has 5 or 6 acute attacks of gout involving multiple joints, which he manages with ibuprofen; the attacks are increasingly debilitating.

On examination, weight is 64.9 kg (143 lb). There are tophi on auricles and distal interphalangeal joints bilaterally. Serum uric acid level is 8 mg/dL, creatinine is 1.7 mg/dL, and hemoglobin A_{1c} is 7.2%.

Which of the following is the most appropriate next step for treating this patient's gout?

(A) Increase the dosage of allopurinol to 400 mg/d and continue ibuprofen for acute attacks.
(B) Decrease the current dosage of allopurinol and continue ibuprofen for acute attacks.
(C) Maintain allopurinol at the current dosage and use prednisone for acute attacks.
(D) Discontinue allopurinol, start febuxostat 40 mg/d, and use prednisone for acute attacks.

12. A 67-year-old man asks about hospice care because he has considerable pain and nausea related to stage 4 pancreatic cancer. He is on chemotherapy, but his condition is declining. His oncologist offers another course of chemotherapy, which would cause uncomfortable adverse effects but possibly increase his life expectancy by 2–3 months. The patient lives at home and is debilitated to the point that he needs assistance to bathe. He is currently enrolled in traditional Medicare Parts A and B. He has no other health insurance.

If the patient switches his insurance status to Medicare hospice benefits, which of the following services will *not* be covered?

(A) Nonpalliative chemotherapy
(B) Home-health aide to assist with bathing
(C) Hospital bed for his home
(D) Grief counseling for his wife

13. A 70-year-old woman comes to the clinic for a routine examination. She lives independently at home. She mentions that she feels unsteady on her feet and now has difficulty getting up from the chair, climbing up and down stairs, and walking a few yards outside of her home to pick up her mail. History includes hypertension, for which she takes hydrochlorothiazide, and obesity. She scores 4 of 15 on the Geriatric Depression Scale (short form), and 28 of 30 on the Mini–Mental State Examination.

On examination, blood pressure is 128/78 mmHg and pulse is 70 beats per minute. Weight is 116 kg (256 lb); over the past year she has gradually gained 11.3 kg (25 lb). BMI is 38 kg/m^2. She gets up from the chair and walks to the examining room slowly. There is no evidence of focal weakness or neurologic deficits. CBC and metabolic profile are normal. Thyrotropin level is 2.3 µU/mL, and vitamin B_{12} level is 712 pg/mL.

Which of the following is the most effective management strategy to improve this patient's physical function and quality of life?

(A) Weight loss by dietary management
(B) Regular exercise
(C) Combined weight loss and regular exercise
(D) Physical therapy for gait and balance training

14. An 80-year-old woman is brought to the office for consultation about depressive symptoms, including social isolation, decreased appetite, and irritability, that have waxed and waned over the past 8 weeks. History includes a diagnosis of probable Alzheimer disease. The patient has been taking sertraline for about 7 weeks, adjusted to a current dosage of 150 mg/d. Her depressive symptoms and signs have not improved, and the medication appears to be associated with nonspecific GI complaints, including nausea.

Which of the following is the most appropriate recommendation for this patient?

(A) Continue the current dosage of sertraline for 3 more weeks.
(B) Increase the dosage of sertraline.
(C) Switch to an antidepressant with a different mechanism of action.
(D) Augment the sertraline with aripiprazole.
(E) Discontinue sertraline and observe for several weeks.

15. A 73-year-old man comes to the office for a routine physical examination. He is in good health and takes no medications. He drinks alcohol daily but has no history of an alcohol use disorder.

Which one of the following is within the daily limit for this patient?

(A) One 1.5-oz glass of whiskey
(B) One 8-oz glass of wine
(C) Two 12-oz beers
(D) One 4-oz glass of sherry

16. With regard to protein and energy requirements of adults >75 years old, which of the following statements is true?

(A) Resting energy expenditure increases in older adults.
(B) Energy expenditure of activity accounts for a significantly greater proportion of total daily energy expenditure for older men than for younger men.
(C) Older adults need proportionally lower amounts of protein in their diets than younger adults.
(D) The most physically active older adults on average lose similar muscle mass over time compared with more sedentary adults.

17. A 79-year-old man is brought to the office because of changes in his behavior. He recently received a diagnosis of Alzheimer disease and has episodic paranoid ideas about his children's interest in taking control of his stock portfolio. He can be reassured and redirected. His MMSE score is 20.

Which of the following is the most appropriate pharmacologic treatment for this patient?

(A) Haloperidol
(B) *Ginkgo biloba*
(C) Memantine
(D) Donepezil
(E) Haloperidol plus donepezil

18. An 81-year-old man is admitted to the coronary care unit with acute kidney injury secondary to decompensated heart failure. History is significant for stage 4 chronic kidney disease, ischemic cardiomyopathy, and moderate dementia. He moved into a nursing home 6 months ago because he had fallen several times and was unable to care for himself. There are no acute indications for dialysis yet, but discussions are started regarding goals of care. The family wants to understand the benefits of renal replacement therapy.

Which of the following statements is true about dialysis for this patient?

(A) Initiation of dialysis will slow further functional decline.
(B) Initiation of dialysis will improve his dementia.
(C) His dementia will not affect his survival on dialysis.
(D) After 6 months on dialysis, his functional status will be preserved.
(E) Dialysis may not affect his survival.

19. A 68-year-old woman comes to the office because she has been bothered by hot flushes for the past 6 months. At age 52, she took estrogen–progestin hormone replacement therapy (HRT) for about 6 years, until publication of the results of the Women's Health Initiative. She abruptly discontinued HRT and experienced hot flushes and insomnia, which decreased over 2 years and finally abated. Now she has episodes of feeling hot and sweating for several minutes during the day, and she awakens 1–3 times at night, throwing her covers off. Thyrotropin level is normal.

Which of the following is the most appropriate next step?

(A) Obtain levels of serum follicle-stimulating hormone and estradiol to check for a hormone-producing tumor.
(B) Prescribe a 3-month trial of estrogen–progestin hormone therapy and ask her to keep a diary of hot flushes.
(C) Refer her to a gynecologist to discuss risks and benefits of HRT.
(D) Review all medications and nutritional supplements.

20. A 72-year-old woman comes to the office for a routine examination. History includes mild hypertension and hypercholesterolemia; last year she was hospitalized for cholecystitis. She has taken an estrogen/progestin combination pill since onset of menopause 20 years ago.

Which of the following is the most appropriate step in regard to the hormone replacement therapy (HRT)?

(A) Continue combination therapy.
(B) Discontinue combination therapy; switch to a progestin-only agent.
(C) Discontinue combination therapy; switch to an estrogen-only agent.
(D) Discontinue hormone replacement therapy.

21. A 72-year-old woman comes to the office because she wants advice before entering a sexual relationship. She has not had intercourse since the death of her partner several years ago. She is now considering intercourse with a companion. She has read extensively about vaginal atrophy and is concerned that this may be an issue for her.

On physical examination, the vulvovaginal area is red and dry. There is difficulty inserting an adult speculum; a pediatric speculum causes slight bleeding due to extreme mucosal friability.

The patient is not willing to start oral hormonal therapy.

Which of the following would be most effective for treating the vaginal atrophy?

(A) Oral diphenhydramine
(B) Topical hydrocortisone cream
(C) Intravaginal petroleum jelly
(D) Intravaginal estrogen tablets

22. An 82-year-old man is admitted to the hospital for treatment of community-acquired pneumonia. He is alert and oriented, interacts appropriately with staff, and provides an accurate medical history. History includes hypertension, hypercholesterolemia, and mild cognitive impairment. Levofloxacin is initiated for treatment of his pneumonia. During the early evening on hospital day 2, nursing staff notes that the patient is agitated. He denies concerns but has obvious difficulty focusing on the questions being asked. He is restless, picks at his bedclothes, and tries to pull out his intravenous line. He insists that he must go home to feed his dog.

On examination, vital signs are stable, and there is no hypoxia. The remainder of the examination is unchanged from admission, including otherwise normal neurologic findings.

Which of the following is the most likely cause of the patient's agitation and cognitive changes?

(A) Progression of mild cognitive impairment
(B) Dementia
(C) Sundowning
(D) Delirium
(E) Major depressive disorder with psychotic features

23. An 85-year-old man comes to the office because he has fallen 3 times in the past 6 months. None of the falls involved dizziness or fainting. One fall occurred while he was walking in his yard; in the other instances, he tripped inside his house. History includes hypertension without postural changes, gout, osteoarthritis, and depression. He takes 5 medications on a regular basis.

Which of his medications is most likely to contribute to his risk of falls?

(A) Acetaminophen
(B) Allopurinol
(C) Hydrochlorothiazide
(D) Lisinopril
(E) Paroxetine

24. A 71-year-old woman comes to the office because she has concerns about entering a sexual relationship. Her husband died 8 years ago, and she has not had intercourse since then. She has had a companion for the past year and she would like to resume having sex. History includes hypertension and osteoarthritis. Medications include losartan/hydrochlorothiazide, ibuprofen as needed, and a multivitamin. She became postmenopausal at age 58 and took combination estrogen/progesterone for 2 years. Hot flushes returned after she stopped hormone therapy, but they abated over time. On questioning, she describes vaginal dryness and itching for the past 4 years, polyuria, and urinary urgency. There is no evidence of depression on administration of the Geriatric Depression Scale.

Which of the following is most likely to interfere with resuming sexual activity?

(A) Decreased libido
(B) Depression related to loss of spouse
(C) Atrophic vaginitis
(D) Medication
(E) Discomfort related to osteoarthritis

25. A 75-year-old woman receives a new diagnosis of type 2 diabetes mellitus. History includes deep-vein thrombosis 5 years ago, hypertension, depression, and generalized anxiety disorder. Medications include hydrochlorothiazide 12.5 mg/d, lisinopril 10 mg/d, citalopram 40 mg/d, and aspirin 81 mg/d. She lives alone in an apartment in a retirement community. She has a history of poor appetite; on a typical day she has toast and coffee for breakfast, fruit and one-half sandwich for lunch, and meat and salad for dinner. She walks 1 mile daily and assists in the community garden.

On physical examination, height is 152 cm (5 ft) and weight is 39 kg (86 lb). Blood pressure is 130/80 mmHg, and pulse is 82 beats per minute.

Laboratory findings:

Fasting glucose	147 mg/dL (change from 152 mg/dL last month)
Serum creatinine	1.0 mg/dL
BUN	16 mg/dL
Hemoglobin A_{1c}	9%

Which of the following would be the best initial approach for the patient's diabetes mellitus?

(A) No therapy needed at this time
(B) Oral metformin 500 mg q12h
(C) Oral glyburide 10 mg/d
(D) Subcutaneous insulin glargine 7 U/d

26. An 86-year-old woman is brought to the emergency room of a local rural community hospital because she has shortness of breath. The previous evening, she had been watching television when, about an hour after dinner, she suddenly felt that she could not catch her breath. The episode spontaneously subsided after 15 minutes. She had no further symptoms until this morning: she awoke feeling normal, but at mid-morning she suddenly became very short of breath. She had no chest pain or palpitations. History includes hypertension and diverticulosis. She has taken hydrochlorothiazide for 12 years. She is physically active and volunteers at the hospital gift shop.

On examination, blood pressure is 100/70 mmHg, pulse is 100 beats per minute, and respirations are 20 breaths per minute; O_2 saturation is 88% on room air. Neck veins have normal carotid upstrokes with 11-mm jugular venous distension. Bibasilar rales are heard. The remainder of the examination is unremarkable.

ECG displays sinus rhythm. There are 3-mm ST-segment convex elevations in the precordial leads (V1-V3), with 1-mm horizontal ST depressions in the inferoapical leads. Laboratory findings include normal CBC and electrolyte levels. Creatinine level is 0.9 mg/dL. High-sensitivity troponin T level is 0.16 ng/mL.

The nearest tertiary care hospital is 30 minutes away.

Which of the following is most appropriate for this patient?

(A) Administer furosemide and schedule a pharmacologic stress test in the morning.
(B) Admit to the hospital telemetry unit and monitor troponin levels.
(C) Arrange urgent transfer to tertiary care hospital for acute mechanical revascularization.
(D) Administer thrombolytic therapy and admit to intensive care.

27. An 82-year-old man is hospitalized with bilobar pneumonia. History includes hypertension and hyperlipidemia. Before development of the pneumonia, he was independent in his basic and instrumental activities of daily living.

Which of the following would be the most appropriate thromboprophylaxis regimen to reduce total mortality in this patient?

(A) Below-knee stockings
(B) Thigh-length stockings
(C) Bilateral lower-extremity intermittent pneumatic compression
(D) Enoxaparin 40 mg/d SC
(E) No prophylaxis treatment has been found to reduce mortality.

28. Which of the following is the most important factor in promoting a culture of resident safety in the nursing home?

(A) Feedback to staff members from supervisors about errors
(B) Staff members' clarity about the organization's goals
(C) Staff members' assessment of their immediate supervisor's leadership ability
(D) Staff members' level of participation in determining processes and practices of resident care
(E) Staff members'opportunities for developing new skills

29. No medications are currently approved by the FDA for psychosis and agitation in patients with dementia. Nonetheless, second-generation antipsychotic agents are frequently prescribed despite their limited efficacy and serious adverse effects, including extrapyramidal adverse effects, metabolic syndrome, and increased mortality and stroke risk. A secondary reanalysis of the Clinical Antipsychotic Trials of Intervention Effectiveness–Alzheimer's Disease (CATIE-AD) study indicated additional concerns.

Which of the following is associated with administration of second-generation antipsychotic agents in patients with dementia?

(A) Atrial fibrillation
(B) Deep-vein thrombosis
(C) Worsening of cognitive function
(D) Bleeding diathesis
(E) Impairment in instrumental activities of daily living (IADLs)

30. A 72-year-old woman comes to the clinic because for the past 2 days she has had dysuria, urinary frequency, and urgency. She reports no fever, vaginal discharge, or genital lesions. History includes hypertension and osteopenia; she received treatment for cystitis 6 months ago. Laboratory findings from a recent visit included a creatinine level of 0.6 mg/dL.

On physical examination, there is no fever. There is mild suprapubic tenderness but no costovertebral angle tenderness. Dipstick urinalysis performed in the office is positive for leukocyte esterase but negative for nitrite.

Nitrofurantoin 100 mg q12h for 5 days is prescribed. The patient inquires about preventive measures to consider for the future.

Which of the following is most likely to help prevent future episodes of cystitis?

(A) Grapefruit juice ≥10 fl oz daily
(B) Cranberry juice ≥10 fl oz daily
(C) Nitrofurantoin 100 mg at bedtime
(D) Trimethoprim/sulfamethoxazole 1 single-strength tablet 3 times/wk
(E) Ciprofloxacin 250 mg/d

31. A 73-year-old man experienced a left hemispheric stroke 2 days ago and has moderate right hemiparesis. He is alert and able to speak, but his speech is somewhat garbled. He has been receiving intravenous fluids for hydration, and he indicates that he is hungry.

Which of the following is the most appropriate initial step in assessing this patient's ability to eat?

(A) Trial of feeding
(B) Bedside assessment of swallowing function
(C) Videofluoroscopy
(D) Fiberoptic endoscopic evaluation
(E) Trial of neuromuscular electrical stimulation

32. An 84-year-old woman is admitted to an inpatient geriatric–orthopedic collaborative care service over the weekend for a suspected hip fracture after a fall. The patient lives in a nursing home. Her daughter witnessed the fall and reported that the patient appeared to slip on the bathroom threshold. Radiography reveals a right intertrochanteric fracture, with no other injury.

History includes mild dementia, hypertension, and atrial fibrillation. The patient takes a diuretic, calcium, and aspirin. She was able to walk without assistance before the fracture, and there is no apparent acute illness or other change in her condition. Echocardiography obtained 12 weeks ago demonstrated left ventricular ejection fraction at 49%; results of ECG, CBC, urinalysis, electrolyte panel, and coagulation studies taken at that time were all at her normal baseline.

Which of the following is an appropriate recommendation?

(A) Delay evaluation by the anesthesiologist until up-to-date echocardiography can be obtained Monday morning.
(B) Contact the hospital discharge planner for possible rehabilitation placement if the patient's nursing home does not offer postoperative rehabilitation.
(C) Limit the patient to partial weight-bearing movement for 6 weeks after surgery to allow fracture healing.
(D) Order nutritional supplements (100 mg protein/d) for several days before surgery.

33. A 70-year-old man comes to the office because he has a rash that started 4–5 months ago with bumps on his back, shoulders, and arms. Now the rash has spread below his belt and the bumps are larger. He reports severe generalized pruritus that is worse at night and awakens him. He stopped using lotions, and then used topical OTC corticosteroids, with no improvement. One month ago, another clinician prescribed a course of oral prednisone that improved the rash, but it worsened again after he stopped taking the corticosteroid. History includes gout and hypertension. He has no pets, lives alone, and recalls no insect bite or contact with anybody with a rash. He takes allopurinol and hydrochlorothiazide.

On physical examination, he has no fever and looks well. He has a symmetric eruption with erythematous papules and excoriations on his back, shoulders, axillae, elbows, flexural wrists, scrotum, and upper legs. There are a few pustulae in the axillae. CBC, renal panel, and liver function tests are normal.

Which of the following is the most appropriate next step?

(A) Prescribe another course of oral corticosteroids.
(B) Examine skin scraping in mineral oil under a light microscope.
(C) Examine skin scraping in potassium hydroxide preparation.
(D) Stop hydrochlorothiazide.
(E) Stop allopurinol.

34. An 88-year-old woman comes to the office because she has chronic pain in both knees, left more than right, which is worse when she walks. She takes acetaminophen 1,000 mg q8h for the pain. Prior radiography demonstrated moderate medial compartment narrowing and subchondral sclerosis in both knees, the left greater than right. She asks whether she can try something other than medicine for pain relief.

On physical examination, there is crepitus in both knees.

Which of the following treatments is most likely to improve the patient's pain?

(A) Acupuncture
(B) Topical capsaicin cream
(C) Topical diclofenac gel
(D) Topical salicylate cream
(E) Transcutaneous electrical nerve stimulation

35. A 72-year-old woman comes to the office because she is depressed and anxious. History includes heart failure. Medications include sertraline 50 mg/d. Two years ago, her husband had a stroke that affected his memory and behavior, and she has had difficulty adjusting to these changes. For example, she is unable to tolerate his dependent behavior and emotional unresponsiveness. She views his neediness as manipulative and threatens him with nursing-home placement. According to her medical record, she often presents herself as acutely depressed and angry, demands treatment for her husband and assistance for herself, and is suspicious of or rejects recommendations.

Screening for depression reveals pervasive dysphoria and irritability, anhedonia, feelings of worthlessness, reduced appetite, poor sleep, and low energy. Her symptoms are not due to current medications or substances. Cognitive examination and thyroid function are normal.

Which of the following should be done next?

(A) Maintain current dosage of sertraline and monitor for adherence.
(B) Discontinue sertraline and begin treatment with a mood-stabilizing agent.
(C) Discontinue sertraline and refer for psychotherapy.
(D) Increase dosage of sertraline and refer for psychotherapy and caregiving respite.

36. An 82-year-old man comes to the clinic for follow-up after recent hospitalization for a transient ischemic attack. History includes hypercholesterolemia, hypertension, diabetes mellitus, gastroesophageal reflux, and benign prostatic hyperplasia. Medications include clopidogrel, simvastatin, lisinopril, metformin, esomeprazole, and doxazosin.

Which of the following pairs of medications has a potential interaction that increases the risk of major cardiovascular events?

(A) Clopidogrel and doxazosin
(B) Lisinopril and metformin
(C) Clopidogrel and esomeprazole
(D) Esomeprazole and lisinopril
(E) Doxazosin and simvastatin

37. An 86-year-old man comes to the office after recent hospitalization for myocardial infarction. History includes diabetes mellitus, hypertension, coronary artery disease, COPD, renal insufficiency, and anemia. Medications include insulin 70/30, lisinopril, metoprolol, aspirin, clopidogrel, simvastatin, mometasone, formoterol, and albuterol. He lives alone; his daughter lives 5 miles away. He is able to do all instrumental activities of daily living and enjoys yard work and fishing.

On examination, weight is 54.4 kg (120 lb) and BMI is 20 kg/m^2. Sitting blood pressure is 98/60 mmHg, and pulse is 60 beats per minute. Cardiovascular and pulmonary examinations are normal.

Laboratory findings include hemoglobin A_{1c} of 8.0% and hemoglobin of 12 g/dL.

Which of the following is the next best step in management of this patient?

(A) Start alendronate weekly with calcium and vitamin D supplements.
(B) Discontinue simvastatin because of limited benefit given life expectancy.
(C) Intensify insulin therapy and glucose monitoring to achieve better glucose control.
(D) Discontinue lisinopril and monitor blood pressure.
(E) Switch insulin to metformin.

38. A 73-year-old man comes to the office because for the past 5 years he has had decreased libido, loss of nocturnal and early-morning erections, and an inability to sustain erections sufficient for intercourse. He has no difficulty with ejaculation. He also reports an overall decrease in energy level. He and his wife of 36 years remain interested in sexual relations. History includes diabetes mellitus, hyperlipidemia, and benign prostatic hyperplasia; he had a myocardial infarction at age 53 with no episodes of chest pain since, and a right-sided stroke with near-complete recovery. Medications include aspirin, simvastatin, combination dutasteride/tamsulosin, metformin, and glimepiride.

On physical examination, blood pressure is 130/75 mmHg, weight is 82.6 kg (182 lb), and height is 172.7 cm (5 ft 8 inches). BMI is 27.7 kg/m². The prostate is borderline enlarged (volume approximately 30 mL), and testicular volume is 20 mL bilaterally. Pedal pulses are diminished (1+). Neurologic function is intact.

Which of the following is the most likely cause of this patient's erectile dysfunction?

(A) Hypogonadism
(B) Medication
(C) Neurologic disease
(D) Vascular disease
(E) Psychogenic issues

39. A 68-year-old man is brought to the office by his sister because she is concerned about changes in his behavior. The patient has always had some limits in his living skills; his Full-Scale Intelligence Quotient (FSIQ) is 62. The sister says that he is sometimes confused and forgetful and gets frustrated easily; he seems sad and lonely, now rarely speaks, and seems to be angrier than in the past. He is sleeping less and has to be urged to shave or shower. His appetite is unchanged, but he has lost weight. He has lived with his sister since his wife died 2 years ago. At the time, he appeared to grieve; after 4 months, he was no longer tearful and ate and slept more regularly. He had been a janitor but no longer works. He takes no medications.

On physical examination, he is thin, but findings are otherwise normal. Laboratory findings are normal.

Which of the following is most appropriate?

(A) Explain that the patient needs more time to grieve.
(B) Prescribe a cholinesterase inhibitor.
(C) Prescribe methylphenidate.
(D) Prescribe aripiprazole.
(E) Prescribe sertraline.

40. A 68-year-old woman comes to the office for a routine physical examination. She generally feels well, but she has had difficulty sleeping over the past few months. She sleeps between 4 and 5 hours each night, and she feels tired. She drinks no caffeine after 10 AM, has not changed her sleep routine, and walks for 30 min most afternoons. She reports no symptoms of depression or anxiety, and asks for advice on whether she should try "natural" therapies to help her sleep.

Which of the following will most likely improve her sleep?

(A) Yoga
(B) Valerian
(C) Acupuncture
(D) Melatonin

41. An 85-year-old woman is evaluated in anticipation of discharge after hospitalization for aspiration pneumonia. She has advanced dementia, is dependent for all activities of daily living, and has been losing weight in the past year. She lives in her own home with a privately paid home attendant. Her daughter, who is the healthcare proxy, says her mother signed a "do not resuscitate" order, had specified that she did not want a "tube" to keep her alive, and wished to remain at home until the end of her life. She has Medicare and AARP health insurance.

Questions

Which of the following is the most appropriate recommendation for her discharge?

(A) Transfer to a nursing facility for long-term care to prevent further aspiration
(B) Referral to a visiting nurse agency to instruct the home attendant on proper feeding techniques and food consistency
(C) Referral to a home hospice program for comprehensive end-of-life care
(D) Transfer to an inpatient hospice unit for care planning

42. An 86-year-old black man is evaluated in preparation for hospital discharge. He was admitted for exacerbation of class IV heart failure and pneumonia. History includes advanced coronary artery disease, diabetes mellitus, and chronic kidney disease. He is frail but ready for discharge. His prognosis remains guarded. Discharge recommendations include completion of advance directives and transfer to a postacute rehabilitation facility. The patient does not want to complete advance directives, and he is upset because the medical resident addressed him by his first name. When his wife arrives, the medical team is not readily available to answer her questions. She believes her husband is in pain that has not been adequately treated. Neither she nor the patient wants him to be transferred to a rehabilitation facility.

Which of the following is the most appropriate next step?

(A) Arrange a patient and family meeting to discuss the patient's wishes and options.
(B) Arrange a family meeting to discuss his urgent need for postacute rehabilitation.
(C) Arrange a family meeting to discuss the need for hospice care.
(D) Meet separately with the patient's wife to discuss her concerns regarding the patient.

43. A 75-year-old man is evaluated in the rehabilitation unit because he has pain on the medial aspect of his left foot. The pain affects his ability to walk. History includes diabetes mellitus, for which he takes metformin.

On examination, there is a thick, mildly erythematous, hyperkeratotic lesion over the medial aspect of the first metatarsal phalangeal joint associated with a severe bunion deformity (hallux valgus).

Which of the following is the most appropriate initial treatment?

(A) Pad the bunion so that the patient may ambulate with less pain.
(B) Have the patient wear a larger, softer shoe to reduce pressure and friction to the bunion.
(C) Start antibiotic therapy.
(D) Debride the lesion and assess for an ulcer.

44. A 72-year-old woman is brought to the office because of a change in her behavior. Over the past year the patient has been calling the police because she believes that a neighbor has been entering her apartment to steal items such as cans of soup and paper towels. The patient lives alone. History includes hypertension and osteoarthritis; there is no history of alcohol or substance abuse. She has no hallucinations or depressive symptoms. She adequately performs daily activities, including managing her finances. Her sister reports that the patient has always tended to be suspicious of others.

Physical examination is normal. MRI of the head is unremarkable.

Which of the following is the most likely explanation for the patient's symptoms?

(A) Delusional disorder
(B) Late-onset schizophrenia
(C) Paranoid personality disorder
(D) Bipolar disease
(E) Alzheimer disease

45. A 68-year-old man comes to the clinic because he has tingling in his hands and forearms. His hands feel clumsy and he has begun to drop things, such as his keys and coffee cup. He is walking unsteadily. Over the past 4 months, he has noticed intermittent lower abdominal pain, decrease in appetite, fatigue, and shortness of breath when climbing stairs. History includes hypertension. He takes lisinopril as well as acetaminophen as needed. He does not smoke or drink.

On examination, weight is 68 kg (150 lb), a decrease from his usual weight of 74.8 kg (165 lb). He is pale, with icteric conjunctiva and skin. He has decreased sensation to light touch in his hands and feet and decreased vibratory sensation in a stocking pattern in his legs. Romberg test is positive (he sways and has near falls); the rest of the neurologic and physical examinations are normal.

Laboratory findings:

WBC	7,000/µL with normal distribution
Hemoglobin	6.3 g/dL
Hematocrit	19%
RBC distribution width	18%
Mean corpuscular volume	124 fL
Mean corpuscular hemoglobin	42 pg/RBC
Mean corpuscular hemoglobin concentration	34 g/dL
Reticulocytes	0.80%
Total bilirubin	3.2 mg/dL
Direct bilirubin	0.7 mg/dL
Lactate dehydrogenase	1,200 U/L

The remaining liver function tests are normal. Electrolytes, glucose, BUN, creatinine, creatine kinase, amylase, magnesium, calcium, and phosphorus are normal.

In order to establish the diagnosis, which of the following should be done next?

(A) CT of the abdomen
(B) MRI of the spine
(C) Bone marrow biopsy and aspirate
(D) Measurement of thyroid function
(E) Measurement of methylmalonic acid and homocysteine levels

46. A 69-year-old man comes to the office because he lost consciousness for about 20 seconds. The episode occurred 1 week ago. The patient's son witnessed it and states that his father was walking across the room, appeared pale, said "I don't feel quite right," and collapsed. The patient says that he felt lightheaded for about 5 seconds before loss of consciousness and felt normal within a few minutes of the event. History includes hyperlipidemia and prostatic hyperplasia.

On examination, blood pressure is 128/56 mmHg with no postural changes. All other findings are normal.

Which of the following is the most appropriate initial diagnostic test?

(A) Two-dimensional echocardiography
(B) Doppler ultrasonography of the carotid artery
(C) Electrocardiography
(D) MRI of the brain
(E) Tilt table test

47. A 75-year-old man undergoes evaluation because within the past month a stage III pressure ulcer has developed on his left buttock. He has lived in a nursing facility for the past 3 years. History includes dementia and stroke. He is hemiparetic on the left side and cannot walk; he usually has no difficulty eating with assistance.

On examination, weight is 72.6 kg (160 lb); he has lost 4.5 kg (10 lb) in the past month. BMI is 20.5 kg/m^2. Laboratory findings include albumin level of 3.2 g/dL and prealbumin level of 14 g/dL. Wound care is started for the pressure ulcer.

Which of the following is most likely to aid in healing the pressure ulcer?

(A) Vitamin C 500 mg q12h
(B) Arginine 17 g/d
(C) Glutamine 40 g/d
(D) Protein 100 g/d

48. A 78-year-old man is admitted to the hospital because he has had cough, shortness of breath, and fever for the past 3–4 days. He was hospitalized 3 months ago for a similar episode; at that time he was treated with ceftriaxone and doxycycline. History includes hypertension, hyperlipidemia, and mild cognitive impairment.

On physical examination, temperature is 38.1°C (100.6°F), and blood pressure is 155/80 mmHg. Heart rate is 101 beats per minute, respiratory rate is 22 breaths per minute, and O_2 saturation is 95% on 2 L of oxygen via nasal cannula. Radiography of the chest shows bilateral lower lobe infiltrates. Laboratory results are normal except for WBC count of 15,700/µL and creatinine level of 1.0 mg/dL.

On admission, the diagnosis is community-acquired pneumonia.

Questions

Which of the following antibiotics would be most effective?

(A) Ceftriaxone
(B) Levofloxacin
(C) Ceftriaxone plus doxycycline
(D) Azithromycin
(E) Doxycycline

49. An 81-year-old man comes to the office for a routine appointment. History includes moderate aortic stenosis for the past 8 years, managed with β-blockers, chronic coronary artery disease, prostate carcinoma (stage 2), and mild COPD. He received a left anterior descending artery stent in 2001. At previous appointments, he reported that he felt well and that he was maintaining his normal, active lifestyle. At this appointment, his daughter notes that her father is much less active than in the past.

Echocardiography undertaken last month was limited by poor echo windows due to COPD, but Doppler imaging detected a peak aortic velocity of 6 m/sec (an increase from 3 m/sec 2 years earlier).

Which of the following is true regarding management of this patient?

(A) Annual echocardiography is sufficient follow-up.
(B) Given that he has no chest pain, syncope, or heart failure, current management is optimal.
(C) Addition of nitrates will alleviate the patient's symptoms.
(D) Valve replacement should be considered in the near future.

50. A frail 85-year-old woman with oxygen-dependent COPD is concerned about potential harms from continuing screening mammography.

Which of the following outcomes from screening mammography is capable of producing the greatest harm to this patient?

(A) Radiation exposure from mammography increases the risk of future cancers in older women.
(B) False-positive mammography results may lead to additional diagnostic tests.
(C) Mammography may lead to the detection and treatment of cancers that would not have caused clinical symptoms.
(D) Mammography may cause significant pain and anxiety that last for several months.

51. A 92-year-old man comes to the office because he believes that his memory loss is making driving more difficult. He has a history of hypertension. His score is 28 of 30 on the Mini–Mental State Examination; neuropsychologic testing is consistent with mild dementia. He has not had any motor vehicle violations, and his wife thinks he is a good driver.

Which of the following is most appropriate?

(A) Tell the patient that he should stop driving.
(B) Refer the patient to the Department of Motor Vehicles (DMV) for a performance-based road test.
(C) Monitor the patient's cognitive impairment every 6 months; report further impairment to the DMV.
(D) Notify the DMV that the patient's driver's license must be revoked.

52. An 83-year-old woman comes to the office for an examination. She has recently returned to her home after a motor vehicle accident that resulted in injuries, a hospital stay complicated by pneumonia, and a nursing-home stay. She is greatly changed since her last office visit: she has lost a lot of weight, moves slowly, and is unable to rise from her chair without using her arms. She previously was an avid golfer and swimmer. She asks what she can do to improve her function now that her injuries have healed.

Which of the following is effective in improving function in frail older adults?

(A) Comprehensive geriatric assessment
(B) Protein supplementation
(C) Anabolic steroids (testosterone, dehydroepiandrosterone)
(D) Exercise
(E) Home visits to evaluate function in the home

53. A 75-year-old woman comes to the office because she has had a gradually increasing sense of imbalance over the past few months. She resides in an independent-living facility.

Which of the following is **least** likely to be identified as the underlying cause?

(A) Visual deficit
(B) Vestibular disorder
(C) Peripheral sensory impairment
(D) Musculoskeletal weakness
(E) Stroke

54. An 80-year-old woman comes to the office because she has mid-epigastric discomfort and heartburn. The symptoms occur daily and are not associated with shortness of breath, diaphoresis, or dizziness. She has been taking aluminum and magnesium hydroxide tablets to relieve the symptoms, but they provide only temporary relief. One month ago, the patient underwent cardiac catheterization with drug-eluting stents for coronary lesions; history also includes diabetes mellitus and hypertension. Medications are clopidogrel, aspirin, metoprolol, lisinopril, pravastatin, and glipizide. She lives with her husband and is independent in all basic and instrumental activities of daily living.

Which of the following is the most appropriate pharmacologic treatment for this patient's symptoms?

(A) Omeprazole
(B) Esomeprazole
(C) Ranitidine
(D) Sucralfate

55. A 68-year-old woman comes to the office because she is experiencing considerable frustration understanding clients in her law practice. She has worn hearing aids since age 50, when severe-to-profound sensorineural hearing impairment developed in each ear. She recently underwent a complete hearing test; hearing status was unchanged, and audiometric test results remained consistent with a sensorineural hearing loss associated with long-standing cochlear damage. Medical history is unremarkable with no history of tinnitus, dizziness, diabetes, cardiovascular disease, or cognitive decline. She recently read about bone-anchored hearing aids and cochlear implants and asks whether either would be appropriate for her.

Which of the following is the best recommendation?

(A) Bone-anchored hearing aid
(B) Cochlear implant in one ear and new hearing aid in the other
(C) Referral to otolaryngologist to exclude an acoustic tumor
(D) Learn sign language

56. An 80-year-old woman comes to the office to request a prescription for an antidepressant. Over the past 2 months she has been sleeping poorly, and her appetite has decreased. She describes feeling miserable all the time, crying often, and fighting with everybody. She has no somatic symptoms. History includes obesity, hypothyroidism, osteoarthritis, and longstanding bipolar disorder. Medications include levothyroxine and acetaminophen as needed. She has been asymptomatic off medication for bipolar disorder for 2 years; shortly before she stopped, she experienced lithium toxicity and required hospitalization. She and her family believe that the bipolar disorder has abated because of her age.

Physical examination is unremarkable. She appears restless, starts to talk of a new hobby, but then switches topic. There is a substantial change from her baseline cognition: she is not sure of the date, and she makes mistakes about events that are familiar to her. CBC and basic chemistry panel are within normal limits. Over the next 24 hours, she becomes increasingly tearful, confused, and restless.

Which of the following is most likely to be true?

(A) Before offering a psychotropic medication, additional tests are needed to exclude a medical illness that may be causing delirium.
(B) Treatment with an antidepressant is likely to improve her symptoms.
(C) The presentation suggests development of dementia with behavioral problems that is unlikely to respond to medications.
(D) A mood stabilizer will slowly improve her confusion resulting from bipolar disorder.
(E) A sedative will improve her anxiety and associated lack of sleep.

57. An 86-year-old woman comes to the office because she has frequent spotting, occasional red blood, and extravaginal discharge that dampen the pads she must now wear. She has no family history of gynecologic, urologic, or GI neoplasia. Her most recent screening colonoscopy was 3 years earlier, and findings were normal.

Which of the following would be the most efficient initial evaluation of her bleeding?

(A) Refer to a gynecologist.
(B) Obtain ultrasonography of the pelvis.
(C) Obtain CT of the abdomen and pelvis.
(D) Perform pelvic examination.
(E) Refer for colonoscopy.

58. A 74-year-old woman comes to the office for preoperative evaluation before cataract surgery. History includes myocardial infarction 10 years ago, and her records state that her ejection fraction is 30%. Medications include extended-release metoprolol, lisinopril, and spironolactone. Dyspnea on exertion is consistent with New York Heart Association (NYHA) functional class II. She has never been hospitalized for heart failure, and has no palpitations or syncope.

ECG shows a 4-beat run of nonsustained ventricular tachycardia.

Which of the following is the most appropriate next step?

(A) Obtain electrophysiologic study (EPS) for risk stratification.
(B) Continue medical therapy alone.
(C) Advise against placement of automatic internal cardiac defibrillator (ICD) because she is >70 years old.
(D) Recommend placement of ICD.

59. An 80-year-old woman is brought to the office because she has hallucinations of children and small animals when she is alone in a room. The hallucinations sometimes disturb and agitate her. Her family also notes that she is having more difficulty walking and has hand tremors when she sits quietly. She has a 9-month history of short-term memory loss; problems with orientation that sometimes worsen dramatically; and difficulty managing her finances, preparing complex meals, and following stories on television. Her score on the Mini–Mental State Examination is 23 of 30.

On physical examination, there are signs of cogwheel rigidity and resting tremors, which have been noted for the past year.

Which of the following is the most likely diagnosis?

(A) Dementia with Lewy bodies
(B) Alzheimer disease
(C) Parkinson disease with dementia
(D) Huntington disease

60. An 81-year-old woman comes to the office because she has had difficulty sleeping for the past 3 years. She falls asleep quickly but wakes up 4–5 times each night. She often goes to the bathroom on awakening, after which it may take her 15–60 minutes to fall asleep again. She is not aware of snoring but has woken up choking a few times. In the morning, she wakes up feeling unrefreshed, and she has significant daytime sleepiness. She reports no shortness of breath or coughing. History includes type 2 diabetes mellitus, osteoarthritis, and cataracts; she has had chronic dry mouth for >5 years. She lives alone, does not smoke or use alcohol, and is retired. She has tried numerous OTC sleep aids with minimal benefit.

On physical examination, BMI is 24 kg/m^2. She has upper and lower dentures.

Which of the following is the most likely cause of the patient's sleep difficulties?

(A) Primary insomnia
(B) Gastroesophageal reflux disease
(C) Nocturnal asthma
(D) Obstructive sleep apnea
(E) Periodic limb movement disorder

61. Each of the following 68-year-old patients has had an episode of syncope. Which one should be assigned the highest priority for admission to the hospital for expedited evaluation?

(A) A woman who reports low energy and feelings of worthlessness
(B) A man whose syncope occurred while urinating in the bathroom
(C) A man with hypertension who had syncope after shoveling snow
(D) A woman with diabetes mellitus who had syncope after standing in line for several hours for tickets to a Broadway show

62. A 75-year-old woman comes to the office for her 6-month follow-up visit. The patient lives independently, and she is independent in instrumental activities of daily living. She reports both a decline in her ability to walk long distances and difficulty crossing streets: the light changes before she can reach the opposite side. She has no numbness, tingling, or changes in sensation in her extremities. During the appointment, she at times uses the wall for support. Physical examination is otherwise unremarkable.

Which of the following is the most appropriate next step?

(A) Refer to social work for long-term care options.
(B) Refer for an individualized, supervised exercise program.
(C) Refer to a neurologist.
(D) Obtain MRI of the head and spine.
(E) Obtain glucose, vitamin B_{12}, and thyroid levels.

63. An 88-year-old woman is brought to the office for evaluation because her son believes that she is unable to remain safely at home without supervision. History includes hypertension, osteoarthritis, and dementia. Her husband, who was her primary caregiver, has had a major stroke and is being admitted to a nursing home. She owns her home and wishes to remain in her community; however, she has consistently refused all home services. She continues to perform activities of daily living but no longer shops or cooks, and occasionally does not remember to eat. Her son manages her finances, which include Social Security and pension benefits. She has Medicare and supplemental medical insurance.

Which of the following is the most appropriate recommendation regarding her living arrangements?

(A) Admission to the same nursing facility as her husband
(B) Referral to an adult day program to ensure a daily meal
(C) Referral to a certified home-healthcare program for help at home
(D) Admission to an assisted-living facility

64. A 77-year-old woman comes to the office for routine follow-up. History includes hypertension, coronary artery disease, emphysema, arthritis, and limited vision. She takes multiple medications. In recent months, she went to the emergency department twice for breathing difficulties, and in the past year, she was admitted to the hospital twice: once to exclude a diagnosis of myocardial infarction, and a second time because of uncontrolled hypertension.

The patient lives alone in a 3-story townhouse. After the last hospital discharge, she received home-health services; the agency discharge note states that the patient is independent in her home, is sometimes confused about her medications, possibly has cognitive impairment, and seems depressed. The patient's daughter would like her to enter an assisted-living facility close to the daughter's house. However, the patient wants to remain at home, is concerned about her finances, and does not want a new primary care physician. She participates in a health maintenance organization (HMO).

Which of the following is the most appropriate next step?

(A) Request that home-health services perform a safety evaluation.
(B) Refer her to the local Program of All-Inclusive Care for the Elderly (PACE).
(C) Enroll her in Guided Care program.
(D) Enroll her in IMPACT (Improving Mood: Promoting Access to Collaborative Treatment for Late-Life Depression) program.

65. Which of the following options is true regarding patients with advanced dementia?

(A) In nursing-home patients with advanced dementia, eating problems are associated with higher 6-month mortality rates than pneumonia.
(B) In patients with advanced dementia, feeding tubes are often placed during a hospital stay.
(C) The proportion of hospice patients with a primary diagnosis of dementia is stable at about 6%, even though the total number of patients served by hospice programs has increased.
(D) Combination therapy with cholinesterase inhibitors and NMDA-receptor modulators has been shown to improve survival in patients with advanced dementia.
(E) Most deaths in patients with advanced dementia are precipitated by catastrophic acute events (eg, myocardial infarction).

66. A 92-year-old woman comes to the office for follow-up. History includes osteoarthritis, well-controlled hypertension, gastroesophageal reflux disease, and a recent cold. Prescribed medications include chlorthalidone and lisinopril.

On examination, blood pressure is 162/70 mmHg and pulse is 76 beats per minute. On further questioning, the patient states that her daughter has been giving her OTC ibuprofen because she has had knee discomfort, which is now resolved. She has also been taking an OTC preparation of pseudoephedrine, 30 mg, three times a day for several days for congestion.

Which of the following is the most likely cause of her high blood pressure?

(A) Pseudoephedrine
(B) Arthritic pain
(C) NSAIDs
(D) Renal artery stenosis

67. An 80-year-old woman comes to the office because the vision in her right eye has suddenly become blurred. The external appearance of the eye is normal. The right pupil does not constrict when a flashlight is shined on it. When the flashlight is swung to the left eye, the right pupil constricts, and when it is swung back to the right eye, the right pupil dilates.

Which one of the following is the most likely explanation for these findings?

(A) Right occipital lobe infarct
(B) Left occipital lobe infarct
(C) Iritis of the right eye
(D) Ischemic optic neuropathy

68. A 77-year-old woman comes to the clinic because she has daytime somnolence and occasional dizziness. History includes osteoporosis (hip fracture 1 year ago), type 2 diabetes mellitus, hypertension, frequent falls, and post-herpetic neuralgia that is controlled. Medications include glipizide 5 mg q12h, extended-release metoprolol 50 mg/d, amlodipine 10 mg/d, pregabalin 200 mg q12h, alendronate 70 mg/wk (started 1 year ago), vitamin D supplement 800 IU/d, calcium carbonate 500 mg q8h, and a multivitamin.

On examination, weight is 62 kg (137 lb). Blood pressure is 140/75 mmHg. Over the past 3 months, blood pressure has ranged from 140 to 150 mmHg systolic and from 70 to 80 mmHg diastolic, with no orthostatic changes. Estimated creatinine clearance is 35 mL/min; it has declined over the past 2 years but has been stable for the past 6 months.

Which of the following would address the patient's most immediate need?

(A) Reduce pregabalin to 150 mg q12h.
(B) Start lisinopril 2.5 mg/d.
(C) Discontinue alendronate.
(D) Start aspirin 81 mg/d.

69. An 82-year-old man comes to the office because he is tired, has lost 4.5 kg (10 lb), and has new-onset back pain. He is eating well and has had no change in appetite. History includes benign prostatic hyperplasia. He reports a modest worsening of hyperplasia-associated symptoms, with more urgency and frequency. He has no other symptoms.

On physical examination, he appears in no distress. The abdomen is soft without masses. There is tenderness to percussion over the low thoracolumbar spine. Genitalia are normal. Rectal examination reveals an enlarged, firm prostate with sidewall fixation. Prostate-specific antigen (PSA) has not been measured in several years; the last measurement was 4.0 ng/mL.

Which of the following is the most appropriate next step?

(A) Measure PSA and refer to a urologist.
(B) Reassure and follow-up in 6 months.
(C) Prescribe a low-dose anticholinergic medication.
(D) Measure PSA and follow-up in 6 months.

70. A 72-year-old man who has metastatic colon cancer is admitted to a hospice inpatient facility because of complete bowel obstruction and failure to thrive. He has been unable to tolerate oral food or fluids for several days because of nausea and vomiting, and he has significant pain throughout the day. The hospice admitting nurse documents a large sacral pressure ulcer measuring 11 cm × 10 cm, with a depth of 4 cm. There is surrounding erythema, exposed muscle, undermining of the edges, and a tunneling tract that extends another 2 cm. Within the ulcer, there is necrotic material and a significant amount of exudate with a foul odor that permeates the room. The treatment plan includes placement of a specialized bed overlay, application of absorptive dressings, and medicine for pain control.

Shortly thereafter, family members tell staff that the wound odor makes spending time in the patient's room very difficult, and they ask if something can be done.

Which of the following is the best next step to reduce odor from the pressure ulcer?

(A) Turn patient every 2 hours.
(B) Apply topical metronidazole gel.
(C) Place potpourri in the room.
(D) Perform surgical debridement.

71. An 80-year-old woman is evaluated because she has erythematous lesions. Initially, the lesions were on her arms and legs; by the end of 1 week, the lesions had spread to her trunk, and several large blisters appeared. The lesions are itchy and cause her to scratch. History includes hypertension and dementia. Medications include atenolol, amlodipine, donepezil, calcium, and vitamin D; she has taken each for several years. The patient lives in a nursing home. A detailed history reveals no specific association with the onset of the rash.

On physical examination, the patient appears frail and in mild distress. She has no fever. There are areas of erythema with tense blisters and serous exudate, occasionally blood tinged. Some blisters have opened in oval erosions with serous exudate; the erosions do not coalesce. Some blisters are healing and covered with scabs. There is no mucosal involvement, and the Nikolsky sign (in which the top layer of skin comes away with gentle rubbing) is negative.

Which of the following is the most likely diagnosis?

(A) Stevens-Johnson syndrome
(B) Toxic epidermal necrolysis
(C) Bullous pemphigoid
(D) Pemphigus vulgaris
(E) Erythema mutiforme

72. A 67-year-old woman comes to the office because she has painless swelling of her right foot 1 day after kicking a trash can. She had a myocardial infarction 3 weeks ago; history also includes diabetes mellitus and severe peripheral neuropathy. Radiography reveals a slightly displaced fracture of the fourth metatarsal bone.

Which of the following is the most appropriate treatment?

(A) Perform open reduction with internal fixation.
(B) Allow patient to walk in a good walking shoe.
(C) Apply a fiberglass cast and have the patient use a wheelchair.
(D) Provide a walking boot and have the patient use a wheelchair.

73. A patient with Parkinson disease comes to the office for follow-up. He has a slow, shuffling gait, has difficulty initiating walking, and occasionally falls. In addition to taking medication, he walks on a treadmill while listening to music to set the pace, and he performs standing balance exercises.

Which of the following is the most efficient way to assess changes in the patient's physical function?

(A) Timed Up and Go test
(B) Standardized balance scale
(C) Number of falls in the past week
(D) Lower-extremity strength using timed chair stands

74. An 89-year-old woman is admitted to the hospital with a urinary tract infection and change in mental status. History includes type 2 diabetes mellitus, depression, and anxiety. She moved in with her daughter 8 months ago because of worsening confusion. Her family notes that her short-term memory is impaired and that she has vivid visual hallucinations of children in the house. They are unaware of any specific diagnosis regarding her cognition.

On examination, temperature is 38°C (100.5°F), blood pressure is 132/78 mmHg, heart rate is 86 beats per minute, and oxygen saturation is 96% on room air. Examination is unremarkable except for a slight resting right hand tremor and that the patient is unable to recite the months of the year or days of the week forward.

Although nonpharmacologic treatment is initiated for delirium, the patient becomes severely agitated overnight.

Which of the following is the most appropriate treatment for this patient's agitation?

(A) Haloperidol
(B) Rivastigmine
(C) Quetiapine
(D) Trazodone
(E) Physical restraints

75. A 77-year-old woman comes to the office because she has episodes of severe dizziness. Evaluation suggests a vestibular problem, and vestibular suppressant treatments are prescribed. At follow-up 1 week later, she reports that the episodes are now mild, but she still has a feeling of imbalance. Vestibular rehabilitation is considered as a possible next management step.

Which of the following is true regarding vestibular rehabilitation and long-term functional recovery?

(A) Vestibular rehabilitation is ineffective in long-term studies.
(B) Combining vestibular rehabilitation with physical repositioning maneuvers improves functional recovery.
(C) Vestibular rehabilitation is effective only for managing vestibular neuritis or Ménière disease.
(D) In patients with benign positional vertigo, vestibular rehabilitation reduces dizziness in short-term rather than long-term studies.

76. A 78-year-old man comes to the office because he has a skin rash and worsening swelling of his legs. History includes hypertension and osteoarthritis. The patient is on a blood pressure medication, but does not recall which one, and he takes multivitamins and an NSAID. He has recently increased the NSAID dosage because of worsening joint pain.

On examination, temperature is 37°C (98.6°F), blood pressure is 138/92 mmHg, and pulse is 78 beats per minute. An S4 gallop is detected. There is a reddish scaly rash on the scalp and on the surface of his elbows and knees. The lower extremities have moderate +2 edema. BUN is 48 mg/dL and serum creatinine is 3.5 mg/dL; levels a year ago were 22 mg/dL and 1.6 mg/dL, respectively. Urinalysis shows many WBCs but no RBCs. Examination of urine sediment shows clumps of WBCs and few WBC casts.

Which of the following is the most likely cause of his acute kidney injury?

(A) Hypertensive nephrosclerosis
(B) Acute tubular necrosis
(C) Prerenal acute kidney injury
(D) Membranoproliferative glomerulonephritis
(E) Acute interstitial nephritis ✓

77. A 63-year-old woman comes to the office because she has difficulty walking. She has noted a significant change in her gait over the last 6 months, and she now uses a walker. She fell 1 month ago while walking on uneven pavement. She has no pain in her lower extremities, but states that her legs "just feel weak and lousy." History includes diabetes mellitus, osteoarthritis, and coronary artery disease. On review of systems, she notes increased urinary urgency, constipation, and difficulty opening jars and buttoning blouses.

On physical examination, there is impairment of fine motor skills of the hands and hyperreflexia in the bilateral ankles and patella. Romberg test is positive.

Which of the following is the most appropriate next evaluation?

(A) Measure creatine kinase level.
(B) Measure serum vitamin B$_{12}$ level.
(C) Obtain electromyography and nerve conduction studies of lower limbs.
(D) Obtain MRI of cervical spine.
(E) Obtain MRI of lumbar spine. ✓

78. An 85-year-old man comes to the office because he has severe pain and blurring of his right eye that improves with blinking or when he rubs the affected eye.

Which of the following is the most likely cause of these symptoms?

(A) Acute angle-closure glaucoma ✓
(B) Anterior uveitis
(C) Keratitis sicca
(D) Chalazion
(E) Allergic conjunctivitis

79. A nursing-home resident has twisted the arm of a nursing assistant who was helping him to the bathroom and appears to have sprained her wrist. The resident has had a number of altercations with staff members and other residents in the past, but this is the first documented injury.

Which of the following is true regarding violent behavior in nursing homes?

(A) Such events are relatively rare.
(B) Most residents who exhibit violent behavior have a previous history of psychiatric illness, such as schizophrenia or bipolar disorder.
(C) Residents with severe dementia are more likely to be verbally than physically abusive toward staff.
(D) The prevalence of resident violence toward staff is probably overestimated.
(E) Most assaults against staff occur during periods of close staff–resident contact, such as when assisting with activities of daily living (ADLs).

80. Accountable care organizations are a key feature of the health reform initiative intended to improve quality of care and reduce costs.

Which of the following best characterizes proposed guidelines for accountable care organizations?

(A) Organizations are based in integrated hospital systems that offer both inpatient and outpatient services.
(B) An organization must employ a sufficient number of primary care physicians and other healthcare professionals to meet the needs of the participating population.
(C) A Medicare beneficiary participating in an accountable care organization may not seek care from providers outside the network.
(D) Organizations that target cost-savings through avoidance of hospitalization and nursing-home placement will be eligible for shared savings by Medicare.
(E) To be eligible for shared savings, an organization must show improved patient/caregiver satisfaction, care coordination, patient safety, preventive health, and management for the at-risk population.

81. Which of the following statements is *not* true about the U.S. population?

(A) The population of adults who are ≥65 years old is projected to more than double between 2010 and 2050.
(B) When the last baby boomer turns 65 in 2029, 19% of adults will be ≥65 years old.
(C) Populations of black and Hispanic adults who are ≥65 years old are growing at equal rates.
(D) By 2032, there will be more people who are ≥65 years old than children who are <15 years old.

82. A 70-year-old man comes to the office because he has recently been having urinary urgency, frequency, nocturia, and hesitancy, with occasional urge incontinence. History includes diabetes mellitus.

On physical examination, the suprapubic area is full, slightly tender, and dull on percussion. Genitalia are normal, and the prostate is small and nontender with a preserved median sulcus and no nodularity. Lower-extremity reflexes and strength are normal. There is decreased sensation to monofilament and reduced 2-point discrimination. Postvoid residual after a normal void is 650 mL.

Serum creatinine is 1.1 mg/dL (stable for this patient). Ultrasonography of the kidneys after voiding shows no hydronephrosis. Urodynamic testing 1 week later reveals large bladder capacity during filling, and poor bladder contraction with low urine flow rate during voiding. There is no evidence of bladder outlet obstruction.

Which of the following is the most appropriate management?

(A) Begin behavioral therapy including Kegel exercises.
(B) Start extended-release oxybutynin.
(C) Perform transurethral resection of the prostate (TURP).
(D) Insert indwelling catheter and arrange with home-health agency for monthly catheter replacement.
(E) Refer for further evaluation and in-and-out catheterization instruction.

83. A 65-year-old man comes to the office because he has had vivid dreams and thrashing movements during sleep for the past 4 years. Most recently, he dreamt that he fended off a thief by punching him. His wife relates that he punched her in his sleep that night, and she has a black eye from the incident. He recalls similar dreams in which he is usually fighting and has punched the headboard. Daytime behavior is normal, and he reports no memory loss. History includes anxiety and depression, which was diagnosed 1 year ago and for which he takes escitalopram. Neurologic examination is normal.

Which of the following is the most appropriate next step?

(A) Refer for polysomnography.
(B) Refer for neuropsychologic testing.
(C) Add ropinirole.
(D) Discontinue escitalopram.

84. An 80-year-old man comes to the office to discuss whether he should undergo colorectal cancer screening. He has well-controlled hypertension and walks 2 miles daily.

Which of the following is the most accurate statement about colorectal screening for this patient?

(A) He is unlikely to benefit from screening.
(B) He is unlikely to tolerate treatment for colorectal cancer, so he should not be screened.
(C) The U.S. Preventive Services Task Force (USPSTF) recommends that adults ≥75 years old not undergo screening for colorectal cancer.
(D) The potential benefits of screening largely balance the related burdens.

85. A 69-year-old woman comes to the clinic because she has GI pain, headaches, and insomnia that have persisted for >3 years and fluctuate daily. When symptoms are severe, they interrupt her daily visit to her mother in a nursing home. History includes hypertension, diabetes mellitus, osteoarthritis, and cataracts. Previous attempts at diagnosis have included upper and lower GI evaluation, neurologic examination, and laboratory studies (thyrotropin, CBC, and comprehensive metabolic panel); all findings were normal. CT of the head was unremarkable. H_2-receptor antagonists, proton-pump inhibitors, and OTC remedies have provided little benefit.

When directly asked, she admits to feeling stressed. She is annoyed that, when she retired 4 years ago, her sisters ceded care of their mother to her. She minimizes these feelings and asserts that she is most distressed by her headaches and GI pain. She does not ruminate about her physical problems, denies depressed mood, enjoys time with her grandchildren, and has no change in appetite or energy level.

Which of the following is the most likely diagnosis?

(A) Major depressive disorder
(B) Undifferentiated somatic symptom disorder
(C) Somatization disorder
(D) Hypochondriasis

√ Assistive devices

86. An 83-year-old man with Parkinson disease has been falling backward for about 2 months, and he occasionally has freezing episodes. He is at his maximal response to medications.

On examination, his gait is stooped, with a forward lean, and there is festination.

Which of the following would be the most appropriate assistive device?

(A) Straight cane
(B) 4-Prong cane
(C) Front-wheeled walker
(D) Pick-up walker
(E) 4-Wheeled walker

87. A 76-year-old woman recently had right total-knee arthroplasty for severe osteoarthritis. Surgery was uneventful, and she has no complicating medical conditions. Before surgery, she was fully independent in activities of daily living (ADLs). She lives with her husband, who is also fully independent in ADLs. She has mild osteoarthritis of her left knee.

Which of the following is the most appropriate rehabilitation strategy after surgery?

(A) Begin inpatient rehabilitation 1 week after surgery.
(B) Delay rehabilitation until the patient has no pain.
(C) Begin rehabilitation at home 2–5 days after surgery.
(D) Arrange for multidisciplinary rehabilitation at a rehabilitation inpatient facility.
(E) Rehabilitation is not necessary.

88. A 65-year-old man comes to the office because he has recurrent anxiety attacks. He describes episodes of intense fear and anxiety that last from 30 minutes to several hours; the episodes are accompanied by physical and autonomic symptoms. He has no other psychiatric symptoms, does not drink, and has no history of alcohol or drug abuse. History includes hypertension, osteoarthritis, and urinary retention related to prostatic hyperplasia. He received a diagnosis of panic disorder as an adult and was prescribed diazepam, but he has not taken the medication for the past 20 years. He is interested in restarting treatment with diazepam.

Physical examination and laboratory evaluation (thyrotropin, CBC, metabolic profile) indicate nothing likely to cause new-onset panic attacks.

Which of the following is the most appropriate treatment?

(A) A benzodiazepine plus an SSRI
(B) A benzodiazepine plus cognitive-behavioral therapy
(C) A benzodiazepine plus nortriptyline
(D) An SSRI plus cognitive-behavioral therapy
(E) Mirtazapine plus an SSRI

Questions

89. A 70-year-old woman comes to the office for routine follow-up. History includes diabetes mellitus, hypertension, and hypercholesterolemia. Medications include aspirin, glipizide, lisinopril, simvastatin, and a multivitamin.

Total cholesterol is 180 mg/dL, low-density lipoprotein level (LDL) is 120 mg/dL, and high-density lipoprotein level (HDL) is 40 mg/dL. She is interested in using therapies other than a statin to improve her cholesterol profile.

Which of the following has the strongest evidence to support its effectiveness in lowering cholesterol?

(A) Valerian
(B) Red yeast rice
(C) Green tea
(D) Viscous fibers (oats, barley, psyllium)

90. A 65-year-old black man comes to the office to establish care. He feels well, does not smoke, and walks 1–2 miles daily. On review of systems, he reports having to get up twice each night to urinate. Family history includes his father's death from prostate cancer at age 55. The risks and benefits of testing and treatment for prostate cancer are discussed with the patient.

A prostate nodule is palpable on digital rectal examination. The physical examination is otherwise unremarkable.

Which of the following is the most appropriate next step?

(A) Recommend no further testing.
(B) Repeat digital rectal examination in 6 months.
(C) Order prostate-specific antigen (PSA) test.
(D) Refer the patient for biopsy of the prostate.
(E) Refer the patient for surgery or radiation therapy.

91. An 85-year-old woman has a history of hypertension controlled with medication. She is independent in instrumental activities of daily living and has no cognitive impairment. She had gone to the emergency department because of nausea, vomiting, and a recent increase in her abdominal girth. On examination, she was found to have a small-bowel obstruction, an adnexal mass, and omental adhesions consistent with stage IV ovarian cancer. The small-bowel obstruction responded to conservative treatment, and the cancer diagnosis was confirmed by biopsy. The standard of care for stage IV ovarian cancer—chemotherapy followed by debulking surgery—has been shown to significantly extend patients' lives. The patient is willing to undergo chemotherapy if it is recommended.

Which of the following is the most appropriate recommendation?

(A) Full-dose chemotherapy followed by debulking surgery
(B) Immediate reduced-dose chemotherapy followed by surgery
(C) Immediate reduced-dose chemotherapy without surgery
(D) Palliative surgery
(E) Enrollment in hospice

92. Which of the following is the most prominent concern when an SSRI is prescribed for an older adult with an anxiety disorder or anxious depression?

(A) The patient may become suicidal.
(B) The patient may stop treatment prematurely because of effects.
(C) Bone loss may accelerate.
(D) The SSRI may cause hyponatremia.
(E) The SSRI may not work.

93. The wife of an 83-year-old man requests help because of her husband's longstanding alcohol abuse. History includes dizziness and falls; he has been prescribed a walker. The wife has forbidden him to drink and has removed all alcoholic beverages from their home. Their adult son takes his father on outings and, in an effort to please him, provides him with alcoholic beverages. The wife must then cope with his gait difficulties and affected demeanor. An appointment is scheduled for the husband, wife, and son to address concerns related to the patient's drinking.

Which of the following is the most appropriate course?

(A) Arrange for a guardian to be appointed who will identify and support the patient's interests and needs.
(B) Inform the family about the risks of falling and likely sequelae if the patient continues to drink.
(C) Inform the wife that she should not allow the son to take the patient out.
(D) Request help from an ethics consultant or family therapist to mediate the family conflict.
(E) Admit the patient to an alcohol rehabilitation facility.

94. A 72-year-old woman comes to the office for a routine physical examination. She lives alone in an apartment in a senior housing complex, drives, and plays bridge twice each week with friends. History includes obesity (BMI 31 kg/m^2), hypertension, and seasonal asthma. Medications include inhaled albuterol as needed, lisinopril, and calcium with vitamin D.

On physical examination, her vital signs are normal and her Mini–Mental State Examination score is 30. She walks 4 m in 6 sec at her usual pace.

Which of the following is accurate regarding her gait speed?

(A) Her gait speed is associated with cognitive decline and cardiovascular mortality.
(B) Her gait speed is not useful as a predictor of adverse outcome, because she has no current functional limitations.
(C) Her gait speed demonstrates that she is aging successfully.
(D) Her gait speed is predictive of lower cardiovascular mortality.

95. A 72-year-old man comes to the office because he has had progressive enlargement of right cervical lymph nodes over the past 5 months. He has also noticed some bilateral enlargement of axillary lymph nodes. He has had no weight loss, night sweats, or fevers.

On physical examination, there is a 6-cm lymph node mass in the right axillary region, as well as multiple 2- to 3-cm lymph nodes in the bilateral cervical region and shotty lymph nodes in the bilateral inguinal region. Spleen tip is palpable on deep inspiration.

Laboratory results:

WBC	50,000/µL
Absolute lymphocytes	34,100/µL
Hemoglobin	12.8 g/dL
Platelets	333,000/µL

In-situ hybridization of peripheral blood leukocytes shows trisomy of chromosome 12.

Which of the following is the most likely diagnosis?

(A) Reactive hyperplasia
(B) Infectious mononucleosis
(C) Hodgkin lymphoma, lymphocyte-predominance type
(D) Poorly differentiated lymphocytic lymphoma
(E) Chronic lymphocytic leukemia

96. A 74-year-old woman is brought to the office by her son because he is concerned about her memory. History includes mild cognitive impairment. She lives alone in her own home, performs all basic and most instrumental activities of daily living (except personal finances and home maintenance, which her son does for her), and drives short distances in the community.

Which of the following is true regarding an evidence-based approach for improving or maintaining her cognitive ability?

(A) Aerobic exercise or resistance training improves cognitive function in older women.
(B) Participation in new stimulating activities, such as taking computer classes, is more effective than exercise in promoting cognitive fitness.
(C) Regular physical activity in older adults will not improve psychomotor processing ability.
(D) Enrollment in a reputable memory program can reduce the likelihood of progression of mild cognitive impairment.

97. An 80-year-old man comes to the office because he has loss of taste, painful ulcerations on his lips and tongue, and soreness in the mouth that hinders chewing. He recently received a diagnosis of stage IV laryngeal cancer and started chemotherapy and radiation therapy 2 weeks ago.

On examination, his oral mucosa is red, raw, and tender, with sloughing tissue.

Which of the following is the most appropriate management?

(A) Refer the patient for biopsy.
(B) Inform the patient that ulcerations are an adverse effect of chemotherapy and no treatment is available.
(C) Initiate supportive treatment for oral mucositis.
(D) Recommend that the patient stop radiation and chemotherapy.

98. An 86-year-old man is admitted to the hospital because he has aspiration pneumonia. This is his third hospitalization for aspiration pneumonia in the last 6 months. History includes Parkinson disease for the past 20 years, moderate cognitive impairment, and progressive dysphagia. He has been bedbound and dependent in all activities of daily living for the past year. The patient has stated repeatedly to his wife and primary physician that he does not want to be "treated with tubes or machines."

Which of the following conditions is required for this patient to qualify for Medicare hospice benefits?

(A) Diagnosis of terminal cancer
(B) "Do not resuscitate" code status
(C) Life expectancy ≤3 months
(D) Life expectancy ≤6 months
(E) Uncontrolled symptoms

99. In January, a 73-year-old nursing-home resident is evaluated because he has had fever, headache, nasal congestion, nonproductive cough, shortness of breath, and malaise since the previous day. A rapid influenza test from a nasal swab is positive for influenza A. Another resident has had similar symptoms for 2 days.

Which of the following should be offered to the other nursing-home residents?

(A) Rimantadine
(B) Amantadine
(C) Oseltamivir
(D) Zanamivir
(E) Peramivir

100. A 91-year-old woman has some new chest discomfort and a poor appetite, which is unusual for her. History includes dementia, hypertension, and diabetes mellitus, and at baseline she walks minimally. Her niece, with whom she lives, provides care for her and is her durable power of attorney for health and finance. The niece contacts her aunt's house-call program, and reports that her aunt needs medical attention. A home visit is arranged.

On examination, blood pressure is 180/100 mmHg, heart rate is 100 beats per minute and regular, respirations are 24 breaths per minute, and O_2 saturation is 92%.

Temperature is normal. Her breathing is more labored than usual, and coarse breath sounds are heard at lung bases. She seems withdrawn but does not appear to be in significant distress. Differential diagnoses include myocardial infarction, congestive heart failure, pulmonary embolus, and pneumonia. The niece states that her aunt wishes to avoid hospitalization and to be cared for at home.

Which of the following is the most appropriate next step?

(A) Call 911 for paramedics to help carry the patient down the stairs so that she can be evaluated at the hospital.
(B) Draw blood for laboratory evaluation of troponin, D-dimer, CBC, and basic metabolic panel; order home chest radiography and portable home ECG.
(C) Begin empiric therapy with antibiotics, sublingual nitroglycerin, and enoxaparin.
(D) Enroll the patient in hospice.

101. An 84-year-old man who lives in a nursing home is seen for his monthly evaluation. History includes moderate dementia, diabetes mellitus, and heart failure. Medications include metformin 1000 mg twice daily with meals and glipizide 10 mg q12h. He undergoes fingerstick monitoring twice daily; values have ranged between 100 and the low 200s for several months. His most recent hemoglobin A_{1c} level was 8.3%.

Which of the following is the most appropriate next step in the management of this patient's diabetes?

(A) Obtain fructosamine level.
(B) Increase glipizide to 20 mg q12h.
(C) Add sitagliptin.
(D) Add NPH insulin at bedtime.
(E) Discontinue fingerstick monitoring.

102. A 68-year-old woman comes to the office because she has periods of shortness of breath and wheezing that have worsened over the past 2 months. The episodes may occur one or two times a week. She does not have cough, chest pain, leg swelling, fever, rash, or rhinorrhea. The patient tried using her grandson's inhaler and believes that it reduced her symptoms. History includes hypercholesterolemia, osteoporosis, and type 2 diabetes mellitus. She does not smoke or drink alcohol. She previously worked as an administrative assistant and is now retired.

Which of the following is the most appropriate initial treatment?

(A) Fluticasone
(B) Tiotropium
(C) Theophylline
(D) Albuterol
(E) Pulmonary rehabilitation

103. An 81-year-old woman comes to the office because she has had lower back pain for 2 weeks. The pain worsens when she sits or stands but is relieved when she lies in bed. History includes vertebral compression fracture 4 years ago and right femoral neck fracture 2 years ago.

On physical examination, straight-leg raise tests are normal bilaterally. Strength of proximal and distal muscles is 5/5 in both legs. There is good mobility of the lumbar spine. The patient describes marked pain when pressure is applied to the sacrum. Radiography of the lumbar spine reveals diffuse osteoporosis and multilevel degenerative disc disease.

Which of the following is the most likely cause of this patient's pain?

(A) Lumbar spinal stenosis
(B) Tumor affecting the lumbar spine
(C) Osteoporotic sacral fracture
(D) Lumbar disc disease
(E) Osteomyelitis of the L4 vertebrae

104. What is the most common cause of death by injury in older adults?

(A) Motor vehicle crash
(B) Fall
(C) Suicide
(D) Fire

105. A 92-year-old man, previously independent, has been gradually losing weight and function after an admission to the hospital for *Clostridium difficile* diarrhea following treatment for a dental abscess. His primary care doctor has found no acute illness. His 70-year-old daughter asks whether her father should undergo a comprehensive geriatric assessment, which is offered by several clinics in his area of the state.

Which of the following is true about comprehensive geriatric assessment?

(A) For frail older adults, the assessment should be performed in a rehabilitation setting.
(B) It is an outpatient evaluation and management service.
(C) Its maximum benefit is attained when the team performing the assessment is also the care provider.
(D) The American Geriatrics Society has defined its scope and components.

106. An 82-year-old man is hospitalized with pneumonia and treated with intravenous antibiotics and oxygen. He has dementia. Before this hospitalization, he used a walker.

Which of the following is most likely to reduce his risk of falling while in the hospital?

(A) Pressure-sensitive bed alarm
(B) Restraint that allows upper-body movement
(C) Scheduled toileting
(D) Physical therapy consultation
(E) Providing educational materials on falls to the family

107. A 70-year-old woman comes to the clinic for a routine examination. History includes mild hypertension, which is well-controlled with hydrochlorothiazide. She takes no other medication, has never smoked, and rarely consumes alcohol. She walks >10 miles each week and works as a school volunteer. A recent dual-energy x-ray absorptiometry (DEXA) scan reveals normal bone density readings at all sites (T scores all ≥–1). The patient asks whether she needs vitamin D supplements.

Which of the following recommendations applies to this patient?

(A) Adults >65 years old should have serum 25(OH)D levels measured as part of routine screening for vitamin D deficiency.
(B) Adults >65 years old should take supplemental vitamin D ≤4,000 IU/d to avoid hypercalcemia.
(C) For adults >70 years old, the recommended dietary allowance (RDA) for vitamin D is 800 IU/d.
(D) Older adults with low serum 25(OH)D levels should receive treatment to achieve a serum level of 40–50 ng/mL (100–125 nmol/L).

108. A 78-year-old man comes to the office because he has difficulty swallowing. The onset has been gradual; he intermittently notices a sensation of fullness in the neck and food regurgitation. He has had no heartburn, recent weight loss, or episodes of choking or coughing after eating. History includes hypertension, hyperlipidemia, and benign prostatic hyperplasia. Physical examination is unremarkable.

Which of the following is the most likely diagnosis?

(A) Parkinson disease
(B) Zenker diverticulum
(C) Oropharyngeal tumor
(D) Achalasia

109. An 82-year-old woman is evaluated because she is frequently incontinent of urine and occasionally incontinent of feces. The patient and her family cannot tell how long she has been incontinent. History includes Alzheimer disease. She was recently admitted to a nursing facility. She is able to feed herself but requires assistance with other basic activities of daily living. She cannot follow a multistep command, yet her answers to simple, direct questions are nearly always accurate. She ambulates slowly with the use of a walker and stand-by assistance.

On physical examination, there is no evidence of severe atrophic vaginitis, pelvic prolapse, or fecal impaction. Catheterization a few minutes after an episode of incontinence reveals a residual volume of 30 mL. Urine is dark yellow;

dipstick analysis shows no leukocyte esterase, nitrites, or hemoglobin.

A 3-day prompted-voiding program is implemented and includes scheduled wet-checks, assistance to the toilet, and praise for successful toileting trips. At baseline, she was wet 60% of the time when checked; after the 3-day program, she was wet 62% of the time.

Which of the following factors indicated that the patient was unlikely to benefit from a prompted-voiding program for urinary continence?

(A) Use of a walker
(B) Degree of cognitive impairment
(C) Poor results in 3-day voiding trial
(D) Increased postvoid residual urine
(E) Fecal incontinence

110. A 75-year-old man comes to the office to establish care because he has difficulty breathing. The breathing difficulty limits his ability to walk 2 blocks to the corner store, and he often has to sleep upright in his recliner. He takes no medication except chewable calcium carbonate tablets for chronic indigestion.

On physical examination, blood pressure is 154/88 mmHg, pulse is 80 beats per minute, and respirations are 16 breaths per minute. There are bibasilar fine crackles. Cardiac examination is notable for normal rhythm with ectopy and a II/VI holosystolic murmur at the apex. There is no peripheral edema. ECG and laboratory evaluation (electrolyte panel and CBC) are ordered. The presumptive diagnosis is heart failure.

Which of the following tests should be ordered next to help establish diagnosis and treatment?

(A) Cardiac catheterization
(B) Echocardiography
(C) Radionuclide ventriculography
(D) MRI
(E) Chest radiography

111. An 85-year-old man with advanced prostate cancer is scheduled to begin therapy with leuprolide acetate injections every 3 months. Baseline bone densitometry is performed to determine his risk of osteoporosis-related fracture; T score of −2.0 at the left femoral neck is reported. He weighs 70 kg (154 lb) and is 172.2 cm (5 ft 8 in.) tall. According to the Fracture Risk Assessment Tool (FRAX ®), his 10-year risk of hip fracture is 4.2%; his risk of any osteoporotic fracture is 9.6%.

To prevent osteoporosis fracture as a complication of gonadotropin-releasing hormone (GnRH) agonist therapy, which of the following antiresorptive therapies is indicated?

(A) Bisphosphonate
(B) Estradiol
(C) Raloxifene
(D) Salmon calcitonin

112. A 72-year-old woman comes to the office because for the past 6 months she has had severe burning pain in her feet that is worse at night. She recently tried gabapentin but discontinued it because it caused gait disturbance. History includes uncontrolled diabetes mellitus, chronic constipation, and mild cognitive impairment. Medications include insulin glargine 20 units at night, lisinopril 20 mg/d, docusate sodium 100 mg q12h, metformin 1,000 mg q12h, and acetaminophen 1,000 mg q8h. Her fingerstick glucose levels have been between 180 and 200 in the morning and in the mid-200s at night.

Which of the following is the most appropriate next step for improving pain control?

(A) Increase insulin dosage.
(B) Refer for sympathectomy.
(C) Start lamotrigine.
(D) Start pregabalin.

113. Dolly, a female domestic sheep, was the first mammal to be cloned by nucleus transfer. The donor was a middle-aged (6-year-old) sheep. Dolly lived for 6 years, which is half the normal lifespan (12 year) that is typical of her species.

Which of the following theories of aging is the most likely explanation for her early death?

(A) Mitochondrial DNA damage
(B) Depletion of stem cell reserves
(C) Loss of chromosomal telomere length
(D) Mutations in gene expression profiles

114. A 68-year-old woman comes to the office because she has shoulder and hip girdle stiffness that is present on awakening and lasts for 90 min. The stiffness began suddenly 2 months ago. She reports intermittent fevers to 38.9°C (102°F) and unintentional weight loss of 3.2 kg (7 lb). History includes hypertension treated with lisinopril and hydrochlorothiazide.

Physical examination is normal, except that strength testing demonstrates impaired effort and strength in her deltoids and hip flexors secondary to pain.

Laboratory results:

Hemoglobin	11.2 g/dL
Hematocrit	34%
Aspartate aminotransferase	54 U/L
Alanine aminotransferase	58 U/L
Alkaline phosphatase	110 U/L
Erythrocyte sedimentation rate	15 mm/h

Treatment is initiated with prednisone 15 mg/d. She returns 1 week later for follow-up and reports no change in her symptoms.

Which of the following is the most appropriate next step?

(A) Obtain autoimmune serology panel, including antihistone antibodies.
(B) Increase prednisone to 1 mg/kg/d and refer for biopsy of the temporal artery.
(C) Evaluate for occult malignancy, including CT of the abdomen.
(D) Measure creatine kinase and aldolase levels and refer for electromyography of hip flexors.

115. A 76-year-old woman comes to the office because she has acute low back pain. History includes hypertension, gastroesophageal reflux disease, angina, and back pain. Medications are enalapril 10 mg/d, hydrochlorothiazide 12.5 mg/d, isosorbide mononitrate 60 mg/d, acetaminophen 500 mg q6h, and calcium citrate 500 mg/d, as well as a daily multivitamin containing vitamin D 400 IU. In addition, she has taken omeprazole 20 mg q12h for 2 years and alendronate 70 mg/wk for 3 months. She eats 3–4 servings of dairy products daily and walks about 1 mile daily. She has not fallen in the past year.

On examination, blood pressure is 120/85 mmHg. Weight is 47.6 kg (105 lb). Serum creatinine level is 0.8 mg/dL, and 25(OH)D level is 34 mcg/L. Radiography of the lumbar spine reveals a vertebral fracture. Dual-energy x-ray absorptiometry of the hip and spine shows bone mineral density T scores of −1.3 and −1.7, respectively.

Which of the following is most likely to improve her bone health?

(A) Reduce omeprazole to 20 mg/d.
(B) Reduce alendronate to 35 mg/wk.
(C) Increase vitamin D supplementation to 1,000 IU/d.
(D) Increase calcium citrate to 500 mg q12h.

116. A 72-year-old man is admitted to the hospital because he has been refusing to eat and has lost approximately 30% of his body weight. History includes multiple sclerosis, which has increased in severity over the last months, and intellectual disability. He has lived in a nursing home for the past 15 years. His only relative was his sister, who visited him almost every day. She died 3 months ago, and since then the patient has deteriorated; he has become incontinent and has stopped eating and participating in social events. He appears to have a psychotic depression. He is physically able to swallow.

Therapy with psychotropic medications is started but then discontinued because of adverse effects. If his nutritional status improves, it may be possible to resume medication or administer electroconvulsive therapy. He refused intravenous feedings but then acquiesced, only to pull out the intravenous line hours later.

An alternative is to perform percutaneous endoscopic gastrostomy (PEG) and discharge the patient to the nursing home.

Which of the following is the most appropriate course for this patient?

(A) Ask the hospital's institutional ethics committee to determine the patient's best interest.
(B) Determine whether the nursing home can accommodate him if he does not undergo PEG.
(C) Ask the hospital for administrative consent to perform PEG.
(D) Ask the hospital to secure a court order to allow PEG.
(E) Enroll the patient in hospice for palliative care.

117. An 89-year-old woman is brought to the office for a routine visit. History includes Alzheimer disease and hypothyroidism that is under control. She lives in an assisted-living facility and has no complaints, except that she does not like the food there. She has lost 2.3 kg (5 lb) in the last 2 months. Her blood pressure has been increasing over the last 5 office visits.

On examination, blood pressure is 177/76 mmHg, consistent with the measurements at the assisted-living facility. Renal function is normal.

Which of the following is the best approach for managing her blood pressure?

(A) Start hydrochlorothiazide.
(B) Start lisinopril.
(C) Start a low-sodium, high-potassium (DASH) diet.
(D) Continue monitoring and treat when the systolic pressure is consistently >180 mmHg.
(E) No treatment is necessary.

118. In discussions with older Hispanic adults about end-of-life decisions, which of the following is commonly a factor?

(A) Older adults tend to make autonomous decisions.
(B) Older adults usually refuse life-sustaining treatments.
(C) Final decisions are usually made by one family member.
(D) Final decisions are usually made by several extended-family members.

119. An 88-year-old man is brought by his daughter to the emergency department because he has fever and lethargy. The daughter believes that he is the victim of physical abuse at the nursing home where he lives. At a later date, the daughter presses formal charges against the nursing home, and the medical chart is subpoenaed and becomes a legal document. The following is the medical record from the emergency department visit, as documented by the admitting physician:

History of present illness: 88-year-old man with a history of coronary artery disease, atrial fibrillation, Parkinson disease, Lewy body dementia admitted from nursing home for agitation and falls. Over last 2 weeks, noted to be more restless, especially in the late afternoon. Over the past 2 days, during bathing and diaper changes, patient was noted to scream and attempt to hit and bite the nursing aides. Decreased appetite. Constipated for 4 days. Patient currently denies chest pain or dyspnea. Remainder of review of systems negative.

History obtained from patient's daughter: Daughter alleges physical abuse at the nursing home. She describes the patient as "wasting away" over the last 3 months. Usually he is alert, recognizes her, and can have simple conversations, but over the last 2 weeks has been more confused.

Medications: Aspirin 81 mg/d, warfarin 2 mg at bedtime, extended-release metoprolol 25 mg/d, lisinopril 10 mg/d, carbidopa/levodopa 25/250 mg q8h, and quetiapine 25 mg at bedtime.

Vital signs: Blood pressure 150/90 mmHg, heart rate 90 beats per minute

Physical exam
General: Patient appears malnourished and agitated.
Eyes, nose, throat: Very dry oral mucous membranes.
Skin: Partially healed abrasion over right cheekbone. On right lateral chest wall, there is a 4 × 8 cm irregular purple ecchymosis that is tender to palpation. On both wrists, there are red and purple ecchymoses that are circumferential and nontender to palpation.
Gait: Normal base, steady without an assistive device.

Which of the following segments of the clinician's note best represents effective medical documentation for suspected abuse?

(A) History of present illness
(B) History obtained from the patient's daughter
(C) Description of the patient's vital signs
(D) Description of patient's behaviors
(E) Description of patient's ecchymoses

120. Which of the following is true regarding patients with Down syndrome and dementia?

(A) Dementia rarely develops in individuals with Down syndrome because of their shortened life span.
(B) Individuals with Down syndrome have beta-amyloid plaques and neurofibrillary tangles years before overt signs of dementia develop.
(C) Most individuals with Down syndrome and dementia live well into their sixties before they die of dementia.
(D) The finding of abnormal telomeres on the chromosomes of individuals with Down syndrome can now be used to diagnose Alzheimer disease years before there are symptoms.
(E) Palliative medications used for patients with Alzheimer disease are appropriate for patients with Down syndrome and dementia.

121. A 79-year-old man comes to the office in preparation for a planned coronary artery bypass graft within the next week. History includes 3-vessel coronary artery disease, hypertension, hypercholesterolemia, stroke, and depression. Findings from preoperative geriatric consultation include a Mini–Mental State Examination (MMSE) score of 29 of 30 and a Geriatric Depression Scale score of 7.

On physical examination, blood pressure is 166/84 mmHg. There is a 2+ holosystolic murmur, and there are 1+ dorsalis pedis pulses bilaterally.

Laboratory findings:

Electrolytes	Normal
BUN	24 mg/dL
Creatinine	1.4 mg/dL
Hematocrit	35.10%
Albumin	3.1 g/dL

The patient and his family have been told that his history of stroke places him at high risk of delirium during his hospitalization. They ask whether there are additional factors that affect his risk.

Which of the following independent variables are significantly associated with postoperative delirium in older adults?

(A) Low albumin and hypertension
(B) Low albumin and anemia
(C) Low albumin and Geriatric Depression Scale score >4
(D) Hypertension and anemia
(E) Hypertension and renal dysfunction

122. A 78-year-old woman comes to the office because she has had lower back pain for 3 weeks. The pain bothers her when she sits or stands and worsens when she moves from sitting to standing positions or when she bends; the pain lessens when she lies down. The pain has become progressively worse, and she has been more fatigued than usual. History includes diabetes mellitus and end-stage renal disease, for which she receives hemodialysis.

On examination, motion of the lumbar spine is limited. She has pain on side flexion to the right and forward flexion of the spine. Side flexion to the left and extension do not produce pain.

Straight-leg raise test is positive at 70 degrees on the right. There is mild weakness of the right great toe extensor, right hip abductor, and right hip extensor. The remainder of the examination is unremarkable.

Hematocrit is 32% and the WBC count is 14,600/µL. Radiography of the lumbar spine reveals multilevel degenerative disc changes but no other abnormalities.

Which of the following diagnoses should be excluded first?

(A) Tumor
(B) Lumbar disc disease
(C) Lumbar spinal stenosis
(D) Infection in the lumbar spine
(E) Vertebral compression fracture

123. A 70-year-old woman comes to the office for a follow-up visit. Last week she went to the local emergency department because she had abdominal pain and diarrhea for >24 hours; while there, she underwent CT of the abdomen. The emergency department physician diagnosed a viral illness. The abdominal symptoms have resolved, and she reports no change in her overall health. History includes hypertension controlled with hydrochlorothiazide.

On physical examination, all findings are normal. The final CT report is now available and refers to the presence of a 2.5-cm left adrenal mass. Electrolyte, blood sugar, and fractionated plasma metanephrine levels are normal, as are results of an overnight dexamethasone suppression test.

Which of the following is the most appropriate next step?

(A) Refer the patient to a surgeon for removal of the adrenal mass.
(B) Refer the patient for fine-needle aspiration biopsy of the adrenal mass.
(C) Obtain MRI.
(D) Schedule repeat CT in 3 months.
(E) Explain to the patient that no follow-up is needed.

124. A 72-year-old woman is brought to the office because she has a bad taste in her mouth and says that her dentures keep falling out. History includes type 2 diabetes mellitus, hypertension, and dementia. Medications are metformin, valsartan, and memantine. Three weeks ago she was given nitrofurantoin for 1 week for a urinary tract infection.

On examination, there are white plaques on the surface of her cheeks, hard palate, and tongue. Wiping off some of the white plaques reveals an erythematous mucosal surface.

Which of the following is the most likely diagnosis?

(A) Hairy leukoplakia
(B) Plaque-type lichen planus
(C) Acute pseudomembranous candidiasis
(D) White sponge nevus

125. A 65-year-old woman comes to the office for her "Welcome to Medicare" preventive visit. She has no history of chronic medical conditions. She experienced menopause at age 50 and did not take hormone replacement therapy. Her only medications are vitamins and supplements, including 2,000 IU omega-3 fish oil capsules, a daily multivitamin, vitamin C 500 mg, vitamin E 400 IU, and calcium 1,000 mg q12h. She performs aerobic weight-bearing exercise for 30 min daily and weight training for 30 min, 3 times per week. She has never smoked, and she drinks only an occasional glass of red wine. She has 3 servings of calcium daily, and her diet is high in fruits and vegetables. She consumes little red meat, and eats organically raised chicken and fish. Family history is significant for her mother's death after hip fracture at age 90.

On physical examination, blood pressure is 120/70 mmHg. She has no documented height loss. CBC, basic comprehensive metabolic panel, and fasting serum lipid levels are normal. Serum calcium is 9.5 mg/dL and 25(OH)D is 30 mcg/L.

On baseline bone densitometry, T scores are −0.9 for lumbar spine, −1.1 for total hip, and −1.2 for left femoral neck. Using FRAX® (Fracture Risk Assessment Tool), her 10-year probability for major osteoporotic fracture is 19%, and for hip fracture, 1.4%.

Which of the following is the most appropriate recommendation?

(A) Prescribe oral ibandronate 150 mg, once each month.
(B) Prescribe oral raloxifene 60 mg/d.
(C) Decrease total calcium intake to 1,200 mg/d.
(D) Recommend supplemental vitamin D_3 800 IU/d.

QUESTIONS, ANSWERS, AND CRITIQUES

Each of the questions or incomplete statements below is followed by four or five suggested answers or completions. For self-assessment question answer sheet to print for use with the *GNRS4* Book version, please visit *GNRS4* on www.geriatricscareonline.org. The table of Normal Laboratory Values on page 551 may be consulted for any of the questions in this book.

1. A 72-year-old man with an 80 pack-year smoking history is admitted to the surgical intensive care unit (SICU) for exacerbation of COPD after elective cholecystectomy. He has no history of dementia, depression, or other cognitive disorder; score on the Mini–Mental State Examination 1 month ago was 30 of 30. He is started on inhaled albuterol prn, fluticasone/salmeterol, intravenous dexamethasone, intravenous ceftriaxone, and supplemental oxygen. He becomes increasingly anxious. Oxygen saturation decreases, and he is started on lorazepam 0.5 mg IV. Oxygen saturation reaches 93% with 35% venturi mask. He improves overnight and into the next day.

At the beginning of day 3 in the SICU, staff notes that he is inattentive and more confused. He becomes fatigued during the day and increasingly confused and hypervigilant toward evening and overnight. He refuses breathing treatments and pulls out intravenous lines; he undergoes intubation for airway protection. On day 12 in the SICU, he undergoes tracheotomy. He is discharged from the SICU on day 15, with symptoms and signs of delirium.

Which of the following may have prevented the prolonged stay in the SICU?

(A) Substituting methylprednisolone for dexamethasone
(B) Substituting haloperidol for lorazepam
(C) Substituting an intravenous opioid for lorazepam
(D) Substituting nonpharmacologic approaches to anxiety for lorazepam
(E) Starting anxiolytics before arrival in the SICU

ANSWER: D

Because medications that activate the CNS are associated with longer stays in the ICU as a result of delirium, alternatives should always be considered. The National Institute for Health and Clinical Excellence (NICE) has released detailed guidelines to prevent delirium. The recommendations include careful and ongoing review of the types and number of medications prescribed for the patient, and establishment of a team of healthcare professionals familiar with the patient who can provide multicomponent strategies (such as reorientation) for assessing and preventing delirium (SOE=A).

Benzodiazepines and opioids produce a 1.64 increase (95% confidence interval: 1.27–2.10) in duration of delirium in the ICU. Haloperidol is associated with an increase in the duration of delirium by a factor of 1.35 (95% confidence interval: 1.21–1.50) (SOE=B).

2. The daughter of an 86-year-old woman wants to discuss her mother's weight loss. The mother had always been moderately obese, but she has steadily lost >10% of her weight over the last 6 months. The patient lives in a dementia-care unit and has slowly progressive, mild to moderate stage dementia.

Which of the following is the best response regarding weight loss in an older adult living in an institutional setting?

(A) Unintended weight loss in an obese adult often improves outcomes.
(B) Unintended weight loss requires evaluation.
(C) The patient should be given protein supplements.
(D) Weight loss in older adults is normal.

ANSWER: B

In an older adult living in an institutional setting, weight loss is usually associated with worse outcomes, including increased mortality, hospitalization, pressure ulcers, infections, and increased healthcare use. Weight loss is a more common problem than weight gain in nursing homes. Recognizing and managing weight loss in nursing-home residents is an important quality indicator. According to the Minimum Data Set, loss of 5% of weight in 1 month or 10% in 6 months is significant. Weight loss should not be viewed as a positive outcome in this case.

Weight loss in an institutional population may be related to medical, social, psychologic, and pharmacologic causes, either alone or in any combination. Careful assessment for correctable causes may reverse, decrease, or prevent further weight loss and may improve outcomes. Protein powder supplementation alone has not been shown to be effective, and supplementation without further investigation would be inappropriate. Although a loss of muscle mass and change in body composition are usual consequences of aging, weight loss is not.

3. Which of the following is true of the 2011 National Institute of Aging and the Alzheimer's Association (NIA–AA) criteria for diagnosis of Alzheimer disease?

(A) Diagnosis of definite Alzheimer disease can be based on neuroimaging findings and markers in cerebrospinal fluid.

(B) Diagnosis of possible Alzheimer disease is reserved for individuals with no memory impairment but with impairment in other cognitive domains.

(C) The criteria now include a formal diagnostic framework for the symptomatic, predementia phase of Alzheimer disease.

(D) Functional decline is not a criterion for Alzheimer disease.

ANSWER: C

In 2011, the National Institute of Aging and the Alzheimer's Association (NIA–AA) published revised criteria for clinical diagnosis of Alzheimer disease. These updated the National Institute of Neurological and Communicative Disorders and Stroke and the Alzheimer's Disease and Related Disorders Association (NINCDS–ADRDA) criteria published in 1984 ("McKhann criteria"), which delineated 3 levels of diagnostic certainty: possible, probable, and definite. The 2011 revised criteria incorporated advances in clinical, laboratory, and imaging assessment that had emerged since 1984. Most notably, the new criteria incorporate biomarkers and formalize different stages of disease.

The 2011 NIA–AA criteria have 3 classifications: probable Alzheimer disease, possible Alzheimer disease, and probable or possible Alzheimer disease with evidence of Alzheimer disease pathophysiologic process (biomarkers). This last classification is currently intended for use only in the research setting; the "probable" and "possible" diagnostic categories are intended for use in all clinical settings. The 2011 criteria do not include the diagnostic category of "definite" Alzheimer disease, which had required histopathologic evidence from biopsy or postmortem examination.

The 2011 NIA–AA criteria do not require memory impairment for probable or possible Alzheimer disease. It has become clear that there are several non–memory-predominant presentations of Alzheimer disease, such as the syndrome of posterior cortical atrophy. The NIA–AA criteria require impairment in ≥2 cognitive domains for diagnosis of all-cause dementia, as well as probable and possible Alzheimer disease. The *Diagnostic and Statistical Manual of Mental Disorders, 4th edition,* criteria continue to require memory impairment for diagnosis of dementia.

The NIA–AA criteria formalize 3 distinct stages of Alzheimer disease: preclinical, defined almost entirely by biomarkers and currently intended for research use only; a symptomatic, predementia phase for mild cognitive impairment; and a dementia phase. The staging system explicitly acknowledges that cognitive function declines gradually across the spectrum of Alzheimer disease, and that there must be a significant degree of cognitive decline before daily activities can no longer be maintained.

In the 2011 NIA–AA criteria, functional impairment continues to be required in the core clinical criteria for all-cause dementia, which must be satisfied before Alzheimer disease–spectrum diagnoses can be applied.

4. An 80-year-old man is brought to the emergency department by police after he was found wandering several blocks from his apartment in the middle of the night. He tells the admitting clinician, "I'm fine. I was taking a walk and got lost." Review of systems is positive only for urinary frequency. When asked about his home medications, he says "it's all there in the chart." His last visit to the primary care clinic was >1 year ago, at which time his medications were listed as glipizide, atenolol, and warfarin. He reports independence in all basic and instrumental activities of daily living (ADLs and IADLs). The patient was evaluated in the emergency department 3 times in the last 3 months for dizziness, back pain, and an INR of 5. He says he has no close family or friends and has no emergency contacts listed in the electronic medical record. Several referrals have been made to home-health agencies, but they report that the patient refuses all nursing and physical therapy visits.

On examination, temperature is 37.7°C (98.0°F), BMI is 16 kg/m^2, blood pressure is 160/90 mmHg, heart rate is 90 beats per minute, and O_2 saturation is 99% on room air. He appears thin and is dressed in a worn bathrobe that smells of urine. Examination of heart, lungs, and abdomen is unremarkable. He becomes irritable and refuses to answer any questions from the Mini–Mental State Examination.

Laboratory findings:

WBC	13,000/µL
Serum glucose	300 mg/dL
Hemoglobin A_{1c}	11%
INR	0.9
Urinalysis	>50 WBC, + nitrites
Urine culture	>100,000 CFU gram-negative rods

The patient is admitted to the hospital, and therapy with antibiotics is initiated for presumed urinary tract infection. His WBC count normalizes, and repeat urinalysis and urine culture are negative. With daily insulin injections and resumption of warfarin, the hyperglycemia resolves and the INR is in the therapeutic range. The patient is medically stable and insists on returning home, but the floor nurse reports that he is unable to self-administer insulin.

Which of the following is the most appropriate next step for determining a safe discharge plan for this patient?

(A) Referral to a home-health agency for evaluation of home safety
(B) Formal evaluation of decision-making capacity
(C) Referral to Adult Protective Services
(D) Evaluation for depression
(E) Evaluation for dementia

ANSWER: B

An appropriate part of evaluation for safe discharge is assessment of the patient's capacity to make decisions. The determination must be made within the context of a particular situation or decision, in this case the patient's ability to participate in discharge planning. To demonstrate decision-making capacity, the patient must show all of the following:

- He is aware of his situation and its consequences.
- He comprehends the discharge options and the risks and benefits of each.
- He is able to express his choice.
- There is reasoning behind his decision.

For patients who are capable of making decisions and if the patient's stated preference is not the result of undue influence or coercion, then the medical team must respect the patient's autonomy and discharge him home despite concerns. The medical team should offer services and pursue interventions that will increase oversight in the home (eg, referral to Adult Protective Services, implementation of home-health care services, and communication with the patient's primary doctor to ensure timely follow-up).

In this case, however, the patient's disregard of his function compromises his ability to understand the risks of returning home and avoiding harm. Because he cannot accurately weigh the risks and benefits of returning home versus going to a facility, he does not have capacity to participate in the discharge-planning process.

This patient exhibits several cardinal features of self-neglect. Behavior is considered self-neglect if ≥1 of the following is present: persistent inattention to personal hygiene or environment, repeated refusal of services that can reasonably be expected to improve quality of life, and self-endangerment through unsafe behaviors. The National Center on Elder Abuse further characterizes self-neglect as the "refusal or failure to provide himself/herself with adequate food, water, clothing, shelter, personal hygiene, needed medications, and safety precautions."

Another referral for home-health services, including a home safety evaluation, would not constitute a safe discharge option for this patient. He has a history of refusing home-care services, and there is evidence of poor self-care and self-management of his multiple chronic illnesses (eg, fluctuating INR, increased hemoglobin A_{1c}, uncontrolled blood pressure). He requires daily insulin injections but is unable to administer them and has no caregiver support.

Referral to Adult Protective Services would not help establish a safe discharge plan for this patient because the agency does not routinely assess patients in the hospital, and he is unsafe to return home. The agency provides services to older or disabled adults who are in danger of mistreatment or neglect, are unable to protect themselves, and have no one to assist them. For patients who can return home with additional monitoring and oversight, a referral to Adult Protective Services would be appropriate. After a referral is made, the agency attempts to visit the patient at home to assess whether there is abuse or neglect. For patients with decision-making capacity, the services are limited to information about available social or health services. Adult Protective Services cannot force patients to accept additional services. If a patient lacks decision-making capacity or is a victim of neglect or abuse (or both), the agency can petition the court to appoint a guardian who may be granted power over the person and his or her property.

Evaluations for depression and dementia are not the next best step in determining a safe discharge plan. Screening for depression is indicated, because treatment of an underlying depression may improve the patient's decision-making capacity in the future. However, in the short-term, antidepressant therapy is unlikely to enable him to participate in discharge planning. Tests of cognition such as the Mini–Mental State Examination often provide useful information to the clinician evaluating the patient's decision-making capacity, but they are not equivalent to a capacity assessment.

5. An 84-year-old woman is admitted to the hospital because of an exacerbation of COPD. Initial therapy included albuterol/ipratropium nebulizer, intravenous corticosteroids, antibiotic therapy, and supplemental oxygen at 2 L/min, but she has become progressively more dyspneic overnight. History includes COPD and hypertension.

On physical examination, respiratory rate is 26 breaths per minute and O_2 saturation is 91%; vital signs are otherwise stable. There is a faint expiratory wheeze and distant breath sounds. She is speaking in partial sentences. Arterial blood gas shows pH of 7.32, pCO_2 of 51 mmHg, and pO_2 of 70 mmHg. Her code status is "Do Not Intubate," but she is willing to go to the intensive care unit.

Which of the following is the most appropriate next step in caring for this patient?

(A) Inhaled corticosteroids via nebulizer
(B) ECG
(C) Noninvasive positive-pressure ventilation
(D) Pulmonary function tests
(E) Repeat measurement of arterial blood gas

ANSWER: C

This patient has progressive exacerbation of COPD that is not responding to therapy with bronchodilators, corticosteroids, and antibiotics. Noninvasive positive-pressure ventilation is the most appropriate next step for a patient with severe dyspnea, respiratory rate ≥25 beats per minute, or pCO_2 between 45 and 60 (SOE=A). Noninvasive positive-pressure ventilation can reduce the rate of intubation and length of stay in patients with pCO_2 as high as 80 mmHg. A variety of protocols can be used. One approach is to initiate therapy with a bilevel device set to an inspiratory positive pressure of 8–12 cm H_2O and expiratory positive pressure of 4 cm H_2O, with the inspiratory and expiratory positive pressure increased in increments of 2 cm H_2O based on patient response, tolerance, and arterial blood gas results (obtained pretreatment, at 1 and 4 hours after initiating therapy, and then as needed). Supplemental oxygen ≤4 L/min can be administered as needed to keep O_2 saturation >90%. There should be continuous monitoring of O_2 saturation, pulse, respiratory rate, and blood pressure.

Relative contraindications to use of noninvasive positive-pressure ventilation include altered mental status (Glasgow coma scale <8), which may carry an increased risk of aspiration. Noninvasive positive-pressure ventilation can cause gastric insufflation, leading to emesis. Emesis in a patient with altered mental status who is wearing a face mask increases the risk of aspiration. Other relative contraindications include copious secretions, craniofacial trauma, and pneumothorax/pneumomediastinum with no chest tube.

Pulmonary function tests are useful to diagnose and monitor COPD but would not be useful in this patient with a known diagnosis of COPD and apparent deterioration. Repeat pulmonary function tests may be appropriate at some point during her hospitalization, but they are unlikely to provide information that will alter therapy during an acute exacerbation. ECG could be useful if the patient had cardiovascular symptoms, but she has none at present and no history of cardiovascular disease. Repeat measures of arterial blood gas can be used to monitor a patient's condition after an intervention or over time but does not have a benefit at this point, because a measure was obtained recently and no new therapy has been initiated since then. Inhaled corticosteroids are unlikely to offer any additional benefit to the intravenous corticosteroids the patient has already received.

6. A 78-year-old man is being discharged to his home from the hospital after treatment for angina. He was hospitalized 3 months ago for a similar illness. History includes hypertension, hyperlipidemia, and mild cognitive impairment.

Which of the following has *not* been shown to reduce risk of readmission?

(A) Comprehensive discharge planning and home follow-up program
(B) Transitions in care/patient coaching intervention
(C) Reengineered discharge intervention
(D) Telehealth discharge intervention

ANSWER: D

There are no randomized controlled trials of telehealth interventions in general medical patients. A trial in patients with heart failure (mean age, 69 years) resulted in a significantly longer time until readmission but did not reduce readmission rates.

A number of interventions have been shown to reduce hospital readmissions in medically ill patients. One effective program comprised comprehensive discharge planning and home follow-up that extended from hospital admission through 4 weeks after discharge. The program included in-hospital patient assessment, ≥2 home visits, and weekly telephone contact. Within 24 weeks of discharge, 20% of patients who participated in the program and 37% of control patients were readmitted at least once (SOE=A). Another strategy involved patient education and reengineered discharge intervention that included a personal health record maintained by the patient and a series of visits and telephone calls with a transition coach. This approach reduced readmissions at 90 days (16.7% versus 22.5% for the control group) (SOE=A).

Another approach focused on medication management and included patient education, comprehensive discharge planning, an after-hospital plan document, and telephone contact with a pharmacist to review medications 2–4 days after discharge. This strategy significantly lowered the rate of hospital use (visits to the emergency department plus readmissions) in the study group (0.314 visits per patient per month) compared with the control group (0.451 visits per patient per month; incidence rate ratio, 0.695 [95% CI, 0.515–0.937]; P=.009]. Readmission within 30 days of hospital discharge occurred in 21.6% of study subjects and in 26.9% of the controls (SOE=B).

7. A 73-year-old woman is admitted to the hospital with shortness of breath and syncope. History is significant for Alzheimer disease, stroke, and seizure disorder. Medications include carbamazepine 300 mg q12h, lisinopril 10 mg/d, aspirin 325 mg/d, citalopram 20 mg/d, and donepezil 23 mg/d.

On examination, blood pressure is 120/75 mmHg and heart rate is 57 beats per minute.

Which of the following is the most likely cause of her symptoms?

(A) Drug interaction between carbamazepine and donepezil
(B) Drug interaction between carbamazepine and citalopram
(C) Adverse effect from donepezil
(D) Adverse effect from lisinopril

ANSWER: C

Donepezil 23 mg was approved for moderate to severe Alzheimer disease in 2010. In a trial comparing 23 mg and 10 mg, patients receiving the higher dose were more likely both to have bradycardia and to discontinue the study because of it. Donepezil and other cholinesterase inhibitors can increase myocardial vagal tone, which may result in bradycardia and syncope (SOE=B). Because these cardiac events were infrequent in the generally healthy individuals recruited for randomized controlled trials of cholinesterase inhibitors, many clinicians may not be aware of possible adverse cardiac effects with cholinesterase use. One study found increased rate of insertion of pacemakers among patients using cholinesterase inhibitors.

Donepezil is metabolized by hepatic enzymes cytochrome P-450 (CYP) 2D6 and 3A4; carbamazepine is an inducer of 3A4. Therefore, a potential drug-drug interaction with donepezil would result in *lower* serum concentrations of donepezil and a lower risk of syncope or bradycardia (SOE=C). A drug-drug interaction between carbamazepine and citalopram is not expected (SOE=C). Carbamazepine, citalopram, and lisinopril are not associated with syncope or bradycardia (SOE=C).

8. An 82-year-old woman comes to the office to establish care. She is accompanied by her daughter, who is concerned that her mother's use of diazepam is related to recent falls and problems with balance. History includes osteoporosis and knee osteoarthritis. Medications include alendronate, calcium, acetaminophen, and diazepam. The patient has been taking diazepam for many years, usually 10 mg q8h. She acknowledges having felt stressed during much of her life but says that she is not anxious or depressed now.

On examination, vital signs are stable, and there are no orthostatic changes in blood pressure. There is some bruising on her elbows and hips, and osteoarthritic changes are noted in both knees. There is no evidence of delirium or cognitive impairment. Her gait is somewhat slow, and she needs to take a couple of steps to make a 180-degree turn. She describes some bilateral knee pain when she rises. She can remain in semi-tandem stance for <10 sec and cannot perform a tandem stance.

Which of the following is the most appropriate first step in addressing the patient's benzodiazepine use?

(A) Refer patient to residential treatment program.
(B) Refer patient for psychiatry consultation.
(C) Recommend gradual taper of the benzodiazepine dosage.
(D) Recommend switch to a shorter-acting benzodiazepine.

ANSWER: C

Most likely, this patient's increased risk of falls is in part related to her use of diazepam. The best option is to taper the dosage of diazepam gradually and to evaluate why she feels stressed to determine appropriate treatment. Discontinuing the benzodiazepine may reduce her fall risk and improve attention.

A meta-analysis of drugs and fall risk in older adults found that benzodiazepines increase the odds of falling by more than 50% (SOE=A). In a study of older adults who wanted to stop using a prescribed benzodiazepine, most of whom had taken the drug for >10 years, 80% successfully withdrew from the medication within 6 months. When compared with patients who remained on benzodiazepines, patients who withdrew had improvements in cognitive and psychomotor tasks up to 1 year later (SOE=C).

Although the patient's dosage is high, there is no evidence that she is abusing diazepam. Therefore, referral to a treatment program or psychiatrist is not appropriate. Switching to a shorter-acting benzodiazepine may pose fewer risks to the patient than remaining on diazepam, but gradual tapering of the diazepam should be the first step.

9. A 75-year-old woman is brought to the office by her daughter. The mother has been falling, most often when rising from the toilet or attempting to climb stairs. History includes sarcopenia and frailty. She has no neurologic or metabolic abnormalities. Exercise was recommended in a previous office visit. Despite the daughter's efforts, the patient is reluctant to spend time and energy on the exercise program. The daughter asks for help prioritizing the exercises; in particular, she wants to know which exercises are most important in preventing falls.

Which of the following is most effective for preventing falls?

(A) Strengthening exercise
(B) Aerobic exercise
(C) Balance exercise
(D) Multicomponent exercise

ANSWER: C

Exercise is beneficial in frailty, yet it is difficult for frail individuals to participate in exercise for a host of reasons. Sarcopenia—loss of muscle with aging—results in a loss of reserve capacity and an increased sense of effort for a given exercise intensity. Lactate threshold increases with age, forcing older adults to exercise at a greater percentage of their maximal capacity. As the perception of effort increases, older individuals become more likely to avoid exercise. Graduated exercises could be prescribed so that an individual participates in the exercise that will benefit him or her most.

Data from the FICSIT trials (Frailty and Injury: Cooperative Studies on Intervention Techniques), performed in the early 1990s, found that exercise prevented 10% of falls across studies, but prevented 20% of falls if balance training was included. Each type of exercise (strength, aerobic, balance) could be beneficial, and the multicomponent exercise could potentially be the most beneficial, yet the case history indicates that the patient resists multicomponent exercise. For this patient, balance exercises are the priority, because they have been found to prevent falls more often than generalized or strengthening exercise (SOE=C).

10. A 74-year-old woman comes to the office for a routine examination. When asked about her hearing, she indicates that she cannot always understand what people are saying because they mumble. This is a problem, especially at work. She appears to struggle to hear the questions, and she seems more withdrawn and confused than in the past.

Which of the following is the most appropriate next step?

(A) Explain that hearing loss is inevitable as people age and there is no effective treatment.
(B) Screen for hearing impairment and hearing handicap.
(C) Screen for dementia.
(D) Refer the patient to an otolaryngologist.

ANSWER: B

When a patient exhibits behavior that suggests hearing impairment, the ear canals should be inspected to confirm that there is no wax buildup, and the patient should undergo screening for hearing impairment or handicap. The AudioScope™ is a hand-held otoscope and audiometer; it delivers pure tones at 40 dBHL at 4 frequencies: 500, 1000, 2000, and 4000 Hz. The AudioScope™ is a sensitive and specific screen for hearing impairment (SOE=A). In addition, the 10-item Hearing Handicap Inventory for the Elderly (HHIE-S) is a sensitive, cost-effective tool for determining whether communication breakdowns due to hearing impairment limit activities or have psychosocial correlates (SOE=A). Inability to hear 2 of 4 test sounds with the AudioScope™ (ie, 1000- and 2000-Hz pure tones at 40 dBHL in both ears) or a score ≥10 on the HHIE-S warrants referral to an audiologist. Hearing aids and communication management strategies can ameliorate the consequences of hearing impairment. Presbycusis cannot be treated medically.

Difficulty hearing often masquerades as impaired cognitive performance, including problems with remembering, comprehending spoken language, or both. Memory and comprehension appear to suffer when the quality of the sound input is reduced by hearing impairment. Because symptoms of untreated hearing impairment can mimic dementia, sensory function must be considered when assessing cognitive function. Hearing loss contributes to or can accelerate clinically significant cognitive decline. In addition, untreated hearing loss is associated with social isolation, withdrawal, and depression. Hearing interventions have been shown to reduce cognitive decline.

Many older adults have a hearing impairment: the prevalence of hearing loss is 63% in individuals >70 years old. Older adults often regard presbycusis—age-related hearing loss—as inevitable and are reluctant to seek help because of cost, vanity, and inconvenience. It is difficult to tease out the effects of age from the contributions of a lifetime of insults to the auditory system from noise damage, genetic susceptibility, and exposure to ototoxic agents. The peripheral and central auditory pathways are affected in presbycusis, and clinical findings often represent a mixture of abnormalities. A classic concern of people with age-related hearing loss is that they can hear others talking but cannot understand what they are saying.

Although the structures of the outer and middle ear undergo age-related changes, they have very little effect on hearing, with the notable exception of cerumen production and impaction, which increase with age. Referral to an otolaryngologist is indicated if the patient has cerumen impaction. Whereas the middle ear is essentially unaffected by aging, the cochlea, auditory brain-stem pathways, and auditory processing center of the brain are dramatically affected. The most prominent element of presbycusis is degeneration of the stria vascularis at the base and apex of the cochlea, which moves medially (mid-cochlea) with age. The stria vascularis is heavily vascularized, and its degeneration is evidence of vascular involvement in age-related hearing loss. Age-related degeneration of the stria vascularis has a substantial effect on the basic physiology of the cochlea. Also, with age, there is a loss of auditory nerve function or poorly synchronized neural activity in the auditory nerve.

11. A 78-year-old man comes to the office to establish care. History includes tophaceous gout, type 2 diabetes mellitus, hypertension, and benign prostatic hyperplasia. He adheres to a low-purine diet and has taken allopurinol for >10 years; his current dosage is 300 mg/d, which he takes exactly as prescribed. Each year he has 5 or 6 acute attacks of gout involving multiple joints, which he manages with ibuprofen; the attacks are increasingly debilitating.

On examination, weight is 64.9 kg (143 lb). There are tophi on auricles and distal interphalangeal joints bilaterally. Serum uric acid level is 8 mg/dL, creatinine is 1.7 mg/dL, and hemoglobin A_{1c} is 7.2%.

Which of the following is the most appropriate next step for treating this patient's gout?

(A) Increase the dosage of allopurinol to 400 mg/d and continue ibuprofen for acute attacks.
(B) Decrease the current dosage of allopurinol and continue ibuprofen for acute attacks.
(C) Maintain allopurinol at the current dosage and use prednisone for acute attacks.
(D) Discontinue allopurinol, start febuxostat 40 mg/d, and use prednisone for acute attacks.

ANSWER: D

This patient requires more aggressive disease management for his chronic tophaceous gout and frequent acute attacks. His serum uric acid level is 8 mg/dL on allopurinol 300 mg/d; using the Cockcroft-Gault equation, estimated creatinine clearance is 39.9 mL/min. Maintaining allopurinol at the current dosage is not an option for a patient who adheres to the management plan but has not reached the target serum uric acid level, which is <6 mg/dL in patients with hyperuricemia and clinical evidence of severe gout (ie, frequent flares, urolithiasis, or tophaceous disease). There is strong evidence that maintaining the serum uric acid level <6 mg/dL decreases the frequency of disease flares and causes regression of tophi (SOE=B). Thus, the main goal for this patient is to lower his serum uric acid level.

Because patients with gout and chronic renal insufficiency are at risk of potentially fatal allopurinol hypersensitivity syndrome, creatinine clearance levels guide allopurinol dosing. Whereas some data indicate that allopurinol can be titrated cautiously in patients with renal insufficiency to achieve a serum uric acid level <6 mg/dL without serious adverse events.

Febuxostat, a potent xanthine oxidase inhibitor, requires no dosage adjustment for patients who have creatinine clearance >30 mL/min, and there are no reported cases of hypersensitivity syndrome.

Given the patient's renal insufficiency, recurrent prolonged courses of ibuprofen are not advisable for acute flares. Brief courses of prednisone may be preferable, because his diabetes mellitus is well controlled.

12. A 67-year-old man asks about hospice care because he has considerable pain and nausea related to stage 4 pancreatic cancer. He is on chemotherapy, but his condition is declining. His oncologist offers another course of chemotherapy, which would cause uncomfortable adverse effects but possibly increase his life expectancy by 2–3 months. The patient lives at home and is debilitated to the point that he needs assistance to bathe. He is currently enrolled in traditional Medicare Parts A and B. He has no other health insurance.

If the patient switches his insurance status to Medicare hospice benefits, which of the following services will *not* be covered?

(A) Nonpalliative chemotherapy
(B) Home-health aide to assist with bathing
(C) Hospital bed for his home
(D) Grief counseling for his wife

ANSWER: A

To qualify for Medicare hospice benefits, two physicians (one of whom is usually the hospice medical director) must certify that the patient has a terminal condition with a life expectancy of ≤6 months. Given the patient's condition and functional status, he has a prognosis of <6 months and would thus qualify for hospice benefits. Once he waives Medicare Part A coverage for the terminal illness and signs up for Medicare hospice benefits, he would be eligible for a number of services not covered under traditional Medicare, including medications related to pain and other uncomfortable symptoms, home-health aides, durable medical equipment such as a hospital bed, physical therapy, occupational therapy, speech therapy, grief counseling for the patient and family, and respite care. The hospice benefits do not cover hospitalization for or curative treatment of the terminal illness; the benefits would possibly cover palliative chemotherapy if it were deemed necessary to reduce the patient's suffering.

13. A 70-year-old woman comes to the clinic for a routine examination. She lives independently at home. She mentions that she feels unsteady on her feet and now has difficulty getting up from the chair, climbing up and down stairs, and walking a few yards outside of her home to pick up her mail. History includes hypertension, for which she takes hydrochlorothiazide, and obesity. She scores 4 of 15 on the Geriatric Depression Scale (short form), and 28 of 30 on the Mini–Mental State Examination.

On examination, blood pressure is 128/78 mmHg and pulse is 70 beats per minute. Weight is 116 kg (256 lb); over the past year she has gradually gained 11.3 kg (25 lb). BMI is 38 kg/m^2. She gets up from the chair and walks to the examining room slowly. There is no evidence of focal weakness or neurologic deficits. CBC and metabolic profile are normal. Thyrotropin level is 2.3 μU/mL, and vitamin B_{12} level is 712 pg/mL.

Which of the following is the most effective management strategy to improve this patient's physical function and quality of life?

(A) Weight loss by dietary management
(B) Regular exercise
(C) Combined weight loss and regular exercise
(D) Physical therapy for gait and balance training

ANSWER: C

The prevalence of obesity is growing among older adults. Obesity is a major cause of functional limitation, most likely due to low muscle mass relative to body weight (relative sarcopenia) (SOE=A). Yet there has been controversy as to the appropriate management of obesity in older adults. Observational studies

Questions/Answers/Critiques

have suggested that weight loss is associated with increased mortality (SOE=B). Other studies have found that the relative health risk associated with increasing BMI declines with aging (SOE=B). Finally, there is concern that weight loss could exacerbate sarcopenia and osteopenia by causing further loss of muscle and bone mass (SOE=C).

It is difficult to distinguish between intentional and unintentional weight loss based on data from observational studies. Follow-up data from 2 randomized controlled trials suggest that intentional weight loss is not significantly associated with increased all-cause mortality (SOE=A). A recent randomized controlled trial provided evidence that successful weight loss (approximately 10%) can be achieved in obese adults (SOE=A). In this study, weight loss alone or exercise alone improved physical function and ameliorated frailty in obese older adults; the combination of weight loss and regular exercise yielded greater improvement in physical function and amelioration of frailty than either intervention alone. Improvement in objective measures of frailty (physical performance test, peak endurance power) was accompanied by subjective improvement in the ability to function (functional status questionnaire, physical-component summary score of the SF-36 quality-of-life questionnaire). Relative sarcopenia improved in response to weight loss alone and exercise alone, but the most positive improvement in body composition occurred in response to their combination. The combination of weight loss and regular exercise resulted in the most consistent improvement in strength, balance, and gait. The need for combined weight loss and regular exercise to maximally improve physical function is also suggested by another study, which showed that exercise alone (without weight loss) was associated with a blunted improvement in physical function in obese older adults (SOE=A). The addition of regular exercise to a weight loss program further improves physical function and attenuates the expected weight loss–induced reduction in lean body mass (from -5% to -3%) and weight loss–induced reduction in bone mass (from 3% to 1%).

Physical therapy for gait imbalance is unlikely to be effective in the context of morbid obesity.

14. An 80-year-old woman is brought to the office for consultation about depressive symptoms, including social isolation, decreased appetite, and irritability, that have waxed and waned over the past 8 weeks. History includes a diagnosis of probable Alzheimer disease. The patient has been taking sertraline for about 7 weeks, adjusted to a current dosage of 150 mg/d. Her depressive symptoms and signs have not improved, and the medication appears to be associated with nonspecific GI complaints, including nausea.

Which of the following is the most appropriate recommendation for this patient?

(A) Continue the current dosage of sertraline for 3 more weeks.
(B) Increase the dosage of sertraline.
(C) Switch to an antidepressant with a different mechanism of action.
(D) Augment the sertraline with aripiprazole.
(E) Discontinue sertraline and observe for several weeks.

ANSWER: E

It is not clear that this patient has severe, persisting major depressive disorder; she has had no response to incremental dosing of sertraline over 7 weeks, and she has continuing, bothersome adverse effects. The clinical features support discontinuing sertraline and observing her over time ("watchful waiting").

Approximately 20% of patients with dementia experience concomitant depression. Research casts doubt on the efficacy of antidepressant agents for this population. Although earlier small studies reported mixed results, a 2002 Cochrane review concluded that there was only weak evidence for the effectiveness of antidepressants in dementia. The 2010 DIADS-2 (Depression in Alzheimer Disease Study–2) reported no benefit of sertraline at 12 and 24 weeks, and a 2011 meta-analysis confirmed that evidence for use of antidepressants in dementia was "equivocal." Finally, a multicenter, randomized, double-blind, placebo-controlled trial was commissioned by the U.K. National Institute for Health Research to test the clinical effectiveness of sertraline, an SSRI, and mirtazapine, a noradrenergic and specific serotonergic antidepressant, as compared with placebo to reduce depression in patients with dementia. The landmark Health Technology Assessment Study of the Use of Antidepressants for Depression in Dementia (HTA-SADD) enrolled 326 participants from 9 geriatric psychiatry centers in England. At 13 weeks, decreases in depression scores did not differ between placebo controls and patients receiving active drugs (SOE=A). The absence of benefit relative to placebo persisted to 39 weeks. Adverse reactions occurred in >40% of patients treated with an antidepressant and in 25% of patients who received placebo. Authors concluded that "antidepressants should not be prescribed as a first-line treatment for people with depression in Alzheimer's disease," because many cases will resolve with usual care without antidepressants. They further suggest a reframing of clinical thinking, with 3 months of observation ("watchful waiting") with stepped psychosocial interventions, after which—if depression has not improved—antidepressants might be considered.

15. A 73-year-old man comes to the office for a routine physical examination. He is in good health and takes no medications. He drinks alcohol daily but has no history of an alcohol use disorder.

Which one of the following is within the daily limit for this patient?

(A) One 1.5-oz glass of whiskey
(B) One 8-oz glass of wine
(C) Two 12-oz beers
(D) One 4-oz glass of sherry

ANSWER: A

For healthy adults ≥65 years old, the National Institutes of Health and the U.S. Department of Health and Human Services recommend that alcohol be limited to ≤3 drinks in a single day and to ≤7 drinks per week (SOE=A). A standard drink in the United States contains about 0.6 fl oz (14 g) of absolute ethanol, which is the equivalent of 12 oz beer, 5 oz wine, 3 oz fortified wine (eg, sherry), or 1.5 oz of 80-proof spirits (eg, whiskey).

16. With regard to protein and energy requirements of adults >75 years old, which of the following statements is true?

(A) Resting energy expenditure increases in older adults.
(B) Energy expenditure of activity accounts for a significantly greater proportion of total daily energy expenditure for older men than for younger men.
(C) Older adults need proportionally lower amounts of protein in their diets than younger adults.
(D) The most physically active older adults on average lose similar muscle mass over time compared with more sedentary adults.

ANSWER: D

Lean body mass (excluding bone) accounts for the majority of energy expenditure at rest (resting metabolic rate) in all age groups. Regardless of whether total body weight remains the same, increases, or declines, lean body mass (especially skeletal muscle mass) and the ratio of lean body mass to total body mass generally decline as people age, especially in adults >75 years old. Consequently, with advanced age, resting metabolic rate declines. Because research findings (based primarily on cross-sectional studies) are inconsistent, there is debate as to whether resting metabolic rate per unit of lean body mass also declines with aging. Longitudinal studies indicate that the decline in resting metabolic rate with advancing age cannot be totally explained by changes in body composition and fat distribution. These studies indicate that there is also a decline in resting energy expenditure per unit weight of body mass, especially lean tissue mass. The decline may be related to any number of qualitative changes in body tissues that occur with age, such as decline in Na–K pump activity, mitochondrial volume density, and oxidative capacity per mitochondrial volume.

There has also been controversy as to whether the loss in lean body mass that occurs with advanced age can be mitigated by remaining highly physically active. Based on a longitudinal study of >300 community-dwelling older adults 70–82 years old, it appears that both men and women who remain physically active (ie, are in the upper third of the population for energy expenditure of activity) have greater fat-free mass than their peers. However, average loss of lean mass with time was similar across tertiles for energy expenditure of activity, which suggests that physical activity is not fully protective. Even among older athletes who adhere to a regular schedule of resistance training, the steady loss of lean body mass with advanced age has been well documented.

Energy expenditure of activity generally declines with age, especially after age 75. There is no evidence that energy expenditure of activity constitutes a significantly greater proportion of total daily energy expenditure in older than in younger adults.

Although there remains some controversy as to the protein requirements of older adults, there is general consensus that the requirements do not decrease with age (SOE=C). Because total energy requirements decline with age, this means that protein should usually make up a proportionally greater part of the diet in older adults.

17. A 79-year-old man is brought to the office because of changes in his behavior. He recently received a diagnosis of Alzheimer disease and has episodic paranoid ideas about his children's interest in taking control of his stock portfolio. He can be reassured and redirected. His MMSE score is 20.

Which of the following is the most appropriate pharmacologic treatment for this patient?

(A) Haloperidol
(B) *Ginkgo biloba*
(C) Memantine
(D) Donepezil
(E) Haloperidol plus donepezil

ANSWER: D

Although it may not be a definitive treatment for this patient's paranoid symptoms, given both the episodic nature of the symptoms and that the patient has Alzheimer disease that was recently diagnosed, donepezil is the optimal and most prudent initial choice (SOE=C). There is some evidence that donepezil can affect cognitive outcomes in the treatment of mild to moderate Alzheimer disease; hence, it is an appropriate first choice for a newly diagnosed patient who has no additional behavioral symptoms. In a review of randomized, placebo-controlled trials that reported a behavioral outcome measure with donepezil, rivastigmine, or galantamine monotherapy, cholinesterase inhibitors were found to be an appropriate pharmacologic strategy for managing behavioral and psychologic symptoms of dementia. However, the researchers cautioned that evidence regarding efficacy is limited, partly because many trials included patients with low symptom base rates or evaluated behavioral and psychologic symptoms only as secondary outcome measures. In an observational treatment study from Spain (SOE=C) that evaluated adverse effects of donepezil as well as neuropsychiatric symptoms as a secondary outcome measure, neuropsychiatric symptoms improved overall by >30% after 6 months.

No antipsychotic agent is approved for treatment of behavioral symptoms of dementia. As with all antipsychotics, haloperidol carries a black box warning about increased cerebrovascular mortality associated with its use in dementia patients, and parkinsonian adverse effects are common. Despite these concerns and the inconsistent reports of efficacy in controlled trials, haloperidol and other antipsychotic agents are regularly prescribed for behavioral symptoms, especially aggression, in dementia patients. The choice of haloperidol as a first-line agent for this patient would be premature for the above reasons and because his paranoid symptoms are erratic, not pervasive. Similarly, combination therapy with haloperidol and donepezil would be premature. If an antipsychotic were to be given, many geriatric psychiatrists would choose a second-generation agent such as risperidone because of its typically more favorable adverse event profile.

Ginkgo biloba has no efficacy in Alzheimer disease. Donepezil should be tried before memantine in early-stage disease. A study in Alzheimer patients with moderate to severe disease found no benefits of donepezil plus memantine versus donepezil alone, on functional or cognitive outcomes, in 1-year follow-up.

18. An 81-year-old man is admitted to the coronary care unit with acute kidney injury secondary to decompensated heart failure. History is significant for stage 4 chronic kidney disease, ischemic cardiomyopathy, and moderate dementia. He moved into a nursing home 6 months ago because he had fallen several times and was unable to care for himself. There are no acute indications for dialysis yet, but discussions are started regarding goals of care. The family wants to understand the benefits of renal replacement therapy.

Which of the following statements is true about dialysis for this patient?

(A) Initiation of dialysis will slow further functional decline.
(B) Initiation of dialysis will improve his dementia.
(C) His dementia will not affect his survival on dialysis.
(D) After 6 months on dialysis, his functional status will be preserved.
(E) Dialysis may not affect his survival.

ANSWER: E

In an older patient with advanced renal failure, initiation of dialysis is often associated with significant functional decline. This is especially true when dialysis is started, as well as for the following 3–6 months. The transition to dialysis is a very vulnerable period and must be managed closely. Studies have shown no slowing of functional decline or improvement in cognitive status with initiation of dialysis (SOE=A). Patients with dementia are at higher risk of morbidity and mortality on initiation of dialysis. In a patient such as this, starting dialysis offers no clear mortality benefit, and conservative medical management may be a better choice.

19. A 68-year-old woman comes to the office because she has been bothered by hot flushes for the past 6 months. At age 52, she took estrogen–progestin hormone replacement therapy (HRT) for about 6 years, until publication of the results of the Women's Health Initiative. She abruptly discontinued HRT and experienced hot flushes and insomnia, which decreased over 2 years and finally abated. Now she has episodes of feeling hot and sweating for several minutes during the day, and she awakens 1–3 times at night, throwing her covers off. Thyrotropin level is normal.

Which of the following is the most appropriate next step?

(A) Obtain levels of serum follicle-stimulating hormone and estradiol to check for a hormone-producing tumor.
(B) Prescribe a 3-month trial of estrogen–progestin hormone therapy and ask her to keep a diary of hot flushes.
(C) Refer her to a gynecologist to discuss risks and benefits of HRT.
(D) Review all medications and nutritional supplements.

ANSWER: D

"Review medication list" is often the best answer in geriatric medicine, and it is particularly applicable in this case. This patient has no reason to be experiencing estrogen withdrawal, unless she had been taking supplements (androgen or estrogen) without a physician's knowledge and then discontinued them. Medications, hyperthyroidism, infection, malignancy, substance abuse, and weight gain must be considered. For example, SSRIs can be used to treat vasomotor symptoms, but paradoxically they can create a hyperthermic feeling and night sweats in some patients. Idiopathic hot flushes can develop in later life and are diagnosed by excluding other causes. A prospective diary helps both the clinician and the patient understand intermittent symptoms.

Although, in the interest of thoroughness, hormone levels may be checked, they are not likely to reveal useful information. A trial of estrogen therapy is not indicated; an older woman who has successfully discontinued HRT is ill advised to resume.

Vasomotor symptoms occur in approximately 85% of women at the time of menopause. They may be mild, moderate, or severe and disabling. They may abate in 6 months, 3 years, or never but almost always improve substantially over time. The reported prevalence of persistent hot flushes is 12%–15% for women in their sixties, and 9% after age 70 years.

The cause of vasomotor symptoms remains unknown. Estrogen withdrawal causes alterations in the hypothalamus that initiate thermoregulatory dysfunction. Any substantial decline in estrogen levels can cause vasomotor symptoms, including a decline from excessively high to normal, as occurs with estrogen injections. The effectiveness of stabilizing hot flushes with a steady estrogen dosage followed by slow tapering is unclear. Rising estrogen levels (such as with rare ovarian tumors) would not cause vasomotor symptoms.

A complaint of vasomotor symptoms appearing, resolving, and reappearing would not be unusual during perimenopause. However, hormone-associated vasomotor symptoms would not occur *de novo* several years after menopause or estrogen discontinuation.

20. A 72-year-old woman comes to the office for a routine examination. History includes mild hypertension and hypercholesterolemia; last year she was hospitalized for cholecystitis. She has taken an estrogen/progestin combination pill since onset of menopause 20 years ago.

Which of the following is the most appropriate step in regard to the hormone replacement therapy (HRT)?

(A) Continue combination therapy.
(B) Discontinue combination therapy; switch to a progestin-only agent.
(C) Discontinue combination therapy; switch to an estrogen-only agent.
(D) Discontinue hormone replacement therapy.

ANSWER: D

Hormone replacement therapy (HRT) is often prescribed to relieve menopausal symptoms, usually for <5 years. In 2002, results of the Women's Health Initiative showed a higher incidence of breast cancer, heart attack, and stroke in women who took HRT (SOE=A). This study followed over 16,000 women for an average of 5.2 years; half took placebo and the other half took a combination of medroxyprogesterone acetate and conjugated equine estrogens. The findings were consistent with those from the United Kingdom (The Million Women Study). The resulting recommendation was that women with normal (not surgical) menopause should take the lowest effective dose of HRT for the shortest possible time to minimize risks (SOE=A).

The increased risk of coronary heart disease associated with HRT varied according to the women's age and years since onset of menopause. Women between the ages of 50 and 59 who used HRT showed a small trend toward lower risk of coronary heart disease, as did women who were within 5 years of onset of menopause. In another study, the incidence of heart attack was reduced in women between the ages of 50 and 59 who took HRT but not for older women (SOE=A).

HRT is indicated for the short-term treatment of menopausal symptoms, such as hot flushes. For most patients, the long-term risks of HRT outweigh its benefits, and HRT should be discontinued in this patient (SOE=A). Most women are able to discontinue HRT either abruptly or by tapering (SOE=B); many experts recommend tapering the dosage over time to minimize recurrence of hot flushes. Progestin by itself offers no health benefit to an older woman. Unopposed estrogen in a woman with an intact uterus increased the risk of endometrial cancer and is not indicated.

21. A 72-year-old woman comes to the office because she wants advice before entering a sexual relationship. She has not had intercourse since the death of her partner several years ago. She is now considering intercourse with a companion. She has read extensively about vaginal atrophy and is concerned that this may be an issue for her.

On physical examination, the vulvovaginal area is red and dry. There is difficulty inserting an adult speculum; a pediatric speculum causes slight bleeding due to extreme mucosal friability.

The patient is not willing to start oral hormonal therapy.

Which of the following would be most effective for treating the vaginal atrophy?

(A) Oral diphenhydramine
(B) Topical hydrocortisone cream
(C) Intravaginal petroleum jelly
(D) Intravaginal estrogen tablets

ANSWER: D

Estrogen in any formulation (oral or vaginal tablets, creams, or rings) improves vaginal atrophy. The creams, tablets, and rings appear to have comparable efficacy (SOE=B), and their use averts the larger systemic impact of oral estrogen. Data suggest that low-dose and even twice-weekly vaginal conjugated estrogen cream has efficacy comparable to that of daily estrogen cream (SOE=B). The cream tends to be less well accepted by patients, because it is messier than tablets or rings and may be less convenient to use. If the patient chooses not to use estrogen at all, a water-based gel or cream that is soluble intravaginally (eg, Replens®, Embrace®, or Astroglide®) would provide vaginal lubrication, although it would do little to reduce inflammation (SOE=C).

Petroleum-based lubricants (eg, Vaseline®) are not water soluble and should not be used. Hydrocortisone cream may reduce topical inflammation but does not treat the underlying cause, and it further reduces skin thickness, which may result in increased friability. Diphenhydramine may relieve the itching but would not affect dryness. It should be avoided, especially in older adults, because of adverse effects, including somnolence, cognitive impairment, and risk of falls.

22. An 82-year-old man is admitted to the hospital for treatment of community-acquired pneumonia. He is alert and oriented, interacts appropriately with staff, and provides an accurate medical history. History includes hypertension, hypercholesterolemia, and mild cognitive impairment. Levofloxacin is initiated for treatment of his pneumonia. During the early evening on hospital day 2, nursing staff notes that the patient is agitated. He denies concerns but has obvious difficulty focusing on the questions being asked. He is restless, picks at his bedclothes, and tries to pull out his intravenous line. He insists that he must go home to feed his dog.

On examination, vital signs are stable, and there is no hypoxia. The remainder of the examination is unchanged from admission, including otherwise normal neurologic findings.

Which of the following is the most likely cause of the patient's agitation and cognitive changes?

(A) Progression of mild cognitive impairment
(B) Dementia
(C) Sundowning
(D) Delirium
(E) Major depressive disorder with psychotic features

ANSWER: D

The most likely explanation for this patient's behavioral and cognitive changes is delirium. Delirium—an acute confusional state with declines in attention and cognition—is characterized by disturbances of consciousness, reduced environmental awareness, and a waxing and waning course. It develops in many older patients during hospitalization. Despite its high prevalence and significant adverse consequences, delirium is unrecognized in up to 70% of older patients who are hospitalized (SOE=B). The Confusion Assessment Method (CAM) provides a useful approach for bedside diagnosis. Delirium is diagnosed if a patient demonstrates an acute, fluctuating change in mental status, inattention, and either disorganized thinking or an altered level of consciousness. The CAM has a sensitivity of 94%–100% and a specificity of 90%–95% in studies using carefully trained personnel and a specific testing protocol (SOE=A).

Other common clinical features of delirium include cognitive deficits, perceptual disturbances such as hallucinations, emotional disturbances, and alteration of the sleep–wake cycle. Psychomotor disturbances are also common, with patients manifesting a hypoactive, hyperactive, or mixed presentation. Hypoactive delirium, most common in older adults, may present as slowed movement, paucity of speech, or even unresponsiveness. Hyperactive periods of delirium range from restlessness to constant movement and agitation.

Mild cognitive impairment is characterized by a change in a single cognitive domain (eg, memory) without significant deficits in other cognitive domains, and no or minimal functional impairment. The changes in this patient's behavior and cognition are not consistent with mild cognitive impairment and are too acute and dramatic to be due to dementia.

Sundowning, a poorly understood cause of behavioral disturbances that occur primarily in the evening or with changes to the person's environment, is most common in older adults with dementia. This patient does not appear to have dementia, and delirium is more likely because of his acute illness.

Major depressive disorder with psychotic features can present with delusions, but it would become evident more gradually and would not explain this patient's sudden onset of inattention.

23. An 85-year-old man comes to the office because he has fallen 3 times in the past 6 months. None of the falls involved dizziness or fainting. One fall occurred while he was walking in his yard; in the other instances, he tripped inside his house. History includes hypertension without postural changes, gout, osteoarthritis, and depression. He takes 5 medications on a regular basis.

Which of his medications is most likely to contribute to his risk of falls?

(A) Acetaminophen
(B) Allopurinol
(C) Hydrochlorothiazide
(D) Lisinopril
(E) Paroxetine

ANSWER: E

Antidepressant agents, including SSRIs, have been shown to increase the risk of falls; thus, paroxetine is most likely to contribute to this patient's risk (SOE=A). In addition, taking ≥4 medications increases an older adult's risk of falls; this patient's drug regimen includes 5 medications.

Acetaminophen and allopurinol are unlikely to affect blood pressure, balance, gait, or mental status. Hydrochlorothiazide and lisinopril reduce blood pressure, and hydrochlorothiazide may reduce intravascular volume and lead to postural changes in blood pressure. However, syncope was not a factor in this patient's falls, and he does not have postural changes in blood pressure.

Review of prescription and OTC medications is an important element of reducing the risk of falls. Medication review should be done at each visit to ensure that patients are taking appropriate medications and correct dosages.

24. A 71-year-old woman comes to the office because she has concerns about entering a sexual relationship. Her husband died 8 years ago, and she has not had intercourse since then. She has had a companion for the past year and she would like to resume having sex. History includes hypertension and osteoarthritis. Medications include losartan/hydrochlorothiazide, ibuprofen as needed, and a multivitamin. She became postmenopausal at age 58 and took combination estrogen/progesterone for 2 years. Hot flushes returned after she stopped hormone therapy, but they abated over time. On questioning, she describes vaginal dryness and itching for the past 4 years, polyuria, and urinary urgency. There is no evidence of depression on administration of the Geriatric Depression Scale.

Which of the following is most likely to interfere with resuming sexual activity?

(A) Decreased libido
(B) Depression related to loss of spouse
(C) Atrophic vaginitis
(D) Medication
(E) Discomfort related to osteoarthritis

ANSWER: C

Vulvovaginal atrophy can occur during perimenopause and progress through menopause (SOE=A). Vaginal dryness and itching and dyspareunia are common symptoms of atrophic vaginitis (inflammation of the vaginal epithelium). The North American Menopause Society estimates that 10%–40% of postmenopausal women have symptoms related to vulvovaginal atrophy (SOE=B). Unlike hot flushes, which tend to abate over time, atrophic vaginitis continues to progress in the absence of estrogen therapy. Because a very low level of estrogen is needed for maintenance of urogenital tissues, vulvovaginal changes tend to occur somewhat later than other postmenopausal symptoms. Vaginal epithelium thins, vascularity decreases, and elastic fibers fragment. Ecchymoses, telangiectasia, mucosal ulceration, and decreased vaginal secretion may contribute to dyspareunia (SOE=A).

The patient does not describe loss of libido, which may occur in some older women, or relationship dissatisfaction, and there is no evidence of depression. The role of medication in sexual dysfunction in women is poorly delineated. Drugs such as SSRIs may cause some combination of anorgasmia, diminished libido, and difficulties in arousal; however, she is not taking this class of medications.

Loss of flexibility and pain due to osteoarthritis may require changing preferred sex positions or practices. However, neither pain nor immobility is among her complaints.

25. A 75-year-old woman receives a new diagnosis of type 2 diabetes mellitus. History includes deep-vein thrombosis 5 years ago, hypertension, depression, and generalized anxiety disorder. Medications include hydrochlorothiazide 12.5 mg/d, lisinopril 10 mg/d, citalopram 40 mg/d, and aspirin 81 mg/d. She lives alone in an apartment in a retirement community. She has a history of poor appetite; on a typical day she has toast and coffee for breakfast, fruit and one-half sandwich for lunch, and meat and salad for dinner. She walks 1 mile daily and assists in the community garden.

On physical examination, height is 152 cm (5 ft) and weight is 39 kg (86 lb). Blood pressure is 130/80 mmHg, and pulse is 82 beats per minute.

glip vs. glyburide

Laboratory findings:

Fasting glucose	147 mg/dL (change from 152 mg/dL last month)
Serum creatinine	1.0 mg/dL
BUN	16 mg/dL
Hemoglobin A_{1c}	9%

Which of the following would be the best initial approach for the patient's diabetes mellitus?

(A) No therapy needed at this time
(B) Oral metformin 500 mg q12h
(C) Oral glyburide 10 mg/d
(D) Subcutaneous insulin glargine 7 U/d

ANSWER: D

According to the American Diabetes Association, older adults who have no functional impairments, are cognitively intact, and have significant life expectancy should receive treatment for diabetes mellitus using goals developed for younger adults. Thus, a target A_{1c} level <7% would be reasonable for this patient, because she has no significant comorbid conditions (SOE=C). A less stringent goal is appropriate if hypoglycemia develops with treatment or if new conditions arise that would affect this patient's life expectancy. A long-acting insulin, such as insulin glargine at 0.2 U/kg, would be appropriate for this patient (SOE=C).

Despite a serum creatinine level of 1.0 mg/dL, the patient's estimated creatinine clearance is 27 mL/min. Creatinine clearance <60 mL/min has usually been considered a contraindication to metformin therapy, although this is controversial and metformin has been used safely at lower doses in patients with renal impairment. In the absence of contraindications, metformin is a first-line agent to start concurrently with lifestyle modification at the time of diagnosis because of its beneficial effect on weight and because it does not cause hypoglycemia. However, in thin older adults, metformin may lead to anorexia and weight loss, which would not be desirable for this patient. In addition, this regimen is not appropriate because the starting dose is too high and may cause adverse GI events (SOE=C). If a sulfonylurea is used, glipizide is preferred over glyburide in older adults because of the lower risk of hypoglycemia (SOE=B). In addition, glyburide 10 mg/d is too high a starting dose.

26. An 86-year-old woman is brought to the emergency room of a local rural community hospital because she has shortness of breath. The previous evening, she had been watching television when, about an hour after dinner, she suddenly felt that she could not catch her breath. The episode spontaneously subsided after 15 minutes. She had no further symptoms until this morning: she awoke feeling normal, but at mid-morning she suddenly became very short of breath. She had no chest pain or palpitations. History includes hypertension and diverticulosis. She has taken hydrochlorothiazide for 12 years. She is physically active and volunteers at the hospital gift shop.

On examination, blood pressure is 100/70 mmHg, pulse is 100 beats per minute, and respirations are 20 breaths per minute; O_2 saturation is 88% on room air. Neck veins have normal carotid upstrokes with 11-mm jugular venous distension. Bibasilar rales are heard. The remainder of the examination is unremarkable.

ECG displays sinus rhythm. There are 3-mm ST-segment convex elevations in the precordial leads (V1-V3), with 1-mm horizontal ST depressions in the inferoapical leads. Laboratory findings include normal CBC and electrolyte levels. Creatinine level is 0.9 mg/dL. High-sensitivity troponin T level is 0.16 ng/mL.

The nearest tertiary care hospital is 30 minutes away.

Which of the following is most appropriate for this patient?

(A) Administer furosemide and schedule a pharmacologic stress test in the morning.
(B) Admit to the hospital telemetry unit and monitor troponin levels.
(C) Arrange urgent transfer to tertiary care hospital for acute mechanical revascularization.
(D) Administer thrombolytic therapy and admit to intensive care.

ANSWER: C

This patient's symptoms and abnormal ECG are consistent with an acute coronary syndrome, specifically ST-elevation myocardial infarction (STEMI). She also has signs of heart failure and possible hemodynamic compromise.

Acute therapy for STEMI entails reperfusion if it is achieved by mechanical revascularization within 2 hours, as well as antithrombin, antiplatelet, anti-ischemic, and cholesterol-lowering therapy (SOE=A). Thrombolytic therapy is an alternative (SOE=C), but it is generally associated with higher bleeding risks and less efficacy for patients who are >80 years old. Thrombolysis in combination with emergent cardiac catheterization (facilitated percutaneous coronary intervention) provides no advantages over emergent catheterization alone and increases bleeding risks.

Key points in this scenario are that the patient may be compromised hemodynamically and that she is within 30 minutes of a medical facility that can provide emergent cardiac catheterization. Her normal kidney function and no increased bleeding risk suggest no obvious contraindications for interventional management.

The risks and benefits of revascularization must be made clear to the patient. If she declines cardiac catheterization, then medical management would still provide benefit. Antithrombin therapy (heparin, bivalirudin, or fondaparinux), antiplatelet therapy (aspirin and thienopyridines), anti-ischemic medications (β-blockers, ACE inhibitors, and nitrates, alone or in combination), and plaque-stabilizing medications (statins) are all associated with clinical benefit (SOE=A).

Coronary artery disease increases with age. Whereas many people regard chest pain as the prototypical manifestation of ischemia, the most common symptom is dyspnea. As the heart struggles with acute ischemia, blood often backs up into the lungs, precipitating acute shortness of breath. Symptoms of ischemia vary and can range from dyspnea to angina to confusion, so it is generally prudent to have a low threshold for suspecting acute coronary syndrome.

27. An 82-year-old man is hospitalized with bilobar pneumonia. History includes hypertension and hyperlipidemia. Before development of the pneumonia, he was independent in his basic and instrumental activities of daily living.

Which of the following would be the most appropriate thromboprophylaxis regimen to reduce total mortality in this patient?

(A) Below-knee stockings
(B) Thigh-length stockings
(C) Bilateral lower-extremity intermittent pneumatic compression
(D) Enoxaparin 40 mg/d SC
(E) No prophylaxis treatment has been found to reduce mortality.

ANSWER: E

Although thromboprophylaxis with low-molecular-weight heparin (LMWH), low-dose unfractionated heparin, or fondaparinux for acutely ill medical patients who are admitted to the hospital with heart failure or severe respiratory disease, or who are confined to bed and have ≥1 additional risk factors can reduce deep-vein thrombosis and pulmonary embolus (SOE=B), prophylaxis does not reduce mortality and the increase in bleeding events balances the decrease in pulmonary embolus and DVT (SOE=A). Thus an individual risk assessment of harms (bleeding) versus benefits (DVT and pulmonary embolus prevention) should be performed for each patient admitted to the hospital, before thromboprophylaxis is initiated with one of these medications.

No differences in benefits or harms are seen with different types of heparin. Mechanical types of prophylaxis have not reduced mortality and cause significant harm (eg, skin damage) to patients with stroke.

28. Which of the following is the most important factor in promoting a culture of resident safety in the nursing home?

(A) Feedback to staff members from supervisors about errors
(B) Staff members' clarity about the organization's goals
(C) Staff members' assessment of their immediate supervisor's leadership ability
(D) Staff members' level of participation in determining processes and practices of resident care
(E) Staff members'opportunities for developing new skills

ANSWER: B

Much evidence suggests that, despite years of regulatory oversight, care in nursing facilities is often suboptimal, with serious implications for the health and safety of residents. Besides general problems of fragmented care and issues around transfers, direct-care workers often indicate that they are assigned too many residents and have too much to do for each resident. Staff turnover is high, and recruiting competent replacements remains a challenge.

Organizational climate has been described as staff members' shared perceptions about the norms—such as approaches to medication errors and other safety issues—that characterize their workplace. The shared perceptions about norms ultimately may determine a nursing-home resident's risk of avoidable adverse events. One recent article examined 9 dimensions of organizational climate (leadership, participation, feedback, competence development, worker engagement, efficiency, goals, work climate, and work stress) and their effect on resident safety culture. Resident safety culture was measured with the Nursing Home Survey on Patient Safety Culture, a version of the Hospital Survey on Patient Safety Culture adapted for nursing facilities. Four of the 9 dimensions—efficiency, work climate, goal clarity, and work stress—emerged as significant predictors (SOE=C) of resident culture safety.

A culture of resident safety fosters more comprehensive and systematic assessments of adverse events as well. For example, a 2009 study examined nursing staff perspectives of person, environment, and interactive circumstances surrounding falls in nursing facilities. Person themes included change in resident health status, decline in resident abilities, and resident behaviors and personality characteristics. Five environment categories were identified: design safety, limited space, obstacles, equipment misuse and malfunction, and staff and organization of care. Only by promoting a culture of safety—emphasizing that safety is the norm and that it is multifactorial—can the long-term care system decrease the occurrence of avoidable adverse events.

29. No medications are currently approved by the FDA for psychosis and agitation in patients with dementia. Nonetheless, second-generation antipsychotic agents are frequently prescribed despite their limited efficacy and serious adverse effects, including extrapyramidal adverse effects, metabolic syndrome, and increased mortality and stroke risk. A secondary reanalysis of the Clinical Antipsychotic Trials of Intervention Effectiveness–Alzheimer's Disease (CATIE-AD) study indicated additional concerns.

Which of the following is associated with administration of second-generation antipsychotic agents in patients with dementia?

(A) Atrial fibrillation
(B) Deep-vein thrombosis
(C) Worsening of cognitive function
(D) Bleeding diathesis
(E) Impairment in instrumental activities of daily living (IADLs)

ANSWER: C

The primary CATIE-AD outcome measure was the time to discontinuation of the initially assigned medication for any reason: this was intended as an overall measure of effectiveness that incorporated the opinions of patients, caregivers, and clinicians, reflecting therapeutic benefits in relation to undesirable effects. Patients were followed for 36 weeks, and cognitive assessments were obtained at baseline and at 12, 24, and 36 weeks.

On average, both active medications and placebo were discontinued after about 8 weeks, indicating no significant differences in effectiveness between the active medications and placebo. Some participants did benefit from treatment as measured by the Clinical Global Impression of Change: between 26% and 32% of those taking the active medications improved (confidence intervals [CI] = 2.7±1.1 and 2.9±1.3, respectively) compared with 21% (CI=3.3±1.5) of those taking placebo. The antipsychotic medications were more often associated with adverse effects, such as sedation, confusion, and weight gain, than placebo. Active medications were discontinued in 15% (CI=1.44–8.91) to 24% (CI=1.84–10.12) of patients because of adverse effects, whereas only 5% of those taking placebo cited adverse effects as the reason for discontinuing use. Study investigators determined the effectiveness of the medications by balancing the associated benefits and risks. They concluded that second-generation antipsychotic medications may be effective against some symptoms of Alzheimer disease compared with placebo, but their tendency to cause intolerable adverse effects offsets their benefits in this vulnerable population.

Secondary reanalysis of cognitive assessment data from the CATIE-AD study showed steady, significant declines over time in most cognitive domains, with cognitive performance declining significantly more in patients receiving second-generation antipsychotic agents than in those given placebo (SOE=A). Over the 9-month study, the magnitude of decline seen with second-generation antipsychotic drugs was equivalent to 1 year of Alzheimer disease progression (about a 2.5-point decrement on the MMSE). The degree of cognitive worsening associated with second-generation antipsychotics is of the same order of magnitude as the therapeutic effects of cholinesterase inhibitors like donepezil.

There was no evidence that use of second-generation antipsychotic agents for symptoms of dementia was associated with atrial fibrillation, deep-vein thrombosis, bleeding diathesis, or further impairment explicitly in IADLs.

30. A 72-year-old woman comes to the clinic because for the past 2 days she has had dysuria, urinary frequency, and urgency. She reports no fever, vaginal discharge, or genital lesions. History includes hypertension and osteopenia; she received treatment for cystitis 6 months ago. Laboratory findings from a recent visit included a creatinine level of 0.6 mg/dL.

On physical examination, there is no fever. There is mild suprapubic tenderness but no costovertebral angle tenderness. Dipstick urinalysis performed in the office is positive for leukocyte esterase but negative for nitrite.

Nitrofurantoin 100 mg q12h for 5 days is prescribed. The patient inquires about preventive measures to consider for the future.

Which of the following is most likely to help prevent future episodes of cystitis?

(A) Grapefruit juice ≥10 fl oz daily
(B) Cranberry juice ≥10 fl oz daily
(C) Nitrofurantoin 100 mg at bedtime
(D) Trimethoprim/sulfamethoxazole 1 single-strength tablet 3 times/wk
(E) Ciprofloxacin 250 mg/d

ANSWER: B

This patient has acute cystitis, her second episode in 6 months. Urinary tract infection is considered recurrent if the patient has had ≥3 episodes in the past year, yet many patients prefer to begin preventive measures after only 1 episode or recurrence. Standard practices should be discussed, such as drinking sufficient water every day, wiping from front to back, taking showers instead of baths, and cleansing the genital area before sexual intercourse. In addition, cranberry juice ≥10 fl oz daily or cranberry extract 500 mg/d has been shown to decrease the frequency of recurrent urinary tract infections in older women (SOE=A). Cranberry juice and extract are inexpensive and well tolerated and do not increase the risk of *Clostridium difficile* infection or antibiotic resistance. Intravaginal or systemic estrogen replacement also helps prevent recurrent urinary tract infections. This patient's only other episode was 6 months ago, however, and the risk of adverse effects from estrogen replacement therapy (such as myocardial infarction, venous thromboembolism, stroke) must be weighed against potential benefits.

Use of antibiotics, including trimethoprim/sulfamethoxazole, nitrofurantoin, and ciprofloxacin, to prevent frequently recurrent urinary tract infections is not recommended because of the possibility of development of resistant organisms, the increased risk of *C difficile* infection, and the risk of adverse drug events. Grapefruit juice has not been shown to prevent recurrent urinary tract infection.

Nitrofurantoin 100 mg q12h for 5 days is an appropriate choice for therapy. Urine culture is not required unless first-line therapy is ineffective (SOE=A).

31. A 73-year-old man experienced a left hemispheric stroke 2 days ago and has moderate right hemiparesis. He is alert and able to speak, but his speech is somewhat garbled. He has been receiving intravenous fluids for hydration, and he indicates that he is hungry.

Which of the following is the most appropriate initial step in assessing this patient's ability to eat?

(A) Trial of feeding
(B) Bedside assessment of swallowing function
(C) Videofluoroscopy
(D) Fiberoptic endoscopic evaluation
(E) Trial of neuromuscular electrical stimulation

ANSWER: B

Stroke guidelines recommend assessment of swallowing function in all patients before beginning feeding. A standardized bedside swallowing test has been shown to detect dysphagia after stroke with a sensitivity of 97% and a specificity of 90% (SOE=B). A trial of feeding without prior assessment of swallowing function would increase the risk of aspiration (SOE=A). Videofluoroscopy and fiberoptic evaluation may be useful if results from the bedside swallowing evaluation are equivocal, but they are expensive and expose the patient to radiation in the first case, and require specialty consultation in the second case. Neuromuscular electrical stimulation may improve swallowing in patients with dysphagia. However, it would be used only after identification of dysphagia in a patient by a bedside assessment and subsequent evaluation by videofluoroscopy.

32. An 84-year-old woman is admitted to an inpatient geriatric–orthopedic collaborative care service over the weekend for a suspected hip fracture after a fall. The patient lives in a nursing home. Her daughter witnessed the fall and reported that the patient appeared to slip on the bathroom threshold. Radiography reveals a right intertrochanteric fracture, with no other injury.

History includes mild dementia, hypertension, and atrial fibrillation. The patient takes a diuretic, calcium, and aspirin. She was able to walk without assistance before the fracture, and there is no apparent acute illness or other change in her condition. Echocardiography obtained 12 weeks ago demonstrated left ventricular ejection fraction at 49%; results of ECG, CBC, urinalysis, electrolyte panel, and coagulation studies taken at that time were all at her normal baseline.

Which of the following is an appropriate recommendation?

(A) Delay evaluation by the anesthesiologist until up-to-date echocardiography can be obtained Monday morning.
(B) Contact the hospital discharge planner for possible rehabilitation placement if the patient's nursing home does not offer postoperative rehabilitation.
(C) Limit the patient to partial weight-bearing movement for 6 weeks after surgery to allow fracture healing.
(D) Order nutritional supplements (100 mg protein/d) for several days before surgery.

ANSWER: B

Recognizing the high prevalence of comorbid conditions and high risk of complications, inpatient geriatric–orthopedic collaborative services focus on improving care and outcomes in older patients with hip fractures. Planning for rehabilitation after discharge is commonly started on the day of admission.

Geriatric–orthopedic collaboration has yielded fewer complications; lower in-hospital costs; and improved patient mobility, function (per SF-36 subscale scores), and affective status (SOE=A). Studies have found shorter hospital stays, lower readmission and long-term mortality rates, decreased costs related to index hospital care, and improved discharge placement (SOE=B). One study also found improved patient and provider satisfaction (SOE=C).

This patient's cardiovascular comorbidity increases her risk of surgical and postoperative complications, yet according to the 2007 perioperative guidelines from the American College of Cardiology/American Heart Association (ACC/AHA), she would not benefit from further cardiac studies that would delay surgery. Observational data indicate that delays in surgery for otherwise stable patients lead to worse outcomes (SOE=B), although it is difficult to differentiate between the adverse effects of delay from the effects of comorbid illnesses. The ACC/AHA guidelines specify more-compromising conditions—including acute coronary syndromes, decompensated heart failure, severe valvular heart disease, and significant arrhythmias—that require full evaluation by anesthesia and cardiology services to optimize surgical and postoperative outcomes (SOE=B).

Mobilizing the patient on the first postoperative day and encouraging weight-bearing movement as tolerated improves postoperative recovery of function and other outcomes. Evidence does not support delaying remobilization to promote healing. Further, complicated rehabilitation regimens that include instructions for partial weight-bearing movement may not be suitable for older patients, particularly those with dementia.

Common postoperative complications—delirium, infection, pain, arrhythmia, renal insufficiency, venous thromboembolism, acute blood loss, and pressure ulcers—can impede functional recovery. Postoperative removal of the urinary catheter lowers risk of subsequent urinary tract infection (SOE=B) and facilitates "detethering" the patient, thereby lessening the likelihood of cascading agitation, use of restraints, and delirium (SOE=A). Similarly, family visits, with food and personal items, appear to help lower the risk of complications (SOE=C).

In older patients who have already had a fragility fracture, secondary prevention of hip fracture is often neglected. Postoperative assessment of osteoporosis and treatment with bisphosphonates are frequently deferred to community primary care physicians who may not institute appropriate evaluations. Vitamin D deficiency is common. Levels of 25(OH)D <25 ng/mL are associated with a nearly 4-fold increase in risk of falls in the year after hip fracture (SOE=B). Vitamin D supplementation may be appropriate for this patient as part of a comprehensive rehabilitation and fall prevention plan.

There is no evidence that outcomes after hip fracture surgery can be improved by increased protein intake.

33. A 70-year-old man comes to the office because he has a rash that started 4–5 months ago with bumps on his back, shoulders, and arms. Now the rash has spread below his belt and the bumps are larger. He reports severe generalized pruritus that is worse at night and awakens him. He stopped using lotions, and then used topical OTC corticosteroids, with no improvement. One month ago, another clinician prescribed a course of oral prednisone that improved the rash, but it worsened again after he stopped taking the corticosteroid. History includes gout and hypertension. He has no pets, lives alone, and recalls no insect bite or contact with anybody with a rash. He takes allopurinol and hydrochlorothiazide.

On physical examination, he has no fever and looks well. He has a symmetric eruption with erythematous papules and excoriations on his back, shoulders, axillae, elbows, flexural wrists, scrotum, and upper legs. There are a few pustulae in the axillae. CBC, renal panel, and liver function tests are normal.

Which of the following is the most appropriate next step?

(A) Prescribe another course of oral corticosteroids.
(B) Examine skin scraping in mineral oil under a light microscope.
(C) Examine skin scraping in potassium hydroxide preparation.
(D) Stop hydrochlorothiazide.
(E) Stop allopurinol.

ANSWER: B

Scabies should be excluded in a patient who has generalized pruritus that is worse at night. In the classic form of scabies, the lesions are symmetric and start as small erythematous papules that can progress to vesicles and pustules. The lesions are located mostly in the web spaces between fingers and toes, flexor surfaces of the wrists, elbows, axillae, male genitalia, and female breasts. Secondary lesions may result from scratching and infection and include excoriations, eczema, and impetigo. The classic burrows may be absent because of patient scratching. Diagnosis is confirmed by examining the skin scraping in mineral oil under a light microscope to identify mites, eggs, eggshell fragments, or mite pellets (scybala). The patient might not recall contact with somebody with a rash, especially if he lives alone. It is sometimes helpful to ask if the patient knows anybody that seems to itch a lot.

Prescribing a course of systemic corticosteroids without a diagnosis would not be appropriate. Repeated courses of systemic corticosteroids can cause immunosuppression. Patients who have scabies and are immunocompromised can develop a severe form of scabies called *crusted scabies* (previously called *Norwegian scabies*). This is an atypical form in which the patient is infected with thousands of mites; it is highly contagious. It appears as a localized or generalized psoriasiform hyperkeratotic dermatosis.

A potassium hydroxide preparation is used when cutaneous candidiasis is suspected. Potassium hydroxide should not be used if scabies is a diagnostic possibility, because it dissolves the excreta. The distribution of this patient's rash is not typical for candidiasis, in which intertriginous sites are most commonly involved. In candidiasis, the surrounding lesions can be papules and are known as *satellite lesions*. They are usually located in sites where there is increased moisture, and are not likely on elbows and wrists, as in this patient.

It is not likely that allopurinol or hydrochlorothiazide is the cause of the rash. There is a rare drug reaction with a pustular eruption that is called *acute generalized exanthematous pustolosis*. Drugs that have been implicated in this reaction are sulfonamides, terbinafine, quinolones, hydroxychloroquine, diltiazem, pristinamycin, ampicillin, and amoxicillin. Usually the reaction occurs within a few days of starting the drug.

34. An 88-year-old woman comes to the office because she has chronic pain in both knees, left more than right, which is worse when she walks. She takes acetaminophen 1,000 mg q8h for the pain. Prior radiography demonstrated moderate medial compartment narrowing and subchondral sclerosis in both knees, the left greater than right. She asks whether she can try something other than medicine for pain relief.

On physical examination, there is crepitus in both knees.

Which of the following treatments is most likely to improve the patient's pain?

(A) Acupuncture
(B) Topical capsaicin cream
(C) Topical diclofenac gel
(D) Topical salicylate cream
(E) Transcutaneous electrical nerve stimulation

ANSWER: C

This patient has chronic pain from osteoarthritis. Osteoarthritis affects >50% of adults >65 years old. Topical diclofenac sodium gel has been approved for treatment of osteoarthritis in the United States. Its efficacy is similar to that of oral diclofenac, and except for application site reactions, it has an adverse effect profile similar to that of placebo. Use of topical diclofenac sodium gel decreases pain and discomfort and improves function (SOE=A).

Topical capsaicin has poor to modest efficacy in patients with osteoarthritis (SOE=B). Because its adverse effects are limited to local irritation, it is not a bad option to try; however, diclofenac gel is more likely to improve the patient's pain.

In patients with osteoarthritis pain, the efficacy of topical salicylates ranges from poor to moderate (SOE=C). Topical methylsalicylate has been associated with severe toxicity and may increase the risk of bleeding for patients on warfarin.

Acupuncture has been shown to provide short-term improvement in osteoarthritis pain when compared with sham control (SOE=B); however, this would not be the next best step. Transcutaneous electrical nerve stimulation thus far has shown little effect in knee osteoarthritis (SOE=C).

35. A 72-year-old woman comes to the office because she is depressed and anxious. History includes heart failure. Medications include sertraline 50 mg/d. Two years ago, her husband had a stroke that affected his memory and behavior, and she has had difficulty adjusting to these changes. For example, she is unable to tolerate his dependent behavior and emotional unresponsiveness. She views his neediness as manipulative and threatens him with nursing-home placement. According to her medical record, she often presents herself as acutely depressed and angry, demands treatment for her husband and assistance for herself, and is suspicious of or rejects recommendations.

Screening for depression reveals pervasive dysphoria and irritability, anhedonia, feelings of worthlessness, reduced appetite, poor sleep, and low energy. Her symptoms are not due to current medications or substances. Cognitive examination and thyroid function are normal.

Which of the following should be done next?

(A) Maintain current dosage of sertraline and monitor for adherence.
(B) Discontinue sertraline and begin treatment with a mood-stabilizing agent.
(C) Discontinue sertraline and refer for psychotherapy.
(D) Increase dosage of sertraline and refer for psychotherapy and caregiving respite.

ANSWER: D

Some older adults have a chronic, unremitting depressive disorder. An inadequately treated mood disorder may be misdiagnosed as a personality disorder if it is longstanding and characterized by irritable mood and an abrasive interpersonal style. In other cases, features of a personality disorder may overshadow depressive symptoms, masking an inadequately treated depression. Distinguishing personality disorder from persisting mood disorder is challenging, and definitive diagnosis may be possible only after the depression is maximally treated (SOE=C). Given this patient's persisting symptoms, she most likely has a major depressive disorder superimposed on comorbid medical illness (ie, heart failure), caregiver burden, and an underlying personality disorder. Maximal use of an antidepressant combined with psychotherapy may be optimal for older depressed patients with comorbid medical illness (SOE=B), and is a promising treatment for depressed older adults with comorbid personality disorder (SOE=C). The goal of treating personality disorders in older adults is not remission but a reduction in the frequency and intensity of symptoms.

Insufficient response to a low dosage of antidepressant may indicate that the current dosage is inadequate. Mood stabilizers can improve mood regulation in some patients with personality disorder (SOE=B), but for this population, psychotropic medication combined with psychotherapy is more effective than either treatment alone. Monitoring for adherence to the current regimen, or discontinuation of medications, would be indicated in patients with a history of nonadherent or self-injurious use of medications.

36. An 82-year-old man comes to the clinic for follow-up after recent hospitalization for a transient ischemic attack. History includes hypercholesterolemia, hypertension, diabetes mellitus, gastroesophageal reflux, and benign prostatic hyperplasia. Medications include clopidogrel, simvastatin, lisinopril, metformin, esomeprazole, and doxazosin.

Which of the following pairs of medications has a potential interaction that increases the risk of major cardiovascular events?

(A) Clopidogrel and doxazosin
(B) Lisinopril and metformin
(C) Clopidogrel and esomeprazole
(D) Esomeprazole and lisinopril
(E) Doxazosin and simvastatin

ANSWER: C

Clopidogrel is a platelet antagonist that targets adenosine diphosphate receptors. It is approved by the FDA for prevention of vascular events such as stroke, acute coronary syndrome, and peripheral artery disease. Clopidogrel is a pro-drug that requires the cytochrome P-450 enzyme pathway for conversion to its active metabolite. Proton-pump inhibitors, specifically esomeprazole and omeprazole, directly inhibit cytochrome P-450, which can reduce the potency of clopidogrel. The American Heart Association/American Stroke Association and the FDA warn that coadministration of clopidogrel and a proton-pump inhibitor may lead to an increased risk of major cardiovascular events such as stroke and myocardial infarction (SOE=B). If an older patient on clopidogrel requires treatment for gastroesophageal reflux disease, an H_2 blocker (eg, ranitidine) or the proton-pump inhibitor pantoprazole, which is least likely to interfere with clopidogrel metabolism, should be used.

Modifying risk factors for stroke is important to prevent future events. The optimal drug regimen for reducing blood pressure includes diuretics or ACE inhibitors such as lisinopril (SOE=A). In addition, glycemic control with, for example, metformin reduces stroke risk. Doxazosin is used in the primary treatment of benign prostatic hyperplasia; it also improves hypertension, although it is not a first-line agent for that purpose. Doxazosin has no known interactions with simvastatin. However, it could further lower blood pressure, which should be monitored closely.

37. An 86-year-old man comes to the office after recent hospitalization for myocardial infarction. History includes diabetes mellitus, hypertension, coronary artery disease, COPD, renal insufficiency, and anemia. Medications include insulin 70/30, lisinopril, metoprolol, aspirin, clopidogrel, simvastatin, mometasone, formoterol, and albuterol. He lives alone; his daughter lives 5 miles away. He is able to do all instrumental activities of daily living and enjoys yard work and fishing.

On examination, weight is 54.4 kg (120 lb) and BMI is 20 kg/m^2. Sitting blood pressure is 98/60 mmHg, and pulse is 60 beats per minute. Cardiovascular and pulmonary examinations are normal.

Laboratory findings include hemoglobin A_{1c} of 8.0% and hemoglobin of 12 g/dL.

Which of the following is the next best step in management of this patient?

(A) Start alendronate weekly with calcium and vitamin D supplements.
(B) Discontinue simvastatin because of limited benefit given life expectancy.
(C) Intensify insulin therapy and glucose monitoring to achieve better glucose control.
(D) Discontinue lisinopril and monitor blood pressure.
(E) Switch insulin to metformin.

BP low

ANSWER: D

Hypotension in an older adult can result in falls and possibly fractures, especially in a thin older man. Treatment with alendronate would not be appropriate without first determining the patient's risk of osteoporosis and possibly bone density imaging. Discontinuation of simvastatin would not improve the patient's hypotension. In addition, the simvastatin is appropriate for a patient with a recent myocardial infarction. Intensifying the insulin regimen would not yield any benefit, given the patient's overall prognosis. Although metformin is first-line treatment of diabetes type II in older adults, the patient has renal disease and has already required insulin for treatment of his diabetes, with a hemoglobin A_{1C} of 8%. Thus, switching to metformin is not appropriate, nor will it address the patient's hypotension.

38. A 73-year-old man comes to the office because for the past 5 years he has had decreased libido, loss of nocturnal and early-morning erections, and an inability to sustain erections sufficient for intercourse. He has no difficulty with ejaculation. He also reports an overall decrease in energy level. He and his wife of 36 years remain interested in sexual relations. History includes diabetes mellitus, hyperlipidemia, and benign prostatic hyperplasia; he had a myocardial infarction at age 53 with no episodes of chest pain since, and a right-sided stroke with near-complete recovery. Medications include aspirin, simvastatin, combination dutasteride/tamsulosin, metformin, and glimepiride.

On physical examination, blood pressure is 130/75 mmHg, weight is 82.6 kg (182 lb), and height is 172.7 cm (5 ft 8 inches). BMI is 27.7 kg/m². The prostate is borderline enlarged (volume approximately 30 mL), and testicular volume is 20 mL bilaterally. Pedal pulses are diminished (1+). Neurologic function is intact.

Which of the following is the most likely cause of this patient's erectile dysfunction?

(A) Hypogonadism
(B) Medication
(C) Neurologic disease
(D) Vascular disease
(E) Psychogenic issues

ANSWER: D

Erectile dysfunction (ED) in older men is caused by vascular disease in >50% of cases (SOE=A). This patient's ED is most likely related to atherosclerotic vascular disease, given his history of diabetes mellitus, hyperlipidemia, and myocardial infarction, as well as his current diminished pedal pulses (SOE=A). Hypertension and smoking are other common risk factors for ED related to vascular disease.

This patient has no sensory or autonomic changes to suggest that the dysfunction is related to neurologic alterations. In about 5% of cases, ED is associated with medication, including antihypertensive agents (SOE=B), antidepressants, anxiolytics, antihistamines, NSAIDs, and anti-androgens such as flutamide and leuprolide (SOE=B). Tamsulosin and other α-blockers are less likely to cause ED than β-blockers or diuretics (SOE=B); 5-α-reductase inhibitors (dutasteride) are not a common cause of ED.

Adequate testicular volume and the extent of somatic disease make hypogonadism or a psychogenic cause unlikely.

39. A 68-year-old man is brought to the office by his sister because she is concerned about changes in his behavior. The patient has always had some limits in his living skills; his Full-Scale Intelligence Quotient (FSIQ) is 62. The sister says that he is sometimes confused and forgetful and gets frustrated easily; he seems sad and lonely, now rarely speaks, and seems to be angrier than in the past. He is sleeping less and has to be urged to shave or shower. His appetite is unchanged, but he has lost weight. He has lived with his sister since his wife died 2 years ago. At the time, he appeared to grieve; after 4 months, he was no longer tearful and ate and slept more regularly. He had been a janitor but no longer works. He takes no medications.

On physical examination, he is thin, but findings are otherwise normal. Laboratory findings are normal.

Which of the following is most appropriate?

(A) Explain that the patient needs more time to grieve.
(B) Prescribe a cholinesterase inhibitor.
(C) Prescribe methylphenidate.
(D) Prescribe aripiprazole.
(E) Prescribe sertraline.

ANSWER: E

An accurate diagnosis may be difficult to ascertain, because this patient's age and intellectual disability are complicating factors. His impaired cognition and behavioral disturbance most likely signify major depressive disorder. In people with an intellectual disability, depression can present differently (SOE=B). The most appropriate treatment option is a trial of an antidepressant that has a low incidence of adverse effects. The dosage should be adjusted for the patient's age and titrated upward to effect (SOE=A for older adults without intellectual disability).

The patient's symptoms may be attributable to early dementia, but there is sufficient evidence of depressive symptoms, including the worsening cognition (SOE=A). Even if dementia and depression are equally likely, the risk-to-benefit assessment of treatment options favors an initial trial of an antidepressant, rather than a cholinesterase inhibitor.

The patient grieved when his wife died and then resumed normal behavior. His current symptoms are unlikely to represent a prolonged grief reaction. Although findings on examination are normal, there are suggestions of physical and psychosocial decline; waiting to see whether his symptoms improve over time is inappropriate.

Prescribing methylphenidate does not address the likely presence of depression. Low-dose stimulants may be used in some situations of apathy (SOE=A) but would not be the first choice for this patient. Similarly, aripiprazole is not a good choice for treating depression. It could be used to augment but should not be used in place of an antidepressant. Aripiprazole may address the patient's anger and agitation, but these are lesser complaints. Second-generation antipsychotics are overused as off-label treatment for many behaviors (SOE=A).

40. A 68-year-old woman comes to the office for a routine physical examination. She generally feels well, but she has had difficulty sleeping over the past few months. She sleeps between 4 and 5 hours each night, and she feels tired. She drinks no caffeine after 10 AM, has not changed her sleep routine, and walks for 30 min most afternoons. She reports no symptoms of depression or anxiety, and asks for advice on whether she should try "natural" therapies to help her sleep.

Which of the following will most likely improve her sleep?

(A) Yoga
(B) Valerian
(C) Acupuncture
(D) Melatonin

ANSWER: A

Although sleep disturbances can be related to medical illness, many patients have chronic insomnia with no underlying medical or psychiatric condition. According to a systematic review of complementary therapies for insomnia, there is supportive evidence that yoga helps with insomnia after 6 months of practice. Yoga combines exercise postures and breathing techniques. There is also supportive evidence for Tai Chi and acupressure. Tai Chi is a low-impact exercise that also focuses on breathing techniques. Acupressure is a manipulative therapy that uses finger pressure to stimulate points along the meridian where energy is thought to flow. Opening the energy blockages is believed to help relieve discomfort and illness.

Unlike acupressure, which relies on finger pressure, acupuncture uses thin needles inserted into meridian points in the body to relieve blockages of energy that are believed to cause illness. Some studies showed acupuncture to be helpful for insomnia, but none included placebo controls.

Valerian is derived from the *Valeriana* plant. Studies have not found valerian more effective than placebo for treatment of insomnia. Melatonin is a hormone secreted by the pineal gland. Levels decrease in older adults. Some studies with melatonin have shown improvement in sleep; other studies have not.

Sedative-hypnotic agents help induce sleep, but they have many potential adverse effects in older patients, including falls and cognitive impairment. They should not be used over long periods.

41. An 85-year-old woman is evaluated in anticipation of discharge after hospitalization for aspiration pneumonia. She has advanced dementia, is dependent for all activities of daily living, and has been losing weight in the past year. She lives in her own home with a privately paid home attendant. Her daughter, who is the healthcare proxy, says her mother signed a "do not resuscitate" order, had specified that she did not want a "tube" to keep her alive, and wished to remain at home until the end of her life. She has Medicare and AARP health insurance.

Which of the following is the most appropriate recommendation for her discharge?

(A) Transfer to a nursing facility for long-term care to prevent further aspiration
(B) Referral to a visiting nurse agency to instruct the home attendant on proper feeding techniques and food consistency
(C) Referral to a home hospice program for comprehensive end-of-life care
(D) Transfer to an inpatient hospice unit for care planning

ANSWER: C

Medicare Part A covers hospice care, which provides end-of-life support for people who are in physical decline, have lost weight, and have multiple comorbidities. Eligibility criteria for patients with dementia that have been proposed by the National Hospice and Palliative Care organization and accepted by Medicare include a Functional Assessment Tool (FAST) score of 7c or worse (ADL dependency and unable to communicate), medical complications (eg, aspiration pneumonia, hospitalization, pressure ulcers), and ongoing weight loss.

This patient meets the criteria for hospice, and she has previously specified that she wants to die at home. In addition, her health insurance would not cover a long-term nursing facility. Visiting nurse services would provide only short-term care. Transfer to an inpatient hospice unit would not address the patient's desire to remain at home until the end of her life.

42. An 86-year-old black man is evaluated in preparation for hospital discharge. He was admitted for exacerbation of class IV heart failure and pneumonia. History includes advanced coronary artery disease, diabetes mellitus, and chronic kidney disease. He is frail but ready for discharge. His prognosis remains guarded. Discharge recommendations include completion of advance directives and transfer to a postacute rehabilitation facility. The patient does not want to complete advance directives, and he is upset because the medical resident addressed him by his first name. When his wife arrives, the medical team is not readily available to answer her questions. She believes her husband is in pain that has not been adequately treated. Neither she nor the patient wants him to be transferred to a rehabilitation facility.

Which of the following is the most appropriate next step?

(A) Arrange a patient and family meeting to discuss the patient's wishes and options.
(B) Arrange a family meeting to discuss his urgent need for postacute rehabilitation.
(C) Arrange a family meeting to discuss the need for hospice care.
(D) Meet separately with the patient's wife to discuss her concerns regarding the patient.

ANSWER: A

Cultural competence is the ability to understand, communicate with, and effectively interact with people across cultures, and elicit what health and illness mean to older adults of many different cultures. For many black Americans, there is limited trust in the healthcare system; longevity may trump quality of life; and advance directives may be perceived as legalized genocide, denial of care, or the cause of premature death. The patient and his wife need to be addressed respectfully and asked about decision-making approaches, their views on end-of-life care, and care preferences. Once the patient's and family's wishes are known, a collaborative treatment approach should follow.

43. A 75-year-old man is evaluated in the rehabilitation unit because he has pain on the medial aspect of his left foot. The pain affects his ability to walk. History includes diabetes mellitus, for which he takes metformin.

On examination, there is a thick, mildly erythematous, hyperkeratotic lesion over the medial aspect of the first metatarsal phalangeal joint associated with a severe bunion deformity (hallux valgus).

Which of the following is the most appropriate initial treatment?

(A) Pad the bunion so that the patient may ambulate with less pain.
(B) Have the patient wear a larger, softer shoe to reduce pressure and friction to the bunion.
(C) Start antibiotic therapy.
(D) Debride the lesion and assess for an ulcer.

ANSWER: D

Foot deformities are common in older adults. A callus is the body's response to pressure or friction and usually develops over a bony prominence. The callus, in turn, adds to the pressure over the bony prominence, and continued pressure may cause the callus to bleed or even ulcerate beneath the surface. Debridement is needed to evaluate for an ulcer that is not visible on the surface of the skin. Furthermore, an abscess may be present. Debridement will also reduce pressure (SOE=C). Clinicians should strongly discourage use of OTC, acid-based callus removers, because they will also break down any exposed, healthy tissue.

Padding the bony prominence and changing the patient's shoes may relieve pain and allow him to resume walking, but debridement is required to evaluate for an ulcer or abscess as well as to reduce pressure. Antibiotics would be necessary only if debridement reveals infection. Ultimately, if the patient is a candidate for surgery, correction of the bony deformity should be considered. If not, custom-molded shoes may be adequate.

44. A 72-year-old woman is brought to the office because of a change in her behavior. Over the past year the patient has been calling the police because she believes that a neighbor has been entering her apartment to steal items such as cans of soup and paper towels. The patient lives alone. History includes hypertension and osteoarthritis; there is no history of alcohol or substance abuse. She has no hallucinations or depressive symptoms. She adequately performs daily activities, including managing her finances. Her sister reports that the patient has always tended to be suspicious of others.

Physical examination is normal. MRI of the head is unremarkable.

Which of the following is the most likely explanation for the patient's symptoms?

(A) Delusional disorder
(B) Late-onset schizophrenia
(C) Paranoid personality disorder
(D) Bipolar disease
(E) Alzheimer disease

ANSWER: A

Delusional disorder is rare, comprising perhaps 2% of all psychotic illnesses in older adults. Findings are mixed regarding its association with hearing loss. The delusions are not bizarre; they involve situations that may occur in real life, such as theft, suffering from a disease, spousal infidelity, or being followed.

Patients with delusional disorder generally do not have prominent auditory or visual hallucinations. (If hallucinations are present, they are related to the delusional theme.) The lack of hallucinations and the maintenance of normal function in areas outside the delusional scope distinguish delusional disorder from schizophrenia.

Delusional disorder is differentiated from dementia by the absence of cognitive impairment. The chronology of symptoms—delusions preceding any mood disturbances—differentiates delusional disorder from mood disorder. Schizotypal and paranoid personality disorders are not associated with delusions; however, these personality disorders are commonly found in delusional disorder.

Poor psychosocial functioning in delusional disorder is related directly to the delusions. Antipsychotic agents often are effective, especially in agitated delusional patients (SOE=C). However, because patients with delusions typically deny their illness, they commonly do not adhere to medication regimens. Cognitive-behavioral therapy may be effective (SOE=D). There have been reports of successful modified electroconvulsive therapy in refractory cases.

45. A 68-year-old man comes to the clinic because he has tingling in his hands and forearms. His hands feel clumsy and he has begun to drop things, such as his keys and coffee cup. He is walking unsteadily. Over the past 4 months, he has noticed intermittent lower abdominal pain, decrease in appetite, fatigue, and shortness of breath when climbing stairs. History includes hypertension. He takes lisinopril as well as acetaminophen as needed. He does not smoke or drink.

On examination, weight is 68 kg (150 lb), a decrease from his usual weight of 74.8 kg (165 lb). He is pale, with icteric conjunctiva and skin. He has decreased sensation to light touch in his hands and feet and decreased vibratory sensation in a stocking pattern in his legs. Romberg test is positive (he sways and has near falls); the rest of the neurologic and physical examinations are normal.

Laboratory findings:

WBC	7,000/µL with normal distribution
Hemoglobin	6.3 g/dL
Hematocrit	19%
RBC distribution width	18%
Mean corpuscular volume	124 fL
Mean corpuscular hemoglobin	42 pg/RBC
Mean corpuscular hemoglobin concentration	34 g/dL
Reticulocytes	0.80%
Total bilirubin	3.2 mg/dL
Direct bilirubin	0.7 mg/dL
Lactate dehydrogenase	1,200 U/L

The remaining liver function tests are normal. Electrolytes, glucose, BUN, creatinine, creatine kinase, amylase, magnesium, calcium, and phosphorus are normal.

In order to establish the diagnosis, which of the following should be done next?

(A) CT of the abdomen
(B) MRI of the spine
(C) Bone marrow biopsy and aspirate
(D) Measurement of thyroid function
(E) Measurement of methylmalonic acid and homocysteine levels

ANSWER: E

This patient presents with paresthesias, ataxia, abdominal pain, jaundice, weight loss, and macrocytic anemia (increased mean corpuscular volume). There are many causes of paresthesias but most do not apply in this case. The patient's ataxia and anemia narrow the focus greatly. His symptoms of shortness of breath and fatigue may be explained by the severe anemia.

On examination, he shows decreased sensation, normal strength, and a positive Romberg test: when he closes his eyes, the positional input from his lower extremities and spinal cord posterior columns is inadequate to maintain balance. Because he does not have signs of hereditary ataxia, infection (tabes dorsalis, leprosy, HIV), diabetes, alcoholism, multiple sclerosis, or multisystem atrophy, nutritional deficiencies are most likely. Inadequate levels of vitamin B_{12}, folate, and vitamin E can cause sensory ataxia. Although other tests can be done to exclude HIV or syphilis, the presence of paresthesias and macrocytic anemia makes vitamin B_{12} or folate deficiency the most likely cause. Severe vitamin B_{12} or folate deficiency causes subacute degeneration of the dorsal columns of the spinal cord and hemolysis, with increased lactate dehydrogenase and total and unconjugated bilirubin levels, as well as nonspecific abdominal pain and weight loss. Hemolysis occurs because of ineffective erythropoiesis, with hemolysis of abnormal megaloblastic erythroid precursors.

Examination of the red cell smear will show hypersegmented neutrophils (>5 lobes), oval macrocytes, and anisocytosis. The patient should have vitamin B_{12} and RBC folate levels checked. However, methylmalonic acid and homocysteine levels can differentiate between vitamin B_{12} and folate deficiency, because methylmalonic acid is increased in both conditions and homocysteine is increased only in folate deficiency.

Causes of vitamin B_{12} deficiency include inadequate diet, pernicious anemia (inadequate intrinsic factor), and infections such as *Helicobacter pylori* and fish tapeworm. Severe deficiency is treated initially with intramuscular vitamin B_{12}.

Abdominal conditions, spinal cord problems, and thyroid disease would not cause the symptoms and signs in this case, and thus assessment for these would not be the best next step. Bone marrow aspirate and biopsy would be abnormal and show signs of megaloblastic anemia; however, it is not necessary to establish the diagnosis.

46. A 69-year-old man comes to the office because he lost consciousness for about 20 seconds. The episode occurred 1 week ago. The patient's son witnessed it and states that his father was walking across the room, appeared pale, said "I don't feel quite right," and collapsed. The patient says that he felt lightheaded for about 5 seconds before loss of consciousness and felt normal within a few minutes of the event. History includes hyperlipidemia and prostatic hyperplasia.

On examination, blood pressure is 128/56 mmHg with no postural changes. All other findings are normal.

Which of the following is the most appropriate initial diagnostic test?

(A) Two-dimensional echocardiography
(B) Doppler ultrasonography of the carotid artery
(C) Electrocardiography
(D) MRI of the brain
(E) Tilt table test

ANSWER: C

Electrocardiography is indicated for all patients who have syncope; the American College of Emergency Physicians considers this a Class A recommendation (SOE=A). It can be performed in the office, is fairly inexpensive, and can be used to discern whether an underlying arrhythmia or conduction abnormality caused the episode. In this case, the sudden loss of consciousness with only a brief prodrome suggests an arrhythmia could be the cause. Normal ECG findings are associated with a more favorable prognosis.

Two-dimensional echocardiography may be useful in the evaluation of syncope, especially when a cardiac cause is suspected. It can be used to identify a low ejection fraction or a valvular disorder causing cardiac outflow obstruction that may have led to the episode. Two-dimensional echocardiography would also reveal a ventricular thrombus that could cause cerebrovascular embolism. However, it would not be the first test to order, particularly in the absence of focal neurologic signs that suggest embolic stroke.

Doppler ultrasonography yields information regarding vessel integrity of the carotid arteries, which provide anterior circulation to the brain. A cerebrovascular cause of syncope, however, would more likely reflect lack of perfusion to the *posterior* circulation (specifically, the reticular activating system in the brain stem), which maintains alertness, which was not the case for this patient. A problem with bihemispheric anterior circulation could also lead to syncope but would involve bilateral simultaneous occlusion of the carotid arteries, an unlikely event.

MRI of the brain can help identify structural abnormalities that may have contributed to the syncope, such as a mass lesion or hydrocephalus. Typically, in the absence of focal neurologic signs or other contributing information, MRI is not ordered for evaluation of syncope, and certainly not as the initial test.

A head-up tilt table test would identify whether autonomic dysfunction contributed to the syncope. This patient provided no information (such as rising from sitting to standing position) to suggest orthostatic syncope. The tilt table test is also more likely to be used once cardiovascular causes are excluded, and thus would not be the initial test in this patient's evaluation.

47. A 75-year-old man undergoes evaluation because within the past month a stage III pressure ulcer has developed on his left buttock. He has lived in a nursing facility for the past 3 years. History includes dementia and stroke. He is hemiparetic on the left side and cannot walk; he usually has no difficulty eating with assistance.

On examination, weight is 72.6 kg (160 lb); he has lost 4.5 kg (10 lb) in the past month. BMI is 20.5 kg/m^2. Laboratory findings include albumin level of 3.2 g/dL and prealbumin level of 14 g/dL. Wound care is started for the pressure ulcer.

Which of the following is most likely to aid in healing the pressure ulcer?

(A) Vitamin C 500 mg q12h
(B) Arginine 17 g/d
(C) Glutamine 40 g/d
(D) Protein 100 g/d

ANSWER: D

Optimal healing of pressure ulcers is influenced by reduction of interface pressure, adequate oxygenation of tissue, protection from bacterial overgrowth, and nutritional support. Evidence is limited, yet the general consensus is that nutritional support is an important part of treatment of pressure ulcers. Adequate calories, protein, fluids, vitamins, and minerals are required by the body to maintain tissue integrity and prevent tissue breakdown. All patients with a pressure ulcer should have a nutritional evaluation (SOE=C).

Having lost >5% of his weight in a short period, this patient is at increased risk of death. Administration of nutrients could potentially reverse undernutrition and thereby promote healing of pressure ulcers. Advisory panels in the United States and Europe recommend provision of adequate protein (1.25–1.5 g/kg) for positive nitrogen balance in an individual with a pressure ulcer (SOE=B).

Vitamin C, a cofactor with iron during hydroxylation of proline and lysine in the production of collagen, is important for tissue repair and regeneration. Deficiency is associated with impaired fibroblastic function and decreased collagen synthesis, which can result in capillary fragility and delayed healing. Physiologic doses of vitamin C are important for nutrition, but no studies have shown that megadoses accelerate healing of pressure ulcers.

Arginine and glutamine are essential amino acids important in cellular processes involved with wound healing. No definitive studies have shown that supplementation with these agents alone improves healing of pressure ulcers.

48. A 78-year-old man is admitted to the hospital because he has had cough, shortness of breath, and fever for the past 3–4 days. He was hospitalized 3 months ago for a similar episode; at that time he was treated with ceftriaxone and doxycycline. History includes hypertension, hyperlipidemia, and mild cognitive impairment.

On physical examination, temperature is 38.1°C (100.6°F), and blood pressure is 155/80 mmHg. Heart rate is 101 beats per minute, respiratory rate is 22 breaths per minute, and O_2 saturation is 95% on 2 L of oxygen via nasal cannula. Radiography of the chest shows bilateral lower lobe infiltrates. Laboratory results are normal except for WBC count of 15,700/µL and creatinine level of 1.0 mg/dL.

On admission, the diagnosis is community-acquired pneumonia.

Which of the following antibiotics would be most effective?

(A) Ceftriaxone
(B) Levofloxacin
(C) Ceftriaxone plus doxycycline
(D) Azithromycin
(E) Doxycycline

ANSWER: B

For patients with community-acquired pneumonia who are admitted to regular inpatient or intensive care units, guideline-concordant antimicrobial therapy (using guidelines jointly developed by the Infectious Diseases Society of America/American Thoracic Society) is associated with lower mortality than guideline-discordant antimicrobial therapy (SOE=B). For patients admitted to regular inpatient units, guideline-concordant care is also associated with both decreased risk of sepsis and renal failure and with shorter hospital stay and duration of parenteral therapy (SOE=B). Several prospective studies have demonstrated comparably high cure rates with a respiratory quinolone alone and with a β-lactam (cefotaxime, ceftriaxone, or ampicillin) plus a macrolide antibiotic (SOE=A). The major determinant in choosing between the 2 regimens is whether the patient has received a β-lactam antibiotic within the previous 3 months. This patient was treated with ceftriaxone and doxycycline 3 months ago, and so levofloxacin is the appropriate choice at this time.

Because of increasing resistance, azithromycin alone cannot be routinely recommended, although its efficacy is supported by 2 randomized controlled trials (SOE=A) and it may be appropriate for carefully selected patients. Doxycycline and ceftriaxone are not recommended for use as single agents for community-acquired pneumonia treated in the hospital.

49. An 81-year-old man comes to the office for a routine appointment. History includes moderate aortic stenosis for the past 8 years, managed with β-blockers, chronic coronary artery disease, prostate carcinoma (stage 2), and mild COPD. He received a left anterior descending artery stent in 2001. At previous appointments, he reported that he felt well and that he was maintaining his normal, active lifestyle. At this appointment, his daughter notes that her father is much less active than in the past.

Echocardiography undertaken last month was limited by poor echo windows due to COPD, but Doppler imaging detected a peak aortic velocity of 6 m/sec (an increase from 3 m/sec 2 years earlier).

Which of the following is true regarding management of this patient?

(A) Annual echocardiography is sufficient follow-up.
(B) Given that he has no chest pain, syncope, or heart failure, current management is optimal.
(C) Addition of nitrates will alleviate the patient's symptoms.
(D) Valve replacement should be considered in the near future.

ANSWER: D

This patient has aortic stenosis, with Doppler echocardiography revealing an increased valvular flow gradient consistent with critical stenosis physiology. Although the patient does not report many symptoms, he has constricted his activity to accommodate the change. Whereas β-blockers are beneficial, valve replacement is indicated when stenosis is significant and there is a high transvalvular gradient (SOE=A). Aortic valve surgery should be considered if the patient is a good candidate. He will need evaluation of cardiac function, coronary artery disease, pulmonary arterial pressures, COPD severity, and renal function.

If surgery is contraindicated, transcatheter aortic valve replacement (TAVR) may be an option. TAVR does not offer the technical advantages of surgery, namely, more surgical control and the ability to integrate valve replacement with coronary artery bypass surgery. Risk of stroke is greater with TAVR, although technology and techniques are rapidly advancing and improved outcomes are anticipated.

Use of nitrates will likely be counter-productive, because nitrates diminish preload filling of the left ventricle (which is severely thickened and stiff because of aortic valve disease) and might thereby lead to reduced cardiac output.

50. A frail 85-year-old woman with oxygen-dependent COPD is concerned about potential harms from continuing screening mammography.

Which of the following outcomes from screening mammography is capable of producing the greatest harm to this patient?

(A) Radiation exposure from mammography increases the risk of future cancers in older women.
(B) False-positive mammography results may lead to additional diagnostic tests.
(C) Mammography may lead to the detection and treatment of cancers that would not have caused clinical symptoms.
(D) Mammography may cause significant pain and anxiety that last for several months.

ANSWER: C

In older patients, the greatest harms from screening come from treating cancers that would never have become clinically significant (SOE=A). As life expectancy decreases, the probability of identifying an inconsequential cancer increases. This patient has a severe, life-limiting comorbidity (end-stage COPD); an asymptomatic lesion detected on screening mammography is unlikely to become symptomatic during her remaining lifetime. Once an asymptomatic lesion is detected, patients often choose to undergo treatment despite the risks of surgery, such as cardiopulmonary complications, chronic wound infections, and pain. Women with severe comorbidity who undergo treatment for an inconsequential lesion have suffered the most serious harm from screening (SOE=A).

The radiation risks associated with mammography in older women are estimated to be small and would not cause serious harm to this patient. A large cohort study of women ≥80 years old found that 11% had a false-positive result from screening mammography. Generally, the most common test after an abnormal result is diagnostic mammography, followed by biopsy, which has a small complication rate (eg, infection or scarring) (SOE=A). Patients with false-positive mammograms experience significant anxiety and other symptoms for months (SOE=A). However, surveys have found that women view the anxiety and pain related to false-positive results as acceptable and not serious consequences of screening.

51. A 92-year-old man comes to the office because he believes that his memory loss is making driving more difficult. He has a history of hypertension. His score is 28 of 30 on the Mini–Mental State Examination; neuropsychologic testing is consistent with mild dementia. He has not had any motor vehicle violations, and his wife thinks he is a good driver.

Which of the following is most appropriate?

(A) Tell the patient that he should stop driving.
(B) Refer the patient to the Department of Motor Vehicles (DMV) for a performance-based road test.
(C) Monitor the patient's cognitive impairment every 6 months; report further impairment to the DMV.
(D) Notify the DMV that the patient's driver's license must be revoked.

ANSWER: B

Some clinicians may be reluctant to refer patients for road tests because the procedures are rarely standardized and the data supporting their use may be limited (SOE=B). However, the ability to demonstrate proficiency behind the wheel in traffic is the method adopted by all 50 states to evaluate novice and medically impaired patients. Therefore, referral for a performance-based road test is the most appropriate next step for this patient.

Because there is no common method of assessing dementia severity in relation to driving fitness, monitoring the patient's cognitive impairment every 6 months would not help to determine driving fitness. Rather, experts recommend that patients with mild dementia or with prominent impairments in key cognitive domains (eg, attention, visuospatial skills) be referred for a performance-based road test (SOE=B), as should patients whose caregivers observe them to be impaired.

An oral or written recommendation for the patient to stop driving is not an appropriate next step.

52. An 83-year-old woman comes to the office for an examination. She has recently returned to her home after a motor vehicle accident that resulted in injuries, a hospital stay complicated by pneumonia, and a nursing-home stay. She is greatly changed since her last office visit: she has lost a lot of weight, moves slowly, and is unable to rise from her chair without using her arms. She previously was an avid golfer and swimmer. She asks what she can do to improve her function now that her injuries have healed.

Which of the following is effective in improving function in frail older adults?

(A) Comprehensive geriatric assessment
(B) Protein supplementation
(C) Anabolic steroids (testosterone, dehydroepiandrosterone)
(D) Exercise
(E) Home visits to evaluate function in the home

ANSWER: D

Exercise is the most common approach to combating frailty. A 2011 systematic review evaluated 47 studies of exercise in older adults and found that, overall, multicomponent exercise in frail older adults results in improved function and fewer adverse health outcomes (SOE=B).

Patients who underwent comprehensive geriatric assessment did not benefit in terms of frailty status or function when they were compared with a control group. Compliance with recommendations was only 40%–60%. Meta-analysis of studies assessing the impact of home visits, overall, did not find improvement in functional status.

In large epidemiologic studies, low protein intake has been associated with incident frailty. Several trials have been done to assess the effect of protein supplements in older adults. A Cochrane review found that weight may be improved and that there was a trend toward reduced mortality, but protein supplementation did not improve function.

Anabolic steroids consistently modify body composition in older adults (more lean mass, less fat mass), but improvements in function are more variable.

53. A 75-year-old woman comes to the office because she has had a gradually increasing sense of imbalance over the past few months. She resides in an independent-living facility.

Which of the following is **least** likely to be identified as the underlying cause?

(A) Visual deficit
(B) Vestibular disorder
(C) Peripheral sensory impairment
(D) Musculoskeletal weakness
(E) Stroke

ANSWER: E

The insidious nature of this patient's symptom points to an ongoing process rather than an acute development such as stroke. Furthermore, in patients presenting with dizziness, vertigo, or imbalance, the proportion of cases attributable to stroke is very low (SOE=A).

The sense of equilibrium is mediated by central integration of multiple inputs from vestibular, visual, and proprioceptive systems. Dysequilibrium is believed to be multifactorial—a variety of disorders can contribute to a subjective sensation of imbalance. For example, the number of vestibular hair cells decreases as people age; although it is unclear what degree of loss yields functional deficits, vestibular hair cell loss is a possible source of this patient's sense of imbalance.

Age-related ocular conditions, such as glaucoma, cataracts, and macular degeneration, may contribute to imbalance. Other possible age-related contributors include disorders of peripheral sensory organs, as found in peripheral vascular disease and diabetes mellitus, and musculoskeletal conditions such as arthritic changes in the cervical spine, knees, and hips.

54. An 80-year-old woman comes to the office because she has mid-epigastric discomfort and heartburn. The symptoms occur daily and are not associated with shortness of breath, diaphoresis, or dizziness. She has been taking aluminum and magnesium hydroxide tablets to relieve the symptoms, but they provide only temporary relief. One month ago, the patient underwent cardiac catheterization with drug-eluting stents for coronary lesions; history also includes diabetes mellitus and hypertension. Medications are clopidogrel, aspirin, metoprolol, lisinopril, pravastatin, and glipizide. She lives with her husband and is independent in all basic and instrumental activities of daily living.

Which of the following is the most appropriate pharmacologic treatment for this patient's symptoms?

(A) Omeprazole
(B) Esomeprazole
(C) Ranitidine
(D) Sucralfate

ANSWER: C

This patient's symptoms are consistent with gastroesophageal reflux disease: the symptoms are relieved with regular use of an antacid, and they are not associated with other angina-equivalent physical findings. All of the options are appropriate treatment for gastroesophageal reflux. However, because she takes clopidogrel, the best choice is ranitidine, an H_2-receptor antagonist.

Many agents, including clopidogrel and omeprazole, require hepatic cytochrome P-450 metabolism to transform into the active form of the drug. In pharmacodynamics studies, omeprazole has been shown to interact with clopidogrel and attenuate its platelet inhibition (SOE=A). Although no interactions between clopidogrel and pantoprazole have been found in pharmacodynamics studies (SOE=A), all proton-pump inhibitors such as omeprazole and pantoprazole have been associated with increased risk of cardiovascular death and of hospitalization for acute coronary syndrome, stroke, or revascularization in patients taking clopidogrel. Yet other studies showed no increased risk of death, stroke, or myocardial infarction in patients treated with a proton-pump inhibitor and clopidogrel. Therefore, it is not clear whether other proton-pump inhibitors such as esomeprazole and pantoprazole will adversely interact with clopidogrel.

Sucralfate has no role in the management of gastroesophageal reflux disease.

55. A 68-year-old woman comes to the office because she is experiencing considerable frustration understanding clients in her law practice. She has worn hearing aids since age 50, when severe-to-profound sensorineural hearing impairment developed in each ear. She recently underwent a complete hearing test; hearing status was unchanged, and audiometric test results remained consistent with a sensorineural hearing loss associated with long-standing cochlear damage. Medical history is unremarkable with no history of tinnitus, dizziness, diabetes, cardiovascular disease, or cognitive decline. She recently read about bone-anchored hearing aids and cochlear implants and asks whether either would be appropriate for her.

Which of the following is the best recommendation?

(A) Bone-anchored hearing aid
(B) Cochlear implant in one ear and new hearing aid in the other
(C) Referral to otolaryngologist to exclude an acoustic tumor
(D) Learn sign language

ANSWER: B

A cochlear implant is an appropriate treatment for severe-to-profound deafness for patients who derive little subjective or objective benefit from hearing aids. Objective benefit is assessed by performance on speech recognition tasks. About 10% of older adults with hearing loss have impairment sufficient to qualify for an implant, yet most of these candidates are not identified or referred. Unlike hearing aids, which work by amplifying sound, cochlear implants bypass damaged areas of the inner ear and transmit signals directly to the brain via undamaged parts of the auditory nerve. The implants replace the function of the damaged hair cells in the cochlea by converting acoustic energy into electric energy, which is picked up by the fibers of the eighth cranial nerve. A cochlear implant consists of a surgically implanted electrode array and a receiver/stimulator. There is an external portion as well, which includes a microphone, speech processor, and transmitter coil.

Cochlear implants have become an accepted treatment for adults with age-related hearing loss or progression of early-onset hearing loss. Healthy older adults can undergo the surgical procedure to receive an implant with minimal risk. A 2010 study demonstrated that a bimodal approach (hearing aid on one ear, cochlear implant for the other ear) provides superior results on tests of speech understanding when compared with a cochlear implant alone (SOE=A). Patients who receive a cochlear implant should continue to wear a hearing aid in the other ear.

In a study that matched 28 adults who received a cochlear implant at age ≥65 years with adults who had received an implant between ages 18 and 64 and had similar pre-implantation hearing test scores, 55 of the 56 total patients showed improvement in hearing 1 year after implantation (SOE=A). Regardless of age at implantation, higher test scores before surgery predicted higher test scores after. However, older patients performed more poorly than younger patients on some speech perception tests at 1-year follow-up. These data suggest that adults with significant progressive presbycusis (age-related hearing loss) might consider undergoing implantation at a younger age, thereby maximizing postimplantation performance.

A bone-anchored hearing aid is appropriate for older adults with single-sided deafness or chronic middle-ear disease that precludes use of hearing aids. The outcome of surgery in older adults is favorable, and the rate of implant loss is comparable to that of the overall population of individuals who undergo surgery for a bone-anchored hearing aid. There appears to be a low risk of severe skin reactions or skin thickening around the implant.

The largest self-help consumer group that focuses on hearing loss and deafness is the Hearing Loss Association of America (HLAA; http://www.hearingloss.org/). Its Web site includes maps to help locate >200 chapters nationwide. HLAA provides support, information about community resources, hearing aids and cochlear implants, tips for coping with hearing loss, and communication strategies. The premise underlying self-help organizations is that participation can facilitate coping and acceptance of chronic conditions. Individuals find relief with others who experience similar frustrations and embarrassment. Recommendations for participating in a support group can be made simultaneous with other interventions to enhance hearing.

The audiometric test results (ie, hearing loss unchanged, results consistent with cochlear site of lesion) and case history results (absence of tinnitus and dizziness) are not indicative of an acoustic tumor.

It is difficult for people who have communicated orally their entire life to begin to learn sign language late in life, because of the cultural, cognitive, and social aspects of communicating via sign language.

56. An 80-year-old woman comes to the office to request a prescription for an antidepressant. Over the past 2 months she has been sleeping poorly, and her appetite has decreased. She describes feeling miserable all the time, crying often, and fighting with everybody. She has no somatic symptoms. History includes obesity, hypothyroidism, osteoarthritis, and longstanding bipolar disorder. Medications include levothyroxine and acetaminophen as needed. She has been asymptomatic off medication for bipolar disorder for 2 years; shortly before she stopped, she experienced lithium toxicity and required hospitalization. She and her family believe that the bipolar disorder has abated because of her age.

Physical examination is unremarkable. She appears restless, starts to talk of a new hobby, but then switches topic. There is a substantial change from her baseline cognition: she is not sure of the date, and she makes mistakes about events that are familiar to her. CBC and basic chemistry panel are within normal limits. Over the next 24 hours, she becomes increasingly tearful, confused, and restless.

Which of the following is most likely to be true?

(A) Before offering a psychotropic medication, additional tests are needed to exclude a medical illness that may be causing delirium.
(B) Treatment with an antidepressant is likely to improve her symptoms.
(C) The presentation suggests development of dementia with behavioral problems that is unlikely to respond to medications.
(D) A mood stabilizer will slowly improve her confusion resulting from bipolar disorder.
(E) A sedative will improve her anxiety and associated lack of sleep.

ANSWER: D

Bipolar disorder is chronic and does not resolve with age, although episodes may present differently in older patients. The patient is currently having a classic mixed episode of bipolar disorder, with a combination of manic symptoms (increased energy, anger, irritability, restlessness, decreased need for sleep or food, new interests, rapid change of attention, and inability to focus) and depressive symptoms (subjectively miserable, tearful, depressed mood). In older patients, the overwhelming excitation caused by manic and mixed states can cause confusion; this frequently is the presenting picture of older patients with bipolar illness.

Lifelong treatment is required for bipolar disorder. There is little more than clinical experience and inference from randomized controlled trials on younger populations to support the use of the same agents in older adults. Expert consensus is that a mood stabilizer is the agent of choice for treatment of mood disorder in older adults (SOE=C). In younger adults, there is strong evidence to support the use of mood stabilizers; lithium, valproic acid, and lamotrigine have the best evidence for efficacy in preventing an acute episode and as maintenance treatment for patients with bipolar illness (SOE=B in younger adults). For an acute episode, the standard of care is to use a mood stabilizer and, if needed, an antipsychotic for sedation until a therapeutic level of the mood stabilizer can be reached. Caution should be used because of the increased risk of adverse effects in older adults, and dosage adjustment is often needed. Supportive measures need to be instituted to ensure patient safety and maintain adequate food and fluid intake. An antipsychotic agent can be used in small doses in the acute phase but should not be used long term because of the increased risk of adverse events.

The development of symptoms in this patient is too rapid to be explained by dementia. Anxiety alone would not cause such a dramatic presentation. It is always prudent to exclude a medical condition, but in the absence of obvious symptoms and signs, this is not the most likely explanation for the onset of confusion.

57. An 86-year-old woman comes to the office because she has frequent spotting, occasional red blood, and extravaginal discharge that dampen the pads she must now wear. She has no family history of gynecologic, urologic, or GI neoplasia. Her most recent screening colonoscopy was 3 years earlier, and findings were normal.

Which of the following would be the most efficient initial evaluation of her bleeding?

(A) Refer to a gynecologist.
(B) Obtain ultrasonography of the pelvis.
(C) Obtain CT of the abdomen and pelvis.
(D) Perform pelvic examination.
(E) Refer for colonoscopy.

ANSWER: D

In any postmenopausal woman who reports vaginal bleeding, evaluation of the urinary, reproductive, and GI tracts must be considered. The most streamlined and cost-effective evaluation starts with a pelvic examination performed by a primary care physician, emergency physician, or skilled nurse. Besides bleeding from the reproductive tract, other possibilities include urethral mucosal prolapse, vulvar ulceration, a rectal polyp, or a foreign body, such as a neglected pessary. A simple pelvic examination will facilitate further evaluation.

From 90% to 95% of postmenopausal bleeding is benign. However, in a geriatric population, statistics such as this can be misleading. Literature regarding postmenopausal bleeding is skewed toward the many younger women whose bleeding is benign. The probability of cancer increases with age in most studies, although the incidence peaked in the seventh decade in one large cohort (SOE=A). A model that used clinical history alone to predict risk of endometrial cancer in postmenopausal women with abnormal uterine bleeding found that nulliparous women with diabetes mellitus who were >70 years old had an 87% risk of complex hyperplasia or endometrial cancer; the risk was 3% in women without any of these characteristics (SOE=B).

Complex endometrial hyperplasia and type I (endometrioid) endometrial cancer are related to greater estrogen exposure, particularly unopposed estrogen. Obesity, oligo-ovulation, nulliparity, lack of progestin-containing contraception, menopause after age 55, diabetes mellitus, and hypertension are risk factors. A recent study found endometrial cancer to be less common in women whose hormone replacement therapy included daily (continuous) progestin than in women who took sequential (intermittent) progestin.

A less common, usually more aggressive type II endometrial cancer is unrelated to estrogen stimulation. Clear cell, papillary serous, and other more aggressive tumors are included in this type. Rarer causes of genital tract bleeding in older women include cervical cancer, uterine sarcoma, and cancers of the fallopian tube and ovary. Bleeding can be neoplastic regardless of a woman's risk factors. All postmenopausal bleeding must be evaluated.

Endometrial biopsy is the preferred modality to evaluate uterine bleeding. Office biopsy will detect about 98% of endometrial cancers. Alternatively, lack of endometrial neoplasia can be inferred from a sonographic finding of a thin endometrial stripe. An endometrial thickness >3 mm requires further investigation. Given the possibility of a false-negative result with all evaluation techniques, unexplained persistent bleeding should be reevaluated.

58. A 74-year-old woman comes to the office for preoperative evaluation before cataract surgery. History includes myocardial infarction 10 years ago, and her records state that her ejection fraction is 30%. Medications include extended-release metoprolol, lisinopril, and spironolactone. Dyspnea on exertion is consistent with New York Heart Association (NYHA) functional class II. She has never been hospitalized for heart failure, and has no palpitations or syncope.

ECG shows a 4-beat run of nonsustained ventricular tachycardia.

Which of the following is the most appropriate next step?

(A) Obtain electrophysiologic study (EPS) for risk stratification.
(B) Continue medical therapy alone.
(C) Advise against placement of automatic internal cardiac defibrillator (ICD) because she is >70 years old.
(D) Recommend placement of ICD.

ANSWER: D

According to the 2009 updated recommendations from the American Heart Association/American College of Cardiology, placement of an ICD is recommended to prevent sudden cardiac death and reduce total mortality in patients who meet the following criteria: nonischemic dilated cardiomyopathy or ischemic heart disease ≥40 days after myocardial infarction, ejection fraction ≤35%, symptoms consistent with NYHA functional class II or III despite ongoing optimal medical management, and expectation of survival >1 year with good functional status (SOE=A). Age is not a contraindication.

The updated recommendation is consistent with the 2008 device-based therapy guidelines from the ACC, AHA, and Heart Rhythm Society. This patient meets the criteria of the original Multicenter Automatic Defibrillator Trial (MADIT), as well as secondary prevention trials such as the Antiarrhythmics Versus Implantable Defibrillators (AVID) trial and the Canadian Implantable Defibrillator Study.

Patients should be informed about the effectiveness, safety, and mortality risks of the ICD shock, and should understand that the therapy does not improve clinical function or delay progression of heart failure. Discussions should also encompass end-of-life preferences and plans related to when the ICD should be disabled.

Continuing with her current medical therapy or undertaking risk stratification using EPS further delays the life-saving measure—ICD placement—in this high-risk patient.

59. An 80-year-old woman is brought to the office because she has hallucinations of children and small animals when she is alone in a room. The hallucinations sometimes disturb and agitate her. Her family also notes that she is having more difficulty walking and has hand tremors when she sits quietly. She has a 9-month history of short-term memory loss; problems with orientation that sometimes worsen dramatically; and difficulty managing her finances, preparing complex meals, and following stories on television. Her score on the Mini–Mental State Examination is 23 of 30.

On physical examination, there are signs of cogwheel rigidity and resting tremors, which have been noted for the past year.

Which of the following is the most likely diagnosis?

(A) Dementia with Lewy bodies
(B) Alzheimer disease
(C) Parkinson disease with dementia
(D) Huntington disease

ANSWER: A

Dementia with Lewy bodies is likely in this patient, given the occurrence of dementia with prominent, distinct visual hallucinations within 1 year of onset of extrapyramidal signs (lead-pipe or cogwheel rigidity, bradykinesia, resting tremor). Affected adults typically have a dementia in which memory impairment in the earlier stages may not be as pronounced as deficits in attention, executive function, and visuospatial ability. According to expert opinion, diagnosis of dementia with Lewy bodies requires the presence of dementia and 2 of 3 core features: fluctuating cognition, parkinsonian features, and recurrent visual hallucinations that are typically well-formed and detailed. Cholinesterase inhibitors may be useful for cognitive impairment and possibly for psychoses (SOE=B). There is no approved treatment for the psychotic symptoms, but if agitation is severe, use of medications with fewer extrapyramidal signs, such as clozapine or quetiapine, may be useful (SOE=C).

Although Parkinson disease presents with extrapyramidal signs, initially these occur without substantial memory loss or psychosis. Hallucinations may occur in patients with Alzheimer disease (typically at mid-stage), but extrapyramidal signs usually occur later in the disease and are generally characterized by bradykinesia and rigidity, not by tremors. Huntington disease is characterized by cognitive impairment and choreiform movement disorder.

60. An 81-year-old woman comes to the office because she has had difficulty sleeping for the past 3 years. She falls asleep quickly but wakes up 4–5 times each night. She often goes to the bathroom on awakening, after which it may take her 15–60 minutes to fall asleep again. She is not aware of snoring but has woken up choking a few times. In the morning, she wakes up feeling unrefreshed, and she has significant daytime sleepiness. She reports no shortness of breath or coughing. History includes type 2 diabetes mellitus, osteoarthritis, and cataracts; she has had chronic dry mouth for >5 years. She lives alone, does not smoke or use alcohol, and is retired. She has tried numerous OTC sleep aids with minimal benefit.

On physical examination, BMI is 24 kg/m2. She has upper and lower dentures.

Which of the following is the most likely cause of the patient's sleep difficulties?

(A) Primary insomnia
(B) Gastroesophageal reflux disease
(C) Nocturnal asthma
(D) Obstructive sleep apnea
(E) Periodic limb movement disorder

ANSWER: D

Obstructive sleep apnea (OSA) occurs in approximately 20% of older adults, a prevalence rate that is nearly double that of younger populations. The presentation of OSA is often more subtle in older adults. Snoring is a common symptom in younger populations, yet many older adults do not have a bed partner and thus cannot provide an accurate history of snoring or nocturnal apneas. In these cases, it can be helpful to ask specifically about whether these symptoms have been noted when travelling to visit family or during group travel (such as a cruise). Other symptoms associated with OSA include insomnia, dry mouth, morning headaches, and daytime sleepiness. Insomnia in the setting of sleep apnea can be associated with higher levels of daytime functional impairment than either condition alone. Edentulous patients are at higher risk of OSA because of changes in the upper airway anatomy associated with the absence of teeth. Normal BMI and an unremarkable physical examination do not exclude OSA. Identification of OSA is important, because it may be linked to higher rates of cognitive impairment, frailty, and mortality.

This patient could possibly have nocturnal asthma, but OSA is more prevalent than nocturnal asthma, and the patient does not have daytime symptoms of asthma. Gastroesophageal reflux may be associated with nocturnal choking, but the patient has no other symptoms of reflux disease. Primary insomnia may cause frequent nocturnal awakenings, but its onset is usually in childhood or young adulthood. Periodic limb movement disorder is not likely in a patient with no history of leg movements at night or leg cramps. In addition, a study examining risk factors for excessive daytime sleepiness in older adults found no significant increased risk of daytime sleepiness from periodic limb movements.

61. Each of the following 68-year-old patients has had an episode of syncope. Which one should be assigned the highest priority for admission to the hospital for expedited evaluation?

(A) A woman who reports low energy and feelings of worthlessness
(B) A man whose syncope occurred while urinating in the bathroom
(C) A man with hypertension who had syncope after shoveling snow
(D) A woman with diabetes mellitus who had syncope after standing in line for several hours for tickets to a Broadway show

ANSWER: C

Syncope that occurs during or after exertion warrants priority hospitalization for evaluation. In the case of the man who shoveled snow, the syncope may be a harbinger of a more serious cardiac condition. Evidence of a cardiovascular cause for syncope from history, examination, or abnormal ECG typically warrants inpatient admission. Hospital evaluation would include telemetry, echocardiography, cardiology consultation, possible surgical evaluation, and close observation.

Priority inpatient admission is also necessary if the syncope may be related to adverse effects of medications, severe orthostatic hypotension, or a possible neurologic disorder, such as stroke.

The woman with low energy may have depression. Her syncope and psychiatric issues need to be addressed but not necessarily in an inpatient setting.

The man whose episode occurred during urination likely has situational syncope. Situational syncope is benign, and the patient's status returns quickly to baseline after the event, without delayed sequelae. Patient education is important. For example, if carotid sinus syncope is suspected, the patient should be informed about possible precipitants of syncope, such as wearing a tight collar. There would be acceptable risk in discharging the patient for follow-up with his primary care physician.

For the woman with diabetes mellitus, the syncope after prolonged standing may be the result of autonomic instability related to her diabetes. Her episode would not need as urgent evaluation as that of the patient with post-exertion syncope. In the former case, arranging for outpatient follow-up with tilt table test would be reasonable.

62. A 75-year-old woman comes to the office for her 6-month follow-up visit. The patient lives independently, and she is independent in instrumental activities of daily living. She reports both a decline in her ability to walk long distances and difficulty crossing streets: the light changes before she can reach the opposite side. She has no numbness, tingling, or changes in sensation in her extremities. During the appointment, she at times uses the wall for support. Physical examination is otherwise unremarkable.

Which of the following is the most appropriate next step?

(A) Refer to social work for long-term care options.
(B) Refer for an individualized, supervised exercise program.
(C) Refer to a neurologist.
(D) Obtain MRI of the head and spine.
(E) Obtain glucose, vitamin B_{12}, and thyroid levels.

ANSWER: B

The patient reports a decline in walking endurance and speed, demonstrated by her inability to cross streets within the time provided by the traffic lights. She reports no changes in peripheral sensation, and there are no neurologic findings. Using the wall for support suggests that her balance is impaired and that she may benefit from use of an assistive device. She is an ideal candidate for a structured, supervised exercise program. An appropriate exercise program would likely result in an improvement in walking endurance, speed, balance, and strength. If improvement does not occur, additional assessments may be needed. According to the ACOVE (Assessing Care of Vulnerable Elders) quality indicators, there should be documentation of a structured or supervised exercise program offered in the previous 6 months or within 3 months after the report of decline to meet high quality-of-care standards (SOE=D).

The patient's symptoms and normal physical examination do not suggest the need for MRI of the head and spine, or referral to a neurologist. Her change in gait speed and balance can be explained by poor endurance alone. Although a stroke, tumor, or other neurologic disease could affect gait and balance, the abnormality would consistently impair her ability to walk. For example, after a stroke in the cerebellum, patients demonstrate an ataxic gait pattern and instability whenever they walk, not just with longer distances, as this patient is demonstrating. She has no symptoms of peripheral neuropathy; hence, laboratory assessment for diabetes mellitus, vitamin B_{12} deficiency, and thyroid disease is not indicated.

The patient's function has declined but not to a degree that warrants a social work referral for consideration of long-term care options.

63. An 88-year-old woman is brought to the office for evaluation because her son believes that she is unable to remain safely at home without supervision. History includes hypertension, osteoarthritis, and dementia. Her husband, who was her primary caregiver, has had a major stroke and is being admitted to a nursing home. She owns her home and wishes to remain in her community; however, she has consistently refused all home services. She continues to perform activities of daily living but no longer shops or cooks, and occasionally does not remember to eat. Her son manages her finances, which include Social Security and pension benefits. She has Medicare and supplemental medical insurance.

Which of the following is the most appropriate recommendation regarding her living arrangements?

(A) Admission to the same nursing facility as her husband
(B) Referral to an adult day program to ensure a daily meal
(C) Referral to a certified home-healthcare program for help at home
(D) Admission to an assisted-living facility

ANSWER: D

Assisted-living facilities provide market-rate housing with studio or 1-bedroom apartments and a basic package of services, such as light housekeeping, linen service, social programs, and 2 or 3 meals daily in a congregate dining room. Additional options are available on an à la carte basis, including services for individuals with dementia. Assisted-living housing would meet the patient's need for nutritional supervision and maintain her privacy in an apartment.

Long-term nursing care is not covered under Medicare and is not yet appropriate for this patient who is ADL independent. Adult day programs do not provide overnight supervision. If a provider specifies that the patient needs nursing, physical therapy, or speech therapy, Medicare will cover certified home-health care for short-term personal care services that will be episodic and short term.

64. A 77-year-old woman comes to the office for routine follow-up. History includes hypertension, coronary artery disease, emphysema, arthritis, and limited vision. She takes multiple medications. In recent months, she went to the emergency department twice for breathing difficulties, and in the past year, she was admitted to the hospital twice: once to exclude a diagnosis of myocardial infarction, and a second time because of uncontrolled hypertension.

The patient lives alone in a 3-story townhouse. After the last hospital discharge, she received home-health services; the agency discharge note states that the patient is independent in her home, is sometimes confused about her medications, possibly has cognitive impairment, and seems depressed. The patient's daughter would like her to enter an assisted-living facility close to the daughter's house. However, the patient wants to remain at home, is concerned about her finances, and does not want a new primary care physician. She participates in a health maintenance organization (HMO).

Which of the following is the most appropriate next step?

(A) Request that home-health services perform a safety evaluation.
(B) Refer her to the local Program of All-Inclusive Care for the Elderly (PACE).
(C) Enroll her in Guided Care program.
(D) Enroll her in IMPACT (Improving Mood: Promoting Access to Collaborative Treatment for Late-Life Depression) program.

ANSWER: C

In the United States, Guided Care is one of a few models of enhanced care that are supported by some degree of evidence. Only Guided Care allows the patient to remain with his or her HMO primary care physician. Guided Care provides proactive, comprehensive health care by physician–nurse teams for patients with multiple chronic conditions who have frequent yet ineffective encounters with the healthcare system. A cluster randomized controlled trial of 14 primary care teams in 3 healthcare organizations showed that Guided Care significantly improved clinicians' knowledge of patients' conditions and communication with chronically ill patients and families; improved patients' and caregivers' ratings of the quality of their health care; and reduced the use of home-health services overall, nursing facility admissions, and number of visits in staff-model HMO practices (SOE=A). Each Guided Care team consists of a registered nurse working with 2 to 5 physicians and other office staff in a primary care site. The team assesses each patient and family caregiver at home, creates care and action plans, monitors the patient's status monthly, promotes self-care, coordinates provider care, provides transitional care (eg, hospital to home) when necessary, educates and supports family caregivers, and facilitates access to community resources. Enrolling this patient in the Guided Care program presents the best available option.

Besides Guided Care, in the United States, the models of enhanced care that are supported by some degree of evidence are Geriatric Resources for Assessment and Care of Elders (GRACE) and Program of All-Inclusive Care for the Elderly (PACE). Each has limited availability. Each provides comprehensive geriatric assessment and team-based complex interventions.

Patients who join PACE must disenroll from their HMO Advantage plan; PACE becomes the plan and provider of integrated services. PACE would not accommodate this patient's preference to remain with her physician. Further, the patient likely would not be eligible for PACE, because she is considered independent at home. Eligibility requirements include meeting the state's standards for needing nursing-home level of care, and qualifying based on income and assets. Because this patient is concerned about preserving her resources, she would be unlikely to pay out-of-pocket for PACE in lieu of the Medicaid share of the capitated monthly payment. Thus, while referral to PACE may be appropriate as her health and circumstances change, it is not the best immediate option.

Depressed older patients in primary care frequently use general medical services, adhere poorly to medical treatments, and are at risk of multiple poor outcomes. Depression is often not recognized, appropriately referred, or effectively treated in primary care settings. Many randomized controlled clinical trials have established the clinical efficacy and cost-effectiveness of collaborative care for depression (SOE=A). IMPACT, one of the more successful and disseminated of the models, is a 1-year stepped collaborative care program provided by a clinical depression specialist (nurse or psychologist care manager) working in a primary care office or clinic in support of the primary care provider. Clinical depression specialists offer patients treatment alternatives, including antidepressant medication and problem-solving therapy. (Problem-solving therapy is a 6- to 8-session psychotherapy program, structured for older primary care patients, that has been found to be similarly effective to antidepressants in treating major depressive disorder.) The clinical depression specialist is trained in pharmacotherapy and problem-solving strategies, adjusts care plans according to a stepped-care treatment algorithm, and is supervised in weekly sessions with a geriatrician and psychiatrist to monitor patient progress.

Compared with usual care of depression, IMPACT shows greater rates of treatment, lower depression severity, more substantial symptom reduction, more satisfaction with depression care, less functional impairment, and better quality of life at 12 months. At 4-year follow-up, mean total healthcare costs were significantly lower for patients who participated in IMPACT than for controls.

This patient could be a candidate for IMPACT services if she meets *Diagnostic and Statistical Manual of Mental Disorders-IV-TR* criteria for current major or minor depressive disorder. Nonetheless, IMPACT focuses on affective status; it does not provide the multidimensional geriatric assessment and management that are part of the GRACE, PACE, and Guided Care approaches.

Previous home-health evaluations have identified several concerns; thus, the most appropriate management needs to go beyond evaluation.

65. Which of the following options is true regarding patients with advanced dementia?

(A) In nursing-home patients with advanced dementia, eating problems are associated with higher 6-month mortality rates than pneumonia.
(B) In patients with advanced dementia, feeding tubes are often placed during a hospital stay.
(C) The proportion of hospice patients with a primary diagnosis of dementia is stable at about 6%, even though the total number of patients served by hospice programs has increased.
(D) Combination therapy with cholinesterase inhibitors and NMDA-receptor modulators has been shown to improve survival in patients with advanced dementia.
(E) Most deaths in patients with advanced dementia are precipitated by catastrophic acute events (eg, myocardial infarction).

ANSWER: B

In a recent secondary analysis that combined Minimum Data Set and Medicare claims files, over two-thirds of feeding tubes were inserted while a patient was in an acute-care hospital (SOE=B). Median survival after tube insertion was 56 days.

Eating problems and infections are widely recognized hallmarks of advanced dementia. In an 18-month prospective study of nursing-home residents with advanced dementia, the probability of ≥1 episode of an eating problem (85.8%) was higher than the probability of ≥1 episode either of pneumonia (41.1%) or of non-pneumonia febrile episode (52.6%). The 6-month mortality (adjusted for age, sex, and time since dementia diagnosis) associated with eating problems was 38.6%; the mortality associated with pneumonia was 46.7%, and with non-pneumonia febrile episodes, 44.5% (SOE=A).

The total number of patients served by hospice has increased annually since 2005. Patients with a primary diagnosis of dementia accounted for 6.8% of hospice cases in 2001, 11.1% in 2008, and 11.2% in 2009 (SOE=D).

In a study examining time to nursing-home placement and death in 943 patients with probable Alzheimer disease who had

≥1-year follow-up evaluation, nursing-home placement was significantly delayed in patients on cholinesterase inhibitors versus in patients who had never received cognition-enhancing medications. This effect was significantly compounded by the addition of memantine to the cholinesterase inhibitor; combination therapy was associated with a 71% reduction in risk of nursing-home placement (SOE=B). The study reported no significant association with time to death, either for cholinesterase inhibitors alone or in combination with memantine. However, a more recent study has shown no benefit of donepezil plus memantine over donepezil alone, in community-dwelling patients with moderate-to-severe dementia, in functional or cognitive outcomes over 1 year follow-up.

Mortality rates are high among patients with advanced dementia. However, dementia is under-recognized as a terminal illness. Mortality and median survival rates for patients with advanced dementia are consistent with rates for patients with commonly recognized end-of-life conditions, such as metastatic cancer and advanced heart failure. In patients with advanced dementia, acute medical conditions with the potential to cause significant change in health status rarely precipitate death. In one study, <5% of patients with advanced dementia who died in a nursing home experienced such sentinel events (SOE=A).

66. A 92-year-old woman comes to the office for follow-up. History includes osteoarthritis, well-controlled hypertension, gastroesophageal reflux disease, and a recent cold. Prescribed medications include chlorthalidone and lisinopril.

On examination, blood pressure is 162/70 mmHg and pulse is 76 beats per minute. On further questioning, the patient states that her daughter has been giving her OTC ibuprofen because she has had knee discomfort, which is now resolved. She has also been taking an OTC preparation of pseudoephedrine, 30 mg, three times a day for several days for congestion.

Which of the following is the most likely cause of her high blood pressure?

(A) Pseudoephedrine
(B) Arthritic pain
(C) NSAIDs
(D) Renal artery stenosis

ANSWER: C

NSAIDs can increase blood pressure in people with and without hypertension (SOE=A). Use of NSAIDs increases the risk of myocardial infarction and stroke and can exacerbate heart failure, especially in patients with known cardiovascular disease (SOE=A). If NSAIDs must be used for pain control, naproxen is the agent of choice (SOE=C). Any use of NSAIDs should be of limited duration in patients with hypertension or patients who have or are at risk of cardiovascular disease.

Although advanced age contributes to an increase in blood pressure, it is unlikely to cause a sudden change in a person with previously controlled hypertension. While the use of pseudoephedrine is often avoided in patients with hypertension, the available data indicates that, when used in therapeutic doses, it has no effect on blood pressure in patients with well-controlled hypertension (SOE=C). Arthritic pain can increase blood pressure, but this patient is not currently in pain. Renal artery stenosis is a secondary cause of hypertension, but it would not be part of the differential diagnosis unless the blood pressure remained increased after the NSAID was discontinued.

67. An 80-year-old woman comes to the office because the vision in her right eye has suddenly become blurred. The external appearance of the eye is normal. The right pupil does not constrict when a flashlight is shined on it. When the flashlight is swung to the left eye, the right pupil constricts, and when it is swung back to the right eye, the right pupil dilates.

Which one of the following is the most likely explanation for these findings?

(A) Right occipital lobe infarct
(B) Left occipital lobe infarct
(C) Iritis of the right eye
(D) Ischemic optic neuropathy

ANSWER: D

The swinging flashlight test is a simple, inexpensive, and reproducible bedside technique for detecting a relative afferent pupillary defect (SOE=B). In this patient, the light shining on the normal left eye results in bilateral constriction of the pupils, but the abnormal right pupil dilates when the normal left eye is no longer responding to the light. A positive test indicates disease in the retina or optic nerve. The test would not be positive if visual loss were caused by an occipital lobe infarct because the pupillary light reflex uses an entirely subcortical pathway. In iritis, a ciliary flush would be seen with injection around the limbus on inspection. Also, the pupil would be small and would not dilate in response to the swinging flashlight.

68. A 77-year-old woman comes to the clinic because she has daytime somnolence and occasional dizziness. History includes osteoporosis (hip fracture 1 year ago), type 2 diabetes mellitus, hypertension, frequent falls, and post-herpetic neuralgia that is controlled. Medications include glipizide 5 mg q12h, extended-release metoprolol 50 mg/d, amlodipine 10 mg/d, pregabalin 200 mg q12h, alendronate 70 mg/wk (started 1 year ago), vitamin D supplement 800 IU/d, calcium carbonate 500 mg q8h, and a multivitamin.

On examination, weight is 62 kg (137 lb). Blood pressure is 140/75 mmHg. Over the past 3 months, blood pressure has ranged from 140 to 150 mmHg systolic and from 70 to 80 mmHg diastolic, with no orthostatic changes. Estimated creatinine clearance is 35 mL/min; it has declined over the past 2 years but has been stable for the past 6 months.

Which of the following would address the patient's most immediate need?

(A) Reduce pregabalin to 150 mg q12h.
(B) Start lisinopril 2.5 mg/d.
(C) Discontinue alendronate.
(D) Start aspirin 81 mg/d.

ANSWER: A

The most immediate issue for this patient is somnolence and dizziness, which may be drug induced. In patients with age- or disease-related renal impairment, dosage adjustments will likely be needed to avoid adverse events from medications that are primarily eliminated by the kidneys. Pregabalin is eliminated by the kidneys as unchanged drug (90%). For patients with creatinine clearance between 30 and 59 mL/min, the recommended dosage of pregabalin is 300 mg/d in 2 or 3 doses. Given her reduced creatinine clearance, this patient's lethargy and dizziness may be related to excessive pregabalin concentrations. Although pregabalin may have been dosed appropriately when started, her worsening renal function may have resulted in higher serum concentrations over time.

Use of an ACE inhibitor or angiotensin-receptor blocker is recommended for initial treatment of hypertension in patients with diabetes mellitus (SOE=C). Although the patient takes metoprolol and amlodipine, her blood pressure is not at goal (<130/80 mmHg) for patients with diabetes mellitus. The American Diabetes Association recognizes that this goal may be too stringent for all patients, and a goal of <140/80 mmHg may be more reasonable. Starting an ACE inhibitor would be appropriate, especially if she has microalbuminuria, but this is not her most immediate need.

According to manufacturers, alendronate and other bisphosphonates are not recommended for patients with severe impairment of renal function (creatinine clearance <35 mL/min) because of lack of experience in this patient population. Many older patients with osteoporosis have age-related changes in the kidneys. Limited evidence suggests that bisphosphonates can be used safely in women with creatinine clearance rates in the range comparable to this patient's rate (SOE=A). There are no data regarding safety of bisphosphonates in more pronounced renal impairment.

In adults with diabetes mellitus, the role of aspirin for primary prevention of cardiovascular events is unclear. The 2010 position statement from the American Diabetes Association indicates that low-dose aspirin would be reasonable for men >50 years old and for women >60 years old who have ≥1 major risk factors (eg, smoking, hypertension, dyslipidemia, family history of premature cardiovascular disease, albuminuria) and who are not at increased risk of bleeding. Thus, adding aspirin for primary prevention could be considered once the immediate patient concern has been resolved.

69. An 82-year-old man comes to the office because he is tired, has lost 4.5 kg (10 lb), and has new-onset back pain. He is eating well and has had no change in appetite. History includes benign prostatic hyperplasia. He reports a modest worsening of hyperplasia-associated symptoms, with more urgency and frequency. He has no other symptoms.

On physical examination, he appears in no distress. The abdomen is soft without masses. There is tenderness to percussion over the low thoracolumbar spine. Genitalia are normal. Rectal examination reveals an enlarged, firm prostate with sidewall fixation. Prostate-specific antigen (PSA) has not been measured in several years; the last measurement was 4.0 ng/mL.

Which of the following is the most appropriate next step?

(A) Measure PSA and refer to a urologist.
(B) Reassure and follow-up in 6 months.
(C) Prescribe a low-dose anticholinergic medication.
(D) Measure PSA and follow-up in 6 months.

ANSWER: A

This patient most likely has metastatic prostate cancer based on his symptoms and the findings on examination. Although the U.S. Preventive Services Task Force (USPSTF) has found little benefit from PSA screening, its recommendations are for asymptomatic men and would not apply to this patient. In this patient, measurement of the PSA would not be considered screening, given the findings and suspicion of underlying malignancy. Advanced prostate cancer can confer significant morbidity and mortality in older men. PSA is believed to have value as a marker for disease stage and response to treatment (SOE=B). This patient is in need of further urologic evaluation, including biopsy of the prostate and staging studies.

Delaying referral for 6 months could have significant impact on disease. While low-dose anticholinergic agents may improve this patient's urinary symptoms, the treatment will not address the main concern of metastatic prostate cancer.

70. A 72-year-old man who has metastatic colon cancer is admitted to a hospice inpatient facility because of complete bowel obstruction and failure to thrive. He has been unable to tolerate oral food or fluids for several days because of nausea and vomiting, and he has significant pain throughout the day. The hospice admitting nurse documents a large sacral pressure ulcer measuring 11 cm × 10 cm, with a depth of 4 cm. There is surrounding erythema, exposed muscle, undermining of the edges, and a tunneling tract that extends another 2 cm. Within the ulcer, there is necrotic material and a significant amount of exudate with a foul odor that permeates the room. The treatment plan includes placement of a specialized bed overlay, application of absorptive dressings, and medicine for pain control.

Shortly thereafter, family members tell staff that the wound odor makes spending time in the patient's room very difficult, and they ask if something can be done.

Which of the following is the best next step to reduce odor from the pressure ulcer?

(A) Turn patient every 2 hours.
(B) Apply topical metronidazole gel.
(C) Place potpourri in the room.
(D) Perform surgical debridement.

ANSWER: B

Severe pressure ulcers tend to have polymicrobial infection with both aerobic and anaerobic bacteria that can cause significant odor. One study sampled tissue from pressure ulcers in patients with advanced cancer on a palliative care unit. Ninety-two species of bacteria were identified in 19 pressure ulcers (79.3% aerobic, 20.7% anaerobic), and bacteria were present in every ulcer cultured. The most common species were *Staphylococcus aureus, S epidermidis, Enterococcus faecalis,* and *Streptococcus pyogenes.* Given the polymicrobial nature of infected pressure ulcers, current National Pressure Ulcer Advisory Panel (NPUAP) guidelines recommend use of topical metronidazole to control pressure ulcer odor associated with anaerobic bacteria and protozoal infections (SOE=C).

A white paper, published in 2010 by the NPUAP and developed in conjunction with its European counterpart (EPUAP), addressed palliative care issues in patients with pressure ulcers. The goals of palliative care are to improve quality of life and reduce suffering for patients with life-threatening or life-limiting illness. Pressure ulcers decrease quality of life physically, emotionally, socially, and mentally.

The goal of pressure ulcer treatment—to promote healing and closure of the wound—may not be possible in patients receiving palliative care. Thus, the focus of care is better directed to reducing or eliminating pain, odor, and infection; to allowing for an environment that can promote ulcer closure; and to supporting the patient's self-image to help prevent social isolation. The guidelines offer many suggestions to help reduce odor, including frequent cleansing of the ulcer and periwound area, routine assessments for wound infection, use of antimicrobial agents, and use of external odor absorbers for the room.

While turning patients every 2 hours is important for healing of pressure ulcers, patients receiving palliative care may be unable to turn frequently because of pain or personal or family preference. Additionally, frequent turning would not directly address the issue of odor in this case.

Placing potpourri in the room or other odor absorbers (vinegar, vanilla, coffee beans, burning candle, and kitty litter under the bed) is also recommended as a measure to control odor (SOE=C), but the absorbers do not directly reduce odor caused by bacteria, and they too can create an odor that overwhelms the room.

Surgical debridement of pressure ulcers is sometimes indicated to remove necrotic material to help reduce growth of bacteria, and by extension odor, but debridement is often invasive and painful, and thus conflicts with the goals of palliative care.

71. An 80-year-old woman is evaluated because she has erythematous lesions. Initially, the lesions were on her arms and legs; by the end of 1 week, the lesions had spread to her trunk, and several large blisters appeared. The lesions are itchy and cause her to scratch. History includes hypertension and dementia. Medications include atenolol, amlodipine, donepezil, calcium, and vitamin D; she has taken each for several years. The patient lives in a nursing home. A detailed history reveals no specific association with the onset of the rash.

On physical examination, the patient appears frail and in mild distress. She has no fever. There are areas of erythema with tense blisters and serous exudate, occasionally blood tinged. Some blisters have opened in oval erosions with serous exudate; the erosions do not coalesce. Some blisters are healing and covered with scabs. There is no mucosal involvement, and the Nikolsky sign (in which the top layer of skin comes away with gentle rubbing) is negative.

Which of the following is the most likely diagnosis?

(A) Stevens-Johnson syndrome
(B) Toxic epidermal necrolysis
(C) Bullous pemphigoid
(D) Pemphigus vulgaris
(E) Erythema mutiforme

ANSWER: C

The most likely diagnosis is bullous pemphigoid, because the bullae are tense—not flaccid—and do not coalesce when they break. Bullous pemphigoid is the most common autoimmune bullous disorder and occurs primarily in older adults. The body produces antibodies against an antigen located in the basement membrane of the dermoepidermal junction. The bullae are tense and resistant to minor trauma because they are subepidermal. Oral involvement is present in about one-third of cases and is rare in drug-induced pemphigoid.

Stevens-Johnson syndrome (SJS) and toxic epidermal necrolysis (TEN) are considered severity variants of the same disease; they are characterized by epidermal detachment. In SJS, the skin detachment affects <30% of body surface area, while in TEN it affects >50%. When skin detachment is between 30% and

50%, the syndrome is considered *SJS or TEN overlap*. Often fever and mucosal involvement develop days before the rash appears. Initial lesions are macular and may form target lesions with purpuric centers. The lesions can coalesce and progress to superficial flaccid bullae. Epidermal necrosis is pathognomonic for SJS/TEN. Usually at least 2 mucous surfaces are involved. SJS and TEN are rare reactions to drugs; >200 drugs have been implicated. The most common are antibiotics, NSAIDs, allopurinol, and anticonvulsants. The patient in this case was not taking any of these medications and did not have flaccid bullae or mucosal involvement.

Erythema multiforme (EM) can present with oral involvement, a generalized eruption with flaccid bullae, and desquamation similar to that of SJS or TEN. Typically, EM is a target lesion with a bulla or dusky discoloration in the center surrounded by an edematous ring and erythema. EM usually follows an episode of herpes simplex outbreak, which had not occurred in this case.

Pemphigus vulgaris also presents with flaccid, easily ruptured intraepidermal blisters. Oral involvement is present in 60% of cases but less common in drug-induced pemphigus. This patient's bullae are tense, and thus unlikely to be pemphigus vulgaris.

Histopathologic examination is essential for definitive diagnosis of bullous disorders.

72. A 67-year-old woman comes to the office because she has painless swelling of her right foot 1 day after kicking a trash can. She had a myocardial infarction 3 weeks ago; history also includes diabetes mellitus and severe peripheral neuropathy. Radiography reveals a slightly displaced fracture of the fourth metatarsal bone.

Which of the following is the most appropriate treatment?

(A) Perform open reduction with internal fixation.
(B) Allow patient to walk in a good walking shoe.
(C) Apply a fiberglass cast and have the patient use a wheelchair.
(D) Provide a walking boot and have the patient use a wheelchair.

ANSWER: D

This patient has foot pain due to a partially displaced fracture. A removable walking boot would provide adequate immobilization and would allow for regular inspection of the skin (SOE=C).

Surgery 3 weeks after myocardial infarction would place the patient at high risk of repeat myocardial infarction or death (SOE=A). The optimal interval between myocardial infarction and surgery has not yet been established, but an interval of 4–6 weeks is recommended with some authors recommending a longer wait.

Allowing the patient to walk without immobilizing the fracture increases the risk of further displacement. A fiberglass cast would immobilize the fracture but would place the patient at risk of pressure ulcers, especially given her severe peripheral neuropathy.

73. A patient with Parkinson disease comes to the office for follow-up. He has a slow, shuffling gait, has difficulty initiating walking, and occasionally falls. In addition to taking medication, he walks on a treadmill while listening to music to set the pace, and he performs standing balance exercises.

Which of the following is the most efficient way to assess changes in the patient's physical function?

(A) Timed Up and Go test
(B) Standardized balance scale
(C) Number of falls in the past week
(D) Lower-extremity strength using timed chair stands

ANSWER: A

For patients with Parkinson disease, often the goal is to maintain the current level of ambulatory function. The advantage of the Timed Up and Go test is that it can be used to assess multiple skills at the same time, including speed, strength, and balance. The test assesses the patient's ability to stand, initiate walking, walk 3 m and turn as quickly as possible, and return to sit back down (SOE=B).

Standardized clinical tests to assess balance and lower-extremity strength could provide additional information about the patient's physical function. Recording the number of falls would provide information helpful to guide treatment, but falls alone are not the best indicator of physical function.

74. An 89-year-old woman is admitted to the hospital with a urinary tract infection and change in mental status. History includes type 2 diabetes mellitus, depression, and anxiety. She moved in with her daughter 8 months ago because of worsening confusion. Her family notes that her short-term memory is impaired and that she has vivid visual hallucinations of children in the house. They are unaware of any specific diagnosis regarding her cognition.

On examination, temperature is 38°C (100.5°F), blood pressure is 132/78 mmHg, heart rate is 86 beats per minute, and oxygen saturation is 96% on room air. Examination is unremarkable except for a slight resting right hand tremor and that the patient is unable to recite the months of the year or days of the week forward.

Although nonpharmacologic treatment is initiated for delirium, the patient becomes severely agitated overnight.

Which of the following is the most appropriate treatment for this patient's agitation?

(A) Haloperidol
(B) Rivastigmine
(C) Quetiapine
(D) Trazodone
(E) Physical restraints

ANSWER: C

No pharmacologic therapy is approved by the FDA for treatment of delirium. This patient's agitation requires management because it places her at risk of harming herself. With her history of memory decline and vivid visual hallucinations, Lewy body dementia is a concern. In patients with Lewy body dementia, Parkinson disease, or extrapyramidal symptoms, quetiapine is the medication of choice because it has a lower risk of causing or exacerbating extrapyramidal symptoms (SOE=B). Quetiapine has a stronger sedation effect than other second-generation antipsychotic agents, which should be considered during prescribing. A reasonable initial dose is 12.5–25 mg/d.

Haloperidol, a first-generation antipsychotic, is commonly used for delirium treatment (SOE=A) (off-label). Studies have found haloperidol to be superior to lorazepam and equivalent to second-generation antipsychotics in treatment of delirium. It has a higher risk of extrapyramidal aadverse effects than second-generation antipsychotic agents.

Rivastigmine, an acetylcholinesterase inhibitor, has also been investigated for treatment of delirium (SOE=B). In an open-label pilot study of stroke patients, rivastigmine decreased delirium severity, but the study was limited by small sample size and uncontrolled design. A double-blind, placebo-controlled randomized trial evaluating the use of rivastigmine as an adjuvant to haloperidol for delirium in the intensive care unit was stopped early because of increased mortality in the rivastigmine group.

Trazodone has been tested in uncontrolled studies and is not recommended for treatment of delirium (SOE=C). Physical restraints are associated with worsening of delirium, injury, and even death. They should be avoided if at all possible.

75. A 77-year-old woman comes to the office because she has episodes of severe dizziness. Evaluation suggests a vestibular problem, and vestibular suppressant treatments are prescribed. At follow-up 1 week later, she reports that the episodes are now mild, but she still has a feeling of imbalance. Vestibular rehabilitation is considered as a possible next management step.

Which of the following is true regarding vestibular rehabilitation and long-term functional recovery?

(A) Vestibular rehabilitation is ineffective in long-term studies.
(B) Combining vestibular rehabilitation with physical repositioning maneuvers improves functional recovery.
(C) Vestibular rehabilitation is effective only for managing vestibular neuritis or Ménière disease.
(D) In patients with benign positional vertigo, vestibular rehabilitation reduces dizziness in short-term rather than long-term studies.

ANSWER: B

Vestibular rehabilitation is an effective means of managing unilateral peripheral vestibular disorders, such as vestibular neuritis, labyrinthitis, Ménière disease, and loss of vestibular function due to ablative surgery (eg, excision of acoustic neuroma) or trauma (eg, temporal bone fracture involving the labyrinth). Rehabilitation involves movement-based training exercises to desensitize the vestibular system and limit associated symptoms. Patients learn to coordinate eye and head movements, to improve balance and walking skills, and to cope with or become more active despite the condition. A Cochrane review of 27 randomized clinical trials showed that vestibular rehabilitation was effective in reducing subjective dizziness and improved participation in life roles and activities of daily living. The exception to these findings was for the group with benign paroxysmal positional vertigo. For this group of patients, comparisons of vestibular rehabilitation with specific physical repositioning maneuvers (eg, Epley maneuver) showed that the repositioning maneuvers more effectively reduced dizziness symptoms, particularly in the short term. Combining the maneuvers with vestibular rehabilitation was effective in improving functional recovery in the longer term. There were no reports of adverse effects after vestibular rehabilitation, and positive effects were maintained in studies with follow-up assessment at 3–12 months (SOE=A).

76. A 78-year-old man comes to the office because he has a skin rash and worsening swelling of his legs. History includes hypertension and osteoarthritis. The patient is on a blood pressure medication, but does not recall which one, and he takes multivitamins and an NSAID. He has recently increased the NSAID dosage because of worsening joint pain.

On examination, temperature is 37°C (98.6°F), blood pressure is 138/92 mmHg, and pulse is 78 beats per minute. An S4 gallop is detected. There is a reddish scaly rash on the scalp and on the surface of his elbows and knees. The lower extremities have moderate +2 edema. BUN is 48 mg/dL and serum creatinine is 3.5 mg/dL; levels a year ago were 22 mg/dL and 1.6 mg/dL, respectively. Urinalysis shows many WBCs but no RBCs. Examination of urine sediment shows clumps of WBCs and few WBC casts.

Which of the following is the most likely cause of his acute kidney injury?

(A) Hypertensive nephrosclerosis
(B) Acute tubular necrosis
(C) Prerenal acute kidney injury
(D) Membranoproliferative glomerulonephritis
(E) Acute interstitial nephritis

ANSWER: E

This patient has been taking NSAIDs, which have caused acute interstitial nephritis. Although he does not have fever, the history of NSAID use and the urinalysis showing WBCs and WBC casts are suggestive of acute interstitial nephritis. This is a well-described complication of NSAID use. Hypertensive nephrosclerosis would explain the chronic kidney disease but not the acute component. The absence of muddy brown casts makes acute tubular necrosis less likely. There is no evidence of a systemic disease or RBCs in the urine to suggest glomerulonephritis. There is nothing in the patient's history to suggest a prerenal etiology for acute kidney injury.

77. A 63-year-old woman comes to the office because she has difficulty walking. She has noted a significant change in her gait over the last 6 months, and she now uses a walker. She fell 1 month ago while walking on uneven pavement. She has no pain in her lower extremities, but states that her legs "just feel weak and lousy." History includes diabetes mellitus, osteoarthritis, and coronary artery disease. On review of systems, she notes increased urinary urgency, constipation, and difficulty opening jars and buttoning blouses.

On physical examination, there is impairment of fine motor skills of the hands and hyperreflexia in the bilateral ankles and patella. Romberg test is positive.

Which of the following is the most appropriate next evaluation?

(A) Measure creatine kinase level.
(B) Measure serum vitamin B_{12} level.
(C) Obtain electromyography and nerve conduction studies of lower limbs.
(D) Obtain MRI of cervical spine.
(E) Obtain MRI of lumbar spine.

ANSWER: D

This patient has cervical cord myelopathy characterized by spinal cord compression that is likely due to narrowing in the sagittal diameter of the cervical spinal canal. This usually occurs from degenerative processes but can also be congenital. Narrowing or canal stenosis can be the result of disc herniation, hypertrophy of the ligamentum flavum, ossification of the ligamentum longitudinale, or spinal cord tumor. The clinical presentation includes subtle gait disturbances, clumsy hands, loss of sense of joint position, and bowel and bladder incontinence. Pain is unusual. Neurologic signs can sometimes be masked by coexisting peripheral articular disease. Careful history and physical examination, including a detailed time course of the symptoms, provide useful clues to the diagnosis. Sudden apoplectic symptoms suggest infarct or hemorrhage; transverse myelitis may occur over days to weeks. Fluctuating symptoms may indicate another diagnosis, such as multiple sclerosis or sarcoidosis. Prompt diagnosis is important before irreversible changes occur. Surgical decompression may help to retard the neurologic effects.

MRI of the cervical spinal cord with and without gadolinium is the modality of choice to establish the diagnosis. For patients unable to undergo MRI, CT myelography is the best alternative.

Measuring creatine kinase levels is not an appropriate next step, because creatine kinase is used to detect myositis, and this patient's symptoms indicate an upper motor neuron lesion. Electromyography is used to assess the electrical potential generated by muscles, and nerve conduction studies are used to assess peripheral conduction of motor and sensory nerves. Both tests are helpful when attempting to diagnose lesions in the peripheral nervous system. Again, this patient has features of an upper motor neuron lesion, as indicated by hyperreflexia and the onset of bladder and bowel dysfunction. Vitamin B_{12} deficiency would not cause changes in bladder and bowel function.

The findings on physical examination of the patient point to an upper motor lesion. MRI of the lumbar spine is not indicated.

78. An 85-year-old man comes to the office because he has severe pain and blurring of his right eye that improves with blinking or when he rubs the affected eye.

Which of the following is the most likely cause of these symptoms?

(A) Acute angle-closure glaucoma
(B) Anterior uveitis
(C) Keratitis sicca
(D) Chalazion
(E) Allergic conjunctivitis

ANSWER: C

With age, tear production decreases, such that older adults are prone to develop keratitis sicca (dry eye), a disorder that presents with redness, foreign body sensation, and reflex tearing. Patients may describe eye discomfort and blurred vision that usually improve with blinking or rubbing the eye. These maneuvers spread the remaining tear film over the cornea, temporarily relieving the symptoms. Improvement in vision after blinking or rubbing the eye would not be expected with glaucoma, uveitis, chalazion, or conjunctivitis (SOE=D). Applying artificial tears a few times daily to both eyes may alleviate the symptoms and improve vision. Topical artificial tears are available without prescription; if the tears do not ease symptoms, the patient should consult his or her eye care provider.

79. A nursing-home resident has twisted the arm of a nursing assistant who was helping him to the bathroom and appears to have sprained her wrist. The resident has had a number of altercations with staff members and other residents in the past, but this is the first documented injury.

Which of the following is true regarding violent behavior in nursing homes?

(A) Such events are relatively rare.
(B) Most residents who exhibit violent behavior have a previous history of psychiatric illness, such as schizophrenia or bipolar disorder.
(C) Residents with severe dementia are more likely to be verbally than physically abusive toward staff.
(D) The prevalence of resident violence toward staff is probably overestimated.
(E) Most assaults against staff occur during periods of close staff–resident contact, such as when assisting with activities of daily living (ADLs).

ANSWER: E

About one-quarter of all workplace violence occurs in the nursing facility. Aggressive and violent behavior includes repetitive demands, verbal outbursts, sexual advances, and physically aggressive acts. Repetitive aggressive disruptive behavior occurs regularly in 43%–85% of nursing facilities surveyed. Prevalence is probably underestimated because many episodes of aggression are not reported.

About 75% of physically aggressive acts occur during close staff–resident contact; up to 33% occur with transfers or turns and 43% with dressing (SOE=B). About 5% of aggressive behavior results in staff injury.

Alzheimer disease is the most common diagnosis associated with residents who are verbally or physically aggressive. The odds ratio for verbal assaults is lower in individuals with severe dementia (1.85 for mild-to-moderate impairment and 1.48 for severe cognitive impairment). This suggests that residents with dementia may be much more likely to exhibit physically aggressive acts without the typical verbal escalation seen in residents with more intact cognition.

Among direct-care staff members who are assaulted, risk factors include increased workload, lower facility staffing patterns, higher staff anger scores on standardized testing, a perception of being poorly trained to manage dementia-driven behaviors, and young age. Some of these factors may make staff members hurry residents to complete ADLs, thus making it more likely that a resident with dementia will become agitated.

An effective intervention to decrease resident-on-staff violence is behavioral management training for staff, which focuses on defining violence and assault, identifying the reasons for violent behavior, enhancing communication techniques, and mentoring de-escalation approaches (SOE=B).

80. Accountable care organizations are a key feature of the health reform initiative intended to improve quality of care and reduce costs.

Which of the following best characterizes proposed guidelines for accountable care organizations?

(A) Organizations are based in integrated hospital systems that offer both inpatient and outpatient services.
(B) An organization must employ a sufficient number of primary care physicians and other healthcare professionals to meet the needs of the participating population.
(C) A Medicare beneficiary participating in an accountable care organization may not seek care from providers outside the network.
(D) Organizations that target cost-savings through avoidance of hospitalization and nursing-home placement will be eligible for shared savings by Medicare.
(E) To be eligible for shared savings, an organization must show improved patient/caregiver satisfaction, care coordination, patient safety, preventive health, and management for the at-risk population.

ANSWER: E

Accountable care organizations offer providers and hospitals financial incentives to provide quality care to Medicare beneficiaries while reducing healthcare costs. In the traditional healthcare model, doctors and hospitals receive fee-for-service payments for tests and procedures performed, irrespective of outcomes. The accountable care model is intended to reduce incentives for providing more services and instead offer incentives for keeping costs down by focusing on prevention and by enhancing care of patients with chronic conditions. Providers would share the savings accrued from keeping patients healthy and out of the hospital.

Accountable care organizations are not limited to integrated hospital systems; a group of providers or a network of individual practices may also qualify. The minimum number of beneficiaries is 5,000 and the minimum duration of participation is 3 years. In order to participate, an organization must demonstrate that there are sufficient numbers of providers within the network to manage the size of the population covered. CMS may ascribe a beneficiary's experience and costs to a local accountable care organization for comparative purposes. Primary care physicians will be required to tell their patients if they are part of an accountable care organization. A Medicare beneficiary seeking care through the organization may also seek care from a provider outside that network.

In addition to demonstrating reduced hospitalization and institutionalization, an accountable care organization must show improvement in other domains before it can be eligible for shared savings. Points have been assigned for 65 quality measures that are grouped into 5 domains: patient/caregiver experience, care coordination, patient safety, preventive health, and management of defined at-risk populations (diabetes, heart failure, coronary artery disease, hypertension, COPD, and frailty). Maximum shared savings occurs when an accountable care organization achieves 90% of the potential points.

81. Which of the following statements is *not* true about the U.S. population?

(A) The population of adults who are ≥65 years old is projected to more than double between 2010 and 2050.
(B) When the last baby boomer turns 65 in 2029, 19% of adults will be ≥65 years old.
(C) Populations of black and Hispanic adults who are ≥65 years old are growing at equal rates.
(D) By 2032, there will be more people who are ≥65 years old than children who are <15 years old.

ANSWER: C

Between 2010 and 2050, the population of older Hispanic adults is projected to increase faster than any other ethnic group, from 3 million to 18 million; the population of older black non-Hispanic adults is projected to grow from 3 million to 10 million. Older white non-Hispanic adults will remain the largest single ethnic group in the United States, but with comparatively slower growth: from 32 million in 2010 to 50 million in 2050. In 2010, white adults constituted 80% of the population of adults who are ≥65 years old; by 2050, they will make up 58% of that population.

As a whole, in the United States the population of adults who are >65 years old is projected to more than double, from 40 million in 2010 to 89 million in 2050. This represents an increase in the percentage of the total population from 13% to 20%. Baby boomers started turning 65 in 2011, and the last baby boomers will turn 65 in 2029; based on U.S. census population projections, adults who are ≥65 years old will make up 19% of the total U.S. population. By 2029, >70 million adults will be ≥65 years old, and by 2032 the number of adults >65 will surpass the number of children <15 years old.

These trends are primarily attributed to decreased birth rates coupled with increased life expectancy in the United States. The shifts in age distribution among the total population will strain public policy programs that were designed for a different distribution. Specifically, with fewer workers to support each retiree, the costs of Social Security and particularly Medicare will grow faster than younger workers can pay into the programs.

82. A 70-year-old man comes to the office because he has recently been having urinary urgency, frequency, nocturia, and hesitancy, with occasional urge incontinence. History includes diabetes mellitus.

On physical examination, the suprapubic area is full, slightly tender, and dull on percussion. Genitalia are normal, and the prostate is small and nontender with a preserved median sulcus and no nodularity. Lower-extremity reflexes and strength are normal. There is decreased sensation to monofilament and reduced 2-point discrimination. Postvoid residual after a normal void is 650 mL.

Serum creatinine is 1.1 mg/dL (stable for this patient). Ultrasonography of the kidneys after voiding shows no hydronephrosis. Urodynamic testing 1 week later reveals large bladder capacity during filling, and poor bladder contraction with low urine flow rate during voiding. There is no evidence of bladder outlet obstruction.

Which of the following is the most appropriate management?

(A) Begin behavioral therapy including Kegel exercises.
(B) Start extended-release oxybutynin.
(C) Perform transurethral resection of the prostate (TURP).
(D) Insert indwelling catheter and arrange with home-health agency for monthly catheter replacement.
(E) Refer for further evaluation and in-and-out catheterization instruction.

ANSWER: E

The initial evaluation of this patient, according to current management guidelines for patients with a postvoid residual >300 mL, includes measuring serum creatinine and referral to a clinician with urologic expertise (SOE=C). The patient may benefit from a self-catheterization regimen for treatment of neurogenic bladder. His urinary symptoms may improve, and his upper tract would be better preserved with regular drainage (SOE=C).

While men with diabetes may have coexisting anatomical obstruction from benign prostate disease, urodynamic testing in this case suggests that the bladder is poorly contractile without evidence of obstruction. With no evidence of obstruction, transurethral resection would be of no benefit. Chronic indwelling catheter placement should not be the initial recommendation because of the risk of urinary tract infection and other complications associated with chronic indwelling catheters (obstruction, urethral meatal damage, urethral strictures, bladder stones, and bladder spasm) (SOE=C). Kegel exercises or extended-release oxybutynin could be useful for urge urinary incontinence and other lower urinary tract symptoms, even in men, and may be helpful if urge incontinence persists after intermittent self-catheterization is under way. Oxybutynin could result in complete urine retention in a patient with untreated increased postvoid residual volume (SOE=A).

83. A 65-year-old man comes to the office because he has had vivid dreams and thrashing movements during sleep for the past 4 years. Most recently, he dreamt that he fended off a thief by punching him. His wife relates that he punched her in his sleep that night, and she has a black eye from the incident. He recalls similar dreams in which he is usually fighting and has punched the headboard. Daytime behavior is normal, and he reports no memory loss. History includes anxiety and depression, which was diagnosed 1 year ago and for which he takes escitalopram. Neurologic examination is normal.

Which of the following is the most appropriate next step?

(A) Refer for polysomnography.
(B) Refer for neuropsychologic testing.
(C) Add ropinirole.
(D) Discontinue escitalopram.

ANSWER: A

This patient's history is consistent with rapid-eye-movement (REM) behavior disorder, which is characterized by complex and often violent motor activity during REM sleep. In this disorder, dreams are often recalled and reflect the actual physical behaviors. Most cases occur with increasing age, typically manifesting when patients are in their 60s or 70s. The disorder is often associated with development of a neurodegenerative disorder, most commonly Parkinson disease or Lewy body dementia. Diagnosis is confirmed by polysomnography, which would reveal the characteristic loss of muscle atonia during REM sleep (SOE=B).

Neuropsychologic testing may be appropriate after confirmation of REM behavior disorder if the patient also has cognitive symptoms. Treatment with ropinirole or pramipexole is not appropriate at this time because the patient's behaviors are not consistent with restless legs syndrome. In addition, his normal neurologic examination excludes a diagnosis of Parkinson disease.

Use of SSRIs (such as escitalopram) and selective norepinephrine-reuptake inhibitors has been associated with REM behavior disorder

(SOE=B). For this patient, however, the onset of symptoms preceded his use of escitalopram.

84. An 80-year-old man comes to the office to discuss whether he should undergo colorectal cancer screening. He has well-controlled hypertension and walks 2 miles daily.

Which of the following is the most accurate statement about colorectal screening for this patient?

(A) He is unlikely to benefit from screening.
(B) He is unlikely to tolerate treatment for colorectal cancer, so he should not be screened.
(C) The U.S. Preventive Services Task Force (USPSTF) recommends that adults ≥75 years old not undergo screening for colorectal cancer.
(D) The potential benefits of screening largely balance the related burdens.

ANSWER: D

For adults 76–85 years old, the USPSTF supports individualized decisions, based on factors such as patient comorbidities, health status, and patient preference, rather than routine screening.

Older adults with a life expectancy of <5 years are unlikely to benefit from colorectal cancer screening. However, the life expectancy for a healthy, active 80-year-old man is >5 years. Recommendations to older patients about colorectal cancer screening should take comorbidity into account, rather than age alone.

The USPSTF does not recommend stopping colorectal cancer screening at age 75; rather, the Task Force recommends individualized treatment decisions for patients 75–84 years old.

85. A 69-year-old woman comes to the clinic because she has GI pain, headaches, and insomnia that have persisted for >3 years and fluctuate daily. When symptoms are severe, they interrupt her daily visit to her mother in a nursing home. History includes hypertension, diabetes mellitus, osteoarthritis, and cataracts. Previous attempts at diagnosis have included upper and lower GI evaluation, neurologic examination, and laboratory studies (thyrotropin, CBC, and comprehensive metabolic panel); all findings were normal. CT of the head was unremarkable. H_2-receptor antagonists, proton-pump inhibitors, and OTC remedies have provided little benefit.

When directly asked, she admits to feeling stressed. She is annoyed that, when she retired 4 years ago, her sisters ceded care of their mother to her. She minimizes these feelings and asserts that she is most distressed by her headaches and GI pain. She does not ruminate about her physical problems, denies depressed mood, enjoys time with her grandchildren, and has no change in appetite or energy level.

Which of the following is the most likely diagnosis?

(A) Major depressive disorder
(B) Undifferentiated somatic symptom disorder
(C) Somatization disorder
(D) Hypochondriasis

ANSWER: B

Undifferentiated somatic symptom disorder is characterized by ≥1 physical complaints that last ≥6 months and are associated with significant distress or functional impairment. The symptoms and impairment are not explained by or exceed what would be expected from medical findings. Psychologic factors are presumed to have a strong role in onset and persistence of the physical symptoms. Undifferentiated somatic symptom disorder is among the most common somatic symptom disorder in late life (SOE=C). For this patient, stress and resentment are temporally associated with physical symptoms, the onset of which appears to relieve her of expectations that she will routinely provide sole care for her mother.

Somatization disorder is also strongly associated with psychologic factors and with physical complaints that are excessive relative to medical findings. Somatization disorder is characterized by onset before age 30, chronicity, and involvement of multiple organ systems (four sites of pain, two GI symptoms, and one sexual and one pseudoneurologic symptom other than pain). Hypochondriasis is a somatic symptom disorder in which a person's fear of having a serious disease persists despite medical evaluation and reassurance. It is based on a misinterpretation of body symptoms and involves anxious rumination. This patient does not ruminate excessively or express fears of having a serious illness.

Somatic preoccupations may mask depression in late life. This patient describes distress and insomnia, not the near-daily depressed mood, anhedonia, or neurovegetative symptoms seen in major depressive disorder. Somatic preoccupation or hypochondriac symptoms that appear in the context of late-life depression and persist after treatment may predict early recurrence of depressive symptoms (SOE=B).

86. An 83-year-old man with Parkinson disease has been falling backward for about 2 months, and he occasionally has freezing episodes. He is at his maximal response to medications.

On examination, his gait is stooped, with a forward lean, and there is festination.

Which of the following would be the most appropriate assistive device?

(A) Straight cane
(B) 4-Prong cane
(C) Front-wheeled walker
(D) Pick-up walker
(E) 4-Wheeled walker

ANSWER: C

This patient would benefit from a front-wheeled walker. It would increase his stability and promote a forward position that would prevent a backward fall. Because all walkers decrease gait speed in patients with Parkinson disease, they should not be used to augment usual gait. Instead, they should be reserved for patients with impaired postural control (backward falls or festination). Walkers do not improve gait freezing (SOE=B).

Because of flexion and internal arm rotation, persons with Parkinson disease tend to turn canes inward; this may cause the patient to trip. A 4-pronged cane may provide more support than a straight cane but entails the same risks. Neither cane is likely to prevent a backward fall, which is a common form of postural instability in Parkinson disease. A pick-up walker promotes an abnormal gait and, when lifted, may cause backward fall. A 4-wheeled walker may be difficult to control (ie, may roll too fast) in a patient with a festinating gait (SOE=B).

87. A 76-year-old woman recently had right total-knee arthroplasty for severe osteoarthritis. Surgery was uneventful, and she has no complicating medical conditions. Before surgery, she was fully independent in activities of daily living (ADLs). She lives with her husband, who is also fully independent in ADLs. She has mild osteoarthritis of her left knee.

Which of the following is the most appropriate rehabilitation strategy after surgery?

(A) Begin inpatient rehabilitation 1 week after surgery.
(B) Delay rehabilitation until the patient has no pain.
(C) Begin rehabilitation at home 2–5 days after surgery.
(D) Arrange for multidisciplinary rehabilitation at a rehabilitation inpatient facility.
(E) Rehabilitation is not necessary.

ANSWER: C

Home rehabilitation appears to be as effective as inpatient rehabilitation after total-knee arthroplasty (SOE=A). Rehabilitation started the day after surgery is associated with better outcomes (SOE=B), so it should not be delayed. Pain medication is helpful in promoting patient participation. Intensive multidisciplinary rehabilitation may not improve functional outcomes when compared with usual care with physical therapy (SOE=B). Medicare will pay for inpatient rehabilitation only if there is bilateral joint replacement.

88. A 65-year-old man comes to the office because he has recurrent anxiety attacks. He describes episodes of intense fear and anxiety that last from 30 minutes to several hours; the episodes are accompanied by physical and autonomic symptoms. He has no other psychiatric symptoms, does not drink, and has no history of alcohol or drug abuse. History includes hypertension, osteoarthritis, and urinary retention related to prostatic hyperplasia. He received a diagnosis of panic disorder as an adult and was prescribed diazepam, but he has not taken the medication for the past 20 years. He is interested in restarting treatment with diazepam.

Physical examination and laboratory evaluation (thyrotropin, CBC, metabolic profile) indicate nothing likely to cause new-onset panic attacks.

Which of the following is the most appropriate treatment?

(A) A benzodiazepine plus an SSRI
(B) A benzodiazepine plus cognitive-behavioral therapy
(C) A benzodiazepine plus nortriptyline
(D) An SSRI plus cognitive-behavioral therapy
(E) Mirtazapine plus an SSRI

ANSWER: D

Panic disorder was identified in about 1% of community-dwelling older adults in a large-scale epidemiologic study. Classic panic disorder (frequent, unexplained panic attacks with marked fear and autonomic symptoms) with first onset in late life appears to be rare. However, panic-like symptoms are common in late life, particularly in the context of cardiac or respiratory illness or Parkinson disease. In addition, because panic disorder, like other anxiety disorders, tends to be chronic and relapsing, its recurrence or persistence in old age is unsurprising (SOE=B).

The best option for this patient is exposure-based cognitive-behavioral therapy, which usually is done by a licensed clinical psychologist who specializes in this type of therapy, combined with a serotoninergic antidepressant (an SSRI or a serotonin-norepinephrine–reuptake inhibitor [SNRI]). Adjunctive treatment with benzodiazepines may be considered until therapeutic levels of the antidepressant are reached, as long as the trial is brief and the patient is aware of the risks (SOE=C). However, the short-term temporary use of benzodiazepines is generally unnecessary.

Benzodiazepines, among the most commonly prescribed medications in older adults, are not first-line treatment for anxiety disorders. Although they are effective in reducing anxiety symptoms, including those related to panic attacks, benzodiazepines are problematic for several reasons. They do not treat the anxiety disorder itself; rather, they provide a temporary reduction in anxiety. The reduction in anxiety is often unhelpful or even countertherapeutic, particularly in the case of panic disorder, for which the focus of psychotherapeutic treatment is exposure and desensitization (arguably the exact opposite of taking a benzodiazepine for quick relief from anxiety). In addition, older adults who take a benzodiazepine are more likely to have falls, fall-related injury, delirium, and cognitive impairment, and chronic use can accelerate cognitive decline (SOE=B). Finally, benzodiazepines can cause dependence in older adults, although the risk is low, particularly if there is no history of alcohol or drug dependence.

Mirtazapine has an anxiolytic effect and is sometimes useful as an alternative agent or to augment an SSRI or SNRI. Mirtazapine is associated with sedation, an adverse event that may be beneficial for some older adults. Mirtazapine is also useful for the small but significant percentage of adults who are unable to tolerate adverse effects of SSRIs and SNRIs. However, there is no evidence-based rationale for starting mirtazapine along with an SSRI.

Like mirtazapine, tricyclic antidepressants have an anxiolytic effect and are sometimes useful as an alternative to or to augment an SSRI or SNRI. However, tricyclic antidepressants also have troublesome anticholinergic adverse events.

89. A 70-year-old woman comes to the office for routine follow-up. History includes diabetes mellitus, hypertension, and hypercholesterolemia. Medications include aspirin, glipizide, lisinopril, simvastatin, and a multivitamin.

Total cholesterol is 180 mg/dL, low-density lipoprotein level (LDL) is 120 mg/dL, and high-density lipoprotein level (HDL) is 40 mg/dL. She is interested in using therapies other than a statin to improve her cholesterol profile.

Which of the following has the strongest evidence to support its effectiveness in lowering cholesterol?

(A) Valerian
(B) Red yeast rice
(C) Green tea
(D) Viscous fibers (oats, barley, psyllium)

ANSWER: D

Viscous fibers, found in oats, barley, beans, and psyllium, help to bind cholesterol and expel it from the body; 5–10 g/d can lower LDL levels by 5%. The evidence is so strong that the Adult Treatment Panel (ATPIII) of the National Cholesterol Education Program recommends adding plant sterols (2 g/d) and viscous fiber (10–25 g/d) to the diet. The FDA allows producers of foods containing sufficient plant sterols, viscous fiber, or soy protein to make claims for reduction in coronary heart disease because of their ability to reduce cholesterol (SOE=A).

Red yeast rice contains a naturally occurring lovastatin. Dosages of 1,800 mg q12h have been shown to lower LDL by 35 mg/dL in 24 weeks in patients with high LDL levels (SOE=B), with fewer of the adverse effects, such as myalgias, associated with statin therapy. The concentration of the active ingredient, monacolins, varies in different preparations of red yeast rice, such that the effectiveness varies by brand.

The antioxidant catechins in green tea could possibly decrease oxidation of LDL and potentially lower the risk of long-term cardiovascular and cerebrovascular events. In 4 randomized studies, green tea flavonoids yielded modest reductions in LDL levels (SOE=B).

Valerian does not lower cholesterol. It is an herbal preparation that has been used for sleep disorders and anxiety.

90. A 65-year-old black man comes to the office to establish care. He feels well, does not smoke, and walks 1–2 miles daily. On review of systems, he reports having to get up twice each night to urinate. Family history includes his father's death from prostate cancer at age 55. The risks and benefits of testing and treatment for prostate cancer are discussed with the patient.

A prostate nodule is palpable on digital rectal examination. The physical examination is otherwise unremarkable.

Which of the following is the most appropriate next step?

(A) Recommend no further testing.
(B) Repeat digital rectal examination in 6 months.
(C) Order prostate-specific antigen (PSA) test.
(D) Refer the patient for biopsy of the prostate.
(E) Refer the patient for surgery or radiation therapy.

ANSWER: C

This man is at high risk of prostate cancer: he is black and he has a first-degree relative who had prostate cancer before age 65. In addition, he has symptoms of urinary frequency. The presence of a nodule means that this is no longer a screening situation. Measurement of PSA is appropriate; biopsy is indicated if the level is >4.0 ng/dL. If he has localized prostate cancer, he would benefit from intervention with surgery or radiation, because his remaining life expectancy is >10 years (SOE=A).

Repeating the digital rectal examination in 6 months is inappropriate, given his risk factors, his symptoms of urinary frequency, and the presence of a nodule.

It is premature to refer the patient for a biopsy before the PSA level is measured. If the level is <4.0 ng/mL, the patient may not need to be exposed to the significant risks of biopsy. If the PSA level is >4.0 ng/mL, the patient should be referred for a 12-needle biopsy. Referral for surgery or radiation is inappropriate without a definitive diagnosis.

91. An 85-year-old woman has a history of hypertension controlled with medication. She is independent in instrumental activities of daily living and has no cognitive impairment. She had gone to the emergency department because of nausea, vomiting, and a recent increase in her abdominal girth. On examination, she was found to have a small-bowel obstruction, an adnexal mass, and omental adhesions consistent with stage IV ovarian cancer. The small-bowel obstruction responded to conservative treatment, and the cancer diagnosis was confirmed by biopsy. The standard of care for stage IV ovarian cancer—chemotherapy followed by debulking surgery—has been shown to significantly extend patients' lives. The patient is willing to undergo chemotherapy if it is recommended.

Which of the following is the most appropriate recommendation?

(A) Full-dose chemotherapy followed by debulking surgery
(B) Immediate reduced-dose chemotherapy followed by surgery
(C) Immediate reduced-dose chemotherapy without surgery
(D) Palliative surgery
(E) Enrollment in hospice

ANSWER: A

This patient has no comorbidities; if treatment is successful, her remaining life expectancy is >5 years. She should therefore be offered the standard of care, including full-dose chemotherapy (SOE=B). There is no evidence that dosage reduction is necessary up front: older patients benefit from full-dose chemotherapy *as much as younge*r patients, and dosages should be reduced only when patients are unable to tolerate higher dosages. Significant toxicities may occur even with reduced dosages. However, the benefits of treatment are gained only with standard-of-care treatment.

The other options mentioned—reduced-dose chemotherapy with or without surgery, palliative surgery, and hospice—represent undertreatment based entirely on this patient's age, an example of ageism. These options should be considered only if the patient prefers to forego standard-of-care treatment.

92. Which of the following is the most prominent concern when an SSRI is prescribed for an older adult with an anxiety disorder or anxious depression?

(A) The patient may become suicidal.
(B) The patient may stop treatment prematurely because of adverse effects.
(C) Bone loss may accelerate.
(D) The SSRI may cause hyponatremia.
(E) The SSRI may not work.

ANSWER: B

To encourage adherence during a trial of antidepressant therapy, patients with an anxiety disorder or anxious depression should receive counseling about potential adverse effects. The emphasis should be on the nature of the adverse effects, ie, adverse effects are possible but not inevitable. If they do occur, they are likely to be benign and short-lived, and often seem to be manifestations of the underlying illness (such as psychic or somatic anxiety symptoms). Patients are usually most concerned that the adverse effect will worsen or is a sign of toxicity. They should be encouraged to call with their concerns (SOE=C). Reassurance is usually sufficient for the patient to continue with the treatment. Discussion about the nature of package inserts—and the list of possible adverse effects—is also useful.

The increased risk of suicidal ideation with antidepressants has been proved in children and in adults <25 years old, but not in older adults (SOE=A); data from the Veterans Administration have shown no relationship after age 60. Accelerated bone loss has been observed in longitudinal epidemiologic studies, but the loss may be the result of poor diet or lack of exercise associated with the depressive disorder for which the antidepressant was indicated. Hyponatremia, due to syndrome of inappropriate antidiuretic hormone (SIADH), occurs in ≤10% of older adults starting treatment with an SSRI, but it is usually transient and clinically insignificant. Still, it should be considered in older adults who have confusion or other concerns immediately after starting treatment.

Lack of response to treatment with an SSRI is possible, but a trial is warranted. Most patients with anxiety disorders or anxious depression can get better, if not well, with the proper use of antidepressants as part of their care.

93. The wife of an 83-year-old man requests help because of her husband's longstanding alcohol abuse. History includes dizziness and falls; he has been prescribed a walker. The wife has forbidden him to drink and has removed all alcoholic beverages from their home. Their adult son takes his father on outings and, in an effort to please him, provides him with alcoholic beverages. The wife must then cope with his gait difficulties and affected demeanor. An appointment is scheduled for the husband, wife, and son to address concerns related to the patient's drinking.

Which of the following is the most appropriate course?

(A) Arrange for a guardian to be appointed who will identify and support the patient's interests and needs.
(B) Inform the family about the risks of falling and likely sequelae if the patient continues to drink.
(C) Inform the wife that she should not allow the son to take the patient out.
(D) Request help from an ethics consultant or family therapist to mediate the family conflict.
(E) Admit the patient to an alcohol rehabilitation facility.

ANSWER: D

The latest edition of *Core Competencies for Health Care Ethics Consultation: The Report of the American Society for Bioethics and Humanities* states that healthcare ethics consultants should help to address value uncertainty or conflict by articulating the specific conflict or question and facilitating a resolution that respects the roles of the involved parties (patients, families, surrogates, healthcare providers). Healthcare ethics consultants can be enlisted to ensure that each party's voice is heard, to assist the parties in clarifying their own values, to facilitate understanding of information, to identify shared values, to identify and support the ethically appropriate decision maker(s), and to apply mediation or other conflict-resolution techniques.

The healthcare ethics consultant or family therapist is able to adapt techniques of mediation and dispute resolution to:

- identify parties to the conflict (most conflicts have more than two sides)
- understand the explicit as well as the unstated interests of the participants
- help participants define their interests
- moderate disparities of power, knowledge, skill, and experience among participants
- search for common ground or areas of consensus
- identify options for conflict resolution that are compatible with principles of bioethics and legal rights of patients and families
- craft a chart note that makes the terms of consensus accessible to all members of the healthcare team, on all shifts
- track implementation of the agreement
- conduct follow-up

In the other options presented, the clinician seeks to resolve the family conflict either by having an outside authority arbitrate or by reverting to "clinician as educator." In each instance, the conflict is avoided by the provider rather than resolved. An effort to manage the conflict by mediating a shared course of action is far more likely to have the desired result.

94. A 72-year-old woman comes to the office for a routine physical examination. She lives alone in an apartment in a senior housing complex, drives, and plays bridge twice each week with friends. History includes obesity (BMI 31 kg/m^2), hypertension, and seasonal asthma. Medications include inhaled albuterol as needed, lisinopril, and calcium with vitamin D.

On physical examination, her vital signs are normal and her Mini–Mental State Examination score is 30. She walks 4 m in 6 sec at her usual pace.

Which of the following is accurate regarding her gait speed?

(A) Her gait speed is associated with cognitive decline and cardiovascular mortality.
(B) Her gait speed is not useful as a predictor of adverse outcome, because she has no current functional limitations.
(C) Her gait speed demonstrates that she is aging successfully.
(D) Her gait speed is predictive of lower cardiovascular mortality.

ANSWER: A

Gait (or walking) speed is a simple, inexpensive, quick, reproducible, and safe assessment tool for identifying adults at greater risk of adverse outcomes. Gait speed as a single-item tool was as accurate as composite tools in predicting these outcomes over time (SOE=A).

Another review looked at 9 cohort studies, each with >400 participants, that included baseline data on gait speed and tracked survival for ≥5 years. The cohorts were diverse and mostly comprised healthy volunteers. When pooled data were analyzed, the relationship of gait speed to survival was continuous across the range of study participants. Gait speed >1 m/sec was associated with healthier aging, while speed <0.6 m/sec was associated with poor health and function (SOE=B).

In a prospective study of independent adults ≥65 years old, slower walking speed was strongly associated with cardiovascular mortality (SOE=A). A smaller prospective study at 4 tertiary-care hospitals enrolled patients ≥70 years old who were scheduled for coronary artery bypass or valve repair or replacement. The study used a composite of in-hospital postoperative mortality and major morbidity as an end point, and follow-up was limited to in-hospital stay. Slow gait speed was an independent predictor of inpatient morbidity and mortality after cardiac surgery (SOE=C).

95. A 72-year-old man comes to the office because he has had progressive enlargement of right cervical lymph nodes over the past 5 months. He has also noticed some bilateral enlargement of axillary lymph nodes. He has had no weight loss, night sweats, or fevers.

On physical examination, there is a 6-cm lymph node mass in the right axillary region, as well as multiple 2- to 3-cm lymph nodes in the bilateral cervical region and shotty lymph nodes in the bilateral inguinal region. Spleen tip is palpable on deep inspiration.

Laboratory results:

WBC	50,000/µL
Absolute lymphocytes	34,100/µL
Hemoglobin	12.8 g/dL
Platelets	333,000/µL

In-situ hybridization of peripheral blood leukocytes shows trisomy of chromosome 12.

Which of the following is the most likely diagnosis?

(A) Reactive hyperplasia
(B) Infectious mononucleosis
(C) Hodgkin lymphoma, lymphocyte-predominance type
(D) Poorly differentiated lymphocytic lymphoma
(E) Chronic lymphocytic leukemia

ANSWER: E

This patient has the classic symptoms and signs of chronic lymphocytic leukemia (CLL), a chronic lymphoproliferative disorder (lymphoid neoplasm). It is characterized by a progressive accumulation of functionally incompetent lymphocytes that are monoclonal in origin. It is the most common leukemia in Western countries and accounts for approximately 30% of all leukemias in the United States. Median age at diagnosis is 70 years. The classic presentation in this patient makes the other options unlikely.

Patients with CLL have a wide range of symptoms and physical and laboratory abnormalities at the time of diagnosis. Most patients consult a physician because they have noticed painless swelling of lymph nodes, often in the cervical area; the swelling spontaneously waxes and wanes but does not altogether disappear. The spleen is the second most frequently enlarged lymphoid organ; it is palpably enlarged in 25%–55% of cases. As with enlarged lymph nodes, an enlarged spleen in CLL is usually painless and nontender to palpation, with a sharp edge and a smooth, firm surface.

Approximately 25% of patients have no symptoms, and CLL is diagnosed when routine blood work reveals an absolute lymphocytosis. Between 5% and 10% of patients present with ≥1 of the typical "B" symptoms of lymphoma: unintentional weight loss ≥10% within the previous 6 months, temperature >38°C (100.5°F) for ≥2 weeks without evidence of infection, drenching night sweats without evidence of infection, and extreme fatigue. The diagnosis is confirmed by demonstration of monoclonal B cells in the peripheral blood with aberrant expression of CD5, typically a marker of T cells. Cytogenetics is typically negative, but in-situ hybridization is needed to identify more aggressive disease biology. This patient has trisomy 12, which is one of the more common features of CLL and associated with an indolent disease course. Occasionally, the presenting features suggest an acquired immunodeficiency disorder, manifested by infections, autoimmune complications such as hemolytic anemia, thrombocytopenia, pure red cell aplasia, or exaggerated reactions to insect stings or bites.

96. A 74-year-old woman is brought to the office by her son because he is concerned about her memory. History includes mild cognitive impairment. She lives alone in her own home, performs all basic and most instrumental activities of daily living (except personal finances and home maintenance, which her son does for her), and drives short distances in the community.

Which of the following is true regarding an evidence-based approach for improving or maintaining her cognitive ability?

(A) Aerobic exercise or resistance training improves cognitive function in older women.
(B) Participation in new stimulating activities, such as taking computer classes, is more effective than exercise in promoting cognitive fitness.
(C) Regular physical activity in older adults will not improve psychomotor processing ability.
(D) Enrollment in a reputable memory program can reduce the likelihood of progression of mild cognitive impairment.

ANSWER: A

Both aerobic exercise and resistance training have been shown to improve cognitive function in older women. A meta-analysis of literature published from 1966 to 2001 concluded unequivocally that aerobic fitness training enhances cognitive function in healthy but sedentary adults, with executive control processes showing the largest benefit. According to the meta-analysis, participants in combined strength and aerobic training regimens improved to a greater degree than those who participated in aerobic training alone; the benefit was greater for women than for men (SOE=A).

A recent Veterans Affairs study examined the effects of aerobic exercise on cognition and on biomarkers associated with Alzheimer disease for 33 older adults (16 men, 17 women) with mild cognitive impairment diagnosed in a memory disorders clinic. After 6 months of graduated aerobic exercise, cardiorespiratory gains were comparable in men and women, but women had greater improvement in executive control abilities. The authors hypothesize that sex differences in cognitive response may relate to metabolic effects of exercise, because glucoregulation and insulin sensitivity improved only in women, and cortisol levels were reduced in women and increased in men (SOE=B). In a Canadian study of 155 community-dwelling women who were between 65 and 75 years old, certain executive cognitive functions (selective attention and conflict resolution) improved after 12 months of once- or twice-weekly resistance training. As previously observed in other studies, the effect was significantly associated with increased gait speed, and the authors concluded that this improvement is a predictor of substantial reduction in mortality from falls and fractures in older women (SOE=A).

Exercise and participation in new activities appear to be equally beneficial. A German study examined the differential effects of complex mental and physical activities on cognitive performance. The participants, 259 healthy women who were between 70 and 93 years old, were randomly assigned to a computer course, an exercise course, or a control group. Both the exercise group and the computer group demonstrated equivalent and sustained improvement in delayed story recall and working memory (SOE=A).

The INVADE study (Intervention Project on Cerebrovascular Diseases and Dementia in the Community of Ebersberg, Bavaria) is a prospective study of 3,903 Bavarians >55 years old who were screened at baseline for cognitive function and for level of physical activity (none, moderate [<3 times/wk], or high [≥3 times/wk]). At 2 years, lack of physical activity had a significant association with incident cognitive impairment, but moderate or high physical activity was independently associated with lower risk (SOE=A). A small study at the University of Pittsburgh used functional MRI (fMRI) to evaluate adults 70–89 years old who had 2 years earlier participated in the Lifestyle Interventions and Independence for Elders Pilot (LIFE-P) study comparing the effectiveness of physical activity and health education. During fMRI, participants performed the Digit Symbol Substitution Test, which assessed psychomotor performance. The group that remained physically active performed the test with shorter response times and greater accuracy; they had greater activation in areas of the brain important for executive control function (SOE=B).

Many studies have found relationships between cognitive function and physical performance in older adults. Some studies looked at cognitive measures as predictors of physical decline, some looked at physical measures as predictors of cognitive decline, and others looked at concurrent decline. In an effort to identify a consistent longitudinal association, investigators in the Women's Health Initiative Memory Study conducted a 6-year study of 1,793 women (mean age 70.3 years) and concluded that cognitive function decrements precede or are concurrent with physical performance declines. The investigators note that this finding needs to be confirmed in a broader population of older adults, because the study included only women, most of whom were white and had at least a high school education (SOE=A).

Memory training programs have not been shown to prevent progression of mild cognitive impairment to dementia.

97. An 80-year-old man comes to the office because he has loss of taste, painful ulcerations on his lips and tongue, and soreness in the mouth that hinders chewing. He recently received a diagnosis of stage IV laryngeal cancer and started chemotherapy and radiation therapy 2 weeks ago.

On examination, his oral mucosa is red, raw, and tender, with sloughing tissue.

Which of the following is the most appropriate management?

(A) Refer the patient for biopsy.
(B) Inform the patient that ulcerations are an adverse effect of chemotherapy and no treatment is available.
(C) Initiate supportive treatment for oral mucositis.
(D) Recommend that the patient stop radiation and chemotherapy.

ANSWER: C

Oral mucositis is due to systemic effects of chemotherapy and to local effects of radiation on the oral mucous membrane (SOE=A). The diffuse ulcerative lesions of the movable mucosa of the mouth and oropharynx can cause severe pain that requires opioid-level analgesics. Oral mucositis occurs in up to 40% of patients undergoing treatment for head and neck cancers and in 10% of patients treated for other cancers.

Symptoms and signs usually start 4–7 days after chemotherapy is administered and about 10 days after radiation therapy. Inflammation develops more frequently in nonkeratinized mucosa (buccal, labial mucosa, and ventral surface of the tongue), which will appear red, raw, and tender with sloughing epithelium

(SOE=B). Early ulcerative changes are often seen by the end of the second week of treatment. The ulcerative lesions associated with severe mucositis are irregular in shape, may be associated with peripheral areas of erythema, and are often covered by a pseudomembrane made up of fibrinous exudates and dead cells. Mucositis at this stage is extremely uncomfortable, causing pain, dysphagia, loss of taste, and difficulty eating (SOE=B).

There are currently no effective options for the prevention or treatment of mucositis in patients receiving chemoradiation therapy for head and neck cancers (SOE=C). Without supportive care, oral mucositis can lead to weight loss, increased propensity for opportunistic infections in the mouth, and decreased quality of life (SOE=B). Options to mitigate pain and discomfort include the following:

- salt and baking soda rinses, topical anesthetics (2% viscous lidocaine), and chlorhexidine without alcohol 0.12%
- half-and-half mixture of diphenhydramine elixir and milk of magnesia
- topical corticosteroids for ulcers
- adequate hydration, oral lubricants, humidified air
- soft food, protein and vitamin supplements, and avoidance of alcohol and tobacco
- zinc supplement to help loss of taste
- cleaning any dentures with an antimicrobial solution

Biopsy is painful and unnecessary because of the condition of the tissue. If lesions persist after the course of chemotherapy, referral to an oral medicine specialist for consideration of a biopsy is recommended (SOE=B). The biopsy sample tissue should be submitted to an oral pathology laboratory to ensure definitive diagnosis (SOE=B).

Interruption of treatment may be considered in unusual cases when oral mucositis cannot be tolerated despite palliative efforts.

98. An 86-year-old man is admitted to the hospital because he has aspiration pneumonia. This is his third hospitalization for aspiration pneumonia in the last 6 months. History includes Parkinson disease for the past 20 years, moderate cognitive impairment, and progressive dysphagia. He has been bedbound and dependent in all activities of daily living for the past year. The patient has stated repeatedly to his wife and primary physician that he does not want to be "treated with tubes or machines."

Which of the following conditions is required for this patient to qualify for Medicare hospice benefits?

(A) Diagnosis of terminal cancer
(B) "Do not resuscitate" code status
(C) Life expectancy ≤3 months
(D) Life expectancy ≤6 months
(E) Uncontrolled symptoms

ANSWER: D

Patients with Medicare Part A are eligible for Medicare hospice benefits if they have a chronic or terminal illness with life expectancy ≤6 months if the disease runs its expected course, as certified by the primary physician and hospice medical director. When a patient chooses hospice care, he or she waives the Medicare Part A coverage that relates to the terminal illness and signs up for Medicare hospice benefits. The benefits cover a variety of services, including care by a multidisciplinary team, durable medical equipment, medical supplies, and palliative medications related to the terminal illness.

Patients are not required to have a diagnosis of cancer to qualify for the benefit. Nor are they required to have a "do not resuscitate" status, although most hospice agencies require or at least recommend the code for their patients, because it reflects the goals of hospice care. Uncontrolled symptoms are not required to qualify for Medicare hospice benefits. The hospice team will address symptoms in the treatment plan for the patient in an ongoing fashion.

99. In January, a 73-year-old nursing-home resident is evaluated because he has had fever, headache, nasal congestion, nonproductive cough, shortness of breath, and malaise since the previous day. A rapid influenza test from a nasal swab is positive for influenza A. Another resident has had similar symptoms for 2 days.

Which of the following should be offered to the other nursing-home residents?

(A) Rimantadine
(B) Amantadine
(C) Oseltamivir
(D) Zanamivir
(E) Peramivir

ANSWER: C

Oseltamivir is a neuraminidase inhibitor that is effective for treatment of influenza if started within 48 hours of symptom onset but is most effective if started within 24 hours (SOE=A). It is the antiviral of choice for influenza outbreaks in long-term care facilities and should be combined with appropriate vaccination strategies (SOE=A). During influenza season, when two residents have signs and symptoms of an influenza-like illness within 72 hours of each other, all residents of the facility should be tested for influenza. Even one positive laboratory result in conjunction with other compatible illnesses in the facility indicates that an outbreak is underway (SOE=A). During documented outbreaks, antiviral chemoprophylaxis for influenza should be offered to all residents, regardless of vaccination status. Ideally, chemoprophylaxis should be implemented on all floors and wards of the facility, because breakthrough cases frequently occur when antiviral medications are administered only to those people on the affected unit or ward and not to all residents in the facility (SOE=A).

Zanamivir is an inhaled neuraminidase inhibitor that can be used for the treatment of influenza or for chemoprophylaxis during an outbreak. However, oseltamivir is preferable, because it is difficult for many older adults to use an inhaler properly.

Peramivir is an experimental neuraminidase inhibitor that is being evaluated for treatment of influenza. The FDA has authorized its emergency use in certain cases of known or suspected pandemic influenza.

Use of the M2 inhibitors rimantadine and amantadine is limited by widespread resistance (>90% of most virulent strains). These agents are not recommended for chemoprophylaxis during an outbreak.

100. A 91-year-old woman has some new chest discomfort and a poor appetite, which is unusual for her. History includes dementia, hypertension, and diabetes mellitus, and at baseline she walks minimally. Her niece, with whom she lives, provides care for her and is her durable power of attorney for health and finance. The niece contacts her aunt's house-call program, and reports that her aunt needs medical attention. A home visit is arranged.

On examination, blood pressure is 180/100 mmHg, heart rate is 100 beats per minute and regular, respirations are 24 breaths per minute, and O_2 saturation is 92%. Temperature is normal. Her breathing is more labored than usual, and coarse breath sounds are heard at lung bases. She seems withdrawn but does not appear to be in significant distress. Differential diagnoses include myocardial infarction, congestive heart failure, pulmonary embolus, and pneumonia. The niece states that her aunt wishes to avoid hospitalization and to be cared for at home.

Which of the following is the most appropriate next step?

(A) Call 911 for paramedics to help carry the patient down the stairs so that she can be evaluated at the hospital.
(B) Draw blood for laboratory evaluation of troponin, D-dimer, CBC, and basic metabolic panel; order home chest radiography and portable home ECG.
(C) Begin empiric therapy with antibiotics, sublingual nitroglycerin, and enoxaparin.
(D) Enroll the patient in hospice.

ANSWER: B

House-call programs have an increasing array of home-based equipment and testing options available to care for acutely ill homebound patients. Most house-call clinicians carry a bag of basic medical equipment and supplies, which usually include equipment for on-site phlebotomy, bladder catheterization, and in some cases, even portable ECG. Many diagnostic tests that are normally performed in an emergency department can now be performed in a home setting. Many communities have agencies that offer portable radiology and portable ECG. Laboratory evaluation and chest radiography can be easily performed in the home to provide more clinical data. Charges for these tests can be submitted to Medicare. Some portable diagnostic agencies may charge additional fees for stairs.

In most situations, an older patient with an acute change in condition might be sent to the emergency department. However, this patient and her niece, as durable power of attorney, have expressly requested to avoid hospitalization. Given the niece's wishes and willingness to care for the patient at home, it would be premature to send the patient to the hospital.

While empiric antibiotics for pneumonia could be started for a homebound patient in whom there is a clinical suspicion of pneumonia, and sublingual nitroglycerin could be useful in this patient with hypertension and chest pain, starting an anticoagulant without further diagnostic evidence carries significant potential risk.

Hospice referral may be appropriate for this patient in the future but would not be the next immediate step in management. Her change in condition may be reversible.

101. An 84-year-old man who lives in a nursing home is seen for his monthly evaluation. History includes moderate dementia, diabetes mellitus, and heart failure. Medications include metformin 1000 mg twice daily with meals and glipizide 10 mg q12h. He undergoes fingerstick monitoring twice daily; values have ranged between 100 and the low 200s for several months. His most recent hemoglobin A_{1c} level was 8.3%.

Which of the following is the most appropriate next step in the management of this patient's diabetes?

(A) Obtain fructosamine level.
(B) Increase glipizide to 20 mg q12h.
(C) Add sitagliptin.
(D) Add NPH insulin at bedtime.
(E) Discontinue fingerstick monitoring.

ANSWER: E

There is little evidence that fingerstick monitoring is beneficial for patients with type 2 diabetes mellitus who do not take insulin. Because glycemic goals for frail older adults are less aggressive than for younger patients, older patients are less likely to benefit from fingerstick monitoring. Such monitoring is often used for hospitalized nursing-home patients, but if the patient has been doing well on stable dosages of hypoglycemic medications, fingerstick monitoring is unlikely to improve outcomes (SOE=B).

The fructosamine level can provide valuable additional information when the hemoglobin A_{1c} level may not be reflective of true glycemic control because of increased turnover of RBCs. However, a hemoglobin A_{1c} measure of 8.3% corresponds to a fingerstick blood glucose level of around 185 mg/dL, which is consistent with this patient's daily glucose values. Thus, it is unlikely that fructosamine levels would provide information that would change management.

Because the macrovascular benefits of intensive glycemic control are realized after approximately 8 years, the primary goal of glycemic control in nursing-home patients, most of whom have limited life expectancy, is to minimize symptoms (eg, malaise, incontinence) rather than to decrease vascular complications. According to guidelines from the Veterans Administration–Department of Defense, the target hemoglobin A_{1c} for frail older adults with diabetes mellitus is 8%–9%. Because this patient's hemoglobin A_{1c} level is at target, increasing the glipizide dosage or adding sitagliptin or NPH insulin is more likely to cause harm by increasing the risk of hypoglycemia (SOE=C).

102. A 68-year-old woman comes to the office because she has periods of shortness of breath and wheezing that have worsened over the past 2 months. The episodes may occur one or two times a week. She does not have cough, chest pain, leg swelling, fever, rash, or rhinorrhea. The patient tried using her grandson's inhaler and believes that it reduced her symptoms. History includes hypercholesterolemia, osteoporosis, and type 2 diabetes mellitus. She does not smoke or drink alcohol. She previously worked as an administrative assistant and is now retired.

Which of the following is the most appropriate initial treatment?

(A) Fluticasone
(B) Tiotropium
(C) Theophylline
(D) Albuterol
(E) Pulmonary rehabilitation

ANSWER: D

Management of new-onset asthma is similar in older and younger patients. Patients with no significant cognitive impairment should be provided with an asthma action plan that includes self-monitoring of peak expiratory flow. Initial therapy with a short-acting β-agonist is recommended (SOE=A) to ascertain patient response. If the patient rarely needs the short-acting agent, then it alone is adequate. If the patient routinely uses the inhaler >2 times in 1 week, inhaled corticosteroids should be added to reduce airway inflammation and delay progression to chronic, fixed obstruction. A short-acting agent alone will not adequately control symptoms in most older adults. Because the amount of systemic exposure to corticosteroids is relatively small with most inhalers, history of osteopenia or osteoporosis is not an absolute contraindication to corticosteroid use.

New-onset asthma is under-recognized in older adults, because it is commonly associated with children. Asthma has a bimodal distribution, peaking in children and then again in older adult populations. The prevalence in older adults is approximately 10%. The mortality rate is higher in older patients—nearly two-thirds of asthma deaths occur in patients >65 years old. The higher mortality rate may be due to the presence of comorbid illness, impaired perception of dyspnea by older patients, and difficulty using asthma medications properly. Risk factors for asthma include exposure to allergens and air pollution, genetic susceptibility, diet, overweight or obese body habitus, adverse effect of medication (seen with β-blockers and NSAIDs), and infections (viral infections, *Mycoplasma).*

Use of combination inhalers (containing both long-acting bronchodilators and inhaled corticosteroids) can reduce the need for multiple inhalers and, in theory, improve adherence. Careful patient instruction in proper inhaler use is essential, especially instruction on distinguishing short-acting from long-acting agents and proper use of inhalers during an acute exacerbation (ie, patient should avoid excessive use of short-acting inhalers and their associated risk of acute hypokalemia and QT prolongation). The patient should be able to demonstrate proper use of the inhaler. A spacer can improve delivery of medication to the pulmonary system and reduce deposition in the oropharynx. A nebulizer-based delivery system may be warranted for adults who are not able to generate adequate inspiratory force to use a dry-powder inhaler properly, or who lack the coordination necessary for an aerosolized inhaler.

This patient's symptoms are consistent with intermittent asthma, and thus use of fluticasone or other inhaled corticosteroids is not indicated for initial treatment. Tiotropium is not warranted, because the patient does not have a diagnosis of COPD. Because theophylline has a low therapeutic index, it is generally used as a last resort for patients who are not responding to other therapies. Pulmonary rehabilitation comprises 10–15 outpatient visits to a pulmonary center, during which patient education and proper exercise technique are emphasized. It may be useful after a patient has started initial therapy, especially in cases of more severe disease.

103. An 81-year-old woman comes to the office because she has had lower back pain for 2 weeks. The pain worsens when she sits or stands but is relieved when she lies in bed. History includes vertebral compression fracture 4 years ago and right femoral neck fracture 2 years ago.

On physical examination, straight-leg raise tests are normal bilaterally. Strength of proximal and distal muscles is 5/5 in both legs. There is good mobility of the lumbar spine. The patient describes marked pain when pressure is applied to the sacrum. Radiography of the lumbar spine reveals diffuse osteoporosis and multilevel degenerative disc disease.

Which of the following is the most likely cause of this patient's pain?

(A) Lumbar spinal stenosis
(B) Tumor affecting the lumbar spine
(C) Osteoporotic sacral fracture
(D) Lumbar disc disease
(E) Osteomyelitis of the L4 vertebrae

ANSWER: C

Sacral insufficiency fracture is a cause of back pain in older adults, most commonly in older women with a history of osteoporosis. Patients report lower back and buttock pain that worsens when they sit or stand and is relieved by lying down. The characteristic physical finding is pain on compression of the sacrum. The fractures are frequently bilateral. There are usually no neurologic abnormalities and no pain on movement of the lumbar spine. Straight-leg raise tests are usually normal, and plain film radiography of the sacrum is typically unrevealing. The fractures are best seen with CT of the pelvis, which shows displacement of the anterior border of the sacrum. Bone scintigraphy often shows H- or butterfly-shaped fractures.

The natural history of sacral insufficiency fractures is favorable. In one study, pain resolved within 4–6 weeks for most patients, and all patients were pain free at 9 weeks. Nonetheless, another study found that mobility declined from preinjury levels for a significant number of patients.

Pain from lumbar spinal stenosis typically improves with sitting and is characterized by neuropathic pain in the lower extremities. There may be associated neurologic findings, such as decreased sensation, in the affected dermatome. Pain from a tumor would be more constant and less affected by change in position; frequently, radiography would show lytic or sclerotic lesions. In addition to its association with lower back pain, lumbar disc disease is often accompanied by pain radiating into one or both legs. The pain is often temporarily relieved by standing, and physical examination may show a positive straight-leg raise. Pain associated with osteomyelitis would be more constant, less affected by changes in position, and often accompanied by systemic symptoms.

104. What is the most common cause of death by injury in older adults?

(A) Motor vehicle crash
(B) Fall
(C) Suicide
(D) Fire

ANSWER: B

Heart disease, cancer, and stroke are the top three causes of death among adults who are ≥65 years old; injury is the eighth most common cause in this age group. About 30% of injury deaths are caused by falls. Motor vehicle crashes are next most common (18%), and suicide by firearm, suffocation, or poisoning accounts for 13%. Men are more likely than women to die from a fall, perhaps because their falls are more catastrophic or because they have more chronic conditions.

The statistics on death from motor vehicle crash include deaths of drivers, passengers, pedestrians, and bicyclists. According to data from the National Highway Traffic Safety Administration, older individuals accounted for 14% of all vehicle occupant fatalities and 18% of all pedestrian fatalities in 2008. By 2030, older drivers are projected to account for up to 25% of all driver fatalities.

Mortality and morbidity due to injuries are preventable and have public health implications. Many interventions exist to prevent falls, motor vehicle accidents, suicide, and other types of injuries among older adults. Deaths due to fire are not as common as those due to falls.

105. A 92-year-old man, previously independent, has been gradually losing weight and function after an admission to the hospital for *Clostridium difficile* diarrhea following treatment for a dental abscess. His primary care doctor has found no acute illness. His 70-year-old daughter asks whether her father should undergo a comprehensive geriatric assessment, which is offered by several clinics in his area of the state.

Which of the following is true about comprehensive geriatric assessment?

(A) For frail older adults, the assessment should be performed in a rehabilitation setting.
(B) It is an outpatient evaluation and management service.
(C) Its maximum benefit is attained when the team performing the assessment is also the care provider.
(D) The American Geriatrics Society has defined its scope and components.

ANSWER: C

Comprehensive geriatric assessment is used to prepare individualized care plans that encompass the medical, psychologic, and functional capabilities of frail older adults. The multidimensional, interdisciplinary assessment can be performed in any healthcare setting, including home, inpatient, and outpatient. Maximum benefit is attained when the team performing the assessment also provides the care (SOE=C). Comprehensive geriatric assessment is not an application of a set of protocols to produce a fixed plan. Instead, the care plans are best seen as works in progress, feeding back on one another. The scope of the assessment differs across settings, and no gold standard has been developed by a professional organization.

Comprehensive assessment improves healthcare outcomes in identifiable groups of frail older adults. However, the data are not consistent across healthcare settings, and no guidelines reliably identify frail or vulnerable older adults. More research is needed to determine whether comprehensive geriatric assessment results in fewer visits to the emergency department, less frequent hospitalization, fewer adverse drug reactions, and reduced costs for acute care. A Cochrane review found that when frail older adults received comprehensive assessment during hospitalization for emergencies, they had improved survival, a higher likelihood of being at home in 6 months, and reduced institutionalization.

Currently there is no explicit Medicare reimbursement for comprehensive geriatric assessment provided by any team member, including physicians. The American Geriatrics Society continues to support reimbursement for comprehensive care for frail older adults with ≥2 chronic illnesses.

106. An 82-year-old man is hospitalized with pneumonia and treated with intravenous antibiotics and oxygen. He has dementia. Before this hospitalization, he used a walker.

Which of the following is most likely to reduce his risk of falling while in the hospital?

(A) Pressure-sensitive bed alarm
(B) Restraint that allows upper-body movement
(C) Scheduled toileting
(D) Physical therapy consultation
(E) Providing educational materials on falls to the family

ANSWER: C

This patient is at high risk of falling in the hospital. He has an acute illness that is being treated with intravenous fluids, antibiotics, and oxygen. In addition, he has dementia, is in a new and disorienting environment, and is at risk of delirium. Before hospitalization, he had impaired gait and balance and required a walker. With bed rest, he is very likely to lose muscle strength. He is not likely to call for help to use the bathroom. Frequent checking on this high-risk patient, with scheduled toileting, will reduce his chance of getting out of bed unsupervised and his risk of falling (SOE=D).

Research on fall prevention in hospitals has been limited by the difficulty of designing randomized controlled trials. A few studies have shown that a multifactorial approach works, but it is not clear which of the interventions in these studies is effective. One component of the interventions is frequent toileting, and it makes empiric sense that this would reduce falls risk.

Bed alarms are widely used in hospitals but have not been shown to reduce the number of hospital falls (SOE=B). Bed alarms signal an exit from bed. Usually by the time the alarm is answered, the patient is already either walking away from the bed or is on the floor. Bed alarms may be turned off when patients are out of bed or off the unit, and staff may forget to turn them on when the patient returns to bed. Restraints, including those that allow upper-body movement, should be avoided in the hospital. Restraints can lead to skin breakdown from reduced movement and may result in injury (SOE=B). A physical therapy consultation might be helpful for exercise and gait training. However, the patient is not likely to be hospitalized long enough to experience a benefit from physical therapy that would translate into a reduced risk of an inpatient fall. This patient has dementia. His family may be able to implement recommendations when the patient is at home, but not while he is in the hospital.

107. A 70-year-old woman comes to the clinic for a routine examination. History includes mild hypertension, which is well-controlled with hydrochlorothiazide. She takes no other medication, has never smoked, and rarely consumes alcohol. She walks >10 miles each week and works as a school volunteer. A recent dual-energy x-ray absorptiometry (DEXA) scan reveals normal bone density readings at all sites (T scores all ≥–1). The patient asks whether she needs vitamin D supplements.

Which of the following recommendations applies to this patient?

(A) Adults >65 years old should have serum 25(OH)D levels measured as part of routine screening for vitamin D deficiency.
(B) Adults >65 years old should take supplemental vitamin D ≤4,000 IU/d to avoid hypercalcemia.
(C) For adults >70 years old, the recommended dietary allowance (RDA) for vitamin D is 800 IU/d.
(D) Older adults with low serum 25(OH)D levels should receive treatment to achieve a serum level of 40–50 ng/mL (100–125 nmol/L).

ANSWER: C

There is considerable controversy regarding the prevalence, definition, and treatment of vitamin D deficiency for all age groups. An Institute of Medicine (IOM) committee charged with determining the population needs for vitamin D and calcium reviewed the strength of evidence causally linking these nutrients to clinically relevant skeletal or extraskeletal outcomes. The committee concluded that the evidence is strong that vitamin D is an important determinant of skeletal health and that the evidence provides a sound basis for determining dietary requirements (SOE=A). It further concluded that, in regard to the effect of vitamin D on extraskeletal outcomes, including cancer, cardiovascular disease, diabetes, and autoimmune disorders, evidence is inconsistent as to causality and insufficient to inform nutritional requirements.

The RDAs for vitamin D represent the estimated intake that would meet the needs of >97.5% of healthy individuals in a given age group with minimal sun exposure. For individuals between the ages of 1 and 70 years, the RDA is 600 IU/d. For adults >70 years old, the RDA is 800 IU/d. These dosages were based on evidence linking bone health with specific serum 25(OH)D levels and then determining the average daily intake of vitamin D that corresponded to these levels. The predominance of evidence indicated that levels of 16 ng/mL (40 nmol/L) meet the needs for optimal bone health in approximately half the population. This amount corresponds to an average vitamin D intake of approximately 400 IU/d for all age groups. Further extrapolation (by taking 2 SD above the median needs) indicated that serum 25(OH)D levels ≥20 ng/mL (≥50 nmol/L) meet the needs of at least 97.5% of the population. The corresponding average daily level of vitamin D intake determined the RDAs for each age group.

The IOM did not find compelling evidence to associate a serum 25(OH)D level >20 ng/mL (>50 nmol/L) or dietary intake above the RDA with greater benefit for bone health or other outcomes. For some conditions, U-shaped associations were observed, with evidence of increased risks at both low and high serum 25(OH)D levels.

The IOM report did not include recommendations on screening for vitamin D deficiency, nor have other groups found evidence supporting routine screening of healthy older adults. Although the IOM committee noted that serum 25(OH)D level may be a valid indicator of the total amount of vitamin D entering the blood from intrinsic (eg, production in the skin) and extrinsic (eg, dietary) sources and that the level may help guide management in some cases, there is a lack of evidence as to benefits or effectiveness of screening for deficiency (SOE=D).

The tolerable upper intake level (UL) is the estimated highest average daily nutrient intake likely to pose no health risk for nearly all people in a particular group. Although the report acknowledged that vitamin D intake <10,000 IU/d has not been associated with an increased risk of hypercalcemia or other acute toxicities, the IOM set the UL for vitamin D at 4,000 IU/d. This level reflects concern about potential adverse effects of long-term intake on chronic disease outcomes and all-cause mortality, as well as emerging concerns about risks at serum 25(OH)D levels >50 ng/mL (>125 nmol/L). Because data are limited regarding the effect of chronic intake on long-term health outcomes, the UL is a conservative estimate designed to guide public health planning.

108. A 78-year-old man comes to the office because he has difficulty swallowing. The onset has been gradual; he intermittently notices a sensation of fullness in the neck and food regurgitation. He has had no heartburn, recent weight loss, or episodes of choking or coughing after eating. History includes hypertension, hyperlipidemia, and benign prostatic hyperplasia. Physical examination is unremarkable.

Which of the following is the most likely diagnosis?

(A) Parkinson disease
(B) Zenker diverticulum
(C) Oropharyngeal tumor
(D) Achalasia

ANSWER: B

Dysphagia, a common problem for older adults, requires evaluation and management to avoid further complications, such as aspiration pneumonia and malnutrition. It is frequently seen in nursing-home residents and probably underdiagnosed in community-dwelling older adults (SOE=B). Zenker diverticulum is a common cause. Symptoms can occur late in life and include food regurgitation and a sensation of fullness in the neck, rather than choking or a sensation of food being stuck. Some patients have recurrent chest infections. Unlike other causes of dysphagia, surgery or endoscopy is curative in Zenker diverticulum (SOE=A).

In patients with Parkinson disease, dysphagia can develop because of abnormalities in oral, pharyngeal, or esophageal stages of swallow. Patients may choke or cough after eating but rarely regurgitate food. This patient has no neurologic findings consistent with Parkinson disease. An oropharyngeal tumor can present gradually and cause a sensation of fullness in the neck, but it does not cause food regurgitation. In addition, this patient does not have the weight loss that can occur with underlying cancer. Some patients with achalasia may sense fullness in the neck, but the dysphagia is intermittent because of lower esophageal ring or esophageal dysmotility.

109. An 82-year-old woman is evaluated because she is frequently incontinent of urine and occasionally incontinent of feces. The patient and her family cannot tell how long she has been incontinent. History includes Alzheimer disease. She was recently admitted to a nursing facility. She is able to feed herself but requires assistance with other basic activities of daily living. She cannot follow a multistep command, yet her answers to simple, direct questions are nearly always accurate. She ambulates slowly with the use of a walker and stand-by assistance.

On physical examination, there is no evidence of severe atrophic vaginitis, pelvic prolapse, or fecal impaction. Catheterization a few minutes after an episode of incontinence reveals a residual volume of 30 mL. Urine is dark yellow; dipstick analysis shows no leukocyte esterase, nitrites, or hemoglobin.

A 3-day prompted-voiding program is implemented and includes scheduled wet-checks, assistance to the toilet, and praise for successful toileting trips. At baseline, she was wet 60% of the time when checked; after the 3-day program, she was wet 62% of the time.

Which of the following factors indicated that the patient was unlikely to benefit from a prompted-voiding program for urinary continence?

(A) Use of a walker
(B) Degree of cognitive impairment
(C) Poor results in 3-day voiding trial
(D) Increased postvoid residual urine
(E) Fecal incontinence

ANSWER: C

Only 25%–40% of patients respond well to prompted voiding (SOE=A). Predicting which residents will benefit from ongoing intervention is an important part of medical and facility-wide management of continence. Responsiveness can generally be determined after a short (3-day) trial (SOE=A). Patients being considered for the program should be able to respond to direct questioning as to whether they are "wet" or "dry." As well, patients should be able to get to the toilet with no more than moderate assistance from one staff member. Patients with dementia or expressive aphasia also can benefit from staff-initiated toileting programs; those who can respond to questions, say their name, or point reliably to an object in the room can be assessed for benefit. Prompted voiding for urinary incontinence can be accompanied by improvement in fecal incontinence as well. Postvoid residual urine of 30 mL is well within acceptable limits for behavioral therapy for urinary incontinence and is normal for older patients (SOE=C).

110. A 75-year-old man comes to the office to establish care because he has difficulty breathing. The breathing difficulty limits his ability to walk 2 blocks to the corner store, and he often has to sleep upright in his recliner. He takes no medication except chewable calcium carbonate tablets for chronic indigestion.

On physical examination, blood pressure is 154/88 mmHg, pulse is 80 beats per minute, and respirations are 16 breaths per minute. There are bibasilar fine crackles. Cardiac examination is notable for normal rhythm with ectopy and a II/VI holosystolic murmur at the apex. There is no peripheral edema. ECG and laboratory evaluation (electrolyte panel and CBC) are ordered. The presumptive diagnosis is heart failure.

Which of the following tests should be ordered next to help establish diagnosis and treatment?

(A) Cardiac catheterization
(B) Echocardiography
(C) Radionuclide ventriculography
(D) MRI
(E) Chest radiography

ANSWER: B

The single most useful diagnostic test in the evaluation of patients with heart failure is 2-dimensional echocardiography to determine the left ventricle ejection fraction as well as structural abnormalities of the left and right ventricles, valves, and pericardium, because it is common for patients to have >1 cardiac abnormality that contributes to the development of heart failure (SOE=C).

Although radionuclide ventriculography can provide highly accurate measurements of left ventricle function and right ventricle ejection fraction, it is unable to directly assess valvular abnormalities or cardiac hypertrophy. MRI or CT may be useful in evaluating chamber size and ventricular mass, detecting right ventricular dysplasia, or recognizing the presence of pericardial disease, but neither is the most appropriate next step for this patient. Because of their low sensitivity and specificity, neither chest radiography nor ECG should form the primary basis for determining the specific cardiac abnormality responsible for the development of heart failure.

111. An 85-year-old man with advanced prostate cancer is scheduled to begin therapy with leuprolide acetate injections every 3 months. Baseline bone densitometry is performed to determine his risk of osteoporosis-related fracture; T score of −2.0 at the left femoral neck is reported. He weighs 70 kg (154 lb) and is 172.2 cm (5 ft 8 in.) tall. According to the Fracture Risk Assessment Tool (FRAX ®), his 10-year risk of hip fracture is 4.2%; his risk of any osteoporotic fracture is 9.6%.

To prevent osteoporosis fracture as a complication of gonadotropin-releasing hormone (GnRH) agonist therapy, which of the following antiresorptive therapies is indicated?

(A) Bisphosphonate
(B) Estradiol
(C) Raloxifene
(D) Salmon calcitonin

ANSWER: A

GnRH agonists inhibit production of sex steroid hormones by the gonads. Men undergoing treatment with GnRH agonists have acute loss of bone when therapy is begun, and bone loss continues with prolonged therapy. Risk of

Questions/Answers/Critiques

osteoporotic fracture increases in men treated with GnRH agonists for prostate cancer. Men at low risk of fracture should be monitored for bone loss with serial measurement of bone mineral density; treatment with a bisphosphonate should be started if bone loss is documented (SOE=A). Therapy with intravenous and oral bisphosphonates has been shown to prevent GnRH agonist–associated bone loss (SOE=A). This patient has a high risk of fracture and should be started on a bisphosphonate.

Estrogens contribute to skeletal homeostasis in healthy men, and higher serum estradiol levels are associated with high bone mineral density of the spine and lower risk of vertebral fracture. However, estrogen therapy is not well tolerated because of its feminization adverse effects. Raloxifene, a selective estrogen-receptor modulator, was found to increase bone mineral density of the hip and spine (SOE=C). However, adverse effects, including increased risk of deep-vein thrombosis and pulmonary embolism, have precluded larger, placebo-controlled studies. Nasal calcitonin has not been studied in men receiving GnRH agonist treatment.

The FRAX® tool has been developed by the World Health Organization to evaluate fracture risk. It is based on individual patient models that integrate the risks associated with clinical risk factors as well as bone mineral density (BMD) at the femoral neck. The FRAX® algorithms give the 10-year probability of hip fracture and the 10-year probability of a major osteoporotic fracture (clinical spine, forearm, hip or shoulder fracture). It is primarily used as a clinical tool to help clinicians assess fracture probability as an aid in identifying which individuals may be candidates for reassurance, bone density evaluation, or pharmacologic treatment.

112. A 72-year-old woman comes to the office because for the past 6 months she has had severe burning pain in her feet that is worse at night. She recently tried gabapentin but discontinued it because it caused gait disturbance. History includes uncontrolled diabetes mellitus, chronic constipation, and mild cognitive impairment. Medications include insulin glargine 20 units at night, lisinopril 20 mg/d, docusate sodium 100 mg q12h, metformin 1,000 mg q12h, and acetaminophen 1,000 mg q8h. Her fingerstick glucose levels have been between 180 and 200 in the morning and in the mid-200s at night.

Which of the following is the most appropriate next step for improving pain control?

(A) Increase insulin dosage.
(B) Refer for sympathectomy.
(C) Start lamotrigine.
(D) Start pregabalin.

ANSWER: D

This patient has painful diabetic neuropathy. A 2009 Cochrane review found that pregabalin has proven efficacy in chronic neuropathic pain conditions (SOE=A). Comparing pregabalin 600 mg/d with placebo for painful diabetic neuropathy, the number needed-to-treat (NNT) for ≥50% pain relief (over baseline pain level) was 5.0 (4.0–6.6).

Increasing the patient's insulin dosage is likely appropriate but will not improve pain control. Surgical or chemical sympathectomy is sometimes performed for neuropathic pain, but its use is based on very little high-quality evidence (SOE=C), and it carries a risk of serious complications. Sympathectomy should likely be used with caution only after other treatment options have failed. So far this patient has tried only gabapentin, and other viable options exist.

Like pregabalin, lamotrigine is an anticonvulsant agent; however, there is no convincing evidence that lamotrigine has efficacy in treating chronic pain, including diabetic neuropathy (SOE=A).

Tricyclic antidepressants are used off-label to treat diabetic neuropathy, and their efficacy has been shown in numerous placebo-controlled studies (SOE=A). However, they are associated with significant anticholinergic adverse effects in older adults, such as confusion, constipation, and urinary retention. If the patient's symptoms do not improve or the patient cannot tolerate pregabalin, low-dosage tricyclic antidepressants are an option.

113. Dolly, a female domestic sheep, was the first mammal to be cloned by nucleus transfer. The donor was a middle-aged (6-year-old) sheep. Dolly lived for 6 years, which is half the normal lifespan (12 year) that is typical of her species.

Which of the following theories of aging is the most likely explanation for her early death?

(A) Mitochondrial DNA damage
(B) Depletion of stem cell reserves
(C) Loss of chromosomal telomere length
(D) Mutations in gene expression profiles

ANSWER: C

Dr. Ian Wilmut of the Roslin Institute in Edinburgh cloned DNA from the mammary cell of an adult sheep with an unfertilized egg from another sheep, which yielded a genetically identical copy of the sheep that was the source of the DNA. It has been suggested that Dolly's death stemmed from a common lung disease and was not related to her cloning. Another possibility is that her genetic age at birth was 6 years. Cellular senescence involves the gradual loss of telomerase activity; with age, it becomes increasingly difficult to maintain sufficient length to the telomere-capping regions of chromosomes for replication.

The other theories listed could help explain or be related to Dolly's death, but they are less likely. Although mitochondrial DNA damage (leading to altered efficiency of respiration/adenosine triphosphate [ATP] production and increased free radicals), altered gene expression profiles (result of cumulative DNA damage), and physical loss of tissue-repairing adult stem cells over time could be factors, they are not as likely when considering the specific age (6 years) of the donor nucleus and its DNA in this case.

114. A 68-year-old woman comes to the office because she has shoulder and hip girdle stiffness that is present on awakening and lasts for 90 min. The stiffness began suddenly 2 months ago. She reports intermittent fevers to 38.9°C (102°F) and unintentional weight loss of 3.2 kg (7 lb). History includes hypertension treated with lisinopril and hydrochlorothiazide.

Physical examination is normal, except that strength testing demonstrates impaired effort and strength in her deltoids and hip flexors secondary to pain.

Laboratory results:

Hemoglobin	11.2 g/dL
Hematocrit	34%
Aspartate aminotransferase	54 U/L
Alanine aminotransferase	58 U/L
Alkaline phosphatase	110 U/L
Erythrocyte sedimentation rate	15 mm/h

Treatment is initiated with prednisone 15 mg/d. She returns 1 week later for follow-up and reports no change in her symptoms.

Which of the following is the most appropriate next step?

(A) Obtain autoimmune serology panel, including antihistone antibodies.
(B) Increase prednisone to 1 mg/kg/d and refer for biopsy of the temporal artery.
(C) Evaluate for occult malignancy, including CT of the abdomen.
(D) Measure creatine kinase and aldolase levels and refer for electromyography of hip flexors.

ANSWER: B

The sudden onset of prolonged morning stiffness of shoulders and hip girdle is typical of polymyalgia rheumatica, yet the patient's symptoms did not respond to a corticosteroid dosage that typically results in rapid, dramatic improvement. The presence of constitutional symptoms (intermittent fever, weight loss) in patients with polymyalgia rheumatica increases the likelihood of giant cell arteritis, even in the absence of increased erythrocyte sedimentation rate, abnormal C-reactive protein levels, or classic giant cell arteritis symptoms, such as headache and jaw claudication. Patients who do not respond to low-dose corticosteroid therapy and have constitutional symptoms should undergo biopsy of the temporal artery (SOE=B). To avoid the risk of sudden, irreversible blindness, patients should be treated with prednisone 1 mg/kg/d while awaiting biopsy. Histopathologic changes supportive of giant cell arteritis remain for weeks to months after initiation of prednisone.

Antihistone antibodies are helpful in diagnosing drug-induced systemic lupus erythematosus, which can be precipitated by hydralazine. This patient's symptoms, however, are consistent with polymyalgia rheumatica and giant cell arteritis, not systemic lupus erythematosus.

Occult malignancy is part of the differential diagnosis for an older adult who has fever and weight loss. CT of the abdomen is unnecessary, however, because the increased ALT and AST levels suggest polymyalgia rheumatica and giant cell arteritis. Although uncommon, polymyalgia rheumatica may occur as a paraneoplastic syndrome; this possibility should be considered if the patient does not respond to high-dose corticosteroid therapy or if her symptoms quickly recur with attempted corticosteroid taper.

Measurement of creatine kinase and aldolase levels and electromyography are indicated for the evaluation of an inflammatory myopathy, such as polymyositis. Patients with polymyositis have proximal muscle weakness, not morning stiffness. This patient's weakness is related to suboptimal effort because of pain.

115. A 76-year-old woman comes to the office because she has acute low back pain. History includes hypertension, gastroesophageal reflux disease, angina, and back pain. Medications are enalapril 10 mg/d, hydrochlorothiazide 12.5 mg/d, isosorbide mononitrate 60 mg/d, acetaminophen 500 mg q6h, and calcium citrate 500 mg/d, as well as a daily multivitamin containing vitamin D 400 IU. In addition, she has taken omeprazole 20 mg q12h for 2 years and alendronate 70 mg/wk for 3 months. She eats 3–4 servings of dairy products daily and walks about 1 mile daily. She has not fallen in the past year.

On examination, blood pressure is 120/85 mmHg. Weight is 47.6 kg (105 lb). Serum creatinine level is 0.8 mg/dL, and 25(OH)D level is 34 mcg/L. Radiography of the lumbar spine reveals a vertebral fracture. Dual-energy x-ray absorptiometry of the hip and spine shows bone mineral density T scores of −1.3 and −1.7, respectively.

Which of the following is most likely to improve her bone health?

(A) Reduce omeprazole to 20 mg/d.
(B) Reduce alendronate to 35 mg/wk.
(C) Increase vitamin D supplementation to 1,000 IU/d.
(D) Increase calcium citrate to 500 mg q12h.

ANSWER: A

According to several epidemiologic studies, proton-pump inhibitors (PPIs) may be associated with increased risk of hip, wrist, and spine fractures (SOE=B). Some studies found that patients at greatest risk of fractures received high doses of PPIs or used them for ≥1 year. Many patients use PPIs as indicated for long-term management of gastroesophageal reflux disease, peptic ulcer disease, and moderate-to-severe dyspepsia. Some patients, however, take a PPI for vague symptoms or because it was initiated as prophylaxis during a hospital stay and was never discontinued. Whenever possible, stepdown therapy should be attempted to the lowest effective dose, or an alternative therapy should be tried, such as H_2-receptor antagonists. Because this patient's gastroesophageal symptoms are presently controlled and did not increase with the start of alendronate therapy, it would be prudent to reduce the omeprazole dosage to 20 mg/d and monitor symptoms.

Although her T score is above the −2.5 threshold, this patient has osteoporosis as evidenced by a vertebral fracture. Alendronate 70 mg/wk is appropriate for treatment (SOE=A); the lower dosage, 35 mg/wk, is indicated for prevention of osteoporosis. The patient's creatinine clearance, calculated by the Cockcroft-Gault equation, is 45 mL/min.

The recommended dietary allowance for vitamin D is 600 IU for adults <70 years old and 800 IU for those ≥71 years old in order to achieve 25(OH)D levels ≥20 ng/mL, which the Institute of Medicine (IOM) defines as adequate to meet the needs of ≥97.5% of the population. (There is some controversy regarding the 25(OH)D target: practice guidelines from the American Association of Clinical Endocrinologists and the National Osteoporosis Foundation, published before release of the IOM report, recommend a target between 30 and 60 ng/mL.) Most multivitamins contain ≥400 IU of vitamin D, and some formulations for older adults contain amounts as high as 1,000 IU. With her diet and multivitamin, her level of 25(OH)D is adequate; thus, there is no need to increase the vitamin D dosage to 1,000 IU (SOE=C). Because the patient achieves the recommended elemental calcium intake of 1,200 mg/d through her diet and current level of supplementation, there is no need to increase that supplement either (SOE=C).

116. A 72-year-old man is admitted to the hospital because he has been refusing to eat and has lost approximately 30% of his body weight. History includes multiple sclerosis, which has increased in severity over the last months, and intellectual disability. He has lived in a nursing home for the past 15 years. His only relative was his sister, who visited him almost every day. She died 3 months ago, and since then the patient has deteriorated; he has become incontinent and has stopped eating and participating in social events. He appears to have a psychotic depression. He is physically able to swallow.

Therapy with psychotropic medications is started but then discontinued because of adverse effects. If his nutritional status improves, it may be possible to resume medication or administer electroconvulsive therapy. He refused intravenous feedings but then acquiesced, only to pull out the intravenous line hours later. An alternative is to perform percutaneous endoscopic gastrostomy (PEG) and discharge the patient to the nursing home.

Which of the following is the most appropriate course for this patient?

(A) Ask the hospital's institutional ethics committee to determine the patient's best interest.
(B) Determine whether the nursing home can accommodate him if he does not undergo PEG.
(C) Ask the hospital for administrative consent to perform PEG.
(D) Ask the hospital to secure a court order to allow PEG.
(E) Enroll the patient in hospice for palliative care.

ANSWER: A

With no relative or friend committed to his welfare, this patient is vulnerable and needs healthcare providers to advocate for his best interest. In such circumstances, it is best to convene a multidisciplinary group to ensure full and robust assessment of the patient's needs and interests.

His refusal to assent to placement of intravenous lines could be interpreted as a choice. Effective informed consent provides ethical as well as legal authorization for the clinician to treat. *Consent,* however, contrasts with *assent.* The latter, a notion with particular relevance in pediatrics, reflects the patient's agreement with a treatment plan, rather than authorization of it. Only when the conditions of disclosure, understanding, and voluntariness have been met in the context of decisional capacity can the patient's consent or refusal be considered truly informed. In this case, it may be that the patient pulls out the intravenous line because of bother or discomfort. It is hard to interpret his wishes because of his limited ability to communicate.

A more stark argument would be that the patient has actually refused artificial nutrition and hydration. The refusal would be legally and ethically adequate if there were evidence that he repeatedly pulled out the line. It is an established principle of law and ethics that a capable patient has the right to refuse any proposed medical treatment, even if the likely consequence is death. Respecting the patient's refusal, like seeking the patient's consent, is an aspect of honoring the patient's autonomy.

However, acting as if the patient is capable of making a decision when he is not abandons the patient to his disabilities.

A patient's refusal of recommended treatment should prompt a discussion about the reasons for the refusal. The patient might not understand the nature of the treatment and its potential risks and benefits, may have fears relating to the treatment that can be addressed, or may have a treatable depression. Because of their profound implications, refusals of life-sustaining treatment in particular should receive heightened scrutiny. This patient is either unwilling or unable to communicate. It may be that he is not really refusing nutrition per se but is so deeply enmeshed in grieving that he avoids all contact with others. Because this is a complicated case and focused psychiatric care will likely be required to address the patient's needs, all interventions that address artificial food and fluid should await a more nuanced and careful assessment of the unaddressed psychiatric needs by a multidisciplinary team. Resolving the issues surrounding PEG as well as referral to hospice care is premature. An open forum, in which the issues can be discussed with staff from the nursing home who know the patient well, can avoid the twin pitfalls of abandonment and arbitrary decision making.

117. An 89-year-old woman is brought to the office for a routine visit. History includes Alzheimer disease and hypothyroidism that is under control. She lives in an assisted-living facility and has no complaints, except that she does not like the food there. She has lost 2.3 kg (5 lb) in the last 2 months. Her blood pressure has been increasing over the last 5 office visits.

On examination, blood pressure is 177/76 mmHg, consistent with the measurements at the assisted-living facility. Renal function is normal.

Which of the following is the best approach for managing her blood pressure?

(A) Start hydrochlorothiazide.
(B) Start lisinopril.
(C) Start a low-sodium, high-potassium (DASH) diet.
(D) Continue monitoring and treat when the systolic pressure is consistently >180 mmHg.
(E) No treatment is necessary.

ANSWER: A

With systolic pressure consistently ≥160 mmHg, this patient has stage 2 hypertension. Hydrochlorothiazide is a first-line agent for systolic hypertension and a good choice for this patient. There is no need to wait to treat her blood pressure, which has been increased on multiple occasions. In the HYVET (Hypertension in the Very Elderly) study, treatment of high blood pressure in adults who were ≥80 years old reduced the incidence of heart failure by 64% and the incidence of stroke by 30% (SOE=A). In that study, the number needed to treat (NNT) for 2 years to prevent 1 stroke was 94; the NNT to reduce 2-year mortality was 40.

The ACE inhibitor lisinopril is not a first-line agent for an older adult with systolic hypertension. A low-sodium, high-potassium DASH diet (www.nhlbi.nih.gov/health/public/heart/hbp/dash/new_dash.pdf) is an important treatment strategy for patients with prehypertension or stage 1 hypertension (systolic pressure between 140 and 159 mmHg; diastolic pressure between 90 and 99 mmHg). Although the DASH diet is appropriate for most hypertensive patients (with or without medication), diet restrictions may have limited value for older patients who are losing weight and have diminished appetite; the restrictions may exacerbate weight loss and may contribute to malnutrition. In addition, a specialized diet may be unavailable in an assisted-living facility.

118. In discussions with older Hispanic adults about end-of-life decisions, which of the following is commonly a factor?

(A) Older adults tend to make autonomous decisions.
(B) Older adults usually refuse life-sustaining treatments.
(C) Final decisions are usually made by one family member.
(D) Final decisions are usually made by several extended-family members.

ANSWER: D

Hispanic adults often confer with several extended-family members in end-of-life discussions, but the final decision usually rests with one family member (SOE=B). End-of-life decision making in minority populations tends to be family centered. For example, when compared with white Americans, Hispanic Americans are more likely to believe that the family—and not the patient—should be told of a terminal prognosis and that the family—not the patient—should make decisions regarding life support (SOE=B).

Among Hispanic Americans, the family's role is meant to remove some of the burden of treatment decisions from the older patient (SOE=B). Hispanics commonly embrace life-sustaining treatments, rather than refuse them. Older Hispanic adults do not tend to make autonomous end-of-life decisions.

119. An 88-year-old man is brought by his daughter to the emergency department because he has fever and lethargy. The daughter believes that he is the victim of physical abuse at the nursing home where he lives. At a later date, the daughter presses formal charges against the nursing home, and the medical chart is subpoenaed and becomes a legal document. The following is the medical record from the emergency department visit, as documented by the admitting physician:

History of present illness: 88-year-old man with a history of coronary artery disease, atrial fibrillation, Parkinson disease, Lewy body dementia admitted from nursing home for agitation and falls. Over last 2 weeks, noted to be more restless, especially in the late afternoon. Over the past 2 days, during bathing and diaper changes, patient was noted to scream and attempt to hit and bite the nursing aides. Decreased appetite. Constipated for 4 days. Patient currently denies chest pain or dyspnea. Remainder of review of systems negative.

History obtained from patient's daughter: Daughter alleges physical abuse at the nursing home. She describes the patient as "wasting away" over the last 3 months. Usually he is alert, recognizes her, and can have simple conversations, but over the last 2 weeks has been more confused.

Medications: Aspirin 81 mg/d, warfarin 2 mg at bedtime, extended-release metoprolol 25 mg/d, lisinopril 10 mg/d, carbidopa/levodopa 25/250 mg q8h, and quetiapine 25 mg at bedtime.

Vital signs: Blood pressure 150/90 mmHg, heart rate 90 beats per minute

Physical exam
General: Patient appears malnourished and agitated.
Eyes, nose, throat: Very dry oral mucous membranes.
Skin: Partially healed abrasion over right cheekbone. On right lateral chest wall, there is a 4 × 8 cm irregular purple ecchymosis that is tender to palpation. On both wrists, there are red and purple ecchymoses that are circumferential and nontender to palpation.
Gait: Normal base, steady without an assistive device.

Which of the following segments of the clinician's note best represents effective medical documentation for suspected abuse?

(A) History of present illness
(B) History obtained from the patient's daughter
(C) Description of the patient's vital signs
(D) Description of patient's behaviors
(E) Description of patient's ecchymoses

ANSWER: E

The description of the patient's ecchymoses represents the most effective documentation for both medical and legal purposes. The abnormal skin findings are described clearly and objectively. Clinicians may be tempted to describe bruises as healing or resolving based on their color. However, in one study, the color of the bruise did not reliably predict its age: 16% of bruises were predominantly yellow on the first day of observation, and reddish coloration was observed throughout the life cycle of the bruises. The location of bruises may be correlated with likelihood of abuse. In the same study, 89% of accidental bruises were located on the extremities. No bruises were observed on the ears, neck, genitalia, buttocks, or soles of the feet.

Effective documentation entails recording objective findings and remaining mindful of the legal implications of information gathered from the history and physical examination. The medical record may provide concrete evidence that affects the outcome of a legal case. When conflicts arise between the medical record and testimony at trial, the medical record may be deemed more credible. Critical components of the medical record include:

- the patient's and caregiver's accounts of the mechanism of injury, timeline of mistreatment, or both, with direct quotes when possible
- detailed description of any injuries, including the type, number, size, location, and color
- documentation of the patient's behavior and appearance
- the clinician's opinion of the adequacy of the explanations provided for any injuries

Inconsistencies between the history and physical examination findings, or between explanations provided by the patient and caregivers, represent red flags for abuse. Body diagrams, photographs, or both can be extremely helpful. The clinician should ask the patient or a surrogate for permission before taking photographs.

For the case described, the history of the present illness does not clearly indicate the source of the information about the patient's recent behavior and provides no report from the nursing-home staff for the patient's injuries. The history lacks a description of the patient's explanation for the bruises on his arms and chest wall. Given the suspicious findings of circumferential bruising around the wrists, the patient should be interviewed alone and asked direct questions about mistreatment.

The description of the patient's behavior would be more effective if it included specific examples (eg, "patient pacing around the room" or "patient getting on and off the bed"), because the term *agitated* is subject to interpretation. Similarly, a more objective assessment of the patient's nutritional status might include his weight and height or BMI, the fit of dentures if he wears them, and the fit of his clothes (SOE=D).

120. Which of the following is true regarding patients with Down syndrome and dementia?

(A) Dementia rarely develops in individuals with Down syndrome because of their shortened life span.
(B) Individuals with Down syndrome have beta-amyloid plaques and neurofibrillary tangles years before overt signs of dementia develop.
(C) Most individuals with Down syndrome and dementia live well into their sixties before they die of dementia.
(D) The finding of abnormal telomeres on the chromosomes of individuals with Down syndrome can now be used to diagnose Alzheimer disease years before there are symptoms.
(E) Palliative medications used for patients with Alzheimer disease are appropriate for patients with Down syndrome and dementia.

ANSWER: B

Various studies have reported that by age 40, virtually all adults with Down syndrome have the classic accumulation of beta-amyloid plaques and neurofibrillary tangles (SOE=B).

There are adults with Down syndrome in whom dementia never develops. In a study from the Netherlands, the prevalence of dementia doubled every 5 years between ages 45 and 59, reaching 25.6% in individuals with Down syndrome who were ≥60 years old. The absence of increased risk after age 60 may be explained by the higher rate of death, seen during 3.3 years of follow-up, among patients with Down syndrome and dementia (44.4%) than among patients with Down syndrome and no dementia (10.7%) (SOE=B).

Most individuals with Down syndrome do not live >60 years. Adults with Down syndrome tend to have premature age-related changes in their health, including conditions that affect skin and hair, earlier-onset menopause, decreased vision and hearing, new-onset seizure disorders, thyroid disorders, diabetes mellitus, obesity, and sleep disorders, particularly obstructive sleep apnea (SOE=B).

Recent advances in positron emission tomography have identified changes in telomeres that facilitate the study of adults with Down syndrome who do and do not have dementia (SOE=C), but the results are not approved for clinical application.

Well-constructed studies have not demonstrated significant palliative effects of standard cholinesterase inhibitors or memantine in patients with Down syndrome and dementia.

121. A 79-year-old man comes to the office in preparation for a planned coronary artery bypass graft within the next week. History includes 3-vessel coronary artery disease, hypertension, hypercholesterolemia, stroke, and depression. Findings from preoperative geriatric consultation include a Mini–Mental State Examination (MMSE) score of 29 of 30 and a Geriatric Depression Scale score of 7.

On physical examination, blood pressure is 166/84 mmHg. There is a 2+ holosystolic murmur, and there are 1+ dorsalis pedis pulses bilaterally.

Laboratory findings:

Electrolytes	Normal
BUN	24 mg/dL
Creatinine	1.4 mg/dL
Hematocrit	35.10%
Albumin	3.1 g/dL

The patient and his family have been told that his history of stroke places him at high risk of delirium during his hospitalization. They ask whether there are additional factors that affect his risk.

Which of the following independent variables are significantly associated with postoperative delirium in older adults?

(A) Low albumin and hypertension
(B) Low albumin and anemia
(C) Low albumin and Geriatric Depression Scale score >4
(D) Hypertension and anemia
(E) Hypertension and renal dysfunction

ANSWER: C

All hospitalized older adults are at risk of delirium, and some patients are at particularly high risk. Predictive models can be used to identify which medical and surgical geriatric patients are at high risk (SOE=A). This patient's risk can be quantified by using a predictive scale from a study evaluating risk factors for delirium in patients ≥60 years old undergoing cardiac surgery. The following were associated with development of postoperative delirium: low MMSE score (≤23 = 2 points, 24–27 = 1 point); history of stroke or transient ischemic attack (1 point); Geriatric Depression Scale score >4 (1 point); and abnormal albumin level (1 point). Compared with individuals with no points, in patients with 1 point the risk of delirium more than doubled. In patients with ≥3 points, the risk of delirium more than quadrupled. For this patient, the combination of a high Geriatric Depression Scale score, history of stroke, and low albumin level indicates that he is at high risk of postoperative delirium.

In a risk stratification system for medical patients, 1 point is assigned to each of the following risk factors: vision impairment, severe illness (a composite of nurse rating and APACHE II [Acute Physiology and Chronic Health Examination] score >16), cognitive impairment (MMSE score <24), and BUN to creatinine ratio ≥18. Patients with no points had a 3%–9% risk of delirium, while those with 3 or 4 points had a risk of 32%–83%.

Among older adults undergoing noncardiac surgery, postoperative delirium was associated with the following independent correlates: age ≥70 years; alcohol abuse; cognitive impairment (as determined by the Telephone Interview for Cognitive Status); severe physical functional impairment (as determined by the American Society of Anesthesiologists physical status classification system); markedly abnormal serum sodium, potassium, or glucose level; noncardiac thoracic surgery; and aortic aneurysm surgery. Adults with no risk factors had a 2% rate of delirium; those with ≥3 factors had a 50% risk of postoperative delirium. In another study, which comprised patients who were ≥70 years old undergoing hip surgery, the following factors were investigated: binocular near vision worse than 20/70 after correction; severe illness (APACHE II score >16); MMSE score <24; and dehydration (BUN to creatinine ratio ≥18). In patients with none of these risk factors, the incidence of postoperative delirium was 3.8%. The incidence increased to 11.1% among individuals with 1 or 2 risk factors, and to 37.1% in patients with ≥3 risk factors.

Renal dysfunction was not included in the predictive scale for older adults undergoing cardiac surgery. Hypertension and anemia have not been identified as useful predictors of delirium in older adults.

122. A 78-year-old woman comes to the office because she has had lower back pain for 3 weeks. The pain bothers her when she sits or stands and worsens when she moves from sitting to standing positions or when she bends; the pain lessens when she lies down. The pain has become progressively worse, and she has been more fatigued than usual. History includes diabetes mellitus and end-stage renal disease, for which she receives hemodialysis.

On examination, motion of the lumbar spine is limited. She has pain on side flexion to the right and forward flexion of the spine. Side flexion to the left and extension do not produce pain. Straight-leg raise test is positive at 70 degrees on the right. There is mild weakness of the right great toe extensor, right hip abductor, and right hip extensor. The remainder of the examination is unremarkable.

Hematocrit is 32% and the WBC count is 14,600/µL. Radiography of the lumbar spine reveals multilevel degenerative disc changes but no other abnormalities.

Which of the following diagnoses should be excluded first?

(A) Tumor
(B) Lumbar disc disease
(C) Lumbar spinal stenosis
(D) Infection in the lumbar spine
(E) Vertebral compression fracture

ANSWER: D

The most common site of spinal infection is the lumbar region, often involving a disc, and its presentation can resemble lumbar disc displacement. This patient's positive straight-leg raise test and mild weakness of L4-5 and L5-S1 innervated leg muscles suggest disc involvement, yet her hemodialysis raises the possibility of spinal infection. Although uncommon, spinal infection occurs more often in older adults and should be considered in any patient with an indwelling venous access catheter, device, or fistula. Risk factors include diabetes mellitus, renal failure requiring hemodialysis, intravenous drug abuse, immunosuppression, and malignancy. Spinal infection most commonly involves *Staphylococcus aureus*. It is believed to arise from hematogenous spread from another site, usually bacterial endocarditis. Because spinal infection can lead to neurologic complications, including paralysis, excluding it from the differential diagnosis is a priority.

In one study of patients with spinal infection, 75% had disc infection; the remainder had isolated vertebral osteomyelitis. Disc infection is usually accompanied by vertebral infection. Back pain is the most common symptom. Up to 50% of patients have no fever; neurologic impairment, such as sensory loss or weakness, is present in ≤33% of cases. Reports of spine tenderness vary: in one study, 66% of patients were affected, in another <20%. The WBC count is increased in only 50%–60% of patients. Erythrocyte sedimentation rate and C-reactive protein levels are increased in >90% of cases.

While this patient's symptoms and signs are consistent with tumor, the presence of a vascular access catheter and the increased WBC count make infection more likely. The increased WBC count is not consistent with either lumbar disc disease or compression fracture, and pain worsened by sitting is not characteristic of lumbar spinal stenosis.

123. A 70-year-old woman comes to the office for a follow-up visit. Last week she went to the local emergency department because she had abdominal pain and diarrhea for >24 hours; while there, she underwent CT of the abdomen. The emergency department physician diagnosed a viral illness. The abdominal symptoms have resolved, and she reports no change in her overall health. History includes hypertension controlled with hydrochlorothiazide.

On physical examination, all findings are normal. The final CT report is now available and refers to the presence of a 2.5-cm left adrenal mass. Electrolyte, blood sugar, and fractionated plasma metanephrine levels are normal, as are results of an overnight dexamethasone suppression test.

Which of the following is the most appropriate next step?

(A) Refer the patient to a surgeon for removal of the adrenal mass.
(B) Refer the patient for fine-needle aspiration biopsy of the adrenal mass.
(C) Obtain MRI.
(D) Schedule repeat CT in 3 months.
(E) Explain to the patient that no follow-up is needed.

ANSWER: D

CT should be repeated 3 months after initial discovery for patients who have an adrenal nodule measuring between 2 and 4 cm, or in whom the initial image is suspicious (SOE=C). For patients who have no history of malignancy and who have small (<2 cm), uniform, hypodense cortical nodules suggesting a benign lesion, repeat imaging in 3–6 months is reasonable. Current practice is to surgically remove any tumor that enlarges by >1 cm in diameter during the follow-up period (SOE=C) or that is >4 cm on initial observation. Glucocorticoid and catecholamine function should be evaluated annually for 4 years in cases in which initial evaluation is negative (SOE=C).

A homogeneous adrenal mass <4 cm in diameter with a smooth border, low attenuation value (<10 HU on unenhanced CT), and rapid contrast medium washout (>50% at 10 minutes) is most likely a benign cortical adenoma. Characteristics suggesting adrenal carcinoma or metastases include irregular shape, diameter >4 cm, inhomogeneous density, high attenuation values (>20 HU on unenhanced CT), delayed contrast medium washout, and tumor calcification. Pheochromocytoma should be excluded in all patients by measuring 24-hour urine fractionated metanephrine and catecholamine levels or plasma fractionated metanephrine levels (SOE=D). Subclinical Cushing syndrome should be excluded with the 1-mg overnight dexamethasone suppression test (SOE=D). In patients with hypertension, primary aldosteronism should be excluded by calculation of the plasma aldosterone to plasma renin activity ratio and plasma potassium concentration (SOE=D).

124. A 72-year-old woman is brought to the office because she has a bad taste in her mouth and says that her dentures keep falling out. History includes type 2 diabetes mellitus, hypertension, and dementia. Medications are metformin, valsartan, and memantine. Three weeks ago she was given nitrofurantoin for 1 week for a urinary tract infection.

On examination, there are white plaques on the surface of her cheeks, hard palate, and tongue. Wiping off some of the white plaques reveals an erythematous mucosal surface.

Which of the following is the most likely diagnosis?

(A) Hairy leukoplakia
(B) Plaque-type lichen planus
(C) Acute pseudomembranous candidiasis
(D) White sponge nevus

ANSWER: C

Acute pseudomembranous candidiasis is an infection of the oral mucosa caused by *Candida albicans*. Use of antibiotics or topical or systemic corticosteroids can contribute to growth of the fungus, as can medications that cause dry mouth, such as those used for depression or endocrine diseases (especially diabetes mellitus). The organisms grow primarily on the epithelial surface as multiple, nonadherent white plaques. Removal of the white plaques reveals an erythematous mucosal surface (SOE=A).

Candidiasis can develop on any oral mucosal site. Patients may note a dry mouth and bad taste. A cytology smear can be prepared from the pseudomembrane debris for diagnosis (SOE=B).

Oral candidiasis can be treated with clotrimazole troches or with nystatin ointment or oral suspension. For chronic candidiasis, systemic antifungals such as ketoconazole, fluconazole, and itraconazole can be used. Itraconazole should be used with caution if the patient is also taking warfarin.

White sponge nevus appears as white, folded, dysplasia lesions and occurs bilaterally on buccal mucosa; it cannot be rubbed off. The lesion presents at birth or childhood and remains unchanged throughout life, although it may become more pronounced during pregnancy. It is asymptomatic (SOE=B).

Hairy leukoplakia appears as adherent white plaques, mostly on the lateral borders of the tongue. The surface of each lesion is wrinkly and rough, and the white plaques cannot be rubbed off. These lesions are seen most often in individuals with compromised immunity (SOE=C).

Plaque-type lichen planus appears as adherent, circumscribed white plaques that cannot be rubbed off. The white plaques are asymptomatic and not usually associated with dry mouth and bad taste (SOE=C).

125. A 65-year-old woman comes to the office for her "Welcome to Medicare" preventive visit. She has no history of chronic medical conditions. She experienced menopause at age 50 and did not take hormone replacement therapy. Her only medications are vitamins and supplements, including 2,000 IU omega-3 fish oil capsules, a daily multivitamin, vitamin C 500 mg, vitamin E 400 IU, and calcium 1,000 mg q12h. She performs aerobic weight-bearing exercise for 30 min daily and weight training for 30 min, 3 times per week. She has never smoked, and she drinks only an occasional glass of red wine. She has 3 servings of calcium daily, and her diet is high in fruits and vegetables. She consumes little red meat, and eats organically raised chicken and fish. Family history is significant for her mother's death after hip fracture at age 90.

On physical examination, blood pressure is 120/70 mmHg. She has no documented height loss. CBC, basic comprehensive metabolic panel, and fasting serum lipid levels are normal. Serum calcium is 9.5 mg/dL and 25(OH)D is 30 mcg/L.

On baseline bone densitometry, T scores are −0.9 for lumbar spine, −1.1 for total hip, and −1.2 for left femoral neck. Using FRAX® (Fracture Risk Assessment Tool), her 10-year probability for major osteoporotic fracture is 19%, and for hip fracture, 1.4%.

Which of the following is the most appropriate recommendation?

(A) Prescribe oral ibandronate 150 mg, once each month.
(B) Prescribe oral raloxifene 60 mg/d.
(C) Decrease total calcium intake to 1,200 mg/d.
(D) Recommend supplemental vitamin D_3 800 IU/d.

ANSWER: C

Calcium supplementation is recommended for prevention and treatment of osteoporosis. However, this patient is taking more than 3,200 mg of calcium daily through diet and supplements. She meets the recommended daily allowance (RDA) of 1,200 mg through diet alone: her 3 servings of calcium daily provide a total of 900 mg/d, and her well-balanced diet provides an additional 300 mg/d. Further supplementation with calcium tablets is not necessary and may be associated with adverse cardiovascular events. There is no increase in cardiovascular events when adequate calcium is taken through diet alone (SOE=C).

In its 2010 report, the Institute of Medicine (IOM) maintained 1,200 mg as the recommended RDA for women >50 years old and men >71 years old. Based on national surveys, adequate calcium intake is achieved through diet for most populations, except for girls 9–19 years old. The IOM report also raised concern about the consequences of excessive calcium intake (eg, kidney stones), especially in postmenopausal woman, including an increase in cardiovascular events (SOE=C).

The IOM noted the lack of evidence regarding high-dose vitamin D supplementation for prevention or treatment of a variety of conditions, including cancer, cardiovascular disease and hypertension, diabetes and metabolic syndrome, falls, immune response, neuropsychologic functioning, physical performance, preeclampsia, and reproductive health. The studies that reported benefit beyond bone health were not considered reliable and had mixed and inconclusive results. A scientifically based threshold was found only for 25(OH)D. The threshold—a serum value of 20 ng/mL—is generally achieved with 400 IU/d in the general population (SOE=C).

Although the patient has low bone mass, she falls below the 10-year probability of a hip fracture ≥3% or a 10-year probability of a major osteoporosis-related fracture of ≥20% on the U.S.-adapted WHO algorithm. Thus, treatment with oral ibandronate or raloxifene is not indicated at this point.

GRS8 EDITORIAL BOARD

CONTRIBUTING CHAPTER AUTHORS

Marc E. Agronin, MD
Associate Professor of Psychiatry
University of Miami Miller School of Medicine
Medical Director for Mental Health and Clinical Research
Miami Jewish Health Systems
Cooper City, FL

Kathleen M. Akgün, MD
Assistant Professor
Yale University School of Medicine
Department of Internal Medicine
Section of Pulmonary and Critical Care Medicine
New Haven, CT
Department of Internal Medicine and General Internal Medicine
VA Connecticut Healthcare System
West Haven, CT

Douglas A. Albreski, DPM
Assistant Professor, Department of Dermatology
University of Connecticut School of Medicine
Director of the Podiatric Dermatology Clinic
Farmington, CT

Cathy A. Alessi, MD, AGSF
Director, Geriatric Research, Education and Clinical Center
Veterans Administration Greater Los Angeles Healthcare System
Professor, David Geffen School of Medicine at UCLA
Los Angeles, CA

Neil B. Alexander, MD
Director, Mobility Research Center
Professor, Department of Internal Medicine,
Division of Geriatric Medicine; Research Professor,
Institute of Gerontology; University of Michigan
Director, VA Ann Arbor Health Care System GRECC
Ann Arbor, MI

Alicia I. Arbaje, MD, MPH
Assistant Professor of Medicine
Associate Director of Transitional Care Research
Division of Geriatric Medicine and Gerontology
Johns Hopkins University School of Medicine
Baltimore, MD

Priscilla F. Bade, MD, FACP, CMD
Professor of Internal Medicine
Sanford School of Medicine at the University of South Dakota
Rapid City, SD

Cynthia Barton, RN, MSN
Geriatric Nurse Practitioner, Memory and Aging Center
Assistant Clinical Professor, School of Nursing
University of California, San Francisco
San Francisco, CA

Sarah D. Berry, MD, MPH
Assistant Professor of Medicine
Harvard Medical School
Research Scientist
Institute for Aging Research
Hebrew SeniorLife
Boston, MA

Marc R. Blackman, MD
Associate Chief of Staff for Research & Development
Washington DC VAMC
Assistant Dean for VA Research
Professor of Medicine and Rehabilitation Medicine
Georgetown University School of Medicine
Professor of Medicine, Biochemistry & Molecular Biology
George Washington University School of Medicine
Washington, DC

Caroline S. Blaum, MD, MS
Diane and Arthur Belfer Professor of Geriatrics
Director, Division of Geriatrics
New York University Langone Medical Center
New York, NY

Cynthia M. Boyd, MD, MPH
Associate Professor
Division of Geriatric Medicine and Gerontology
Department of Medicine
Johns Hopkins School of Medicine
Baltimore, MD

Cynthia J. Brown, MD, MSPH
Associate Professor of Medicine
University of Alabama at Birmingham
Veterans Affairs Medical Center GRECC
Birmingham, AL

Julie C. Chapman, PsyD
Director of Neuroscience
War Related Illness & Injury Study Center (WRIISC)
Washington, DC Veterans Affairs Medical Center
Assistant Professor of Neurology
Georgetown University School of Medicine
Washington, DC

Gurkamal S. Chatta, MD
Staff Physician, Hematology-Oncology
Virginia Mason Medical Center
Cancer Institute
Seattle, WA

Colleen Christmas, MD
Program Director, Internal Medicine
Johns Hopkins Bayview Medical Center
Associate Professor of Medicine
Division of Geriatric Medicine and Gerontology
Johns Hopkins University
Baltimore, MD

Anne L. Coleman, MD, PhD
The Fran and Ray Stark Professor of Ophthalmology
Professor of Epidemiology
Jules Stein Eye Institute
UCLA David Geffen School of Medicine
Los Angeles, CA

Leo M. Cooney, Jr, MD
Humana Foundation Professor of Geriatric Medicine
Yale University School of Medicine
New Haven, CT

Grace A. Cordts, MD, MPH, MS
Medical Director, Palliative Care Consult Service
Medical Director, Care Management
Johns Hopkins Medical Center
Baltimore, MD

Steven R. Counsell, MD, AGSF
Mary Elizabeth Mitchell Professor
Director, IU Geriatrics
Scientist, IU Center for Aging Research
Indiana University School of Medicine
Indianapolis, IN

G. Willy Davila, MD
Chairman, Department of Gynecology
Head, Section of Urogynecology and Reconstructive Pelvic Surgery
Cleveland Clinic Florida
Weston, FL

Maria L. Diaz, MD
Head, Section of Ambulatory Gynecology
Department of Gynecology
Cleveland Clinic Florida
Weston, FL

Margaret A. Drickamer, MD
Professor
Yale University School of Medicine
New Haven, CT

Catherine E. DuBeau, MD
Professor of Medicine
Clinical Chief, Division of Geriatric Medicine
Departments of Medicine and Family Medicine and Community Health, and Obstetrics & Gynecology
University of Massachusetts Medical School
UMassMemorial Medical Center
Worcester, MA

Neal S. Fedarko, PhD
Professor, Division of Geriatric Medicine and Gerontology
Department of Medicine
Co-Director, Biology of Healthy Aging Program
Director, Translational Research Training Program in Gerontology & Geriatrics
Johns Hopkins University
Baltimore, MD

Mark H. Fleisher, MD, FAPA
Professor of Psychiatry & Vice Chair for Clinical Services
Department of Psychiatry
Director, Neurodevelopmental Psychiatry Services
Professor of Pediatrics (Courtesy), UNMC
Professor, Munroe-Meyer Institute (Courtesy), UNMC
University of Nebraska College of Medicine
Omaha, NE

Kathleen T. Foley, PhD, OTR/L
Assistant Professor
Department of Occupational Therapy
The University of Alabama at Birmingham
Birmingham, AL

Linda P. Fried, MD, MPH, AGSF
Dean and DeLamar Professor of Public Health
Columbia University Mailman School of Public Health
Professor of Epidemiology and Medicine
Senior Vice President, Columbia University Medical Center
New York, NY

Terry Fulmer, PhD, RN, FAAN, AGSF
Dean of the Bouvé College of Health Sciences
Northeastern University
College of Health Sciences
Boston, MA

Joseph E. Gaugler, PhD
Associate Professor, McKnight Presidential Fellow
University of Minnesota
School of Nursing
Center on Aging, Center for Gerontological Nursing
Minneapolis, MN

Allan C. Gelber, MD, MPH, PhD
Associate Professor of Medicine
Director, Rheumatology Fellowship Program
Johns Hopkins University School of Medicine
Baltimore, MD

Angela Gentili, MD
Associate Professor of Internal Medicine
Director, Geriatrics Fellowship Training Program
VAMC/Virginia Commonwealth University
Richmond, VA

JoAnn A. Giaconi, MD
Assistant Clinical Professor of Ophthalmology
Jules Stein Eye Institute
UCLA David Geffen School of Medicine and the
Veterans Administration of Greater Los Angeles
Jules Stein Eye Institute
Los Angeles, CA

Thomas M. Gill, MD
Humana Foundation Professor of Geriatric Medicine
Professor of Medicine, Epidemiology & Investigative Medicine
Yale School of Medicine
New Haven, CT

Suzanne M. Gillespie, MD, RD, CMD, FACP
Instructor of Medicine
Division of Geriatrics/Aging
University of Rochester School of Medicine and Dentistry
Rochester, NY

Jane M. Grant-Kels, MD
Assistant Dean of Clinical Affairs
University of Connecticut Health Center
Professor and Chair, Department of Dermatology
Dermatology Residency Director
Director of Dermatopathology
Director of the Cutaneous Oncology and Melanoma Program
Farmington, CT

Lisa J. Granville, MD, FACP, AGSF
Professor and Associate Chair
Department of Geriatrics
Florida State University College of Medicine
Tallahassee, FL

David A. Gruenewald, MD
Associate Professor of Medicine
Division of Gerontology and Geriatric Medicine
Department of Medicine
University of Washington School of Medicine
Geriatrics/Extended Care Service
VA Puget Sound Health Care System
Seattle, WA

Ihab Hajjar, MD, MS, FACP
Assistant Professor of Medicine
University of Southern California
Department of Medicine, Divisions of GHPGIM
Section of Geriatrics
Los Angeles, CA

Paul R. Katz, MD, CMD, AGSF
Vice President, Medical Services
Baycrest Health Science Centre
Professor of Medicine
University of Toronto
Toronto, ON

Gary J. Kennedy, MD
Professor of Psychiatry and Behavioral Science
Albert Einstein College of Medicine
Director, Division of Geriatric Psychiatry
Montefiore Medical Center
Bronx, NY

Anne M. Kenny, MD
Professor of Medicine
Center on Aging
University of Connecticut Health Center
Farmington, CT

Douglas P. Kiel, MD, MPH
Professor of Medicine
Harvard Medical School
Director Musculoskeletal Research Center
Institute for Aging Research
Hebrew SeniorLife
Boston, MA

Melinda S. Lantz, MD
Chief of Geriatric Psychiatry
Beth Israel Medical Center
New York, NY

Susan W. Lehmann, MD
Associate Professor
Department of Psychiatry and Behavioral Sciences
Johns Hopkins University School of Medicine
Baltimore, MD

Seema S. Limaye, MD
Primary Care Attending
Jesse Brown VA Medical Center
Chicago, IL

Courtney H. Lyder, ND, GNP, FAAN
Dean and Professor, School of Nursing
Assistant Director for Academic Nursing
Ronald Reagan UCLA Medical Center
University of California, Los Angeles
Los Angeles, CA

Kenneth W. Lyles, MD, AGSF
Professor of Medicine
Medical Director, Medicine Site-Based Research
Duke University School of Medicine
VA Medical Center
Durham, NC

Edward R. Marcantonio, MD, SM
Professor of Medicine
Harvard Medical School
Section Chief for Research
Director, Aging Research Program
Division of General Medicine and Primary Care
Beth Israel Deaconess Medical Center
Boston, MA

Alvin M. Matsumoto, MD
Professor of Medicine
Acting Head, Division of Gerontology & Geriatric Medicine
Department of Medicine
University of Washington School of Medicine
Associate Director, Geriatric Research, Education, and Clinical Center
VA Puget Sound Health Care System
Seattle, WA

Donovan Maust, MD
University of Pennsylvania
Geriatric Psychiatry Section
Philadelphia, PA

Robert McCann, MD, AGSF
Professor of Medicine
University of Rochester School of Medicine and Dentistry
Highland Hospital Department of Medicine
Rochester, NY

Matthew K. McNabney, MD
Associate Professor of Medicine
Johns Hopkins University
Fellowship Program Director, Geriatrics
Medical Director, Hopkins ElderPlus
Baltimore, MD

Supriya Mohile, MD, MS
Associate Professor of Medicine
Director of Geriatric Oncology
University of Rochester Medical Center
Rochester, NY

Thomas Mulligan, MD, AGSF
Director, Center on Aging and
Medical Director, Senior Services
St. Bernards Healthcare
Jonesboro, AR

Daniel L. Murman, MD, MS
Director, Behavioral and Geriatric Neurology Program
Associate Professor, Department of Neurological Sciences College of Medicine
University of Nebraska Medical Center
Omaha, NE

Aman Nanda, MD
Associate Professor of Medicine
Program Director
Geriatric Medicine Fellowship Program
Alpert Medical School of Brown University
Division of Geriatrics
Rhode Island Hospital
Providence, RI

Judith Neugroschl, MD
Medical Director, Mount Sinai School of Medicine Alzheimer's Disease Research Center Clinical Core
Co-Director, ADRC Education and Information Transfer Core
New York, NY

David W. Oslin, MD
VA Associate Chief of Staff for Behavioral Health
Director, VISN 4 MIRECC
Professor
Geriatric and Addiction Psychiatry
Perelman School of Medicine
University of Pennsylvania
Philadelphia, PA

James T. Pacala, MD, MS, AGSF
Associate Professor and Associate Head
Distinguished University Teaching Professor
Department of Family Practice and Community Health
University of Minnesota Medical School
Minneapolis, MN

Sanjeevkumar R. Patel, MD, MS
Associate Professor
Division of Nephrology
University of Michigan Medical School
Ann Arbor, MI

Sushmitha Patibandla, MD
Cardiovascular Disease–Electrophysiology
Arizona Cardiology Group
Phoenix, AZ

Vyjeyanthi S. Periyakoil, MD
Clinical Associate Professor
Director, Palliative Care Education & Training
Director, eCampus Geriatrics
VA Palo Alto Health Care System &
Stanford University School of Medicine
Stanford, CA

Edgar Pierluissi, MD
Professor of Medicine, University of California at San Francisco
Medical Director, Acute Care for Elders (ACE) Unit
San Francisco General Hospital
San Francisco, CA

Margaret Pisani, MD, MPH
Associate Professor
Yale University School of Medicine
Pulmonary & Critical Care Medicine
New Haven, CT

James S. Powers, MD, AGSF
Associate Professor of Medicine
Vanderbilt University Medical Center
Associate Clinical Director, TVHS GRECC
Nashville, TN

Michael W. Rich, MD, AGSF
Professor of Medicine
Washington University School of Medicine
Cardiovascular Division
St. Louis, MO

David Sarraf, MD
Associate Clinical Professor of Ophthalmology
Retinal Disorders and Ophthalmic Genetics Division
Jules Stein Eye Institute, UCLA School of Medicine
Los Angeles, CA

Mara A. Schonberg, MD, MPH
Assistant Professor in Medicine
Beth Israel Deaconess Medical Center
Harvard Medical School
Brookline, MA

Todd P. Semla, MS, PharmD, BCPS, FCCP, AGSF
National PBM Clinical Pharmacy Program
Manager–Mental Health & Geriatrics
Pharmacy Benefits Management Services
Department of Veterans Affairs
Associate Professor
Departments of Medicine, and Psychiatry and Behavioral Sciences
The Feinberg School of Medicine
Northwestern University
Evanston, IL

Kenneth Shay, DDS, MS
Director of Geriatrics Programs
VA Office of Geriatrics and Extended Care
Ann Arbor VA Medical Center
Ann Arbor, MI

Win-Kuang Shen, MD
Professor of Medicine
Mayo Clinic College of Medicine
Chair, Division of Cardiovascular Diseases
Mayo Clinic Arizona
Phoenix, AZ

Roy E. Smith, MD
Professor of Medicine
Hematology-Oncology
University of Pittsburgh
Pittsburgh, PA

Peter G. Snell, PhD
Adjunct Associate Professor of Medicine
Department of Internal Medicine
Division of Cardiology
UT Southwestern Medical Center
Dallas, TX

Margarita Sotelo, MD
Assistant Clinical Professor
Divisions of Geriatrics and Hospital Medicine
University of California San Francisco
San Francisco, CA

Richard G. Stefanacci, DO, MGH, MBA, AGSF, CMD
Associate Professor
Health Policy & Public Health
University of the Sciences
Philadelphia, PA

H. Keipp Talbot, MD, MPH
Assistant Professor
Department of Medicine
Division of Infectious Diseases
Vanderbilt University
Nashville, TN

Alexander W. Threlfall, MD, MA
Associate Chief, MH - SFVAMC CBOC's
Acting Director, Mental Health Service Santa Rosa CBOC
Clinical Instructor
Department of Geriatric Psychiatry
University of California, San Francisco
San Francisco, CA

George Triadafilopoulos, MD, DSc
Clinical Professor of Medicine
Division of Gastroenterology and Hepatology
Stanford University School of Medicine
Editor-in-Chief Emeritus, Gastrointestinal Endoscopy
Stanford, CA

Jocelyn E. Wiggins, MA, BM, BCh, MRCP
Assistant Professor
Division of Geriatrics
University of Michigan Medical School
Ann Arbor, MI

Kyle Widmer, MD
Assistant Professor of Medicine
Department of Internal Medicine
Sections of General Internal Medicine and Infectious Diseases
Tulane University School of Medicine
Southeast Louisiana Veterans Healthcare System
New Orleans, LA

Loren Martinez Wilkerson, MD
Medical Instructor
Department of Medicine, Division of Geriatrics
Duke University School of Medicine
Durham, NC

Jennifer L. Wolff, PhD
Associate Professor
Department of Health Policy and Management
Johns Hopkins Bloomberg School of Public Health
Baltimore, MD

Kristine Yaffe, MD
Scola Endowed Professor of Psychiatry
Associate Chair for Research
Professor, Psychiatry, Neurology and Epidemiology
University of California, San Francisco
Director, Memory Disorders Program
San Francisco VA Medical Center
San Francisco, CA

CONTRIBUTING QUESTION AUTHORS

Emaad Abdel-Rahman, MD, PhD, FASN
Professor
Division of Nephrology
University of Virginia Health System
Charlottesville, VA

R. Morgan Bain, MD
Medical Director, Palliative Care Program
Section on General Internal Medicine
Section on Gerontology and Geriatric Medicine
Wake Forest University School of Medicine
Winston-Salem, NC

Angela Catic, MD
Instructor of Medicine
Harvard Medical School
Boston, MA

Rebecca Boxer, MD, MS
Assistant Professor of Medicine
Department of Medicine
Case Western Reserve University
Harrington Heart and Vascular Institute
University Hospitals/Case Medical Center
Cleveland, OH

Rachelle Bernacki, MD, MS
Director of Quality Initiatives
Department of Psychosocial Oncology and Palliative Care
Dana Farber Cancer Institute
Division of Aging
Brigham and Women's Hospital
Boston, MA

Kenneth Brummel-Smith, MD, AGSF
Charlotte Edwards Maguire Professor and Chair
Department of Geriatrics
Florida State University College of Medicine
Tallahassee, FL

Morgan Carlson, PhD
Assistant Professor, UConn Center on Aging
Department of Genetics and Developmental Biology
University of Connecticut Health Center
Farmington, CT

Susan Charette, MD
Associate Clinical Professor
Division of Geriatrics
Department of Medicine
UCLA Medical Center
Los Angeles, CA

Carl I. Cohen, MD
SUNY Distinguished Service Professor & Director
Division of Geriatric Psychiatry
SUNY Downstate Medical Center
Brooklyn, NY

Leo M. Cooney, Jr, MD
Humana Foundation Professor of Geriatric Medicine
Yale University School of Medicine
New Haven, CT

M.E. Csuka, MD, FACP
Professor
Division of Rheumatology
Department of Medicine
Medical College of Wisconsin
Milwaukee, WI

William Dale, MD, PhD
Chief, Section of Geriatrics & Palliative Medicine
Director, Specialized Oncology Care & Research in the Elderly (SOCARE) Clinic
Chicago, IL

Ann R. Datunashvili, MD
Clinical Instructor in Medicine (Geriatrics)
Yale University School of Medicine
New Haven, CT

Nancy Neveloff Dubler, LL.B.
Senior Associate Montefiore-Einstein Bioethics Center
Consultant for Ethics New York City Health and Hospitals Corporation
Bronx, NY

Shahrooz Eshaghian, MD, FACP
Clinical Instructor
David Geffen School of Medicine at UCLA
Division of Hematology/Oncology
Cedars Sinai Medical Center
Los Angeles, CA

David V. Espino, MD, FAAFP, AGSF, CAQ-Geriatrics
Professor and Coordinator of Family Medicine Geriatrics Training
Division of Community Geriatrics
Department of Family & Community Medicine
University of Texas Health Science Center at San Antonio
San Antonio, TX

Mark H. Fleisher, MD
Professor of Psychiatry & Vice Chair for Clinical Services
Department of Psychiatry
Director, Neurodevelopmental Psychiatry Services
Professor of Pediatrics (Courtesy), UNMC
Professor, Munroe-Meyer Institute (Courtesy), UNMC
University of Nebraska College of Medicine
Omaha, NE

Daniel E. Forman, MD, FACC, FAHA
Associate Professor of Medicine, Harvard Medical School
Director, Exercise Testing Laboratory and Cardiac Rehabilitation, Brigham and Women's Hospital
Director, Cardiac Rehabilitation, VA Boston Healthcare System
Physician Scientist, New England Geriatric Research, Education, and Clinical Center
Boston, MA

Susan M. Friedman, MD, MPH, AGSF
Associate Professor of Medicine
Research Director, Geriatric Fracture Center
University of Rochester School of Medicine and Dentistry
Highland Hospital
Rochester, NY

Steven R. Gambert, MD, FACP, AGSF
Professor of Medicine
University of Maryland School of Medicine
Department of Medicine-Geriatrics
Baltimore, MD

Nalaka Gooneratne, MD
Associate Professor of Medicine
University of Pennsylvania School of Medicine
Philadelphia, PA

Angela Gentili, MD
Associate Professor of Internal Medicine
Director, Geriatrics Fellowship Program
VA Medical Center/Virginia Commonwealth University
Richmond, VA

Shelly L. Gray, PharmD, MS
Professor and Vice Chair for Curriculum and Instruction
Director, Geriatric Program and Plain Certificate
School of Pharmacy
University of Washington
Seattle, WA

Debra Greenberg, MSW, PhD
Instructor
Albert Einstein School of Medicine
Senior Social Worker
Geriatrics Division
Montefiore Medical Center
Bronx, NY

Blaine S. Greenwald, MD
Vice Chairman, Combined Department of Psychiatry
Long Island Jewish Medical Center/North Shore University Hospital
Director, Geriatric Psychiatry Division
The Zucker Hillside Hospital
Glen Oaks, NY

Namirah Jamshed, MD
Assistant Professor of Clinical Medicine
Geriatric Education Director
MedStar Washington Hospital Center
Washington DC

Theodore M. Johnson II, MD, MPH
Professor of Medicine
Emory School of Medicine
Director, Division of General Medicine and Geriatrics
Director, Emory Center for Health in Aging
Atlanta Site Director, Birmingham/Atlanta VA GRECC
Atlanta, GA

Fran E. Kaiser, MD, AGSF, FGSA
Adjunct Professor of Medicine
St. Louis University School of Medicine
St. Louis, MO
Executive Medical Director
Region Medical Director Program
Merck and Co., Inc
Upper Gwynedd, PA

Helen Kao, MD
University of California, San Francisco
Division of Geriatrics
San Francisco, CA

Catherine McVearry Kelso, MD, MS
Associate Professor of Internal Medicine
Virginia Commonwealth University
Acting, ACOS Geriatrics and Extended Care
Medical Director, Community Living Center
Medical Director, Hospice and Palliative Care
Site Director, HPM Fellowship
Ethics Consultation Coordinator, Integrated Ethics
Richmond, VA

Anne Kenny, MD
Professor of Medicine
Center on Aging
University of Connecticut Health Center
Farmington, CT

Mary B. King, MD
Geriatrician
Williamstown Medical Associates
Williamstown, MA

Tia Kostas, MD
Associate Physician, Brigham and Women's Hospital
Staff Physician, GRECC, VA Boston Healthcare System
Instructor of Medicine, Harvard Medical School
Boston, MA

Stephen Krieger, MD
Assistant Professor of Neurology
Mount Sinai Medical Center
New York, NY

Lorand Kristof, MD, MSc
William Osler Health System
Ontario, Canada

Larry W. Lawhorne, MD
Chair, Department of Geriatrics
Boonshoft School of Medicine
Wright State University
Dayton, OH

Sei J. Lee, MD, MAS
Assistant Professor
University of California, San Francisco
Senior Scholar
San Francisco VA Quality Scholars Fellowship
Division of Geriatrics
San Francisco, CA

Eric Lenze, MD
Professor
Department of Psychiatry
Washington University School of Medicine
St. Louis, MO

Michael C. Lindberg, MD, FACP
Chairman, Department of Medicine
Hartford Hospital
Hartford, CT

Hannah I. Lipman, MD, MS
Associate Director, Montefiore-Einstein Center for Bioethics
Chief, Bioethics Consultation Service
Associate Professor of Clinical Medicine
Divisions of Geriatrics and Cardiology
Montefiore-Einstein Center for Bioethics
Bronx, NY

Vera P. Luther, MD
Associate Program Director for Subspecialty Education,
Internal Medicine Residency Program
Assistant Professor of Medicine
Section on Infectious Diseases
Department of Internal Medicine
Wake Forest University Health Sciences
Winston-Salem, NC

Mary Ann McLaughlin, MD, MPH
Associate Professor of Medicine
Division of Cardiology
Mount Sinai School of Medicine
New York, NY

Daniel Ari Mendelson, MS, MD, FACP, CMD, AGSF
Associate Professor of Medicine, Division of Geriatrics
University of Rochester School of Medicine & Dentistry
Highland Hospital, Department of Medicine
Rochester, NY

Diana V. Messadi, DDS, MMSc, DMSc
Professor and Chair
Section of Oral Medicine and Orofacial Pain
Division of Oral Biology & Medicine
UCLA School of Dentistry
Los Angeles, CA

Karen L. Miller, MD
Adjunct Associate Professor
Department of Obstetrics and Gynecology
University of Utah
Salt Lake City, UT

Alison A. Moore, MD, MPH
Professor of Medicine and Psychiatry
David Geffen School of Medicine at UCLA
Division of Geriatric Medicine
Los Angeles, CA

Karin M. Ouchida, MD
Assistant Professor of Medicine
Division of Geriatrics and Gerontology
Weill Cornell Medical College/NY Presbyterian Hospital
New York, NY

Joseph G. Ouslander, MD, AGSF
Professor and Associate Dean for Geriatric Programs
Charles E. Schmidt College of Medicine
Professor (Courtesy), Christine E. Lynn College of Nursing
Florida Atlantic University
Executive Editor, Journal of the American Geriatrics Society
Boca Raton, FL

James T. Pacala, MD, MS, AGSF
Associate Professor and Associate Head
Distinguished University Teaching Professor
Department of Family Practice and Community Health
University of Minnesota Medical School
Minneapolis, MN

Kourosh Parham, MD, PhD
Associate Professor
Assistant Program Director
Director of Research
Division of Otolaryngology, Department of Surgery
University of Connecticut Health Center
Farmington, CT

Donna J. Parker, MD
Assistant Professor of Medicine
Department of Internal Medicine, Geriatrics and Palliative Care
University of New Mexico
Albuquerque, NM

Birju B. Patel, MD, FACP
Director, Bronze Geriatric Outpatient Clinic
Director, Mild Cognitive Impairment Clinic
Atlanta Veterans Affairs Medical Center
Assistant Professor of Medicine
Division of General Medicine and Geriatrics
Emory University School of Medicine
Atlanta, GA

Claire Peel, PhD, PT, FAPTA
Dean, School of Health Professions
University of North Texas Health Science Center
Ft. Worth, TX

Edgar Pierluissi, MD
Professor of Medicine, University of California at San Francisco
Medical Director, Acute Care for Elders (ACE) Unit
San Francisco General Hospital
San Francisco, CA

Anitha Rao-Frisch MD, MA
Department of Neurology
University Hospital Case Medical Center
Cleveland, OH

Julie Robison, PhD
Associate Professor of Medicine
Center on Aging
University of Connecticut Health Center
Farmington, CT

Mitchell H. Rosner, MD
Henry B. Mulholland Professor of Medicine
Chairman, Department of Medicine
University of Virginia Health System
Charlottesville, VA

Amy E. Sanders, MD, MS
Assistant Professor of Neurology
Saul R. Korey Department of Neurology
Albert Einstein College of Medicine
Bronx, NY

Alessandra Scalmati, MD
Director Montefiore Aging and Memory Center
Assistant Professor of Psychiatry and Behavioral Sciences
Albert Einstein College of Medicine
Associate Director Fellowship in Geriatric Psychiatry
Montefiore Medical Center
Bronx, NY

Gary J. Schiller, MD
Professor, Department of Medicine
Director, Hematological Malignancy/Stem Cell Transplant Program
David Geffen School of Medicine at UCLA
Division of Hematology/Oncology
UCLA School of Medicine
Los Angeles, CA

Jodie Sengstock, DPM
Past President
Michigan Podiatric Medical Association
Canton, MI

David Sengstock, MD, MS
Program Director
Fellowship in Geriatric Medicine
Oakwood Hospital
Assistant Professor
Wayne State University
Dearborn, MI

Jagat Shetty, MD
Sleep Medicine Department
University of Michigan
Ann Arbor, MI

Gwen K. Sterns, MD
Chief, Department of Ophthalmology
Rochester General Hospital
Clinical Professor of Ophthalmology
University of Rochester School of Medicine and Dentistry
Rochester, NY

Winnie Suen, MD, MSc
Assistant Professor of Medicine
Department of Internal Medicine, Section of Geriatrics
Boston University School of Medicine
Boston, MA

Dennis H. Sullivan, MD, AGSF
Director, Geriatric Research Education and Clinical Center
Central Arkansas Veterans Healthcare System
Professor, Geriatrics and Internal Medicine
Donald W. Reynolds Department of Geriatrics
University of Arkansas for Medical Sciences
Little Rock, AR

George Taler, MD
Director, Long Term Care
Washington Hospital Center
Professor, Clinical Medicine, Geriatrics and Long Term Care
Georgetown University School of Medicine
Washington, DC

John A. Taylor, III, MD, MS
Associate Professor of Surgery, Division of Urology
Chairman, Cancer Committee
University of Connecticut Health Center
Farmington, CT

Helen Torabzadeh, DDS
Lecturer
Oral Medicine and Orofacial Pain Section
UCLA School of Dentistry
Los Angeles, CA

Dennis T. Villareal, MD, FACP, FACE
Professor and Chief, Geriatrics
New Mexico VA Health Care System
University of New Mexico School of Medicine
Albuquerque, NM

Louise C. Walter, MD
Associate Professor of Medicine
Division of Geriatrics
University of California, San Francisco
San Francisco VA Medical Center
San Francisco, CA

Debra Kaye Weiner, MD
Professor of Medicine, Anesthesiology & Psychiatry
Program Director, Geriatric Medicine Fellowship
University of Pittsburgh
Staff Physician, VA Pittsburgh GRECC
University of Pittsburgh Medical Center
Pittsburgh, PA

Barbara E. Weinstein, PhD
Professor and Executive Officer
Health Sciences Doctoral Programs
The Graduate Center
The City University of New York
New York, NY

Peter J. Whitehouse, MD, PhD
Professor
Case Western Reserve University
Physician, University Hospitals Case Medical Center
Cleveland, OH

G. Darryl Wieland, PhD, MPH
Research Director–Geriatrics Services
Palmetto Health Richland Hospital
Columbia, SC

Michi Yukawa, MD, MPH
Medical Director for Community Living Center
San Francisco VA Medical Center
San Francisco, CA

Fariba S. Younai, DDS
Professor of Clinical Dentistry
Oral Medicine and Orofacial Pain
Vice Chair, Division of Oral Biology and Medicine
UCLA School of Dentistry
Los Angeles, CA

Phyllis C. Zee, MD, PhD
Professor of Neurology, Neurobiology and Physiology
Director Sleep Disorders Center
Chicago, IL

Richard Zweig, PhD
Director, Ferkauf Older Adult Program
Associate Professor of Psychology
Ferkauf Graduate School of Yeshiva University
Bronx, NY

DISCLOSURE OF FINANCIAL INTERESTS

As an accredited provider of Continuing Medical Education, the American Geriatrics Society continuously strives to ensure that the education activities planned and conducted by our faculty meet generally accepted ethical standards as codified by the ACCME, the Food and Drug Administration, and the American Medical Association's Guide for Gifts to Physicians. To this end, we have implemented a process wherein everyone who is in a position to control the content of an educational activity has disclosed to us all relevant financial relationships with any commercial interests within the past 12 months as related to the content of their presentations and under which we work to resolve any real or apparent conflicts of interest. Conflicts of interest in this particular CME activity have been resolved by having the presentation content independently peer reviewed before publication by the Editorial Board and Question Review Committee.

The following contributors (and/or their spouses/partners) have reported real or apparent conflicts of interest that have been resolved through a peer review content validation process.

Marc E. Agronin, MD
Dr. Agronin serves as a paid consultant for Eli Lilly and is a member of the speaker's bureau for Accera, Assure Rx, and Novartis.

Cathy A. Alessi, MD, AGSF
Dr. Alessi serves as a paid consultant for Optum Rx, Inc.

Priscilla F. Bade, MD, FACP, CMD
Dr. Bade works with the following commercial entities: Golden Living, Hospice of the Hills, and Internal Medicine and Geriatrics Associates, LLP.

R. Morgan Bain, MD
Dr. Bain receives grant support from the Donald W. Reynolds Foundation.

Rebecca Boxer, MD, MS
Dr. Boxer serves a paid consultant for David and Young law firm and has received grant support from the NIH and Montefiore Nursing Facility.

Cynthia M. Boyd, MD, MPH
Dr. Boyd is a paid author for UpToDate.

Cynthia J. Brown, MD, MSPH
Dr. Brown receives grant support from NIH, VA, Donald W. Reynolds Foundation, and John A. Hartford Foundation.

Julie C. Chapman, PsyD
Dr. Chapman receives grant support from the Institute for Clinical Research (ICR).

G. Willy Davila, MD
Dr. David serves as a paid consultant for AMS, CL Medical and Astellas and serves on the speaker's bureau for AMS, Astellas, and Warner-Chilcott.

Catherine E. DuBeau, MD
Dr. DuBeau serves as a paid consultant for Pfizer and UpToDate.

Mark H. Fleisher, MD, FAPA
Dr. Fleisher receives grant support from Novartis Pharmaceutical-Research.

Linda P. Fried, MD, MPH, AGSF
Dr. Fried is a paid consultant for Sanofi Aventis.

Susan M. Friedman, MD, MPH, AGSF
Dr. Friedman receives grant support from the Donald W. Reynolds Foundation and teaches courses for AO North America.

Terry Fulmer, PhD, RN, FAAN, AGSF
Dr. Fulmer is a paid consultant for Senior Bridge.

John D. Gazewood, MD, MSPH
Dr. Gazewood is a paid author for Elsevier Publishing.

Allan C. Gelber, MD, MPH, PhD
Dr. Gelber receives grant support from NIH/NIAMS, ACR/REF, Human Genome Sciences and Amgen.

Angela Gentili, MD
Dr. Gentili receives grant support from VHA Rehabilitation Research and Development.

JoAnn A. Giaconi, MD
Dr. Giaconi is a paid consultant for Allergan Inc.

Nalaka Gooneratne, MD
Dr. Gooneratne receives grant support from Respironics, Inc.

Theodore M. Johnson, II, MD, MPH
Dr. Johnson receives grant support from the NIH, Department of Veteran Affairs, and Pfizer. He is a paid consultant for Pfizer, Ferring, and Johnson & Johnson.

Fran E. Kaiser, MD, AGSF, FGSA
Dr. Kaiser holds significant shares and is an employee of Merck & Co., Inc.

Gary J. Kennedy, MD
Dr. Kennedy receives grant support from Forest Laboratories and Pfizer.

Douglas P. Kiel, MD, MPH
Dr. Kiel is a paid consultant for Merck, Novartis, Amgen, and Lilly. He receives grant support from Merck, Amgen, and Lilly.

Eric Lenze, MD
Dr. Lenze receives grant support from Lundbeck, Roche, and Johnson & Johnson.

Courtney H. Lyder, ND, GNP, FAAN
Dr. Lyder serves as a paid consultant and is a member of the Speaker's Bureau for ConvaTec and Hill-Rom Inc. He receives grant support from ConvaTec and Hill-Rom.

Kenneth W. Lyles, MD, AGSF
Dr. Lyles receives research support from Novartis, Alliance for Better Bone Health, and Amgen. He is a paid consultant for Novartis, Procter & Gamble, Merck, Amgen, Kirin Pharmaceutical, GTx, Lilly, GSK, Bone Medical Ltd, Wyeth, and Osteologix. He is co-inventor of US Patent Application: "Methods for preventing or reducing secondary fractures after hip fracture," Number 20050272707; inventor of US Patent Application: "Medication Kits and Formulations for Preventing, Treating or Reducing Secondary Fractures After Previous Fracture," Number 12532285; and is co-inventor of US Patent Application: "Bisphosphonate Compositions and Methods for Treating Heart Failure."

Alvin M. Matsumoto, MD
Dr. Matsumoto received grant support from AbbVie (formerly Abbott) Pharmaceuticals and GlaxoSmithKline. He was a paid consultant for EliLilly Pharmaceuticals and GTx, Inc.

Robert McCann, MD, AGSF
Dr. McCann receives grant support from Donald W. Reynolds Foundation.

Karen L. Miller, MD
Dr. Miller is employed part-time by Juneau Biosciences, LLC, for women's health genetics research.

Daniel L. Murman, MD, MS
Dr. Murman has received grant support from Janssen Alzheimer's Immunotherapy, Inc. They do not have any commercially available products at this time.

Aman Nanda, MD
Dr. Nanda is a paid consultant for Kindred Health Care, Inc.

Joseph G. Ouslander, MD, AGSF
Dr. Ouslander receives grant support from Medine Industries and Point Click Care.

Margaret Pisani, MD, MPH
Dr. Pisani receives grant support from NIH.

James S. Powers, MD, AGSF
Dr. Powers serves as a paid consultant for Health Spring Pharmacy Advisory Committee.

Mitchell H. Rosner, MD
Dr. Rosner is a paid consultant for Johnson & Johnson and Astute Medical.

David Sarraf, MD
Dr. Sarraf is an investigator and paid consultant for Genentech and receives grant support from Genentech and Regeneron.

Gary J. Schiller, MD
Dr. Schiller receives grant support from Celgene Corp, Envision Communications, L&M Healthcare Communications and Millenium Selva Group. He is a member of the Speaker's Bureau for Celgene and Millenium.

Todd P. Semla, MS, PharmD, BCPS, FCCP, AGSF
Dr. Semla has received honoraria/royalties from Omnicare, Inc, LexiComp, Inc., and AARP, and his spouse is an employee and shareholder of Abbott Labs.

Richard G. Stefanacci, DO, MGH, MBA, AGSF, CMD
Dr. Stefanacci has received grant support from Avanir and is on the speaker's bureau for Amgen, BI, and Avanir. He holds significant shares of TabSafe.

Dennis H. Sullivan, MD, AGSF
Dr. Sullivan is a paid consultant for Abbott Nutrition.

Keipp Talbot, MD
Dr. Talbot receives grant support from SanofiPasteur and MedImmune/AstraZeneca.

George Taler, MD
Dr. Taler is on the speaker's bureau of Merck and Co, Inc for a non-commercial educational program.

Belinda A. Vicioso, MD, AGSF
Dr. Vicioso holds significant shares in Abbott Laboratories, Amgen, Biotech Holders Trust, Glaxosmithkline, Johnson & Johnson, Nestle, Pfizer, Procter and Gamble, Unilever, and Wyeth.

Jocelyn E. Wiggins, MA, BM, BCh, MRCP
Dr. Wiggins receives grant support from NIH.

Jennifer L. Wolff, PhD
Dr. Wolff receives grant support from NIH and AARP.

Kristine Yaffe, MD
Dr. Yaffe serves on the data safety monitoring board of Takeda and receives grant support from NIH, DOD, Alzheimer's Association, and AHAF.

Phyllis C. Zee, MD, PhD
Dr. Zee serves as a paid consultant for Takeda, UCB, Phillips/Respironics, Jazz, Purdue, and Merck and receives grant support from Phillips/Respironics. She holds significant shares in Teva and has a significant financial relationship with Zeo.

The following contributors have returned disclosure forms indicating that they (and/or their spouses/partners) have no affiliation with, or financial interest in, any commercial interest that may have direct interest in the subject matter of their chapters/questions:

Emaad Abdel-Rahman, MD, PhD, FASN
Kathleen M. Akgün, MD
Douglas A. Albreski, DPM
Neil B. Alexander, MD
Alicia I. Arbaje, MD, MPH
Cynthia Barton, RN, MSN
Judith L. Beizer, PharmD, CGP, FASCP
Rachelle Bernacki, MD, MS
Sarah D. Berry, MD, MPH
Marc R. Blackman, MD
Caroline S. Blaum, MD, MS
Marie Boltz, PhD, RN, GNP-BC
Kenneth Brummel-Smith, MD, AGSF
Elizabeth Capezuti, PhD, RN, FAAN
Morgan Carlson, PhD
Deirdre M. Carolan, CRNP, PhD
Angela Catic, MD
Susan Charette, MD
Gurkamal S. Chatta, MD
Colleen Christmas, MD
Carl I. Cohen, MD
Anne L. Coleman, MD, PhD
Leo M. Cooney, Jr, MD
Grace A. Cordts, MD, MPH, MS
Steven R. Counsell, MD, AGSF
M. E. Csuka, MD, FACP
William Dale, MD, PhD
Ann R. Datunashvili, MD
Maria L. Diaz, MD
Margaret A. Drickamer, MD
Nancy Neveloff Dubler, LL.B.
Samuel C. Durso, MD, MBA, AGSF
Shahrooz Eshaghian, MD, FACP
David V. Espino, MD, FAAFP, AGSF, CAQ-Geriatrics
Neal S. Fedarko, PhD
Ellen Flaherty, PhD, APRN, AGSF
Kathleen T. Foley, PhD, OTR/L
Daniel E. Forman, MD, FACC, FAHA
Elizabeth Galik, PhD, CRNP
Steven R. Gambert, MD, FACP, AGSF
Joseph E. Gaugler, PhD
Angela Gentili, MD
Thomas M. Gill, MD
Suzanne M. Gillespie, MD, RD
Jane M. Grant-Kels, MD
Lisa J. Granville, MD, FACP, AGSF
Shelly L. Gray, PharmD, MS
Debra Greenberg, MSW, PhD
Blaine S. Greenwald, MD
David A. Gruenewald, MD
Ihab Hajjar, MD, MS, FACP
Namirah Jamshed, MD
Helen Kao, MD
Paul R. Katz, MD, AGSF
Catherine McVearry Kelso, MD, MS
Laurie Kennedy-Malone, PhD, GNP-BC
Anne M. Kenny, MD
Mary B. King, MD
Tia Kostas, MD
Stephen Krieger, MD
Melinda S. Lantz, MD
Larry W. Lawhorne, MD
Sei J. Lee, MD, MAS
Susan W. Lehmann, MD
Michael C. Lindberg, MD, FACP
Seema S. Limaye, MD
Hannah I. Lipman, MD, MS
Vera P. Luther, MD
Edward R. Marcantonio, MD, SM
Donovan Maust, MD
Mary Ann McLaughlin, MD, MPH
Matthew McNabney, MD
Annette Medina-Walpole, MD, AGSF
Daniel Ari Mendelson, MS, MD, FACP, AGSF
Diana V. Messadi, DDS, MMSc, DMSc
Supriya Mohile, MD, MS
Alison A. Moore, MD, MPH
Thomas Mulligan, MD, AGSF
Judith Neugroschl, MD
David W. Oslin, MD
Karin M. Ouchida, MD
James T. Pacala, MD, MS, AGSF
Kourosh Parham, MD, PhD
Donna J. Parker, MD
Birju B. Patel, MD, FACP
Sanjeevkumar R. Patel, MD, MS
Sushmitha Patibandia, MD
Claire Peel, PhD, PT, FAPTA
Edgar Pierluissi, MD
Vyjeyanthi S. Periyakoil, MD
Anitha Rao-Frisch, MD, MA
Barbara Resnick, PhD, CRNP, FAAN, FAANP, AGSF
Michael W. Rich, MD, AGSF
Julie Robison, PhD
Amy E. Sanders, MD
Alessandra Scalmati, MD
Mara A. Schonberg, MD
David Sengstock, MD, MS
Jodie Sengstock, DPM
Kenneth Shay, DDS, MS
Win-Kuang Shen, MD
Jagat Shetty, MD
Roy E. Smith, MD
Peter G. Snell, PhD
Rainier Patrick Soriano, MD
Margarita Sotelo, MD
Gwen K. Sterns, MD
Winnie Suen, MD, MSc
Gail M. Sullivan, MD, MPH, AGSF
John A. Taylor, III, MD, MS
Alexander W. Threlfall, MD, MA
Helen S. Torabzadeh, DDS
George Triadafilopoulos, MD, DSc
Dennis T. Villareal, MD, FACP, FACE

Louise C. Walter, MD
Debra Kaye Weiner, MD
Barbara E. Weinstein, PhD
Peter J. Whitehouse, MD, PhD
Kyle Widmer, MD
G. Darryl Wieland, PhD, MPH
Loren Martinez Wilkerson, MD
Michi Yukawa, MD, MPH
Fariba S. Younai, DDS
Richard Zweig, PhD

INDEX

NOTE: References followed by *t* and *f* indicate tables and figures, respectively. Numbers preceded by "Q" indicate question numbers and critiques.

Abandonment, 97, 99*t*
Abciximab, 381
Abdominal aortic aneurysm, 391
    indications for repair, 392
    screening for, 72*t*, 75
Abdominal ultrasonography, 72*t*
ABI (ankle-brachial index), 355
Abiraterone, 549
Abnormal Involuntary Movement Scale (AIMS), 325
Abstinence
    from nicotine, 343
    pharmacotherapy support for, 340–341, 342*t*
    from substances of abuse, 336–337
Abuse. *See* Mistreatment
ACA (Affordable Care Act), 35, 38, 39, 40, 47, 162
    Independence at Home Act, Q100
Acamprosate, 340–341, 342*t*
Acarbose (Precose), 526*t*
ACC. *See* American College of Cardiology
Accidents, 3–4, 5*t*
Accountable Care Organizations, 35, Q80
Acculturation, 60–61
Accumulation theories of aging, 10
ACE (Acute Care for Elders), 137
Acetaminophen (Tylenol)
    for delirium, 280, 281*t*
    for musculoskeletal pain, 458
    for persistent pain, 124*t*, 126
    for persistent pain in cognitively impaired, 133–134
Achalasia, Q108
Acid excretion, 421*t*
Aclidinium, 375*t*
ACOG (American College of Obstetricians and Gynecology), 431
Acoustic therapy, 305
Acquired immunodeficiency syndrome (AIDS), 155, 502–503
Acral lentiginous melanoma, 360, 361*f*
ACSM. *See* American College of Sports Medicine
ACTH (adrenocorticotropic hormone) stimulation test, 514
Actinic cheilitis, 359
Actinic keratoses, 359, 359*f*
Action tremor, 489
Active Choices program, 69
Active Living Every Day program, 69
Activities of daily living (ADLs), 49–50, 49*t*, 132
    Barthel ADL Index, 141*t*, 145
Activity theory, 9
ACTOplus met (pioglitazone and metformin), 527*t*
Actos (pioglitazone), 527*t*
Acupuncture, 93, 94, Q34, Q40
Acute care, 156. *See also* Hospital care
Acute Care for Elders (ACE), 137
Acute colonic pseudo-obstruction, 418
Acute confusional state, 276
Acute coronary syndromes, 380–382, Q26
Acute functional decline, 53
Acute generalized exanthematous pustolosis, Q33
Acute glomerulonephritis, 425–426
Acute interstitial nephritis, 425, Q76
Acute ischemic stroke, 482–483
Acute kidney injury, 424–426, Q18, Q76
Acute mental status change, 276
Acute myeloid leukemia, 549
Acute pain, 119
Acute Physiology and Chronic Health Evaluation scoring system (APACHE III), 31–32
Acute pseudomembranous candidiasis, Q124
Acute renal failure, 426, Q18
Acute tubular necrosis, 425
Adaptive behavioral difficulties, 347
Adaptive methods, 149, 151–152
Addiction, 128, 336–343
    alcohol, Q15
    definition of, 120*t*
    drug, Q8
    magnitude of the problem, 337–338
    pseudoaddiction, 120*t*, 128
    substance abuse, 336–337
    treatment of, 340–341, 342*t*
Adenoma, cortical, Q123
ADEs. *See* Adverse drug events
ADLs. *See* Activities of daily living
Administration on Aging (AoA), 20
Adrenal androgens, 515–516
Adrenal cortex disorders, 514–516
Adrenal incidentalomas, 515, 515*t*
Adrenal insufficiency, 516
Adrenal neoplasms, 515
Adrenal nodules, Q123
α-Adrenergic agonists, 190, 191*t*
β-Adrenergic agonists, 374, 375*t*
α-Adrenergic antagonists or blockers
    adverse drug events, 86, 86*t*
    for benign prostatic hyperplasia, 438, 438*t*
    for hypertension, 406
β-Adrenergic antagonists. *See* β-Blockers
β-Adrenergic receptors, 214*t*
Adrenocorticotropic hormone stimulation test, 514
ADT (androgen-deprivation therapy), 549
Adult day care, 169
Adult foster care, 171
Adult Protective Services (APS), 101, Q4
Advance care plans, 28. *See also* Advance directives
Advance directives, 28, 33–34, 62, 160, 215
    living wills, 29
    recommendations for, 73*t*, 78
Adverse drug events, 85–86, 86*t*, Q7
    definition of, 85
    in-hospital, 134–135
    risk factors for, 85, 85*t*
Aerobic activity recommendations, 64, 65–66, 66*t*, 317
AF. *See* Atrial fibrillation
Affordable Care Act (ACA), 35, 38, 39, 40, 47, 162
    Independence at Home Act, Q100
African Americans. *See* Black Americans
Age-related changes, 11–16, 12*t*, 209–210
    in auditory system, 192
    in body composition, 209
    in bone formation, 244
    bone remodeling and bone loss, 244
    in calcium homeostasis, 510, 510*t*
    in cancer, 540–541
    cardiovascular, 378, 379*t*
    in eating, 216
    in energy requirements, 209
    in female sexuality, 446
    in fluid needs, 210
    in immune function, 494, 495*t*
    in kidney function, 420, 421*t*
    in lower urinary tract, 221
    in macronutrient needs, 210
    in male sexuality, 448
    in micronutrient requirements, 209–210
    in oral tissues, 362, 363*t*
    in pharmacodynamics, 83–84
    in pharmacokinetics, 81–83
    pulmonary, 371
    in salivary function, 365
    in salivary glands, 362, 363*t*
    in skin, 350
    in sleep, 285–286, 287*t*
    in swallowing, 216
    in taste, 368
    in teeth, 362, 363*t*
Age-related hyporeninemic hypoaldosteronism, 514

Age-related macular degeneration (ARMD), 187–188
rehabilitation for, 191
symptoms and treatment of, 184t
Age-related pathologies, 16, 16t
Agency for Health Care Policy and Research (AHCPR), 342
Agency for Healthcare Research and Quality (AHRQ)
guidelines for management of pressure ulcers, 300
guidelines for preventing pressure ulcers, 298
Aggression. *See also* Behavioral problems
in dementia, 275
intermittent, 275
management of, Q79
in nursing homes, Q79
Aging
accumulation theories of, 10
antagonistic pleiotropy theory of, 9
current issues in, 1–47
definition of, 8
demography of, 1–7
endocrine theory of, 11
epigenetic theory of, 10–11
error catastrophe theory of, 10
evolutionary theories of, 8–9
free radical theory of, 10
global trends, 1
hematopoietic response with, 530–531
hematopoietic stem cells and, 530
homeostasis and, 16–17
immune theory of, 11
mitochondrial DNA (mtDNA) theory of, 9
mutation accumulation theory of, 8
normal, 16
organ system changes of, 11–16, 12t
photoaging, 350
physiologic changes of, 11–16, 12t
physiologic theories of, 9–11
psychosocial theories of, 9
rate of living theory of, 10
stem cell/progenitor cell theory of, 11
telomere theory of, 9–10
theories of, 8–11, Q113
Agitated delirium, 282, 283t
Agitation, Q74
Cohen-Mansfield Agitation Inventory (CMAI), 268
in dementia, 267–268, 275
intermittent, 275
Agoraphobia, 320, 322t
AGS. *See* American Geriatrics Society
AHA. *See* American Heart Association
Aid to Capacity Evaluation (ACE), 28
AIDS (acquired immunodeficiency syndrome), 155, 502–503
AIMS (Abnormal Involuntary Movement Scale), 325
AKI (acute kidney injury), 424–426, Q18, Q76
Albumin, 211
Albuterol, 374, 375t, Q102
Alcohol
benefits of consumption, 338
and delirium, 281t
nutrient interactions, 211, 211t
and risk of osteoporosis, 246, 246t
Alcohol abuse, Q93
at-risk drinking, 336, 340–341, 342t
clinical settings, 338
counseling interventions for, 73t, 76
cultural and demographic factors, 338
heavy drinking, 337
low-risk or moderate drinking, 337
magnitude of the problem, 337–338
Michigan Alcoholism Screening Test (MAST)—Geriatric Version, 339
problem drinking, 340–341, 342t, Q15
Alcohol addiction, Q15
Alcohol consumption, Q15
Alcohol dependence, 340–341, 342t, Q15
Alcohol detoxification, 340–341, 342t
Alcohol-related dementia, 339
Alcohol Use Disorders Identification Test (AUDIT), 76
Alcohol Use Disorders Identification Test-Consumption (AUDIT-C) questions, 339, 341t
Alcoholics Anonymous, 340
Alcoholics Victorious, 340
Alendronate, 250, 251t, 252, Q68, Q115
ALFs (assisted-living facilities), 154, 170–171, Q63
Allergic conjunctivitis, 184–185, 185–186, 185t
Allodynia, 120t
Allopurinol hypersensitivity syndrome, Q11
Alosetron, 416–417
α-Adrenergic agonists, 86, 86t, 190, 191t
α-Adrenergic antagonists or blockers
adverse drug events, 86, 86t
for benign prostatic hyperplasia, 438, 438t
for hypertension, 406
Alprazolam, 87, 281t
Alprostadil, 451–452, 451t
ALS (amyotrophic lateral sclerosis), 490–491
Alteplase, 482–483
Altered mental status, 276
Alternative medicine, 90–96, 91t
Alvimopan (Entereg), 414t
Alzheimer disease, 256, Q7
agitation in, Q29
Behavioral Pathology in Alzheimer Disease Rating Scale (BEHAVEAD), 268
behavioral symptoms of, Q17, Q79
deaths due to, 3–4, 5t
dementia associated with, 94
depression in, Q14
diagnostic criteria for, Q3
diagnostic features and treatment of, 259t
differential diagnosis of, 259–260
extrapyramidal signs, Q59
familial, 257
psychosis of, Q29
risk factors for, 257
Alzheimer disease caregivers, 19–20
Alzheimer's Association, 263, 266
AMA (American Medical Association), 52–53
Amantadine, Q99
and delirium, 281t
for influenza, 499
for Parkinson disease, 486
Amaryl (glimepiride), 526t
Ambulance services, 38t
Ambulatory blood pressure monitoring, 403
Ambulatory electrocardiographic monitoring, 206–207
Ambulatory function, Q73
American Academy of Family Practitioners, 212
American Academy of Ophthalmology, 183
American Academy of Otolaryngology–Head and Neck Surgery, 371–372
American Academy of Pediatrics (AAP), 174
American Association of Family Physicians (AAFP), 174
American Association of Sex Educators, Counselors, and Therapists, 447
American Cancer Society, 440
American College of Cardiology (ACC)
cardiac risk assessment for noncardiac surgery, 103, 105f
guidelines for preoperative cardiac assessment, 102–103
American College of Chest Physicians, 136
American College of Obstetricians and Gynecology (ACOG), 431
American College of Physicians (ACP), 104, 174
American College of Sports Medicine (ACSM)
Exercise is Medicine Initiative, 68
Exercise Management for Chronic Diseases and Disabilities, 68
recommendations for physical activity, 65, 67
American Diabetes Association, 520
American Dietetic Association, 212

American Geriatrics Society (AGS), 70
clinical practice guidelines for care of nursing-home residents, 160
guidelines for care of older adults with diabetes mellitus, 523
guidelines for prevention of falls, 239–240, 240–242
guidelines for research on cognitively impaired older adults, 30, 30*t*
resources, 266
American Heart Association (AHA)
cardiac risk assessment for noncardiac surgery, 103, 105*f*
guidelines for preoperative cardiac assessment, 102–103
recommendations for dental treatment of older adults, 369
recommendations for physical activity, 65, 67
recommendations for treatment of acute ischemic stroke, 483
American Indian and Alaska Natives, 542
American Medical Association (AMA), 52–53
American Medical Directors Association, 160
American Osteopathic Association (AOA), 174
American Recovery and Reinvestment Act, 47
American Society of Anesthesiologists, 102–103, 104*t*
American Urogynecologic Association, 434
American Urological Association, 440
Amiodarone, 388
Amitiza (lubiprostone), 414*t*
Amitriptyline, 281*t*
AML (acute myeloid leukemia), 549
Ammonium excretion, 421*t*
Amoxicillin
drug interactions, 87, 87*t*
for Lyme disease, 504
Amputation
assessment of, 149
in diabetes mellitus, 524
epidemiology of, 149
leg, 149
rehabilitation for, 149
Amyloid precursor protein (APP), 257
Amyotrophic lateral sclerosis, 490–491
Anagrelide, 539
Analgesia. *See also* Pain management; Palliative care
definition of, 120*t*
narcotic, 211, 458
nonopioid adjuvant, 128–129
preemptive, 109
Three-Step Analgesic Ladder (WHO), 126, 127*f*
ANAs (antinuclear antibodies), 454
Androgen ablation, 442*t*, 444
Androgen deficiency, 516
Androgen deprivation, 442*t*
Androgen-deprivation therapy, 549
Androgen receptors, 214*t*
Androgen replacement therapy, 516, 517
Androgens, adrenal, 515–516
Anemia, 531–536
of chronic disease, 533–535
diagnostic criteria for, 531
evaluation of, 531–532
hemolytic, 532, 532*t*, 536
hypoproliferative, 532–535, 532*t*, 533*f*, 534*f*
ineffective, 532, 532*t*
of inflammation, 533–534
iron therapy for, 533
laboratory evaluation of, 532, 533*f*, 534*f*
macrocytic, Q45
management of, 427
physiologic classification of, 532, 532*t*
and rehabilitation, 143
sideroblastic, 535
valve-associated, 536
Aneurysms, abdominal aortic (AAA), 391
indications for repair, 392
screening for, 72*t*, 75
Angina
interventions to reduce risk of readmission, Q6
unstable, 380
Angiodysplasia, 417
Angiotensin-converting enzyme (ACE), 214*t*
Angiotensin-converting enzyme (ACE) inhibitors
for acute coronary syndrome, 381, 382
adverse drug events, 86, 86*t*
for chronic CAD, 383
drug interactions, 87, 87*t*
for heart failure, 397, 397*t*
for hypertension, 405
for peripheral arterial disease, 392
Angiotensin-receptor blockers (ARBs)
for acute coronary syndrome, 381, 382
adverse drug events, 86, 86*t*
for chronic CAD, 383
drug interactions, 87, 87*t*
for heart failure, 397, 397*t*
for hypertension, 405
for peripheral arterial disease, 392
Angular cheilitis, 367, 367*f*
Ankle, 478–479
Ankle-brachial index (ABI), 355, 391
Anorexia, 116
Antacids
adverse drug events, 86, 86*t*
for nausea, 115*t*
nutrient interactions, 211, 211*t*
Antagonistic pleiotropy theory of aging, 9
Antalgic gait, 229–230, 229*t*
Anterior ischemic optic neuropathy, 190–191, 191*f*
Anthropometrics, 210
Antiandrogens, 443*t*
Antianxiety agents, 333
Antiarrhythmics
for acute coronary syndrome, 381–382
adverse drug events, 86, 86*t*
for atrial fibrillation, 388
Antibiotics
for community-acquired pneumonia, Q48
minimum criteria for initiation in long-term care settings, 496–497, 497*t*
nutrient interactions, 211, 211*t*
for prostatitis, 445
Anticholinergics
adverse drug events, 86, 86*t*, 224
for COPD, 374, 375*t*
and delirium, 280, 281*t*
for nausea, 115*t*
for Parkinson disease, 486
Anticoagulation therapy
adverse drug events, 86, 86*t*
cessation before surgery, 103, 107*t*
Anticonvulsants
adverse drug events, 86, 86*t*
and delirium, 281*t*
for persistent pain, 124*t*, 129
for seizures, 490, 491*t*
to stabilize mood in mania and bipolar depression, 316*t*
Antidepressants
adverse drug events, 86, 86*t*, 270–271
for alcohol detoxification, 340–341, 342*t*
for anxiety disorders, 322
for anxiety or anxious depression, Q92
and delirium, 281*t*
for dementia, 265
for depression, 312, 314*t*–315*t*
for depression in dementia, Q14
for depression in terminally ill, 117
for depressive features of behavioral disturbances in dementia, 270, 271*t*
indications for, 309, 309*t*
interventions for preventing falls with, 241*t*
for persistent pain, 124*t*, 128–129
for personality disorders, 333
sedating, 293, 294*t*
tricyclic, 124*t*, 270–271, 271*t*, 281*t*, 315*t*, Q88
Antidiuretic hormone, inappropriate, syndrome of, 422, 513
Antihistamines
adverse drug events, 86, 86*t*
and delirium, 281*t*
for nausea, 115*t*
sedating, 290, 294–295, 294*t*

Antihypertensives, 86, 86t
Antimicrobial management, 496–497
Antimuscarinics, 224, 226
Antinuclear antibodies (ANAs), 454
Antiparkinsonian agents
adverse drug events, 86, 86t
and delirium, 281t
Antiplatelet therapy
adverse drug events, 86, 86t
for thrombocytosis, 538
Antipsychotics
adverse drug events, 86, 86t, Q29
and delirium, 280, 281t
dosing and adverse events of, 325, 326t
for hypersexuality, 274–275
interventions for preventing falls with, 241t
for personality disorders, 333
for psychosis in dementia, 272–274, 273t
second generation, 281t, Q29
sedating, 293
to stabilize mood in mania and bipolar depression, 312–313, 316t
Antiretroviral therapy, highly active, 503
Antisecretory medications, 116, 116t
Antisocial personality disorder
features of, 329, 330t
therapeutic strategies for, 332, 332t
Antispasmodic medications, 116, 116t
Antithrombotics
for ACS, 381
for stroke prophylaxis in AF, 389
Anxiety attacks, Q88
Anxiety disorders, 319–323, Q88, Q92
classes of, 319–321
comorbidity, 321–322
depression with anxiety, 321
features of anxious or fearful behaviors, 329, 330t
generalized anxiety disorder, 321, 322t
marked anxiety, 321
and medical disorders, 321–322, 322t
nonpharmacologic approaches to, Q1
pharmacologic management of, 322–323
psychologic management of, 323
treatment strategies for, 322, 322t
Aortic regurgitation (AR), 384
clinical features and treatment of, 386t
diagnosis of, 385
epidemiology of, 384–385
Aortic stenosis (AS), 384, Q49
clinical features and treatment of, 386t
diagnosis of, 385
prevalence of, 384
Aortic valve surgery, Q49
APACHE III (Acute Physiology and Chronic Health Evaluation scoring system), 31–32
Apathetic thyrotoxicosis, 508
Aphthous ulcers, 367–368, 368f
Apidra (insulin glulisine), 528t
Apixaban, 389
Apolipoprotein E gene *(APOE)*, 257
Appetite stimulants, 214
APS (Adult Protective Services), 101
Aqueous outflow facilitators, 191t
Aqueous suppressants, 191t
AR. *See* Aortic regurgitation
ARBs. *See* Angiotensin-receptor blockers
Area Agencies on Aging, 266
Arformoterol, 375t
Arginine, Q47
Aripiprazole
dosing and adverse events of, 325, 326t
for psychosis in dementia, 272–273, 273t
to stabilize mood in mania and bipolar depression, 316t
ARMD (age-related macular degeneration), 187–188
rehabilitation for, 191
symptoms and treatment of, 184t
Aromatherapy, 94–95, 323
Arousal, 18
Arrhythmias
bradyarrhythmias, 390
cardiac, 385–391
indications for permanent pacemaker implantation, 390, 391t
supraventricular, 389
ventricular, 389–390
Arterial ulcers, 355–356, 356t
Arteriosclerotic parkinsonism, 230
Arteriovenous malformation, 417
Arthritic pain, Q66
Arthritis, 453
differential diagnosis of, 453, 454t
of elbow, 455
exercise for, 457
of foot, 479
general management of, 457, 458–459
of knee, 456
osteoarthritis, 458–459, 459f, Q24, Q34
prevalence of symptoms, 3, 4f
psoriatic, 355
rheumatoid arthritis, 459–460
of wrist, 455
Arthritis Foundation, 123
Arthrocentesis, 454, 461–462
Arthroplasty, total hip and knee, 147–148
Arthroscopic debridement, 459
Artificial feeding, 215
Artificial sphincter, 225
Artificial tears, Q78
AS. *See* Aortic stenosis
ASA (American Society of Anesthesiologists), 102–103, 104t
Asenapine
dosing and adverse events of, 325, 326t
for psychosis in dementia, 273t
Asian Americans
burning mouth syndrome in, 367
cancer incidence, 542
end-of-life care, 111
nursing-home population, 153
Aspiration, 217
Aspiration pneumonia, 143, 217
Aspirin therapy, Q68
for acute coronary syndrome, 381, 382
adverse drug events, 86, 86t
for atrial fibrillation, 388
for chronic CAD, 383
for diabetes mellitus, 523
low-dose, 539
for peripheral arterial disease, 392
preventive, 73t, 79
for stroke prevention, 482
Assaults on staff, Q79
Assessment, 48–53. *See also* Screening
of ambulatory function, Q73
of amputation, 149
of behavioral problems in dementia, 268–269
Berg Balance Test, 238
brown-bag evaluation, 88
of cancer patients, 543
cardiac risk assessment for noncardiac surgery, 103, 105f
cognitive, 51
comprehensive eye examination, 183
comprehensive geriatric assessment (CGA), 77, 144–145, 173–174, Q105
Confusion Assessment Method (CAM), 134, 276, 277, 277t
Confusion Assessment Method for the Intensive Care Unit (CAM-ICU), 276–277, 277t
daily evaluation of hospitalized patients, 137
of decisional capacity, 27
driving performance tests, Q51
of eating ability, Q31
executive function testing, 51
falls risk assessment, 73t
of frailty, 179–180
of gait speed, Q94
of hearing loss, 194
of hip, 141t, 145, 147
in home care, 167
at hospital admission, 131, 131t
of hospitalized older patients, 130–137
MacArthur Competency Assessment Tool, 28
medication assessment, 51

Mini-Cog Assessment Instrument for Dementia, 51, 77, 133, 258, 258*t*
Mini-Nutritional Assessment (MNA), 212
Mini-Nutritional Assessment, short form (MNA-SF), 209
Mini–Mental State Examination (MMSE), 27–28, 51, 77, 133, 258, 258*t*, Q4
Montreal Cognitive Assessment (MoCA), 51, 258, 258*t*
of nutrition, 210–212
of older drivers, 52–53
Outcome and Assessment Information Set (OASIS), 141, 166
Patient Health Questionnaire (PHQ-2), 51
Performance-Oriented Mobility Assessment (POMA), 50, 231, 238
of persistent pain, 119–121
physical, 49–51
of physical activity, 68
preoperative, 102–106
of pressure ulcers, 300–301
psychologic, 51–52
Rapid Assessment of Physical Activity, 68
rapid screening followed by, 48, 49*t*
rolling, 48
Short Form-36 Health Survey (SF-36), 52
Simplified Nutrition Assessment Questionnaire, 212
social, 52
St. Louis University Mental Status (SLUMS) examination, 51, 258, 258*t*
St. Thomas's Risk Assessment Tool (STRATIFY), 238
of swallowing, Q31
systematic, 131, 131*t*
Timed Up and Go (TUG) test, 50, 231, 236–238
of urinary incontinence, 225–226
vertebral fracture assessment (VFA), 248–249
vision testing, 73*t*, 77–78, 183
Assessment instruments, 141*t*
Assisted-living facilities, 154, 170–171, Q63
Assistive devices, 5–6, 149–150
Assistive listening devices, 195
costs of, 197, 197*t*
Asthma, 372–373, Q102
Asthma action plans, 373, 373*t*
At-risk drinking, 338, 340–341, 342*t*
At-risk substance use, 336
Atherosclerosis
in diabetes mellitus, 523–524
prevention and management of, 523–524
ATN (acute tubular necrosis), 425
Atorvastatin, 381
Atrial fibrillation, 387–389
clinical features, 387
diagnosis of, 387
in hospitalized patients, 131*t*
interventions for, 131*t*
management of, 387–389
prevalence of, 387
Atrial natriuretic hormone, 514
Atrioventricular block, 390, 391*t*
Atrophic vaginitis, Q24
Atrophy
multiple system, 487, 487*t*
urogenital, 432–433
Attention
inattention, 276, 277*t*
tests of, 276, 277*t*
Attention Screening Examination, 277
Attitudes
regarding disclosure and consent, 62
toward advance directives, 62–63
toward North American health services, 60–61
Audiometry screening, 73*t*, 78, 193–194
AudioScope™, Q10
AUDIT (Alcohol Use Disorders Identification Test), 76
AUDIT-C (Alcohol Use Disorders Identification Test-Consumption), 339, 341*t*
Auditory system changes, 192
Autoimmune skin conditions, 350–355
Automobile accidents, 52–53, Q104
Autonomy, 21
in dementia, 33
respect for, 26
Avanafil, 450–451, 451*t*
Avandamet (rosiglitazone and metformin), 527*t*
Avandaryl (rosiglitazone and glimepiride), 527*t*
Avandia (rosiglitazone), 527*t*
Aventyl (nortriptyline), 124*t*
Avoidant personality disorder
features of, 329, 330*t*
therapeutic strategies for, 332, 332*t*
Azilsartan, 397*t*
Azithromycin, 87, 87*t*, Q48
Azotemia, prerenal, 424–425

B-cell lymphoma, 549–550
Back pain, 457, 465–469, Q103, Q115, Q122
CAM for, 93
conditions causing, 465, 466*t*
laboratory tests and imaging, 468–469
management of, 469
nonsystemic causes of, 465–467
physical examination of, 468, 468*t*
systemic causes of, 465
Bacteremia, 497
Bacterial keratitis, 183, 185*t*
Bacterial meningitis, 503
Bacteriuria, 226–227
asymptomatic, 499
Balance assessment, 50, Q73
Berg Balance Scale (Test), 231, 238
Balance impairment, 241*t*, Q53, Q62
Balance screening, 73*t*
Balance training, 66, 66*t*, Q9
Balanced Budget Act of 1997 (BBA 97), 43, 46, 141
Balanced Budget Revision Act of 1999, 46
Barbiturates, 281*t*
Barthel ADL Index, 141*t*, 145
Basal cell carcinoma, 359–360, 360*f*
Baseline activity, 64
Bathing, 292
Beclomethasone diproprionate, 375*t*
Bed alarms, Q106
Bed-positioning devices, 300
Bedsores, 297. *See also* Pressure ulcers
BEHAVEAD (Behavioral Pathology in Alzheimer Disease Rating Scale), 268
Behavior changes
with delusional disorder, Q44
rapid-eye-movement (REM) behavior disorder, Q83
Behavioral health management, 317*t*
Behavioral interventions. *See also* Cognitive behavioral therapy
for dementia care, 269–270, 270*t*
for depression, 317*t*, 318
for frailty, 181
for insomnia, 274, 274*t*
for sleep problems, 291–292
for urinary incontinence, 223–224, 226
Behavioral Pathology in Alzheimer Disease Rating Scale (BEHAVEAD), 268
Behavioral problems
assessment of, 268–269
clinical features of, 267–268
in dementia, 267–275, 271*t*, Q17, Q29, Q79
differential diagnosis of, 268–269
disorders in aging adults with intellectual disability, 347
manic-like features of, 271–272, 272*t*
medications to treat depressive features of, 270, 271*t*
treatment of, 269–270, 270–275
Behavior(s)
adaptive, 347
anxious or fearful, 329, 330*t*
challenging, 345
dramatic, emotional, or erratic, 329, 330*t*
healthy behaviors, 25
maladaptive, 347
odd or eccentric, 329, 330*t*
pain behaviors in cognitively impaired, 121–122, 123*t*

self-injurious, 346
socially inappropriate, 33
violent, Q79
Beliefs, self-efficacy, 22
physical and mental health impacts of, 22, 22*t*
strategies effective for strengthening, 22
Bell's palsy (facial nerve palsy), 504
Benazepril, 397*t*
Beneficence, 26, 28*t*, 29
Benign growths, 358–359
Benign paroxysmal positional vertigo (BPPV), 199
diagnostic criteria for, 202
self-treatment of, 202*f*, 203
Benign prostatic hyperplasia, 437–439
CAM for, 95
diagnosis of, 438
epidemiology of, 437
management options for, 438, 438*t*
medical treatment of, 438–439
treatment of, 438
Benzodiazepines
adverse drug events, 86, 86*t*
adverse effects of, Q1
for alcohol detoxification, 340–341, 342*t*
for anxiety disorders, 322, 322*t*, Q88
chronic use of, 290, 294
and delirium, 280, 281*t*
dependency on, 340–341, 342*t*
drug interactions, 87, 87*t*
fall risk, Q8
for insomnia, 293, 294*t*
interventions for preventing falls with, 241*t*
for panic disorder, Q88
for sleep problems, 290, 293, 294*t*
Benztropine, 281*t*
Bereavement therapy, 313–317, 317*t*
Berg Balance Scale (Test), 231, 238
Best-interest standard, 29
β-Adrenergic agonists, 374, 375*t*
β-Adrenergic receptors, 214*t*
β-Blockers
for acute coronary syndrome, 382
adverse drug events, 86, 86*t*, 191*t*
for anxiety disorders, 322, 322*t*
for atrial fibrillation, 387
for chronic CAD, 383
for heart failure, 397–398, 397*t*
for hypertension, 406
β-Carotene, 187, 213
Betamethasone, 461–462
Bevacizumab, 187–188
Bi-level positive airway pressure (biPAP), 288
Bibliotherapy, 313–317, 317*t*
Biguanides, 525, 526*t*
Biliary disease, 412
Bio-identical hormonal products, 432
Bioavailability, 81
Biofeedback, 93–94
Biologic therapy, 545
Biologically based methods, 91, 91*t*
Biology, 8–17, Q16, Q113
Bipolar depression, 313, 316*t*
Bipolar disorder, 310–311, Q56
type 1, 310
type 2, 310
Bisacodyl (Dulcolax), 414*t*
Bisoprolol, 397*t*
Bisphosphonates
adverse drug events, 86, 86*t*, 251–252
for osteoporosis prevention and treatment, 250–252, 251*t*
for persistent pain, 129
to prevent osteoporotic fracture, Q111
renal safety of, Q68
special concerns, 253–254
Bivalirudin, 381
Black Americans, Q42, Q81
alcohol use, 338
cancer diagnosis and survival, 542
cancer incidence, 542
diabetes mellitus, 520
dual eligibles, 40
end-of-life care, 111–112
hypertension, 402
leading causes of death, 3–4, 5*t*
life expectancy, 2, 2*t*
nursing-home population, 153
oral cancer, 366
perceived health, 3, 4*t*
poverty rates, 2
pressure ulcers, 298
self-reported functional limitations, 5
social status, 21
Black cohosh, 95
Black hairy tongue, 368, 368*f*
Bladder, neurogenic, Q82
Bladder contractions, uninhibited, 221
Bladder diaries, 223
Bladder obstruction, 221
Bladder training, 223–224
Bleeding
gastrointestinal, 417
vaginal, 435–436, 436*t*, Q57
Bleeding diatheses, 537
Blepharitis, 184–185, 185*t*
Blindness
causes of, 183, 184*t*
definition of, 183
irreversible, 184*t*
reversible, 184*t*
Blood glucose screening, 72*t*
Blood pressure. *See also* Hypertension; Hypotension
classification of, 402, 402*t*
management of, Q117
screening, 72*t*
Blood pressure monitoring, Q37, Q68
ambulatory, 403
indirect or cuff, 403
Blood values, normal, 551
BMI (body mass index), 78, 210
Body-based methods, 90, 91
Body composition changes, 209
Body language, 60
Body mass index (BMI), 78, 210
Body size classification, 210
Body weight, 67
Bone
age-related changes, 12*t*, 13, 16*t*
musculoskeletal complaints, 453
Bone-anchored hearing aids (BAHA), 198, Q55
Bone disease
calcium, phosphorus, and renal bone disease, 427–428
Paget disease of bone, 512–513
Bone formation changes, 244
Bone infections, 502
Bone loss, 244. *See also* Osteoporosis
Bone mineral density testing, 247–248
diagnostic criteria for osteoporosis, 243
indications for, 248, 248*t*
recommendations for, 248
serial measurement, 254
WHO definitions, 243, 244*t*
Bone remodeling, 244
Bone-specific alkaline phosphatase, 246, 247*t*
Bone turnover, 249
Borderline personality disorder
features of, 329, 330*t*
therapeutic strategies for, 332, 332*t*
Bordetella pertussis infection, 372
Boston Naming Test, 260
Botulinum toxin, 225
Bowel incontinence, 413–415
with developmental disabilities, 348*t*, 349
Bowel obstruction
medications for, 116, 116*t*
in terminal illness, 115–116
Brachytherapy, 442*t*, 443–444
Braden Scale, 298
Bradyarrhythmias, 390
Bradycardia, 390, 391*t*
Bradykinesia, 485
Brain imaging studies, 258–259, Q46
Breast cancer, 546–547
adjunct hormonal treatment of, 547
CAM for, 95–96
characteristics of, 541–542
ethnic and racial differences in incidence, 540
hormonal therapy for, 544
metastatic, 547
racial differences in diagnosis and survival, 540
screening for, 71
Breast self-examination (BSE), 71
Breathing disorders, sleep-related, 287–288, 290
Breathlessness, 117–118
Bright light, 289, 290, 291–292, 292*t*
Brimonidine, 191*t*

British Geriatrics Society (BGS), 239–240, 240–242
Bronchodilators, inhaled, 374, 375*t*, Q102
Brown-bag review, 88, 279
BSE (breast self-examination), 71
Budesonide, 375*t*
Bulk laxatives, 414*t*
Bullous pemphigoid, 353, 353*f*, Q71
Bunion (hallux valgus), 472*t*, 474, Q43
Bunions, 472*t*
Buprenorphine, 340–341, 342*t*
Bupropion, 270–271, 271*t*, 312, 315*t*
Burch operation (colposuspension), 225
Burning mouth syndrome, 368
Bursitis, 453
  olecranon, 455
  subacromial, 455
Buspirone
  for anxiety disorders, 322, 322*t*
  for depression, 312, 315*t*
Busulfan, 539
Butorphanol, 129
Bydureon (long-acting exenatide), 527*t*
Byetta (exenatide), 527*t*
Bypass surgery, 384

C difficile–associated diarrhea, 418, 504
C-reactive protein, 380
Cachexia, 116
CAD. *See* Coronary artery disease
Caffeine, 241*t*
CAGE (Cut down, Annoy, Guilt, Eye-opener) questionnaire, 76, 339, 341*t*
Calcaneal spur, 472*t*
Calcitonin, 251*t*, 252, Q111
Calcitriol, 245
Calcium, Q125
  coronary artery content, 380
  deficiency of, 245
  dietary intake, 249–250
  disorders of metabolism of, 510–513
  drug interactions, 211, 211*t*
  foods that contain, 249–250, 250*t*
  homeostasis changes, 510, 510*t*
  RDIs for adults ≥71 years old, 210*t*, 213–214
  recommended dietary intakes, 510
  and renal bone disease, 427–428
Calcium channel blockers
  adverse drug events, 86, 86*t*, 211
  for chronic CAD, 383
  drug interactions, 87, 87*t*
  for hypertension, 406
  and incontinence, 225
Calcium-containing antacids, 86, 86*t*
Calcium pyrophosphate dihydrate deposition disease, 461–462
Calcium supplements, Q125
  for osteoporosis prevention and treatment, 246, 246*t*, 253
  preventive, 73*t*, 79
California Healthcare Foundation, 523
Callus, Q43
CAM. *See* Complementary and alternative medicine
CAM (Confusion Assessment Method), 134, 276, 277, 277*t*, Q22
Canalith repositioning procedure, 202*f*, 203
Cancer, 540
  biologic therapy for, 545
  biology of, 540–542
  breast cancer, 71, 546–547, Q50
  CAM for, 95–96
  cervical cancer, 74
  characteristics of, 541–542
  chemotherapy for, 543–544, 544*t*
  colon cancer, 71–74, 418–419, 541, 548, Q70
  colorectal cancer, 418–419, 540, 546, Q84
  endometrial cancer, Q57
  esophageal cancer, 410–411
  ethnic differences in incidence, 542
  hormonal therapy for, 544
  incidence of, 540
  laryngeal cancer, Q97
  leukemia, 542, 549, Q95
  lip cancer, 366
  lung cancer, 540, 547–548
  mortality of, 540
  oral cancer, 365–366
  ovarian cancer, 74, Q91
  physical activity recommendations for, 66*t*
  prevalence of, 3, 4*f*, 541
  principles of management of, 542–546, 550
  prostate cancer, 74, 439–444, 540, 546, 548–549, Q69, Q90, Q111
  pseudodisease, 71
  quality-of-life issues, 546
  racial differences in diagnosis and survival of, 542
  radiation therapy for, 545–546
  skin cancer, 74, 359–361
  surgery for, 443, 546, Q91
  survival of, 540
  thyroid cancer, 509–510
  treatment options, 543
  of vulva, 434
Cancer screening, 543, Q50, Q84
  counseling on, 79–80
  recommendations for, 72*t*
  tests, 70–74
Candesartan, 397*t*
Candidiasis
  acute pseudomembranous, Q124
  oral, 367, 367*f*
  skin, 352, 353*f*, 357–358
Canes, 150, 150*t*
Capacity for consent, 26, 27–30
Capsaicin cream, 458
Capsicum frutescens (cayenne), 93
Captopril, 397*t*
Carbamazepine (Tegretol, Epitol)
  adverse drug events, 86, 86*t*
  for alcohol detoxification, 340–341, 342*t*
  for behavioral disturbances in dementia with manic-like features, 272, 272*t*
  for dementia, 265
  for epilepsy, 491*t*
  for persistent pain, 124*t*, 129
  to stabilize mood in mania and bipolar depression, 316*t*
Carbidopa-levodopa
  for Parkinson disease, 485
  for periodic limb movement disorder, 289
  for restless legs syndrome, 289
Carbonic anhydrase inhibitors, 191*t*
Cardiac arrhythmias, 385–391
Cardiac assessment, preoperative, 102–103
Cardiac disease
  deaths due to, 3–4, 5*t*
  with developmental disabilities, 348*t*, 349
  prevalence of, 3, 4*f*
Cardiac rehabilitation
  for acute coronary syndrome, 382
  for chronic CAD, 384
Cardiac resynchronization therapy, 400
Cardiac risk assessment for noncardiac surgery, 103, 105*f*
Cardiac stress testing, preoperative, 103
Cardiac syncope, 206, 206*t*
Cardioembolic stroke, 482
Cardiovascular diseases and disorders, 378–394, Q26, Q49
  activity recommendations for, 66*t*
  CAM for, 93–94
  epidemiology of, 378, 378*t*
  prevalence of, 378, 378*t*
Cardiovascular events, Q7
  major, Q36
  prevention of, Q68
Cardiovascular risk factors, 379–380, 391–392
Cardiovascular system
  age-related changes in, 12*t*, 13–14, 378, 379*t*
  age-related pathologies, 16*t*
  indications for revascularization, 103, 104*t*
  postoperative management of problems, 106–107
  preoperative assessment and management of, 102–103
Care Area Assessments, 215
Care plans, 56
Care systems, 130–176
Care transitions, 162*f*
  barriers to safety, 162
  communication for, 164
  definition of, 161
  discharge destinations, 163

planning for, 109
questions to assist with, 164
steps to improve, 164
suboptimal, 161–162
target measures for improvement, 164
venues of care, 163
Caregiver Abuse Screen, 78
Caregivers, Q85
communication with, 164
dementia caregiver counseling, 313–317, 317*t*
education of, 263
family caregivers, 6, 156
role of older adult with, 100
support for, 168, 263, 266
Caregiving, 19–20
risk factors for inadequate or abusive caregiving, 97, 98*t*
Carotid sinus hypersensitivity, 241*t*
Carpal tunnel syndrome, 455–456
Carvedilol, 397*t*, 406
Castrate-resistant prostate cancer, 549
Cataracts, 184*t*, 186–187, 241*t*
Catastrophic insurance, 39
Catechol-*O*-methyltransferase inhibitors, 486
Catheter care, 226–227
Catheters, 226–227
Cavus foot, 471–473
CBE (clinical breast examination), 71
CBT. *See* Cognitive behavioral therapy
CCRCs (continuing-care retirement communities), 171
Ceftriaxone, 504, Q48
Celecoxib (Celebrex), 124*t*
Cellular senescence, Q113
Center for Medicare and Medicaid Innovations (CMI), 35, 40, 47
Center of Excellence on Elder Abuse & Neglect, 97
Centers for Medicare and Medicaid Services (CMS), 35
Federal Coordinated Health Care Office, 40
Medicare Prescription Drug Plan Finder, 39
Quality Indicator Survey (QIS) process, 157
quality measures for nursing homes, 156–157, 157*t*
Central artery occlusion, 185*t*
Central pain, 120*t*
Central sleep apnea, 287
Cephalexin, 87, 87*t*
Cerebral insufficiency, 265
Cerebrovascular disease, 480–483
deaths due to, 3–4, 5*t*
large-vessel disease, 481–482
small-vessel disease, 481
Cerumen impaction, 194
Cervical cancer screening, 74
Cervical myelopathy, 232, Q77
CGA. *See* Comprehensive geriatric assessment
Chalazion, 185*t*
Charles Bonnet syndrome, 327
Checklist of Nonverbal Pain Indicators, 122
Chemical restraints, 33
Chemoprophylaxis, 73*t*, 79
Chemosensory perception, oral, 368–369
Chemotherapy, 543–544, 544*t*
adverse effects of, Q97
Medicare benefits, Q12
for ovarian cancer, Q91
Cherry angiomas, 358–359
Chest pain, Q26
Cheynes-Stokes breathing, 287
Chinese culture, 111
Chiropractic services, 90–91
Chloral hydrate, 281*t*
Chlordiazepoxide, 281*t*
Chloride channel activators, 414*t*
Cholecalciferol (vitamin D_3)
supplements, Q125
to reduce risk of osteoporosis, 246, 246*t*
for vitamin D deficiency, 511
Cholesterol, 211, Q89
Cholesterol screening, 72*t*
Cholestyramine
adverse drug events, 86, 86*t*
for diarrhea, 115
Choline magnesium trisalicylate, 458
Cholinesterase inhibitors, Q65
adverse drug events, 86, 86*t*
for dementia, 264
Chondrocalcinosis, 461, 461*f*
Chondroitin, 92
Chorea, 488
Choroidal neovascularization, 187, 188*f*
Chromosomal telomere length, Q113
Chronic benzodiazepine use, 290, 294
Chronic constipation, 413, 413*t*
Chronic coronary artery disease, 382–384
medical therapy for, 382–384
presentation and diagnosis of, 382
Chronic cough, 372
Chronic diarrhea, 415
Chronic disease, anemia of, 533–535
Chronic dislocated metatarsal phalangeal joint, 474, 475*f*
Chronic hospitalization, 163
Chronic hypnotic use, 293–294
Chronic kidney disease, 426–428
classification of, 426
management of, 426–428
medication use in, 427
Chronic leg ulcers, 355
Chronic lower respiratory disease, 3–4, 5*t*
Chronic lymphocytic leukemia, 549, Q95
Chronic myeloproliferative disorders, 538–539
Chronic obstructive pulmonary disease, 373–374
anxiety and, 321
diagnostic criteria for, 373–374, 374*t*
exacerbation of, Q5
GOLD guidelines for, 373–374, 374*t*
inhaled bronchodilators for, 374, 375*t*
therapy for, 374, 375*t*
Chronic pain, 119, Q34. *See also* Persistent pain
Chronic pain syndromes with developmental disabilities, 348*t*, 349
Chronic subdural hematoma, 483
Chronulac (lactulose), 414*t*
Cilostazol, 392
Cimetidine, 115*t*
Ciprofloxacin
for diverticulitis, 416
drug interactions, 87, 87*t*
Circadian rhythm sleep disorders, 289
Circumduction, 229*t*
Citalopram, 270, 271*t*, 312, 314*t*
Citroma (magnesium citrate), 414*t*
Citrucel (methylcellulose), 414*t*
Clarithromycin, 87, 87*t*
Clinical breast examination (CBE), 71
Clinical feasibility, 56
Clinical management, 54
Clinical settings
promoting physical activity in, 68
rehabilitation services, 140*t*
Clinicians
in home care, 166–167
in nursing home, 159–160
Clinker theory, 10
Clock-drawing test, 51, 77
Clomipramine, 322, 322*t*
Clonazepam (Klonopin)
for persistent pain, 124*t*, 129
for REM sleep behavior disorder, 289
Clonidine, 406, 432
Clopidogrel
for acute coronary syndrome, 381
for chronic CAD, 383
drug interactions, Q36
metabolism of, Q54
for peripheral arterial disease, 392
for stroke prevention, 482
Clostridium difficile infection, 418, 504
Clotting factor deficiencies, 538
Clozapine
and delirium, 281*t*
dosing and adverse events of, 325, 326*t*
for Parkinson disease and hallucinations, 327
for psychosis in dementia, 272–273, 273*t*
CMAI (Cohen-Mansfield Agitation Inventory), 268

CMI (Center for Medicare and Medicaid Innovations), 35, 40, 47
CMS. *See* Centers for Medicare and Medicaid Services
Coaching, patient, Q6
Coagulation, 537–538. *See also* Anticoagulation
Cochlear implants, 198, 198*t*, Q55
Cockcroft-Gault equation, 83, 104–106, 420
Code of Federal Regulations, 156
Coenzyme Q_{10}, 91, 92*t*, 93
Cognitive assessment, 51
  Mini-Cog Assessment Instrument for Dementia, 51, 77, 133, 258, 258*t*
  Mini–Mental State Examination (MMSE), 27–28, 51, 77, 133, 258, 258*t*, Q4
  Montreal Cognitive Assessment (MoCA), 51, 258, 258*t*
  rapid screening followed by assessment and management, 48, 49*t*
  screening instruments for, 258, 258*t*
  St. Louis University Mental Status (SLUMS) examination, 51, 258, 258*t*
Cognitive behavioral therapy
  for anxiety disorders, 322, 322*t*
  for depression, 317*t*, 318
  for pain, 123
  for panic disorder, Q88
  for sleep problems, 291, 292*t*, 294
Cognitive bibliotherapy, 313–317, 317*t*
Cognitive enhancers, 265
Cognitive impairment, Q96
  AGS guidelines for research on cognitively impaired older adults, 30, 30*t*
  in dementia, 260, 261*t*
  in hospitalized patients, 131*t*, 133–134
  interventions for, 131*t*, 134
  interventions for preventing falls, 241*t*
  mild, 259, 259*t*, Q22
  pain assessment and treatment in, 121–122
  pain behaviors in, 121–122, 123*t*
  postoperative decline, 109
  screening for, 73*t*, 77
  sexuality and, 34
Cognitive rehabilitation, 262
Cognitive restructuring, 323
Cognitive training, 262
Cohen-Mansfield Agitation Inventory (CMAI), 268
Colace (docusate), 414*t*
Colchicine
  for gouty attacks, 460
  nutrient interactions, 211, 211*t*
Cold therapy, 457
Colitis, pseudomembranous, 418
Collagen, 225
Collapsing pes plano valgus foot, 471–473
Colon, 412–419
Colon cancer, 418–419, 548, Q70
  CAM for, 96
  prevalence of, 541
Colon cancer screening, 71–74, 72*t*
Colonic angiodysplasia, 417
Colonic ischemia, 418
Colonic polyps, 418
Colonic pseudo-obstruction, acute, 418
Colonoscopy, 71, 72*t*
Colorectal cancer, 418–419, 540, 546, Q84
  ethnic and racial differences in incidence, 540
  racial differences in diagnosis and survival, 540
Colposuspension (Burch operation), 225
Combunox (oxycodone, immediate release), 125*t*
Communication
  addressing the healthcare provider, 59
  addressing the patient, 59
  discussing death, 112
  discussing serious news, 113–114, 115*t*
  end-of-life decision-making conversations, 114
  framework for, 113–114, 115*t*
  with hearing-impaired people, 194–195, 194*t*, Q55
  key techniques, 59
  patient-clinician, 48
  respectful nonverbal communication, 60
  strategies to enhance, 48, 49*t*, 194–195, 194*t*
  strategies to facilitate, 48
  teach-back method, 59
  in transitional care, 164
  unspoken challenges, 61
Community-acquired pneumonia, 498, Q48
Community-based care, 166–172, Q63, Q100
  services not requiring change in residence, 169–170
  services requiring change of residence, 170–171
Community Care Transitions Program, 43
Community-dwelling older Americans, 236, 237*f*
Competence
  MacArthur Competency Assessment Tool, 28
  testamentary, 27
Complementary and alternative medicine, 90–96, Q40, Q89
  definition of, 90
  diversity of modalities, 90
  efficacy of, 92
  for managing illness in older adults, 92–96
  safety issues, 91–92
  usage patterns, 91, 91*t*
Complicated grief therapy, 313–317, 317*t*
Comprehensive eye examination, 183
Comprehensive geriatric assessment (CGA), 77, Q105
  in primary care, 173–174
  in rehabilitation, 144–145
Compulsions, 320, 322, 322*t*
Computed tomography, 455
COMT (catechol-*O*-methyltransferase) inhibitors, 486
Conduction disturbances, 390, 391*t*
Confusion Assessment Method (CAM), 134, 276, 277, 277*t*, Q22
Confusion Assessment Method for the Intensive Care Unit (CAM-ICU), 276–277, 277*t*
Conivaptan, 422
Conjunctivitis
  allergic, 184–185, 185–186, 185*t*
  viral, 184–185, 185*t*
Consciousness: altered level of, 276, 277*t*
Consent
  attitudes regarding, 62
  capacity for, 26, 27–30
  informed consent for research, 30
Conservatorships, 29
Constipation, 412–413
  management of chronic constipation, 413, 413*t*
  medications that may relieve, 413, 414*t*
  opioid-induced, 128
  postoperative, 108
  in terminal illness, 114–115
Consultation
  outpatient, 173–174
  proactive, 283
Continuing-care retirement communities (CCRCs), 171
Continuity theory, 9
Continuous passive-motion (CPM) machines, 148
Continuous positive airway pressure (CPAP), 287, 288, 290, 376
Control-relevant intervention, 313–317, 317*t*
Conversion disorder, 333
COPD. *See* Chronic obstructive pulmonary disease
Coping strategies, 22–23
Copper, 211, 211*t*
Corneal ulcers, 184, 185*t*, 186
Coronary artery calcium content, 380
Coronary artery disease, 380, Q26, Q89
  chronic, 382–384
  epidemiology of, 380
  medical therapy for, 382–384
  presentation and diagnosis of, 382
Coronary revascularization, 103, 104*t*

Cortical adenoma, Q123
Corticosteroids
- for asthma, Q102
- for COPD, 374, 375*t*
- for CPPD, 461–462
- for idiopathic pulmonary fibrosis, 376
- inhaled, 374, 375*t*
- ophthalmic, 186
- perioperative, 109
- for persistent pain, 129
- stress doses, 109

Costs
- of assisted-living residences, 171
- of assistive listening devices, 197, 197*t*
- of dementia care, 256
- exercise benefits, 65
- of glaucoma, 189
- of health care, 35–47
- of hearing aids, 197, 197*t*
- of nursing-home care, 155
- of preventive health measures, 70, 72*t*–73*t*
- of suboptimal care transitions, 161

Cough
- chronic, 372
- in terminal illness, 118

Councils on Aging, 266
Counseling
- on cancer screening and preventive health, 79–80
- dementia caregiver counseling, 313–317, 317*t*
- family counseling, 282, Q93
- grief counseling, Q12
- healthy lifestyle counseling, 72*t*–73*t*, 76
- for increasing physical activity, 68

COX-2 inhibitors
- for musculoskeletal pain, 458
- for persistent pain, 127

CPAP (continuous positive airway pressure), 287, 288, 290, 376
CPM (continuous passive-motion) machines, 148
CPPD (calcium pyrophosphate dihydrate deposition disease), 461–462
Cranberry juice, Q30
Creatinine clearance, 83, 420, Q115
Crepitus, Q34
Cross-cultural health care, 58
Cross-over toe deformity, 474, 475*f*
CRT (cardiac resynchronization therapy), 400
Crusted scabies (Norwegian scabies), Q33
Crutches, 150
Cruzan v. *Director, Department of Health of Missouri,* 30–31
CSA (central sleep apnea), 287
Cultural aspects of care, 21, 58–63, 111–112
- alcohol use, 338

Cultural differences, 27
Cultural identity, 59
Culturally competent care, Q42, Q118
Culture, 61
- of resident safety, Q28

Curanderos, 91
Custodial care, 38*t*
Cutaneous horn, 359
Cymbalta (duloxetine), 124*t*
Cyproheptadine, 214
Cystic erosion, 472*t*
Cystitis, Q30
Cysts, epidermal inclusion, 477
Cytochrome P450, 87, 87*t*
Cytokine-modulating agents, 214
Cytokines, inflammatory, 214*t*

Dabigatran
- adverse drug events, 86, 86*t*
- for stroke prophylaxis in AF, 389

Daily evaluation, 137
Dalteparin, 381
Dance, 262
Darifenacin, 224
Day care, 156
Day hospitals, 169
DDIs (drug-drug interactions), 87, 87*t*, 490, Q36
Death
- ability to predict time of, 31–32
- interventions that can hasten, 31
- leading causes and numbers of, 3–4, 5*t*
- overall care near, 111

Death with Dignity Act (Oregon), 31–32
Debridement, 301, 303*t*
- arthroscopic, 459

Decision making
- about institutionalization, 168–169
- approaches to, 61–62
- cultural aspects, 58–64, 111–112
- end-of-life, 30–33, 62
- ETHNICS mnemonic, 62–63
- in extended-care settings, 32–33
- family decisions, 111–112
- hierarchy of strategies, 28, 28*t*
- for patients who lack decisional capacity, 28–29
- role of incapacitated patient in, 29–30
- treatment decisions, 32–33

Decisional capacity, 26, 27–30, Q4
- assessment of, 27
- decision making for those who lack, 28–29
- elements of, 27, 28*t*
- standardized tests of, 27–28
- temporary loss of, 30

Decubitus ulcers, 297
Deep brain stimulation, 487
Deep venous thrombosis (DVT), 392, Q27
Deep venous thrombosis prophylaxis
- guidelines for, 107, 108*t*
- in hospitalized patients, 131*t*, 136
- Padua Prediction Score, 136

Defecography, 413
Defibrillators, Q58
Degenerative joint disease, 348*t*, 349
Dehydration, 210
Dehydroepiandrosterone (DHEA), 93
- safety issues, 91, 92*t*
- supplements, 515–516

Delirium, 276–284
- agitated, 282, 283*t*
- clinical features of, Q22
- and dementia, 279
- diagnosis of, 276–278, 277*t*
- differential diagnosis of, 276–278
- drugs to reduce or eliminate in management of, 280, 281*t*
- evaluation of, 279–282
- guideline for, 283–284, 284*t*
- in hospitalized patients, 134
- incidence of, 276
- management of, 279–283, 280*t*
- models of care for, 282–283
- neuropathophysiology of, 278
- pharmacologic therapy for, 282, 283*t*
- postoperative, 109, 279, Q121
- preoperative assessment and management of, 106
- prevention of, Q1
- prognosis for, 276
- psychotic symptoms in, 326
- quiet, 278
- in rehabilitation, 143–144
- reversible causes of, 278, 278*t*
- risk factors for, 278
- spectrum of, 278
- in terminal illness, 116–117
- treatment of, Q74

Delirium Abatement Program, 283
Delusional disorder, 326, Q44
Delusions, 311
- antipsychotic medications for, 272–274, 273*t*
- definition of, 324
- in dementia, 272–274, 273*t*
- evaluation of patient with, 324
- of infidelity, 326
- mood-congruent, 326
- of poverty, 326
- somatic, 326

Dementia, 256–266, Q3, Q7
- advanced, Q65
- aggression or agitation in, 275
- alcohol-related, 339
- of Alzheimer disease, 94
- assessment of, 257–259
- associated with Parkinson disease, 486
- behavior problems in, Q17, Q29, Q79
- behavioral interventions for, 269–270, 270*t*
- behavioral problems in, 267–275
- CAM for, 94
- criteria for hospice care, Q41
- definition of, 259

delirium and, 279
delusions in, 272–274, 273*t*
depression in, 267–268, 270–271, 271*t*, Q14
diagnostic features of, 259, 259*t*
differential diagnosis of, 257–259
differentiating types of, 259–262
in Down syndrome, Q120
driving risk in, Q51
end-stage, 134
epidemiology of, 256
ethical issues in, 33–34
etiology of, 256–257
frontotemporal, 256–257, 259*t*, 260
general progression of, 260, 261*t*
hallucinations in, 272–274, 273*t*
in hospitalized patients, 134
with intellectual disability, 346–347
with Lewy bodies, 487, 487*t*, Q59, Q74
Lewy body, 256–257, 259*t*, 260, 327
management of, 262–266
manic-like behavioral syndromes in, 271–272
Mini-Cog Assessment Instrument for Dementia, 51, 77, 133, 258, 258*t*
mixed, 256
mood disturbances in, 270–271
in nursing-home population, 153
pharmacologic treatment of, 264–265
prevention of, 72*t*–73*t*, 257
psychosis in, 272–274, 273*t*, 326–327, Q29
pugilistic, 346
and rehabilitation, 144
resources for, 266
reversible, 276
risk factors for, 257
safety concerns, 263–264
screening for, 77
sleep disturbances in, 274, 289–290
societal impact of, 256
supportive therapy for, 262
treatment of, 259, 259*t*, 262–266
and urinary incontinence, 221
vascular, 256, 259*t*, 260
Dementia caregiver counseling, 313–317, 317*t*
Demographics, Q81, Q104
Demography
of aging, 1–7
of nursing-home population, 153–154
Denosumab (RANK ligand inhibitor), 251*t*, 253
Dental anatomy, 362, 362*f*
Dental caries, 362–363
Dental decay, 362–363
Dental/oral conditions with developmental disabilities, 348*t*, 349
Dental pulp changes, 362, 363*t*
Dental treatment, 369–370
Denture stomatitis, 367, 367*f*
Dentures, 364–365
Dependence
alcohol, 340–341, 342*t*
benzodiazepine, 340–341, 342*t*
definition of, 336
nicotine, 340–341, 342*t*
opioid, 340–341, 342*t*
physical, 127
psychological, 128
substance, 336
tobacco, 76, 341–343
Dependent personality disorder
features of, 329, 330*t*
therapeutic strategies for, 332, 332*t*
Depression, 308–318
activity recommendations for, 66*t*
in Alzheimer disease, Q14
anxious, Q92
bipolar, 313
CAM for, 94
in chronic kidney disease, 428
clinical presentation of, 308–311
in dementia, 267–268, 270–271, Q14
with developmental disabilities, 348*t*, 349
diagnosis of, 308–311
electroconvulsive therapy for, 312, 313
epidemiology of, 308
Geriatric Depression Scale, 51, 309–310, 310*t*
in hospitalized patients, 131*t*, 133
indications to start antidepressant therapy based on PHQ-9, 309, 309*t*
interventions for, 131*t*, 133
interventions for preventing falls, 241*t*
late-life, geriatric syndrome of, 308–309
major depressive disorder, Q35, Q85
major depressive disorder with psychotic features, Q22
major depressive disorder without mania but with hypomania, 310
mania with or without, 310
with marked anxiety, 321
minor, 308, 311
in nursing-home population, 153
pharmacotherapy for, 270–271, 271*t*, 312
prescriber response guidelines based on PHQ-9 and the STAR*D studies for, 309, 310*t*
psychosocial interventions for, 313–318
psychotherapy for, 313–317, 317*t*
psychotic, 311
rapid screening followed by assessment and management of, 48, 49*t*
recommended preventive measures for, 73*t*
and rehabilitation, 143–144
remission of, 309
with severe anxiety, 322, 322*t*
subclinical, 311
subsyndromal, 308, 311
in terminal illness, 117
treatment of, 311–318, Q35, Q39, Q92
Depression care management, 313–317, 317*t*
Depression screening, 73*t*, 77, 309–310
Dermatitis
neurodermatitis, 352
seborrheic, 350–351, 351*f*
stasis dermatitis, 355
Dermatofibromas, 477
Dermatologic diseases and disorders, 350–361, Q33, Q71
skin and nail disorders of foot, 476–478
skin cancer, 359–361
skin infections, 496–497, 497*t*
Dermatomyositis, 463–464
Desipramine (Norpramin)
for depression, 315*t*
for depressive features of behavioral disturbances in dementia, 270–271, 271*t*
for persistent pain, 124*t*
Desvenlafaxine, 271*t*, 314*t*
DETERMINE checklist, 212
Detoxification, 340–341, 342*t*
Detrusor hyperactivity with impaired contractility (DHIC), 220
Detrusor overactivity, 221
Detrusor underactivity, 221
Developmental disabilities, 344–349
and health problems, 348*t*, 349
with intellectual disability, 349
Developmental disability, Q120
Device therapy, 399–400
DHEA. *See* Dehydroepiandrosterone
DHIC (detrusor hyperactivity with impaired contractility), 220
Diabetes mellitus, 520–529, Q4, Q82
activity recommendations for, 66*t*
atherosclerotic complications of, 523–524
blood pressure monitoring in, Q68
CAM for, 95
and cardiovascular risk, 379
classification of, 520
clinical evaluation of, 521–522
deaths due to, 3–4, 5*t*
diagnosis of, 521–522
education and self-management support, 528–529
evaluation of, 521–522

and foot, 478–479
guidelines for care of older adults with, 523
hyperglycemia in, 528
hypoglycemia in, 528
management of, 522–528, Q101
microvascular complications of, 524
non-insulin agents for, 525, 526*t*–527*t*
in nursing-home population, 153
pathophysiology of, 520–521
postoperative management of, 108–109
prediabetes, 520–521
prevalence of, 3, 4*f*
and rehabilitation, 144
screening for, 75
self-management support for, 528–529
syncope with, Q61
type 1, 520
type 2, 520, 521, Q25, Q37, Q101
Diabetic neuropathy, painful, Q112
Diabetic retinopathy, 184*t*, 188–189, 190*f*
Diagnostic and Statistical Manual of Mental Disorders, 5th edition (DSM-5™), 319, 333
criteria for bipolar disorder type 1, 310
descriptions of personality disorders, 329
Diagnostic and Statistical Manual of Mental Disorders, 5th edition, Text Revision (DSM-5™)
criteria for intellectual disability, 344
Diagnostic imaging, 38*t*
Diagnostic laboratory tests
in falls, 238
health insurance coverage for, 38*t*
Diagnostic-related groups (DRGs), 166
Dialectical behavior therapy, 313–317, 317*t*
Dialysis, renal, 428–429, 428*t*
Diarrhea
C difficile–associated, 418, 504
chronic, 415
infectious, 504–505
postoperative, 108
in terminal illness, 115
Diazepam, 87, 281*t*, Q7, Q8, Q88
Diaβeta (glyburide), 526*t*
DIC (disseminated intravascular coagulation), 536
Diclofenac sodium, 124*t*
Dicyclomine, 225
Diet
altered consistencies, 217, 218*t*
and cancer, 96
for chronic kidney disease, 428
Modified Diet in Renal Disease (MDRD) formula, 83, 104–106, 420
for pressure ulcers, 302
Dietary management
of cholesterol levels, Q89
Dietary reference intakes (DRIs), 209–210
Dietary Supplement Health and Education Act (DSHEA), 91
Dietary supplements, 213–214
for pressure ulcers, 302
safety issues, 91, 92*t*
Dietitians, 142, 143*t*
Diffuse large B-cell lymphoma, 549–550
Digestive problems. *See* Gastrointestinal diseases and disorders
Digestive system
age-related changes, 12*t*, 14–15
age-related pathologies, 16*t*
Digit flexus, 472*t*
Digit quinti varus, 472*t*
Digital rectal examination, 440, Q90
Digoxin
adverse drug events, 86, 86*t*, 211
drug interactions, 87, 87*t*
for heart failure, 398–399
nutrient interactions, 211, 211*t*
Dihydropyridines, 211
Dilaudid (hydromorphone), 125*t*
Diltiazem
adverse drug events, 86, 86*t*
for atrial fibrillation, 387
Dilutional hyponatremia, 422
Diphenhydramine
adverse drug events, 86, 86*t*, 295
and delirium, 281*t*
for nausea, 115*t*
Dipivefrin, 191*t*
Diplopia, 183, 185*t*
Disability
excess, 338–339
International Classification of Functioning, Disability, and Health (ICF) (WHO), 139
preclinical, 50
trends in, 4–5
Disability accommodation, 5–6
Disabled dual eligibles, 40
Disalcid (salsalate), 125*t*
Discharge destinations, 163
Discharge medication regimen, 163
Discharge planning
reengineered discharge intervention, Q6
telehealth discharge interventions, Q6
Disclosure, 62
Discontinuing interventions, 30–31
DISCUS (Dyskinesia Identification System Condensed User Scale), 325
Disease management, 175–176
Disease-modifying anti-inflammatory drugs (DMARDs), 460
Disengagement theory, 9
Dislocation
of lesser metatarsal phalangeal joint, 472*t*
of metatarsal phalangeal joint, 474, 475*f*
Disorganized thinking, 276, 277*t*
Disseminated intravascular coagulation, 536
Disulfiram, 340–341, 342*t*
Diuretics
adverse drug events, 86, 86*t*
drug interactions, 87, 87*t*
for heart failure, 398
for hypertension, 405
loop, 398
nutrient interactions, 211, 211*t*
thiazide-type, 405
Divalproex sodium
for behavioral disturbances in dementia with manic-like features, 272, 272*t*
for personality disorders, 332–333
to stabilize mood in mania and bipolar depression, 312–313, 316*t*
Diverticular disease, 415–416
Dix-Hallpike test, 202, 230
Dizziness, 199–203, Q53, Q75
classification of, 199–201, 201*t*
diagnostic testing for, 203
drug-induced, Q68
evaluation of, 201–203
history, 201
management of, 203
mixed, 199, 201*t*
physical examination of, 201–202
prevalence of, 199
DMARDs (disease-modifying anti-inflammatory drugs), 460
DO (detrusor overactivity), 221
"Do-not-hospitalize" orders, 160
Do-not-resuscitate ("DNR") bracelets, 29
Docetaxel, 544, 549
Docusate (Colace), 414*t*
Donepezil, 264, 346–347
adverse effects of, Q7
for paranoia, Q17
Doorway thoughts in cross-cultural health care, 58
Dopamine agonists
and delirium, 281*t*
for Parkinson disease, 486
for periodic limb movement disorder, 289
for restless legs syndrome, 289
Dopamine antagonists, 115*t*
Doppler ultrasonography, Q46
Dorzolamide, 191*t*
Double crush phenomenon, 455–456
Double effect, rule of, 31
Down syndrome, 344, 346, Q120
Doxazosin, Q36
Doxepin
and delirium, 281*t*
for insomnia, 293, 294*t*
Doxycycline, 504, Q48
DPP-4 enzyme inhibitors, 525, 526*t*

Dramatic, emotional, or erratic
behaviors, 329, 330*t*
Dressings for pressure ulcers, 301–302, 304*t*
DRGs (diagnostic-related groups), 166
Drinking. *See* Alcohol
DRIs (dietary reference intakes), 209–210
Driving
ethical issues, 33
risk factors for automobile accidents, 52–53
Driving assessment, 52–53
driving performance tests, Q51
recommendations for, 73*t*, 78
Dronabinol, 214
Dronedarone, 388
Drug abuse. *See also* Substance abuse
addiction, Q8
magnitude of the problem, 337
Drug-disease interactions, 490
Drug-drug interactions (DDIs), 87, 87*t*, 490, Q36
Drug holidays, 252
Drug-induced esophageal injury, 410
Drug-induced movement disorders, 488–489
Drug-nutrient interactions, 211, 211*t*
Drug regimen review, 89
Drugs. *See also* Pharmacotherapy; *specific drugs*
absorption of, 81–82
adverse drug events, 85*t*, 86, 86*t*, 321–322, Q68
for anxiety disorders, 322–323, 322*t*
to avoid in older adults, 129
in chronic kidney disease, 427
clearance of, 82–83
for depressive features of behavioral disturbances in dementia, 270, 271*t*
discontinuing, 88
distribution of, 82
elimination of, 82–83
guidelines for prevention of falls, 239
half-life of, 82–83
health insurance coverage for, 38*t*
hydrophilic, 82
inappropriate/overprescribed and underprescribed medications/ classes, 84, 84*t*, 85
for incontinence, 224–225
interventions for preventing falls, 241*t*
lipophilic, 82
Medicare Prescription Drug Plan Finder (CMS), 39
metabolism of, 82
nonadherence to regimens, 89
outpatient, 38*t*
outpatient care, 38*t*
to reduce or eliminate in management of delirium, 280, 281*t*
risk of falls with, Q23
sleeping medications, 290
to stabilize mood in mania and bipolar depression, 316*t*
to support abstinence, 340–341, 342*t*
that can increase risk of osteoporosis, 246, 246*t*
that interfere with gustation (taste) and olfaction (smell), 368, 369*t*
that may relieve constipation, 413, 414*t*
Dry eye, 184–185, 185*t*, Q78
Dry mouth, 365
DSHEA (Dietary Supplement Health and Education Act), 91
Dual eligibles, 40, 45
Dual energy x-ray absorptiometry (DXA)
criteria for osteoporosis, 72*t*, 243
screening for osteoporosis, 427–428
Dual tasking, 231
Duetact (pioglitazone and glimepiride), 527*t*
Dulcolax (bisacodyl), 414*t*
Duloxetine (Cymbalta)
for depression, 314*t*
for depressive features of behavioral disturbances in dementia, 271*t*
for incontinence, 225
for persistent pain, 124*t*, 129
Durable medical equipment, 38*t*
Durable power of attorney for healthcare, 160
Duragesic (transdermal fentanyl), 126*t*
DVT (deep venous thrombosis), 392, Q27
DXA. *See* Dual energy x-ray absorptiometry
Dysequilibrium, 199–201, 201*t*, Q53
Dysesthesia, 120*t*
Dyskinesia Identification System Condensed User Scale (DISCUS), 325
Dyslipidemia, 379
Dyspareunia, 446, 447, 448*t*
Dyspepsia, 411
Dysphagia, 216–217, 408–409, Q31, Q108
classification of, 216
esophageal, 217
oral, 216
oropharyngeal, 217
pharyngeal, 216–217
Dyspnea, 372, Q26
in terminal illness, 117–118
Dystonia, 488, 489
Ears: age-related changes, 12*t*, 14, 16*t*
Eating assessment, Q31
Eating changes, 216
Eating problems, 216–219
Eccentric behaviors, 329, 330*t*
Ecchymoses, Q119
Echinacea, 91, 92*t*
Echocardiography, 207, Q110
transesophageal, 501
two-dimensional, Q46
Eczema, 477
Eczema craquelé, 352, 352*f*
Eden Alternative, 159
Edentulism, 364–365
Education, 3. *See also* Patient education
Effexor (venlafaxine), 124*t*
EGSYS (Evaluation of Guidelines in Syncope Study) score, 206, 206*t*
Elbow pain, 455
Elder abuse, Q4, Q119
Elder mistreatment. *See* Mistreatment
Elderly onset lupus, 463
Electrical stimulation, 304
Electrocardiography, Q46
ambulatory monitoring, 206–207
implantable loop recorders, 207
in syncope, 206–207
Electroconvulsive therapy, 312, 313
for depression in terminally ill, 117
for depressive features of behavioral disturbances in dementia, 271
Electrolyte balance, 514
Electrolyte disorders, 420–423
postoperative management of, 107
Electronic health records, 47
Electrophysiologic studies, 207
EM (erythema multiforme), Q71
Emergency care, 38*t*
hypertensive emergencies and urgencies, 407
Emotion-oriented psychotherapy, 262
Emotional behaviors, 329, 330*t*
Emotionally supportive interventions, 313–317, 317*t*
Emphysema, 373–374, 374*t*, 375*t*
Employment, 2–3
Enalapril, 397*t*
Encephalopathy, toxic or metabolic, 276
End-of-life care, 62, Q41, Q118
cultural aspects of, 111–112
financing, 45–46
for heart failure, 401
palliative care, 111–119
preventive health measures in, 72*t*–73*t*
End-of-life decisions, 30–33, 62
continuum of, 32
conversations, 114
cultural issues, 111–112
variables that should be considered, 32
End-stage kidney disease, 428–430
Endocarditis, infective, 501–502

Endocrine disorders, 506–519, Q123
postoperative management of, 108–109
Endocrine Society, 447
Endocrine system: age-related changes, 12*t*, 15–16, 16*t*
Endocrine theory of aging, 11
Endometrial cancer, 544, Q57
Endoscopic palliation, 410–411
Enemas, 413, 413*t*
Energy intake, 211
Energy requirements, 209, Q16
Energy therapy, 90, 91*t*, 93
Enhanced primary care, 174–175
Enoxaparin, 381
Entacapone, 486
Entereg (alvimopan), 414*t*
Entrapment syndrome, 472*t*
Environmental modifications
for dementia, 263
home care, 167
for preventing falls, 240, 241*t*
for rehabilitation, 149, 151–152
Epidermal inclusion cysts, 477
Epigenetic theory of aging, 10–11
Epilepsy, 489–490
Epinephrine, 191*t*
Eplerenone, 398
Epley maneuver, 202*f*, 203
Eprosartan, 397*t*
Eptifibatide, 381
Equinovarus, 229*t*
Equinus deformity, 471–473, 472*t*
Erectile dysfunction, 448–452, Q38
causes of, 448–450, 449*t*
evaluation of, 450
treatment options for, 450–452, 451*t*
Ergocalciferol (vitamin D_2) supplements, 511
Erratic behaviors, 329, 330*t*
Error catastrophe theory of aging, 10
Erythema, Q71
Erythema multiforme (EM), Q71
Erythrocyte sedimentation rate (ESR), 454
Erythroleukemia, 536
Erythromycin, 224
drug interactions, 87, 87*t*
Erythroplakia, 366, 366*f*
Erythropoiesis, ineffective, 535
Erythropoietin therapy
for anemia, 534–535
Medicare guidelines for, 427
Escitalopram, 271*t*, 314*t*, Q83
Esomeprazole, Q36
Esophageal cancer, 410–411
Esophageal dysphagia, 217
Esophagus, 408–411
drug-induced injury to, 410
gastroesophageal reflux disease, 409–410, Q54
ESR (erythrocyte sedimentation rate), 454
Essential thrombocythemia, 538, 539
Essential tremor, 489
Estrogen deficiency, 245
Estrogen therapy, 518
adverse effects of, Q111
for female sexual dysfunction, 447
for incontinence, 225
for menopausal symptoms, 432
for osteoporosis, 251*t*, 252–253
for urogenital atrophy, 432–433
for vaginal atrophy, Q21
vaginal estrogen tablets, Q21
Eszopiclone, 293, 294*t*
ET (essential thrombocythemia), 538, 539
Ethical issues, 26–34, Q116
in dementia, 33–34
in home care, 168–169
in malnutrition, 214–215
medical ethics, 26–27
normative ethics, 26
Ethics consultants, Q93
Ethnic differences: cancer, 540
ETHNICS mnemonic, 62–63
Euthanasia, 31
Evaluation of Guidelines in Syncope Study (EGSYS) score, 206, 206*t*
Evidence, 55
Evolutionary theories of aging, 8–9
Exalgo (hydromorphone, extended release), 125*t*
Exanthematous pustolosis, acute generalized, Q33
Executive function testing, 51
Executive Interview, 28
Exenatide (Byetta), 525, 527*t*
long-acting (Bydureon), 527*t*
Exercise
aerobic, Q96
cognitive benefits of, Q96
counseling for, 73*t*, 76
for dementia, 262
for depression, 317
for frailty, Q52
for gait disorders, 231–232
for musculoskeletal diseases and disorders, 457
for older adults with low fitness or low functional ability, 69
for osteoporosis prevention and treatment, 249
pelvic muscle, 223–224
for peripheral arterial disease, 392
for preventing falls, 239, 241*t*
for preventing functional decline, Q62
recommendations for, 65–67, 66*t*
to reduce risk of osteoporosis, 246, 246*t*
relative exercise intensity, 64
for sleep problems, 292
vestibular rehabilitation therapy (VRT), 203
Exercise: A Guide from the National Institute on Aging, 69
Exercise intensity, 64, 65*t*
Exercise is Medicine Initiative (ACSM), 68
Exercise Management for Chronic Diseases and Disabilities (ACSM), 68
Exercise programs, Q62
Exercise volume, 64, 65*t*
Exhaustion, 179*t*
Exploitation, 97, 99, 99*t*
Extended-care settings, 32–33
External beam radiation therapy, 442*t*
Extracellular fluid volume
contracted, 421–422
expanded, 422
normal, 422
Eye conditions, 183–186, 184*t*, 185*t*
Eye drops, 190, 191*t*
Eyes
age-related changes, 12*t*, 14, 16*t*
comprehensive examination of, 183

F-tags, 156, 225–226
FACES Pain Rating Scale with Foreign Translations, 120
Faces Pain Scale, 120, 121*f*, 306
Facial nerve palsy (Bell's palsy), 504
Factitious disorders, 333
Factor VIII, 538
Failure to thrive, 181–182
Falls, 234–242
activity recommendations for, 66*t*
causes of, 234–238
clinical guidelines for prevention of, 239–240, 240–242
history in, 236–238
in hospitalized patients, 131*t*, 132
interventions for, 131*t*, 132, 239–240, 241*t*
laboratory and diagnostic tests for, 238
mortality due to, Q104
physical examination in, 236–238
prevalence and morbidity of, 234
prevention of, 77, 236, 237*f*, 238–240, 240–242, 241*t*, Q8, Q9, Q23, Q106
risk assessment for, 73*t*, 77
risk factors for, 239–240, 241*t*
screening for, 238
treatment of, 238–240
Familial Alzheimer's disease, 257
Family caregivers, 6, 156, 256
Family counseling, 282, Q93
Family decisions, 111, 263
Family-focused therapy, 317*t*, 318
Famotidine, 115*t*
Fearful behaviors, 329, 330*t*
Febuxostat, Q11
Fecal impaction, 413
Fecal incontinence, 413–415, Q109
with developmental disabilities, 348*t*, 349
Fecal occult blood testing, 417
recommendations for, 71–74, 72*t*

Federal Coordinated Health Care Office, 40
Federal financing of health care, 46–47
Fee-for-service (FFS) care
discounted FFS, 42
home-health care, 44
inpatient care, 43
Medicare, 35, 36–37, 38*t*, 41–42, 42*t*
Medicare Advantage, 42, 43*t*
nursing-home care, 45
outpatient care, 41–42
postacute rehabilitation, 43–44
private plans, 37
Feeding, 217–219
artificial, 215
hand, 217
tube, 217, 218
Feeding problems, 216–219
Feeding tubes, 215, 217, 218, Q65
Female sexual dysfunction, 446–447
evaluation of, 447
treatment options for, 447, 448*t*
Female sexuality, 446
Fentanyl, transdermal (Duragesic), 126*t*
Fesoterodine, 224
Festination, 229*t*, 485
Fever
antibiotic therapy for, 496–497, 497*t*
evaluation of, 504*t*, 505
in frail, older residents of long-term care facilities, 495–496, 496*t*
in older nursing-home residents, 495–496
of unknown origin, 504*t*, 505
FFS care. *See* Fee-for-service care
Fiber, 413, 413*t*
FiberCon (polycarbophil), 414*t*
Fibers, viscous, Q89
Fibrinolytic therapy, 381
Fibromyalgia, 120, 456–457
Fidaxomicin, 504
FIM (Functional Independence Measure), 140–141, 142*t*
Financial assessment, 99
Financial mistreatment, 99
Financing, Q12, Q80
for assisted living, 171
costs of hearing aids, 197, 197*t*
end-of-life care, 45–46
federal, 46–47
health care, 35–47
home-health care, 44–45
for house calls, 168
inpatient care, 42–43
nursing-home care, 45, 155
outpatient care, 41–42
personal, 27, 28*t*
postacute rehabilitation, 43–44
for rehabilitation services, 139–140, 140*t*
Fingerstick monitoring, Q101
Firearms, 33
Fitness, low, 69
"Five A's" for smoking cessation, 342
Five Wishes, 29, 29*t*
Flashes, 185*t*
Flat foot, 473
Flavor enhancement, 368
Flavoxate, 225
Fleet (sodium phosphate/biphosphate emollient enema), 414*t*
Flexibility activity recommendations, 66, 66*t*
Flexible sigmoidoscopy, 71
Floaters, 183, 185*t*
Flu shots, 72*t*
Fluconazole, 87, 87*t*
Fludarabine, 544
Fludrocortisone, 241*t*
Fluid needs, 210
Fluoxetine, 224
for depression, 314*t*
for depressive features of behavioral disturbances in dementia, 270, 271*t*
to stabilize mood in mania and bipolar depression, 316*t*
Flurazepam, 281*t*
Fluticasone, 375*t*
Folate
drug interactions, 211, 211*t*
RDIs for adults ≥71 years old, 210*t*
Folate deficiency, 532, 534*f*, Q45
Folic acid, 213
Folic acid replacement, 537
Follicular lymphoma, 550
Folstein Mini–Mental State Examination (MMSE), 27–28, 51, 77, 133, 258, 258*t*, Q4
Fondaparinux, 381, 393–394
Food and Nutrition Board, Institute of Medicine, 209–210
Foods, calcium-containing, 249–250, 250*t*
Foot care, 471
Foot diseases and disorders, 471–479, 472*t*
associated deformities, 473–475, Q43
in diabetes mellitus, 524
guidelines for prevention of falls, 239–240
skin and nail disorders, 476–478
surgical considerations for deformities, 476
systemic diseases, 478–479
treatment strategies for, 475–476
Foot drop, 229–230, 229*t*
Foot examination, 524
Foot fracture, Q72
Foot slap, 229*t*
Foot ulcers, 478, Q43
Footwear
for preventing falls, 239–240
shoe terms, 476*t*
shoes, 476
Forgoing and discontinuing interventions, 30–31
Formality, 59
Formoterol fumarate, 375*t*
Fortamet (metformin), 526*t*
Fosinopril, 397*t*
Foster care, 171
Fracture risk assessment model (FRAX™) (WHO), 243, 245*t*, 246, 248, Q111
Fractures
diagnosis of, 246–249
foot, Q72
fragility, 243
of hip, 146–147, Q32
osteoporotic sacral fractures, 467, Q103, Q111
osteoporotic vertebral compression fractures, 466–467
prediction of, 246–249
prevention of, Q111
risk factors for, 245*t*, 246
sacral insufficiency fracture, Q103
secondary causes of, 246–247
vertebral, 248–249, 254–255
Fragility fracture, 243
Frail older adults
activity recommendations for, 66*t*
preventive health measures for, 72*t*–73*t*
residents of long-term care facilities, 495–496, 496*t*
Frailty, 177–182, Q9, Q52
assessment of, 179–180
and associated vulnerability, 177
behavioral prevention or treatment of, 181
causes of, 178–179, 180*f*
as clinical syndrome, 177–179
as core clinical concept, 177
criteria that define, 178, 179*t*
cycle of, 178, 178*f*
evidence-based findings, 177–179
and failure to thrive, 181–182
management strategies for, 180–181
palliative care for, 182
pharmacologic treatments for, 181
prevention of, 181
primary, 177, 179
screening measures for, 179–180
secondary, 177, 179
FRAX™ (fracture risk assessment model) (WHO), 243, 245*t*, 246, 248, Q111
Free radical theory of aging, 10
Free water deficit, 423
Freezing of gait, 229*t*, 485
Frontotemporal dementia
diagnostic features and treatment of, 259*t*
differential diagnosis of, 260
etiology of, 256–257
Frozen shoulder, 455
Fructosamine, Q101
Fukuda stepping test, 202

Functional Activities Questionnaire, 258
Functional Ambulation Classification scale, 231
Functional Independence Measure (FIM), 140–141, 142*t*
Functional reach test, 236–238
Functional status
acute decline, 53
assessment of, 49–50, 141*t*
with developmental disabilities, 348*t*, 349
impairments in hospitalized patients, 131*t*, 132
International Classification of Functioning, Disability, and Health (ICF) (WHO), 139
interventions for, 131*t*
limitations of Medicare enrollees, 3, 5*f*
low fitness or low functional ability, older adults with, 69
of nursing-home population, 153
performance-based assessment of, 231
prevention of decline in, Q62
rapid screening followed by assessment and management of, 48, 49*t*
trends in, 3–4
Fungal infections, 477–478, 477*f*
FUO (fever of unknown origin), 504*t*, 505
Furosemide, 211
Futility, 136–137
Future issues, 6–7

Gabapentin (Neurontin, Gralise)
for epilepsy, 491*t*
for persistent pain, 124*t*, 129
for restless legs syndrome, 289
for vasomotor symptoms, 432
Gait abnormalities, 229–230, 229*t*
antalgic gait, 229–230, 229*t*
festinating, 229*t*, 485
freezing, 229*t*, 485
steppage gait, 229*t*
Trendelenburg gait, 229–230, 229*t*
Gait and balance screening, 73*t*
Gait apraxia, 230
Gait impairment, 50, 228–233, Q62, Q73
assessment of, 229–231
conditions that contribute to, 228–229
epidemiology of, 228
history and physical examination of, 230
interventions for preventing falls, 241*t*
interventions to reduce disorders, 231–233
laboratory and imaging assessments of, 230–231
performance-based functional assessment of, 231
Gait speed, 50, 231, Q94
Gait training, 241*t*
Galantamine, 264, 346–347
Gallstones, 412
Gambling, 343
Gammopathy, monoclonal, of uncertain significance, 550
Gastroesophageal reflux disease, 409–410, Q54
Gastrointestinal bleeding, 417
Gastrointestinal diseases and disorders, 408–419, Q54, Q108
with developmental disabilities, 348*t*, 349
infections, 504
Gastrointestinal system, 108
Gastrostomy
contraindications to, 218
percutaneous endoscopic, 218
Gastrostomy tube placement, 218
GEM (geriatric evaluation and management) units, 137, 174
Gemcitabine, 544
Gender differences
cultural aspects, 62
in drug metabolism, 82
in urinary incontinence, 221
Generalized anxiety disorder, 321, 322*t*
Genetic damage, 9
Genu recurvatum, 229*t*
"Geographical Practices Cost Indices," 166
GERD (gastroesophageal reflux disease), 409–410, Q54
Geriatric Depression Scale, 51, 77, 309–310, 310*t*
Geriatric evaluation and management (GEM) units, 137, 174
Geriatric Resource Nurse (GRN) Model, 138
Geriatric Resources for Assessment and Care of Elders (GRACE), 174–175, Q64
Geriatric specialty care, 173
Geriatric syndrome of late-life depression. *See* Depression
Gerotranscendence theory, 9
GFR. *See* Glomerular filtration rate
Giant cell arteritis, 462, Q114
headache due to, 484
signs and symptoms of, 183, 185*t*
Ginkgo biloba, 94, Q17
for dementia, 265
safety issues, 91, 92*t*
Glaucoma, 189–190
angle-closure, 183, 184, 185*t*
definition of, 189–190
eye drops for, 190, 191*t*
narrow-angle, 184*t*
open-angle, 184*t*, 189–190
screening for, 78
symptoms and treatment of, 184*t*
types of, 189–190
Gleason grading system, 441
Glimepiride (Amaryl)
for diabetes mellitus, 526*t*
pioglitazone and glimepiride (Duetact), 527*t*
rosiglitazone and glimepiride (Avandaryl), 527*t*
Glipizide (Glucotrol, Glucotrol XL), 526*t*, Q25, Q101
Glipizide and metformin (METAGLIP), 527*t*
Global aging trends, 1
Global Initiative for Chronic Obstructive Lung Disease (GOLD), 373–374, 374*t*
Glomerular filtration rate (GFR), 104–106
age-related changes in, 83, 421*t*
estimating (eGFR), 83
Glomerulonephritis, acute, 425–426
Glucocorticoid hypersecretion, subclinical, 515
Glucocorticoids
adverse drug events, 86, 86*t*
and bone loss, 247
for dermatomyositis, 464
for giant cell arteritis, 462
for knee pain, 459
for musculoskeletal pain, 458
for polymyositis, 464
Glucophage (metformin), 526*t*
Glucophage XR (metformin), 526*t*
Glucosamine, 91, 92, 92*t*
Glucose intolerance, 521
Glucose monitoring, Q101
Glucose screening, 72*t*
α-Glucosidase inhibitors, 525, 526*t*
Glucotrol (glipizide), 526*t*
Glucotrol XL (glipizide), 526*t*
Glucovance (glyburide and metformin), 527*t*
Glumetza (metformin), 526*t*
Glutamine, Q47
Glyburide (Diaβeta, Micronase)
for diabetes mellitus, 526*t*
micronized (Glynase), 526*t*
Glyburide and metformin (Glucovance), 527*t*
Glycemic control, 524–525, Q101
Glycoprotein IIb/IIIa inhibitors, 381
Glycopyrrolate
for bowel obstruction, 116*t*
for loud respirations, 118
Glynase (micronized glyburide), 526*t*
Glyset (miglitol), 526*t*
GnRH (gonadotropin-releasing hormone) agonist therapy, Q111
Gout, 460–461, Q11
GRACE (Geriatric Resources for Assessment and Care of Elders), 174–175, Q64
Grading of Recommendations Assessment, Development and Evaluation working group (GRADE), 56

Gralise (gabapentin), 124*t*
Grand mal seizures, 489
Granisetron, 115*t*
Granulocyte colony-stimulating factor, 544*t*
Granulocyte-macrophage colony-stimulating factor, 544*t*
Green House Model, 159
Green Prescription (New Zealand), 68
Green tea, Q89
Grief, 20, Q39
Grief counseling, Q12
Grief therapy, 313–317, 317*t*
Group exercise, 231–232
Group homes, 171
Growth factors, 296, 305
Growth hormone, 214, 518–519
Growth hormone deficiency, 518–519
Growth retardation, 348*t*, 349
Guardians, 29
Guided Care, 175, Q64
Gustatory dysfunction
  medications that cause, 368, 369*t*
  nonpharmacologic causes of, 368, 369*t*
Gynecologic diseases and disorders, 431–436, Q19, Q21, Q24, Q57, Q91

H_2-receptor antagonists
  adverse drug events, 211
  and delirium, 280, 281*t*
  for nausea, 115*t*
HAART (highly active antiretroviral therapy), 503
Haemophilus influenzae, 498
Haglund deformity, 472*t*
Hairy leukoplakia, Q124
Hairy tongue, 368, 368*f*
Half-life, 82
Hallucinations, Q59
  antipsychotic medications for, 272–274, 273*t*
  definition of, 324
  in dementia, 272–274, 273*t*
  in dementia associated with Lewy bodies, 327
  evaluation of patients with, 324
  isolated, 327
Hallux abducto valgus, 472*t*, 475*f*
Hallux limitus, 472*t*, 474
Hallux rigidus, 472*t*
Hallux valgus, 472*t*, 474, Q43
Haloperidol
  adverse effects of, Q1
  for agitated delirium, 282, 283*t*
  for delirium, Q74
  dosing and adverse events of, 325, 326*t*
  for nausea, 115*t*
  for psychosis in dementia, 273*t*
Hammertoe, 472*t*, 474
Hand feeding, 217
Hand osteoarthritis, 458–459, 459*f*
Handoffs, 161
Handovers, 161
Harpagophytum procumbens (devil's claw), 93
Harris Hip Questionnaire, 141*t*, 145, 147
Hartford Institute for Geriatric Nursing, 48
Hayflick's limit, 9–10
Head-thrust test, 202
Headaches, 483–484
Healers, 63, 91
Healing
  cascade of, 296–297
  monitoring, 305
  Pressure Ulcer Scale for Healing, 305
Health beliefs, 60–61
Health care
  attitudes toward North American health services, 60–61
  costs of, 35–47
  coverage of, 35–47
  federal financing of, 46–47
  financing of, 35–47
  flow of funds for, 35, 36*f*
  GRACE model, 174–175, Q64
  trends in, 3–4
Health insurance
  coverage for older Americans, 35–47, 38*t*
  coverage for rehabilitation, 140–141
Health literacy, 3, 59
Health Maintenance Organizations (HMOs), 37, Q64
Healthcare agent or proxy, 28, 78
Healthcare Employers' Data Information System (HEDIS), 46
Healthcare providers
  addressing, 59
  Medicare Advantage plan payments, 42, 43*t*
  primary, 166–167
  response guidelines based on PHQ-9 and STAR*D studies, 309, 310*t*
  role in home care, 166–167
Healthy behaviors, 25
Healthy lifestyle counseling, 72*t*–73*t*, 76
Hearing
  age-related changes in, 192
  health insurance coverage for services, 38*t*
  normal, 192
Hearing aids, 195–197, Q55
  bone-anchored (BAHA), 198
  caring for, 198
  costs of, 197, 197*t*
  styles of, 196, 196*t*
Hearing Handicap Inventory for the Elderly—Screening Version (HHIE-S), 193–194, Q10
Hearing impairment, 192–198
  assessment of, 50–51
  clinical presentation of, 193–194
  effects of, 195, 196*t*
  epidemiology of, 192–193, Q10
  prevalence of, Q10
  rapid screening followed by assessment and management of, 48, 49*t*
  recommended preventive measures for, 73*t*, 78
  rehabilitation of, 195, 196*t*
  screening for, 73*t*, 78, 193–194, Q10
  sensorineural, Q55
  strategies to improve communication, 194–195, 194*t*
  treatment of, 194–198
Hearing Loss Association of America (HLAA), Q55
Heart: age-related changes, 12*t*, 13–14, 16*t*
Heart disease
  deaths due to, 3–4, 5*t*
  in nursing-home population, 153
  prevalence of, 3, 4*f*
  and rehabilitation, 144
  valvular, 384–385
Heart failure, 395–401, Q26, Q58
  Cheynes-Stokes breathing pattern of, 287
  classification of, 398, 398*t*
  clinical features of, 395–396
  device therapy for, 399–400
  diagnosis of, 396, Q110
  diastolic, 399
  end-of-life care for, 401
  epidemiology of, 395
  etiology of, 395
  management of, 396–400
  pathophysiology of, 395
  prognosis, 401
  recurrent hospitalization for, 400
  systolic, 399
Heart rate abnormalities, 239
Heat therapy, 457
Heavy drinking, 337
HEDIS (Healthcare Employers' Data Information System), 46
Heel pain, 475
Heel pressure ulcers, 300, 300*t*
Heel spur, 472*t*
Height measurement, 72*t*, 78
Helicobacter pylori infection, 411
HELP (Hospitalized Elderly Longitudinal Project), 111, 137–138, 283
Hemangioma, 477
Hematologic diseases and disorders, 530–539, Q45, Q95
  malignancies, 549–550
Hematoma, subdural, 483
Hematopoiesis, 530–531
Hematopoietic stem cells, 530

Hemodialysis, 428–429, 428*t*
Hemoglobin, replacement, 427
Hemoglobin A_{1c}, Q101
Hemolytic anemia, 532, 532*t*, 536
Hemorrhage
intracerebral, 483
subconjunctival, 184–185, 185*t*, 186
Hemostasis, 296
Heparin, 393–394
Hepatitis A vaccine, 495, 496*t*
Hepatitis B vaccine, 495, 496*t*
Herbal medicine, 90–91
for low back pain, 93
for sleep problems, 294–295
Herpes simplex, 367–368, 368*f*
Herpes simplex keratitis, 184, 185*t*
Herpes zoster ("shingles"), 185*t*, 186, 356–357, 357*f*, 504
Herpes zoster ophthalmicus
signs and symptoms of, 184, 185*t*
treatment of, 185*t*, 186
Herpes zoster vaccine
immunization schedule for adults ≥65 years old, 495, 496*t*
recommendations for, 72*t*, 79
HF. *See* Heart failure
HHIE-S (Hearing Handicap Inventory for the Elderly), Q10
HHRGs (home-health–related groups), 166
HHS (U.S. Department of Health and Human Services), 66, 67
High T_4 syndrome, 508
Highly active antiretroviral therapy (HAART), 503
Hip fracture, 146–147
epidemiology of, 146–147
prevention of recurrence, 147
rehabilitation after, 147, Q32
surgical care of, 146–147
Hip joint assessment, 141*t*, 145, 147
Hip pain, 456
Hip protectors, 240
Hip surgery
for hip fracture, 146–147
rehabilitation after, 232–233
total hip and knee arthroplasty, 147–148
Hispanic Americans, Q81, Q118
alcohol use, 338
cancer incidence, 542
diabetes mellitus, 520
dual eligibles, 40
leading causes of death, 3–4, 5*t*
nursing-home population, 153
perceived health, 3, 4*t*
poverty rates, 2
self-reported functional limitations, 5
History of immigration or migration, 60
History of traumatic experiences, 60
Histrionic personality disorder
features of, 329, 330*t*
therapeutic strategies for, 332, 332*t*
HIV infection, 155, 502–503
HIV screening, 72*t*, 76
HLAA (Hearing Loss Association of America), Q55
Hmong, 21
Hoarding disorder, 320
Hodgkin disease, 542, 550
Home care, 166–169, Q64
angina follow-up, Q6
ethical issues in, 168–169
fee-for-service, 44
financing, 44–45, Q12
health insurance coverage for, 38*t*
liability and legal issues, 168
limitations of, 168
managed care, 45
patient assessment, 167
physician's role in, 166–167
preventing falls, 240, 241*t*
prospective payment system for, 166
rehabilitation services, 140*t*, 141–142, Q87
technologic innovations in, 171
Home-delivered meals, 213
Home-health–related groups (HHRGs), 166
Home hospice care, Q41
Home hospital, 138, 170
Home safety evaluation, 240, 241*t*
Home visits, Q100
Homeostasis, 16–17
Homocysteine, 537, Q45
Hormonal regulation
influences in men, 245–246
screening tests for hypersecretion, 515, 515*t*
of water and electrolyte balance, 513–514
Hormone therapy, Q19, Q20
for breast cancer, 544, 547
for cancer, 544
for endometrial cancer, 544
for erectile dysfunction, 452
estrogen therapy, 518
for female sexual dysfunction, 447, 516
growth hormone supplementation, 518–519
for incontinence, 225
for menopausal symptoms, 432
for osteoporosis, 251*t*, 252–253
preventive, 73*t*, 79
for prostate cancer, 544
testosterone replacement therapy, 516–517
testosterone supplementation, 516–518, 517, 517*t*
for urogenital atrophy, 432–433
Horner syndrome, 482
Hospice, 112–113
criteria for, Q41
cultural aspects, 21, 111
for dementia, Q65
for end-stage kidney disease, 429–430
health insurance coverage for, 38*t*
home care, Q41
Medicare benefits, Q12, Q41, Q98
services, 112, 112*t*
Hospital-acquired pneumonia, 498–499
Hospital-acquired pressure ulcers
incidence of, 135
prevention of, 131*t*, 135
Hospital-at-home care, 138
Hospital care, 130–138, Q27, Q106
alternatives to, 138
daily evaluation, 137
day hospitals, 169
fall prevention during, Q106
geriatric evaluation and management (GEM) units, 137, 174
hazards and opportunities commonly overlooked in, 131–132, 131*t*
health insurance coverage for, 38*t*
home hospitals, 170
priority admission, Q61
recurrent, 400
rehabilitation hospitals, 140–141, 140*t*
systematic assessment on admission, 131, 131*t*
Hospital Elder Life Program (HELP), 137–138, 283
Hospitalization, chronic, 163
Hospitalized Elderly Longitudinal Project (HELP), 111
Hospitalized patients
assessment of, 130–137
daily evaluation, 137
management of, 130–137
sleep disturbances in, 290
systems of care for, 137–138
Hot flushes, 432, Q19
House calls, 167, Q100
choosing patients for, 167–168
financial considerations, 168
office-based programs, 167–168
Housing and Urban Development programs, 171
HRT (hormone replacement therapy), Q19, Q20
HSDD (hypoactive sexual desire disorder), 447
Humalog (insulin lispro), 528*t*
Human growth hormone, 214
Human immunodeficiency virus (HIV) infection, 155, 502–503
Human immunodeficiency virus (HIV) screening, 72*t*, 76
Humulin (insulin), 528*t*
Huntington disease, 488
Hurley Discomfort Scale, 122
Hutchinson sign, 186, 356, 360
Hydralazine, 399, 406
Hydrocephalus, normal-pressure (NPH), 232

Hydrochlorothiazide, 405, Q117
Hydrocodone (Lorcet, Lortab, Vicodin, Norco, Vicoprofen), 125*t*
Hydrocortisone, 109
Hydromorphone (Dilaudid, Hydrostat), 125*t*, 127
  extended release (Exalgo), 125*t*
Hydrophilic drugs, 82
Hydroxychloroquine, 463
Hydroxyurea, 538, 539
Hydroxyzine, 115*t*
Hyoscyamine, 225
  for bowel obstruction, 116*t*
  for loud respirations, 118
Hyperadrenocorticoidism, 514–515
Hyperalgesia, 120*t*
Hypercalcemia, 511–512, 512*t*
Hypercalciuria, idiopathic, 246
Hyperglycemia
  in diabetes mellitus, 528
  management of, 524–528
  perioperative, 109
Hypericum perforatum (St. John's wort), 94
  for depression, 315*t*
  safety issues, 91, 92*t*
Hyperkalemia, 423
Hyperkinetic movement disorders, 488
Hyperlipidemia, 75–76
Hypernatremia, 422–423
Hyperparathyroidism, 511–512, 512*t*
  screening for secondary osteoporosis in, 246–247, 247*t*
  secondary, 245
Hyperpathia, 120*t*
Hypersexuality, 274–275
Hypertension, 402–407, Q61, Q117
  CAM for, 93–94
  and cardiovascular risk, 379
  causes of, Q66
  classification of, 402, 402*t*
  clinical evaluation of, 403
  emergencies and urgencies, 407
  epidemiology and physiology of, 402–403
  follow-up visits, 406–407
  in long-term care setting, 407
  pharmacologic treatment of, 404–406
  prehypertension, 402, 402*t*
  prevalence of, 3, 4*f*
  recommended preventive measures for, 72*t*
  screening for, 75
  special considerations for, 407
  stages, 402*t*
  treatment of, 403–407, 405*t*
  white-coat, 403
Hyperthyroidism, 508–509
  subclinical, 509
Hypertonic saline, 422
Hypnotics
  chronic use of, 293–294
  and delirium, 281*t*
  interventions for preventing falls with, 241*t*
  for sleep problems, 290
Hypoactive sexual desire disorder (HSDD), 447
Hypoadrenocorticoidism, 514
Hypoaldosteronism, hyporeninemic, 514
Hypoalgesia, 120*t*
Hypochondriasis, Q85
Hypoglycemia, 528
Hypogonadism, 245–246
  male, 449–450, 449*t*, 516
  screening for secondary osteoporosis in, 247, 247*t*
  testosterone preparations available for, 516–517, 517*t*
Hypokalemia, 423
Hypomania, 310
Hyponatremia, 421
  dilutional, 422
  hypotonic, 421–422
  treatment of, 422
Hypophonic speech, 485
Hypoproliferative anemia, 532–535, 532*t*
  due to iron deficiency, 532–533, 533*f*
  due to vitamin B_{12} or folate deficiency, 532, 534*f*
Hyporeninemic hypoaldosteronism, age-related, 514
Hypotension, Q37
  postural, 207–208, 239, 241*t*
Hypothyroidism, 507–508
  secondary, 507–508
  subclinical, 507
Hypotonic hyponatremia, 421–422

IADLs. *See* Instrumental activities of daily living
Ibandronate, 251*t*, 252
IBS (irritable bowel syndrome), 413, 416–417
Ibuprofen
  for musculoskeletal pain, 458
  for persistent pain, 125*t*, 126–127
ICD-9 (International Classification of Diseases), 166
ICDs (implantable cardiac defibrillators), 399–400, Q58
Identity, cultural, 59
Idiopathic myelofibrosis, 538
Idiopathic pulmonary fibrosis, 376
Iliotibial band syndrome, 456
Illness anxiety disorder, 333
Iloperidone
  dosing and adverse events of, 325, 326*t*
  for psychosis in dementia, 273*t*
ILRs (implantable loop recorders), 207
Imaging
  abdominal ultrasonography, 72*t*
  brain imaging studies, 258–259
  of gait impairment, 230–231
Imbalance, Q53
IMF (idiopathic myelofibrosis), 538
Imipramine, 225, 281*t*
Immigration status, 60
Immobility
  in hospitalized patients, 131*t*, 132
  interventions for, 131*t*, 132
Immune function changes, 494, 495*t*
Immune system
  age-related changes, 12*t*, 15
  age-related pathologies, 16*t*
Immune theory of aging, 11
Immune thrombocytopenia, 537
Immunizations, 72*t*, 78–79
  for hospitalized patients, 131*t*, 136
  interventions for, 131*t*
  recommendations for, 78–79
  schedule for adults ≥65 years old, 495, 496*t*
Immunosenescence, 494
IMPACT (Improving Mood—Promoting Access to Collaborative Treatment), 175–176, Q64
Implantable cardiac defibrillators (ICDs), 399–400, Q58
Implantable loop recorders (ILRs), 207
Implants, cochlear, 198, Q55
  characteristics of older candidates for, 198, 198*t*
Improving Mood—Promoting Access to Collaborative Treatment (IMPACT), 175–176, Q64
Inattention, 276, 277*t*
Incompetence, 27
Incontinence
  with developmental disabilities, 348*t*, 349
  fecal, 413–414
  and rehabilitation, 143
  urinary, 73*t*, 77, 95, 220–227, Q82, Q109
Independence at Home Act, Q100
Ineffective anemia, 532, 532*t*
Ineffective erythropoiesis, 535
Infections
  antimicrobial management of, 496–497
  bone and joint, 502
  diagnosis and management of, 495–497
  fungal, 477–478, 477*f*
  gastrointestinal, 504
  HIV and AIDS, 502–503
  predisposition to, 494–495
  presentation of, 495–496
  in pressure ulcers, 305–306
  prevention of, 497
  prosthetic device infections, 502
  sexually transmitted, 76
  skin problems, 356–358
  spinal, Q122
  vulvovaginal, 433
Infectious diarrhea, 504–505
Infectious diseases, 494–505, Q30, Q48

Infectious Diseases Society of America, 498
Infectious syndromes, 497–505
Infective endocarditis, 501–502
Infestations, 356–358
Infidelity, 326
Inflammation
  anemia of, 533–534
  vulvovaginal, 433
Inflammatory cytokines, 214*t*
Inflammatory skin conditions, 350–355
Influenza, 499, Q99
  deaths due to, 3–4, 5*t*
  immunization schedule for adults ≥65 years old, 495, 496*t*
  recommended immunizations for, 72*t*, 78–79
  vaccination against, 72*t*, 78–79, 136
Information guidelines for prevention of falls, 240
Informed consent, Q116
  for research, 30
Ingrown nails, 477
INH (isoniazid), 501
Inhaled bronchodilators, 374, 375*t*
Inhalers, 374, Q102
Injectable agents, 527*t*
Injury, Q104
  deaths due to unintentional injuries, 3–4, 5*t*
  preventing, 78
Inpatient care
  fee for service, 43
  financing, 42–43
  managed care, 43
  rehabilitation care, 142
Insomnia, 286–287, Q40
  behavioral management of, 274, 274*t*, 291
  epidemiology of, 285
  nonpharmacologic interventions for, 292
  prescription medications for, 292–293, 294*t*
  prevalence of, 286
Institute for Healthcare Improvement, 298
Institute of Medicine Food and Nutrition Board, 209–210
Institutional mistreatment, 100
Institutional settings, Q2
Institutionalization decisions, 156
Instrumental activities of daily living (IADLs), 49–50, 49*t*, 132
  self-reported limitations, 5
Insulin
  for diabetes, 525–528, Q112
  preparations, 525–528, 528*t*, Q25, Q101
Insulin aspart (NovoLog), 528*t*
Insulin aspart protamine and insulin aspart (NovoLog Mix 70/30), 528*t*
Insulin detemir (Levemir), 528*t*
Insulin glargine (Lantus), 528*t*, Q25
Insulin glulisine (Apidra), 528*t*
Insulin-like growth factor 1, 214*t*
Insulin lispro (Humalog), 528*t*
Insurance coverage, 35–47, 38*t*
Integrative medicine, 90
Intellectual development disorder, 344
Intellectual disability, 344–349, Q39, Q120
  definition of, 344
  with developmental disabilities, 348*t*, 349
  diagnostic issues, 345
  medical disorders with, 348–349
  mental disorders with, 344–345, 346–348
  prevalence of, 344–345
  social conditions with, 349
  treatment issues, 345
Intensive care
  Confusion Assessment Method for the Intensive Care Unit (CAM-ICU), 276–277, 277*t*
  of critically ill, 136–137
Interferon, 539, 545
Interleukin-2, 545
Interleukin-6, 531
Intermittent clean catheterization, 226
Internal carotid artery disease, 481–482
International Classification of Diseases (ICD-9), 166
International Classification of Functioning, Disability, and Health (ICF) (WHO), 139
International Continence Society, 434
International Society of Clinical Densitometry, 248
Interpreters, 59–60
Interstitial nephritis, acute, 425, Q76
Intertrigo, 352, 353*f*
Intracerebral hemorrhage, 483
Investigational agents, 254
Ipratropium bromide
  adverse drug events, 211
  for COPD, 374, 375*t*
Irbesartan, 397*t*
Iron, 210*t*
Iron-containing antacids, 86, 86*t*
Iron deficiency, 427, 532–533, 533*f*
Iron therapy
  for anemia, 533
  drug interactions, 211, 211*t*
  for restless legs syndrome, 289
Irritable bowel syndrome, 413, 416–417
Ischemic optic neuropathy, 183, 185*t*
Ischemic stroke
  acute, 482–483
  prevention of, 482
Isoflavones, 95
Isoniazid (INH), 211, 211*t*, 501
Isosorbide dinitrate, 399
Isosorbide mononitrate, 383
Ivermectin, 358
Jaeger cards, 50, 133
Janumet (sitagliptin and metformin), 527*t*
Januvia (sitagliptin), 526*t*
Japanese Americans, 153
Jehovah's Witness, 26
Jejunostomy, percutaneous endoscopic, 218
Jentadueto (linagliptin and metformin), 527*t*
Joint disease, degenerative, 348*t*, 349
Joint infections, 502
Joint Principles of the PCMH (AAP, ACP, AAFP, AOA), 174
Joint replacement
  knee replacement, 232–233
  total hip and knee arthroplasty, 147–148
Judgment, substituted, 26, 28–29, 28*t*
Justice, 26–27

Kadian (morphine, sustained release), 125*t*
Kava, 295
KDOQI (Kidney Disease Outcomes Quality Initiative), 83
Keratitis, bacterial, 183, 185*t*
Keratitis sicca, 184–185, Q78
Keratotic lesions, 476
Ketoconazole, 224
Ketorolac, 125*t*
Kidney Disease Outcomes Quality Initiative (KDOQI), 83
Kidney diseases and disorders, 420–430, Q18, Q76
  acute kidney injury, 424–426, Q18, Q76
  chronic kidney disease, 426–428
  end-stage kidney disease, 428–430
  impaired kidney function, 83
  intrinsic renal disease, 425–426
  Modified Diet in Renal Disease (MDRD) formula, 83, 104–106, 420
  monitoring, 420
  postoperative management of, 107
  renal function impairment, 83
Kidney transplantation, 429
Kidney(s)
  age-related changes, 83, 420, 421*t*
  preoperative assessment and management of, 104–106
Klebsiella, 498
Klonopin (clonazepam), 124*t*
Knee osteoarthritis, 458–459, 459*f*, Q34
Knee pain, 456, Q34
Knee replacement
  rehabilitation after, 232–233, Q87
  total hip and knee arthroplasty, 147–148
Kombiglyze XR (saxagliptin and metformin), 527*t*
Korean Americans, 153
Kyphoplasty, 254–255

Labetalol, 406
Labor force participation, 2–3, 20–21
Laboratory testing, 211
in anemia, 532, 533*f*, 534*f*
in falls, 238
in gait impairment, 230–231
health insurance coverage for, 38*t*
in lower back pain, 468–469
normal values, 551
in osteoporosis, 246–247, 247*t*
Lactulose (Chronulac), 414*t*
Lacunar disease, 481
Lamotrigine, Q112
for behavioral disturbances in dementia with manic-like features, 272, 272*t*
for bipolar depression, 316*t*
for depression, 315*t*
for epilepsy, 491*t*
Language, 59
body language, 60
Wong-Baker FACES Pain Rating Scale with Foreign Translations, 120
Lansoprazole, 115*t*
Lantus (insulin glargine), 528*t*
Laryngeal cancer, Q97
Laryngoscopy, nasopharyngeal, 217
Laser therapy, 186
Last will and testament, 27, 28*t*
Latanoprost, 191*t*
Laxatives
bulk, 414*t*
for chronic constipation, 413, 413*t*
nutrient interactions, 211, 211*t*
osmotic, 414*t*
saline, 414*t*
stimulant, 414*t*
surfactant, 414*t*
LDLs (low-density lipoproteins), Q89
Left ventricular ejection fraction, 395
Leg-length discrepancies, 230
Legal issues, 26–34, Q93, Q116
decisional capacity, 26, 27–30
in home care, 168
informed consent for research, 30
in malnutrition, 214–215
Legionella pneumophila, 498
Legislation, 156–158
Length of stay, 155
Lentigo maligna, 360
Lesser metatarsal phalangeal joint dislocation, 472*t*
Leukemia, 549
acute, 542
acute myeloid leukemia, 549
chronic lymphocytic leukemia, 549, Q95
Leukoaraiosis, 230
Leukoplakia, 366, 366*f*
hairy, Q124
Leuprolide acetate, 274–275
Levalbuterol, 375*t*
Levemir (insulin detemir), 528*t*
Levetiracetam, 491*t*
Levodopa, 211, 211*t*
Levodopa-carbidopa
and delirium, 281*t*
for Parkinson disease, 485
Levofloxacin, 87, 87*t*, Q48
Lewy body dementia, 327, Q59, Q74
diagnostic features and treatment of, 259*t*
differential diagnosis of, 260
early features that distinguish, 487, 487*t*
epidemiology of, 256
etiology of, 256–257
Liability, 168
Libido, Q24
decreased, 446–447, 448*t*
Lice, 358
Lichen planus, 434, Q124
Lichen sclerosus, 433, 434
Lichen simplex chronicus, 352, 434
Lid abnormalities, 186
Lid malposition/exposure, 184–185, 185*t*
Life-course theory, 9
Life expectancy, 2, 2*t*
on dialysis, 428–429, 428*t*
Life review, 313–317, 317*t*
Life space assessment, 50
Lifestyle modification
for benign prostatic hyperplasia, 438, 438*t*
healthy lifestyle counseling, 73*t*, 76
for hypertension, 404–405
for urinary incontinence, 223
Light therapy, 291–292, 292*t*
Limb movements
periodic limb movements during sleep, 288–289
restless legs syndrome, 288–289
Linagliptin (Tradjenta), 526*t*
Linagliptin and metformin (Jentadueto), 527*t*
Lip cancer, 366
Lipid abnormalities, 524
Lipid-binding resins, 211, 211*t*
Lipid-lowering therapy, 524
Lipophilic drugs, 82
Liraglutide (Victoza), 527*t*
Lisinopril, 397*t*, Q36, Q68
Literacy, 3, 59
Lithium
for behavioral disturbances in dementia with manic-like features, 272, 272*t*
for depression, 312
drug interactions, 87, 87*t*
for personality disorders, 332–333
to stabilize mood in mania and bipolar depression, 313, 316*t*
Living arrangements, 3, 3*t*
Living wills, 29
Long lie, 234
Long-term care. *See also* Assisted-living facilities; Nursing-home care
fever in frail, older residents, 495–496, 496*t*
hypertension in, 407
interface with acute care, 156
managed long-term care programs (MLTC), 170
minimum criteria for initiation of antibiotic therapy in, 496–497, 497*t*
urinary incontinence in, 225–226
Loop diuretics
drug interactions, 87, 87*t*
for heart failure, 398
Lorazepam, 282, 283*t*, Q1
Lorcet (hydrocodone), 125*t*
Lortab (hydrocodone), 125*t*
Losartan, 397*t*
Loss and grief, 20
Louse infestations, 358
Low back pain, Q103, Q115, Q122
Low-density lipoproteins (LDLs), Q89
Low T_3 syndrome, 507–508
Low T_4 syndrome, 507–508
Low thyrotropin, 508
Low-vision aids, 191
Low-vision rehabilitation, 191
Lower back pain, 465
assessment of, 467–469, 467*t*
CAM for, 93
history, 467–468
laboratory tests and imaging, 468–469
physical examination of, 468, 468*t*
Lower extremities, 466, 466*t*
Lower respiratory disease, chronic, 3–4, 5*t*
Lower urinary tract
age-related changes in, 221
pathophysiology in UI, 221
Lower urinary tract symptoms (LUTS), 220, 437
Lubiprostone (Amitiza), 414*t*
Lubrication, decreased, 447, 448*t*
Lumbar spinal stenosis, 232, 465–466
Lumbar spine, unstable, 466
Lumpectomy, 547
Lung cancer, 547–548
CAM for, 96
ethnic and racial differences in incidence, 540
racial differences in diagnosis and survival, 540
Lung disease, 372–377
chronic obstructive pulmonary disease, 321, 373–374
with developmental disabilities, 348*t*, 349
Lurasidone
dosing and adverse events of, 325, 326*t*
for psychosis in dementia, 273*t*
LUT. *See* Lower urinary tract
Lutein, 96
Luteinizing hormone-releasing hormone (LHRH) agonists, 442*t*, 444

LUTS (lower urinary tract symptoms), 220, 437
Lyme disease, 504
Lymphadenectomy, pelvic, 441
Lymphoma, 549–550
diffuse large B-cell lymphoma, 549–550
follicular lymphoma, 550
non-Hodgkin lymphoma, 549–550
Lyrica (pregabalin), 124*t*

M2 inhibitors, 499
M6 leukemia, 536
MA. *See* Medicare Advantage
MacArthur Competency Assessment Tool, 28
Macronutrient guidelines, 209
Macronutrient needs, 209
Macular degeneration, age-related, 184*t*, 187–188
rehabilitation for, 191
symptoms and treatment of, 184*t*
Magnesium
drug interactions, 211, 211*t*
RDIs for adults ≥71 years old, 210*t*
Magnesium citrate (Citroma), 414*t*
Magnesium-containing antacids, 86, 86*t*
Magnesium hydroxide (Milk of Magnesia), 414*t*
Magnetic resonance imaging (MRI), 454–455, Q46
Maladaptive behaviors, 347
Malassezia furfur, 350
Male hypogonadism, 449–450, 449*t*, 516
Male sexuality, 448–452
Malignancy
deaths due to, 3–4, 5*t*
hematologic malignancies, 549–550
humoral hypercalcemia of, 511–512, 512*t*
occult, Q114
Malignant melanoma, 477
Malnutrition, 209–215, Q2, Q16, Q107
Mammography, 71, 72*t*, Q50
Managed care
home-health care, 45
inpatient care, 43
nursing-home care, 45
outpatient care, 43
postacute rehabilitation, 44
Managed long-term care programs (MLTC), 170
Mandibular torus, 366–367, 367*f*
Mania
DSM-5™ criteria for, 310
hypomania, 310
late-onset, 310–311
medications to stabilize mood in, 316*t*
pharmacotherapy for, 312–313, 316*t*
Manic-like behavioral syndromes
in dementia, 268, 271–272
mood stabilizers for, 271–272, 272*t*
treatment of, 271–272
Manipulative and body-based methods, 90, 91*t*
Marche a petits pas, 230
Marital status of community-dwelling older Americans, 3, 3*t*
Masked facies, 485
Massage, 90–91
for musculoskeletal pain, 457
MAST (Michigan Alcoholism Screening Test)—Geriatric Version, 339
McGill Pain Questionnaire, 120, 306
MDRD (Modified Diet in Renal Disease) formula, 83, 104–106, 420
MDS. *See* Minimum Data Set; Myelodysplastic syndromes
Meals-on-Wheels, 266
"Meaningful Use" standard, 47
Mechanical loading, 299–300
Mechanical revascularization, acute, Q26
Meclizine, 115*t*
Mediators, 21–22
Medicaid, 2, 35, 38*t*, 39–40
advantages and disadvantages of, 41–42, 42*t*
assisted-living benefits, 171
continuing-care retirement community benefits, 171
day care benefits, 169
dual eligibles, 40, 45
future directions, 47
glaucoma-related payments, 189
hearing aid benefits, 197
hospice benefits, 112–113
residential-care benefits, 6
Medicaid Home and Community-Based Services waiver, 175
Medical decisions, 27, 28*t*
Medical ethics, 26–27
Medical homes, 35, 174–175
Medical interpreters, 59–60
Medical-legal interface, 101
Medical records, Q119
Medical savings accounts (MSAs), 37
Medicare, 2, 35–41
assisted-living benefits, 171
care venues, 163
cochlear implant coverage, 198
continuing-care retirement community benefits, 171
day hospital benefits, 169
dual eligibles, 40, 45
fee-for-service (FFS), 35, 36–37, 38*t*, 41–42, 42*t*
functional limitations of enrollees, 3, 5*f*
future directions, 47
"Geographical Practices Cost Indices," 166
glaucoma-related payments, 189
guidelines for erythropoietin therapy, 427
hearing aid benefits, 197
home-care benefits, 168
home-health benefits, 141
hospice benefits, 31–32, 112–113, Q98
house-call benefits, 168, Q100
mobility-related device benefits, 151
nursing-home care benefits, 155
out-of-pocket expenses, 37
Part A, 35–37, 38*t*, 140*t*, 141, Q41
Part B, 35–37, 38*t*, 46, 140, 140*t*
Part C, 35 (*See also* Medicare Advantage)
Part D, 35, 38–39, 38*t*, 40, 47, 80
postacute care benefits, 141
preventive health benefits, 78, 80, Q125
Program of All-Inclusive Care for the Elderly (PACE), 45, 169–170, Q64
prospective payment system (PPS), 43–44, 155, 166
prospective reimbursement, 141, 141*t*
rehabilitation benefits, 139–140, 140*t*, 141
requirements for rehabilitation sites, 140*t*
skilled-nursing-facility benefits, 155
transitions in care, 161
"Welcome to Medicare" visits, 41, 80, Q125
Medicare Administrative Contractors, 36
Medicare Advantage (MA), 35, 37–38, 38*t*
advantages and disadvantages of, 41–42, 42*t*
fee-for-service, 42, 43*t*
healthcare provider payments, 42, 43*t*
types of plans, 37
Medicare Health Maintenance Organizations (HMOs), 37, Q64
Medicare Health Outcomes Survey, 46
Medicare Personal Plan Finder, 40, 46
Medicare Prescription Drug Improvement and Modernization Act, 46–47
Medicare Prescription Drug Plan Finder (CMS), 39
Medicated urethral system for erection (MUSE), 451*t*, 452
Medication assessment, 51. *See also* Medication review
Medication-induced parkinsonism, 487, 487*t*
Medication Regimen Complexity Index, 56
Medication review, 51, Q19, Q23
for angina, Q6

annual drug regimen review, 89
brown-bag evaluation, 88, 279
discharge medication regimen, 163
at hospital admission, 131, 131*t*, 135
for preventing falls, 241*t*
screening tool of older persons' potentially inappropriate prescriptions (STOPP), 134–135
Medication trays, 89
Medications. *See* Drugs; Pharmacotherapy; *specific medications*
Medigap, 35, 38*t*, 39
advantages and disadvantages of, 41–42, 42*t*
Megestrol, 214
Meglitinides, 526*t*
Melanoma, 360–361, 361*f*
acral lentiginous, 360, 361*f*
malignant, 477
superficial spreading, 360, 361*f*
Melatonin, 290, 295, 519, Q40
Melatonin receptor agonists, 293, 294*t*
Memantine, 265
Memory loss, Q51, Q96
Memory problems. *See also* Cognitive impairment; Dementia
three-item recall test for, 77
Memory retraining, 262
Men
alcohol use among, 338
cardiovascular disease in, 378, 378*t*
erectile dysfunction in, 448–452
functional limitations of Medicare enrollees, 3, 5*f*
gallstones in, 412
hormonal influences in, 245–246
indications for osteoporosis screening, 248, 248*t*
leading causes of death for, 3–4, 5*t*
life expectancy of, 2, 2*t*
marital status and living arrangements of, 3, 3*t*
osteoporosis in, 247
prostate disease, 437–445
RDIs for micronutrients, 209–210, 210*t*
recommended requirements of vitamin D, 249–250
sexual problems, 76
stroke in, 480
testosterone supplementation for, 516–518, 517*t*
urinary tract infections in, 499, 500
Mendelson syndrome, 217
Meniere disease, 197, 199, Q75
Meningitis, bacterial, 503
Meningococcal vaccination, 495, 496*t*
Meniscus, 461, 461*f*
Menopausal symptoms, Q19, Q20
CAM for, 95
treatment of, 432
Menopause, 432
Mental health
acute status change, 276, 277*t*
health insurance coverage for outpatient care, 38*t*
rehabilitation and, 143–144
self-efficacy beliefs and, 22, 22*t*
social networks and, 23–24, 24*t*
Mental health problems, 339
diagnosis and treatment of, 347–348
intellectual disability with, 344–345, 346–348
Meperidine, 129, 281*t*
Metabolic disorders, 506–519, Q123
Metabolic encephalopathy, 276
Metabolism
age-associated changes in, 82
of drugs, 82
preoperative assessment and management of, 104–106
METAGLIP (glipizide and metformin), 527*t*
Metamucil (psyllium), 414*t*
Metastatic breast cancer, 547
Metatarsal phalangeal joint dislocation, 472*t*, 474, 475*f*
Metatarsalgia, 472*t*
Metformin (Glucophage, Riomet, Glucophage XR, Fortamet, Glumetza), Q25, Q36
for diabetes mellitus, 525, 526*t*
glipizide and metformin (METAGLIP), 527*t*
glyburide and metformin (Glucovance), 527*t*
linagliptin and metformin (Jentadueto), 527*t*
nutrient interactions, 211, 211*t*
pioglitazone and metformin (ACTOplus met), 527*t*
repaglinide and metformin (PrandiMet), 527*t*
rosiglitazone and metformin (Avandamet), 527*t*
saxagliptin and metformin (Kombiglyze XR), 527*t*
sitagliptin and metformin (Janumet), 527*t*
Methadone, 340–341, 342*t*
Methicillin-resistant *Staphylococcus aureus* (MRSA), 498–499
Methylcellulose (Citrucel), 414*t*
Methyldopa, 432
Methylmalonic acid, 537, Q45
Methylnaltrexone (Relistor), 414*t*
Methylphenidate, 117, 270–271, 315*t*
Methylprednisolone
for CPPD, 461–462
for dermatomyositis, 464
for giant cell arteritis, 462
for gout, 460
for polymyositis, 464
Metoclopramide
adverse drug events, 86, 86*t*
for nausea, 115*t*
Metolazone, 398
Metoprolol, 397*t*
Metronidazole, Q70
for *C difficile* colitis, 418
for diverticulitis, 416
Mexican Curanderos, 91
Mexiletine (Mexitil), 124*t*
MGUS (monoclonal gammopathy of uncertain significance), 550
Michigan Alcoholism Screening Test (MAST)—Geriatric Version, 339
Micrographia, 485
Micronase (glyburide), 526*t*
Micronutrient requirements
age-related changes in, 209–210
recommended dietary intakes, 209–210, 211*t*
Micronutrient supplements, 213–214
Microvascular complications of diabetes mellitus, 524
Midodrine, 241*t*
Miglitol (Glyset), 526*t*
Migraine headache, 484
Migration history, 60
Mild cognitive impairment, Q22
diagnostic features and treatment of, 259*t*
differential diagnosis of, 259
Milk of Magnesia (magnesium hydroxide), 414*t*
Milnacipran (Savella), 124*t*
Milwaukee shoulder, 455
Mind-body interventions, 90, 91, 91*t*, 96
Mineral oil, 211, 211*t*
Mini-Cog Assessment Instrument for Dementia, 51, 77, 133, 258, 258*t*
Mini–Mental State Examination (MMSE), 27–28, 51, 77, 133, 258, 258*t*, Q4
Mini-Nutritional Assessment (MNA), 212
Mini-Nutritional Assessment, short form (MNA-SF), 209
Minimum Data Set (MDS), 156–157, 210, 225
quality measures for nursing homes based on, 156–157, 157*t*
sections related to nutritional status, 215
Minoxidil, 406
Miotics, 191*t*
Mirabegron, 225
Miralax (polyethylene glycol), 414*t*
Mirror therapy, 146
Mirtazapine, Q88
for depression, 312, 315*t*
for depressive features of behavioral disturbances in dementia, 270–271, 271*t*
for insomnia, 265, 293, 294*t*
for sleep disturbances in dementia, 274
for undernutrition, 214

Mistreatment, 97–100, Q4, Q119
definition of, 97
financial, 99
incidence of, 97
institutional, 100
interventions for, 100–101
medical-legal interface, 101
physical, 98
prevalence of, 97
prevention of, 97
psychological abuse, 98–99
questions to guide intervention for, 100
risk factors for, 97, 98*t*
screening for, 78, 98, 99*t*
signs of abuse, 98, 99*t*
Mistreatment history, 98
Mitochondrial DNA (mtDNA) theory of aging, 9
Mitral regurgitation, 385, 386*t*
Mitral stenosis, 385, 386*t*
Mixed dementia, 256
Mixed UI, 220, 221
MLTC (managed long-term care programs), 170
MMSE (Mini–Mental State Examination), 27–28, 51, 77, 133, 258, 258*t*, Q4
Mnemonic for reversible causes of delirium, 278*t*
Mobility, 300
Mobility aids, 149–150, 150–151, 150*t*
for gait disorders, 233
Mobility assessment
activities of daily living (ADLs), 49–50, 49*t*
Performance-Oriented Mobility Assessment (POMA), 50, 231, 238
rapid screening followed by assessment and management of, 48, 49*t*
Mobility training, 241*t*
MoCA (Montreal Cognitive Assessment), 51, 258, 258*t*
Modafinil, 315*t*
Moderators, 23–25
Modified Diet in Renal Disease (MDRD) formula, 83, 104–106, 420
Moexipril, 397*t*
Mometasone furoate, 375*t*
Mono-Gesic (salsalate), 125*t*
Monoamine oxidase inhibitors, 314*t*
Monoclonal antibodies, 545
Monoclonal gammopathy of uncertain significance, 550
Montreal Cognitive Assessment (MoCA), 51, 258, 258*t*
Mood-congruent delusions, 326
Mood disorders, 308–318, Q35, Q56
with developmental disabilities, 348*t*, 349
psychotic symptoms in, 326
Mood disturbances
in dementia, 270–271
treatment of, 270–271
Mood stabilizers, Q56
for alcohol detoxification, 340–341, 342*t*
for behavioral disturbances in dementia with manic-like features, 271–272, 272*t*
for mania and bipolar depression, 312, 316*t*
for personality disorders, 332–333
Moraxella catarrhalis, 498
Morbidity, 5
Morning stiffness, Q114
Morpheaform basal cell carcinoma, 360
Morphine, immediate release (MSIR, Roxanol), 125*t*
Morphine, sustained release (MSContin, Kadian), 125*t*
Morse Fall Scale, 238
Mortality, 3–4
Morton neuroma/syndrome, 472*t*, 475
Motor neuron disease, 490–491
Motorized scooters, 151
Movement disorders, 484–489
drug-induced, 488–489
hyperkinetic, 488
Movement therapy, 90
MR (mitral regurgitation), 385, 386*t*
MRSA (methicillin-resistant *Staphylococcus aureus*), 498–499
MS (mitral stenosis), 385, 386*t*
MSAs (medical savings accounts), 37
MSContin (morphine, sustained release), 125*t*
MSIR (morphine, immediate release), 125*t*
Mucositis, oral, Q97
Multimorbidity, 54–57, Q37
approach for optimal management of, 54, 55*f*
guiding principles, 54–56
in nursing-home population, 153–154
relevant domains, 54
Multiple myeloma, 550
Multiple system atrophy, 487, 487*t*
Multivitamin supplements, 73*t*, 79
Munchausen syndrome, 334
Muscle-strengthening activity recommendations, 64, 66, 66*t*
Musculoskeletal diseases and disorders, 453–464, Q11, Q114
CAM for, 92–93
comorbid conditions, 457
diagnostic approach to, 453–455
diagnostic testing, 453–454
evaluation of, 455–457
exercise for, 457
general management strategies for, 457–458
nonpharmacologic strategies for, 457
and rehabilitation, 144
Musculoskeletal system: age-related changes, 12*t*, 13, 16*t*
Music therapy, 94, 323
Mutation accumulation theory of aging, 8
Mycobacterium tuberculosis, 500, 501
Myelodysplastic syndromes, 535–536
Myelofibrosis, idiopathic, 538
Myelopathy, 492
cervical, 232, Q77
Myelosuppressive agents, 538
Myelotoxicity, chemotherapy-related, 544, 544*t*
Myocardial infarction
indications for permanent pacemaker implantation, 390, 391*t*
management of, Q37
non-ST-elevation (NSTEMI), 380, 382
ST-elevation (STEMI), 380, 381, Q26
Myofascial pain, 121, 122*t*
Myopathy, 493
Myostatin, 214*t*
MyPlate (USDA), 209

Nabumetone (Relafen), 125*t*
Nail disorders, 477–478
Nails, ingrown, 477
Naloxone, 128
Naltrexone, 340–341, 342*t*
Naproxen, 125*t*, Q66
Narcissistic personality disorder
features of, 329, 330*t*
therapeutic strategies for, 332, 332*t*
Narcotics
adverse drug events, 211
for musculoskeletal pain, 458
Narcotics Anonymous, 340
Nasal calcitonin, Q111
Nasal pillows, 376
Nasopharyngeal laryngoscopy, 217
Nateglinide (Starlix), 526*t*
National Adult Protective Services Association, 101
National Center on Elder Abuse, 101
National Council on Aging, Inc.
Nutrition Screening Initiative, 212
Web site, 68–69
National Hospice and Palliative Care Organization, 31–32
National Institute for Health and Clinical Excellence (NICE), 284, 284*t*
National Institute of Aging and the Alzheimer's Association (NIA–AA), Q3
National Institute on Aging
Exercise: A Guide from the National Institute on Aging, 69
strategies to facilitate communication with older patients, 48

National Institutes of Health (NIH)
guidelines regarding body size classification based on BMI, 210
Stroke Scale, 145–146, 480, 480*t*, 483
National Kidney Foundation
guidelines for renal replacement therapy, 429
Kidney Disease Outcomes Quality Initiative (KDOQI), 83
National Osteoporosis Foundation, 246
National Pressure Ulcer Advisory Panel (NPUAP), 301, 303*t*
National Transitions of Care Coalition, 164
Native Americans, 21
burning mouth syndrome, 367
cancer incidence, 542
nursing-home population, 153
traditional medicine, 91
Natural products, 90
Nausea and vomiting
medications for nausea, 115*t*
opioid-induced, 128
postoperative nausea, 108
in terminal illness, 115
NBRAs (nonbenzodiazepine-benzodiazepine receptor agonists), 293, 294*t*
NCSE (nonconvulsive status epilepticus), 490
Neck pain, 469–470
assessment of, 470
causes of, 469–470
diagnostic imaging of, 470
management of, 470
Negative-pressure wound therapy, 305
Neglect. *See also* Mistreatment
risk factors for inadequate caregiving, 97, 98*t*
self-neglect, 100, 320
signs of, 98, 99*t*
Neoplasia
adrenal, 515
skin, 476–477
vulvar, 434
Nephritis
acute interstitial, 425
deaths due to, 3–4, 5*t*
Nephritis, acute interstitial, Q76
Nephrosis, 3–4, 5*t*
Nephrotic syndrome, 423
deaths due to, 3–4, 5*t*
Nervous system: age-related changes, 11–13, 12*t*, 16*t*
Neuraminidase inhibitors, 499
Neuregulins, 214*t*
Neurodermatitis, 352, 434
Neurogenic bladder, Q82
Neurologic diseases and disorders, 480–493, Q77, Q86
CAM for, 94–95
Neurologic testing, 207
Neuroma, 475
Neuromuscular electrical stimulation, 457
Neurontin (gabapentin), 124*t*
Neuropathic pain, 121, 122*t*
Neuropsychiatric concerns, preoperative, 106
Neuropsychiatric Inventory (NPI), 268
Neuropsychologic testing, Q83
Neurosyphilis, 503–504
New York Heart Association classification of HF, 398, 398*t*
New Zealand, 68
Niacin
drug interactions, 211, 211*t*
RDIs for adults ≥71 years old, 210*t*
NICHE (Nurses Improving Care of Health System Elders), 138
Nicotine dependence, 340–341, 342*t*
Nicotine replacement, 340–341, 342*t*
Nifedipine, 87
NIH Stroke Scale, 145–146, 480, 480*t*, 483
Nikolsky sign, Q71
Nitrates, Q49
adverse drug events, 86, 86*t*
for chronic CAD, 383
Nitrofurantoin, Q30
NMDA-receptor modulators, Q65
NMES (neuromuscular electrical stimulation), 457
Nociceptive pain, 121, 122*t*
Nociceptors, 120*t*
Nocturia, 221
Nodular basal cell carcinoma, 359
Nodular melanoma, 360
Nodular thyroid disease, 509–510
Non-Hodgkin lymphoma, 549–550
Nonadherence to medication regimens, 89
Nonbenzodiazepine-benzodiazepine receptor agonists (NBRAs), 293, 294*t*
Nonconvulsive status epilepticus, 490
Noninvasive positive-pressure ventilation, Q5
Nonmaleficence, 26
Nonsteroidal anti-inflammatory drugs (NSAIDs), Q66, Q76
adverse drug events, 86, 86*t*, 211
drug interactions, 87, 87*t*
gastric complications, 411
and incontinence, 225
for musculoskeletal pain, 458
for persistent pain, 124*t*–125*t*, 126–127
for polymyalgia rheumatica, 462
Nonthyroidal illness syndromes, 507–508
Nonverbal communication, respectful, 60
Norco (hydrocodone), 125*t*
Normative ethics, 26
Norpramin (desipramine), 124*t*
Norton Scale, 298
Nortriptyline (Aventyl, Pamelor)
for depression, 312, 315*t*
for depressive features of behavioral disturbances in dementia, 270–271, 271*t*
for persistent pain management, 124*t*
Norwegian scabies (crusted scabies), Q33
Novolin (insulin), 528*t*
Novolin 70/30 (isophane insulin + regular insulin), 528*t*
NovoLog (insulin aspart), 528*t*
NovoLog Mix 70/30 (insulin aspart protamine and insulin aspart), 528*t*
Noxious stimulus, 120*t*
NPH insulin (Humulin, Novolin), 528*t*, Q101
NPI (Neuropsychiatric Inventory), 268
NPUAP (National Pressure Ulcer Advisory Panel), 301, 303*t*
NSAIDs. *See* Nonsteroidal anti-inflammatory drugs
Nucynta (tapentadol), 126*t*
Nucynta ER (tapentadol extended release), 126*t*
Numeric Rating Scale, 120
Nurse practitioners, 38*t*
in home care, 166–167
in nursing home, 159–160
rehabilitation team role, 142, 143*t*
Nurses Improving Care of Health System Elders (NICHE), 138
Nursing, 142, 143*t*
Nursing facilities, 6
staffing patterns, 155
Nursing-home care, 153–160
availability of, 154–155
clinical practice guidelines for, 160
clinician practice in, 159–160
culture of resident safety in, Q28
for dementia, Q65
fee-for-service, 45
fever in, 496–497
financing, 45, 155
health insurance coverage for, 38*t*, 45*t*
for influenza, Q99
legislation influencing, 156–158
length of stay in, 154
managed care, 45
medical care issues, 158–159
occupancy rates, 154
organizational climate, Q28
placement factors, 156
population, 153–154
postacute care, 154–155
for pressure ulcers, Q47
quality issues, 156–158
quality measures for, 156–157, 157*t*
rehabilitation care, Q32
sleep in, 290–291
staffing patterns, 155
standards of care, 215

unacceptable weight loss, 214–215
urinary incontinence in, 221, 225–226
violent behavior in, Q79
Nursing-home–acquired pneumonia, 498–499
Nutrition
for chronic kidney disease, 428
drug-nutrient interactions, 211, 211*t*
for hospitalized patients, 131*t*
intake, 210–211
interventions, 131*t*, 213–214
malnutrition, 209–215
oral, 213–214
for prevention of pressure ulcers, 299
to reduce risk of osteoporosis, 246, 246*t*
risk factors for poor status, 212, 212*t*
standards of care for, 215
syndromes, 212–213
undernutrition, 212
Nutrition assessment, 50, 210–212
multi-item tools for, 212
rapid screening followed by assessment and management, 48, 49*t*
screening evaluations, 78
threshold to trigger, 215
Nutrition Screening Initiative, 212
Nutritional deficits, Q45, Q107
in hospitalized patients, 135–136
Nutritional supplements, 213–214
for pressure ulcers, 302
safety issues, 91, 92*t*

OASIS (Outcome and Assessment Information Set), 141, 166
Obesity, 212–213
cardiovascular risk, 380
management of, Q13
prevalence of, 212–213
recommendations for, 78
OBRA (Omnibus Budget Reconciliation Act), 100, 153, 156–157, 157–158, 214–215
Obsessions, 320
Obsessive-compulsive disorder, 320
features of, 329, 330*t*
treatment strategies for, 322, 322*t*, 323, 332, 332*t*
Obstruction
acute colonic pseudo-obstruction, 418
bowel, 115–116, 116*t*
postrenal ARF, 426
Obstructive pulmonary disease, chronic, 373–374
anxiety and, 321
exacerbation of, Q5
Obstructive sleep apnea, 287–288, 290, 375–376, Q60
Occupational therapy (OT), 38*t*
for pain, 457
rehabilitation team role, 142, 143*t*
Octreotide, 116*t*
Odd or eccentric behaviors, 329, 330*t*
Odor control, Q70
Office-based house-call programs, 167–168
Office visits, 48, 262
25(OH)D levels, 250, 510
Olanzapine, Q29
for agitated delirium, 282, 283*t*
for depression, 312
dosing and adverse events of, 325, 326*t*
for psychosis in dementia, 272–273, 273*t*
to stabilize mood in mania and bipolar depression, 316*t*
Olanzapine/fluoxetine, 316*t*
Older Americans Act, 171, 213, 266
Olfactory dysfunction
medications that cause, 368, 369*t*
nonpharmacologic causes of, 368, 369*t*
Olivopontocerebellar atrophy, 487
Olmesartan, 397*t*
Omega-3 fatty acids, 91, 92*t*, 93
Omeprazole, 115*t*, Q54, Q115
Omnibus Budget Reconciliation Act (OBRA), 100, 153, 156–157, 157–158, 214–215
Oncology, 540–550. *See also* Cancer
Ondansetron, 115*t*
Onglyza (saxagliptin), 526*t*
Onychocryptosis, 477
Onychomycosis, 477–478, 477*f*
Operative therapy. *See also* Surgical care
iatrogenic complications, 106
preoperative assessment and management of, 102–106
Ophthalmic corticosteroids, 186
Opioid antagonists, 414*t*
Opioids
adverse drug events, 86, 86*t*
adverse effects of, 128, Q1
barriers to using, 127–128
and delirium, 280, 281*t*
dependence on, 340–341, 342*t*
for dyspnea, 117
for persistent pain, 125*t*–126*t*, 127
Optic neuropathy, ischemic, 183, 185*t*, 190–191, 191*f*, Q67
Optimizing therapies and care plans, 56
Oral appliances, 288
Oral diseases and disorders, 362–370, Q97, Q124
cancer, 365–366
candidiasis, 367, 367*f*, Q124
dental decay, 362–363
edentulism, 364–365
lesions, 365–368
mucositis, Q97
Oral dysphagia, 216
Oral nutrition, 213–214
Oral tissues, 362, 363*t*
Orchiectomy, 442*t*
Oregon
adult foster care, 171
Death with Dignity Act, 31–32
physician-assisted suicide in, 31
Organ systems: age-related changes, 11–16, 12*t*, 16*t*
Organic brain syndrome, 276
Organizational climate, Q28
Oropharyngeal carcinoma, 365–366
Oropharyngeal dysphagia, 217
Oropharyngeal tumors, Q108
Orthoses, 475–476
Orthotics
for gait disorders, 233
for rehabilitation, 149, 151–152
OSA (obstructive sleep apnea), 287–288, 290, 375–376, Q60
Oseltamivir, 499, Q99
Osmotic laxatives, 414*t*
Osteoarthritis, 458–459, 459*f*
activity recommendations for, 66*t*
CAM for, 92
interventions for preventing falls, 241*t*
knee, Q34
nonpharmacologic strategies for, 457
and sexual activity, Q24
Osteoblasts, 244
Osteodystrophy, renal, 427–428
Osteomyelitis, 502
Osteopenia, 348*t*, 349
definition of, 244*t*
Osteoporosis, 243–255
activity recommendations for, 66*t*
CAM for, 92–93
definition of, 243, 244*t*
with developmental disabilities, 348*t*, 349
diagnosis of, 243
epidemiology of, 243–244
fractures of, 466–467, Q103, Q111, Q115
impact of, 243–244
investigational agents for, 254
laboratory testing in, 246, 247*t*
modifications to reduce risk of, 246, 246*t*
pathogenesis of, 244–246
pharmacologic options for, 250–254, 251*t*
physical examination in, 247
prevention of, 249–254, Q125
prevention of fractures, Q111
risk factors for, 245*t*, 246
sacral fractures of, 467, Q103
screening for, 72*t*, 75, 243
secondary, 243, 246–247, 247*t*
treatment of, 249–254, Q125
vertebral compression fractures of, 466–467
OT. *See* Occupational therapy

Outcome and Assessment Information Set (OASIS), 141, 166
Outpatient care, Q105
 fee-for-service (FFS) care, 41–42
 financing, 41–42
 health insurance coverage for, 38*t*
 managed care, 43
 medications, 38*t*
 mental health care, 38*t*
 options for, Q64
 patient selection for interventions, 176
 rehabilitation services, 140*t*, 142
 systems of care, 173–176
Outpatient consultation, 173–174
Ovarian cancer, 74, Q91
Overprescribing, 84–85, 84*t*, 85*t*, 88
Overweight, 383
Oxandrolone, 214
Oxcarbazepine, 491*t*
Oxybutynin
 and delirium, 281*t*
 for incontinence, 224, 226
Oxycodone
 immediate release (OxyIR, Percocet, Percodan, Tylox, Combunox), 125*t*
 for persistent pain, 127
 sustained release (OxyContin), 126*t*
Oxygen therapy, Q5
 for COPD, 374, 375*t*
 for dyspnea, 118
OxyIR (oxycodone, immediate release), 125*t*

PACE (Program of All-inclusive Care of the Elderly), 45, 169–170, Q64
Pacemakers, 208
 indications for, 390, 391*t*
PAD. *See* Peripheral arterial disease
Padua Prediction Score, 136
Paget disease of bone, 512–513
Pain
 acute, 119
 arthritic, Q66
 back pain, 465–469
 central, 120*t*
 chronic, 119, 348*t*, 349, Q34
 in cognitively impaired adults, 121–122, 123*t*
 definition of, 119
 diffuse, 456–457
 evaluation of, 455–457
 heel pain, 475
 low back pain, Q122
 mixed or unspecified, 121, 122*t*
 myofascial, 121, 122*t*
 neck pain, 469–470
 neuropathic, 121, 122*t*
 nociceptive, 121, 122*t*
 persistent, 119–129
 phantom limb pain, 149
 somatic, 121, 122*t*
 terms used in care of patients in, 120*t*
 total, 119
 types of, 121, 122*t*
 visceral, 121, 122*t*
 wind-up, 120*t*
Pain Disability Scale, 120
Pain intensity scales, 120
Pain management, 122–129
 in cognitively impaired, 133–134
 knee pain, Q34
 nonpharmacologic therapy, 122–123, 457
 pharmacologic therapy, 123–129, 458
 postoperative, 109–110
 in vertebral compression fractures, 254–255
Painful diabetic neuropathy, Q112
Paliperidone
 dosing and adverse events of, 325, 326*t*
 for psychosis in dementia, 272–273, 273*t*
Palliative care, 111–118
 cultural aspects of, 111–112
 endoscopic palliation, 410–411
 ethnographic data, 111–112
 for frailty, 182
 hospice, 112–113, Q41, Q98
 overall care near death, 111
 quality indicators for, 113
 for terminally ill, 114–118
Palsy, progressive supranuclear, 487–488, 487*t*
Pamelor (nortriptyline), 124*t*
Panic attacks/disorder, 319–320, 322, 322*t*, Q88
Pantoprazole, Q54
Pantothenic acid, 210*t*
PaO_2, 371
Pap smear, 72*t*, 74
Papaverine, 451–452, 451*t*
Paranoia, Q17
Paranoid personality disorder
 features of, 329, 330*t*
 therapeutic strategies for, 332, 332*t*
Parathyroid hormone (teriparatide)
 for osteoporosis prevention and treatment, 251*t*, 253
 and renal bone disease, 427
 secondary hyperparathyroidism, 245
Parathyroid hormone-related peptide (PTHrp), 512
Parathyroid metabolism disorders, 510–513
Parathyroid surgery, 511–512
Paresthesias, Q45
Parkinson disease, 484–487
 assistive devices for, Q86
 CAM for, 94
 dysphagia with, Q108
 early features that distinguish, 487*t*
 extrapyramidal signs of, Q59
 functional assessment, Q73
 interventions for preventing falls, 241*t*
 psychosis in, 327
Parkinson plus syndromes, 487–488
Parkinsonian syndromes, 487–488, 487*t*
Parkinsonism
 medication-induced, 487, 487*t*
 vascular, 487, 487*t*
Paronychia, 477
Paroxetine, Q23
 for depression, 270, 314*t*
 for depressive features of behavioral disturbances in dementia, 271*t*
 drug interactions, 87, 87*t*
Past medical history, 131, 131*t*
PATH (problem adaptation therapy), 313–317, 317*t*
Patient-centered medical homes (PCMHs), 35, 174
Patient coaching, Q6
Patient education
 about diabetes, 528–529
 guidelines for prevention of falls, 240
Patient Health Questionnaire (PHQ), 51–52
 indications to start antidepressant therapy based on, 309, 309*t*
 response guidelines based on, 309, 310*t*
 screening questions and complete assessment, 309, 309*t*
Patient preferences, 55
Patient safety. *See* Safety
Patient Self-Determination Act (PSDA), 45–46
Pay for performance, 47
PCI. *See* Percutaneous coronary intervention
PCMH (patient-centered medical home), 174
PDGF (platelet-derived growth factor), 303–304
PE. *See* Pulmonary embolism
Peak expiratory flow meters and inhalers, 374
Pediculosis capitis, 358
Pediculosis corporis, 358
Pediculosis pubis, 358
Pegaptanib sodium, 187–188
Pelvic examination, 431–432, Q57
Pelvic floor support disorders, 434–435
Pelvic lymphadenectomy, 441
Pelvic muscle exercises, 223–224
Pelvic organ prolapse, 434–435, 434*t*
Pelvic Organ Prolapse Quantification, 434
Pemphigus vulgaris, Q71
Penile prosthesis, 451*t*, 452
Peptic ulcer disease, 411–412
Peramivir, Q99
Percocet (oxycodone, immediate release), 125*t*
Percodan (oxycodone, immediate release), 125*t*

Percutaneous coronary intervention (PCI)
for acute coronary syndrome, 382
for chronic CAD, 384
Percutaneous endoscopic gastrostomy or jejunostomy, 218
Performance-based functional assessment, 231
Performance-Oriented Mobility Assessment (POMA), 50, 231, 238
Perimenopause, Q19
Perindopril, 397*t*
Periodic limb movements during sleep, 288–289
Periodontal anatomy, 362, 362*f*
Periodontal ligament, 363
Periodontitis, 363
Periodontium, 363–364
Perioperative care, 102–110, Q1, Q121
Periostitis, 472*t*
Peripheral arterial disease, 391–392
diagnosis of, 391
and foot, 479
treatment of, 391–392
Peripheral neuropathy, 492–493
Peripheral vascular disease, 144
Peroxisome proliferator-activated receptor-delta, 214*t*
Peroxisome proliferator-activated receptor-gamma coactivator 1-α, 214*t*
Perphenazine
dosing and adverse events of, 325, 326*t*
for nausea, 115*t*
for psychosis in dementia, 273*t*
Persistent pain, 119–129, Q34, Q112
assessment of, 119–121
nonopioid adjuvant medications for, 128–129
pharmacotherapy for, 123, 124*t*–126*t*
treatment of, 122–129
Personality disorders, 329–333
diagnostic challenges, 330–331
differential diagnosis of, 331
epidemiology of, 329–330
features of, 329, 330*t*
long-term course, 331
not otherwise specified, 329
therapeutic strategies for, 332, 332*t*
treatment of, Q35
Personhood, 33–34
Pes cavus, 472*t*
Pes planus, 471–473, 472*t*
Pes valgo planus, 472*t*
Pessaries, 225, 435
Phantom limb pain, 149
Pharmacodynamics
age-associated changes in, 83–84
chemotherapy issues, 544, 544*t*
Pharmacokinetics
age-associated changes in, 81–83
chemotherapy issues, 544, 544*t*
Pharmacotherapy, 81–89. *See also specific drugs*
adverse drug events, 85*t*, 86, 86*t*, 321–322, Q68
for agitated delirium, 282, 283*t*
anticonvulsant therapy, 491*t*
for anxiety disorders, 322–323
for benign prostatic hyperplasia, 438, 438*t*
brown-bag evaluation of, 88
for dementia, 264–265
for depression, 312
for diastolic HF, 399
drug addictions, Q8
drug interactions, Q36
for frailty, 181
for hypertension, 404–406
inappropriate prescribing, 84–85, 84*t*, 85*t*
investigational agents for osteoporosis, 254
for mania, 312–313, 316*t*
non-insulin agents for diabetes mellitus, 525, 526*t*–527*t*
nonadherence to regimens, 89
optimizing, 56, 84–85
for osteoporosis, 250–254, 251*t*
for pain, 123–129, 458
for persistent pain, 123, 124*t*–126*t*
polypharmacy, 56
prescribing cascade, 86
principles of prescribing, 88, 88*t*
to reduce or eliminate in management of delirium, 280, 281*t*
for sarcopenia, 214, 214*t*
for schizophrenia and schizophrenia-like syndromes, 325–326
screening tool of older persons' potentially inappropriate prescriptions (STOPP), 134–135
for sleep problems, 292–293, 294*t*
suboptimal, 131*t*, 134
for substance abuse, 340–341
that may relieve constipation, 413, 414*t*
for undernutrition syndromes, 214
Pharyngeal dysphagia, 216–217
Phenobarbital, 281*t*, 491*t*
Phentolamine, 451–452, 451*t*
Phenytoin
adverse drug events, 211
and delirium, 281*t*
drug interactions, 87, 87*t*
for epilepsy, 491*t*
nutrient interactions, 211, 211*t*
Phlebotomy, 538
Phobia
social, 322, 322*t*
specific, 320, 322, 322*t*
treatment strategies for, 322, 322*t*
Phosphodiesterase type 5 inhibitors, 86, 86*t*
Phosphorus, 427–428
Photoaging, 350
Phototherapy, 305
PHQ (Patient Health Questionnaire), 51–52, 309, 309*t*
Physical activity, 64–69. *See also* Exercise
assessing, 68
baseline activity, 64
benefits of, 64–65
for chronic constipation, 413, 413*t*
cognitive benefits of, Q96
counseling for, 68, 73*t*, 76
criteria that define frailty, 179*t*
for dementia, 262
economic benefits of, 65
guidelines for plans, 68
for obesity, Q13
for pain, 123
prescription for, 68
preventive health benefits of, 64–65
promoting, 67–69
providing assistance in increasing, 68–69
Rapid Assessment of Physical Activity, 68
recommendations for, 65–67, 66*t*
relative exercise intensity, 64
risks of, 69
screening for, 67
therapeutic benefits of, 65
Physical Activity Guidelines Advisory Committee, 67
2008 Physical Activity Guidelines for Americans (HHS), 66, 67
Physical assessment, 49–51
Physical dependence, 127
Physical disability
excess, 338–339
International Classification of Functioning, Disability, and Health (ICF) (WHO), 139
Physical disability accommodation, 5–6
Physical examination
daily evaluation, 137
foot examination, 524
gynecologic, 431–432
at hospital admission, 131, 131*t*
in mistreatment, 98
in osteoporosis, 247
with urinary incontinence, 222
Physical health
self-efficacy beliefs and, 22, 22*t*
social networks and, 23–24, 24*t*
Physical mistreatment, 98
Physical restraints, 33, Q74
Physical status, 102–103, 104*t*
Physical therapy (PT), 38*t*
for gait disorders, 231–232
for pain, 123, 457
for Parkinson disease, 94
for preventing falls, 241*t*
rehabilitation team role, 142, 143*t*
Physician-assisted suicide, 31

Physician Orders for Life-Sustaining Treatment (POLST), 29
Physician Quality Reporting System (PQRS), 47
Physicians
health insurance coverage for, 38*t*
rehabilitation team role, 142, 143*t*
role in home care, 166–167
The Physician's Guide to Assessing and Counseling Older Drivers (AMA), 52–53
Physiologic theories of aging, 9–11
Phytoestrogens, 93, 95
Pick disease, 260, 269
Pilates, 66*t*, 90
Pilocarpine, 191*t*
Pink eye, 185
Pioglitazone (Actos), 527*t*
Pioglitazone and glimepiride (Duetact), 527*t*
Pioglitazone and metformin (ACTOplus met), 527*t*
Pirbuterol, 375*t*
Planning for transitions, 110
Plantar fasciitis, 472*t*, 475
Plantar verruca, 476–477
Plaque, 363
Plaque-type lichen planus, Q124
Plasma values, 551
Platelet-derived growth factor (PDGF), 303–304
Platelet function disorders, 537–538
Platelets, 537–538
PLMS (periodic limb movements during sleep), 288–289
PMR (polymyalgia rheumatica), 462
Pneumococcal pneumonia, 217
Pneumococcal vaccination
in hospitalized patients, 131*t*, 136
immunization schedule for adults ≥65 years old, 495, 496*t*
recommendations for, 72*t*, 79, 499
Pneumonia, 498–499
antibiotic treatment of, Q48
aspiration, 217
community-acquired, 498, Q48
deaths due to, 3–4, 5*t*
guidelines for therapy, 498
hospital-acquired, 498–499
nursing-home–acquired, 498–499
pneumococcal, 217
and rehabilitation, 143
thromboprophylaxis for, Q27
Political correctness, 58
Polycarbophil (FiberCon, others), 414*t*
Polycythemia vera, 538–539
Polyethylene glycol (Miralax), 414*t*
Polymyalgia rheumatica, 462, Q114
Polymyositis, 463–464
Polypharmacy, 56
Polyps, colonic, 418
Polysomnography, Q83
POMA (Performance-Oriented Mobility Assessment), 50, 231, 238
Positional vertigo, benign paroxysmal, 199, 202, 202*f*, 203
Positive-pressure ventilation, noninvasive, Q5
Post-herpetic neuralgia, 186, 356, 357
Postacute care, 141
health insurance coverage for, 38*t*
nursing-home care, 154–155
Postacute rehabilitation
fee-for-service (FFS) care, 43–44
financing, 43–44
managed care, 44
Posterior tibial tendon dysfunction, 473–474, 473*f*
Posterior uveitis, 184, 185*t*
Postimpairment syndrome, 348*t*
Postoperative delirium, 279
Postoperative management, 106–110
Posttraumatic stress disorder, 320–321, 322, 322*t*
Postural abnormalities, 485
Postural hypotension, 207–208
guidelines for prevention of falls, 239
interventions for preventing falls, 241*t*
Postural stability tests, 236–238
Postvoid residual (PVR)
increased, 220, 221, 223
testing, 223
Potassium, 210*t*
Potassium balance disorders, 423
Potassium-sparing diuretics
adverse drug events, 86, 86*t*
drug interactions, 87, 87*t*
Potassium supplements
adverse drug events, 86, 86*t*, 211
drug interactions, 211, 211*t*
Poverty, 326
Poverty rates, 2
Power mobility devices, 151
PPD (purified-protein derivative) skin tests, 501
PPOs (preferred provider organizations), 37
PPS (prospective payment system), 155, 166
Pra (Probability of Repeated Admission) Questionnaire, 176
Pramipexole, Q83
for Parkinson disease, 486
for periodic limb movement disorder, 289
for restless legs syndrome, 289
Pramlintide (Symlin), 527*t*
PrandiMet (repaglinide and metformin), 527*t*
Prandin (repaglinide), 526*t*
Prasugrel, 381, 382
Prealbumin, 211
Preclinical disability, 50
Precose (acarbose), 526*t*
Prediabetes, 520–521
Prednisolone
drug interactions, 87
for giant cell arteritis, 462
Prednisone
for dermatomyositis, 464
for giant cell arteritis, 462
for gout, 460, Q11
for musculoskeletal pain, 458
for polymyalgia rheumatica, 462, Q114
for polymyositis, 464
for rheumatoid arthritis, 460
Preferred provider organizations (PPOs), 37
Pregabalin, Q68, Q112
Pregabalin (Lyrica)
for epilepsy, 491*t*
for persistent pain, 124*t*, 129
Prehabilitative approach, 137
Prehypertension, 402, 402*t*
Preoperative assessment and management, 102–106
Presbycusis, 193
Presbyesophagus, 216
Prescribing
inappropriate, 84–85, 84*t*, 85*t*
optimizing, 56, 84–85
principles of, 88, 88*t*
screening tool of older persons' potentially inappropriate prescriptions (STOPP), 134–135
Prescribing cascade, 86
Prescription drugs. *See* Drugs; Pharmacotherapy
Presenilin 1 (PS1), 257
Presenilin 2 (PS2), 257
Pressure Sore Status Tool, 305
Pressure stockings, 241*t*
Pressure Ulcer Scale for Healing, 305
Pressure ulcers, 297–307
assessment of, 300–301, 302*t*
avoidable, 306–307
Braden Scale, 298
complications from, 306
control of infections in, 305–306
definition of, 297
dressings for, 301–302, 304*t*
epidemiology of, 297–298
guidelines for management of, 300
guidelines for preventing, 298
hospital-acquired, 135
management of, 300–306, 302*t*, Q47, Q70
monitoring healing of, 305
new or unproven therapies for, 303–306
Norton Scale, 298
odor control for, Q70
prevention of, 131*t*, 135, 298–300, 300*t*
and rehabilitation, 142–143
risk-assessment scales, 298
risk factors for, 298
staging system for, 301, 303*t*
support surfaces for older adults at risk of, 300, 301*t*
surgical repair of, 302
unavoidable, 306–307

Presyncope, 199, 201*t*
Prevention, 70–80
aspirin therapy, 73*t*, 79
of atherosclerotic complications of diabetes mellitus, 523–524
available health measures for, 70, 72*t*–73*t*
of cardiovascular events, Q68
counseling on, 79–80
of cystitis, Q30
of delirium, Q1
of falls, 236, 237*f*, 238–240, 240–242, 241*t*, Q8, Q9, Q23, Q106
of fracture, Q111
of frailty, 181
of functional decline, Q62
health insurance coverage for services, 38*t*
of hip fracture recurrence, 147
HIV, 503
of infections, 497
Medicare benefits, Q125
of microvascular complications of diabetes mellitus, 524
of mistreatment, 97
of osteoporosis, 249–254, Q125
physical activity benefits for, 64–65
of pressure ulcers, 131*t*, 135, 298–300, 300*t*
recommended measures for, 70, 72*t*–73*t*
of stroke, 480–481, 482
of venous thromboembolism, 131*t*, 136
"Welcome to Medicare" visits, 41, 80, Q125
Primary care
comprehensive geriatric assessment (CGA) in, 173–174
enhanced, 174–175
geriatrics in, 173–176
GRACE model of, 174–175, Q64
Primidone, 281*t*
Private FFS plans, 37
Probability of Repeated Admission Questionnaire (Pra), 176
Probenecid, 461
Problem adaptation therapy (PATH), 313–317, 317*t*
Problem drinking, 340–341, 342*t*
Problem-solving therapy, 313–317, 317*t*
Problem substance use, 336
Prochlorperazine, 115*t*
Productivity, 23
Progesterone, 274–275
Progestins, 432
Prognosis, 55–56
Program of All-inclusive Care of the Elderly (PACE), 45, 169–170, Q64
Progressive supranuclear palsy, 487–488, 487*t*
Prokinetic agents, 115*t*
Prolapse
pelvic organ, 434–435, 434*t*
surgery for, 435
Promethazine, 115*t*
Prompted voiding, 223, 224, 225, Q109
Propantheline, 225
Propulsion, 229*t*
Prospective payment system (PPS), 43–44, 155, 166
Prostaglandins, 190, 191*t*
Prostate cancer, 439–444, 546, 548–549, Q69, Q90, Q111
advanced, 442*t*, 444
CAM for, 96
castrate-resistant, 549
diagnostic tests, 440–441
ethnic and racial differences in incidence, 540
expectant or conservative management of, 443
grading, 441
hormonal therapy for, 544
incidence and epidemiology of, 439
locally advanced, 442*t*, 444
management approaches for, 442*t*, 443–444
staging, 441, 441*t*
surveillance, 443
symptoms of, 439
Prostate cancer screening, 440–441
controversy, 440
recommendations for, 74
Prostate disease, 437–445
Prostate-specific antigen (PSA), Q69, Q90
Prostate-specific antigen testing, 440–441
recommendations for, 72*t*, 74
Prostatectomy, radical, 442*t*, 443
Prostatic hyperplasia, benign, 437–439
CAM for, 95
Prostatism, 437
Prostatitis, 444–445
Prostheses, penile, 451*t*, 452
Prosthetic device infections, 502
Prosthetic rehabilitation, 149
Prosthetists, 142, 143*t*
Protein-energy undernutrition, 212
Protein requirements, Q16, Q47
Proton-pump inhibitors, Q54, Q115
adverse drug events, 211
for GERD, 409–410
for nausea, 115*t*
Provider-sponsored organizations (PSOs), 37
Proxy, 28
Pruritus, 353–354, Q33
Pseudo-obstruction, acute colonic, 418
Pseudoaddiction, 120*t*, 128
Pseudoclaudication, 466
Pseudodisease, 71
Pseudoephedrine, Q66
Pseudogout, 461
Pseudomembranous candidiasis, acute, Q124
Pseudomembranous colitis, 418
Psoriasis, 354–355, 354*f*
PSOs (provider-sponsored organizations), 37
PSP (progressive supranuclear palsy), 487–488, 487*t*
Psychiatric disorders
in aging adults with intellectual disability, 346–348
CAM for, 94
diagnosis and treatment of, 347–348
Psychiatry, 308–349
Psychoactive medications, 265
Psychodynamic therapy, 313–317, 317*t*
Psychologic assessment, 51–52
Psychologic interventions, 123
Psychological abuse, 98–99
Psychological assessment, 98–99
Psychological dependence, 128
Psychological factors affecting medical conditions, 333
Psychological mistreatment, 98–99
Psychosis
antipsychotic medications for, 272–274, 273*t*
in dementia, 267, 272–274, 273*t*, Q29
late-onset, 325
major depressive disorder with, Q22
in Parkinson disease, 327
Psychosocial interventions
for dementia, 262
for depression, 313–318
Psychosocial issues, 18–25
Psychosocial theories of aging, 9
Psychotherapy, Q35
for alcohol dependence, 340–341, 342*t*
for anxiety disorders, 323
for depression, 313–317, 317*t*
emotion-oriented, 262
Psychotic depression, 311
Psychotic disorders, 324–328, Q44, Q59
Psychotic symptoms
definition of, 324
in delirium and delusional disorder, 326
in dementia, 326–327
in mood disorders, 326
Psychotropic medications, 333
Psyllium (Metamucil), 414*t*
PT (physical therapy), 38*t*
for gait disorders, 231–232
for pain, 123, 457
for Parkinson disease, 94
for preventing falls, 241*t*
rehabilitation team role, 142, 143*t*
PTHrp (parathyroid hormone-related peptide), 512
Pulmonary disease, 372–377
chronic obstructive pulmonary disease, 321, 373–374
with developmental disabilities, 348*t*, 349

guidelines for risk assessment and perioperative management of, 104
Pulmonary embolism, Q27
differential diagnosis of, 393
guidelines for prophylaxis, 107, 108*t*
Pulmonary fibrosis, idiopathic, 376
Pulmonary system: age-related changes, 12*t*, 14, 16*t*, 371
Pulmonary thromboembolism, 376–377
Pupillary defects, relative afferent, Q67
Pure red cell aplasia, 535
Purified-protein derivative (PPD) skin tests, 501
PV (polycythemia vera), 538–539
PVD (peripheral vascular disease), 144
PVR. *See* Postvoid residual
Pyelonephritis, 500
Pyrazinamide, 501

Quality Improvement System for Managed Care (QISMC), 46
Quality Indicator Survey (QIS), 157
Quality of care, 156–158
Quality of life
assessment of, 52
with cancer, 546
Quetiapine, Q29, Q74
for agitated delirium, 282, 283*t*
dosing and adverse events of, 325, 326*t*
for Parkinson disease and hallucinations, 327
for psychosis in dementia, 272–273, 273*t*
to stabilize mood in mania and bipolar depression, 316*t*
Quinapril, 397*t*

Racial differences: cancer, 540
Radiation therapy
for cancer, 545–546
external beam, 442*t*, 443–444
postoperative, after lumpectomy, 547
for prostate cancer, 442*t*, 443–444
Radical prostatectomy, 442*t*, 443
Radiculopathy, 492
Radiographs, 454–455
Raloxifene, 251*t*, 252, Q111
Ramelteon, 293, 294*t*
Ramipril, 397*t*
Ramping technique, 376
Ramsay Hunt syndrome, 356
Ranibizumab, 187–188
Ranitidine, 115*t*, Q54
RANK ligand inhibitor (denosumab), 251*t*, 253
Ranolazine, 383–384
Rapid Assessment of Physical Activity, 68
Rapid-eye-movement (REM) behavior disorder, Q83
Rapid screening, 48, 49*t*
Rasagiline, 486
Rate of living theory of aging, 10
Rational Recovery, 340
Raynaud phenomenon, 463
RDAs (recommended dietary allowances), 209–210
Reality orientation, 262
Recall test, three-item, 77
Recombinant tissue-plasminogen activator (alteplase), 482–483
Recommended dietary allowances (RDAs), 209–210
Rectal examination, digital, Q90
Red eye, 183, 184–186, 185*t*
Red yeast rice, Q89
5α-Reductase inhibitors, 438–439, 438*t*
Reflex syncope, 207–208
Reflux, gastroesophageal, 409–410, Q54
Refractive error, 186–187
Refusal of treatment, 26, Q116
forgoing and discontinuing interventions, 30–31
right to, 30–31
Rehabilitation, 139–152, Q31, Q32, Q87
adaptive methods for, 151–152
for amputation, 149
approaches and interventions, 144
cardiac, 382, 384
cognitive, 262
comorbid conditions and, 142–144
comprehensive assessment of, 144–145
conceptual model for, 140
coverage and services, 140–141
environmental modifications for, 149, 151–152
goals of, 144, 145
of hearing loss, 195, 196*t*
after hip fracture, 147, Q32
after hip or knee replacement, 232–233
low-vision, 191
nursing home care, Q32
outcomes, 141–142
postacute, 43–44
prosthetic, 149
sites of care, 139–140, 140–141, 140*t*, 141–142
for stroke, 145–146
after surgery, Q87
teams and roles, 142, 143*t*
total hip arthroplasty, 148
vestibular, Q75
vestibular rehabilitation therapy (VRT), 203
Rehabilitation Engineering and Assistive Technology Society of North America Wheelchair Service Guide, 151
Rehabilitation hospitals, 140–141, 140*t*
Relafen (nabumetone), 125*t*
Relative exercise intensity, 64
Relaxation techniques
for anxiety disorders, 323
for sleep problems, 292*t*
Relaxation therapy, 93
Relaxation training, 323
Religion, 61
Religious identity, 59
Religious involvement, 24–25
Relistor (methylnaltrexone), 414*t*
REM (rapid-eye-movement) behavior disorder, Q83
REM sleep behavior disorder, 289
Reminiscence therapy, 262, 313–317, 317*t*
Remitting seronegative symmetrical synovitis with pitting edema ("RS3PE" syndrome), 460
Renal artery stenosis, Q66
Renal bone disease, 427–428
Renal diseases and disorders. *See* Kidney diseases and disorders
Renal replacement therapy, 428–429
Renin inhibitors, 405–406
Renovascular angioplasty, 424
Renovascular disease, 424
Repaglinide (Prandin), 526*t*
Repaglinide and metformin (PrandiMet), 527*t*
Reperfusion therapy, 382
Research
on cognitively impaired older adults, 30, 30*t*
informed consent for, 30
Resident Assessment Protocols, 215
Residential-care facilities, 6
Resistance training, Q96
interventions for preventing falls, 241*t*
recommendations for, 64, 66*t*
Resource utilization group system (RUGS), 43–44
Respect for life, 111
Respectful nonverbal communication, 60
Respiration, loud, 118
Respiratory diseases and disorders, 371–377, Q5, Q102
antibiotic therapy for infections, 496–497, 497*t*
chronic lower respiratory disease, 3–4, 5*t*
preoperative assessment and management of, 104
pulmonary disease, 372–377
symptoms and complaints, 371–372
Restless legs syndrome, 288–289
Restraints, 33, 137, Q74
for behavioral problems in dementia, 275
Retinal detachment, 183, 185*t*
Retinopathy, diabetic, 184*t*, 188–189, 190*f*
Retropulsion, 229*t*

Revascularization
for chronic CAD, 384
mechanical, Q26
for peripheral arterial disease, 392
Review of systems at hospital admission, 131, 131*t*
Rheumatic mitral stenosis, 385
Rheumatoid arthritis, 459–460
Rheumatoid factor, 454
Rheumatologic diseases, 458–464
Rhinosinusitis, 371–372
Rhythm abnormalities, 239
Riboflavin, 210*t*
Rifampin, 501
Rimantadine, 499, Q99
Riomet (metformin), 526*t*
Risedronate, 250, 251*t*
Risperidone, Q29
for agitated delirium, 282, 283*t*
dosing and adverse events of, 325, 326*t*
for psychosis in dementia, 272–273, 273*t*
to stabilize mood in mania and bipolar depression, 316*t*
Rituximab, 545
Rivaroxaban
adverse drug events, 86, 86*t*
for stroke prophylaxis in AF, 389
Rivastigmine, Q74
for dementia, 264
for dementia with intellectual disability, 346–347
for dementia with Parkinson disease, 486
RLS (restless legs syndrome), 288–289
Road tests, Q51
Role loss and acquisition, 20–21
Rollators, 151
Rolling assessment, 48
Romberg test, 230, Q45
Ropinirole, Q83
for Parkinson disease, 486
for periodic limb movement disorder, 289
for restless legs syndrome, 289
Rosacea, 351–352, 351*f*
Rosiglitazone (Avandia), 525, 527*t*
Rosiglitazone and glimepiride (Avandaryl), 527*t*
Rosiglitazone and metformin (Avandamet), 527*t*
Rotigotine, 486
Roxanol (morphine, immediate release), 125*t*
"RS3PE" syndrome (remitting seronegative symmetrical synovitis with pitting edema), 460
RUGS (resource utilization group system), 43–44
Rule of double effect, 31

S-adenosylmethionine (SAM-e), 91, 92*t*, 94
Sacral fractures, osteoporotic, 467, Q103, Q111
Sacral insufficiency fracture, Q103
Sacral nerve neuromodulation, 226
Safe Return, 263
Safety, 78
attention to, 263–264
of CAM therapies, 91–92
and dementia, 263–264
of dietary supplements, 91, 92*t*
home safety evaluation, 241*t*
preventing injury, 78
resident, Q28
staff, Q79
in transitions, 162
Salflex (salsalate), 125*t*
Salicylates, 211, 211*t*, Q34
Saline laxatives, 414*t*
Salivary function, 365
Salivary glands, 362, 363*t*
Salix alba (white willow bark), 93
Salmeterol, 374, 375*t*
Salsalate (Disalcid, Mono-Gesic, Salflex), 125*t*
Salt depletion, primary, 421–422
SAM-e (S-adenosylmethionine), 91, 92*t*, 94
Sarcopenia, 212
activity recommendations for, 66*t*
definition of, 212
drug treatment of, 214, 214*t*
Sarcoptes scabiei var *hominis*, 358
Satellite lesions, Q33
Savella (milnacipran), 124*t*
Saw palmetto *(Serenoa repens)*
for benign prostatic hyperplasia, 439
safety issues, 91, 92*t*
Saxagliptin (Onglyza), 526*t*
Saxagliptin and metformin (Kombiglyze XR), 527*t*
Scabies, 358, Q33
Scheduled toileting, Q106
Schizoid personality disorder
features of, 329, 330*t*
therapeutic strategies for, 332, 332*t*
Schizophrenia and schizophrenia-like syndromes, 324–326
clinical characteristics of, 325
definition of, 324
epidemiology of, 325
late-onset schizophrenia, 324, 325
treatment and management of, 325–326
Schizophrenia-like psychosis
late-onset, 325
very-late-onset, 324
Schizotypal personality disorder
features of, 329, 330*t*
therapeutic strategies for, 332, 332*t*
Sciatica, 466
Scissoring, 229*t*
Scleritis, 183–184, 185*t*
Scooters, motorized, 151
Scopolamine
for bowel obstruction, 116*t*
for nausea, 115*t*
Screening, 74–76
for breast cancer, Q50
for cancer, 70–74, 543, Q50, Q84
for cognitive assessment, 258, 258*t*
for colorectal cancer, Q84
criteria for recommending, 70
for depression, 309–310
for frailty, 179–180
for hearing loss, 193–194, Q10
for hormone hypersecretion with adrenal incidentalomas, 515, 515*t*
for mistreatment, 98, 99*t*
nutrition, 78, 210–212
for osteoporosis, 243
PHQ-9 questions, 309, 309*t*
physical activity, 67
for prostate cancer, 440–441
rapid, 48, 49*t*
recommendations for, 70, 72*t*
for risk of falls, 238
for urinary incontinence, 73*t*, 222, 225–226
for vitamin D deficiency, 213
Screening tool of older persons' potentially inappropriate prescriptions (STOPP), 134–135
Seborrheic dermatitis, 350–351, 351*f*
Seborrheic keratoses, 358, 359*f*
Section 8, Housing and Urban Development programs, 171
Sedating antidepressants, 293, 294*t*
Sedating antihistamines, 290, 294–295, 294*t*
Sedating antipsychotics, 293
Sedative/hypnotics, Q40
adverse drug events, 86, 86*t*
chronic use, 293–294
interventions for preventing falls with, 241*t*
for sleep problems, 290, 292–293, 294*t*
Seizures, 489–490
anticonvulsant therapy for, 490, 491*t*
with developmental disabilities, 348*t*, 349
Selective estrogen-receptor modulators, 251*t*, 252
Selective norepinephrine-reuptake inhibitors (SNRIs), Q83, Q88
for anxiety disorders, 322, 322*t*
for depression, 314*t*
for depressive features of behavioral disturbances in dementia, 271*t*
Selective serotonin-reuptake inhibitors (SSRIs)
adverse drug events, 86, 86*t*, 211, Q83, Q92
for anxiety disorders, 322, 322*t*, Q92
for depression, 312, 314*t*, Q92

for depressive features of behavioral disturbances in dementia, 270, 271*t*
for panic disorder, Q88
for vasomotor symptoms or hot flushes, 432
Selegiline
for depression, 314*t*
for Parkinson disease, 486
Selenium, 210*t*
Self-care, 49–50, 49*t*
Self-care decisions, 27, 28*t*
Self-efficacy beliefs, 22
physical and mental health impacts of, 22, 22*t*
strategies effective for strengthening, 22
Self-injurious behavior, 346
Self-management support, 528–529
Self-neglect, 100, 320, Q4
Self-prayer, 91, 91*t*
Senescence, 494
Senile chorea, 488
"Senile" gait disorder, 229
Senile squalor syndrome, 320
Senior Health Clinic (SHC), 173
Senna (Senokot), 414*t*
Sensory impairment
with developmental disabilities, 348*t*, 349
hearing impairment, 192–198
in hospitalized patients, 131*t*, 132–133
interventions for, 131*t*
and rehabilitation, 144
smell dysfunction, 368, 369*t*
taste dysfunction, 368, 369*t*
vision impairment, 183–191, 241*t*
Sepsis, 497
Septicemia, 3–4, 5*t*
Sequenced Treatment Alternatives to Relieve Depression (STAR*D), 309, 310*t*
Serenoa repens (saw palmetto)
for benign prostatic hyperplasia, 439
safety issues, 91, 92*t*
Serotonin antagonists, 115*t*
Serotonin-norepinephrine–reuptake inhibitors (SNRIs), Q83, Q88
Serotonin syndrome, 271, 271*t*
Sertraline, 270, 271*t*, 312, 314*t*, Q14, Q35, Q39
Serum values, 551
Sex hormone-binding globulin, 516
Sex therapy, 451*t*, 452
Sexual activity, 76, Q24
Sexual function disorders, 446–452, Q24, Q38
counseling for, 73*t*, 76
female dysfunction, 446–447
male dysfunction, 448–450, 449*t*, Q38
Sexual satisfaction, 446–447
Sexuality
and cognitive impairment, 34
female, 446
male, 448–452
Sexually transmitted infections (STIs), 76
SF-36 (Short Form-36 Health Survey), 52, 145
SHBG (sex hormone-binding globulin), 516
SHC (Senior Health Clinic), 173
Sheltered housing, 171
"Shingles" (herpes zoster), 185*t*, 186, 356–357, 357*f*, 504
Shoe problems, 239–240
Shoe terms, 476*t*
Shoes, 476
Short Form-36 Health Survey (SF-36), 52, 145
Shoulder pain, 455
Shy-Drager syndrome, 487
SIADH (syndrome of inappropriate antidiuretic hormone), 422, 513
Sicca symptoms, 464
Sick sinus syndrome, 387, 390–391
Sideroblastic anemia, 535
Sight problems. *See* Visual impairment
Sigmoidoscopy, 71
Sign language, Q55
Sildenafil, 450–451, 451*t*
Simplified Nutrition Assessment Questionnaire, 212
Simvastatin, Q36
Sitagliptin (Januvia), 526*t*
Sitagliptin and metformin (Janumet), 527*t*
Sites of care, 163
6-minute walk test, 231
Sjögren syndrome, 464
Skeletal system: age-related changes, 12*t*, 16*t*
Skilled nursing facilities (SNFs), 38*t*, 140*t*, 141, 142
Skin: age-related changes, 12*t*, 13, 16*t*, 350
Skin care, 298–299
Skin equivalents, 305
Skin problems
autoimmune conditions, 350–355
benign growths, 358–359
cancer, 74, 359–361
dermatologic diseases and disorders, 350–361
on foot, 476–478
infections, 356–358, 496–497, 497*t*
infestations, 356–358
inflammatory conditions, 350–355
neoplasms, 476–477
rash, Q33
Sleep problems, 285–295
age-related changes, 285–286, 287*t*
CAM for, 94–95
central sleep apnea, 287
in dementia, 274, 289–290
drug-induced somnolence, Q68
epidemiology of, 285
evaluation of, 286
in hospitalized patients, 131*t*, 135, 290
interventions for, 131*t*, 135
management of, 291–295, Q40, Q60
measures to improve sleep hygiene, 291, 291*t*
nonpharmacologic interventions for, 291–292, 292*t*
in nursing home, 290–291
obstructive sleep apnea, 287–288, 290, 375–376
periodic limb movements, 288–289
pharmacotherapy for, 292–293
rapid-eye-movement (REM) behavior disorder, Q83
sleep apnea, 287–288
treatment of, 274
Sleep-related breathing disorders, 287–288, 290
Sleep restriction, 292*t*
Sleeping medications, 290, 294–295
Slings, 225
Slowness, 179*t*
SLUMS (St. Louis University Mental Status) examination, 51, 258, 258*t*
Smell dysfunction
medications that cause, 368, 369*t*
nonpharmacologic causes of, 368, 369*t*
odor control, Q70
Smoking cessation
and cardiovascular risk, 379–380
"Five A's" for, 342
to reduce risk of osteoporosis, 246, 246*t*
Smoking cessation counseling, 76
recommendations for, 73*t*
Snellen charts, 50
SNFs (skilled nursing facilities), 38*t*, 140*t*, 141
SNRIs. *See* Selective norepinephrine-reuptake inhibitors
Social assessment, 52
Social conditions, 349
Social history, 131, 131*t*
Social involvement, 23
Social networks, 23–24, 24*t*
Social phobia, 322, 322*t*
Social rhythm therapy, 317*t*, 318
Social Security, 2
Social Services Block Grant programs, 171
Social status, 21
Social support, 313–317, 317*t*
Social workers, 142, 143*t*
Socially inappropriate behaviors, 33
Socioeconomic status, 2–3
Sodium, 422
Sodium balance disorders, 421–423
Sodium conservation, 421*t*
Sodium deficit, 422

Sodium excretion, 421*t*
Sodium phosphate/biphosphate
emollient enema (Fleet), 414*t*
Soft-tissue infections, 496–497, 497*t*
Solifenacin, 224
Somatic delusions, 326
Somatic pain, 121, 122*t*
Somatic symptom and related disorders, 333–335, Q85
clinical characteristics and causes of, 334
diagnostic criteria for, 333
other or unspecified, 333
treatment of, 334–335
undifferentiated, Q85
Somatization disorder, Q85
Sorbitol 70%, 414*t*
Soy products, 93, 95
Special needs, 47
Special needs plans, 37
Specialty care, geriatric, 173
Speech, hypophonic, 485
Speech therapy, 38*t*
rehabilitation team role, 142, 143*t*
Spinal cord compression, Q77
Spinal cord dysfunction, 492
Spinal cord tumors, Q77
Spinal deformities, 348*t*, 349
Spinal infections, Q122
Spinal manipulation, 93
Spirituality, 24–25, 63
Spironolactone, 398
Squamous cell carcinoma, 360
oral, 365–366
oropharyngeal, 365–366
Squamous hyperplasia, 434
SSI (Supplemental Security Income), 171
SSRIs. *See* Selective serotonin-reuptake inhibitors
ST (speech therapy), 38*t*, 142, 143*t*
St. John's wort *(Hypericum perforatum)*, 94
for depression, 315*t*
safety issues, 91, 92*t*
St. Louis University Mental Status (SLUMS) examination, 51, 258, 258*t*
St. Thomas's Risk Assessment Tool (STRATIFY), 238
ST-elevation myocardial infarction (STEMI), 380, 381, Q26
Stabilization, 340
Staff assaults, Q79
Staffing patterns, 155
Staphylococcus aureus, 498–499
STAR*D (Sequenced Treatment Alternatives to Relieve Depression), 309, 310*t*
Starlix (nateglinide), 526*t*
Stasis dermatitis, 355
State Veterans Homes, 154
Statins
for acute coronary syndrome, 382
for atherosclerotic complications of diabetes mellitus, 524
for chronic CAD, 383
Stem cell/progenitor cell theory of aging, 11
Stem cells, hematopoietic, 530
Steppage gait, 229*t*
Stevens-Johnson syndrome, Q71
Stiffness, morning, Q114
Stimulant laxatives, 414*t*
Stimulants, 315*t*
Stimulation-oriented treatment, 262
Stimulus control, 292*t*
STIs (sexually transmitted infections), 76
Stomach disorders, 411–412
Stomatitis, denture, 367, 367*f*
STOPP (screening tool of older persons' potentially inappropriate prescriptions), 134–135
STRATIFY (St. Thomas's Risk Assessment Tool), 238
Strength testing, Q73
Streptococcus pneumoniae, 498
Stress
mediators, 21–22
moderators, 23–25
posttraumatic stress disorder, 320–321, 322, 322*t*
Stress incontinence, 220
and impaired urethral sphincter support, 221
minimally invasive procedures for, 225
surgery for, 225
treatment of, 225
Stress management, 96
Stress process models, 18
Stress testing, preoperative, 103
Stressors, 18–21
Striatonigral degeneration, 487
Stroke
acute ischemic, 482–483
approach to management of, 145–146
cardioembolic, 482
follow-up management, Q31
goals of rehabilitation after, 145
guidelines for rehabilitation after, 145–146
incidence of, 480
NIH Stroke Scale, 145–146, 480, 480*t*, 483
in nursing-home population, 153
prevalence of, 3, 4*f*
prevention of, 388, 480–481, 482
rehabilitation after, 145–146
risk factors for, 480–481
Stroke Impact Scale, 141*t*, 145
Strontium ranelate, 254
Subclinical depression, 311
Subclinical glucocorticoid hypersecretion, 515
Subclinical hyperthyroidism, 509
Subclinical hypothyroidism, 507
Subconjunctival hemorrhage, 184–185, 185*t*, 186
Subdural hematoma, 483
Subluxation, foot, 472*t*
Suboptimal care transitions, 161–162
Substance abuse
at-risk use, 336
counseling interventions for, 73*t*
definition of, 336–337
identifying substance-use disorders, 339
outpatient management of, 340
pharmacotherapy for, 340–341
risks and benefits of, 338–339
treatment of, 339–343
Substance dependence, 336
Substituted judgment, 26, 28–29, 28*t*
Sucralfate, Q54
Suicide
physician-assisted, 31
prevention of, 313–317, 317*t*
Sulfonylureas, 2nd-generation, 525, 526*t*
Sundowning, Q22
Superficial basal cell carcinoma, 360
Superficial spreading melanoma, 360, 361*f*
Supplemental Security Income (SSI), 171
Supplements, 213–214. *See also specific hormones, minerals, vitamins*
for pressure ulcers, 302
safety issues, 91, 92*t*
Supplies, 38*t*
Support surfaces, 300, 301*t*
Supraventricular arrhythmias, 389
Supraventricular tachycardia, 390–391
Surfactant laxatives, 414*t*
Surgical care
aortic valve, Q49
for benign prostatic hyperplasia, 438*t*, 439
bypass surgery, 384
for cancer, 443, 546, Q91
cardiac risk assessment for, 103, 105*f*
for epilepsy, 490
for foot deformities, 476
for gait disorders, 232
for hip fracture, 146–147
iatrogenic complications, 106
for incontinence, 226
knee replacement, Q87
noncardiac, 103, 105*f*
for osteoarthritis, 459
for ovarian cancer, Q91
parathyroid, 511–512
perioperative care, 102–110
postoperative delirium, 279, Q121
postoperative management, 106–110, Q87
preoperative assessment and management, 102–106
for pressure ulcers, 302
for prolapse, 435
for prostate cancer, 443

rehabilitation after, Q87
for stress incontinence, 228
total hip and knee arthroplasty, 147–148
for vertebral compression fractures, 254–255
Surveillance, 443
Suspiciousness, isolated, 327
Swallowing, 216–217, Q31, Q108
Swinging flashlight test, 183, Q67
Symlin (pramlintide), 527*t*
Sympathectomy, Q112
Syncope, 204–208
causes of, 204
diagnosis of, 204, Q46
evaluation of, 205–207
history in, 205–206
indications for permanent pacemaker implantation, 390, 391*t*
natural history of, 204
during or after exertion, Q61
pathophysiology of, 204–205
physical examination of, 206–207
predictors of, 206, 206*t*
prognosis for, 204
reflex, 207–208
situational, Q61
treatment of, 207–208
vasovagal, 204
Syndrome of inappropriate antidiuretic hormone, 422, 513
Syndromes, 177–307
Synovitis, 460
Syphilis, 503–504
Systematic assessment, 131, 131*t*
Systemic lupus erythematosus, 463
Systems of care, 130–176
Systems review, 131, 131*t*

T-score, 247–248
T_3. *See* Triiodothyronine
T_4. *See* Thyroxine
Tachy-brady syndrome, 390–391
Tadalafil, 450–451, 451*t*
Tai Chi, Q40
for frailty, 181
for pain, 123
for preventing falls, 67, 238, 241*t*
recommendations for, 66*t*, 76
for sleep problems, 292
Tailor's bunion, 472*t*
Tamoxifen, 87, 87*t*
Tapentadol (Nucynta), 126*t*, 129
Tapentadol extended release (Nucynta ER), 126*t*
Tardive dyskinesia (TD), 325–326, 489
Tardive dystonia, 489
Target theory of genetic damage, 9
Tarsal tunnel syndrome, 472*t*
Task Force on Community Preventive Services, 68
Taste dysfunction
age-related changes, 368
medications that cause, 368, 369*t*
nonpharmacologic causes of, 368, 369*t*
TCAs. *See* Tricyclic antidepressants
TD (tardive dyskinesia), 325–326, 489
Teach-back method, 59
Teams, rehabilitation, 142, 143*t*
Technetium bone scan, 468
Technologic innovations, 170
Teeth
age-related changes in, 362, 363*t*
anatomy of, 362, 362*f*
Tegretol (carbamazepine), 124*t*
Telecoil, 196–197
Telehealth discharge interventions, Q6
Telephone quit lines, 73*t*
Telmisartan, 397*t*
Telomere length, Q113
Telomere theory of aging, 9–10
Temazepam, 293, 294*t*
Temporal arteritis, 462
headache due to, 484
Temporal artery, Q114
Tendinitis, 453, 455
Tenosynovitis, 472*t*
TENS (transcutaneous electrical nerve stimulation), 457
Teriparatide (parathyroid hormone), 251*t*, 253
Terminal illness
anorexia in, 116
bowel obstruction in, 115–116
cachexia in, 116
constipation in, 114
cough in, 118
delirium in, 116
depression in, 116–117
diarrhea in, 114–115
dyspnea in, 117–118
nausea and vomiting in, 114
palliative care, 114–118
Terminology
glossary of gait abnormalities, 229*t*
preferred terms for cultural or religious identity, 59
shoe terms, 476*t*
terms used in care of patients in pain, 120*t*
Testamentary competence, 27
Testosterone, 516–518
Testosterone replacement therapy, 516–517
Testosterone supplementation
available preparations, 517, 517*t*
benefits and risks for men, 516–518, 517*t*
for erectile dysfunction, 452
for female sexual dysfunction, 447, 516
Tetanus, diphtheria, pertussis (Td/Tdap), 495, 496*t*
Tetanus booster, 72*t*, 79
Theophylline
adverse drug events, 211
drug interactions, 87, 87*t*
Theories of aging, 8–11
Thiamine, 210*t*
Thiazide-type diuretics, 405
Thiazolidinediones, 525, 526*t*–527*t*
Thinking problems. *See* Cognitive impairment
32P, 539
Thought disorder, 324
Thrombocythemia, essential, 538, 539
Thrombocytopenia, 537
Thromboembolism
pulmonary, 376–377
venous, 107, 108*t*, 392–394
Thrombopathy, 537–538
Thromboprophylaxis
guidelines for, 107, 108*t*, 136
in hospitalized patients, 131*t*, 136
regimens, Q27
Thrombotic thrombocytopenic purpura, 536
Thrush, 367, 367*f*
Thyroid disorders, 506–510
cancer, 509–510
with developmental disabilities, 348*t*, 349
nodular, 509–510
screening for, 74
Thyroid hormone replacement, 507–508
Thyroid-stimulating hormone (thyrotropin), 506
Thyroid ultrasonography, 509–510, 510*t*
Thyrotoxicosis
apathetic, 508
triiodothyronine (T_3), 508
Thyrotropin (thyroid-stimulating hormone), 506
low thyrotropin, 508
screening test, 72*t*, 506–507
Thyroxine (T_4)
high T_4 syndrome, 508
low T_4 syndrome, 507–508
replacement therapy, 508
Tiagabine, 491*t*
Tibialis posterior dysfunction, 472*t*, 473, 473*f*
Tilt-table testing, 207, Q46
Time of death, 31–32
Timed Up and Go (TUG) test, 50, 231, 236–238, Q73
Timolol, 191*t*
Tinnitus, 193
Tiotropium bromide, 374, 375*t*
Tirofiban, 381
Tissue plasminogen activator (tPA), recombinant (alteplase), 482–483
TMP (trimethoprim), 211, 211*t*
TMP-SMX (trimethoprim-sulfamethoxazole)
drug interactions, 87, 87*t*
for UTIs, 500
Tobacco dependence, 76, 341–343
α-Tocopherol (vitamin E)
for dementia, 265
RDIs for adults ≥71 years old, 210*t*
Toileting, scheduled, Q106

Tolerance, 127
Tolterodine, 224
Tolvaptan, 422
Tongue, black hairy, 368, 368*f*
Toothlessness, 364–365
Topiramate, 491*t*
Total hip and knee arthroplasty, 147–148
 cause and surgical care of, 147–148
 management of, 148
 rehabilitation after, 148
Total knee replacement, Q87
Toxic encephalopathy, 276
Toxic epidermal necrolysis (TEN), Q71
Toxicity, chemotherapy, 544, 544*t*, 545
Tradition, 60–61
Traditional Chinese medicine, 90
Traditional Native American medicine, 91
Tradjenta (linagliptin), 526*t*
Tramadol (Ultram), 126*t*, 129
Trandolapril, 397*t*
Transcatheter aortic valve replacement (TAVR), Q49
Transcutaneous electrical nerve stimulation, 457, Q34
Transdermal fentanyl (Duragesic), 126*t*
Transesophageal echocardiography, 501
Transfer skills impairment, 241*t*
Transfers, 161
Transient ischemic attack, 481
Transitional care, 161–165, Q6, Q32
Transitions in care, 162*f*
 barriers to safety, 162
 communication for, 164
 discharge destinations, 163
 planning for, 110
 steps/strategies to improve, 163, 164
 suboptimal, 161–162
 venues of care, 163
Transplantation, kidney, 429
Tranylcypromine, 312, 314*t*
Trastuzumab, 545
Trauma
 history of traumatic experiences, 60
 posttraumatic stress disorder, 320–321, 322, 322*t*
Trazodone, Q74
 adverse drug events, 86, 86*t*
 for depression, 315*t*
 for depressive features of behavioral disturbances in dementia, 271*t*
 for insomnia, 265, 293, 294*t*
 for sleep disturbances in dementia, 274
Treatment decisions
 ETHNICS mnemonic, 63
 in extended-care settings, 32–33
Treatment initiation programs, 313–317, 317*t*
Tremors
 action tremor, 489
 essential tremor, 489
Trendelenburg gait, 229–230, 229*t*
Trends, 3–4
Triamcinolone acetonide, 375*t*, 461–462
Triamterene, 86, 86*t*
Triazolam, 281*t*
Tricyclic antidepressants (TCAs), Q88, Q112
 adverse drug events, 86, 86*t*, 270–271
 and delirium, 281*t*
 for depression, 315*t*
 for depressive features of behavioral disturbances in dementia, 270–271, 271*t*
 for persistent pain, 124*t*, 128–129
Triiodothyronine (T_3), 312, 315*t*
 low T_3 syndrome, 507–508
Triiodothyronine (T_3) thyrotoxicosis, 508
Trimethoprim (TMP), 211, 211*t*
Trimethoprim-sulfamethoxazole (TMP-SMX)
 drug interactions, 87, 87*t*
 for UTIs, 500
Trospium, 224
Truth telling, 33
Try This, 48
TTP (thrombotic thrombocytopenic purpura), 536
Tube feeding, 217, 218
Tuberculosis, 500–501
Tubular necrosis, acute, 425
TUG (Timed Up and Go) test, 50, 231, 236–238, Q73
Tumors
 oropharyngeal, Q108
 spinal cord, Q77
Turn en bloc, 229*t*
Tylenol (acetaminophen), 124*t*
Tylox (oxycodone, immediate release), 115*t*

UI. *See* Urinary incontinence
Ulcers, 355–356
 aphthous ulcers, 367–368, 368*f*
 arterial ulcers, 355–356, 356*t*
 chronic leg ulcers, 355
 corneal, 184, 185*t*, 186
 decubitus ulcer, 297
 foot ulcers, 478, Q43
 NSAID-induced, 411
 peptic ulcer disease, 411–412
 pressure ulcers, 297–307, Q47, Q70
 venous ulcers, 355–356, 356*t*
Ultram (tramadol), 126*t*
Ultrasound
 abdominal, 72*t*
 therapeutic, 457
 thyroid, 509–510, 510*t*
Undernutrition, 212, 214
Underprescribing, 84, 84*t*, 85
Unspoken challenges, 61
Unstable lumbar spine, 467
Urethral sphincter support, impaired, 221
Urge incontinence, 220
 with detrusor overactivity (uninhibited bladder contractions), 221
 minimally invasive procedures for, 225
Urgencies, hypertensive, 407
Urinary incontinence (UI), 220–227, Q82
 assessment of, 225–226
 behavioral therapies for, 223–224, 226
 CAM for, 95
 comorbid conditions that can cause or worsen, 221
 with developmental disabilities, 348*t*, 349
 evaluation of, 222–223
 functional, 220
 history in, 222
 with impaired bladder emptying, 221
 from incomplete emptying, 220
 lower urinary tract pathophysiology in, 221
 management of, 223–225, Q109
 minimally invasive procedures for, 225
 mixed UI, 220, 221
 in nursing-home residents, 225–226
 pathophysiology of, 221
 physical examination with, 222
 prevalence and impact of, 220
 prevention of, 77
 prompted voiding for, Q109
 red flag symptoms, 222
 risk factors for, 221
 screening for, 73*t*, 222, 225–226
 stress UI, 220, 221
 supportive care for, 225
 surgery for, 225
 testing for, 223
 transient, 220
 treatment of, 223–225
 types of, 220
 urge UI, 220, 221
Urinary system: age-related changes, 12*t*, 15, 16*t*
Urinary tract infections, 499–500
 antibiotic therapy for, 496–497, 497*t*
 in men, 499, 500
 recurrent, Q30
 in women, 499–500
Urine values, 551
Urodynamic testing, 223
Urogenital atrophy, 432–433
U.S. Department of Agriculture (USDA), 209
U.S. Department of Health and Human Services (HHS), 66, 67

U.S. Preventive Services Task Force (USPSTF), 67, 68, 70, 71–74, 75, 76
indications for osteoporosis screening, 248, 248*t*
recommendations for BMD testing, 248
recommendations for prostate cancer screening, 440
USDA (U.S. Department of Agriculture), 209
USPSTF. *See* U.S. Preventive Services Task Force
Uveitis, 184, 185*t*

Vaccinations
herpes zoster, 72*t*, 79, 495, 496*t*
for hospitalized patients, 131*t*, 136
influenza, 499
for influenza, 72*t*, 78–79, 136
in nursing-home care, 159–160
pneumococcal, 72*t*, 79, 131*t*, 136, 499
Vacuum tumescence devices, 451, 451*t*
Vaginal atrophy, 446, Q21, Q24
Vaginal bleeding, postmenopausal, 435–436, 436*t*, Q57
Vaginal dryness, 95
Vaginal estrogen tablets, Q21
Vaginal prolapse
classification of, 434–435, 434*t*
surgery for, 435
Vaginitis, atrophic, Q24
Valerian, 295, Q40, Q89
Valerian root, 94
Valgus position, 472*t*
Valproic acid (valproate, divalproex), 265, 491*t*
Valsartan, 397*t*
Valve-associated anemia, 536
Valve replacement, Q49
Valvular heart disease, 384–385
clinical features and treatment of, 386*t*
diagnosis of, 385
epidemiology of, 384–385
Vancomycin, 418
Vardenafil, 450–451, 451*t*
Varenicline, 340–341, 342*t*
Varicella immunization, 495, 496*t*
Varicella-zoster virus, 504
Varus position, 472*t*
Vascular dementia
diagnostic features and treatment of, 259*t*
differential diagnosis of, 260
epidemiology of, 256
Vascular disease
cardiovascular disease, 378–394
cerebrovascular disease, 3–4, 5*t*
peripheral vascular disease, 144
Vascular ectasia, 417
Vascular endothelial growth factor inhibitors, 187–188
Vascular parkinsonism, 487, 487*t*
Vasculature: age-related changes, 12*t*, 13–14, 16*t*
Vasodilators, 406
Vasomotor symptoms, 432, Q19
Vasovagal syncope, 204
VDE (videofluoroscopic deglutition examination), 216, 217
VDRL (Venereal Disease Research Laboratory) test, 503–504
VEGF Trap-Eye, 188
Venereal Disease Research Laboratory (VDRL) test, 503–504
Venlafaxine (Effexor)
for depression, 312, 314*t*
for depressive features of behavioral disturbances in dementia, 270–271, 271*t*
for persistent pain, 124*t*
Venous thromboembolic disease, 392–394
Venous thrombosis prophylaxis
guidelines for, 107, 108*t*
in hospitalized patients, 131*t*, 136
Venous ulcers, 355–356, 356*t*
Ventricular arrhythmias, 389–390
Ventricular tachycardia, Q58
Venues for care, 163
Verapamil
adverse drug events, 86, 86*t*
for atrial fibrillation, 387
drug interactions, 87, 87*t*
Verbal Descriptor Scale, 120
Vertebral fracture assessment (VFA), 248–249
Vertebral fractures
compression fractures, 254–255
management of, 254–255
osteoporotic, Q115
osteoporotic compression fractures, 466–467
Vertebroplasty, 254–255
Vertigo, 199, 201*t*
benign paroxysmal positional vertigo (BPPV), 199, 202, 202*f*, 203
VES-13 (Vulnerable Elders Survey-13), 176
Vestibular neuritis, Q75
Vestibular rehabilitation, Q75
Vestibular rehabilitation therapy (VRT), 203
Veterans Administration (VA), 40–41, 175
Veterans Affairs, Department of
guidelines for rehabilitation after stroke, 145–146
hearing aid benefits, 197
VFA (vertebral fracture assessment), 248–249
Vicodin (hydrocodone), 125*t*
Vicoprofen (hydrocodone), 125*t*
Victoza (liraglutide), 527*t*
Videofluoroscopic deglutition examination (VDE), 216, 217
Vilazodone
for depression, 315*t*
for depressive features of behavioral disturbances in dementia, 271*t*
VIN (vulvar intraepithelial neoplasia), 434
Vinorelbine, 544
Violent behavior, Q79
Viral conjunctivitis, 184–185, 185*t*
Visceral pain, 121, 122*t*
Vision services, 38*t*
Vision testing, 73*t*, 77–78, 183
Visual Analog Scale, 306
Visual hallucinations, Q59
Visual imagery, 323
Visual impairment, 183–191, Q67, Q78
assessment of, 50–51
definition of, 183
low-vision rehabilitation, 191
preventing falls with, 239, 241*t*
rapid screening followed by assessment and management of, 48, 49*t*
screening for, 73*t*, 77–78
signs and symptoms requiring immediate referral, 183–184, 185*t*
sudden decrease in vision, 183, 185*t*
symptoms and treatment of common eye diseases, 184*t*, 185*t*
Vitamin A
drug interactions, 211, 211*t*
RDIs for adults ≥71 years old, 210*t*
Vitamin B_1, 211, 211*t*
Vitamin B_2, 211, 211*t*
Vitamin B_6
drug interactions, 211, 211*t*
RDIs for adults ≥71 years old, 210*t*
Vitamin B_6 supplements, 213
Vitamin B_{12}
drug interactions, 211, 211*t*
RDIs for adults ≥71 years old, 210*t*
Vitamin B_{12} deficiency, 532, Q45
hypoproliferative anemia due to, 532, 534*f*
Vitamin B_{12} replacement, 537
Vitamin B_{12} supplements, 213
Vitamin C, Q47
for AMD, 187
RDIs for adults ≥71 years old, 210*t*
Vitamin D, Q107, Q115
drug interactions, 211, 211*t*
for malnutrition, 213
for osteoporosis, 249–250, 253
for prevention of falls, 239, 241*t*
preventive, 73*t*, 79
RDIs for adults ≥71 years old, 210*t*, 213–214
recommended dietary intakes, 510
for vitamin D deficiency, 511
Vitamin D deficiency, 510–511, Q107
in hospitalized patients, 135
screening for, 213

Vitamin D insufficiency, 245
Vitamin D_2 (ergocalciferol) supplements, 511
Vitamin D_3 (cholecalciferol)
supplements, Q125
to reduce risk of osteoporosis, 246, 246*t*
for vitamin D deficiency, 511
Vitamin E (α-tocopherol)
for ARMD, 187
for dementia, 265
drug interactions, 211, 211*t*
Vitamin E supplements, 213–214
Vitamin K
drug interactions, 211, 211*t*
RDIs for adults ≥71 years old, 210*t*
Vitamin therapy
for ARMD, 187
multivitamin supplements, 73*t*, 79
Volume depletion, 514
Vomiting. *See* Nausea and vomiting
VTED (venous thromboembolic disease), 392–394
Vulnerability, 177
Vulnerable Elders Survey-13 (VES-13), 176
Vulvar disorders, 433–434
Vulvar excoriation, 433
Vulvar intraepithelial neoplasia, 434
Vulvar lesions, nonneoplastic, 433–434
Vulvar neoplasia, 434
Vulvodynia, 433
Vulvovaginal atrophy, 433, 446–447, Q24
Vulvovaginal infection and inflammation, 433

Walkers, 150–151, 150*t*, Q86
Walking, 66*t*
limitations in, 228
6-minute walk test, 231
Walking boots, Q72
Walking (gait) speed, Q94
Wandering, 33
Warfarin therapy
for acute coronary syndrome, 382
adverse drug events, 86, 86*t*
for atrial fibrillation, 388
drug interactions, 87, 87*t*
recommendations for cessation before surgery, 103, 107*t*
for stroke prevention, 482
for venous thromboembolic disease, 393–394
Watchful waiting, 442*t*, 443
Water balance, 514
Weakness, 179*t*
Weight loss
anorexia, 116
for chronic CAD, 383
criteria that define frailty, 179*t*
definition of, 210
for musculoskeletal diseases and disorders, 457
unacceptable, 214–215
unintended, Q2
Weight management, 67
Weight screening, 72*t*, 78
Westergren erythrocyte sedimentation rate, 454
Wheelchairs, 151
Wheezing, 372, 373
WHI (Women's Health Initiative), 518
Whisper-voice test, 51, 78, 133
White Americans
alcohol use, 338
cancer diagnosis and survival, 542
cancer incidence, 542
diabetes mellitus, 520
end-of-life care, 111
hypertension, 402
leading causes of death, 3–4, 5*t*
life expectancy, 2, 2*t*
nursing-home population, 153
oral lesions, 366
perceived health, 3, 4*t*
pressure ulcers, 298
self-reported functional limitations, 5
social status, 21
White sponge nevus, Q124
WHO. *See* World Health Organization
Widower's syndrome, 449*t*
Wind-up pain, 120*t*
Withholding or withdrawing therapy, 30–31
Women
alcohol use, 338
cardiovascular disease, 378, 378*t*
dual eligibles, 40
estrogen deficiency, 245
functional limitations of Medicare enrollees, 3, 5*f*
gallstones in, 412
gynecologic diseases and disorders, 431–436
history and physical examination, 431–432
indications for osteoporosis screening, 248, 248*t*
leading causes of death, 3–4, 5*t*
life expectancy, 2, 2*t*
marital status and living arrangements, 3, 3*t*
menopausal symptoms, 95, Q19, Q20
ovarian cancer, 74, Q91
postmenopausal symptoms, Q24
preventive hormone therapy, 73*t*
RDIs for micronutrients, 209–210, 210*t*
recommendations for BMD testing, 248
recommendations for dietary calcium intake, 249–250
recommendations for vitamin D, 249–250
sexual dysfunction, 76, 446–447
stroke in, 480
urinary tract infections in, 499–500
vaginal atrophy, Q21
vaginal bleeding, Q57
Women's Health Initiative (WHI), 518
Wong-Baker FACES Pain Rating Scale with Foreign Translations, 120
World Health Organization (WHO)
BMD definitions, 243, 244*t*
definition of osteoporosis, 243, 244*t*
diagnostic criteria for anemia, 531
fracture risk assessment model (FRAX™), 243, 245*t*, 246, 248, Q111
International Classification of Functioning, Disability, and Health (ICF), 139
Three-Step Analgesic Ladder, 126, 127*f*
Wound care, 296–307, Q47
odor control, Q70
Wound healing
cascade of, 296–297
inflammatory phase, 296
maturation phase, 297
monitoring, 305
Pressure Ulcer Scale for Healing, 305
proliferative phase, 296
Wrist pain
chondrocalcinosis of, 461, 461*f*
evaluation of, 455–456

Xerosis, 352, 477

Yergason sign, 455
Yoga, 66, 66*t*, Q40

Z-score, 247–248
Zaleplon
for insomnia, 293, 294*t*
for sleep disturbances in dementia, 274
Zanamivir, 499, Q99
Zenker diverticulum, Q108
Zinc
for AMD, 187
drug interactions, 211, 211*t*
RDIs for adults ≥71 years old, 210*t*
Ziprasidone
dosing and adverse events of, 325, 326*t*
for psychosis in dementia, 272–273, 273*t*
Zoledronic acid, 250–251, 251*t*, 252
Zolpidem
and delirium, 281*t*
drug interactions, 87, 87*t*
for insomnia, 293, 294*t*
for sleep disturbances in dementia, 274
Zonisamide, 491*t*